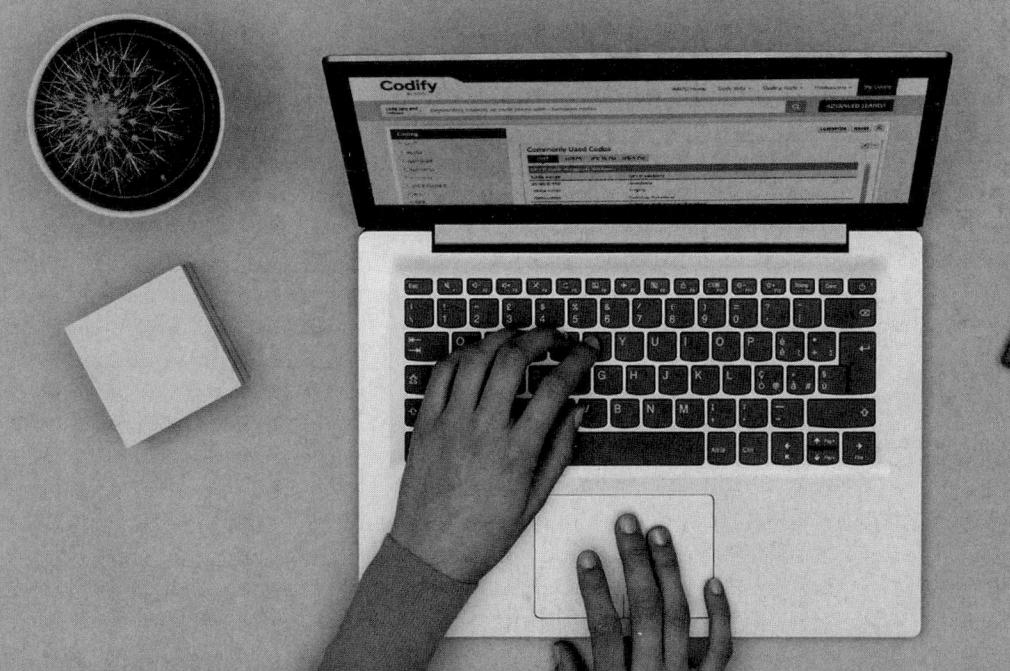
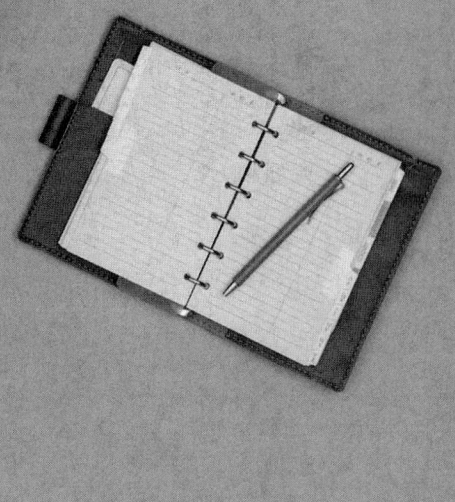

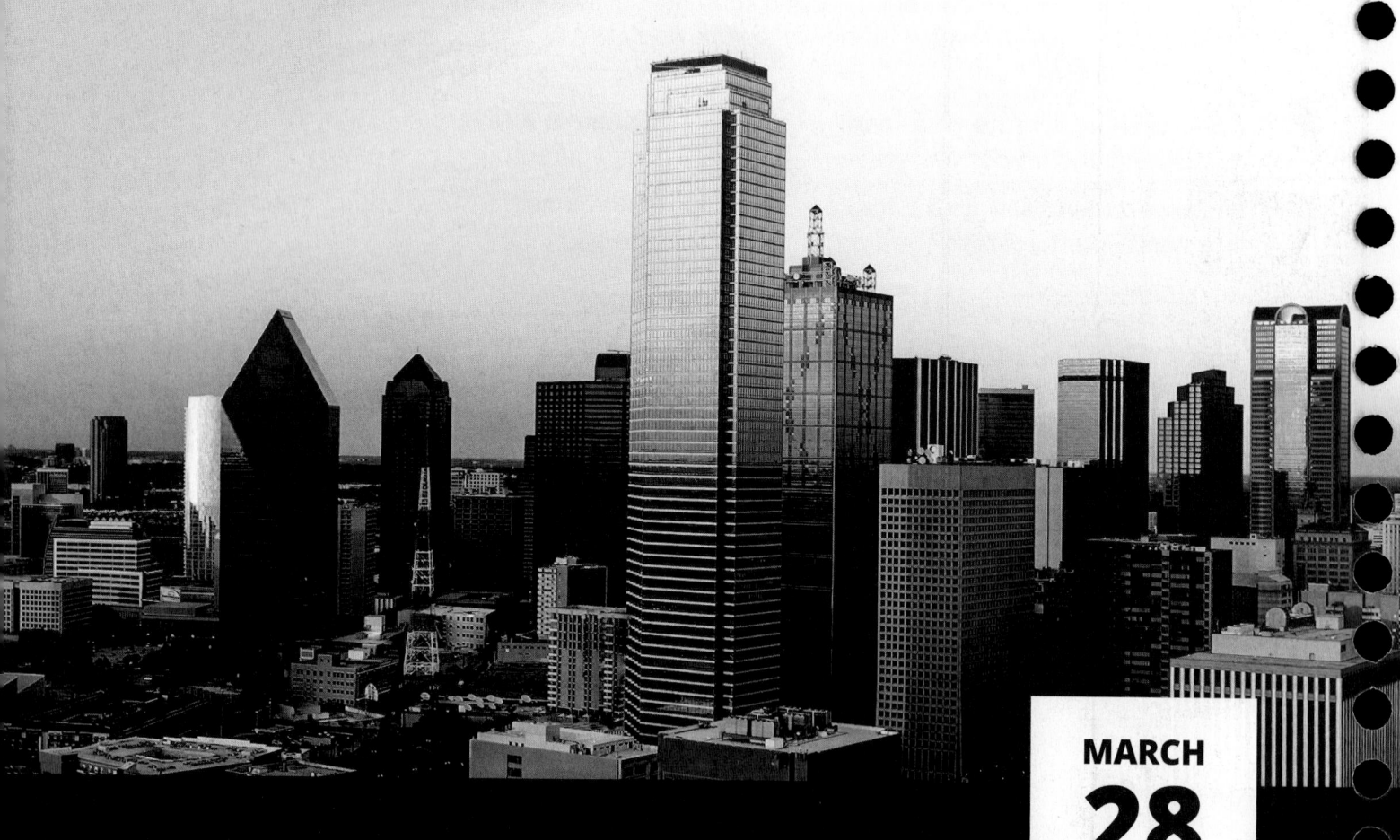

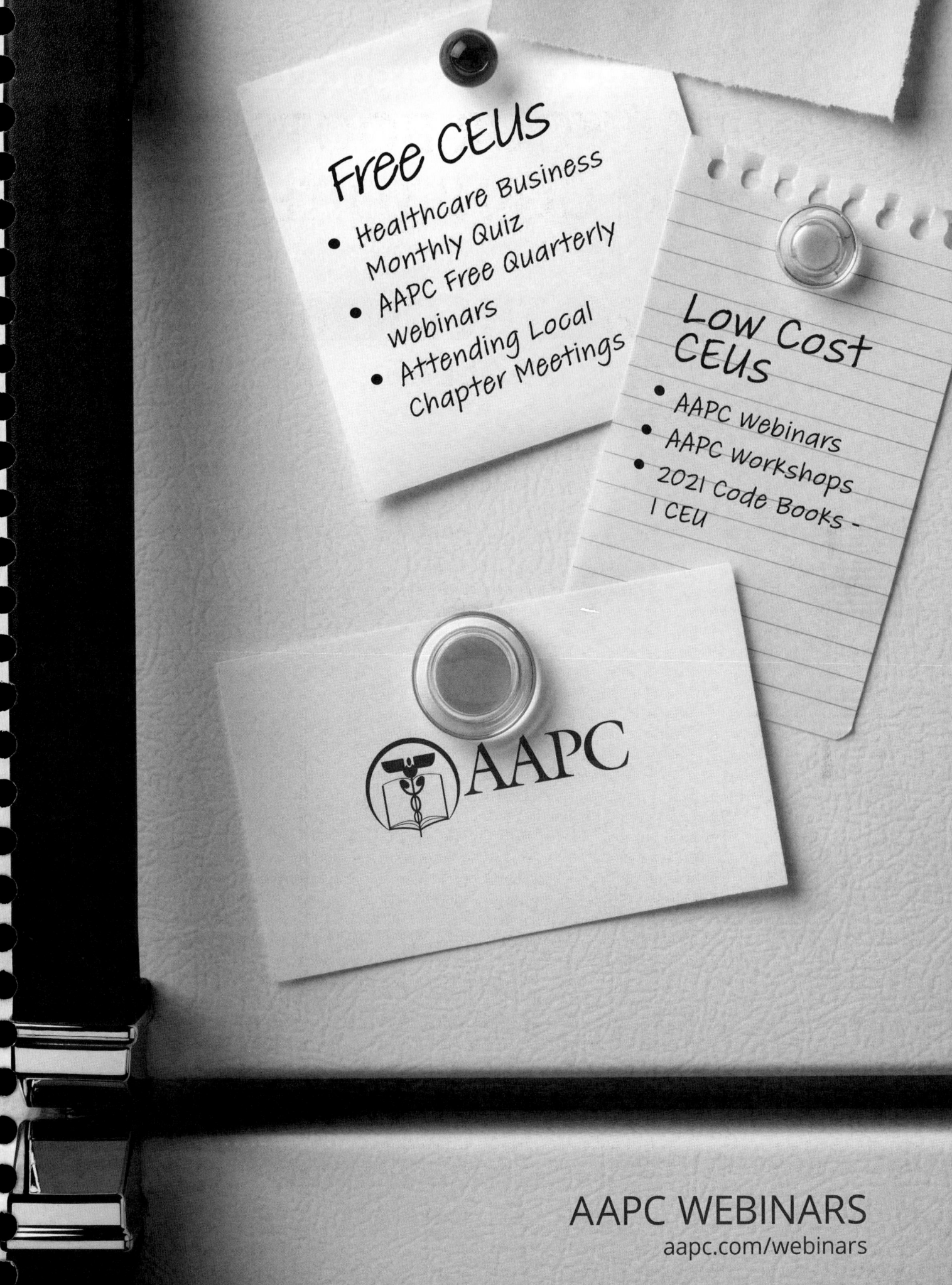

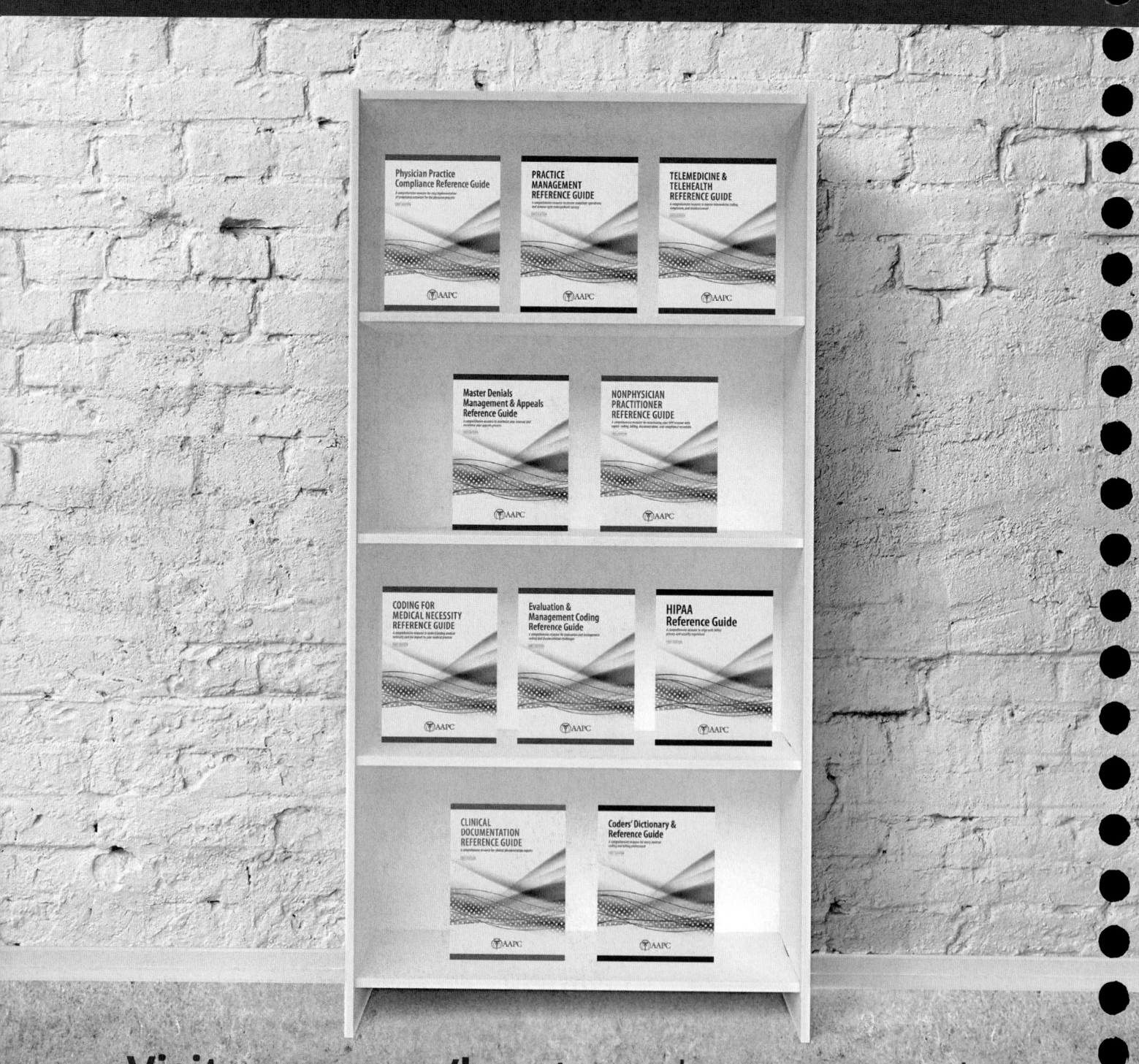

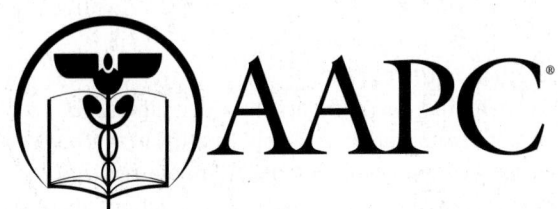

ICD-10
PCS
EXPERT

Inpatient Procedure Codes
for Facilities

2021

PUBLISHER'S NOTICE

Coding, billing, and reimbursement decisions should not be made based solely upon information within this ICD-10-PCS code book. Application of the information in this book does not imply or guarantee claims payment. Make inquiries of your local carriers' bulletins, policy announcements, etc., to resolve local billing requirements. Finally, the law, applicable regulations, payers' instructions, interpretations, enforcement, etc., of ICD-10-PCS codes may change at any time in any particular area. Information in this book is solely based on ICD-10-PCS rules and regulations.

This ICD-10-PCS is designed to be an accurate and authoritative source regarding coding, and every reasonable effort has been made to ensure accuracy and completeness of content. However, this publisher makes no guarantee, warranty, or representation that this publication is complete, accurate, or without errors. It is understood that this publisher is not rendering any legal or professional services or advice in this code book and bears no liability for any results or consequences arising from use of this ICD-10-PCS code book.

AAPC'S COMMITMENT TO ACCURACY

This publisher is committed to providing our members accurate and reliable materials. However, codes and the guidelines by which they are applied change or are reinterpreted through the year. This book contains data from Medicare Code Edits (v. 37.1), proposed MS-DRG v. 38. Definitions Manual, updates for CMS for symbols and appendices, along with the 2021 PCS code set in the Tables which was the latest information available at the time of printing. Check www.aapc.com periodically for updates. To report corrections and updates, please contact AAPC Customer Service via 1-800-626-2633 or via email to code.books@aapc.com.

ACKNOWLEDGEMENT

Jaspal Arora	**Himanshu Arora,** BE	**Chandrashekhar Boreda,** CPC
Sushanta Das, MBA	**Leesa A. Israel,** BA, CPC, CUC, CEMC, CPPM, CMBS	**Rahul Jain,** MDSE
Prashant Kumar, MBA	**Lisa Meaney,** BS	**Sabyasachi Nath,** MS
Ganesh Prasad Sahoo	**Harshita Sharma,** PT, PhD	**Rajendra Sharma,** RN, CPC

Get updates, coding tips, and corrections for this book at www.aapc.com/codebook_updates.

Images/illustrations by the following artists at shutterstock.com:

stockshoppe - 180896807, 99671552, 180896810, 187162193, 180896855, 180896738, 177790997, 177791516, 180896873 | Blamb - 786347626, 24129706 | Alila Medical Media - 76386163, 72231811, 149230337, 149230217, 228843253, 155445671, 147789479, 228843103, 88094230, 155445686, 101696095, 96426923, 97755608, 147943922, 147943910, 155445662, 147943874, 106263593, 106263560, 125891585, 228843262 | Designua - 430118209, 180938618, 135935735, 165084413 | Suwin - 405537832 | Vecton - 661087531 | Sakurra - 676139677 | stihii - 109588457, 129969767, 124562680, 121824442, 129804629, 225637774, 505306105, 505306069 | DeryaDraws - 557609659 | Naeblys - 650014342 | NatthapongSachan - 416973331, 452997697 | udaix - 502058023, 108531449 | ducu59us- 104022683, 125200733 | BlueRingMedia- 141161404, 141162229, 141161560 | joshya - 261971498 | Della_Liner- 324447776 | snapgalleria - 142194094 | okili77- 156466463 | lotan - 186878060 | Alexander_P - 404964388 | udaix - 1336924949

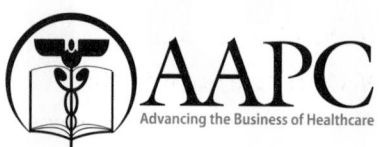

Table of Contents

Preface

Thank you for your purchase! We are pleased to offer you the 2021 ICD-10-PCS official code set in this book.

This code book goes beyond the basics to help you code accurately and efficiently. In addition to including the official Alphabetic Index, Tables, and ICD-10-PCS Official Guidelines, we've crafted a select set of bonus features based on requests from coders in the field as well as the recommendations of our core group of veteran coding educators.

Our goal was to apply our unique approach to focusing on the practical application of the codes to this procedure coding code book.

A few of the other features you'll benefit from page after page include the following:

- Colorful illustrations of body systems and disease processes at the front of the book so you don't have to search for these images

- An Approach Table at the front of the book listing each approach, its definition, and examples

- Medicare Code Edits, including gender edits and edits for limited coverage, noncovered procedures, HAC-associated procedures, combination clusters, non-OR procedures affecting MS-DRG assignment, and questionable obstetric admission

- Intuitive color-coded symbols and alerts to identify critical coding and reimbursement issues quickly

- A list of non-OR procedures NOT affecting MS-DRG assignment

- A full list of adhesive tabs to label your book for quick and easy access to specific sections

See the complete List of Features to learn about everything this code book has to offer.

Rely on Our Combination of Official Sources and Experience

This code book includes the official ICD-10-PCS 2021 Alphabetic Index and Tables. We've also included the 2021 ICD-10-PCS Official Guidelines.

Our dedicated team drew on their years of experience using code books to develop this book's user-friendly features and layout, all designed to help you find the information you need quickly.

Let Us Know What You Think

Our goal for this code book is to support those involved in the business side of healthcare, helping them to do their jobs well. We'd appreciate your feedback, including your suggestions for what you'd like to see in an ICD-10-PCS resource, so we can be sure our code books serve your needs. Thank you.

Changes for 2021

FY 2021 Update Summary

Change Summary Table

2020 Total	New Codes	Revised Titles	Deleted Codes	2021 Total
77,559	544	0	0	**78,103**

ICD-10-PCS Code FY 2021 Totals, By Section

Medical and Surgical	67,655
Obstetrics	304
Placement	861
Administration	1,336
Measurement and Monitoring	421
Extracorporeal or Systemic Assistance and Performance	51
Extracorporeal or Systemic Therapies	46
Osteopathic	100
Other Procedures	78
Chiropractic	90
Imaging	2,973
Nuclear Medicine	463
Radiation Therapy	2,087
Physical Rehabilitation and Diagnostic Audiology	1,380
Mental Health	30
Substance Abuse Treatment	59
New Technology	169
Total	**78,103**

List of FY 2021 Files

Note: All 2021 ICD-10-PCS data files can be found on the CMS website at https://www.cms.gov/medicare/icd-10/2021-icd-10-pcs

Descriptions of these data files are as follows:

2021 Official ICD-10-PCS Coding Guidelines

- New Guidelines B3.18 and B5.2b added in response to public comment.
- Guidelines B3.1b and B3.10c revised in response to public comment and internal review.
- Downloadable PDF, file name **pcs_guidelines_2021.pdf**

2021 ICD-10-PCS Code Tables and Index (zip file)

- Code tables for use beginning October 1, 2020.
- Downloadable PDF, file name is **pcs_2021.pdf**

- Downloadable xml files for developers, file names are **icd10pcs_tables_2021.xml, icd10pcs_index_2021.xml, icd10pcs_definitions_2021.xml**
- Accompanying schema for developers, file names are **icd10pcs_tables.xsd, icd10pcs_index.xsd, icd10pcs_definitions.xsd**

2021 ICD-10-PCS Codes File (zip file)

- ICD-10-PCS Codes file is a simple format for non-technical uses, containing the valid FY 2021 ICD-10-PCS codes and their long titles.
- File is in text file format, file name is **icd10pcs_codes_2021.txt**
- Accompanying documentation for codes file, file name is **icd10pcsCodesFile.pdf**
- Codes file addenda in text format, file name is **codes_addenda_2021.txt**

2021 ICD-10-PCS Order File (Long and Abbreviated Titles) (zip file)

- ICD-10-PCS order file is for developers, provides a unique five-digit "order number" for each ICD-10-PCS table and code, as well as a long and abbreviated code title.
- ICD-10-PCS order file name is **icd10pcs_order_2021.txt**
- Accompanying documentation for tabular order file, file name is **icd10pcsOrderFile.pdf**
- Tabular order file addenda in text format, file name is **order_addenda_2021.txt**

2021 ICD-10-PCS Final Addenda (zip file)

- Addenda files in downloadable PDF, file names are **tables_addenda_2021.pdf, index_addenda_2021.pdf, definitions_addenda_2021.pdf**
- Addenda files also in machine readable text format for developers, file names are **tables_addenda_2021.txt, index_addenda_2021.txt, definitions_addenda_2021.txt**

2021 ICD-10-PCS Conversion Table (zip file)

- ICD-10-PCS code conversion table is provided to assist users in data retrieval, in downloadable Excel spreadsheet, file name is **icd10pcs_conversion_table.xlsx**
- Conversion table also in machine readable text format for developers, file name is **icd10pcs_conversion_table.txt**
- Accompanying documentation for code conversion table, file name is **icd10pcsConversionTable.pdf**

List of Features

ICD-10-PCS is essential for reporting services rendered, and accurate codes mean better outcomes for the patient, your claims, and your facility.

You can count on this code book to help you choose and report the right ICD-10-PCS code. Unique features, intuitive design, and expert details that coders developed ensure this code book will keep your coding on target.

This code book includes the ICD-10-PCS Alphabetic Index and ICD-10-PCS Tables for procedures, effective October 1, 2020 (FY 2021 code set).

To help you make the most of this code book, we include the following features:

- ICD-10-PCS Official Conventions and additional conventions and symbols

- ICD-10-PCS Official Guidelines for Coding and Reporting, effective October 1, 2020 (FY 2021)

- Approach Table with each approach, definition, and example listed at the front of the book for quick reference

- Colorful illustrations of body systems and disease processes at the front of the book for easy look-up

- Medicare Code Edits symbols, including gender edits and edits for limited coverage, noncovered procedures, hospital acquired conditions (HAC-) associated procedures, combination clusters, non-OR procedures affecting MS-DRG assignment, and questionable obstetric admission

- Intuitive color-coded symbols and alerts for quick identification of coding and reimbursement issues

- Adhesive tabs for specific sections of the book to find specific sections quickly and easily

- Appendices for root operations definitions in alphabetical order by Tables, body part key, device key and aggregation table, character meaning, substance key, combination clusters, and non-OR procedures not affecting MS-DRG assignment

- A user-friendly page design, including dictionary-style headers, colored bleed tabs, and legend keys

Official Conventions and Additional Conventions Specific to This ICD-10-PCS Book

This code book includes the procedure code set from the International Classification of Diseases, 10th Revision, Procedure Coding System (ICD-10-PCS). Hospitals and third-party payers use these codes to classify inpatient procedures.

Official Conventions

Index

Refer to the ICD-10-PCS Index to identify the appropriate Tables in the code book. The Index mirrors the structure of the Tables, so it follows a consistent pattern of organization and use of hierarchies. The Index is organized as an alphabetic lookup.

Two types of main terms are listed in the Index:

- Those based on the value of the third character, such as a root operations (excision, insertion)
- Those listing common procedures

Main Terms

For the Medical and Surgical and related sections, the root operation values are used as main terms in the Index. In other sections, the values representing the general type of procedure performed, such as nuclear medicine or imaging type, are listed as main terms.

For the Medical and Surgical and related sections, values such as Excision, Bypass, and Transplantation are included as main terms in the Index. The applicable body system entries are listed beneath the main term and refer to a specific table. For the ancillary sections, values such as Fluoroscopy and Positron Emission Tomography, are listed as main terms.

To find the code to cross-reference to the Tables, search for the root operation for the procedure in the Index, followed by the subterm for the anatomic site or the subterm that further describes the procedure. Locate the partial code, and cross-reference it to the Table that matches the first three characters of the code.

Tables

The Tables are organized in alphanumeric order in a series by Section, which is the first character of a code. Tables that begin with 0 to 9 are listed first, then Tables beginning with B-D, then letters F-X, are listed next.

The same convention is followed within each Table for the second through the seventh characters — numeric values in order first, followed by alphabetical values.

The Medical and Surgical section (first character 0) is organized by body system values. Each body system subdivision in the Medical and Surgical section contains Tables that list the valid root operations for that body system. These are the root operation Tables that form the system. These Tables provide the valid choices of values available to construct a code.

The root operation Tables consist of four columns and a varying number of rows, as in the following example of the root operation Insertion, in the Subcutaneous Tissue and Fascia body system.

The values for characters 1 through 3 are provided at the top of each Table.

Character 1:	0: MEDICAL AND SURGICAL (Section)
Character 2:	J: SUBCUTANEOUS TISSUE AND FASCIA (Body System)
Character 3:	H: INSERTION: Putting in a nonbiological appliance that monitors, assists, performs, or prevents a physiological function but does not physically take the place of a body part (Root Operation)

The Table itself contains four columns with the applicable values for characters 4 through 7.

Body Part	Approach	Device	Qualifier
Character 4	**Character 5**	**Character 6**	**Character 7**
S Subcutaneous Tissue and Fascia, Head and Neck **V** Subcutaneous Tissue and Fascia, Upper Extremity **W** Subcutaneous Tissue and Fascia, Lower Extremity	**0** Open **3** Percutaneous	**1** Radioactive Element **3** Infusion Device **Y** Other Device	**Z** No Qualifier
T Subcutaneous Tissue and Fascia, Trunk	**0** Open **3** Percutaneous	**1** Radioactive Element **3** Infusion Device **V** Infusion Device, Pump **Y** Other Device	**Z** No Qualifier

A Table may be separated into rows to specify the valid choices of values in characters 4 through 7. A code built using values from more than one row of a Table is not a valid code.

Refer to the ICD-10-PCS Official Guidelines for Coding and Reporting in this code book for detailed guidance on assigning ICD-10-PCS codes.

'See' Reference

The *see* reference directs you to go elsewhere in the Index to find the root operation that you need.

'Use' Reference

The *use* reference directs you to a character value selection as an additional reference.

Additional Conventions

Additional conventions that you will find in the Tables in this manual include Medicare Code Edits - Symbols and colored font.

Medicare Code Edits – Symbols Applied to 4th Characters

LC Limited Coverage

Procedures that are medically complex and serious in nature that incur extraordinary associated costs. Medicare limits coverage to a portion of the cost.

NC Noncovered

Procedures for which Medicare does not typically reimburse.

HAC HAC-associated Procedure

Procedures that are associated with hospital-acquired conditions (HAC).

CC Combination Cluster

The procedure is part of a procedure code combination, or cluster, listed in Appendix G of this code book. Medicare does not typically pay for these procedures unless you report them with other specific procedures.

DRG Non-OR-Affecting MS-DRG Assignment

Non-operating room procedures which affect MS-DRG assignment for claims reporting.

New/Revised Text in **Orange**

Procedure text was new or revised from the last version of the code set. For new codes, orange text will be shown for all characters in the code. New codes may be shown as their own row in a Table and characters 4-7 may be shown in a row that is separate from other characters within that Table.

♂ Male

Male procedure only

♀ Female

Female procedure only

QOA Questionable Obstetric Admission

Procedure codes for cesarean or vaginal delivery that are considered questionable unless reported with a corresponding secondary diagnosis describing the outcome of delivery.

Code Lists

Codes that are applicable to each type of symbol in the book are listed after each Table.

Notes Pages

Notes pages are included between sections within the Tables.

ICD-10-PCS Official Guidelines for Coding and Reporting 2021

The Centers for Medicare and Medicaid Services (CMS) and the National Center for Health Statistics (NCHS), two departments within the U.S. Federal Government's Department of Health and Human Services (DHHS) provide the following guidelines for coding and reporting using the International Classification of Diseases, 10th Revision, Procedure Coding System (ICD-10-PCS). These guidelines should be used as a companion document to the official version of the ICD-10-PCS as published on the CMS website. The ICD-10-PCS is a procedure classification published by the United States for classifying procedures performed in hospital inpatient health care settings.

These guidelines have been approved by the four organizations that make up the Cooperating Parties for the ICD-10-PCS: the American Hospital Association (AHA), the American Health Information Management Association (AHIMA), CMS, and NCHS.

These guidelines are a set of rules that have been developed to accompany and complement the official conventions and instructions provided within the ICD-10-PCS itself. They are intended to provide direction that is applicable in most circumstances. However, there may be unique circumstances where exceptions are applied. The instructions and conventions of the classification take precedence over guidelines. These guidelines are based on the coding and sequencing instructions in the Tables, Index and Definitions of ICD-10-PCS, but provide additional instruction. Adherence to these guidelines when assigning ICD-10-PCS procedure codes is required under the Health Insurance Portability and Accountability Act (HIPAA). The procedure codes have been adopted under HIPAA for

hospital inpatient healthcare settings. A joint effort between the healthcare provider and the coder is essential to achieve complete and accurate documentation, code assignment, and reporting of diagnoses and procedures. These guidelines have been developed to assist both the healthcare provider and the coder in identifying those procedures that are to be reported. The importance of consistent, complete documentation in the medical record cannot be overemphasized. Without such documentation accurate coding cannot be achieved.

Table of Contents

Conventions

A1

ICD-10-PCS codes are composed of seven characters. Each character is an axis of classification that specifies information about the procedure performed. Within a defined code range, a character specifies the same type of information in that axis of classification.

Example: The fifth axis of classification specifies the approach in sections 0 through 4 and 7 through 9 of the system.

A2

One of 34 possible values can be assigned to each axis of classification in the seven- character code: they are the numbers 0 through 9 and the alphabet (except I and O because they are easily confused with the numbers 1 and 0). The number of unique values used in an axis of classification differs as needed.

Example: Where the fifth axis of classification specifies the approach, seven different approach values are currently used to specify the approach.

A3

The valid values for an axis of classification can be added to as needed.

Example: If a significantly distinct type of device is used in a new procedure, a new device value can be added to the system.

A4

As with words in their context, the meaning of any single value is a combination of its axis of classification and any preceding values on which it may be dependent.

Example: The meaning of a body part value in the Medical and Surgical section is always dependent on the body system value. The body part value 0 in the Central Nervous body system specifies Brain and the body part value 0 in the Peripheral Nervous body system specifies Cervical Plexus.

A5

As the system is expanded to become increasingly detailed, over time more values will depend on preceding values for their meaning.

Example: In the Lower Joints body system, the device value 3 in the root operation Insertion specifies Infusion Device and the device value 3 in the root operation Replacement specifies Ceramic Synthetic Substitute.

A6

The purpose of the alphabetic index is to locate the appropriate table that contains all information necessary to construct a procedure code. The PCS Tables should always be consulted to find the most appropriate valid code.

A7

It is not required to consult the index first before proceeding to the tables to complete the code. A valid code may be chosen directly from the tables.

A8

All seven characters must be specified to be a valid code. If the documentation is incomplete for coding purposes, the physician should be queried for the necessary information.

A9

Within a PCS table, valid codes include all combinations of choices in characters 4 through 7 contained in the same row of the table. In the example below, 0JHT3VZ is a valid code, and 0JHW3VZ is *not* a valid code.

A10

"And," when used in a code description, means "and/or," except when used to describe a combination of multiple body parts for which separate values exist for each body part (e.g., Skin and Subcutaneous Tissue used as a qualifier, where there are separate body part values for "Skin" and "Subcutaneous Tissue").

Example: Lower Arm and Wrist Muscle means lower arm and/or wrist muscle.

A11

Many of the terms used to construct PCS codes are defined within the system. It is the coder's responsibility to determine what the documentation in the medical record equates to in the PCS definitions. The physician is not expected to use the terms used in PCS code descriptions, nor is the coder required to query the physician when the correlation between the documentation and the defined PCS terms is clear.

Example: When the physician documents "partial resection" the coder can independently correlate "partial resection" to the root operation Excision without querying the physician for clarification.

Section:	0 Medical and Surgical
Body System:	J Subcutaneous Tissue and Fascia
Operation:	H Insertion: Putting in a nonbiological appliance that monitors, assists, performs, or prevents a physiological function but does not physically take the place of a body part

Body Part	Approach	Device	Qualifier
S Subcutaneous Tissue and Fascia, Head and Neck V Subcutaneous Tissue and Fascia, Upper Extremity W Subcutaneous Tissue and Fascia, Lower Extremity	0 Open 3 Percutaneous	1 Radioactive Element 3 Infusion Device Y Other Device	Z No Qualifier
T Subcutaneous Tissue and Fascia, Trunk	0 Open 3 Percutaneous	1 Radioactive Element 3 Infusion Device V Infusion Pump Y Other Device	Z No Qualifier

Medical and Surgical Section Guidelines (Section 0)

B2. Body System

General guidelines

B2.1a

The procedure codes in Anatomical Regions, General, Anatomical Regions, Upper Extremities and Anatomical Regions, Lower Extremities can be used when the procedure is performed on an anatomical region rather than a specific body part, or on the rare occasion when no information is available to support assignment of a code to a specific body part.

Examples: Chest tube drainage of the pleural cavity is coded to the root operation Drainage found in the body system Anatomical Regions, General.

Suture repair of the abdominal wall is coded to the root operation Repair in the body system Anatomical Regions, General.

Amputation of the foot is coded to the root operation Detachment in the body system Anatomical Regions, Lower Extremities.

B2.1b

Where the general body part values "upper" and "lower" are provided as an option in the Upper Arteries, Lower Arteries, Upper Veins, Lower Veins, Muscles and Tendons body systems, "upper" or "lower "specifies body parts located above or below the diaphragm respectively.

Example: Vein body parts above the diaphragm are found in the Upper Veins body system; vein body parts below the diaphragm are found in the Lower Veins body system.

B3. Root Operation

General guidelines

B3.1a

In order to determine the appropriate root operation, the full definition of the root operation as contained in the PCS Tables must be applied.

B3.1b

Components of a procedure specified in the root operation definition or explanation as integral to that root operation are not coded separately. Procedural steps necessary to reach the operative site and close the operative site, including anastomosis of a tubular body part, are also not coded separately.

Examples: Resection of a joint as part of a joint replacement procedure is included in the root operation definition of Replacement and is not coded separately.

Laparotomy performed to reach the site of an open liver biopsy is not coded separately. In a resection of sigmoid colon with anastomosis of descending colon to rectum, the anastomosis is not coded separately.

Multiple procedures

B3.2

During the same operative episode, multiple procedures are coded if:

a. The same root operation is performed on different body parts as defined by distinct values of the body part character.

    Examples: Diagnostic excision of liver and pancreas are coded separately.

    Excision of lesion in the ascending colon and excision of lesion in the transverse colon are coded separately.

b. The same root operation is repeated in multiple body parts, and those body parts are separate and distinct body parts classified to a single ICD-10-PCS body part value.

    Examples: Excision of the sartorius muscle and excision of the gracilis muscle are both included in the upper leg muscle body part value, and multiple procedures are coded.

    Extraction of multiple toenails are coded separately.

c. Multiple root operations with distinct objectives are performed on the same body part.

    Example: Destruction of sigmoid lesion and bypass of sigmoid colon are coded separately.

d. The intended root operation is attempted using one approach but is converted to a different approach.

    Example: Laparoscopic cholecystectomy converted to an open cholecystectomy is coded as percutaneous endoscopic Inspection and open Resection.

Discontinued or incomplete procedures

B3.3

If the intended procedure is discontinued or otherwise not completed, code the procedure to the root operation performed. If a procedure is discontinued before any other root operation is performed, code the root operation Inspection of the body part or anatomical region inspected.

Example: A planned aortic valve replacement procedure is discontinued after the initial thoracotomy and before any incision is made in the heart muscle, when the patient becomes hemodynamically unstable. This procedure is coded as an open Inspection of the mediastinum.

Biopsy procedures

B3.4a

Biopsy procedures are coded using the root operations Excision, Extraction, or Drainage and the qualifier Diagnostic.

Examples: Fine needle aspiration biopsy of fluid in the lung is coded to the root operation Drainage with the qualifier Diagnostic.

Biopsy of bone marrow is coded to the root operation Extraction with the qualifier Diagnostic.

Lymph node sampling for biopsy is coded to the root operation Excision with the qualifier Diagnostic

Biopsy followed by more definitive treatment

B3.4b

If a diagnostic Excision, Extraction, or Drainage procedure (biopsy) is followed by a more definitive procedure, such as Destruction, Excision or Resection at the same procedure site, both the biopsy and the more definitive treatment are coded.

Example: Biopsy of breast followed by partial mastectomy at the same procedure site, both the biopsy and the partial mastectomy procedure are coded.

Overlapping body layers

B3.5

If root operations such as Excision, Extraction, Repair or Inspection are performed on overlapping layers of the musculoskeletal system, the body part specifying the deepest layer is coded.

Example: Excisional debridement that includes skin and subcutaneous tissue and muscle is coded to the muscle body part.

Bypass procedures

B3.6a

Bypass procedures are coded by identifying the body part bypassed "from" and the body part bypassed "to." The fourth character body part specifies the body part bypassed from, and the qualifier specifies the body part bypassed to.

Example: Bypass from stomach to jejunum, stomach is the body part and jejunum is the qualifier.

B3.6b

Coronary artery bypass procedures are coded differently than other bypass procedures as described in the previous guideline. Rather than identifying the body part bypassed from, the body part identifies the number of coronary arteries bypassed to, and the qualifier specifies the vessel bypassed from.

Example: Aortocoronary artery bypass of the left anterior descending coronary artery and the obtuse marginal coronary artery is classified in the body part axis of classification as two coronary arteries, and the qualifier specifies the aorta as the body part bypassed from.

B3.6c

If multiple coronary arteries are bypassed, a separate procedure is coded for each coronary artery that uses a different device and/or qualifier.

Example: Aortocoronary artery bypass and internal mammary coronary artery bypass are coded separately.

Control vs. more definitive root operations

B3.7

The root operation Control is defined as, "Stopping, or attempting to stop, postprocedural or other acute bleeding." If an attempt to stop postprocedural or other acute bleeding is unsuccessful, and to stop the bleeding requires performing a more definitive root operation, such as Bypass, Detachment, Excision, Extraction, Reposition, Replacement, or Resection, then the more definitive root operation is coded instead of Control.

Example: Resection of spleen to stop bleeding is coded to Resection instead of Control.

Excision vs. Resection

B3.8

PCS contains specific body parts for anatomical subdivisions of a body part, such as lobes of the lungs or liver and regions of the intestine. Resection of the specific body part is coded whenever all of the body part is cut out or off, rather than coding Excision of a less specific body part.

Example: Left upper lung lobectomy is coded to Resection of Upper Lung Lobe, Left rather than Excision of Lung, Left.

Excision for graft

B3.9

If an autograft is obtained from a different procedure site in order to complete the objective of the procedure, a separate procedure is coded, except when the seventh character qualifier value in the ICD-10-PCS table fully specifies the site from which the autograft was obtained.

Examples: Coronary bypass with excision of saphenous vein graft, excision of saphenous vein is coded separately.

Replacement of breast with autologous deep inferior epigastric artery perforator (DIEP) flap, excision of the DIEP flap is not coded separately. The seventh character qualifier value Deep Inferior Epigastric Artery Perforator Flap in the Replacement table fully specifies the site of the autograft harvest.

Fusion procedures of the spine

B3.10a

The body part coded for a spinal vertebral joint(s) rendered immobile by a spinal fusion procedure is classified by the level of the spine (e.g. thoracic). There are distinct body part values for a single vertebral joint and for multiple vertebral joints at each spinal level.

Example: Body part values specify Lumbar Vertebral Joint, Lumbar Vertebral Joints, 2 or More and Lumbosacral Vertebral Joint.

B3.10b

If multiple vertebral joints are fused, a separate procedure is coded for each vertebral joint that uses a different device and/or qualifier.

Example: Fusion of lumbar vertebral joint, posterior approach, anterior column and fusion of lumbar vertebral joint, posterior approach, posterior column are coded separately.

B3.10c

Combinations of devices and materials are often used on a vertebral joint to render the joint immobile. When combinations of devices are used on the same vertebral joint, the device value coded for the procedure is as follows:

- If an interbody fusion device is used to render the joint immobile (containing bone graft or bone graft substitute), the procedure is coded with the device value Interbody Fusion Device

- If bone graft is the only device used to render the joint immobile, the procedure is coded with the device value Nonautologous Tissue Substitute or Autologous Tissue Substitute
- If a mixture of autologous and nonautologous bone graft (with or without biological or synthetic extenders or binders) is used to render the joint immobile, code the procedure with the device value Autologous Tissue Substitute

Examples: Fusion of a vertebral joint using a cage style interbody fusion device containing morsellized bone graft is coded to the device Interbody Fusion Device.

Fusion of a vertebral joint using a bone dowel interbody fusion device made of cadaver bone and packed with a mixture of local morsellized bone and demineralized bone matrix is coded to the device Interbody Fusion Device.

Fusion of a vertebral joint using both autologous bone graft and bone bank bone graft is coded to the device Autologous Tissue Substitute.

Inspection procedures

B3.11a
Inspection of a body part(s) performed in order to achieve the objective of a procedure is not coded separately.

Example: Fiberoptic bronchoscopy performed for irrigation of bronchus, only the irrigation procedure is coded.

B3.11b
If multiple tubular body parts are inspected, the most distal body part (the body part furthest from the starting point of the inspection) is coded. If multiple non-tubular body parts in a region are inspected, the body part that specifies the entire area inspected is coded.

Examples: Cystoureteroscopy with inspection of bladder and ureters is coded to the ureter body part value.

Exploratory laparotomy with general inspection of abdominal contents is coded to the peritoneal cavity body part value.

B3.11c
When both an Inspection procedure and another procedure are performed on the same body part during the same episode, if the Inspection procedure is performed using a different approach than the other procedure, the Inspection procedure is coded separately.

Example: Endoscopic Inspection of the duodenum is coded separately when open Excision of the duodenum is performed during the same procedural episode.

Occlusion vs. Restriction for vessel embolization procedures

B3.12
If the objective of an embolization procedure is to completely close a vessel, the root operation Occlusion is coded. If the objective of an embolization procedure is to narrow the lumen of a vessel, the root operation Restriction is coded.

Examples: Tumor embolization is coded to the root operation Occlusion, because the objective of the procedure is to cut off the blood supply to the vessel.

Embolization of a cerebral aneurysm is coded to the root operation Restriction, because the objective of the procedure is not to close off the vessel entirely, but to narrow the lumen of the vessel at the site of the aneurysm where it is abnormally wide.

Release procedures

B3.13
In the root operation Release, the body part value coded is the body part being freed and not the tissue being manipulated or cut to free the body part.

Example: Lysis of intestinal adhesions is coded to the specific intestine body part value.

Release vs. Division

B3.14
If the sole objective of the procedure is freeing a body part without cutting the body part, the root operation is Release. If the sole objective of the procedure is separating or transecting a body part, the root operation is Division.

Examples: Freeing a nerve root from surrounding scar tissue to relieve pain is coded to the root operation Release.

Severing a nerve root to relieve pain is coded to the root operation Division.

Reposition for fracture treatment

B3.15
Reduction of a displaced fracture is coded to the root operation Reposition and the application of a cast or splint in conjunction with the Reposition procedure is not coded separately. Treatment of a nondisplaced fracture is coded to the procedure performed.

Examples: Casting of a nondisplaced fracture is coded to the root operation Immobilization in the Placement section.

Putting a pin in a nondisplaced fracture is coded to the root operation Insertion.

Transplantation vs. Administration

B3.16
Putting in a mature and functioning living body part taken from another individual or animal is coded to the root operation Transplantation. Putting in autologous or nonautologous cells is coded to the Administration section.

Example: Putting in autologous or nonautologous bone marrow, pancreatic islet cells or stem cells is coded to the Administration section.

Transfer procedures using multiple tissue layers

B3.17
The root operation Transfer contains qualifiers that can be used to specify when a transfer flap is composed of more than one tissue layer, such as a musculocutaneous flap. For procedures involving

transfer of multiple tissue layers including skin, subcutaneous tissue, fascia or muscle, the procedure is coded to the body part value that describes the deepest tissue layer in the flap, and the qualifier can be used to describe the other tissue layer(s) in the transfer flap.

Example: A musculocutaneous flap transfer is coded to the appropriate body part value in the body system Muscles, and the qualifier is used to describe the additional tissue layer(s) in the transfer flap.

Excision/Resection followed by replacement

B3.18
If an excision or resection of a body part is followed by a replacement procedure, code both procedures to identify each distinct objective, except when the excision or resection is considered integral and preparatory for the replacement procedure.

Examples: Mastectomy followed by reconstruction, both resection and replacement of the breast are coded to fully capture the distinct objectives of the procedures performed.

Maxillectomy with obturator reconstruction, both excision and replacement of the maxilla are coded to fully capture the distinct objectives of the procedures performed. Excisional debridement of tendon with skin graft, both the excision of the tendon and the replacement of the skin with a graft are coded to fully capture the distinct objectives of the procedures performed. Esophagectomy followed by reconstruction with colonic interposition, both the resection and the transfer of the large intestine to function as the esophagus are coded to fully capture the distinct objectives of the procedures performed.

Examples: Resection of a joint as part of a joint replacement procedure is considered integral and preparatory for the replacement of the joint and the resection is not coded separately. Resection of a valve as part of a valve replacement procedure is considered integral and preparatory for the valve replacement and the resection is not coded separately.

B4. Body Part

General guidelines

B4.1a
If a procedure is performed on a portion of a body part that does not have a separate body part value, code the body part value corresponding to the whole body part.

Example: A procedure performed on the alveolar process of the mandible is coded to the mandible body part.

B4.1b
If the prefix "peri" is combined with a body part to identify the site of the procedure, and the site of the procedure is not further specified, then the procedure is coded to the body part named. This guideline applies only when a more specific body part value is not available.

Examples: A procedure site identified as perirenal is coded to the kidney body part when the site of the procedure is not further specified.

A procedure site described in the documentation as peri-urethral, and the documentation also indicates that it is the vulvar tissue and not the urethral tissue that is the site of the procedure, then the procedure is coded to the vulva body part.

A procedure site documented as involving the periosteum is coded to the corresponding bone body part.

B4.1c
If a procedure is performed on a continuous section of a tubular body part, code the body part value corresponding to the furthest anatomical site from the point of entry.

Example: A procedure performed on a continuous section of artery from the femoral artery to the external iliac artery with the point of entry at the femoral artery is coded to the external iliac body part.

Branches of body parts

B4.2
Where a specific branch of a body part does not have its own body part value in PCS, the body part is typically coded to the closest proximal branch that has a specific body part value. In the cardiovascular body systems, if a general body part is available in the correct root operation table, and coding to a proximal branch would require assigning a code in a different body system, the procedure is coded using the general body part value.

Examples: A procedure performed on the mandibular branch of the trigeminal nerve is coded to the trigeminal nerve body part value.

Occlusion of the bronchial artery is coded to the body part value Upper Artery in the body system Upper Arteries, and not to the body part value Thoracic Aorta, Descending in the body system Heart and Great Vessels.

Bilateral body part values

B4.3
Bilateral body part values are available for a limited number of body parts. If the identical procedure is performed on contralateral body parts, and a bilateral body part value exists for that body part, a single procedure is coded using the bilateral body part value. If no bilateral body part value exists, each procedure is coded separately using the appropriate body part value.

Examples: The identical procedure performed on both fallopian tubes is coded once using the body part value Fallopian Tube, Bilateral.

The identical procedure performed on both knee joints is coded twice using the body part values Knee Joint, Right and Knee Joint, Left.

Coronary arteries

B4.4
The coronary arteries are classified as a single body part that is further specified by number of arteries treated. One procedure code specifying multiple arteries is used when the same procedure is performed, including the same device and qualifier values.

Examples: Angioplasty of two distinct coronary arteries with placement of two stents is coded as Dilation of Coronary Artery, Two Arteries with Two Intraluminal Devices.

Angioplasty of two distinct coronary arteries, one with stent placed and one without, is coded separately as Dilation of Coronary Artery, One Artery with Intraluminal Device, and Dilation of Coronary Artery, One Artery with no device.

Tendons, ligaments, bursae and fascia near a joint

B4.5
Procedures performed on tendons, ligaments, bursae and fascia supporting a joint are coded to the body part in the respective body system that is the focus of the procedure. Procedures performed on joint structures themselves are coded to the body part in the joint body systems.

Examples: Repair of the anterior cruciate ligament of the knee is coded to the knee bursa and ligament body part in the bursae and ligaments body system.

Knee arthroscopy with shaving of articular cartilage is coded to the knee joint body part in the Lower Joints body system.

Skin, subcutaneous tissue and fascia overlying a joint

B4.6
If a procedure is performed on the skin, subcutaneous tissue or fascia overlying a joint, the procedure is coded to the following body part:

- Shoulder is coded to Upper Arm
- Elbow is coded to Lower Arm
- Wrist is coded to Lower Arm
- Hip is coded to Upper Leg
- Knee is coded to Lower Leg
- Ankle is coded to Foot

Fingers and toes

B4.7
If a body system does not contain a separate body part value for fingers, procedures performed on the fingers are coded to the body part value for the hand. If a body system does not contain a separate body part value for toes, procedures performed on the toes are coded to the body part value for the foot.

Example: Excision of finger muscle is coded to one of the hand muscle body part values in the Muscles body system.

Upper and lower intestinal tract

B4.8
In the Gastrointestinal body system, the general body part values Upper Intestinal Tract and Lower Intestinal Tract are provided as an option for the root operations Change, Inspection, Removal and Revision. Upper Intestinal Tract includes the portion of the gastrointestinal tract from the esophagus down to and including the duodenum, and Lower Intestinal Tract includes the portion of the gastrointestinal tract from the jejunum down to and including the rectum and anus.

Example: In the root operation Change table, change of a device in the jejunum is coded using the body part Lower Intestinal Tract.

B5. Approach

Open approach with percutaneous endoscopic assistance

B5.2a
Procedures performed using the open approach with percutaneous endoscopic assistance are coded to the approach Open.

Example: Laparoscopic-assisted sigmoidectomy is coded to the approach Open.

Percutaneous endoscopic approach with extension of incision

B5.2b
Procedures performed using the percutaneous endoscopic approach, with incision or extension of an incision to assist in the removal of all or a portion of a body part or to anastomose a tubular body part to complete the procedure, are coded to the approach value Percutaneous Endoscopic.

Examples: Laparoscopic sigmoid colectomy with extension of stapling port for removal of specimen and direct anastomosis is coded to the approach value percutaneous endoscopic.

Laparoscopic nephrectomy with midline incision for removing the resected kidney is coded to the approach value percutaneous endoscopic.

Robotic-assisted laparoscopic prostatectomy with extension of incision for removal of the resected prostate is coded to the approach value percutaneous endoscopic.

External approach

B5.3a
Procedures performed within an orifice on structures that are visible without the aid of any instrumentation are coded to the approach External.

Example: Resection of tonsils is coded to the approach External.

B5.3b
Procedures performed indirectly by the application of external force through the intervening body layers are coded to the approach External.

Example: Closed reduction of fracture is coded to the approach External.

Percutaneous procedure via device

B5.4
Procedures performed percutaneously via a device placed for the procedure are coded to the approach Percutaneous.

Example: Fragmentation of kidney stone performed via percutaneous nephrostomy is coded to the approach Percutaneous.

B6. Device

General guidelines

B6.1a
A device is coded only if a device remains after the procedure is completed. If no device remains, the device value No Device is coded. In limited root operations, the classification provides the qualifier values Temporary and Intraoperative, for specific procedures involving clinically significant devices, where the purpose of the device is to be utilized for a brief duration during the procedure or current inpatient stay. If a device that is intended to remain after the procedure is completed requires removal before the end of the operative episode in which it was inserted (for example, the device size is inadequate or a complication occurs), both the insertion and removal of the device should be coded.

B6.1b
Materials such as sutures, ligatures, radiological markers and temporary post-operative wound drains are considered integral to the performance of a procedure and are not coded as devices.

B6.1c
Procedures performed on a device only and not on a body part are specified in the root operations Change, Irrigation, Removal and Revision, and are coded to the procedure performed.

Example: Irrigation of percutaneous nephrostomy tube is coded to the root operation Irrigation of indwelling device in the Administration section.

Drainage device

B6.2
A separate procedure to put in a drainage device is coded to the root operation Drainage with the device value Drainage Device.

Obstetric Section Guidelines (Section 1)

C. Obstetrics Section

Products of conception

C1
Procedures performed on the products of conception are coded to the Obstetrics section. Procedures performed on the pregnant female other than the products of conception are coded to the appropriate root operation in the Medical and Surgical section.

Example: Amniocentesis is coded to the products of conception body part in the Obstetrics section. Repair of obstetric urethral laceration is coded to the urethra body part in the Medical and Surgical section.

Procedures following delivery or abortion

C2
Procedures performed following a delivery or abortion for curettage of the endometrium or evacuation of retained products of conception are all coded in the Obstetrics section, to the root operation Extraction and the body part Products of Conception, Retained.

Diagnostic or therapeutic dilation and curettage performed during times other than the postpartum or post-abortion period are all coded in the Medical and Surgical section, to the root operation Extraction and the body part Endometrium.

Radiation Therapy Section Guidelines (Section D)

D. Radiation Therapy Section

Brachytherapy

D1.a
Brachytherapy is coded to the modality Brachytherapy in the Radiation Therapy section. When a radioactive brachytherapy source is left in the body at the end of the procedure, it is coded separately to the root operation Insertion with the device value Radioactive Element.

Example: Brachytherapy with implantation of a low dose rate brachytherapy source left in the body at the end of the procedure is coded to the applicable treatment site in section D, Radiation Therapy, with the modality Brachytherapy, the modality qualifier value Low Dose Rate, and the applicable isotope value and qualifier value. The implantation of the brachytherapy source is coded separately to the device value Radioactive Element in the appropriate Insertion table of the Medical and Surgical section. The Radiation Therapy section code identifies the specific modality and isotope of the brachytherapy, and the root operation Insertion code identifies the implantation of the brachytherapy source that remains in the body at the end of the procedure.

Exception: Implantation of Cesium-131 brachytherapy seeds embedded in a collagen matrix to the treatment site after resection of brain tumor is coded to the root operation Insertion with the device value Radioactive Element, Cesium-131 Collagen Implant. The procedure is coded to the root operation Insertion only, because the device value identifies both the implantation of the radioactive element and a specific brachytherapy isotope that is not included in the Radiation Therapy section tables.

D1.b
A separate procedure to place a temporary applicator for delivering the brachytherapy is coded to the root operation Insertion and the device value Other Device.

Examples: Intrauterine brachytherapy applicator placed as a separate procedure from the brachytherapy procedure is coded to Insertion of Other Device, and the brachytherapy is coded separately using the modality Brachytherapy in the Radiation Therapy section.

Intrauterine brachytherapy applicator placed concomitantly with delivery of the brachytherapy dose is coded with a single code using the modality Brachytherapy in the Radiation Therapy section.

New Technology Section Guidelines (Section X)

E. New Technology Section

General guidelines

E1.a
Section X codes fully represent the specific procedure described in the code title, and do not require additional codes from other sections of ICD-10-PCS. When section X contains a code title which fully describes a specific new technology procedure, and it is the only procedure performed, only the section X code is reported for the procedure.

There is no need to report an additional code in another section of ICD-10-PCS. Example: XW04321 Introduction of Ceftazidime-Avibactam Anti-infective into Central Vein, Percutaneous Approach, New Technology Group 1, can be coded to indicate that Ceftazidime-Avibactam Anti-infective was administered via a central vein. A separate code from table 3E0 in the Administration section of ICD-10-PCS is not coded in addition to this code.

E1.b
When multiple procedures are performed, New Technology section X codes are coded following the multiple procedures guideline.

Examples: Dual filter cerebral embolic filtration used during transcatheter aortic valve replacement (TAVR), X2A5312 Cerebral Embolic Filtration, Dual Filter in Innominate Artery and Left Common Carotid Artery, Percutaneous Approach, New Technology

Group 2, is coded for the cerebral embolic filtration, along with an ICD-10-PCS code for the TAVR procedure.

Magnetically controlled growth rod (MCGR) placed during a spinal fusion procedure, a code from table XNS, Reposition of the Bones is coded for the MCGR, along with an ICD-10-PCS code for the spinal fusion procedure.

F. Selection of Principal Procedure

The following instructions should be applied in the selection of principal procedure and clarification on the importance of the relation to the principal diagnosis when more than one procedure is performed:

1. Procedure performed for definitive treatment of both principal diagnosis and secondary diagnosis
   a. Sequence procedure performed for definitive treatment most related to principal diagnosis as principal procedure.

2. Procedure performed for definitive treatment and diagnostic procedures performed for both principal diagnosis and secondary diagnosis.
   a. Sequence procedure performed for definitive treatment most related to principal diagnosis as principal procedure

3. A diagnostic procedure was performed for the principal diagnosis and a procedure is performed for definitive treatment of a secondary diagnosis.
   a. Sequence diagnostic procedure as principal procedure, since the procedure most related to the principal diagnosis takes precedence.

4. No procedures performed that are related to principal diagnosis; procedures performed for definitive treatment and diagnostic procedures were performed for secondary diagnosis
   a. Sequence procedure performed for definitive treatment of secondary diagnosis as principal procedure, since there are no procedures (definitive or nondefinitive treatment) related to principal diagnosis.

This page intentionally left blank

Anatomical Illustrations

Circulatory System — Arteries and Veins

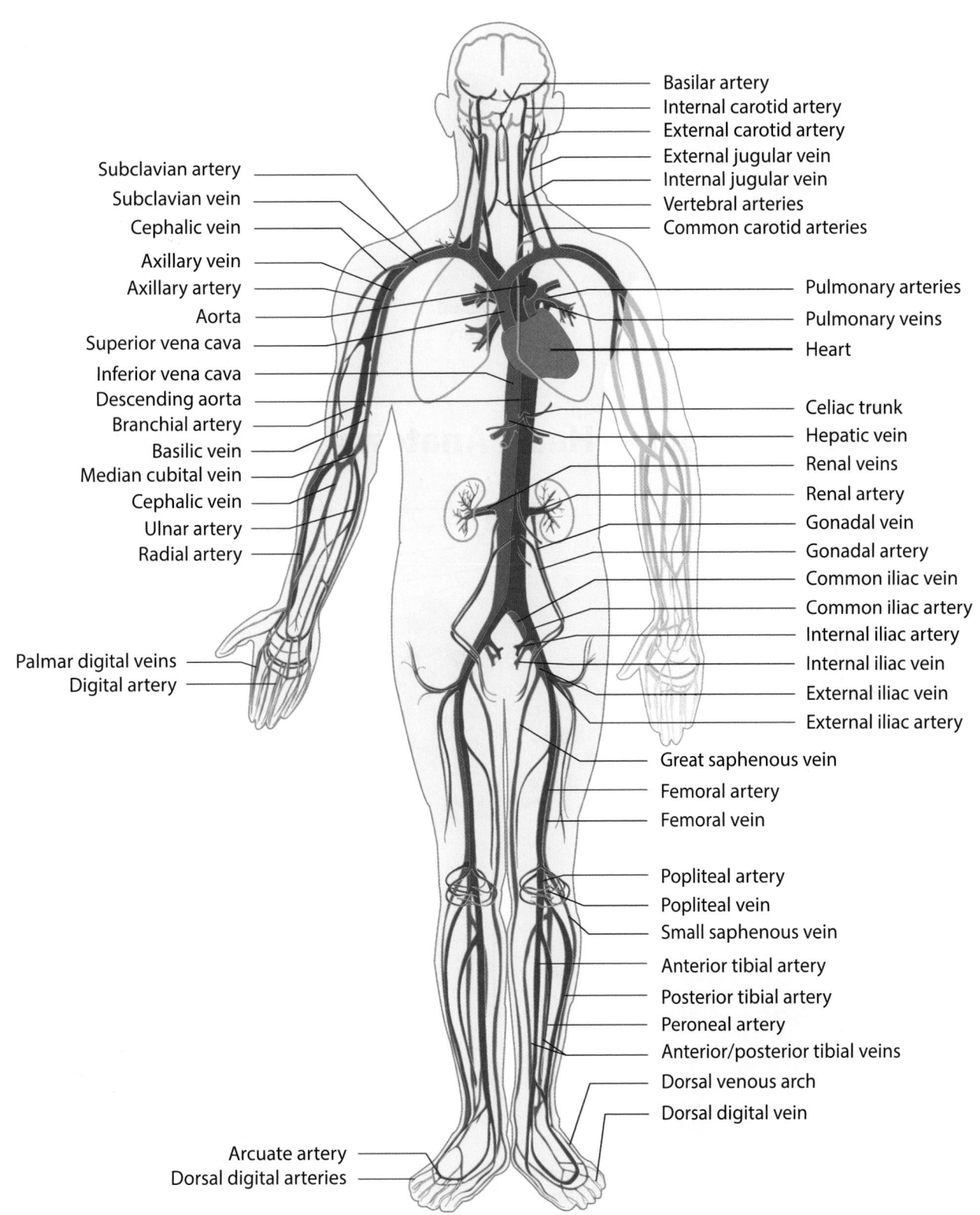

Subclavian artery
Subclavian vein
Cephalic vein
Axillary vein
Axillary artery
Aorta
Superior vena cava
Inferior vena cava
Descending aorta
Branchial artery
Basilic vein
Median cubital vein
Cephalic vein
Ulnar artery
Radial artery

Palmar digital veins
Digital artery

Basilar artery
Internal carotid artery
External carotid artery
External jugular vein
Internal jugular vein
Vertebral arteries
Common carotid arteries

Pulmonary arteries
Pulmonary veins
Heart

Celiac trunk
Hepatic vein
Renal veins
Renal artery
Gonadal vein
Gonadal artery
Common iliac vein
Common iliac artery
Internal iliac artery
Internal iliac vein
External iliac vein
External iliac artery

Great saphenous vein
Femoral artery
Femoral vein

Popliteal artery
Popliteal vein
Small saphenous vein
Anterior tibial artery
Posterior tibial artery
Peroneal artery
Anterior/posterior tibial veins
Dorsal venous arch
Dorsal digital vein

Arcuate artery
Dorsal digital arteries

ANATOMICAL ILLUSTRATIONS

Circulatory System — Artery and Vein Anatomy

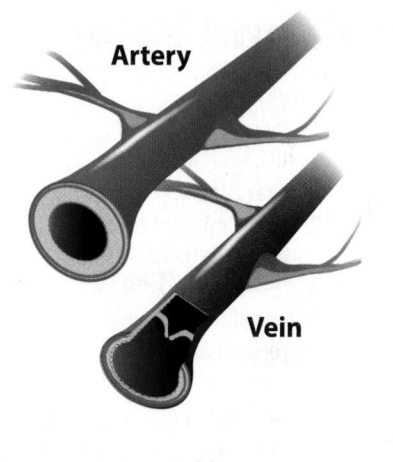

Artery

Vein

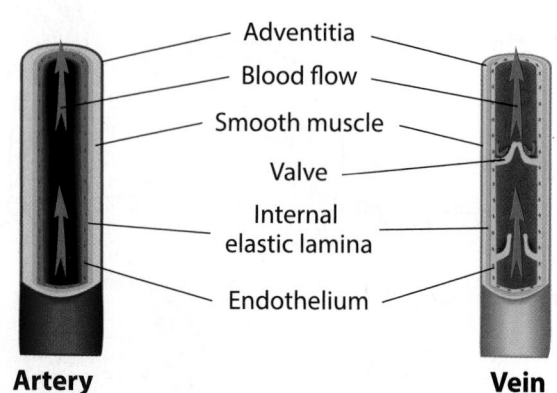

Adventitia
Blood flow
Smooth muscle
Valve
Internal elastic lamina
Endothelium

Artery

Vein

Circulatory System — Heart Anatomy and Cardiac Cycle

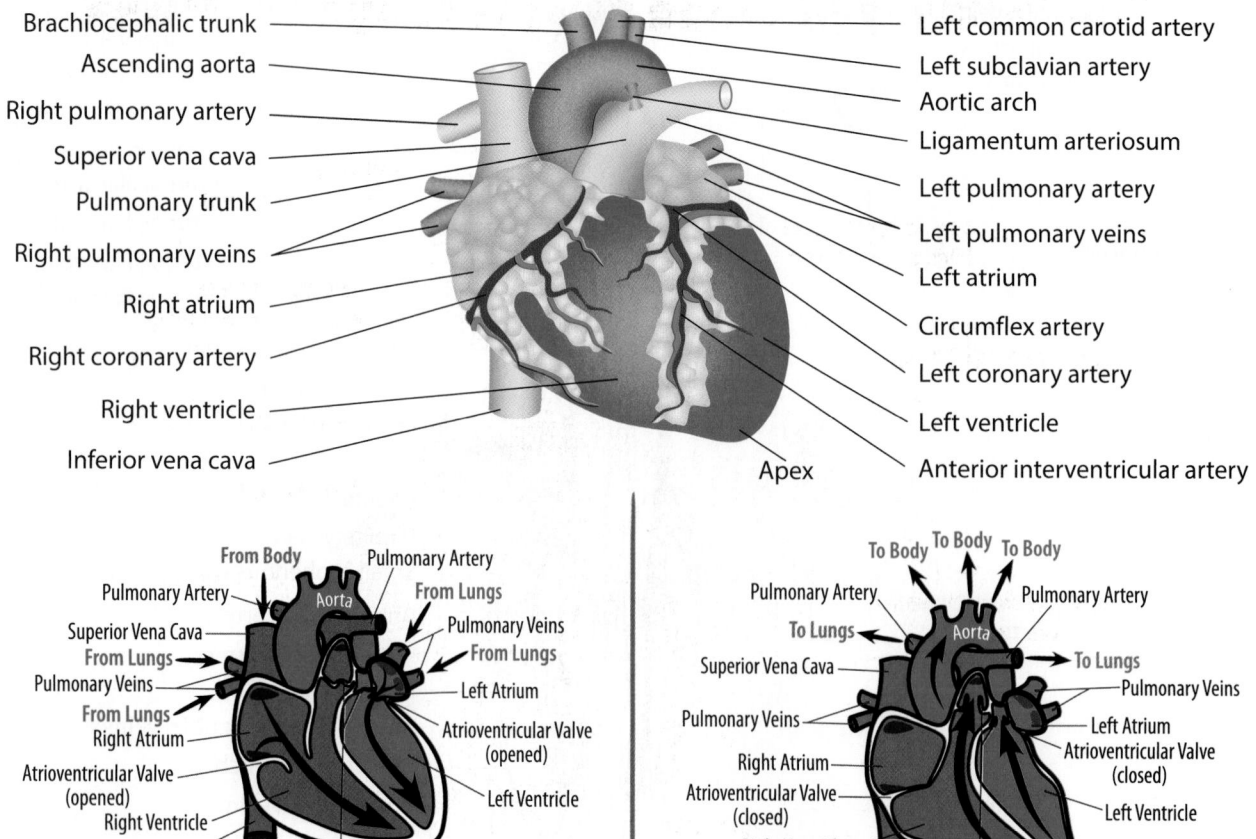

Brachiocephalic trunk
Ascending aorta
Right pulmonary artery
Superior vena cava
Pulmonary trunk
Right pulmonary veins
Right atrium
Right coronary artery
Right ventricle
Inferior vena cava

Left common carotid artery
Left subclavian artery
Aortic arch
Ligamentum arteriosum
Left pulmonary artery
Left pulmonary veins
Left atrium
Circumflex artery
Left coronary artery
Left ventricle
Apex
Anterior interventricular artery

From Body
Pulmonary Artery
Pulmonary Artery
From Lungs
Aorta
Superior Vena Cava
Pulmonary Veins
From Lungs
From Lungs
From Lungs
Left Atrium
Right Atrium
Atrioventricular Valve (opened)
Atrioventricular Valve (opened)
Right Ventricle
Left Ventricle
Inferior Vena Cava
Semilunar Valves (closed)
From Body

Diastole (Filling)

To Body   To Body   To Body
Pulmonary Artery
Pulmonary Artery
To Lungs
Aorta
Superior Vena Cava
To Lungs
Pulmonary Veins
Pulmonary Veins
Left Atrium
Right Atrium
Atrioventricular Valve (closed)
Atrioventricular Valve (closed)
Left Ventricle
Right Ventricle
Inferior Vena Cava
Semilunar Valves (opened)

Systole (Pumping)

Electrical Conducting System of the Heart

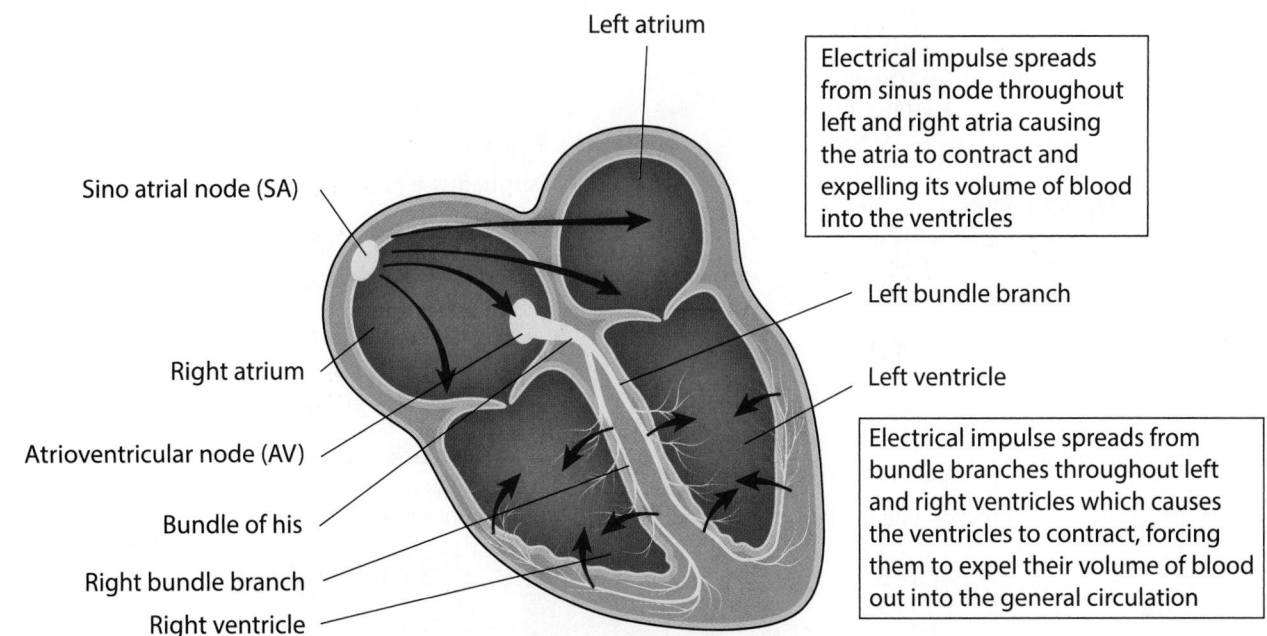

Left atrium

Sino atrial node (SA)

Right atrium

Atrioventricular node (AV)

Bundle of his

Right bundle branch

Right ventricle

Left bundle branch

Left ventricle

Electrical impulse spreads from sinus node throughout left and right atria causing the atria to contract and expelling its volume of blood into the ventricles

Electrical impulse spreads from bundle branches throughout left and right ventricles which causes the ventricles to contract, forcing them to expel their volume of blood out into the general circulation

The Pathway of Blood Flow Through the Heart

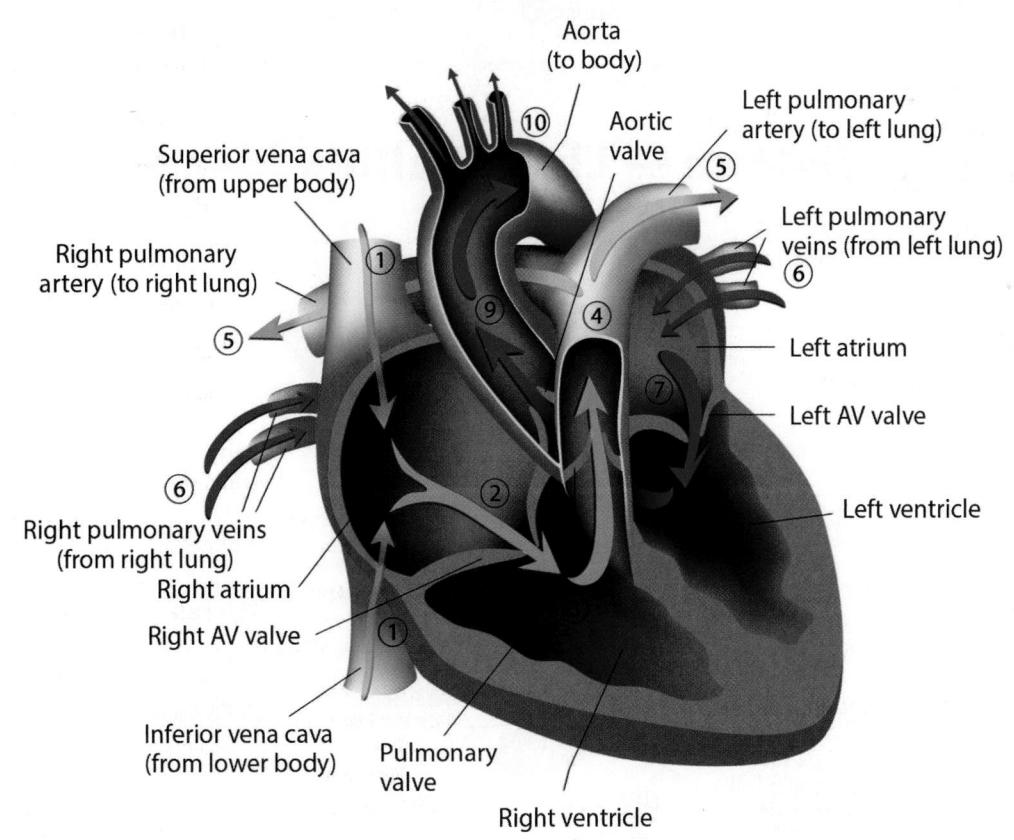

Aorta
(to body)

Aortic
valve

Left pulmonary
artery (to left lung)

Superior vena cava
(from upper body)

Right pulmonary
artery (to right lung)

Left pulmonary
veins (from left lung)

Left atrium

Left AV valve

Left ventricle

Right pulmonary veins
(from right lung)

Right atrium

Right AV valve

Inferior vena cava
(from lower body)

Pulmonary
valve

Right ventricle

Digestive System Anatomy

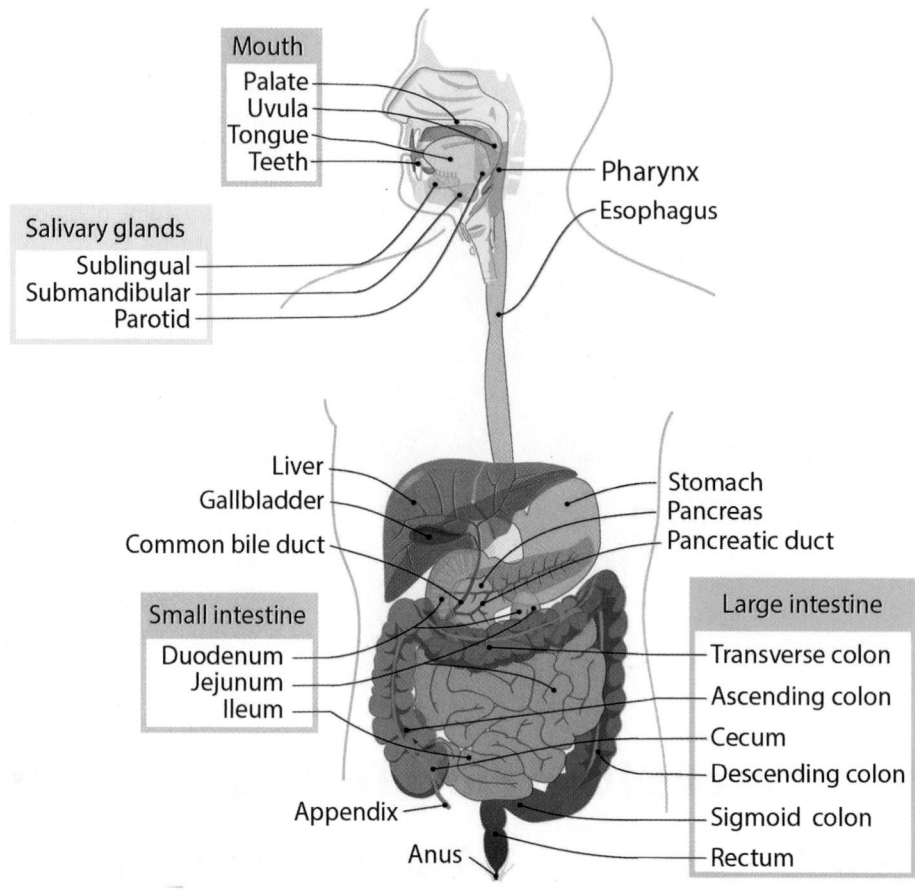

Title: Diagram of the gastrointestinal tract, **Author:** Mariana Ruiz (Lady of Hats), Jmarchn, **Source:** Own work, **License:** Public domain, **URL link:** https://en.wikiversity.org/wiki/File:Digestive_system_diagram_en.svg

Digestive System — Liver, Gallbladder, Pancreas

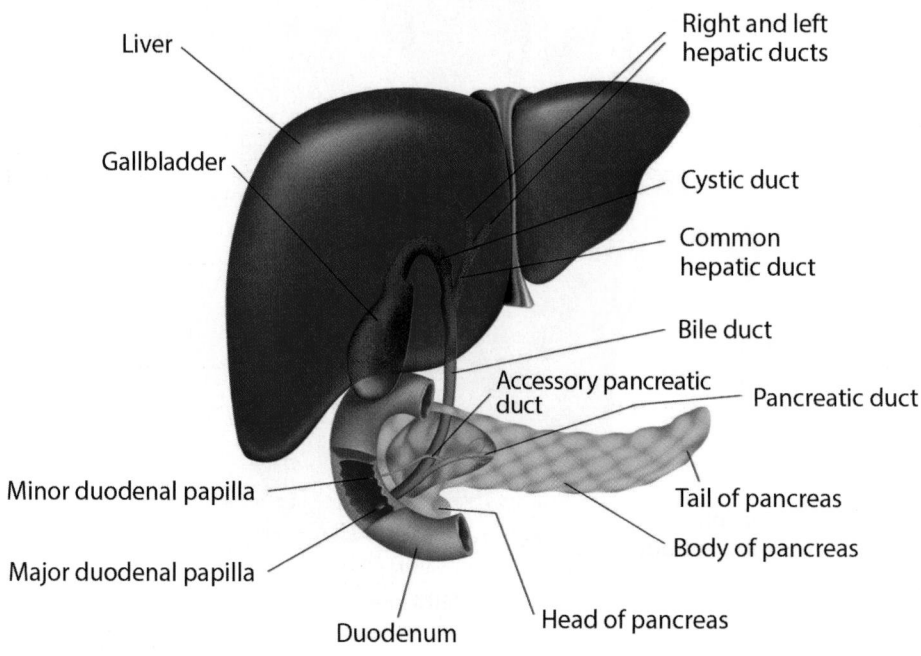

Digestive System — Mouth Anatomy

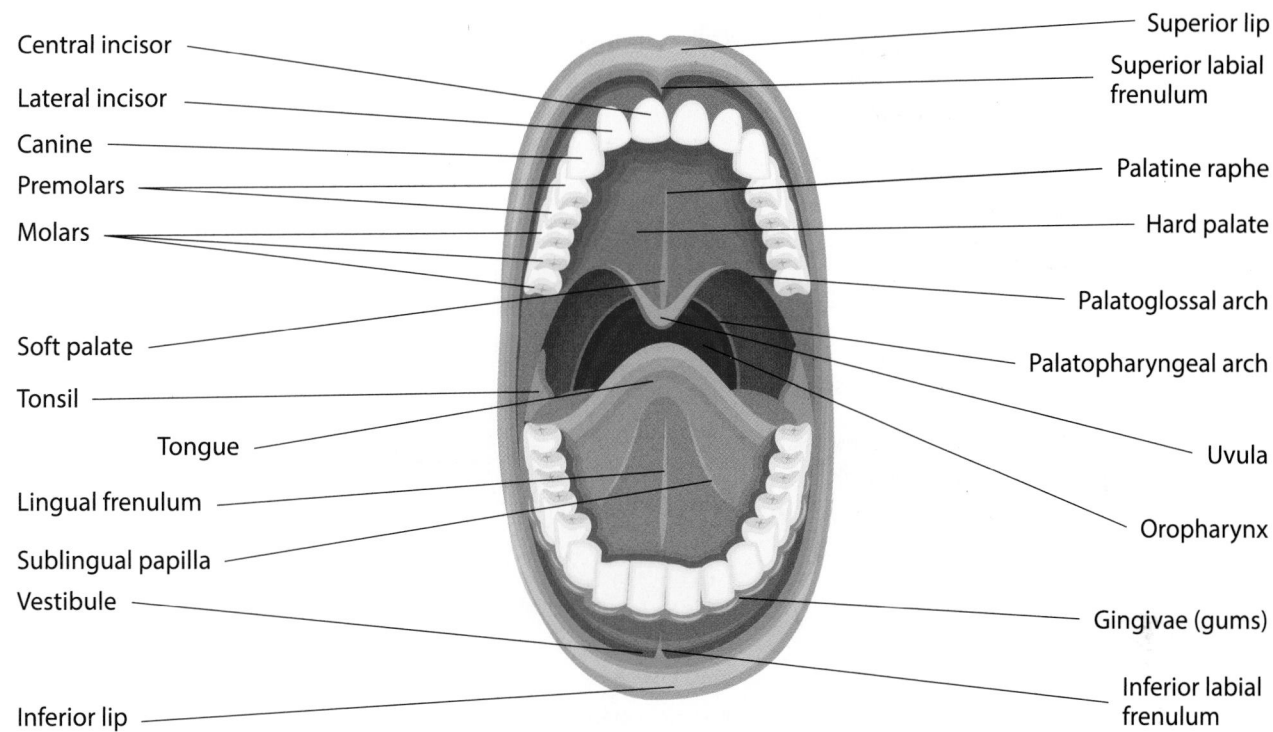

Central incisor

Lateral incisor

Canine

Premolars

Molars

Soft palate

Tonsil

Tongue

Lingual frenulum

Sublingual papilla

Vestibule

Inferior lip

Superior lip

Superior labial frenulum

Palatine raphe

Hard palate

Palatoglossal arch

Palatopharyngeal arch

Uvula

Oropharynx

Gingivae (gums)

Inferior labial frenulum

Digestive System — Tongue Anatomy

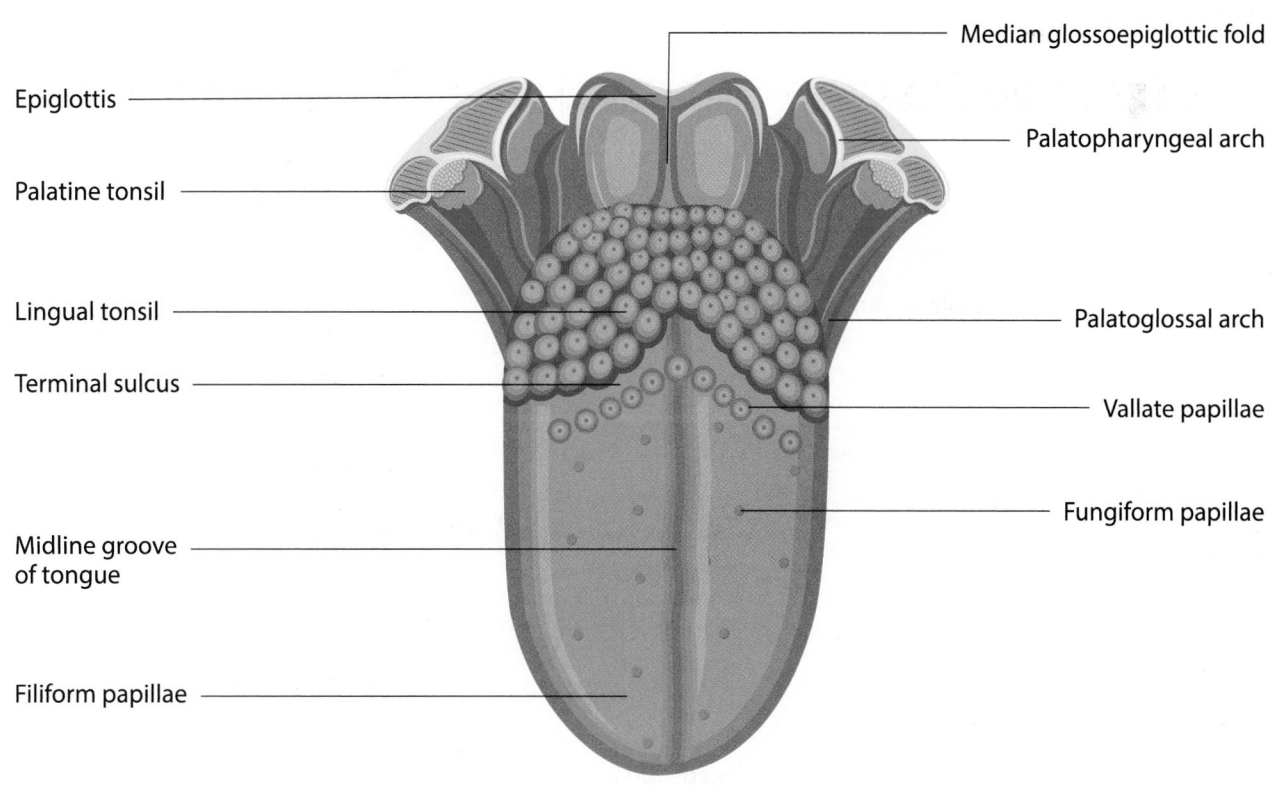

Epiglottis

Palatine tonsil

Lingual tonsil

Terminal sulcus

Midline groove of tongue

Filiform papillae

Median glossoepiglottic fold

Palatopharyngeal arch

Palatoglossal arch

Vallate papillae

Fungiform papillae

Digestive System — Stomach Anatomy

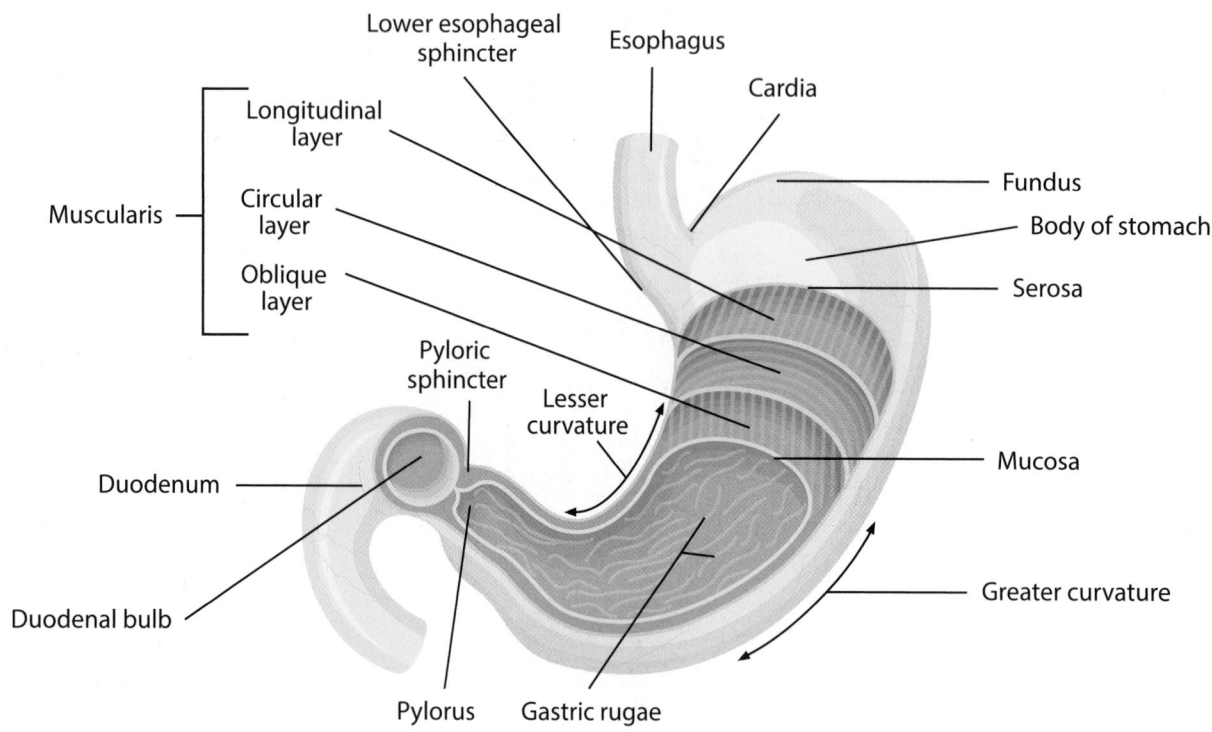

Digestive System — Small Intestine Anatomy

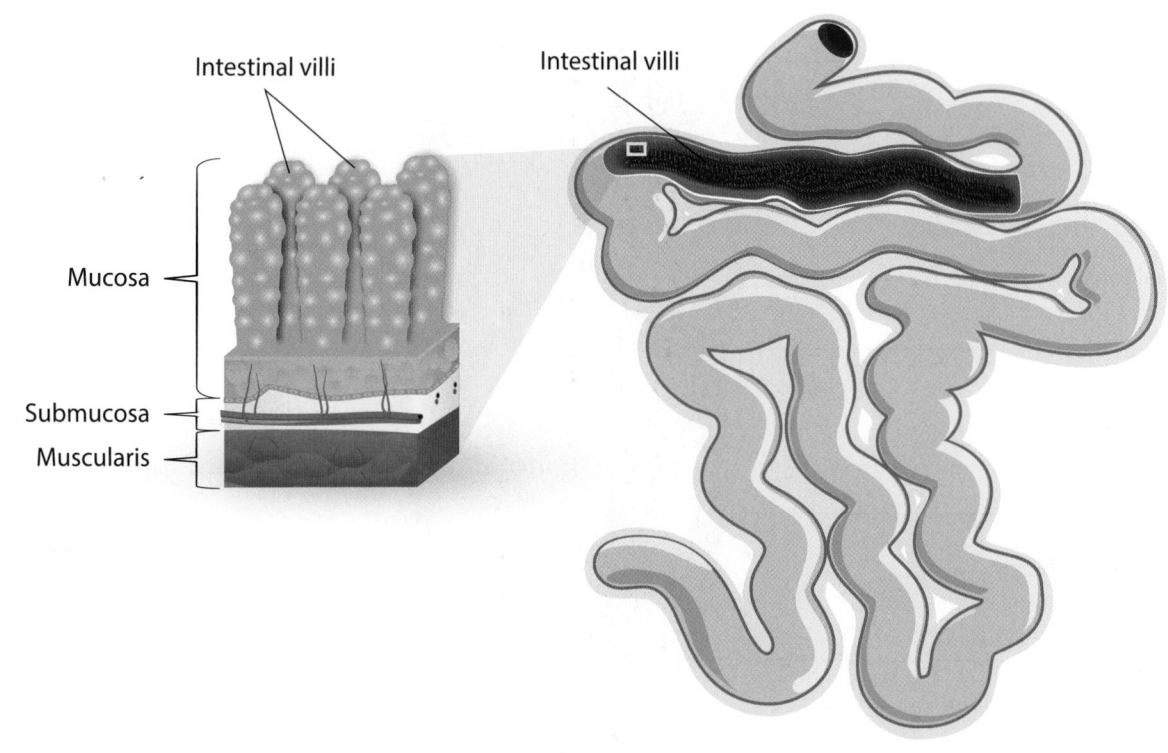

Digestive System — Large Intestine Anatomy

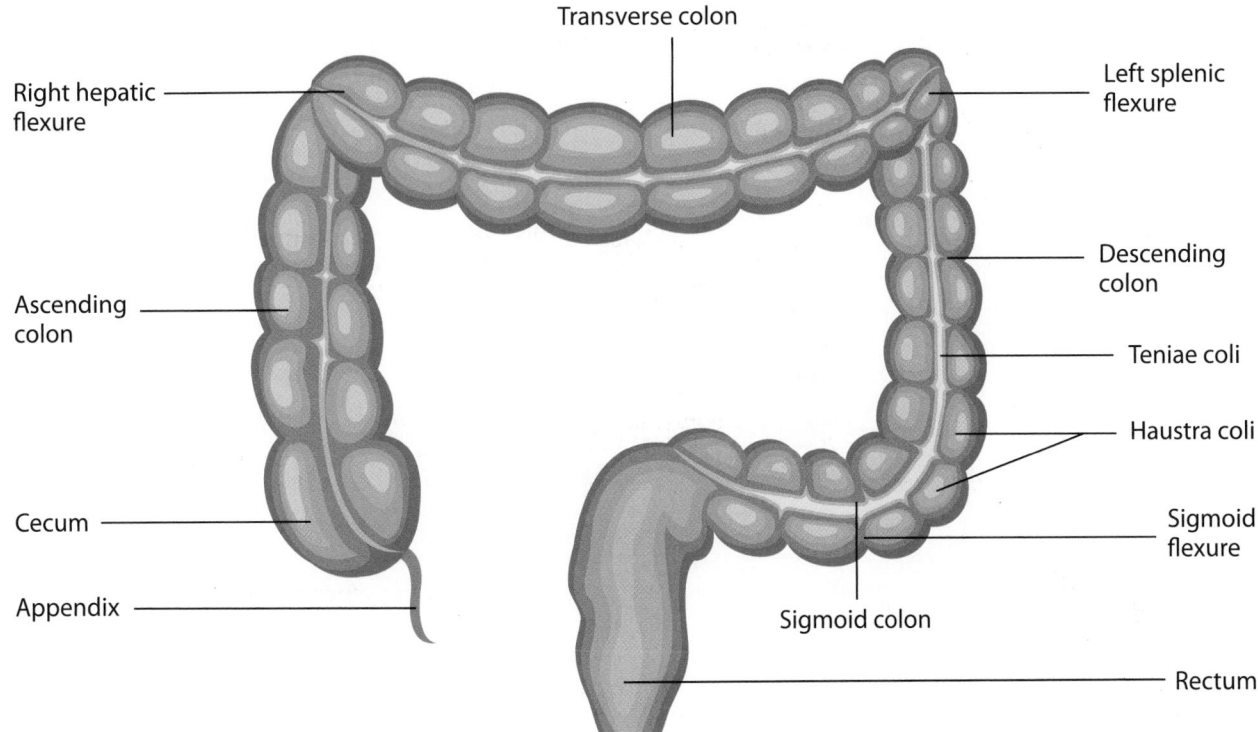

Digestive System — Rectum Anatomy

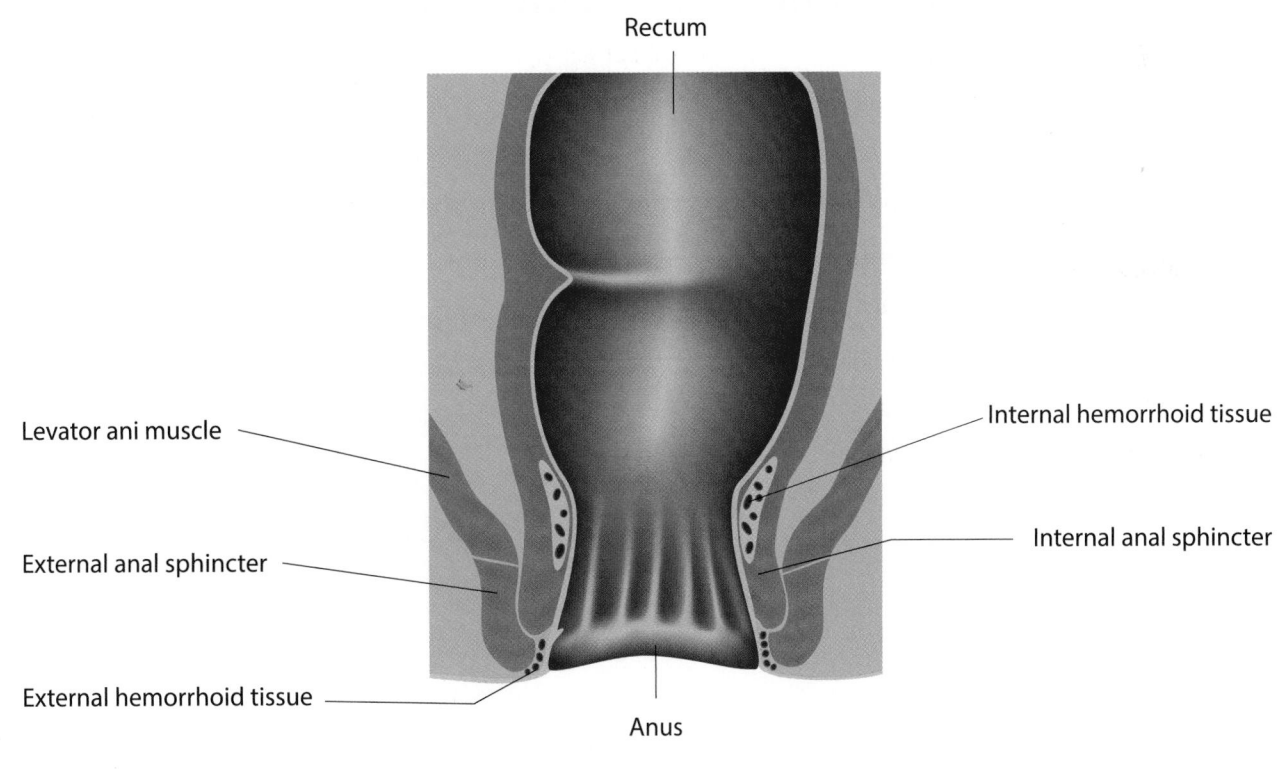

Ear Anatomy

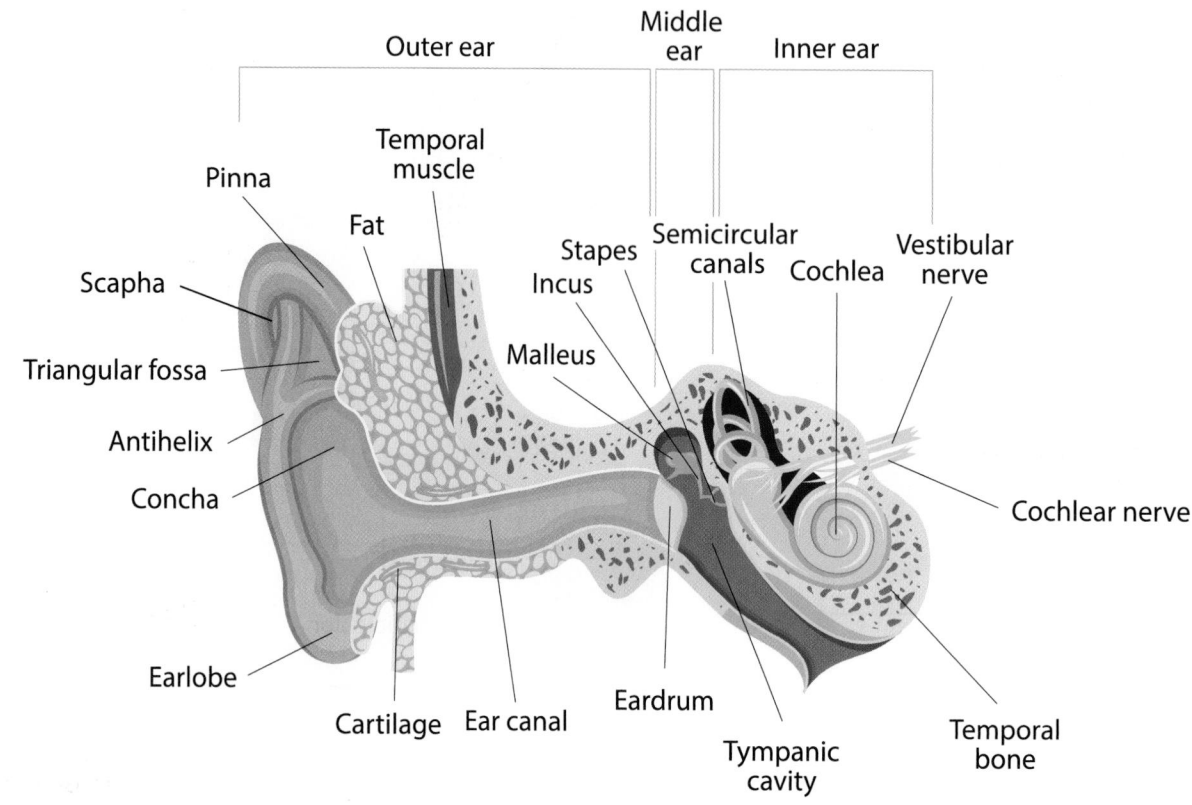

Ear Anatomy - Cochlea (Inner Ear)

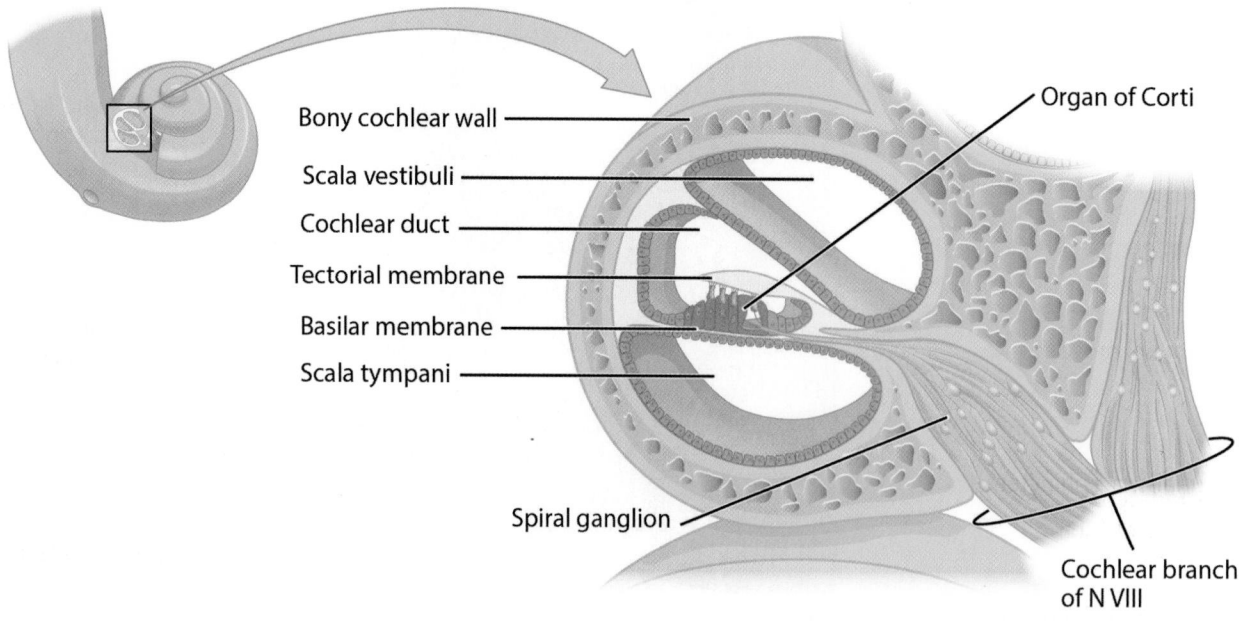

Title: 1406 Cochlea.jpg, **Author:** OpenStax, **Source:** https://cnx.org/contents/FPtK1zmh@8.25:fEl3C8Ot@10/Preface, **License/Permission:** This file is licensed under the Creative Commons Attribution 4.0 International license., **URL link:** https://en.wikiversity.org/wiki/File:1406_Cochlea.jpg

Endocrine System Anatomy and Hormones

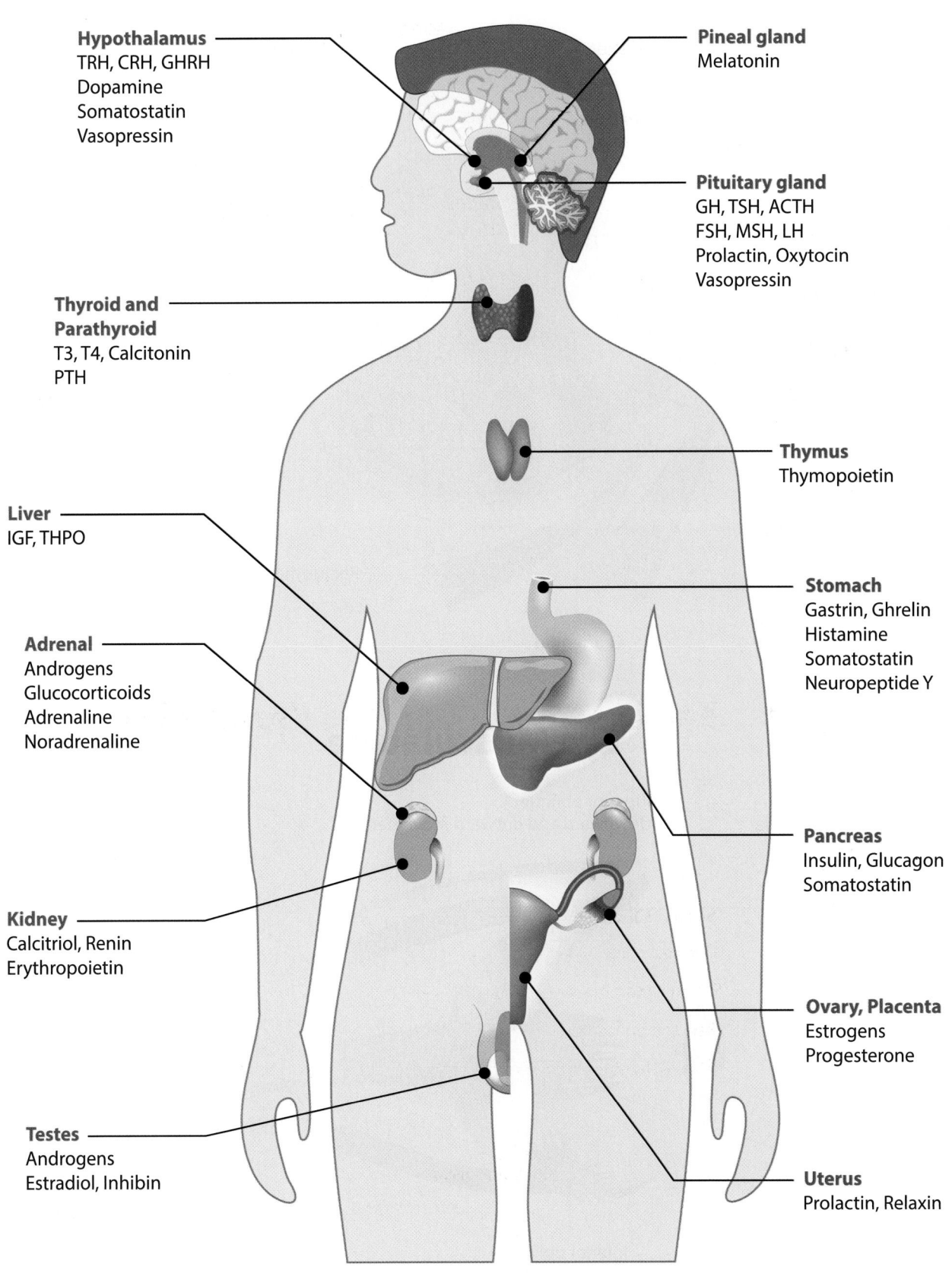

Hypothalamus
TRH, CRH, GHRH
Dopamine
Somatostatin
Vasopressin

Pineal gland
Melatonin

Pituitary gland
GH, TSH, ACTH
FSH, MSH, LH
Prolactin, Oxytocin
Vasopressin

Thyroid and Parathyroid
T3, T4, Calcitonin
PTH

Thymus
Thymopoietin

Liver
IGF, THPO

Stomach
Gastrin, Ghrelin
Histamine
Somatostatin
Neuropeptide Y

Adrenal
Androgens
Glucocorticoids
Adrenaline
Noradrenaline

Pancreas
Insulin, Glucagon
Somatostatin

Kidney
Calcitriol, Renin
Erythropoietin

Ovary, Placenta
Estrogens
Progesterone

Testes
Androgens
Estradiol, Inhibin

Uterus
Prolactin, Relaxin

Eye Anatomy

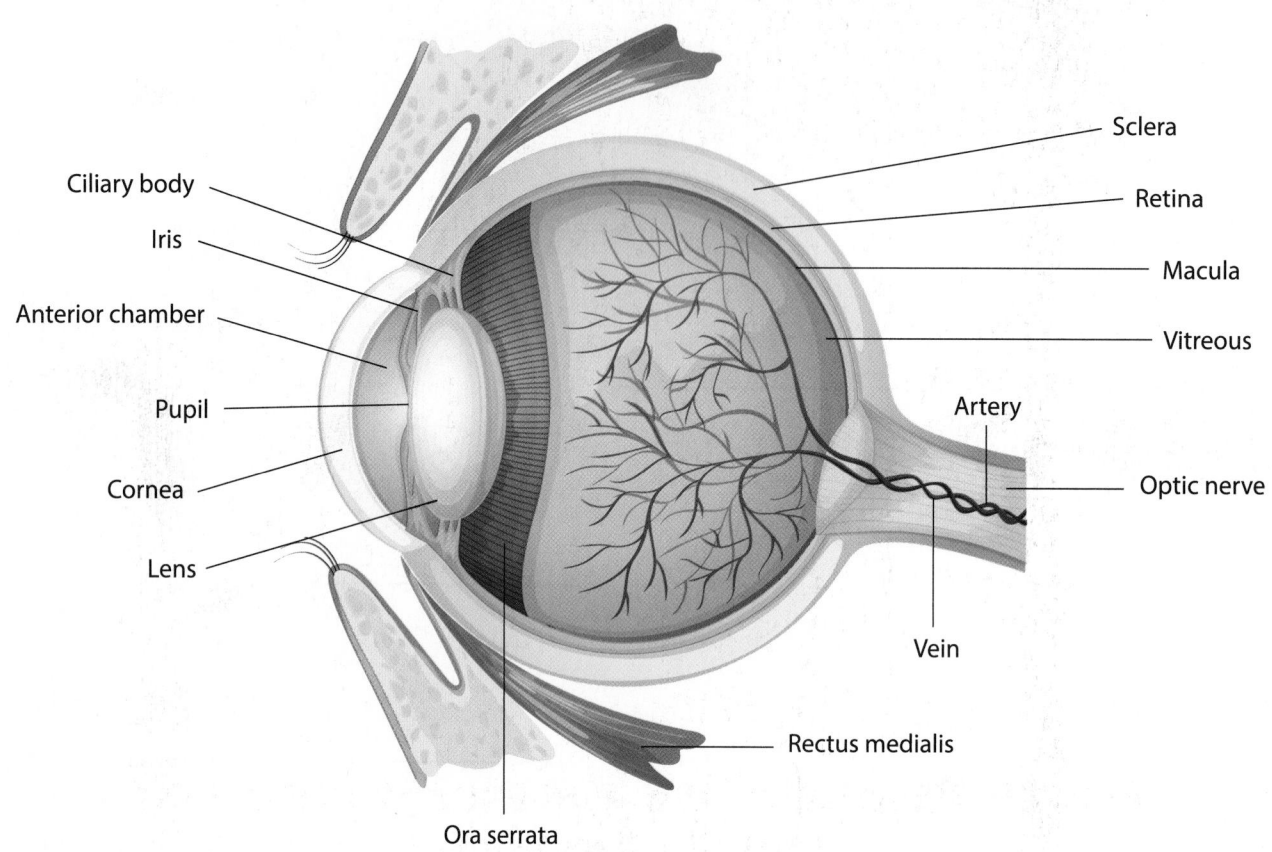

Eye Musculature

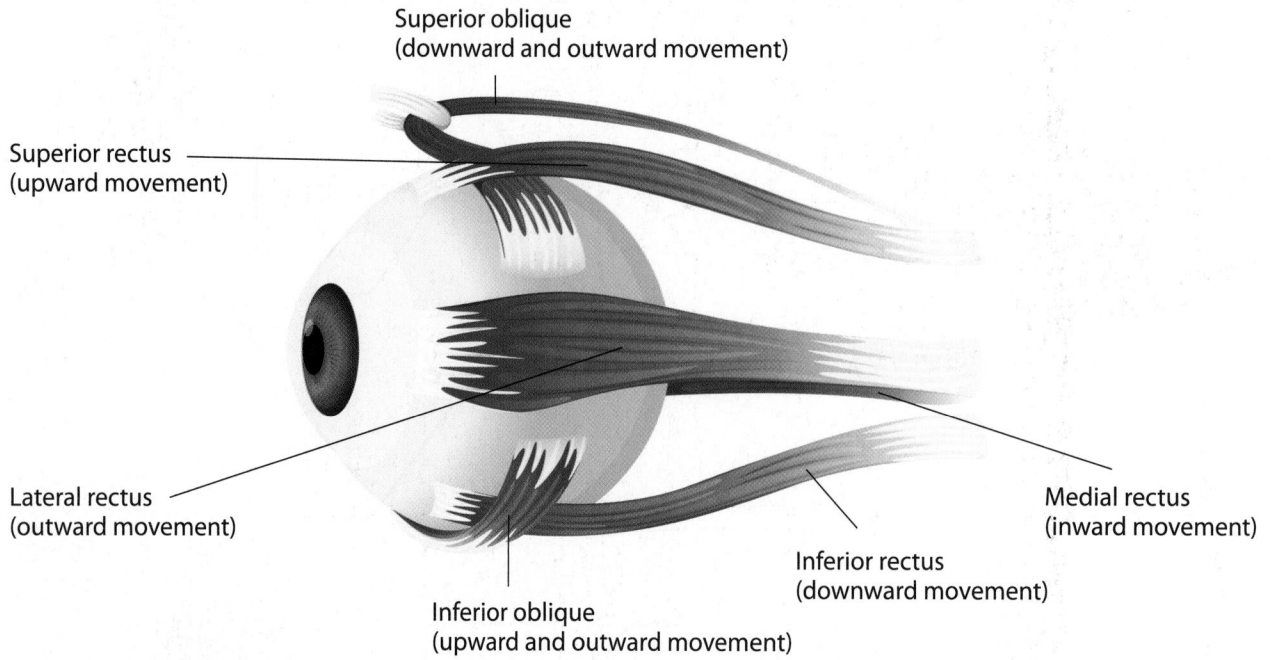

Female Reproductive System Anatomy

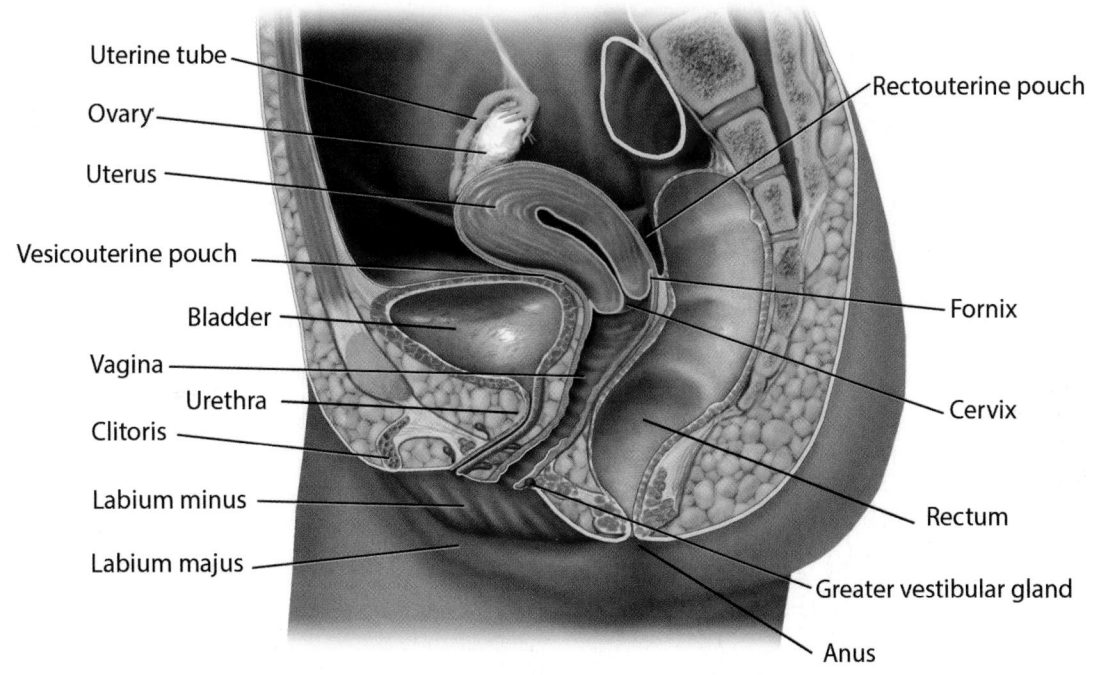

Title: Blausen 0400 FemaleReproSystem 02b.png, **Author:** BruceBlaus., **Source:** Blausen.com staff (2014). "Medical gallery of Blausen Medical 2014". *WikiJournal of Medicine* **1** (2). DOI:10.15347/wjm/2014.010. ISSN 2002-4436.Modified by User:ArnoldReinhold who released mods under CC0, **License/Permission:** This file is licensed under the Creative Commons Attribution 3.0 Unported license., **URL link:** https://commons.wikimedia.org/wiki/File:Blausen_0400_FemaleReproSystem_02b.png

Female Reproductive System — Uterus and Adnexa Anatomy

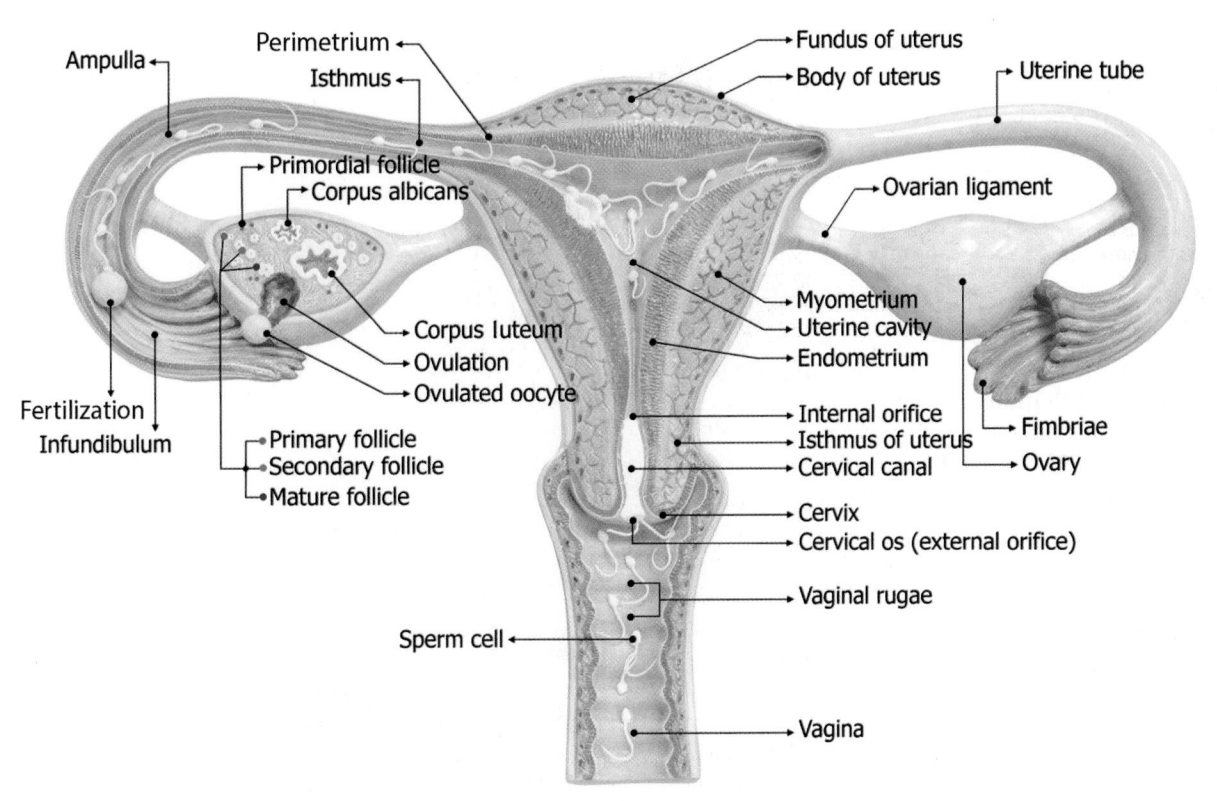

Female Reproductive System — Breast Anatomy

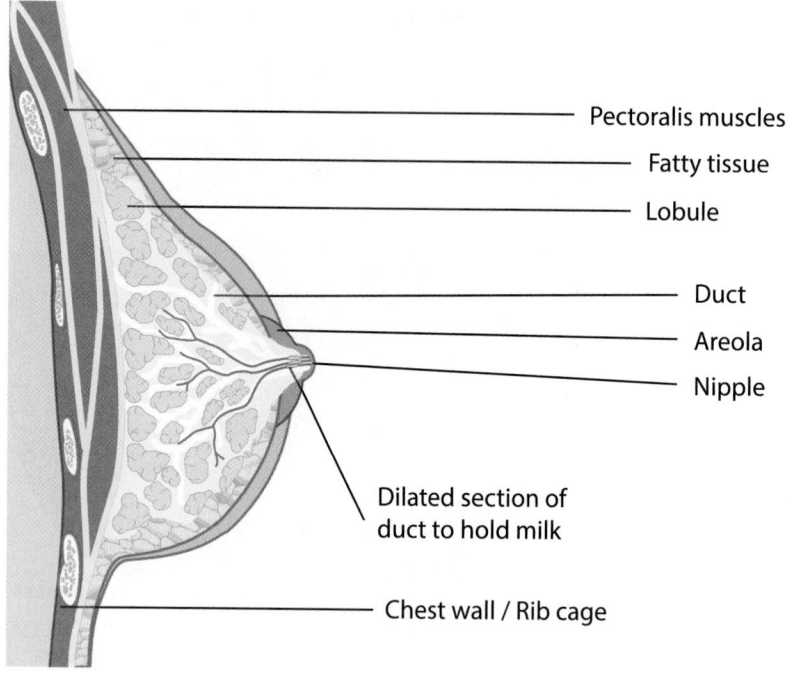

- Pectoralis muscles
- Fatty tissue
- Lobule
- Duct
- Areola
- Nipple
- Dilated section of duct to hold milk
- Chest wall / Rib cage

Female Reproductive System — Perineum Anatomy

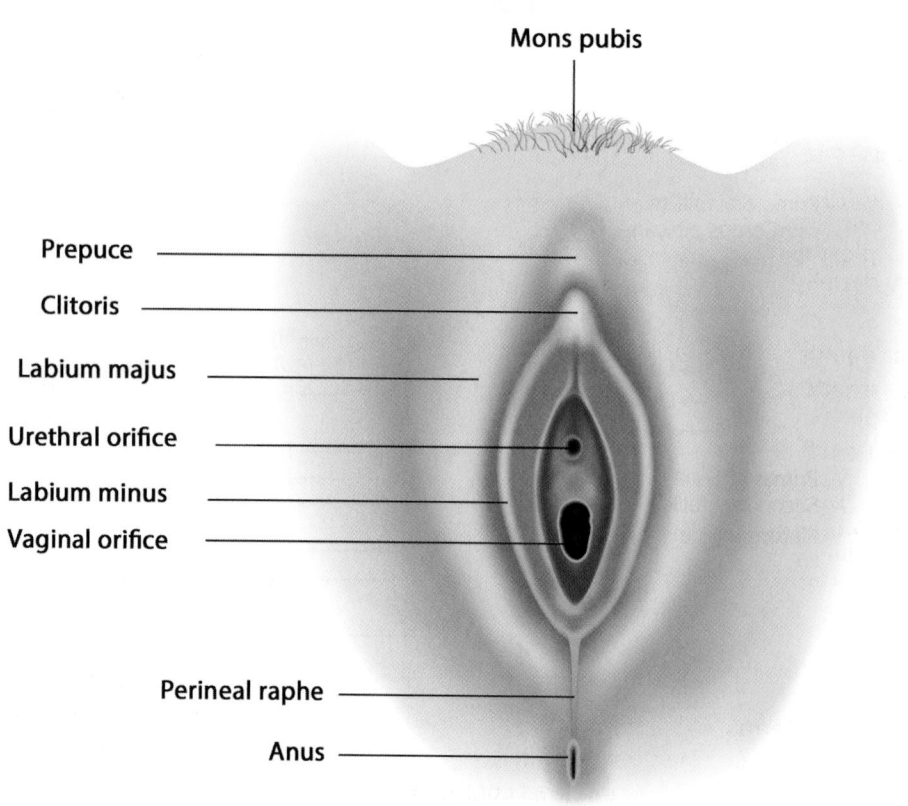

- Mons pubis
- Prepuce
- Clitoris
- Labium majus
- Urethral orifice
- Labium minus
- Vaginal orifice
- Perineal raphe
- Anus

Integumentary System Anatomy

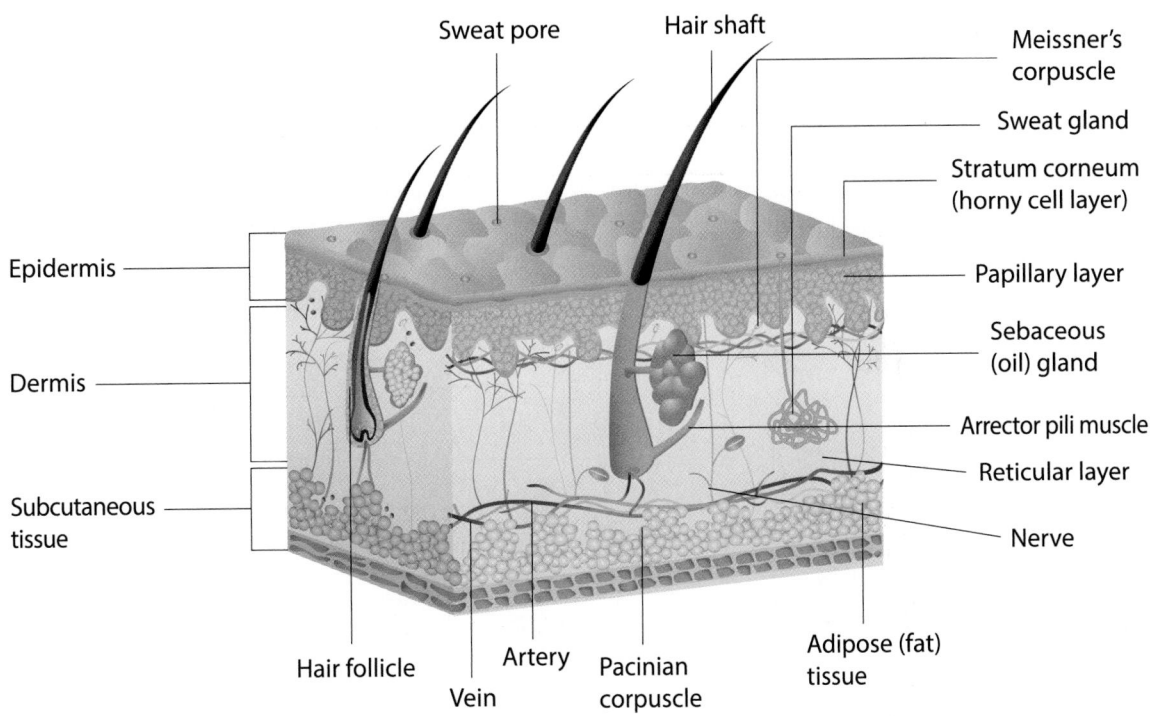

Sweat pore
Hair shaft
Meissner's corpuscle
Sweat gland
Stratum corneum (horny cell layer)
Epidermis
Papillary layer
Dermis
Sebaceous (oil) gland
Arrector pili muscle
Reticular layer
Subcutaneous tissue
Nerve
Hair follicle
Vein
Artery
Pacinian corpuscle
Adipose (fat) tissue

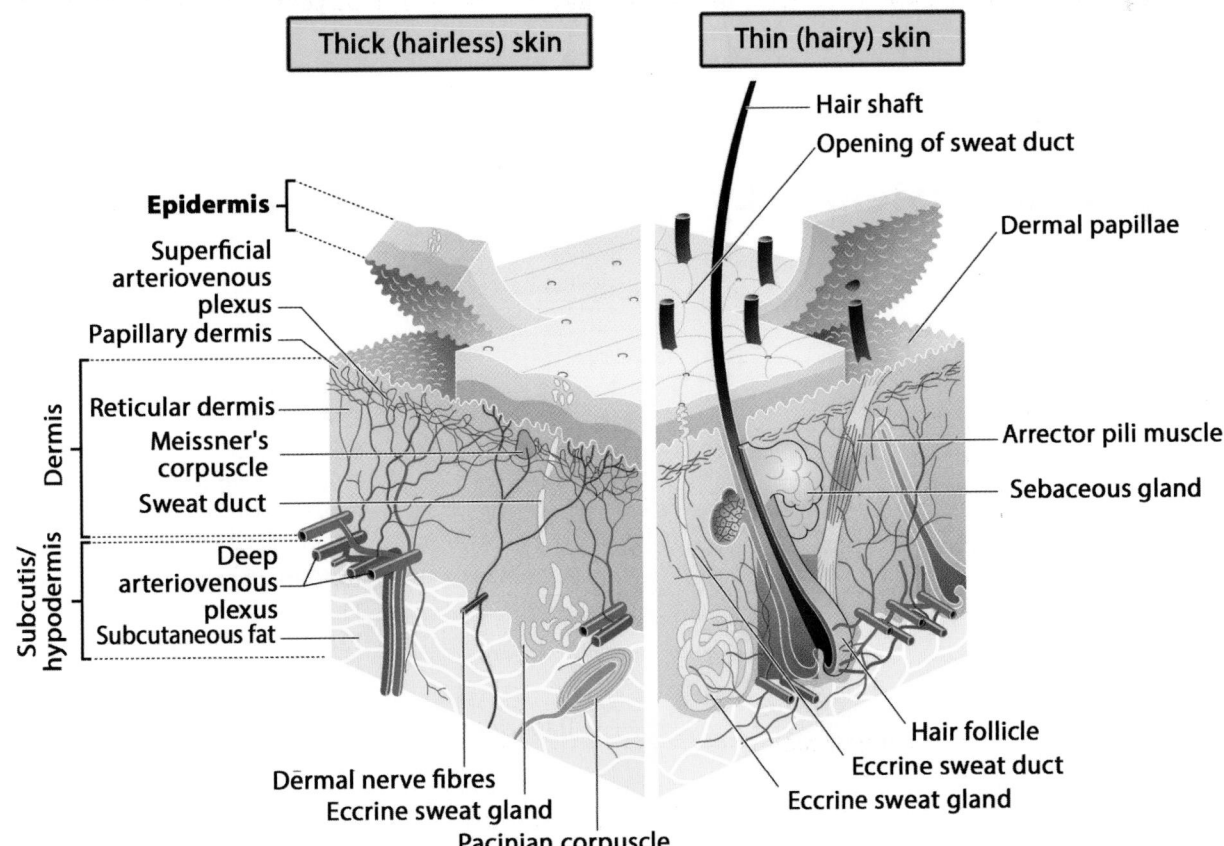

Thick (hairless) skin
Thin (hairy) skin

Hair shaft
Opening of sweat duct
Epidermis
Dermal papillae
Superficial arteriovenous plexus
Papillary dermis
Dermis
Reticular dermis
Arrector pili muscle
Meissner's corpuscle
Sebaceous gland
Sweat duct
Subcutis/hypodermis
Deep arteriovenous plexus
Subcutaneous fat
Hair follicle
Eccrine sweat duct
Dermal nerve fibres
Eccrine sweat gland
Eccrine sweat gland
Pacinian corpuscle

ANATOMICAL ILLUSTRATIONS

Lymphatic System Anatomy

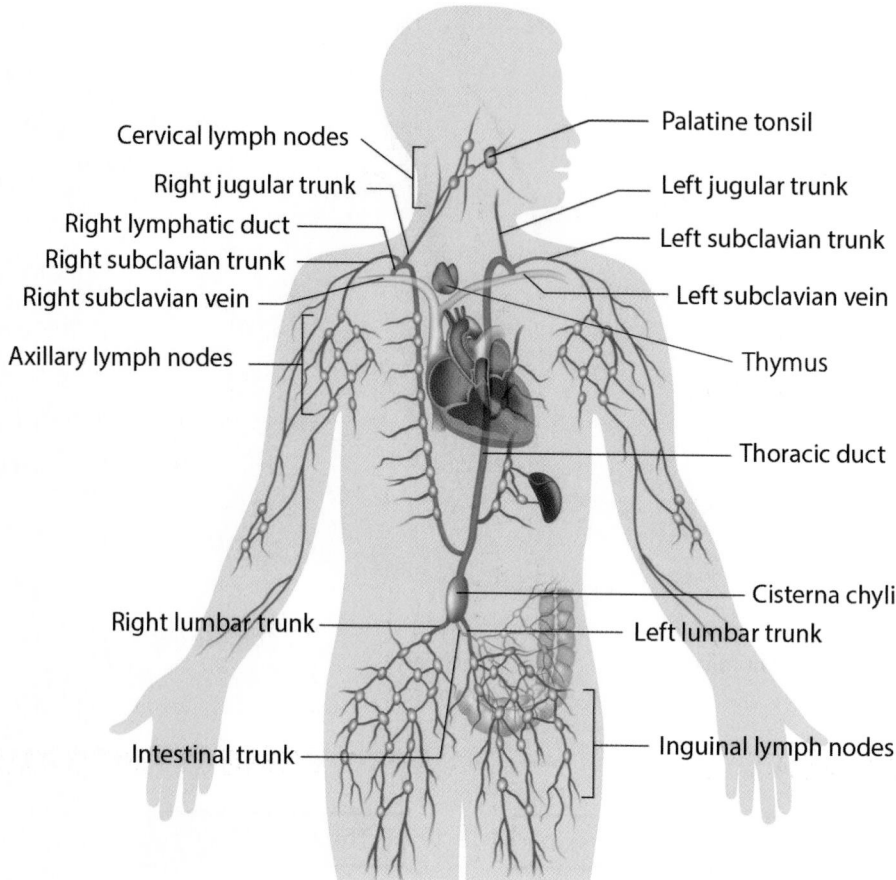

Lymphatic System — Lymph Nodes of the Head and Neck

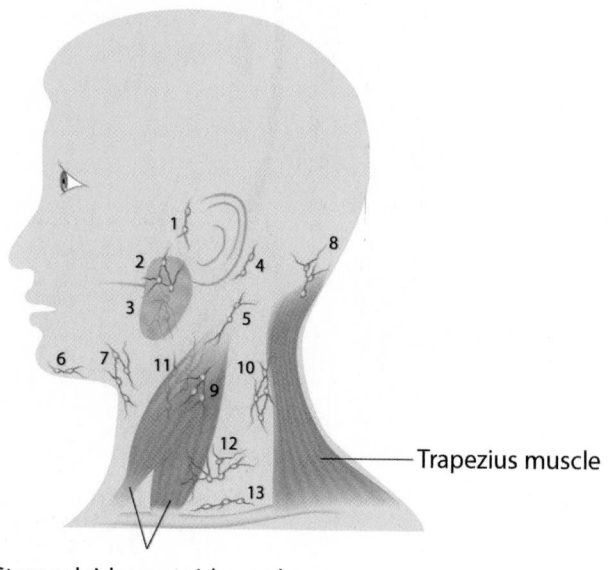

1. Preauricular
2. Superficial parotid
3. Deep parotid
4. Posterior auricular
5. Mastoid
6. Submental
7. Submandibular
8. Occipital
9. Superficial anterior cervical
10. Superficial posterior cervical
11. Superior deep cervical
12. Inferior deep cervical
13. Supraclavicular

Lymphatic System — Humoral Immunity

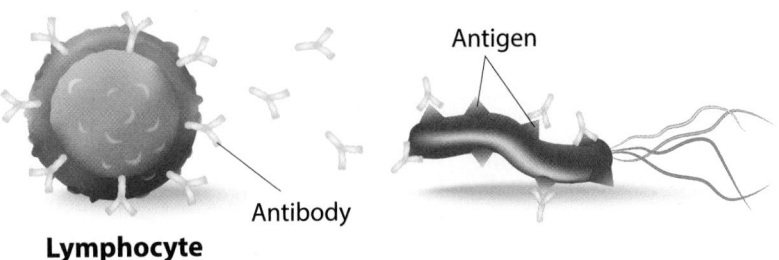

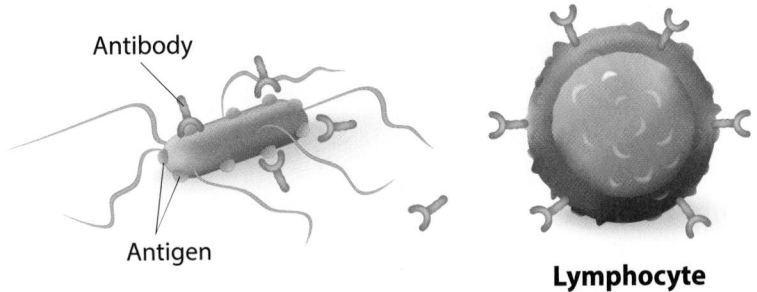

Lymphatic System — Lymph Node Anatomy

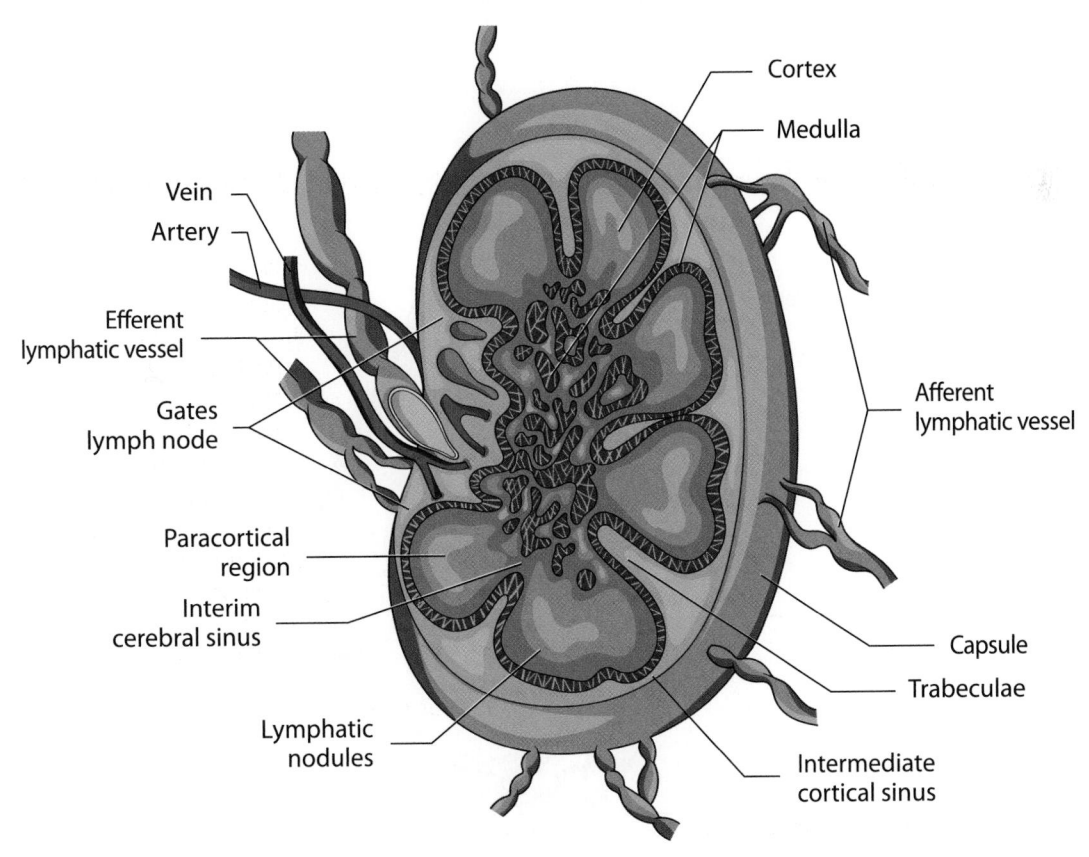

Male Reproductive System Anatomy

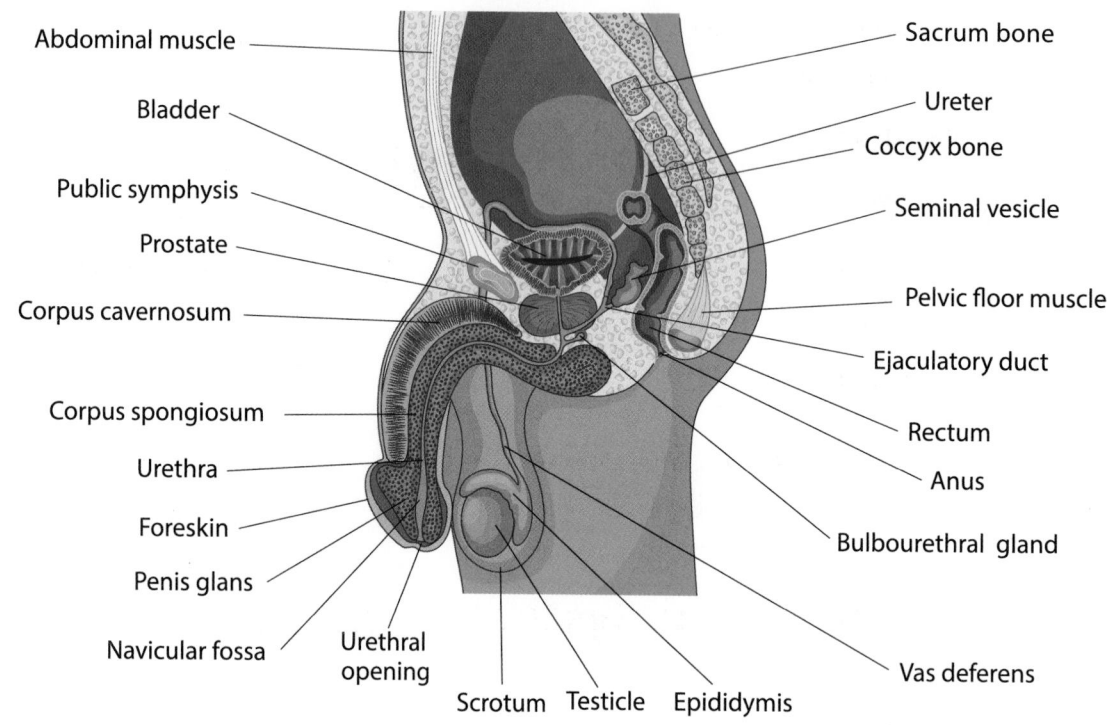

Abdominal muscle
Bladder
Public symphysis
Prostate
Corpus cavernosum
Corpus spongiosum
Urethra
Foreskin
Penis glans
Navicular fossa
Urethral opening
Scrotum   Testicle   Epididymis

Sacrum bone
Ureter
Coccyx bone
Seminal vesicle
Pelvic floor muscle
Ejaculatory duct
Rectum
Anus
Bulbourethral gland
Vas deferens

Male Reproductive System — Testicle

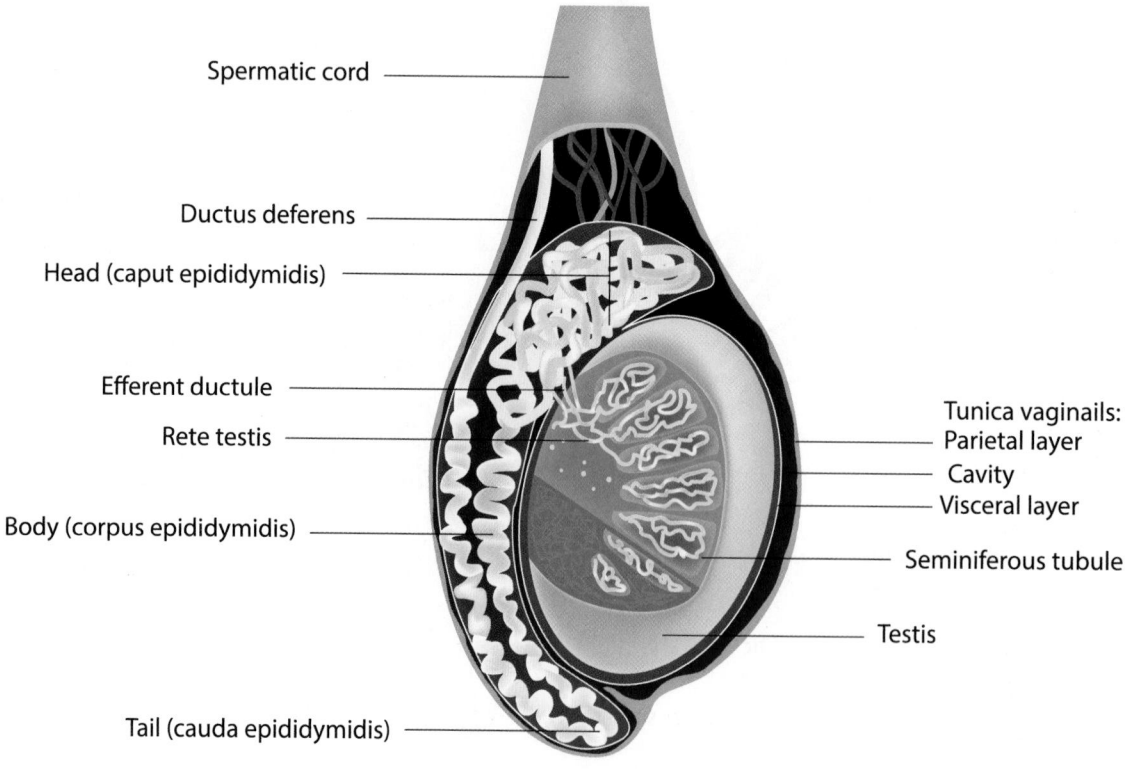

Spermatic cord
Ductus deferens
Head (caput epididymidis)
Efferent ductule
Rete testis
Body (corpus epididymidis)
Tail (cauda epididymidis)

Tunica vaginails:
Parietal layer
Cavity
Visceral layer
Seminiferous tubule
Testis

Male Reproductive System — Penis Anatomy

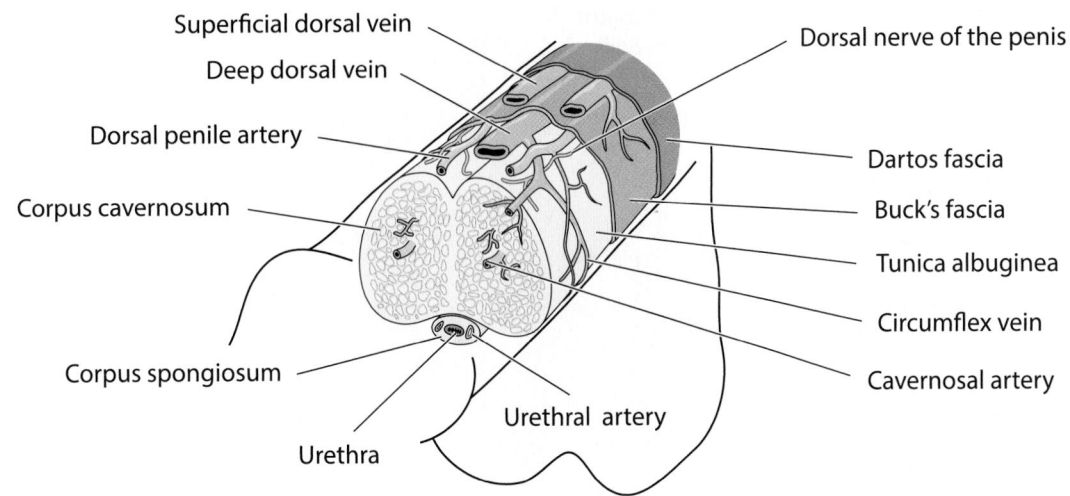

Superficial dorsal vein
Deep dorsal vein
Dorsal penile artery
Corpus cavernosum
Corpus spongiosum
Urethra
Urethral artery
Dorsal nerve of the penis
Dartos fascia
Buck's fascia
Tunica albuginea
Circumflex vein
Cavernosal artery

Muscular System Anatomy

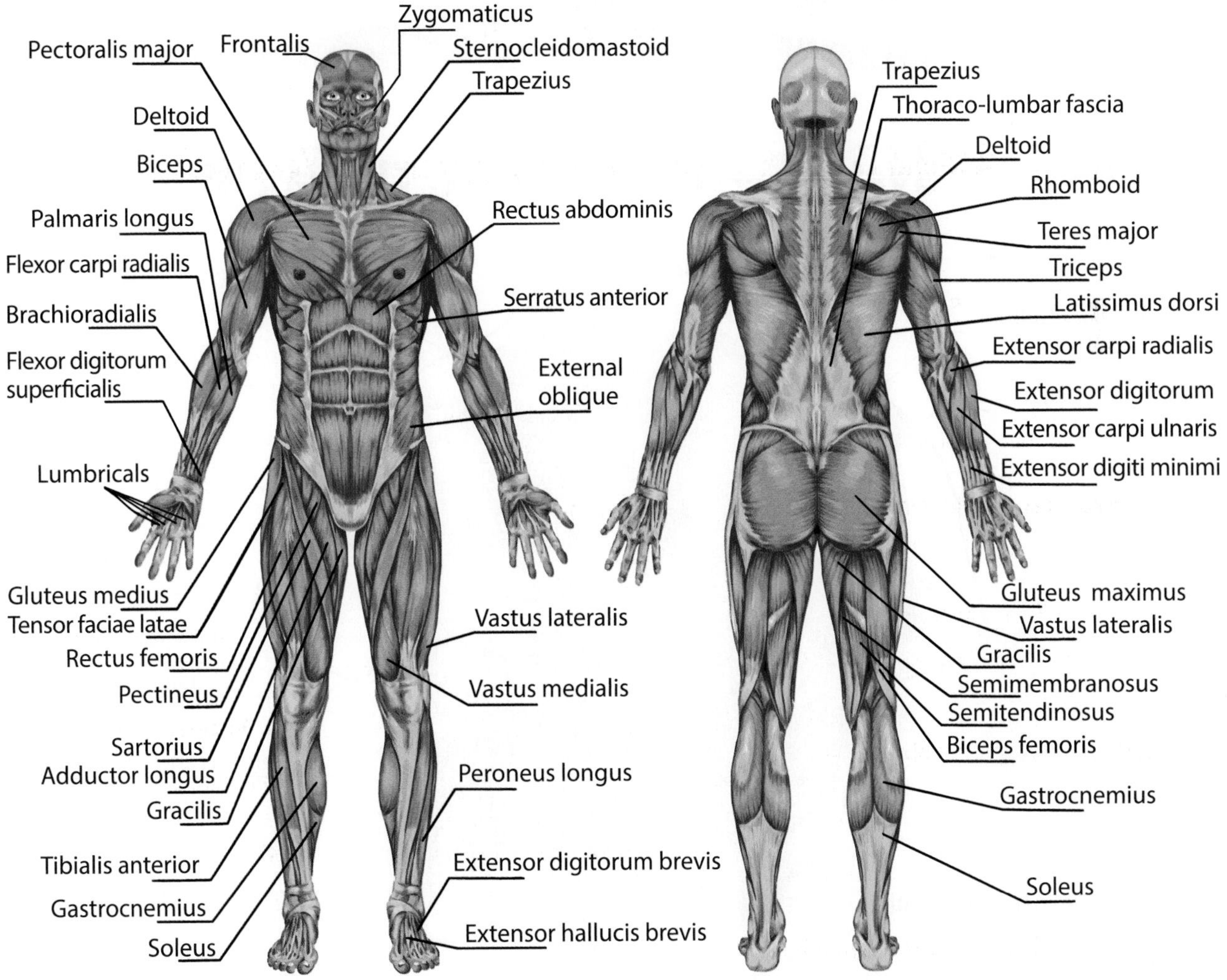

Zygomaticus
Pectoralis major   Frontalis
Sternocleidomastoid
Trapezius
Deltoid
Biceps
Palmaris longus
Flexor carpi radialis
Brachioradialis
Flexor digitorum superficialis
Rectus abdominis
Serratus anterior
External oblique
Lumbricals
Gluteus medius
Tensor faciae latae
Rectus femoris
Pectineus
Sartorius
Adductor longus
Gracilis
Tibialis anterior
Gastrocnemius
Soleus
Vastus lateralis
Vastus medialis
Peroneus longus
Extensor digitorum brevis
Extensor hallucis brevis

Trapezius
Thoraco-lumbar fascia
Deltoid
Rhomboid
Teres major
Triceps
Latissimus dorsi
Extensor carpi radialis
Extensor digitorum
Extensor carpi ulnaris
Extensor digiti minimi
Gluteus maximus
Vastus lateralis
Gracilis
Semimembranosus
Semitendinosus
Biceps femoris
Gastrocnemius
Soleus

Muscular System — Face Muscles

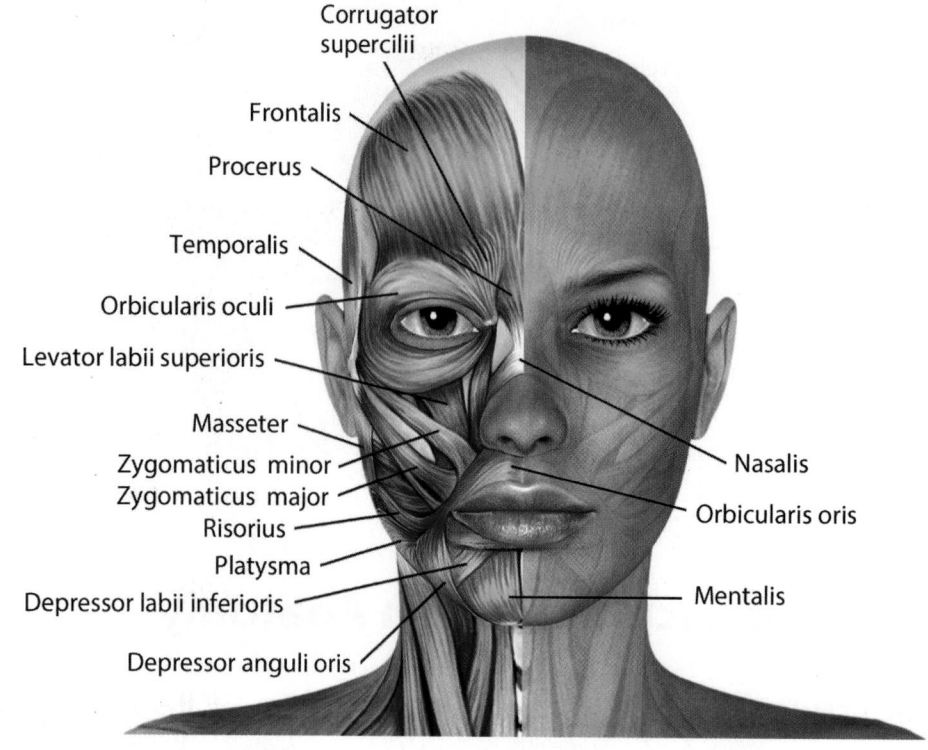

Corrugator supercilii

Frontalis

Procerus

Temporalis

Orbicularis oculi

Levator labii superioris

Masseter

Zygomaticus minor

Zygomaticus major

Risorius

Platysma

Depressor labii inferioris

Depressor anguli oris

Nasalis

Orbicularis oris

Mentalis

Muscular System — Neck, Chest, Thorax Muscles

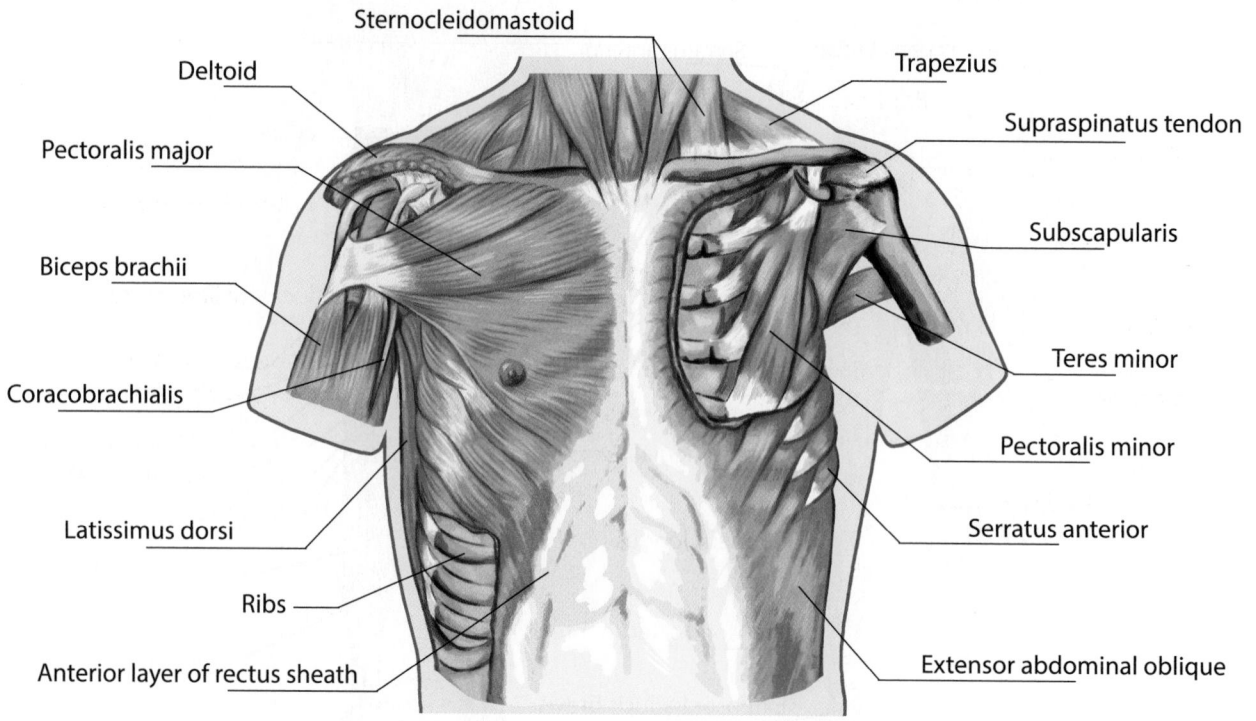

Sternocleidomastoid

Deltoid

Pectoralis major

Biceps brachii

Coracobrachialis

Latissimus dorsi

Ribs

Anterior layer of rectus sheath

Trapezius

Supraspinatus tendon

Subscapularis

Teres minor

Pectoralis minor

Serratus anterior

Extensor abdominal oblique

Muscular System — Shoulder (Rotator Cuff) Muscles

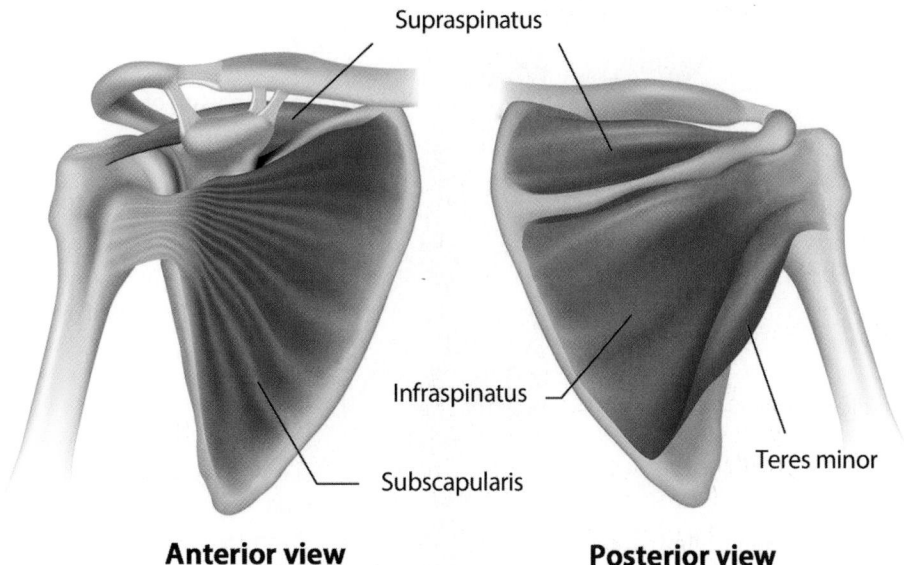

Supraspinatus

Infraspinatus

Subscapularis

Teres minor

Anterior view   **Posterior view**

Muscular System — Forearm Muscles (Right Arm, Posterior Compartment)

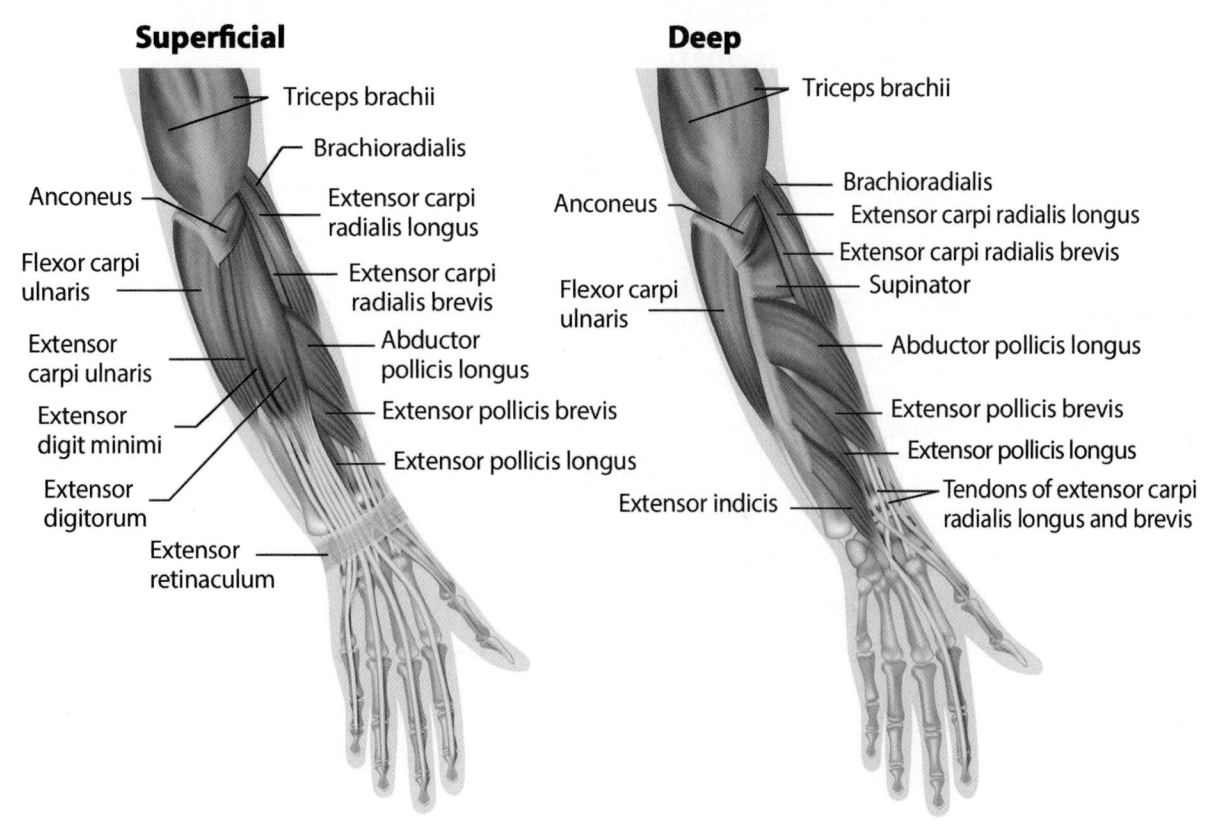

Superficial

Triceps brachii

Brachioradialis

Anconeus

Extensor carpi radialis longus

Flexor carpi ulnaris

Extensor carpi radialis brevis

Extensor carpi ulnaris

Abductor pollicis longus

Extensor digit minimi

Extensor pollicis brevis

Extensor digitorum

Extensor pollicis longus

Extensor retinaculum

Deep

Triceps brachii

Brachioradialis

Anconeus

Extensor carpi radialis longus

Extensor carpi radialis brevis

Flexor carpi ulnaris

Supinator

Abductor pollicis longus

Extensor pollicis brevis

Extensor pollicis longus

Extensor indicis

Tendons of extensor carpi radialis longus and brevis

ANATOMICAL ILLUSTRATIONS

Muscular System — Muscles of the Hand
(right hand, dorsal view)

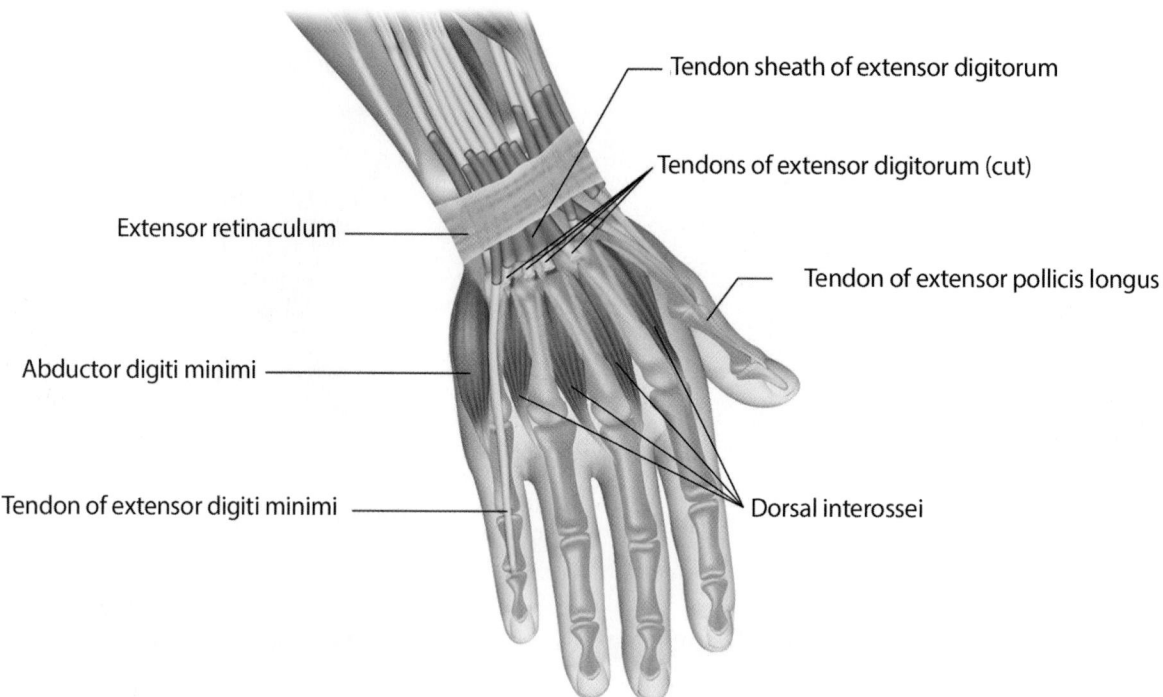

- Tendon sheath of extensor digitorum
- Tendons of extensor digitorum (cut)
- Extensor retinaculum
- Tendon of extensor pollicis longus
- Abductor digiti minimi
- Tendon of extensor digiti minimi
- Dorsal interossei

Muscular System — Muscles of the Hand
(right hand, palmar view)

Deep

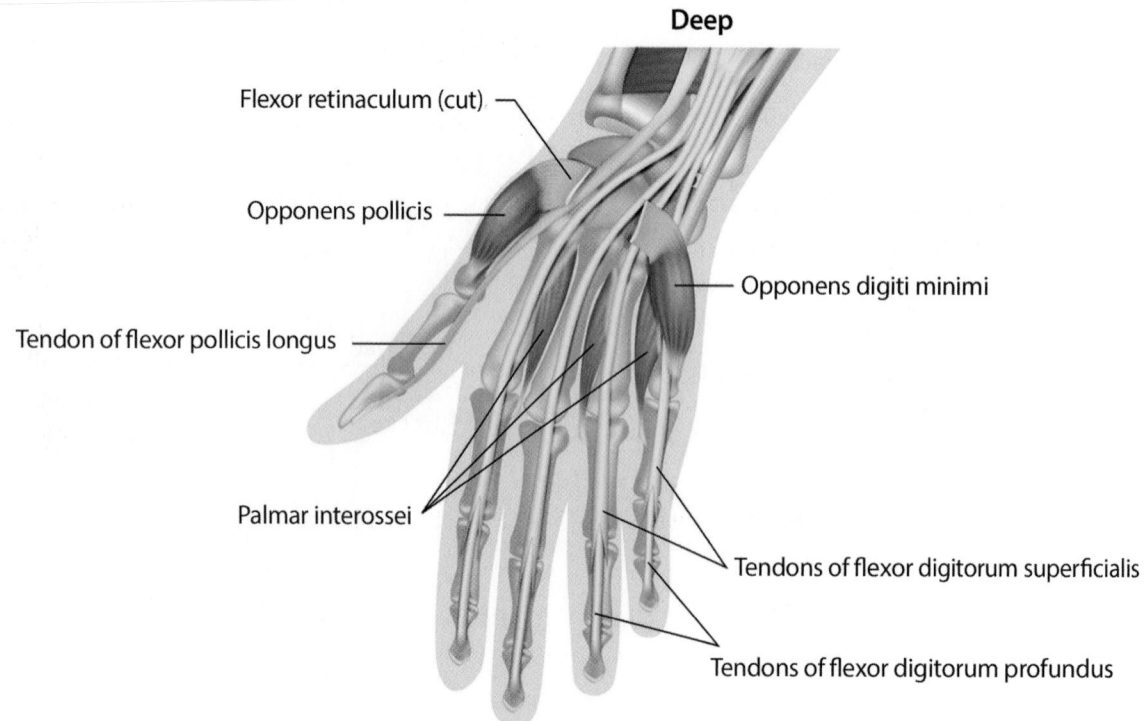

- Flexor retinaculum (cut)
- Opponens pollicis
- Opponens digiti minimi
- Tendon of flexor pollicis longus
- Palmar interossei
- Tendons of flexor digitorum superficialis
- Tendons of flexor digitorum profundus

Muscular System — Leg Muscles

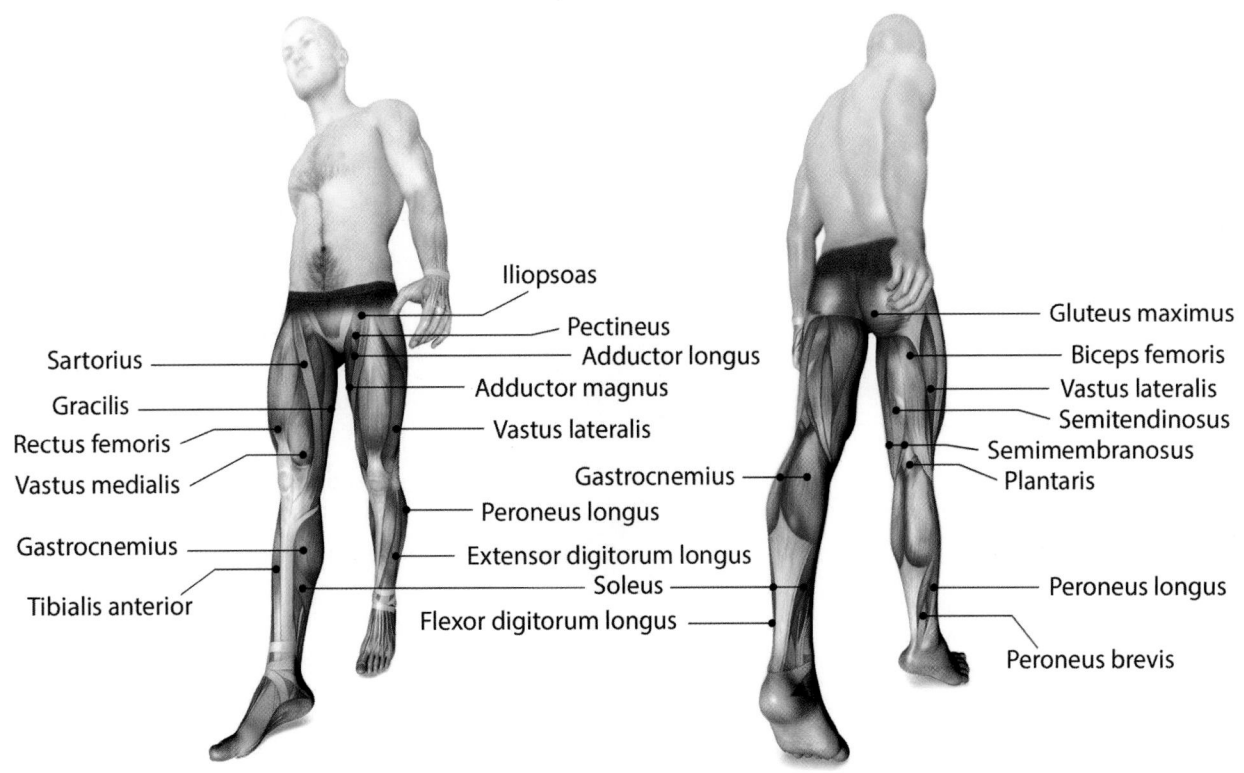

Iliopsoas
Pectineus
Adductor longus
Adductor magnus
Vastus lateralis
Sartorius
Gracilis
Rectus femoris
Vastus medialis
Gastrocnemius
Peroneus longus
Gastrocnemius
Tibialis anterior
Extensor digitorum longus
Soleus
Flexor digitorum longus

Gluteus maximus
Biceps femoris
Vastus lateralis
Semitendinosus
Semimembranosus
Plantaris
Peroneus longus
Peroneus brevis

Muscular System — Knee and Leg

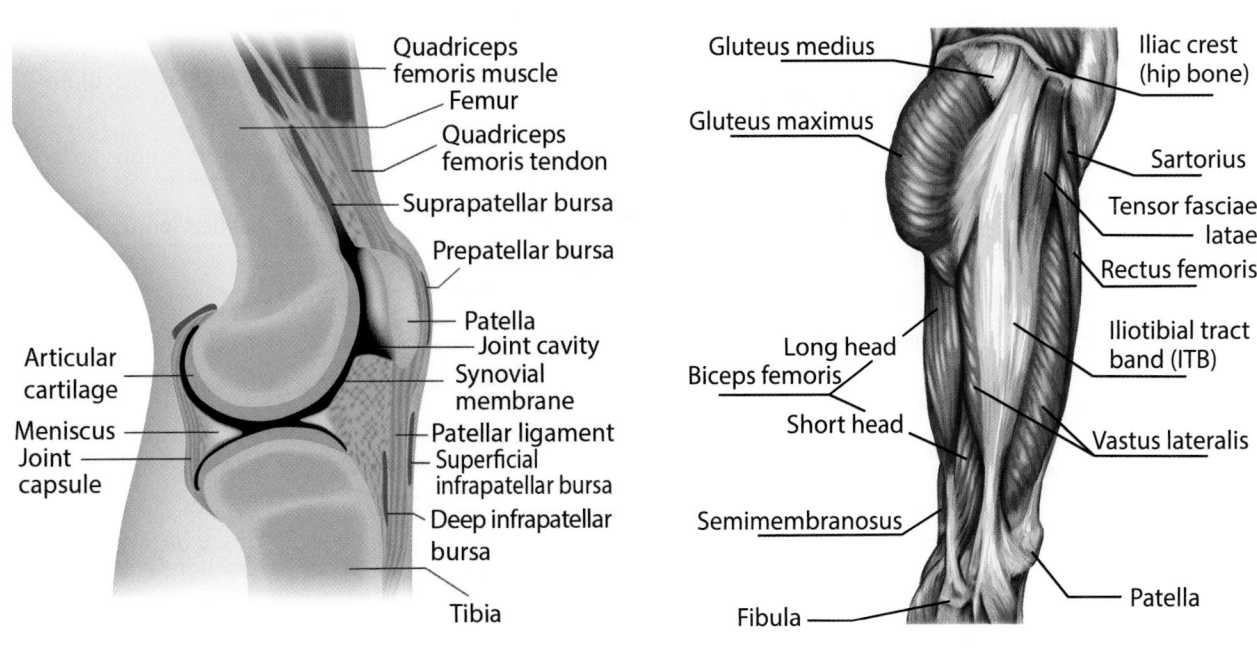

Quadriceps femoris muscle
Femur
Quadriceps femoris tendon
Suprapatellar bursa
Prepatellar bursa
Patella
Joint cavity
Synovial membrane
Articular cartilage
Patellar ligament
Superficial infrapatellar bursa
Meniscus
Joint capsule
Deep infrapatellar bursa
Tibia

Gluteus medius
Gluteus maximus
Iliac crest (hip bone)
Sartorius
Tensor fasciae latae
Rectus femoris
Iliotibial tract band (ITB)
Long head
Biceps femoris
Short head
Vastus lateralis
Semimembranosus
Patella
Fibula

Muscular System — Foot Muscles

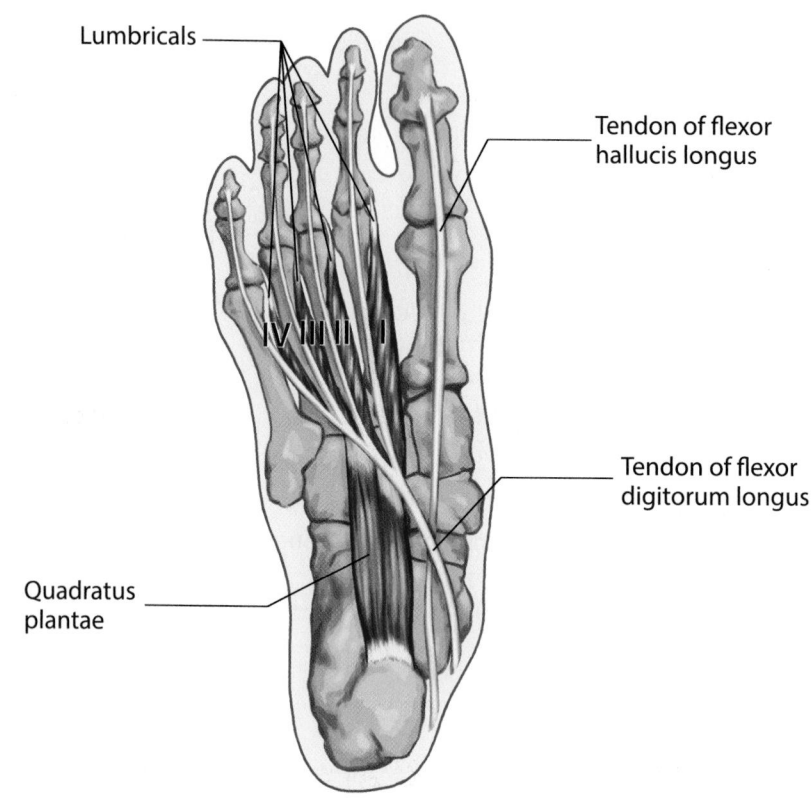

Lumbricals

Tendon of flexor hallucis longus

Tendon of flexor digitorum longus

Quadratus plantae

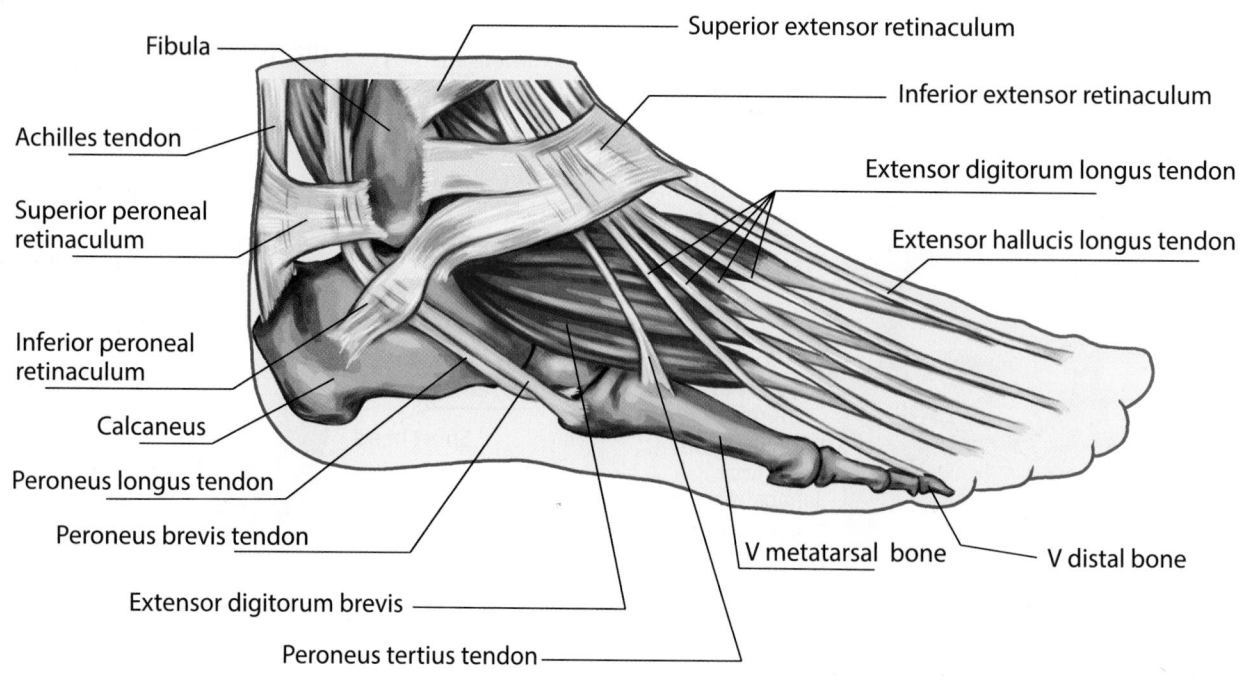

Fibula

Superior extensor retinaculum

Inferior extensor retinaculum

Achilles tendon

Extensor digitorum longus tendon

Superior peroneal retinaculum

Extensor hallucis longus tendon

Inferior peroneal retinaculum

Calcaneus

Peroneus longus tendon

Peroneus brevis tendon

Extensor digitorum brevis

V metatarsal bone

V distal bone

Peroneus tertius tendon

Musculoskeletal System — Shoulder Joint Structure

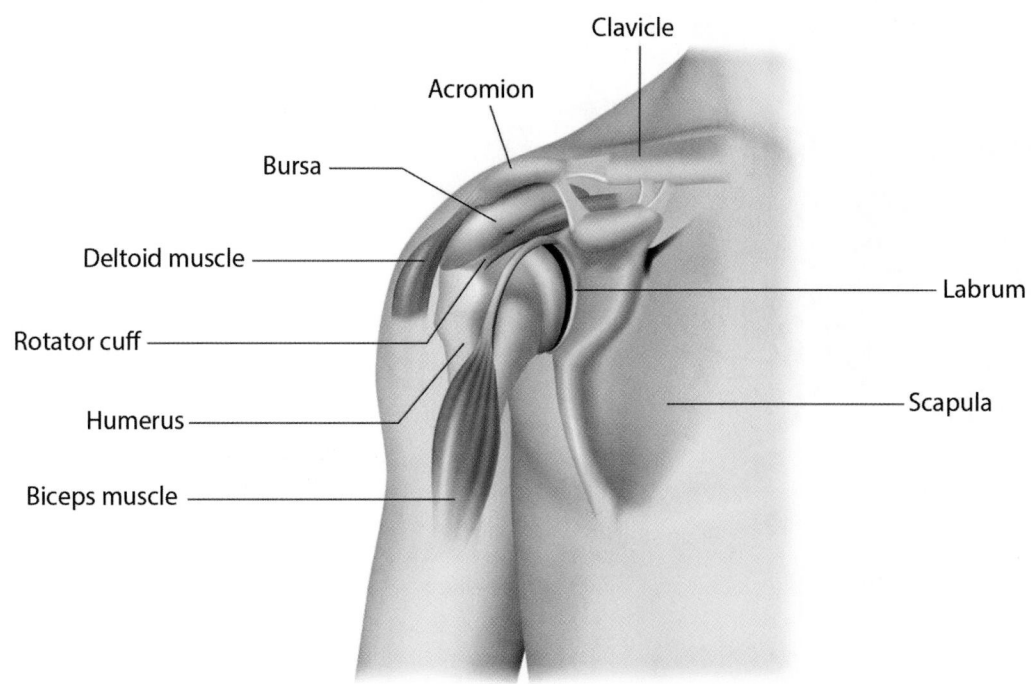

Clavicle

Acromion

Bursa

Deltoid muscle

Rotator cuff

Humerus

Biceps muscle

Labrum

Scapula

Nervous System Anatomy

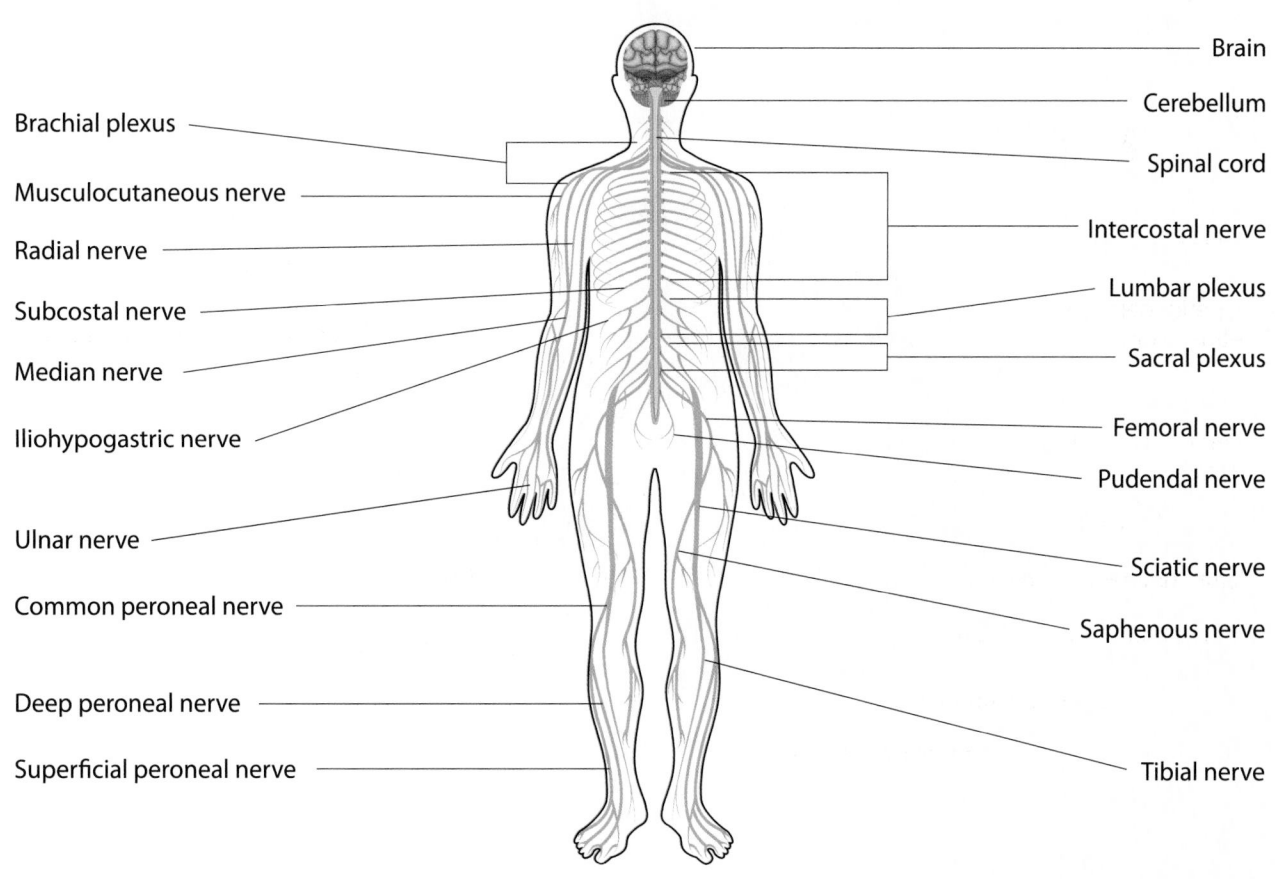

Brachial plexus

Musculocutaneous nerve

Radial nerve

Subcostal nerve

Median nerve

Iliohypogastric nerve

Ulnar nerve

Common peroneal nerve

Deep peroneal nerve

Superficial peroneal nerve

Brain

Cerebellum

Spinal cord

Intercostal nerve

Lumbar plexus

Sacral plexus

Femoral nerve

Pudendal nerve

Sciatic nerve

Saphenous nerve

Tibial nerve

Nervous System — Brain Anatomy

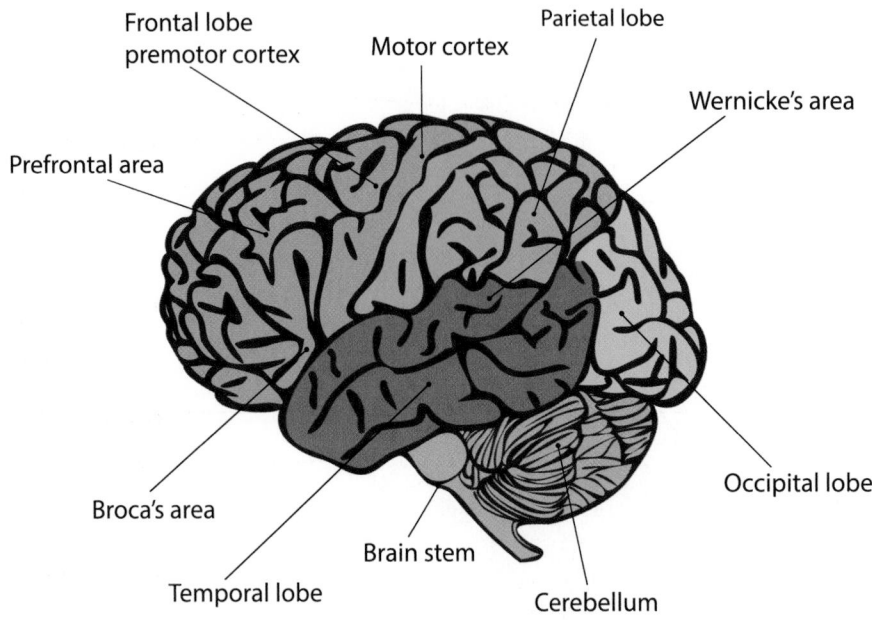

Nervous System — Median Section of the Brain

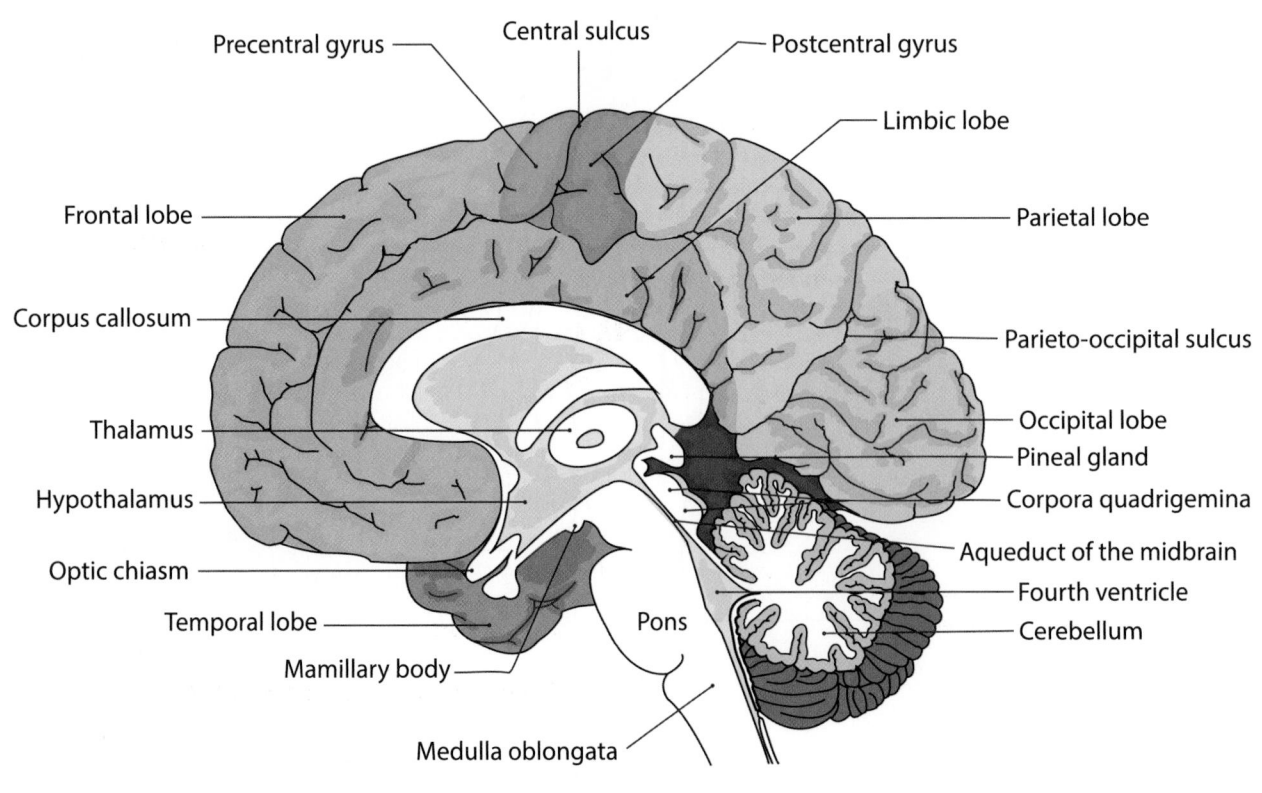

Nervous System — Cranial Nerves

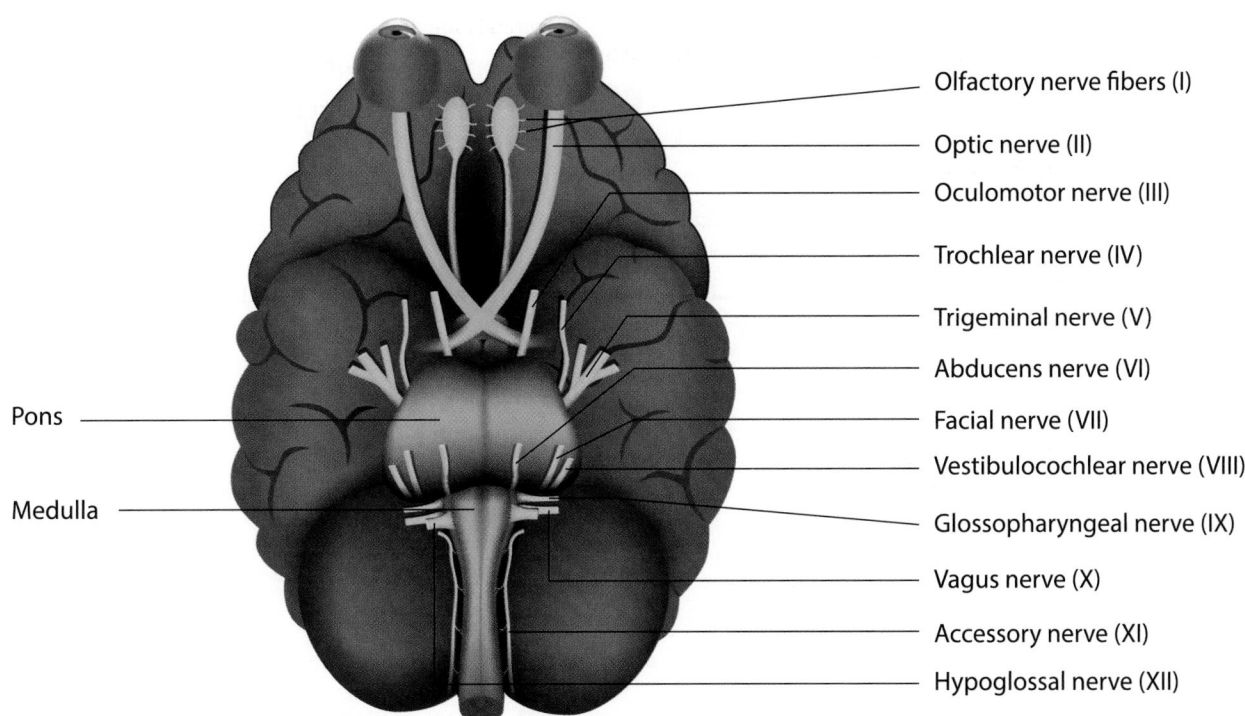

Olfactory nerve fibers (I)
Optic nerve (II)
Oculomotor nerve (III)
Trochlear nerve (IV)
Trigeminal nerve (V)
Abducens nerve (VI)
Facial nerve (VII)
Vestibulocochlear nerve (VIII)
Glossopharyngeal nerve (IX)
Vagus nerve (X)
Accessory nerve (XI)
Hypoglossal nerve (XII)

Pons

Medulla

Nervous System — Nerve Anatomy

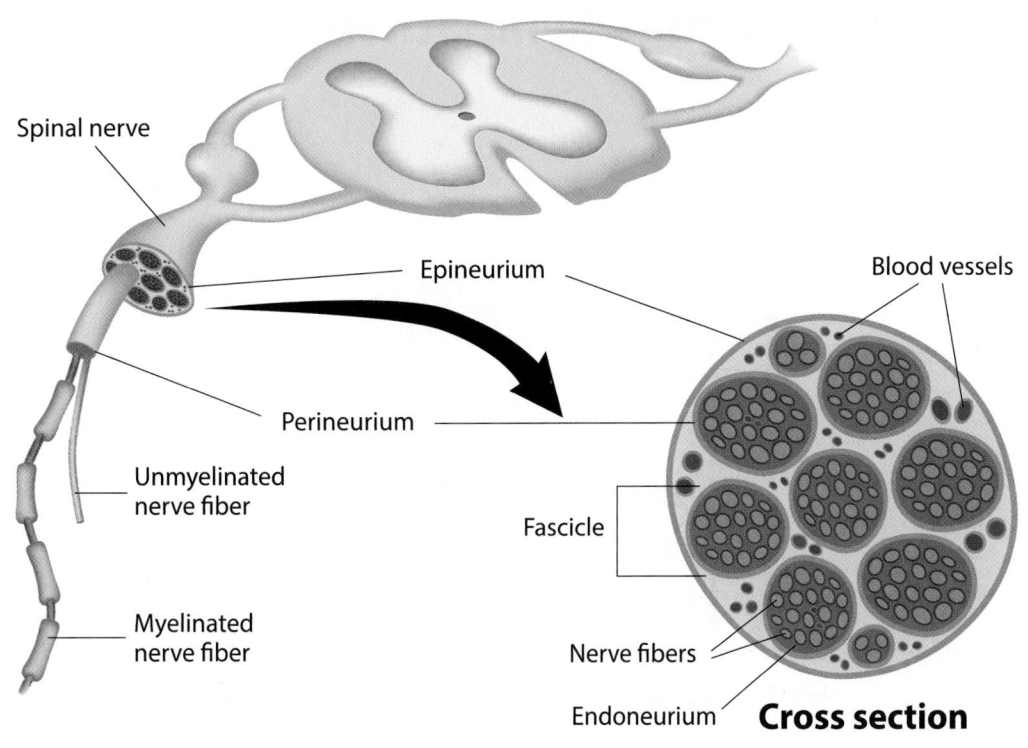

Spinal nerve

Epineurium

Blood vessels

Perineurium

Unmyelinated
nerve fiber

Fascicle

Myelinated
nerve fiber

Nerve fibers

Endoneurium

Cross section

Nervous System — Parasympathetic System Anatomy

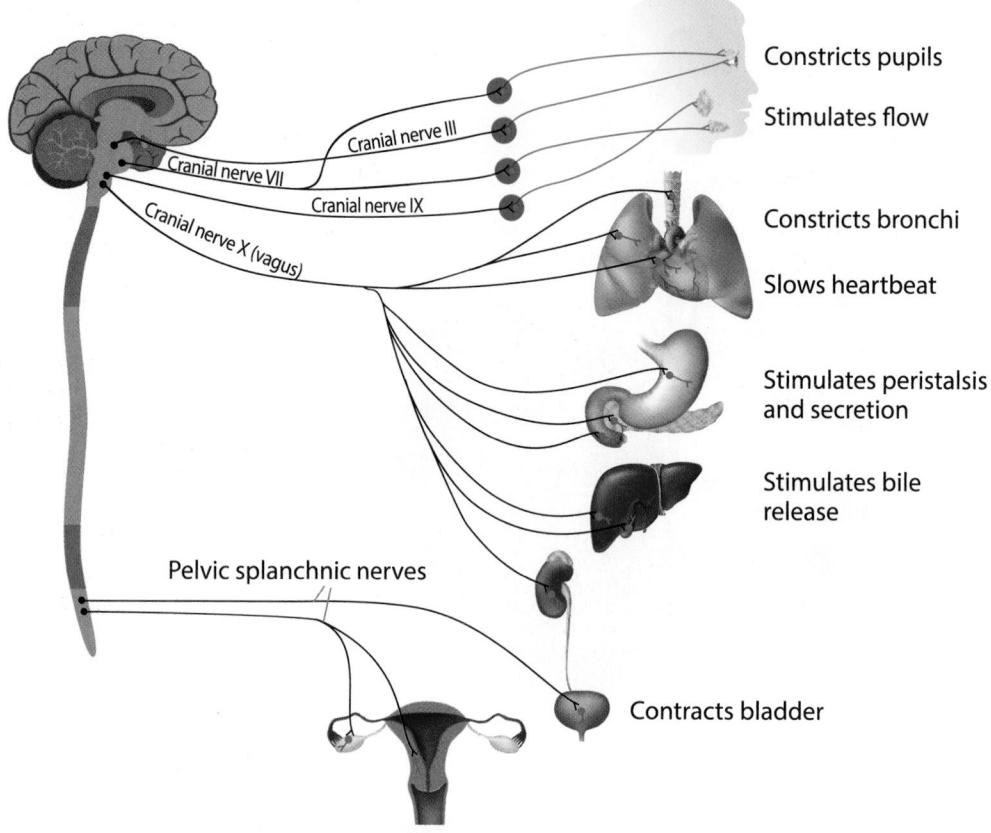

Cranial nerve III

Cranial nerve VII

Cranial nerve IX

Cranial nerve X (vagus)

Constricts pupils

Stimulates flow

Constricts bronchi

Slows heartbeat

Stimulates peristalsis and secretion

Stimulates bile release

Pelvic splanchnic nerves

Contracts bladder

Nervous System — Sympathetic System Anatomy

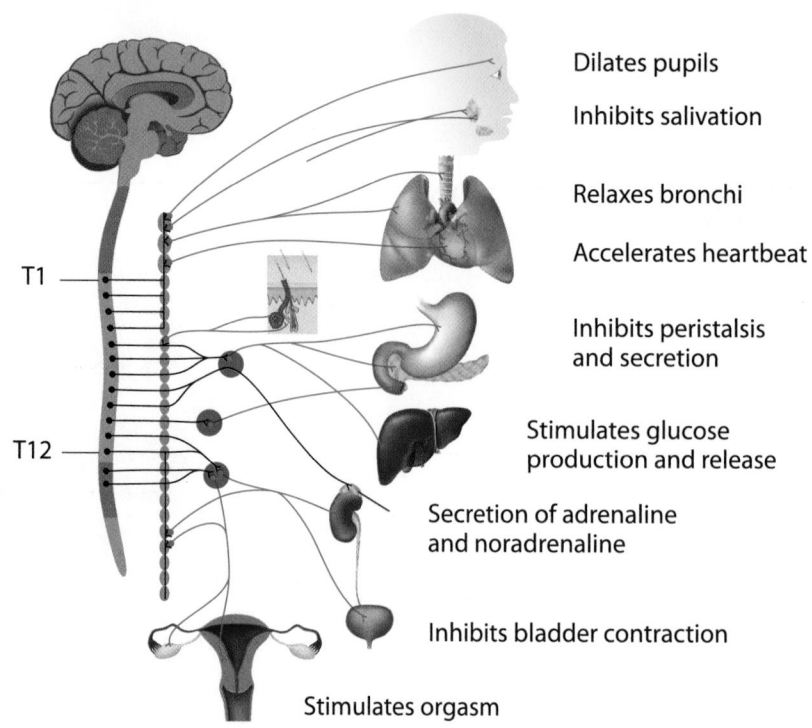

T1

T12

Dilates pupils

Inhibits salivation

Relaxes bronchi

Accelerates heartbeat

Inhibits peristalsis and secretion

Stimulates glucose production and release

Secretion of adrenaline and noradrenaline

Inhibits bladder contraction

Stimulates orgasm

Respiratory System Anatomy

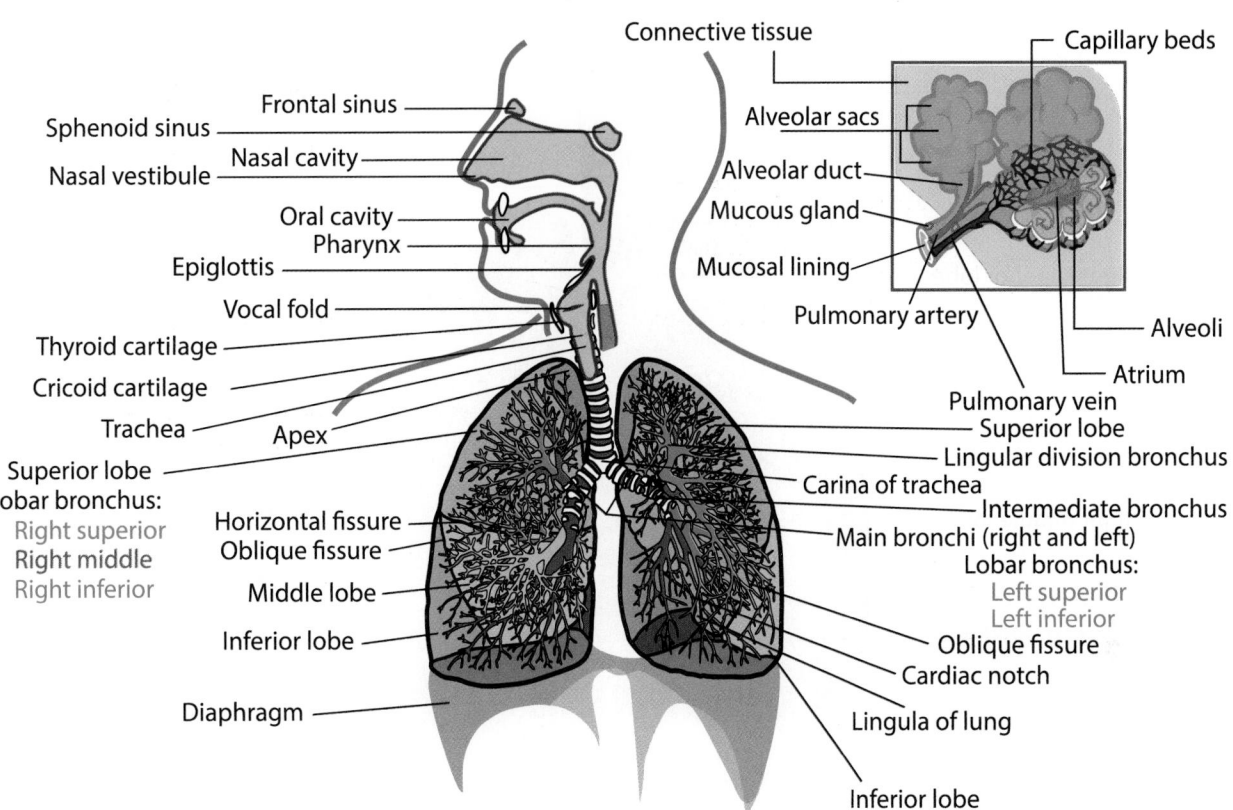

Respiratory System — Larynx Anatomy

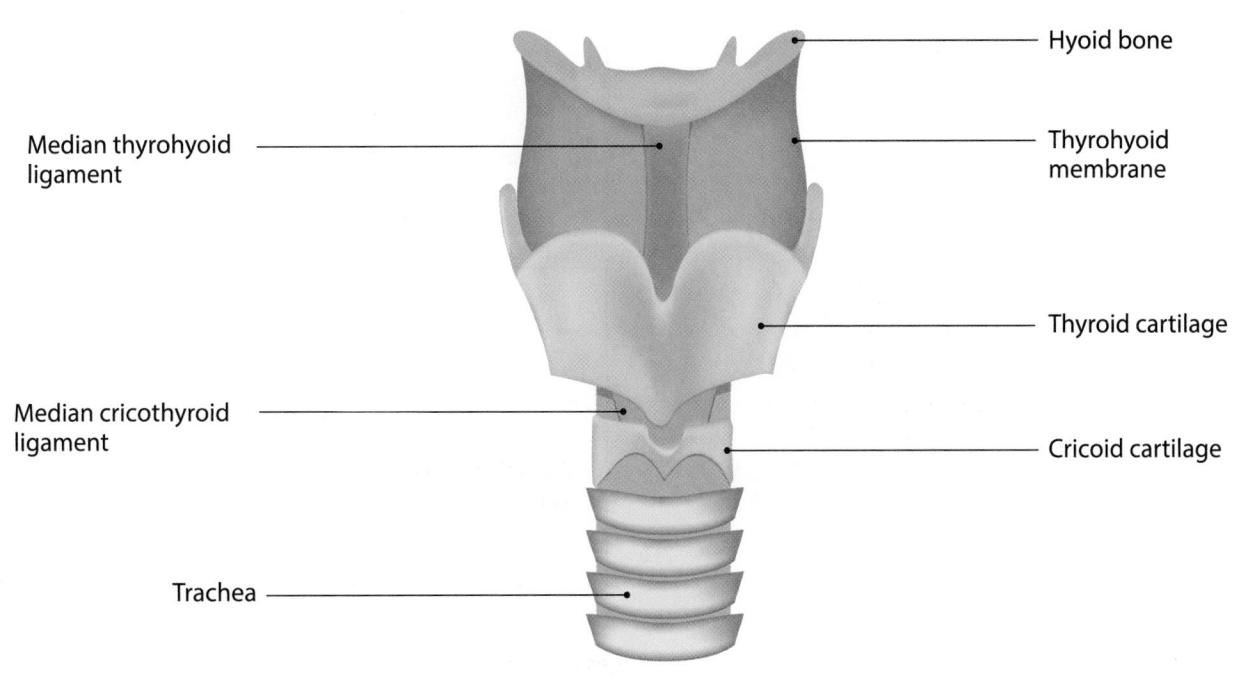

Respiratory System — Lung Anatomy

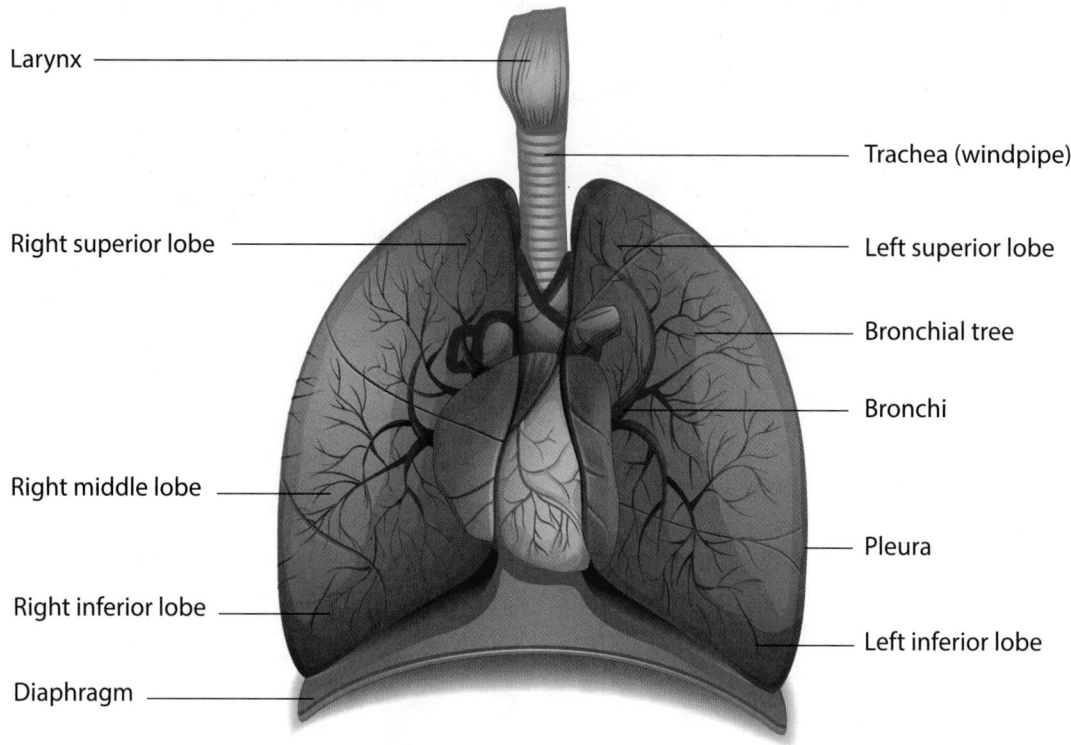

Larynx

Trachea (windpipe)

Right superior lobe

Left superior lobe

Bronchial tree

Bronchi

Right middle lobe

Right inferior lobe

Pleura

Left inferior lobe

Diaphragm

Respiratory System Function

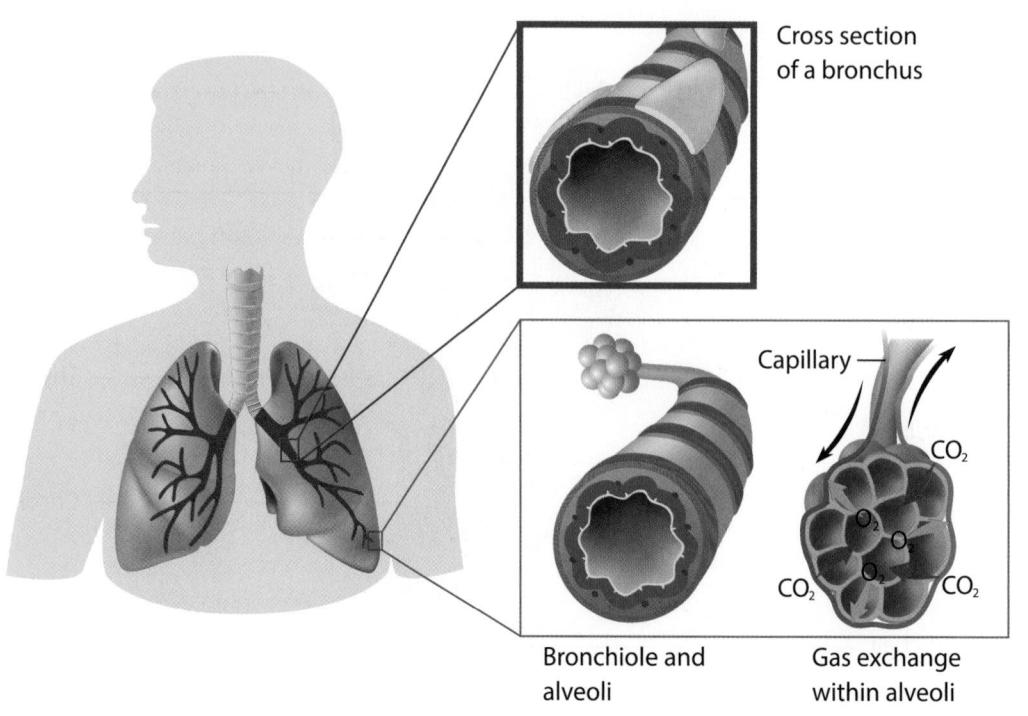

Cross section
of a bronchus

Capillary

CO_2

O_2 O_2

CO_2 O_2 CO_2

Bronchiole and
alveoli

Gas exchange
within alveoli

Respiratory System — Nose Anatomy

Respiratory System — Sinus Anatomy

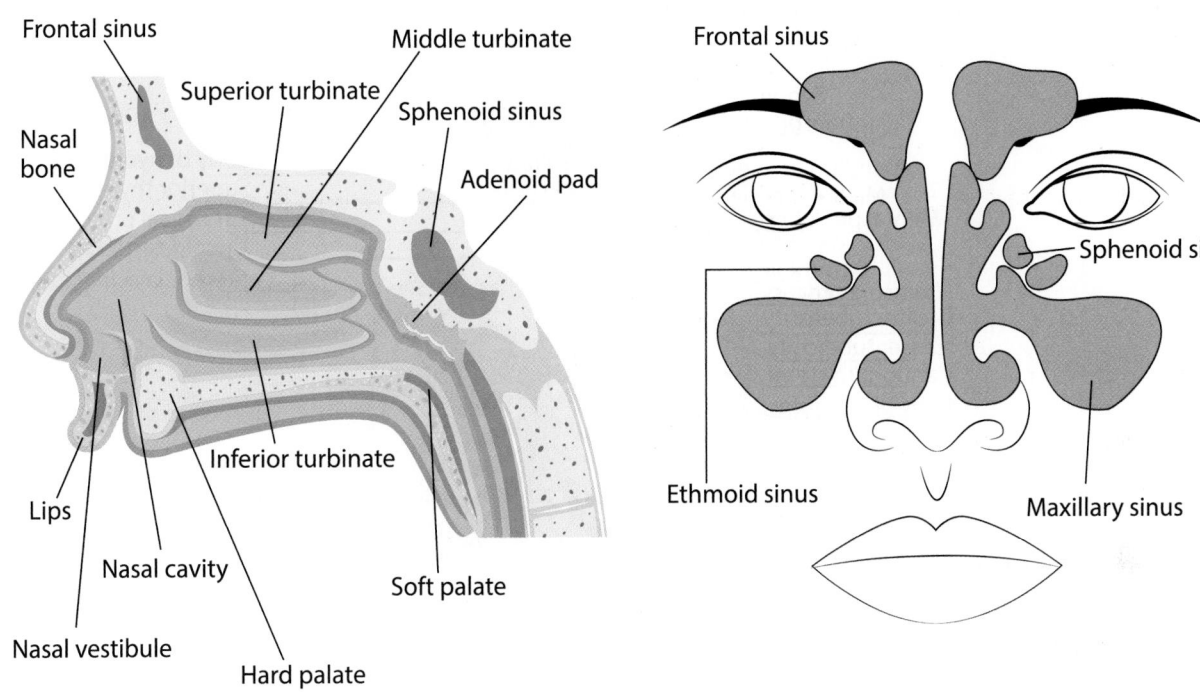

Respiratory System — Throat Anatomy

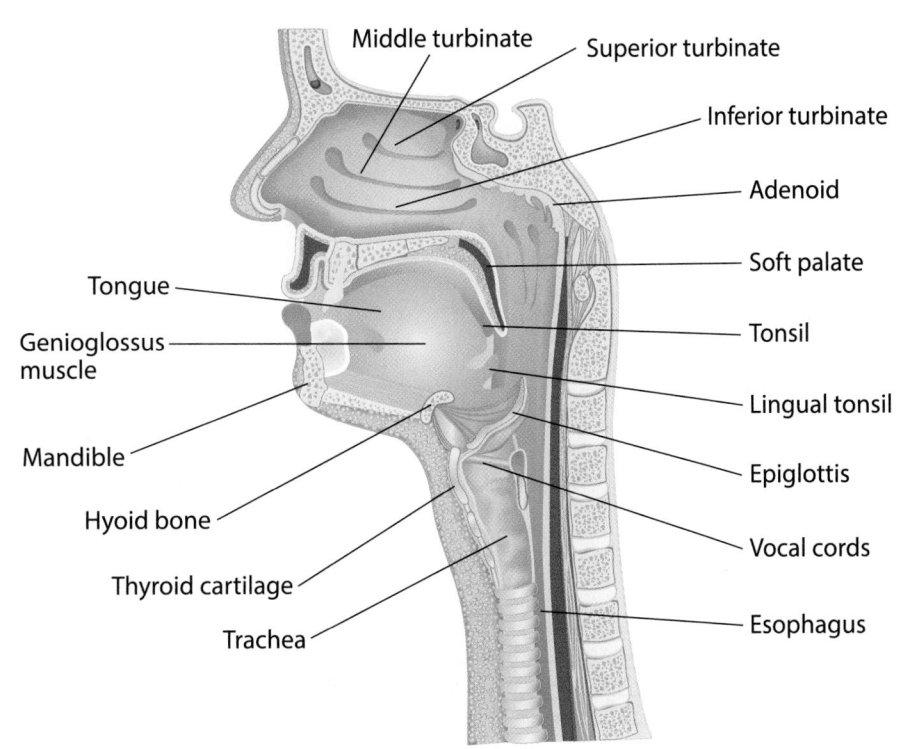

Skeletal System Anatomy

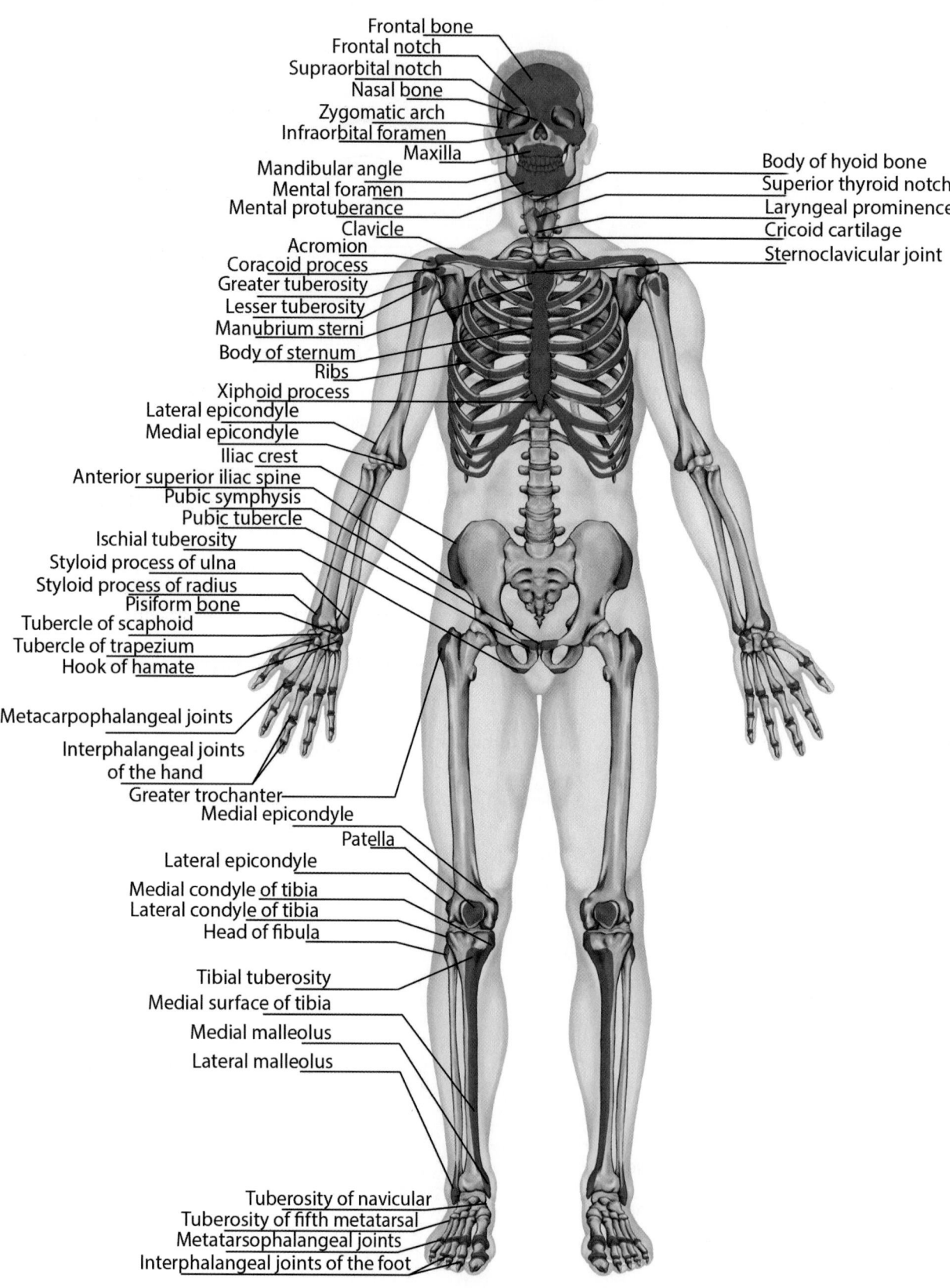

Frontal bone
Frontal notch
Supraorbital notch
Nasal bone
Zygomatic arch
Infraorbital foramen
Maxilla
Mandibular angle
Mental foramen
Mental protuberance
Clavicle
Acromion
Coracoid process
Greater tuberosity
Lesser tuberosity
Manubrium sterni
Body of sternum
Ribs
Xiphoid process
Lateral epicondyle
Medial epicondyle
Iliac crest
Anterior superior iliac spine
Pubic symphysis
Pubic tubercle
Ischial tuberosity
Styloid process of ulna
Styloid process of radius
Pisiform bone
Tubercle of scaphoid
Tubercle of trapezium
Hook of hamate

Metacarpophalangeal joints

Interphalangeal joints
of the hand
Greater trochanter
Medial epicondyle
Patella
Lateral epicondyle
Medial condyle of tibia
Lateral condyle of tibia
Head of fibula

Tibial tuberosity
Medial surface of tibia

Medial malleolus

Lateral malleolus

Tuberosity of navicular
Tuberosity of fifth metatarsal
Metatarsophalangeal joints
Interphalangeal joints of the foot

Body of hyoid bone
Superior thyroid notch
Laryngeal prominence
Cricoid cartilage
Sternoclavicular joint

Skeletal System — Bone Structure

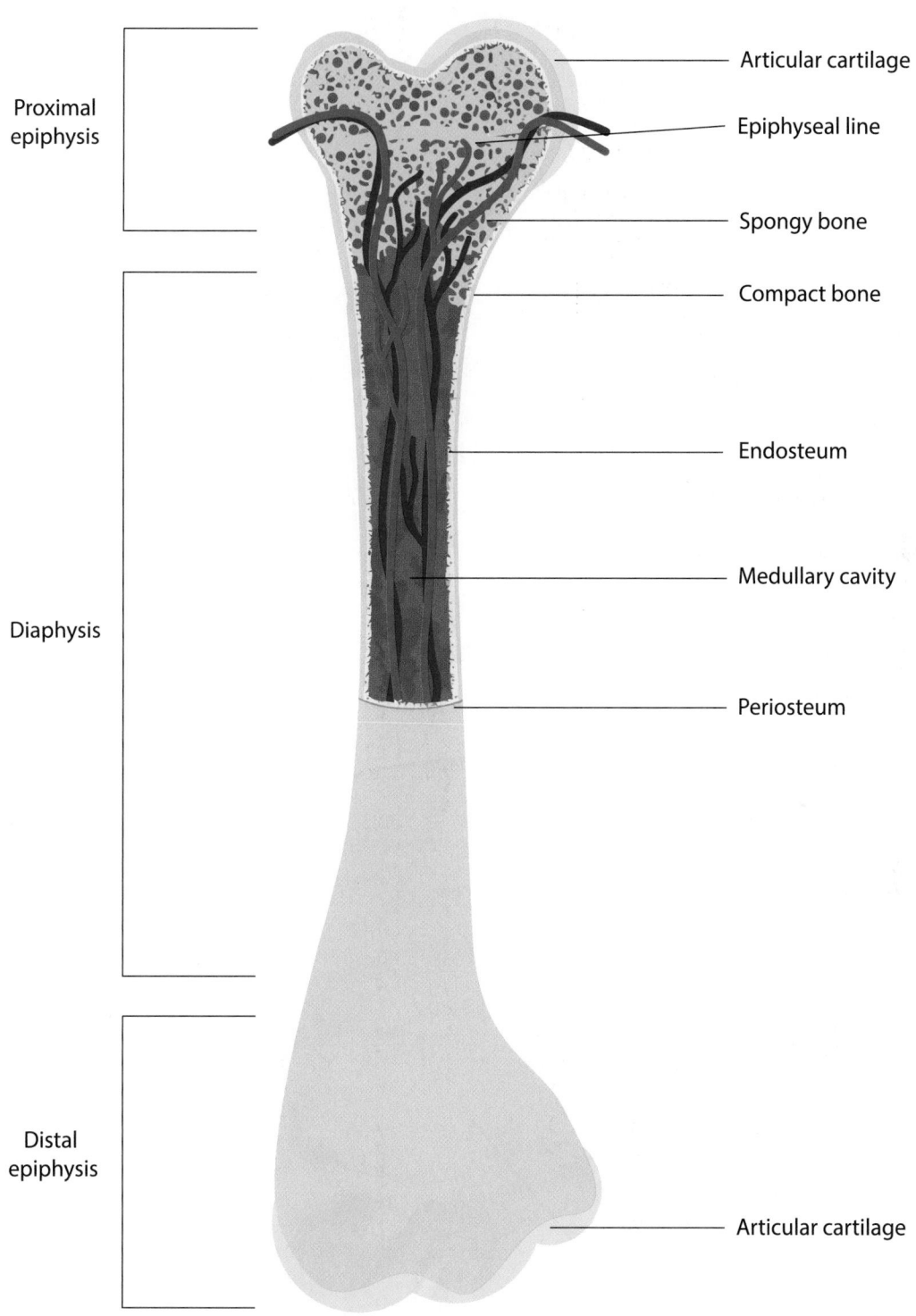

Proximal epiphysis

Diaphysis

Distal epiphysis

Articular cartilage

Epiphyseal line

Spongy bone

Compact bone

Endosteum

Medullary cavity

Periosteum

Articular cartilage

Skeletal System — Skull

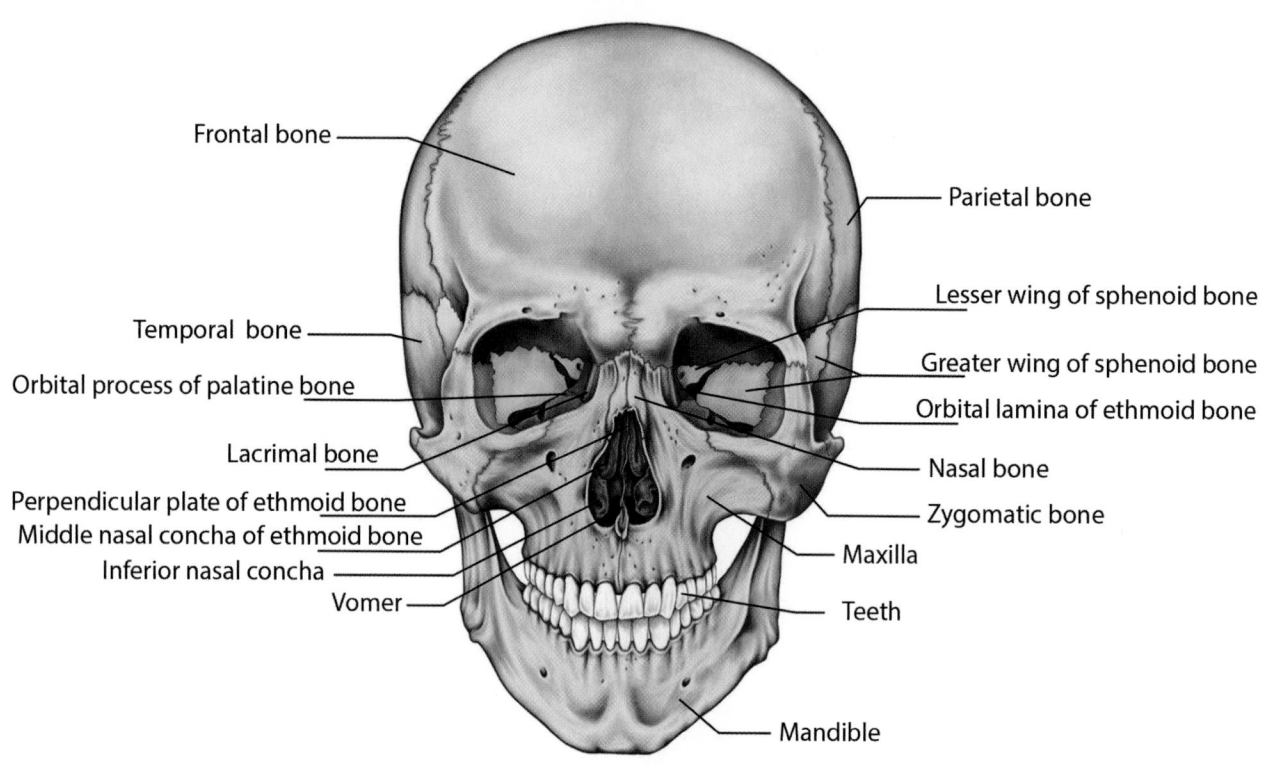

Frontal bone

Parietal bone

Lesser wing of sphenoid bone

Temporal bone

Greater wing of sphenoid bone

Orbital process of palatine bone

Orbital lamina of ethmoid bone

Lacrimal bone

Nasal bone

Perpendicular plate of ethmoid bone

Zygomatic bone

Middle nasal concha of ethmoid bone

Maxilla

Inferior nasal concha

Vomer

Teeth

Mandible

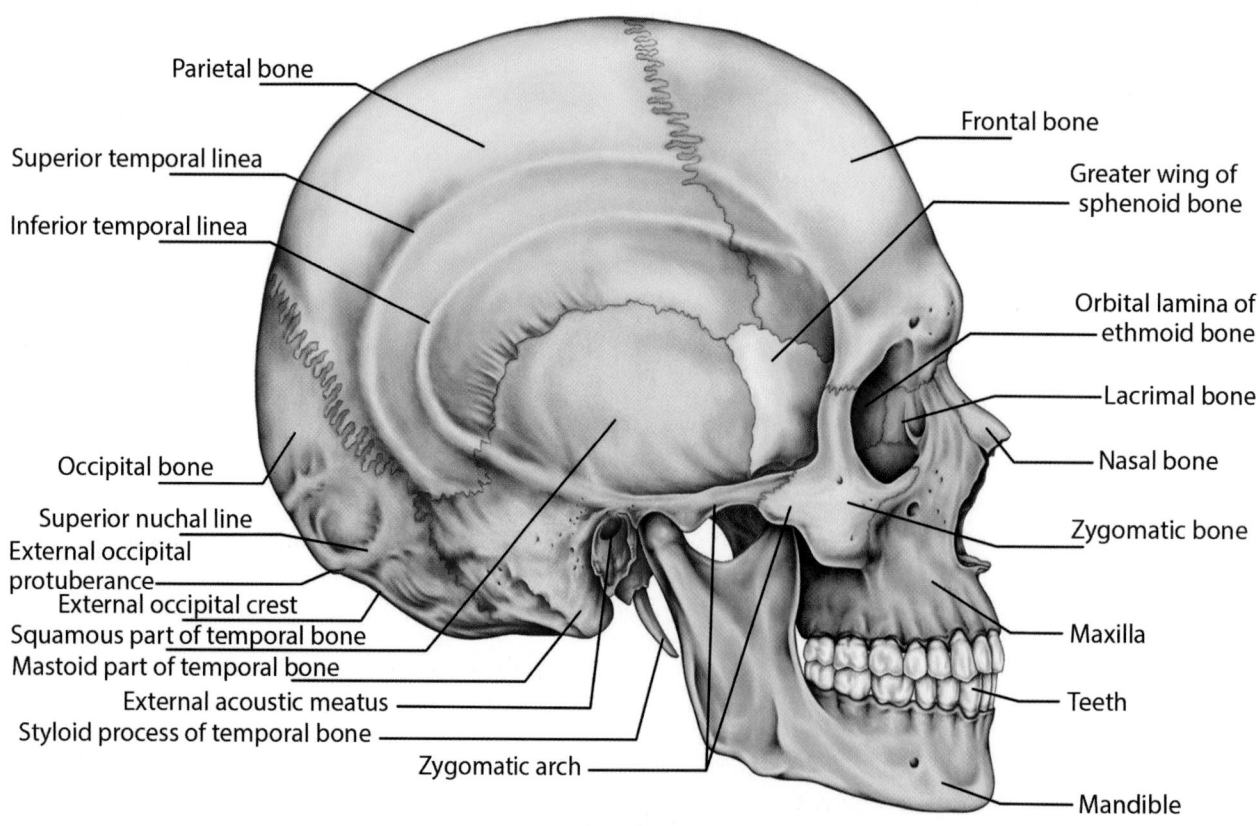

Parietal bone

Frontal bone

Superior temporal linea

Greater wing of sphenoid bone

Inferior temporal linea

Orbital lamina of ethmoid bone

Lacrimal bone

Nasal bone

Occipital bone

Superior nuchal line

Zygomatic bone

External occipital protuberance

External occipital crest

Squamous part of temporal bone

Maxilla

Mastoid part of temporal bone

External acoustic meatus

Teeth

Styloid process of temporal bone

Zygomatic arch

Mandible

Skeletal System — Cervical, Thoracic, and Lumbar Spine

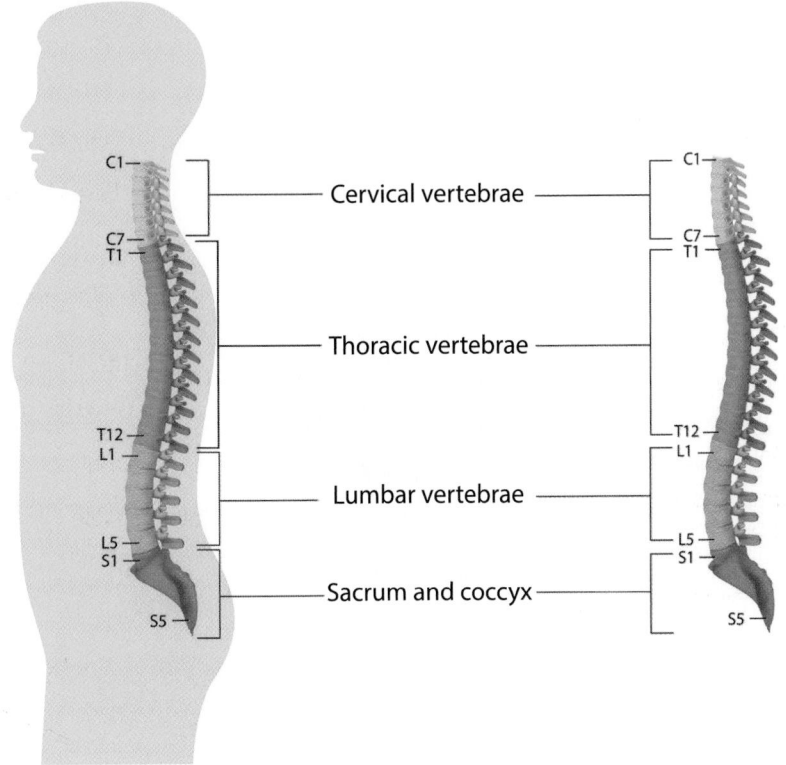

Skeletal System — Pelvic Girdle

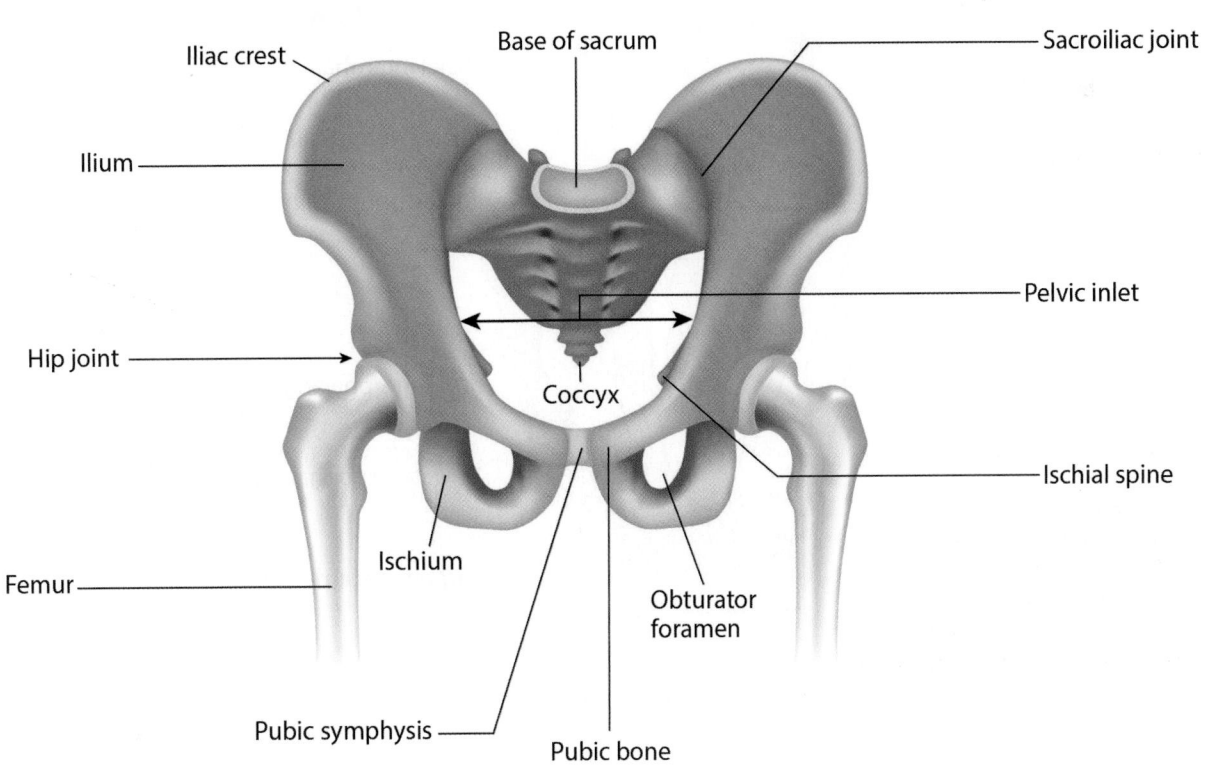

Skeletal System — Elbow Joint Structure

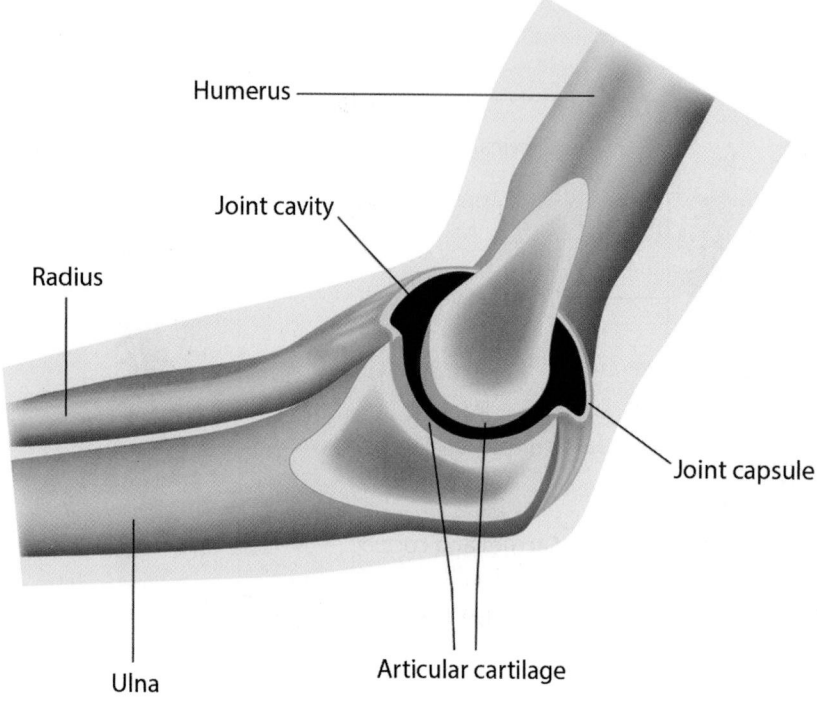

Humerus

Joint cavity

Radius

Joint capsule

Ulna

Articular cartilage

Skeletal System — Hand Bones

Bones

Joints

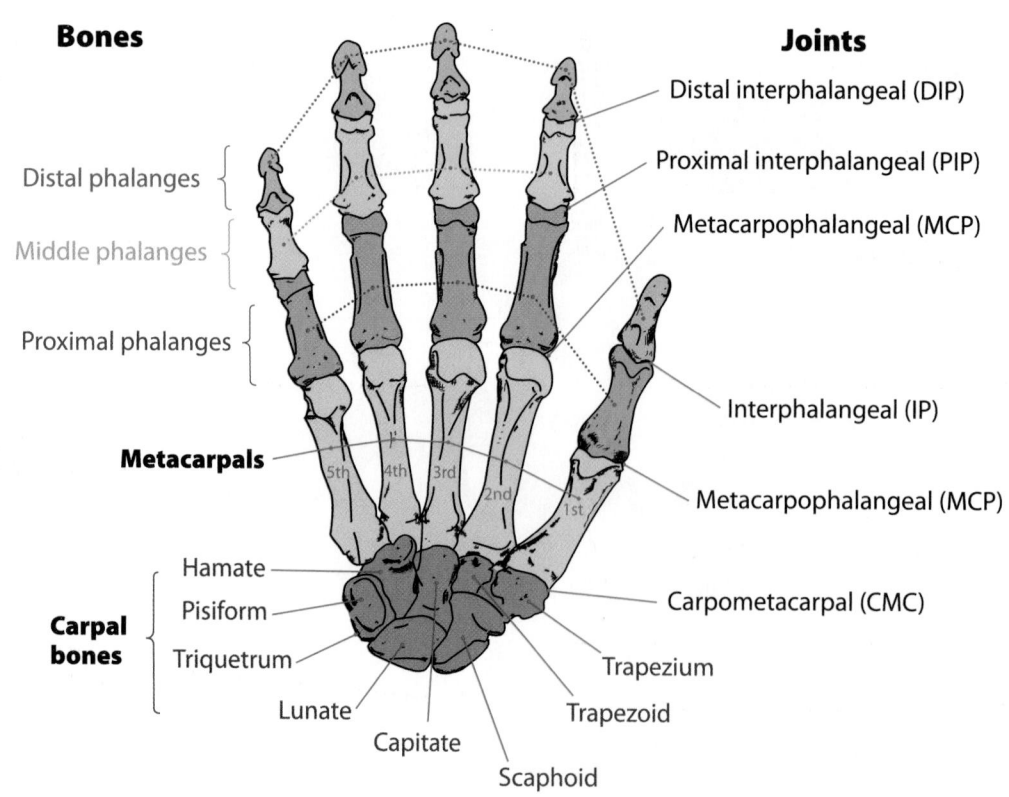

Distal interphalangeal (DIP)

Proximal interphalangeal (PIP)

Metacarpophalangeal (MCP)

Distal phalanges

Middle phalanges

Proximal phalanges

Interphalangeal (IP)

Metacarpals

5th 4th 3rd 2nd 1st

Metacarpophalangeal (MCP)

Hamate

Pisiform

Triquetrum

Carpal bones

Carpometacarpal (CMC)

Trapezium

Trapezoid

Lunate

Capitate

Scaphoid

Skeletal System — Foot Bones
(Right Foot, Lateral View)

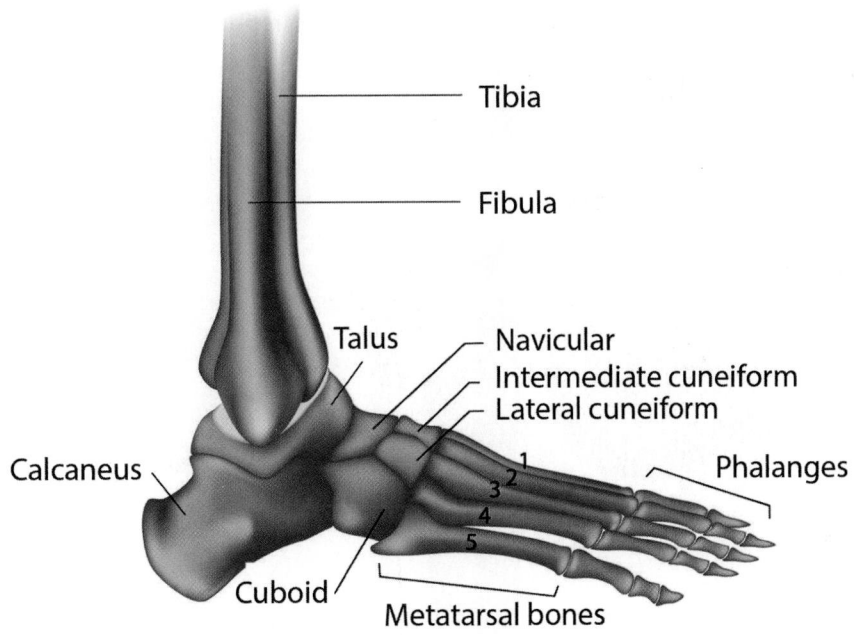

- Tibia
- Fibula
- Talus
- Navicular
- Intermediate cuneiform
- Lateral cuneiform
- Calcaneus
- Phalanges
- Cuboid
- Metatarsal bones

Urinary System Anatomy

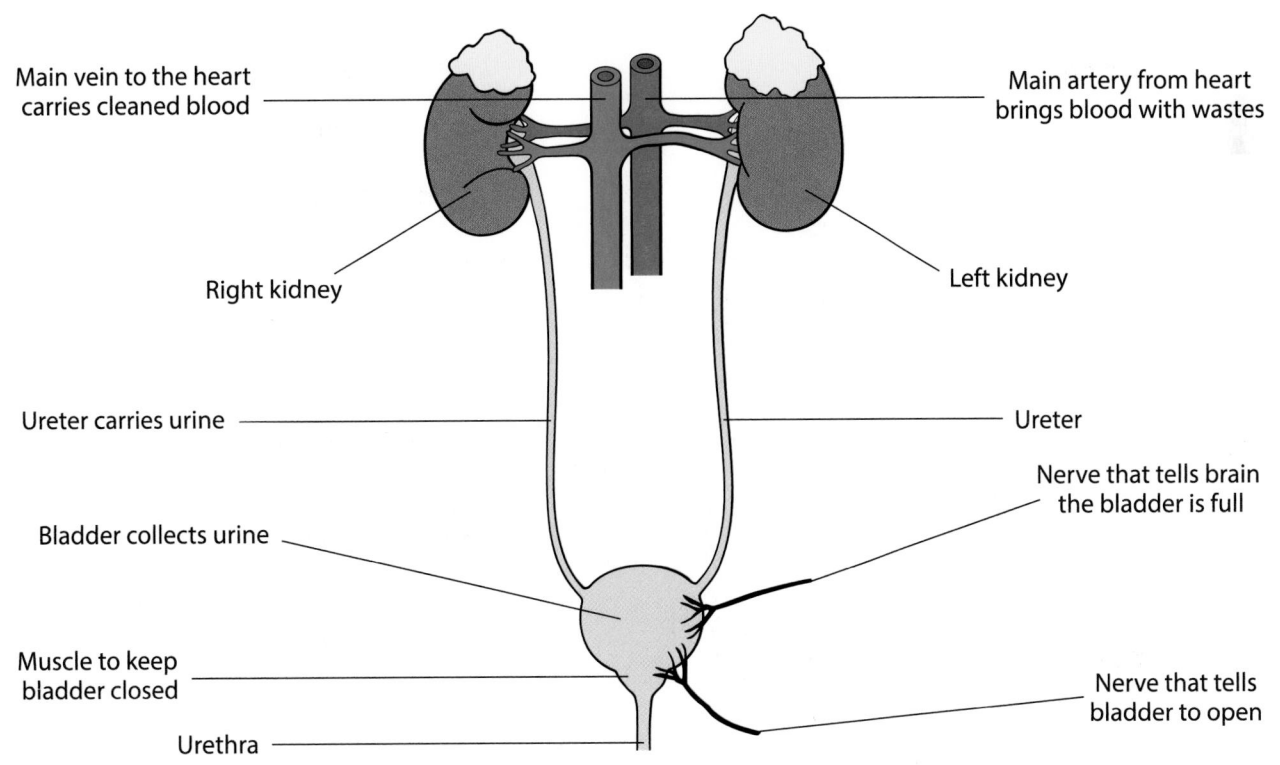

- Main vein to the heart carries cleaned blood
- Main artery from heart brings blood with wastes
- Right kidney
- Left kidney
- Ureter carries urine
- Ureter
- Nerve that tells brain the bladder is full
- Bladder collects urine
- Muscle to keep bladder closed
- Nerve that tells bladder to open
- Urethra

Urinary System — Kidney Anatomy

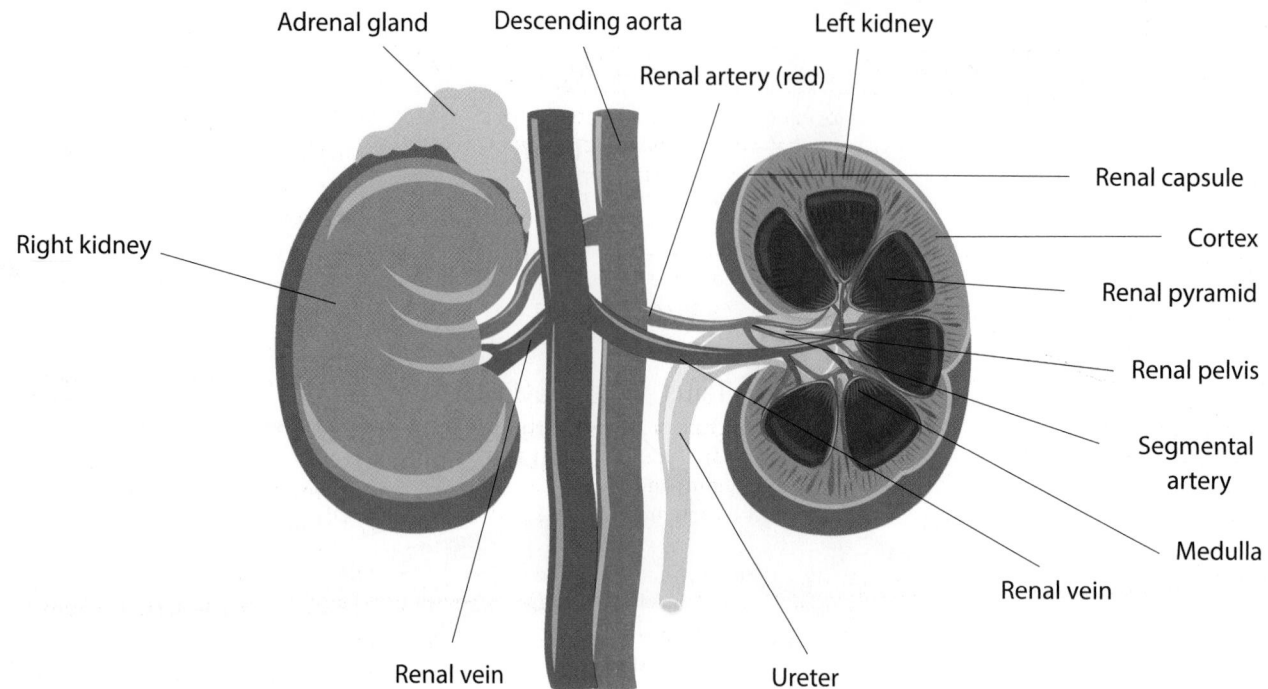

Approach Table

Section 0 - Medical and Surgical
Character 5 - Approach

Approach	5th Character	Definition	Examples
External	X	Procedures performed directly on the skin or mucous membrane and procedures performed indirectly by the application of external force through the skin or mucous membrane	• Cauterization of epistaxis • Reduction of a dislocated shoulder • Destruction of renal calculi with lithotripsy
Open	0	Cutting through the skin or mucous membrane and any other body layers necessary to expose the site of the procedure	• Open reduction and internal fixation of a fracture • Abdominal appendectomy • Open coronary artery bypass graft
Percutaneous	3	Entry, by puncture or minor incision, of instrumentation through the skin or mucous membrane and/or any other body layers necessary to reach the site of the procedure	• Percutaneous paracentesis • Tracheostomy formation with tracheostomy tube placement • Needle biopsy of breast mass
Percutaneous, Endoscopic	4	Entry, by puncture or minor incision, of instrumentation through the skin or mucous membrane and/or any other body layers necessary to reach and visualize the site of the procedure	• Shoulder arthroscopy • Autograft nerve graft to right median nerve • Mapping of left cerebral hemisphere
Via Natural or Artificial Opening	7	Entry of instrumentation through a natural or artificial external opening to reach the site of the procedure	• Placement of a Foley catheter • Endotracheal intubation • Transvaginal cervical cerclage
Via Natural or Artificial Opening, Endoscopic	8	Entry of instrumentation through a natural or artificial external opening to reach and visualize the site of the procedure	• Colonoscopy • Bronchoscopy • Esophagogastroduodenoscopy (EGD)
Via Natural or Artificial Opening, with Percutaneous Endoscopic Assistance	F	Entry of instrumentation through a natural or artificial external opening to reach and visualize the site of the procedure, and entry, by puncture or minor incision, of instrumentation through the skin or mucous membrane and any other body layers necessary to aid in the performance of the procedure	• Resections of the female reproductive system • Laparoscopic-assisted vaginal salpingo-oophorectomy and hysterectomy

This page intentionally left blank

3

3f (Aortic) Bioprosthesis valve
use Zooplastic Tissue in Heart and Great Vessels

A

Abdominal aortic plexus
use Abdominal Sympathetic Nerve
Abdominal esophagus
use Esophagus, Lower
Abdominohysterectomy
see Resection, Uterus 0UT9
Abdominoplasty
see Alteration, Abdominal Wall 0W0F
see Repair, Abdominal Wall 0WQF
see Supplement, Abdominal Wall 0WUF
Abductor hallucis muscle
use Foot Muscle, Right
use Foot Muscle, Left
AbioCor® Total Replacement Heart
use Synthetic Substitute
Ablation
see Control bleeding in
see Destruction
Abortion
Abortifacient 10A07ZX
Laminaria 10A07ZW
Products of Conception 10A0
Vacuum 10A07Z6
Abrasion
see Extraction
Absolute Pro Vascular (OTW) Self-Expanding Stent System
use Intraluminal Device
Accelerate PhenoTest™ BC XXE5XN6
Accessory cephalic vein
use Cephalic Vein, Right
use Cephalic Vein, Left
Accessory obturator nerve
use Lumbar Plexus
Accessory phrenic nerve
use Phrenic Nerve
Accessory spleen
use Spleen
Acculink (RX) Carotid Stent System
use Intraluminal Device
Acellular Hydrated Dermis
use Nonautologous Tissue Substitute
Acetabular cup
use Liner in Lower Joints
Acetabulectomy
see Excision, Lower Bones 0QB
see Resection, Lower Bones 0QT
Acetabulofemoral joint
use Hip Joint, Right
use Hip Joint, Left
Acetabuloplasty
see Repair, Lower Bones 0QQ
see Replacement, Lower Bones 0QR
see Supplement, Lower Bones 0QU
Achilles tendon
use Lower Leg Tendon, Right
use Lower Leg Tendon, Left
Achillorrhaphy
see Repair, Tendons 0LQ
Achillotenotomy, achillotomy
see Division, Tendons 0L8
see Drainage, Tendons 0L9
Acoustic Pulse Thrombolysis
see Fragmentation, Artery

Acromioclavicular ligament
use Shoulder Bursa and Ligament, Right
use Shoulder Bursa and Ligament, Left
Acromion (process)
use Scapula, Right
use Scapula, Left
Acromionectomy
see Excision, Upper Joints 0RB
see Resection, Upper Joints 0RT
Acromioplasty
see Repair, Upper Joints 0RQ
see Replacement, Upper Joints 0RR
see Supplement, Upper Joints 0RU
ACTEMRA®
use Tocilizumab
Activa PC neurostimulator
use Stimulator Generator, Multiple Array in 0JH
Activa RC neurostimulator
use Stimulator Generator, Multiple Array Rechargeable in 0JH
Activa SC neurostimulator
use Stimulator Generator, Single Array in 0JH
Activities of Daily Living Assessment F02
Activities of Daily Living Treatment F08
ACUITY™ Steerable Lead
use Cardiac Lead, Pacemaker in 02H
use Cardiac Lead, Defibrillator in 02H
Acupuncture
Breast
Anesthesia 8E0H300
No Qualifier 8E0H30Z
Integumentary System
Anesthesia 8E0H300
No Qualifier 8E0H30Z
Adductor brevis muscle
use Upper Leg Muscle, Right
use Upper Leg Muscle, Left
Adductor hallucis muscle
use Foot Muscle, Right
use Foot Muscle, Left
Adductor longus muscle
use Upper Leg Muscle, Right
use Upper Leg Muscle, Left
Adductor magnus muscle
use Upper Leg Muscle, Right
use Upper Leg Muscle, Left
Adenohypophysis
use Pituitary Gland
Adenoidectomy
see Excision, Adenoids 0CBQ
see Resection, Adenoids 0CTQ
Adenoidotomy
see Drainage, Adenoids 0C9Q
Adhesiolysis
see Release
Administration
Blood products *see* Transfusion
Other substance *see* Introduction of substance in or on
Adrenalectomy
see Excision, Endocrine System 0GB
see Resection, Endocrine System 0GT
Adrenalorrhaphy
see Repair, Endocrine System 0GQ
Adrenalotomy
see Drainage, Endocrine System 0G9
Advancement
see Reposition
see Transfer
Advisa (MRI)
use Pacemaker, Dual Chamber in 0JH
AFX® Endovascular AAA System
use Intraluminal Device

AIGISRx Antibacterial Envelope
use Anti-Infective Envelope
Alar ligament of axis
use Head and Neck Bursa and Ligament
Alfieri Stitch Valvuloplasty
see Restriction, Valve, Mitral 02VG
Alimentation
see Introduction of substance in or on
Alteration
Abdominal Wall 0W0F
Ankle Region
Left 0Y0L
Right 0Y0K
Arm
Lower
Left 0X0F
Right 0X0D
Upper
Left 0X09
Right 0X08
Axilla
Left 0X05
Right 0X04
Back
Lower 0W0L
Upper 0W0K
Breast
Bilateral 0H0V
Left 0H0U
Right 0H0T
Buttock
Left 0Y01
Right 0Y00
Chest Wall 0W08
Ear
Bilateral 0902
Left 0901
Right 0900
Elbow Region
Left 0X0C
Right 0X0B
Extremity
Lower
Left 0Y0B
Right 0Y09
Upper
Left 0X07
Right 0X06
Eyelid
Lower
Left 080R
Right 080Q
Upper
Left 080P
Right 080N
Face 0W02
Head 0W00
Jaw
Lower 0W05
Upper 0W04
Knee Region
Left 0Y0G
Right 0Y0F
Leg
Lower
Left 0Y0J
Right 0Y0H
Upper
Left 0Y0D
Right 0Y0C
Lip
Lower 0C01X
Upper 0C00X

Alteration — *continued*
　Nasal Mucosa and Soft Tissue 090K
　Neck 0W06
　Perineum
　　Female 0W0N
　　Male 0W0M
　Shoulder Region
　　Left 0X03
　　Right 0X02
　Subcutaneous Tissue and Fascia
　　Abdomen 0J08
　　Back 0J07
　　Buttock 0J09
　　Chest 0J06
　　Face 0J01
　　Lower Arm
　　　Left 0J0H
　　　Right 0J0G
　　Lower Leg
　　　Left 0J0P
　　　Right 0J0N
　　Neck
　　　Left 0J05
　　　Right 0J04
　　Upper Arm
　　　Left 0J0F
　　　Right 0J0D
　　Upper Leg
　　　Left 0J0M
　　　Right 0J0L
　Wrist Region
　　Left 0X0H
　　Right 0X0G
Alveolar process of mandible
　use Mandible, Right
　use Mandible, Left
Alveolar process of maxilla
　use Maxilla
Alveolectomy
　see Excision, Head and Facial Bones 0NB
　see Resection, Head and Facial Bones 0NT
Alveoloplasty
　see Repair, Head and Facial Bones 0NQ
　see Replacement, Head and Facial
　　Bones 0NR
　see Supplement, Head and Facial
　　Bones 0NU
Alveolotomy
　see Division, Head and Facial Bones 0N8
　see Drainage, Head and Facial Bones 0N9
Ambulatory cardiac monitoring 4A12X45
Amniocentesis
　see Drainage, Products of Conception 1090
Amnioinfusion
　see Introduction of substance in or on,
　　Products of Conception 3E0E
Amnioscopy 10J08ZZ
Amniotomy
　see Drainage, Products of Conception 1090
AMPLATZER® Muscular VSD Occluder
　use Synthetic Substitute
Amputation
　see Detachment
AMS 800® Urinary Control System
　use Artificial Sphincter in Urinary System
Anal orifice
　use Anus
Analog radiography
　see Plain Radiography
Analog radiology
　see Plain Radiography
Anastomosis
　see Bypass
Anatomical snuffbox
　use Lower Arm and Wrist Muscle, Right
　use Lower Arm and Wrist Muscle, Left

Andexanet Alfa, Factor Xa Inhibitor
　Reversal Agent
　use Coagulation Factor Xa, Inactivated
Andexxa
　use Coagulation Factor Xa, Inactivated
AneuRx® AAA Advantage®
　use Intraluminal Device
Angiectomy
　see Excision, Heart and Great Vessels 02B
　see Excision, Upper Arteries 03B
　see Excision, Lower Arteries 04B
　see Excision, Upper Veins 05B
　see Excision, Lower Veins 06B
Angiocardiography
　Combined right and left heart *see*
　　Fluoroscopy, Heart, Right and Left B216
　Left Heart *see* Fluoroscopy, Heart,
　　Left B215
　Right Heart *see* Fluoroscopy, Heart,
　　Right B214
　SPY system intravascular fluorescence *see*
　　Monitoring, Physiological Systems 4A1
Angiography
　see Plain Radiography, Heart B20
　see Fluoroscopy, Heart B21
Angioplasty
　see Dilation, Heart and Great Vessels 027
　see Repair, Heart and Great Vessels 02Q
　see Replacement, Heart and Great
　　Vessels 02R
　see Supplement, Heart and Great
　　Vessels 02U
　see Dilation, Upper Arteries 037
　see Repair, Upper Arteries 03Q
　see Replacement, Upper Arteries 03R
　see Supplement, Upper Arteries 03U
　see Dilation, Lower Arteries 047
　see Repair, Lower Arteries 04Q
　see Replacement, Lower Arteries 04R
　see Supplement, Lower Arteries 04U
Angiorrhaphy
　see Repair, Heart and Great Vessels 02Q
　see Repair, Upper Arteries 03Q
　see Repair, Lower Arteries 04Q
Angioscopy
　02JY4ZZ
　03JY4ZZ
　04JY4ZZ
Angiotensin II
　use Synthetic Human Angiotensin II
Angiotripsy
　see Occlusion, Upper Arteries 03L
　see Occlusion, Lower Arteries 04L
Angular artery
　use Face Artery
Angular vein
　use Face Vein, Right
　use Face Vein, Left
Annular ligament
　use Elbow Bursa and Ligament, Right
　use Elbow Bursa and Ligament, Left
Annuloplasty
　see Repair, Heart and Great Vessels 02Q
　see Supplement, Heart and Great
　　Vessels 02U
Annuloplasty ring
　use Synthetic Substitute
Anoplasty
　see Repair, Anus 0DQQ
　see Supplement, Anus 0DUQ
Anorectal junction
　use Rectum
Anoscopy 0DJD8ZZ
Ansa cervicalis
　use Cervical Plexus
Antabuse therapy HZ93ZZZ

Antebrachial fascia
　use Subcutaneous Tissue and Fascia, Right
　　Lower Arm
　use Subcutaneous Tissue and Fascia, Left
　　Lower Arm
Anterior (pectoral) lymph node
　use Lymphatic, Right Axillary
　use Lymphatic, Left Axillary
Anterior cerebral artery
　use Intracranial Artery
Anterior cerebral vein
　use Intracranial Vein
Anterior choroidal artery
　use Intracranial Artery
Anterior circumflex humeral artery
　use Axillary Artery, Right
　use Axillary Artery, Left
Anterior communicating artery
　use Intracranial Artery
Anterior cruciate ligament (ACL)
　use Knee Bursa and Ligament, Right
　use Knee Bursa and Ligament, Left
Anterior crural nerve
　use Femoral Nerve
Anterior facial vein
　use Face Vein, Right
　use Face Vein, Left
Anterior intercostal artery
　use Internal Mammary Artery, Right
　use Internal Mammary Artery, Left
Anterior interosseous nerve
　use Median Nerve
Anterior lateral malleolar artery
　use Anterior Tibial Artery, Right
　use Anterior Tibial Artery, Left
Anterior lingual gland
　use Minor Salivary Gland
Anterior medial malleolar artery
　use Anterior Tibial Artery, Right
　use Anterior Tibial Artery, Left
Anterior spinal artery
　use Vertebral Artery, Right
　use Vertebral Artery, Left
Anterior tibial recurrent artery
　use Anterior Tibial Artery, Right
　use Anterior Tibial Artery, Left
Anterior ulnar recurrent artery
　use Ulnar Artery, Right
　use Ulnar Artery, Left
Anterior vagal trunk
　use Vagus Nerve
Anterior vertebral muscle
　use Neck Muscle, Right
　use Neck Muscle, Left
Antibacterial Envelope (TYRX) (AIGISRx)
　use Anti-Infective Envelope
Antigen-free air conditioning
　see Atmospheric Control, Physiological
　　Systems 6A0
Antihelix
　use External Ear, Right
　use External Ear, Left
　use External Ear, Bilateral
Antimicrobial envelope
　use Anti-Infective Envelope
Antitragus
　use External Ear, Right
　use External Ear, Left
　use External Ear, Bilateral
Antrostomy
　see Drainage, Ear, Nose, Sinus 099
Antrotomy
　see Drainage, Ear, Nose, Sinus 099
Antrum of Highmore
　use Maxillary Sinus, Right
　use Maxillary Sinus, Left

Aortic annulus
   use Aortic Valve
Aortic arch
   use Thoracic Aorta, Ascending/Arch
Aortic intercostal artery
   use Upper Artery
Aortography
   see Plain Radiography, Upper Arteries B30
   see Fluoroscopy, Upper Arteries B31
   see Plain Radiography, Lower Arteries B40
   see Fluoroscopy, Lower Arteries B41
Aortoplasty
   see Repair, Aorta, Thoracic,
      Descending 02QW
   see Repair, Aorta, Thoracic, Ascending/
      Arch 02QX
   see Replacement, Aorta, Thoracic,
      Descending 02RW
   see Replacement, Aorta, Thoracic,
      Ascending/Arch 02RX
   see Supplement, Aorta, Thoracic,
      Descending 02UW
   see Supplement, Aorta, Thoracic,
      Ascending/Arch 02UX
   see Repair, Aorta, Abdominal 04Q0
   see Replacement, Aorta,
      Abdominal 04R0
   see Supplement, Aorta, Abdominal 04U0
Apalutamide Antineoplastic XW0DXJ5
Apical (subclavicular) lymph node
   use Lymphatic, Right Axillary
   use Lymphatic, Left Axillary
Apneustic center
   use Pons
Appendectomy
   see Excision, Appendix 0DBJ
   see Resection, Appendix 0DTJ
Appendicolysis
   see Release, Appendix 0DNJ
Appendicotomy
   see Drainage, Appendix 0D9J
Application
   see Introduction of substance in or on
Aquablation therapy, prostate XV508A4
Aquapheresis 6A550Z3
Aqueduct of Sylvius
   use Cerebral Ventricle
Aqueous humour
   use Anterior Chamber, Right
   use Anterior Chamber, Left
Arachnoid mater, intracranial
   use Cerebral Meninges
Arachnoid mater, spinal
   use Spinal Meninges
Arcuate artery
   use Foot Artery, Right
   use Foot Artery, Left
Areola
   use Nipple, Right
   use Nipple, Left
AROM (artificial rupture of membranes)
   10907ZC
Arterial canal (duct)
   use Pulmonary Artery, Left
Arterial pulse tracing
   see Measurement, Arterial 4A03
Arteriectomy
   see Excision, Heart and Great Vessels 02B
   see Excision, Upper Arteries 03B
   see Excision, Lower Arteries 04B
Arteriography
   see Plain Radiography, Heart B20
   see Fluoroscopy, Heart B21
   see Plain Radiography, Upper Arteries B30
   see Fluoroscopy, Upper Arteries B31
   see Plain Radiography, Lower Arteries B40
   see Fluoroscopy, Lower Arteries B41

Arterioplasty
   see Repair, Heart and Great Vessels 02Q
   see Replacement, Heart and Great
      Vessels 02R
   see Supplement, Heart and Great
      Vessels 02U
   see Repair, Upper Arteries 03Q
   see Replacement, Upper Arteries 03R
   see Supplement, Upper Arteries 03U
   see Repair, Lower Arteries 04Q
   see Replacement, Lower Arteries 04R
   see Supplement, Lower Arteries 04U
Arteriorrhaphy
   see Repair, Heart and Great Vessels 02Q
   see Repair, Upper Arteries 03Q
   see Repair, Lower Arteries 04Q
Arterioscopy
   see Inspection, Great Vessel 02JY
   see Inspection, Artery, Upper 03JY
   see Inspection, Artery, Lower 04JY
Arthrectomy
   see Excision, Upper Joints 0RB
   see Resection, Upper Joints 0RT
   see Excision, Lower Joints 0SB
   see Resection, Lower Joints 0ST
Arthrocentesis
   see Drainage, Upper Joints 0R9
   see Drainage, Lower Joints 0S9
Arthrodesis
   see Fusion, Upper Joints 0RG
   see Fusion, Lower Joints 0SG
Arthrography
   see Plain Radiography, Skull and Facial
      Bones BN0
   see Plain Radiography, Non-Axial Upper
      Bones BP0
   see Plain Radiography, Non-Axial Lower
      Bones BQ0
Arthrolysis
   see Release, Upper Joints 0RN
   see Release, Lower Joints 0SN
Arthropexy
   see Repair, Upper Joints 0RQ
   see Reposition, Upper Joints 0RS
   see Repair, Lower Joints 0SQ
   see Reposition, Lower Joints 0SS
Arthroplasty
   see Repair, Upper Joints 0RQ
   see Replacement, Upper Joints 0RR
   see Supplement, Upper Joints 0RU
   see Repair, Lower Joints 0SQ
   see Replacement, Lower Joints 0SR
   see Supplement, Lower Joints 0SU
Arthroplasty, radial head
   see Replacement, Radius, Right 0PRH
   see Replacement, Radius, Left 0PRJ
Arthroscopy
   see Inspection, Upper Joints 0RJ
   see Inspection, Lower Joints 0SJ
Arthrotomy
   see Drainage, Upper Joints 0R9
   see Drainage, Lower Joints 0S9
Articulating Spacer (Antibiotic)
   use Articulating Spacer in Lower Joints
Artificial anal sphincter (AAS)
   use Artificial Sphincter in Gastrointestinal
      System
Artificial bowel sphincter (neosphincter)
   use Artificial Sphincter in Gastrointestinal
      System
Artificial Sphincter
   Insertion of device in
      Anus 0DHQ
      Bladder 0THB
      Bladder Neck 0THC
      Urethra 0THD

Artificial Sphincter — *continued*
   Removal of device from
      Anus 0DPQ
      Bladder 0TPB
      Urethra 0TPD
   Revision of device in
      Anus 0DWQ
      Bladder 0TWB
      Urethra 0TWD
Artificial urinary sphincter (AUS)
   use Artificial Sphincter in Urinary System
Aryepiglottic fold
   use Larynx
Arytenoid cartilage
   use Larynx
Arytenoid muscle
   use Neck Muscle, Right
   use Neck Muscle, Left
Arytenoidectomy
   see Excision, Larynx 0CBS
Arytenoidopexy
   see Repair, Larynx 0CQS
Ascenda Intrathecal Catheter
   use Infusion Device
Ascending aorta
   use Thoracic Aorta, Ascending/Arch
Ascending palatine artery
   use Face Artery
Ascending pharyngeal artery
   use External Carotid Artery, Right
   use External Carotid Artery, Left
Aspiration, fine needle
   Fluid or gas *see* Drainage
   Tissue biopsy
      see Excision
      see Extraction
Assessment
   Activities of daily living *see* Activities
      of Daily Living Assessment,
      Rehabilitation F02
   Hearing *see* Hearing Assessment,
      Diagnostic Audiology F13
   Hearing aid *see* Hearing Aid Assessment,
      Diagnostic Audiology F14
   Intravascular perfusion, using indocyanine
      green (ICG) dye *see* Monitoring,
      Physiological Systems 4A1
   Motor function *see* Motor Function
      Assessment, Rehabilitation F01
   Nerve function *see* Motor Function
      Assessment, Rehabilitation F01
   Speech *see* Speech Assessment,
      Rehabilitation F00
   Vestibular *see* Vestibular Assessment,
      Diagnostic Audiology F15
   Vocational *see* Activities of Daily Living
      Treatment, Rehabilitation F08
Assistance
   Cardiac
      Continuous
         Balloon Pump 5A02210
         Impeller Pump 5A0221D
         Other Pump 5A02216
         Pulsatile Compression 5A02215
      Intermittent
         Balloon Pump 5A02110
         Impeller Pump 5A0211D
         Other Pump 5A02116
         Pulsatile Compression 5A02115
   Circulatory
      Continuous
         Hyperbaric 5A05221
         Supersaturated 5A0522C
      Intermittent
         Hyperbaric 5A05121
         Supersaturated 5A0512C

Assistance — *continued*
Respiratory
24-96 Consecutive Hours
Continuous Negative Airway Pressure 5A09459
Continuous Positive Airway Pressure 5A09457
High Nasal Flow/Velocity 5A0945A
Intermittent Negative Airway Pressure 5A0945B
Intermittent Positive Airway Pressure 5A09458
No Qualifier 5A0945Z
Continuous, Filtration 5A0920Z
Greater than 96 Consecutive Hours
Continuous Negative Airway Pressure 5A09559
Continuous Positive Airway Pressure 5A09557
High Nasal Flow/Velocity 5A0955A
Intermittent Negative Airway Pressure 5A0955B
Intermittent Positive Airway Pressure 5A09558
No Qualifier 5A0955Z
Less than 24 Consecutive Hours
Continuous Negative Airway Pressure 5A09359
Continuous Positive Airway Pressure 5A09357
High Nasal Flow/Velocity 5A0935A
Intermittent Negative Airway Pressure 5A0935B
Intermittent Positive Airway Pressure 5A09358
No Qualifier 5A0935Z
Assurant (Cobalt) stent
use Intraluminal Device
Atezolizumab Antineoplastic XW0
Atherectomy
see Extirpation, Heart and Great Vessels 02C
see Extirpation, Upper Arteries 03C
see Extirpation, Lower Arteries 04C
Atlantoaxial joint
use Cervical Vertebral Joint
Atmospheric Control 6A0Z
AtriClip LAA Exclusion System
use Extraluminal Device
Atrioseptoplasty
see Repair, Heart and Great Vessels 02Q
see Replacement, Heart and Great Vessels 02R
see Supplement, Heart and Great Vessels 02U
Atrioventricular node
use Conduction Mechanism
Atrium dextrum cordis
use Atrium, Right
Atrium pulmonale
use Atrium, Left
Attain Ability® lead
use Cardiac Lead, Pacemaker in 02H
use Cardiac Lead, Defibrillator in 02H
Attain StarFix® (OTW) lead
use Cardiac Lead, Pacemaker in 02H
use Cardiac Lead, Defibrillator in 02H
Audiology, diagnostic
see Hearing Assessment, Diagnostic Audiology F13
see Hearing Aid Assessment, Diagnostic Audiology F14
see Vestibular Assessment, Diagnostic Audiology F15
Audiometry
see Hearing Assessment, Diagnostic Audiology F13

Auditory tube
use Eustachian Tube, Right
use Eustachian Tube, Left
Auerbach's (myenteric) plexus
use Abdominal Sympathetic Nerve
Auricle
use External Ear, Right
use External Ear, Left
use External Ear, Bilateral
Auricularis muscle
use Head Muscle
Autograft
use Autologous Tissue Substitute
Autologous artery graft
use Autologous Arterial Tissue in Heart and Great Vessels
use Autologous Arterial Tissue in Upper Arteries
use Autologous Arterial Tissue in Lower Arteries
use Autologous Arterial Tissue in Upper Veins
use Autologous Arterial Tissue in Lower Veins
Autologous vein graft
use Autologous Venous Tissue in Heart and Great Vessels
use Autologous Venous Tissue in Upper Arteries
use Autologous Venous Tissue in Lower Arteries
use Autologous Venous Tissue in Upper Veins
use Autologous Venous Tissue in Lower Veins
Autotransfusion
see Transfusion
Autotransplant
Adrenal tissue *see* Reposition, Endocrine System 0GS
Kidney *see* Reposition, Urinary System 0TS
Pancreatic tissue *see* Reposition, Pancreas 0FSG
Parathyroid tissue *see* Reposition, Endocrine System 0GS
Thyroid tissue *see* Reposition, Endocrine System 0GS
Tooth *see* Reattachment, Mouth and Throat 0CM
Avulsion
see Extraction
Axial Lumbar Interbody Fusion System
use Interbody Fusion Device in Lower Joints
AxiaLIF® System
use Interbody Fusion Device in Lower Joints
Axicabtagene Ciloeucel
use Engineered Autologous Chimeric Antigen Receptor T-cell Immunotherapy
Axillary fascia
use Subcutaneous Tissue and Fascia, Right Upper Arm
use Subcutaneous Tissue and Fascia, Left Upper Arm
Axillary nerve
use Brachial Plexus
AZEDRA®
use Iobenguane I-131 Antineoplastic

B

BAK/C® Interbody Cervical Fusion System
use Interbody Fusion Device in Upper Joints
BAL (bronchial alveolar lavage), diagnostic
see Drainage, Respiratory System 0B9

Balanoplasty
see Repair, Penis 0VQS
see Supplement, Penis 0VUS
Balloon atrial septostomy (BAS) 02163Z7
Balloon Pump
Continuous, Output 5A02210
Intermittent, Output 5A02110
Bamlanivimab Monoclonal Antibody XW0
Bandage, Elastic
see Compression
Banding
see Occlusion
see Restriction
Banding, esophageal varices
see Occlusion, Vein, Esophageal 06L3
Banding, laparoscopic (adjustable) gastric
Initial procedure 0DV64CZ
Surgical correction *see* Revision of device in, Stomach 0DW6
Bard® Composix® (E/X)(LP) mesh
use Synthetic Substitute
Bard® Composix® Kugel® patch
use Synthetic Substitute
Bard® Dulex™ mesh
use Synthetic Substitute
Bard® Ventralex™ hernia patch
use Synthetic Substitute
Baricitinib XW0
Barium swallow
see Fluoroscopy, Gastrointestinal System BD1
Baroreflex Activation Therapy® (BAT®)
use Stimulator Lead in Upper Arteries
use Stimulator Generator in Subcutaneous Tissue and Fascia
Barricaid® Annular Closure Device (ACD)
use Synthetic Substitute
Bartholin's (greater vestibular) gland
use Vestibular Gland
Basal (internal) cerebral vein
use Intracranial Vein
Basal metabolic rate (BMR)
see Measurement, Physiological Systems 4A0Z
Basal nuclei
use Basal Ganglia
Base of Tongue
use Pharynx
Basilar artery
use Intracranial Artery
Basis pontis
use Pons
Beam Radiation
Abdomen DW03
Intraoperative DW033Z0
Adrenal Gland DG02
Intraoperative DG023Z0
Bile Ducts DF02
Intraoperative DF023Z0
Bladder DT02
Intraoperative DT023Z0
Bone
Other DP0C
Intraoperative DP0C3Z0
Bone Marrow D700
Intraoperative D7003Z0
Brain D000
Intraoperative D0003Z0
Brain Stem D001
Intraoperative D0013Z0
Breast
Left DM00
Intraoperative DM003Z0
Right DM01
Intraoperative DM013Z0
Bronchus DB01
Intraoperative DB013Z0
Cervix DU01
Intraoperative DU013Z0

Beam Radiation — *continued*
Chest DW02
Intraoperative DW023Z0
Chest Wall DB07
Intraoperative DB073Z0
Colon DD05
Intraoperative DD053Z0
Diaphragm DB08
Intraoperative DB083Z0
Duodenum DD02
Intraoperative DD023Z0
Ear D900
Intraoperative D9003Z0
Esophagus DD00
Intraoperative DD003Z0
Eye D800
Intraoperative D8003Z0
Femur DP09
Intraoperative DP093Z0
Fibula DP0B
Intraoperative DP0B3Z0
Gallbladder DF01
Intraoperative DF013Z0
Gland
Adrenal DG02
Intraoperative DG023Z0
Parathyroid DG04
Intraoperative DG043Z0
Pituitary DG00
Intraoperative DG003Z0
Thyroid DG05
Intraoperative DG053Z0
Glands
Salivary D906
Intraoperative D9063Z0
Head and Neck DW01
Intraoperative DW013Z0
Hemibody DW04
Intraoperative DW043Z0
Humerus DP06
Intraoperative DP063Z0
Hypopharynx D903
Intraoperative D9033Z0
Ileum DD04
Intraoperative DD043Z0
Jejunum DD03
Intraoperative DD033Z0
Kidney DT00
Intraoperative DT003Z0
Larynx D90B
Intraoperative D90B3Z0
Liver DF00
Intraoperative DF003Z0
Lung DB02
Intraoperative DB023Z0
Lymphatics
Abdomen D706
Intraoperative D7063Z0
Axillary D704
Intraoperative D7043Z0
Inguinal D708
Intraoperative D7083Z0
Neck D703
Intraoperative D7033Z0
Pelvis D707
Intraoperative D7073Z0
Thorax D705
Intraoperative D7053Z0
Mandible DP03
Intraoperative DP033Z0
Maxilla DP02
Intraoperative DP023Z0
Mediastinum DB06
Intraoperative DB063Z0
Mouth D904
Intraoperative D9043Z0

Beam Radiation — *continued*
Nasopharynx D90D
Intraoperative D90D3Z0
Neck and Head DW01
Intraoperative DW013Z0
Nerve
Peripheral D007
Intraoperative D0073Z0
Nose D901
Intraoperative D9013Z0
Oropharynx D90F
Intraoperative D90F3Z0
Ovary DU00
Intraoperative DU003Z0
Palate
Hard D908
Intraoperative D9083Z0
Soft D909
Intraoperative D9093Z0
Pancreas DF03
Intraoperative DF033Z0
Parathyroid Gland DG04
Intraoperative DG043Z0
Pelvic Bones DP08
Intraoperative DP083Z0
Pelvic Region DW06
Intraoperative DW063Z0
Pineal Body DG01
Intraoperative DG013Z0
Pituitary Gland DG00
Intraoperative DG003Z0
Pleura DB05
Intraoperative DB053Z0
Prostate DV00
Intraoperative DV003Z0
Radius DP07
Intraoperative DP073Z0
Rectum DD07
Intraoperative DD073Z0
Rib DP05
Intraoperative DP053Z0
Sinuses D907
Intraoperative D9073Z0
Skin
Abdomen DH08
Intraoperative DH083Z0
Arm DH04
Intraoperative DH043Z0
Back DH07
Intraoperative DH073Z0
Buttock DH09
Intraoperative DH093Z0
Chest DH06
Intraoperative DH063Z0
Face DH02
Intraoperative DH023Z0
Leg DH0B
Intraoperative DH0B3Z0
Neck DH03
Intraoperative DH033Z0
Skull DP00
Intraoperative DP003Z0
Spinal Cord D006
Intraoperative D0063Z0
Spleen D702
Intraoperative D7023Z0
Sternum DP04
Intraoperative DP043Z0
Stomach DD01
Intraoperative DD013Z0
Testis DV01
Intraoperative DV013Z0
Thymus D701
Intraoperative D7013Z0
Thyroid Gland DG05
Intraoperative DG053Z0

Beam Radiation — *continued*
Tibia DP0B
Intraoperative DP0B3Z0
Tongue D905
Intraoperative D9053Z0
Trachea DB00
Intraoperative DB003Z0
Ulna DP07
Intraoperative DP073Z0
Ureter DT01
Intraoperative DT013Z0
Urethra DT03
Intraoperative DT033Z0
Uterus DU02
Intraoperative DU023Z0
Whole Body DW05
Intraoperative DW053Z0
Bedside swallow F00ZJWZ
Berlin Heart Ventricular Assist Device
use Implantable Heart Assist System in Heart and Great Vessels
Bezlotoxumab Monoclonal Antibody XW0
Biceps brachii muscle
use Upper Arm Muscle, Right
use Upper Arm Muscle, Left
Biceps femoris muscle
use Upper Leg Muscle, Right
use Upper Leg Muscle, Left
Bicipital aponeurosis
use Subcutaneous Tissue and Fascia, Right Lower Arm
use Subcutaneous Tissue and Fascia, Left Lower Arm
Bicuspid valve
use Mitral Valve
Bili light therapy
see Phototherapy, Skin 6A60
Bioactive embolization coil(s)
use Intraluminal Device, Bioactive in Upper Arteries
Biofeedback GZC9ZZZ
BioFire® FilmArray® Pneumonia Panel XXEBXQ6
Biopsy
see Drainage with qualifier Diagnostic
see Excision with qualifier Diagnostic
see Extraction with qualifier Diagnostic
BiPAP
see Assistance, Respiratory 5A09
Bisection
see Division
Biventricular external heart assist system
use Short-term External Heart Assist System in Heart and Great Vessels
Blepharectomy
see Excision, Eye 08B
see Resection, Eye 08T
Blepharoplasty
see Repair, Eye 08Q
see Replacement, Eye 08R
see Reposition, Eye 08S
see Supplement, Eye 08U
Blepharorrhaphy
see Repair, Eye 08Q
Blepharotomy
see Drainage, Eye 089
Blinatumomab Antineoplastic Immunotherapy XW0
Block, Nerve, anesthetic injection 3E0T3BZ
Blood glucose monitoring system
use Monitoring Device
Blood pressure
see Measurement, Arterial 4A03
BMR (basal metabolic rate)
see Measurement, Physiological Systems 4A0Z

Body of femur
  use Femoral Shaft, Right
  use Femoral Shaft, Left
Body of fibula
  use Fibula, Right
  use Fibula, Left
Bone anchored hearing device
  use Hearing Device, Bone Conduction
    in 09H
  use Hearing Device in Head and Facial
    Bones
Bone bank bone graft
  use Nonautologous Tissue Substitute
Bone Growth Stimulator
  Insertion of device in
    Bone
      Facial 0NHW
      Lower 0QHY
      Nasal 0NHB
      Upper 0PHY
    Skull 0NH0
  Removal of device from
    Bone
      Facial 0NPW
      Lower 0QPY
      Nasal 0NPB
      Upper 0PPY
    Skull 0NP0
  Revision of device in
    Bone
      Facial 0NWW
      Lower 0QWY
      Nasal 0NWB
      Upper 0PWY
    Skull 0NW0
Bone marrow transplant
  see Transfusion, Circulatory 302
Bone morphogenetic protein 2 (BMP 2)
  use Recombinant Bone Morphogenetic
    Protein
**Bone screw (interlocking)(lag)(pedicle)
  (recessed)**
  use Internal Fixation Device in Head and
    Facial Bones
  use Internal Fixation Device in Upper
    Bones
  use Internal Fixation Device in Lower Bones
Bony labyrinth
  use Inner Ear, Right
  use Inner Ear, Left
Bony orbit
  use Orbit, Right
  use Orbit, Left
Bony vestibule
  use Inner Ear, Right
  use Inner Ear, Left
Botallo's duct
  use Pulmonary Artery, Left
Bovine pericardial valve
  use Zooplastic Tissue in Heart and Great
    Vessels
Bovine pericardium graft
  use Zooplastic Tissue in Heart and Great
    Vessels
BP (blood pressure)
  see Measurement, Arterial 4A03
Brachial (lateral) lymph node
  use Lymphatic, Right Axillary
  use Lymphatic, Left Axillary
Brachialis muscle
  use Upper Arm Muscle, Right
  use Upper Arm Muscle, Left
Brachiocephalic artery
  use Innominate Artery
Brachiocephalic trunk
  use Innominate Artery

Brachiocephalic vein
  use Innominate Vein, Right
  use Innominate Vein, Left
Brachioradialis muscle
  use Lower Arm and Wrist Muscle, Right
  use Lower Arm and Wrist Muscle, Left
Brachytherapy
  Abdomen DW13
  Adrenal Gland DG12
  Back
    Lower DW1LBB
    Upper DW1KBB
  Bile Ducts DF12
  Bladder DT12
  Bone Marrow D710
  Brain D010
  Brain Stem D011
  Breast
    Left DM10
    Right DM11
  Bronchus DB11
  Cervix DU11
  Chest DW12
  Chest Wall DB17
  Colon DD15
  Cranial Cavity DW10BB
  Diaphragm DB18
  Duodenum DD12
  Ear D910
  Esophagus DD10
  Extremity
    Lower DW1YBB
    Upper DW1XBB
  Eye D810
  Gallbladder DF11
  Gastrointestinal Tract DW1PBB
  Genitourinary Tract DW1RBB
  Gland
    Adrenal DG12
    Parathyroid DG14
    Pituitary DG10
    Thyroid DG15
  Glands, Salivary D916
  Head and Neck DW11
  Hypopharynx D913
  Ileum DD14
  Jejunum DD13
  Kidney DT10
  Larynx D91B
  Liver DF10
  Lung DB12
  Lymphatics
    Abdomen D716
    Axillary D714
    Inguinal D718
    Neck D713
    Pelvis D717
    Thorax D715
  Mediastinum DB16
  Mouth D914
  Nasopharynx D91D
  Neck and Head DW11
  Nerve, Peripheral D017
  Nose D911
  Oropharynx D91F
  Ovary DU10
  Palate
    Hard D918
    Soft D919
  Pancreas DF13
  Parathyroid Gland DG14
  Pelvic Region DW16
  Pineal Body DG11
  Pituitary Gland DG10
  Pleura DB15
  Prostate DV10
  Rectum DD17

Brachytherapy — continued
  Respiratory Tract DW1QBB
  Sinuses D917
  Spinal Cord D016
  Spleen D712
  Stomach DD11
  Testis DV11
  Thymus D711
  Thyroid Gland DG15
  Tongue D915
  Trachea DB10
  Ureter DT11
  Urethra DT13
  Uterus DU12
Brachytherapy seeds
  use Radioactive Element
Brachytherapy, CivaSheet®
  see Brachytherapy with qualifier
    Unidirectional Source
  see Insertion with device Radioactive
    Element
Breast procedures, skin only
  use Skin, Chest
Brexanolone XW0
Brexucabtagene Autoleucel
  use Brexucabtagene Autoleucel
    Immunotherapy
**Brexucabtagene Autoleucel
  Immunotherapy** XW2
Broad ligament
  use Uterine Supporting Structure
Bronchial artery
  use Upper Artery
Bronchography
  see Plain Radiography, Respiratory
    System BB0
  see Fluoroscopy, Respiratory System BB1
Bronchoplasty
  see Repair, Respiratory System 0BQ
  see Supplement, Respiratory System 0BU
Bronchorrhaphy
  see Repair, Respiratory System 0BQ
Bronchoscopy 0BJ08ZZ
Bronchotomy
  see Drainage, Respiratory System 0B9
Bronchus Intermedius
  use Main Bronchus, Right
BRYAN® Cervical Disc System
  use Synthetic Substitute
Buccal gland
  use Buccal Mucosa
Buccinator lymph node
  use Lymphatic, Head
Buccinator muscle
  use Facial Muscle
Buckling, scleral with implant
  see Supplement, Eye 08U
Bulbospongiosus muscle
  use Perineum Muscle
Bulbourethral (Cowper's) gland
  use Urethra
Bundle of His
  use Conduction Mechanism
Bundle of Kent
  use Conduction Mechanism
Bunionectomy
  see Excision, Lower Bones 0QB
Bursectomy
  see Excision, Bursae and Ligaments 0MB
  see Resection, Bursae and Ligaments 0MT
Bursocentesis
  see Drainage, Bursae and Ligaments 0M9
Bursography
  see Plain Radiography, Non-Axial Upper
    Bones BP0
  see Plain Radiography, Non-Axial Lower
    Bones BQ0

Bursotomy
  see Division, Bursae and Ligaments 0M8
  see Drainage, Bursae and Ligaments 0M9
BVS 5000 Ventricular Assist Device
  use Short-term External Heart Assist
    System in Heart and Great Vessels
Bypass
  Anterior Chamber
    Left 08133
    Right 08123
  Aorta
    Abdominal 0410
    Thoracic
      Ascending/Arch 021X
      Descending 021W
  Artery
    Anterior Tibial
      Left 041Q
      Right 041P
    Axillary
      Left 03160
      Right 03150
    Brachial
      Left 03180
      Right 03170
    Common Carotid
      Left 031J0
      Right 031H0
    Common Iliac
      Left 041D
      Right 041C
    Coronary
      Four or More Arteries 0213
      One Artery 0210
      Three Arteries 0212
      Two Arteries 0211
    External Carotid
      Left 031N0
      Right 031M0
    External Iliac
      Left 041J
      Right 041H
    Femoral
      Left 041L
      Right 041K
    Foot
      Left 041W
      Right 041V
    Hepatic 0413
    Innominate 03120
    Internal Carotid
      Left 031L0
      Right 031K0
    Internal Iliac
      Left 041F
      Right 041E
    Intracranial 031G0
    Peroneal
      Left 041U
      Right 041T
    Popliteal
      Left 041N
      Right 041M
    Posterior Tibial
      Left 041S
      Right 041R
    Pulmonary
      Left 021R
      Right 021Q
    Pulmonary Trunk 021P
    Radial
      Left 031C
      Right 031B
    Splenic 0414
    Subclavian
      Left 03140
      Right 03130

Bypass — *continued*
  Artery — *continued*
    Temporal
      Left 031T0
      Right 031S0
    Ulnar
      Left 031A
      Right 0319
  Atrium
    Left 0217
    Right 0216
  Bladder 0T1B
  Cavity, Cranial 0W110J
  Cecum 0D1H
  Cerebral Ventricle 0016
  Colon
    Ascending 0D1K
    Descending 0D1M
    Sigmoid 0D1N
    Transverse 0D1L
  Duct
    Common Bile 0F19
    Cystic 0F18
    Hepatic
      Common 0F17
      Left 0F16
      Right 0F15
    Lacrimal
      Left 081Y
      Right 081X
    Pancreatic 0F1D
      Accessory 0F1F
  Duodenum 0D19
  Ear
    Left 091E0
    Right 091D0
  Esophagus 0D15
    Lower 0D13
    Middle 0D12
    Upper 0D11
  Fallopian Tube
    Left 0U16
    Right 0U15
  Gallbladder 0F14
  Ileum 0D1B
  Intestine
    Large 0D1E
    Small 0D18
  Jejunum 0D1A
  Kidney Pelvis
    Left 0T14
    Right 0T13
  Pancreas 0F1G
  Pelvic Cavity 0W1J
  Peritoneal Cavity 0W1G
  Pleural Cavity
    Left 0W1B
    Right 0W19
  Spinal Canal 001U
  Stomach 0D16
  Trachea 0B11
  Ureter
    Left 0T17
    Right 0T16
  Ureters, Bilateral 0T18
  Vas Deferens
    Bilateral 0V1Q
    Left 0V1P
    Right 0V1N
  Vein
    Axillary
      Left 0518
      Right 0517
    Azygos 0510
    Basilic
      Left 051C
      Right 051B

Bypass — *continued*
  Vein — *continued*
    Brachial
      Left 051A
      Right 0519
    Cephalic
      Left 051F
      Right 051D
    Colic 0617
    Common Iliac
      Left 061D
      Right 061C
    Esophageal 0613
    External Iliac
      Left 061G
      Right 061F
    External Jugular
      Left 051Q
      Right 051P
    Face
      Left 051V
      Right 051T
    Femoral
      Left 061N
      Right 061M
    Foot
      Left 061V
      Right 061T
    Gastric 0612
    Hand
      Left 051H
      Right 051G
    Hemiazygos 0511
    Hepatic 0614
    Hypogastric
      Left 061J
      Right 061H
    Inferior Mesenteric 0616
    Innominate
      Left 0514
      Right 0513
    Internal Jugular
      Left 051N
      Right 051M
    Intracranial 051L
    Portal 0618
    Renal
      Left 061B
      Right 0619
    Saphenous
      Left 061Q
      Right 061P
    Splenic 0611
    Subclavian
      Left 0516
      Right 0515
    Superior Mesenteric 0615
    Vertebral
      Left 051S
      Right 051R
  Vena Cava
    Inferior 0610
    Superior 021V
  Ventricle
    Left 021L
    Right 021K
Bypass, cardiopulmonary 5A1221Z

C

Caesarean section
  see Extraction, Products of
    Conception 10D0
Calcaneocuboid joint
  use Tarsal Joint, Right
  use Tarsal Joint, Left

Calcaneocuboid ligament
  use Foot Bursa and Ligament, Right
  use Foot Bursa and Ligament, Left
Calcaneofibular ligament
  use Ankle Bursa and Ligament, Right
  use Ankle Bursa and Ligament, Left
Calcaneus
  use Tarsal, Right
  use Tarsal, Left
Cannulation
  see Bypass
  see Dilation
  see Drainage
  see Irrigation
Canthorrhaphy
  see Repair, Eye 08Q
Canthotomy
  see Release, Eye 08N
Capitate bone
  use Carpal, Right
  use Carpal, Left
Caplacizumab XW0
Capsulectomy, lens
  see Excision, Eye 08B
Capsulorrhaphy, joint
  see Repair, Upper Joints 0RQ
  see Repair, Lower Joints 0SQ
Cardia
  use Esophagogastric Junction
Cardiac contractility modulation lead
  use Cardiac Lead in Heart and Great Vessels
Cardiac event recorder
  use Monitoring Device
Cardiac Lead
  Defibrillator
    Atrium
      Left 02H7
      Right 02H6
    Pericardium 02HN
    Vein, Coronary 02H4
    Ventricle
      Left 02HL
      Right 02HK
  Insertion of device in
    Atrium
      Left 02H7
      Right 02H6
    Pericardium 02HN
    Vein, Coronary 02H4
    Ventricle
      Left 02HL
      Right 02HK
  Pacemaker
    Atrium
      Left 02H7
      Right 02H6
    Pericardium 02HN
    Vein, Coronary 02H4
    Ventricle
      Left 02HL
      Right 02HK
  Removal of device from, Heart 02PA
  Revision of device in, Heart 02WA
Cardiac plexus
  use Thoracic Sympathetic Nerve
Cardiac Resynchronization Defibrillator Pulse Generator
  Abdomen 0JH8
  Chest 0JH6
Cardiac Resynchronization Pacemaker Pulse Generator
  Abdomen 0JH8
  Chest 0JH6
Cardiac resynchronization therapy (CRT) lead
  use Cardiac Lead, Pacemaker in 02H
  use Cardiac Lead, Defibrillator in 02H

Cardiac Rhythm Related Device
  Insertion of device in
    Abdomen 0JH8
    Chest 0JH6
  Removal of device from, Subcutaneous Tissue and Fascia, Trunk 0JPT
  Revision of device in, Subcutaneous Tissue and Fascia, Trunk 0JWT
Cardiocentesis
  see Drainage, Pericardial Cavity 0W9D
Cardioesophageal junction
  use Esophagogastric Junction
Cardiolysis
  see Release, Heart and Great Vessels 02N
CardioMEMS® pressure sensor
  use Monitoring Device, Pressure Sensor in 02H
Cardiomyotomy
  see Division, Esophagogastric Junction 0D84
Cardioplegia
  see Introduction of substance in or on, Heart 3E08
Cardiorrhaphy
  see Repair, Heart and Great Vessels 02Q
Cardioversion 5A2204Z
Caregiver Training F0FZ
Caroticotympanic artery
  use Internal Carotid Artery, Right
  use Internal Carotid Artery, Left
Carotid (artery) sinus (baroreceptor) lead
  use Stimulator Lead in Upper Arteries
Carotid glomus
  use Carotid Body, Left
  use Carotid Body, Right
  use Carotid Bodies, Bilateral
Carotid sinus
  use Internal Carotid Artery, Right
  use Internal Carotid Artery, Left
Carotid sinus nerve
  use Glossopharyngeal Nerve
Carotid WALLSTENT® Monorail® Endoprosthesis
  use Intraluminal Device
Carpectomy
  see Excision, Upper Bones 0PB
  see Resection, Upper Bones 0PT
Carpometacarpal ligament
  use Hand Bursa and Ligament, Right
  use Hand Bursa and Ligament, Left
Casting
  see Immobilization
CAT scan
  see Computerized Tomography (CT Scan)
Catheterization
  see Dilation
  see Drainage
  see Insertion of device in
  see Irrigation
  Heart *see* Measurement, Cardiac 4A02
  Umbilical vein, for infusion 06H033T
Cauda equina
  use Lumbar Spinal Cord
Cauterization
  see Destruction
  see Repair
Cavernous plexus
  use Head and Neck Sympathetic Nerve
CBMA (Concentrated Bone Marrow Aspirate)
  use Concentrated Bone Marrow Aspirate
CBMA (Concentrated Bone Marrow Aspirate) injection, intramuscular XK02303
CD24Fc Immunomodulator XW0
Cecectomy
  see Excision, Cecum 0DBH
  see Resection, Cecum 0DTH

Cecocolostomy
  see Bypass, Gastrointestinal System 0D1
  see Drainage, Gastrointestinal System 0D9
Cecopexy
  see Repair, Cecum 0DQH
  see Reposition, Cecum 0DSH
Cecoplication
  see Restriction, Cecum 0DVH
Cecorrhaphy
  see Repair, Cecum 0DQH
Cecostomy
  see Bypass, Cecum 0D1H
  see Drainage, Cecum 0D9H
Cecotomy
  see Drainage, Cecum 0D9H
Cefiderocol Anti-infective XW0
Ceftazidime-Avibactam Anti-infective XW0
Ceftolozane/Tazobactam Anti-infective XW0
Celiac (solar) plexus
  use Abdominal Sympathetic Nerve
Celiac ganglion
  use Abdominal Sympathetic Nerve
Celiac lymph node
  use Lymphatic, Aortic
Celiac trunk
  use Celiac Artery
Central axillary lymph node
  use Lymphatic, Right Axillary
  use Lymphatic, Left Axillary
Central venous pressure
  see Measurement, Venous 4A04
Centrimag® Blood Pump
  use Short-term External Heart Assist System in Heart and Great Vessels
Cephalogram BN00ZZZ
Ceramic on ceramic bearing surface
  use Synthetic Substitute, Ceramic in 0SR
Cerclage
  see Restriction
Cerebral aqueduct (Sylvius)
  use Cerebral Ventricle
Cerebral Embolic Filtration
  Dual Filter X2A5312
  Extracorporeal Flow Reversal Circuit X2A
  Single Deflection Filter X2A6325
Cerebrum
  use Brain
Cervical esophagus
  use Esophagus, Upper
Cervical facet joint
  use Cervical Vertebral Joint
  use Cervical Vertebral Joints, 2 or more
Cervical ganglion
  use Head and Neck Sympathetic Nerve
Cervical interspinous ligament
  use Head and Neck Bursa and Ligament
Cervical intertransverse ligament
  use Head and Neck Bursa and Ligament
Cervical ligamentum flavum
  use Head and Neck Bursa and Ligament
Cervical lymph node
  use Lymphatic, Right Neck
  use Lymphatic, Left Neck
Cervicectomy
  see Excision, Cervix 0UBC
  see Resection, Cervix 0UTC
Cervicothoracic facet joint
  use Cervicothoracic Vertebral Joint
Cesarean section
  see Extraction, Products of Conception 10D0
Cesium-131 Collagen Implant
  use Radioactive Element, Cesium-131 Collagen Implant in 00H

Change device in
Abdominal Wall 0W2FX
Back
  Lower 0W2LX
  Upper 0W2KX
Bladder 0T2BX
Bone
  Facial 0N2WX
  Lower 0Q2YX
  Nasal 0N2BX
  Upper 0P2YX
Bone Marrow 072TX
Brain 0020X
Breast
  Left 0H2UX
  Right 0H2TX
Bursa and Ligament
  Lower 0M2YX
  Upper 0M2XX
Cavity, Cranial 0W21X
Chest Wall 0W28X
Cisterna Chyli 072LX
Diaphragm 0B2TX
Duct
  Hepatobiliary 0F2BX
  Pancreatic 0F2DX
Ear
  Left 092JX
  Right 092HX
Epididymis and Spermatic Cord 0V2MX
Extremity
  Lower
    Left 0Y2BX
    Right 0Y29X
  Upper
    Left 0X27X
    Right 0X26X
Eye
  Left 0821X
  Right 0820X
Face 0W22X
Fallopian Tube 0U28X
Gallbladder 0F24X
Gland
  Adrenal 0G25X
  Endocrine 0G2SX
  Pituitary 0G20X
  Salivary 0C2AX
Head 0W20X
Intestinal Tract
  Lower 0D2DXUZ
  Upper 0D20XUZ
Jaw
  Lower 0W25X
  Upper 0W24X
Joint
  Lower 0S2YX
  Upper 0R2YX
Kidney 0T25X
Larynx 0C2SX
Liver 0F20X
Lung
  Left 0B2LX
  Right 0B2KX
Lymphatic 072NX
  Thoracic Duct 072KX
Mediastinum 0W2CX
Mesentery 0D2VX
Mouth and Throat 0C2YX
Muscle
  Lower 0K2YX
  Upper 0K2XX
Nasal Mucosa and Soft Tissue 092KX
Neck 0W26X
Nerve
  Cranial 002EX
  Peripheral 012YX

Change device in — *continued*
Omentum 0D2UX
Ovary 0U23X
Pancreas 0F2GX
Parathyroid Gland 0G2RX
Pelvic Cavity 0W2JX
Penis 0V2SX
Pericardial Cavity 0W2DX
Perineum
  Female 0W2NX
  Male 0W2MX
Peritoneal Cavity 0W2GX
Peritoneum 0D2WX
Pineal Body 0G21X
Pleura 0B2QX
Pleural Cavity
  Left 0W2BX
  Right 0W29X
Products of Conception 10207
Prostate and Seminal Vesicles 0V24X
Retroperitoneum 0W2HX
Scrotum and Tunica Vaginalis 0V28X
Sinus 092YX
Skin 0H2PX
Skull 0N20X
Spinal Canal 002UX
Spleen 072PX
Subcutaneous Tissue and Fascia
  Head and Neck 0J2SX
  Lower Extremity 0J2WX
  Trunk 0J2TX
  Upper Extremity 0J2VX
Tendon
  Lower 0L2YX
  Upper 0L2XX
Testis 0V2DX
Thymus 072MX
Thyroid Gland 0G2KX
Trachea 0B21
Tracheobronchial Tree 0B20X
Ureter 0T29X
Urethra 0T2DX
Uterus and Cervix 0U2DXHZ
Vagina and Cul-de-sac 0U2HXGZ
Vas Deferens 0V2RX
Vulva 0U2MX
Change device in or on
Abdominal Wall 2W03X
Anorectal 2Y03X5Z
Arm
  Lower
    Left 2W0DX
    Right 2W0CX
  Upper
    Left 2W0BX
    Right 2W0AX
Back 2W05X
Chest Wall 2W04X
Ear 2Y02X5Z
Extremity
  Lower
    Left 2W0MX
    Right 2W0LX
  Upper
    Left 2W09X
    Right 2W08X
Face 2W01X
Finger
  Left 2W0KX
  Right 2W0JX
Foot
  Left 2W0TX
  Right 2W0SX
Genital Tract, Female 2Y04X5Z
Hand
  Left 2W0FX
  Right 2W0EX

Change device in or on — *continued*
Head 2W00X
Inguinal Region
  Left 2W07X
  Right 2W06X
Leg
  Lower
    Left 2W0RX
    Right 2W0QX
  Upper
    Left 2W0PX
    Right 2W0NX
Mouth and Pharynx 2Y00X5Z
Nasal 2Y01X5Z
Neck 2W02X
Thumb
  Left 2W0HX
  Right 2W0GX
Toe
  Left 2W0VX
  Right 2W0UX
Urethra 2Y05X5Z
Chemoembolization
  see Introduction of substance in or on
Chemosurgery, Skin 3E00XTZ
Chemothalamectomy
  see Destruction, Thalamus 0059
Chemotherapy, Infusion for cancer
  see Introduction of substance in or on
Chest x-ray
  see Plain Radiography, Chest BW03
Chiropractic Manipulation
  Abdomen 9WB9X
  Cervical 9WB1X
  Extremities
    Lower 9WB6X
    Upper 9WB7X
  Head 9WB0X
  Lumbar 9WB3X
  Pelvis 9WB5X
  Rib Cage 9WB8X
  Sacrum 9WB4X
  Thoracic 9WB2X
Choana
  use Nasopharynx
Cholangiogram
  see Plain Radiography, Hepatobiliary
    System and Pancreas BF0
  see Fluoroscopy, Hepatobiliary System and
    Pancreas BF1
Cholecystectomy
  see Excision, Gallbladder 0FB4
  see Resection, Gallbladder 0FT4
Cholecystojejunostomy
  see Bypass, Hepatobiliary System and
    Pancreas 0F1
  see Drainage, Hepatobiliary System and
    Pancreas 0F9
Cholecystopexy
  see Repair, Gallbladder 0FQ4
  see Reposition, Gallbladder 0FS4
Cholecystoscopy 0FJ44ZZ
Cholecystostomy
  see Bypass, Gallbladder 0F14
  see Drainage, Gallbladder 0F94
Cholecystotomy
  see Drainage, Gallbladder 0F94
Choledochectomy
  see Excision, Hepatobiliary System and
    Pancreas 0FB
  see Resection, Hepatobiliary System and
    Pancreas 0FT
Choledocholithotomy
  see Extirpation, Duct, Common Bile 0FC9
Choledochoplasty
  see Repair, Hepatobiliary System and
    Pancreas 0FQ

Choledochoplasty — *continued*
　　see Replacement, Hepatobiliary System
　　　　and Pancreas 0FR
　　see Supplement, Hepatobiliary System and
　　　　Pancreas 0FU
Choledochoscopy 0FJB8ZZ
Choledochotomy
　　see Drainage, Hepatobiliary System and
　　　　Pancreas 0F9
Cholelithotomy
　　see Extirpation, Hepatobiliary System and
　　　　Pancreas 0FC
Chondrectomy
　　see Excision, Upper Joints 0RB
　　see Excision, Lower Joints 0SB
　　Knee *see* Excision, Lower Joints 0SB
　　Semilunar cartilage *see* Excision, Lower
　　　　Joints 0SB
Chondroglossus muscle
　　use Tongue, Palate, Pharynx Muscle
Chorda tympani
　　use Facial Nerve
Chordotomy
　　see Division, Central Nervous System and
　　　　Cranial Nerves 008
Choroid plexus
　　use Cerebral Ventricle
Choroidectomy
　　see Excision, Eye 08B
　　see Resection, Eye 08T
Ciliary body
　　use Eye, Right
　　use Eye, Left
Ciliary ganglion
　　use Head and Neck Sympathetic Nerve
Circle of Willis
　　use Intracranial Artery
Circumcision 0VTTXZZ
Circumflex iliac artery
　　use Femoral Artery, Right
　　use Femoral Artery, Left
CivaSheet®
　　use Radioactive Element
CivaSheet® Brachytherapy
　　see Brachytherapy with qualifier
　　　　Unidirectional Source
　　see Insertion with device Radioactive
　　　　Element
**Clamp and rod internal fixation system
(CRIF)**
　　use Internal Fixation Device in Upper Bones
　　use Internal Fixation Device in Lower Bones
Clamping
　　see Occlusion
Claustrum
　　use Basal Ganglia
Claviculectomy
　　see Excision, Upper Bones 0PB
　　see Resection, Upper Bones 0PT
Claviculotomy
　　see Division, Upper Bones 0P8
　　see Drainage, Upper Bones 0P9
Clipping, aneurysm
　　see Occlusion using Extraluminal Device
　　see Restriction using Extraluminal Device
Clitorectomy, clitoridectomy
　　see Excision, Clitoris 0UBJ
　　see Resection, Clitoris 0UTJ
Clolar
　　use Clofarabine
Closure
　　see Occlusion
　　see Repair
Clysis
　　see Introduction of substance in or on
Coagulation
　　see Destruction

Coagulation Factor Xa, Inactivated XW0
**Coagulation Factor Xa, (Recombinant)
Inactivated**
　　use Coagulation Factor Xa, Inactivated
**COALESCE® radiolucent interbody fusion
device**
　　use Interbody Fusion Device, Radiolucent
　　　　Porous in New Technology
CoAxia NeuroFlo catheter
　　use Intraluminal Device
**Cobalt/chromium head and polyethylene
socket**
　　use Synthetic Substitute, Metal on
　　　　Polyethylene in 0SR
Cobalt/chromium head and socket
　　use Synthetic Substitute, Metal in 0SR
Coccygeal body
　　use Coccygeal Glomus
Coccygeus muscle
　　use Trunk Muscle, Right
　　use Trunk Muscle, Left
Cochlea
　　use Inner Ear, Right
　　use Inner Ear, Left
**Cochlear implant (CI), multiple channel
(electrode)**
　　use Hearing Device, Multiple Channel
　　　　Cochlear Prosthesis in 09H
**Cochlear implant (CI), single channel
(electrode)**
　　use Hearing Device, Single Channel
　　　　Cochlear Prosthesis in 09H
Cochlear Implant Treatment F0BZ0
Cochlear nerve
　　use Acoustic Nerve
COGNIS® CRT-D
　　use Cardiac Resynchronization Defibrillator
　　　　Pulse Generator in 0JH
**COHERE® radiolucent interbody fusion
device**
　　use Interbody Fusion Device, Radiolucent
　　　　Porous in New Technology
Colectomy
　　see Excision, Gastrointestinal System 0DB
　　see Resection, Gastrointestinal System 0DT
Collapse
　　see Occlusion
Collection from
　　Breast, Breast Milk 8E0HX62
　　Indwelling Device
　　　　Circulatory System
　　　　　　Blood 8C02X6K
　　　　　　Other Fluid 8C02X6L
　　　　Nervous System
　　　　　　Cerebrospinal Fluid 8C01X6J
　　　　　　Other Fluid 8C01X6L
　　Integumentary System, Breast
　　　　Milk 8E0HX62
　　Reproductive System, Male,
　　　　Sperm 8E0VX63
Colocentesis
　　see Drainage, Gastrointestinal System 0D9
Colofixation
　　see Repair, Gastrointestinal System 0DQ
　　see Reposition, Gastrointestinal System 0DS
Cololysis
　　see Release, Gastrointestinal System 0DN
Colonic Z-Stent®
　　use Intraluminal Device
Colonoscopy 0DJD8ZZ
Colopexy
　　see Repair, Gastrointestinal System 0DQ
　　see Reposition, Gastrointestinal System 0DS
Coloplication
　　see Restriction, Gastrointestinal
　　　　System 0DV

Coloproctectomy
　　see Excision, Gastrointestinal System 0DB
　　see Resection, Gastrointestinal System 0DT
Coloproctostomy
　　see Bypass, Gastrointestinal System 0D1
　　see Drainage, Gastrointestinal System 0D9
Colopuncture
　　see Drainage, Gastrointestinal System 0D9
Colorrhaphy
　　see Repair, Gastrointestinal System 0DQ
Colostomy
　　see Bypass, Gastrointestinal System 0D1
　　see Drainage, Gastrointestinal System 0D9
Colpectomy
　　see Excision, Vagina 0UBG
　　see Resection, Vagina 0UTG
Colpocentesis
　　see Drainage, Vagina 0U9G
Colpopexy
　　see Repair, Vagina 0UQG
　　see Reposition, Vagina 0USG
Colpoplasty
　　see Repair, Vagina 0UQG
　　see Supplement, Vagina 0UUG
Colporrhaphy
　　see Repair, Vagina 0UQG
Colposcopy 0UJH8ZZ
Columella
　　use Nasal Mucosa and Soft Tissue
Common digital vein
　　use Foot Vein, Right
　　use Foot Vein, Left
Common facial vein
　　use Face Vein, Right
　　use Face Vein, Left
Common fibular nerve
　　use Peroneal Nerve
Common hepatic artery
　　use Hepatic Artery
Common iliac (subaortic) lymph node
　　use Lymphatic, Pelvis
Common interosseous artery
　　use Ulnar Artery, Right
　　use Ulnar Artery, Left
Common peroneal nerve
　　use Peroneal Nerve
Complete (SE) stent
　　use Intraluminal Device
Compression
　　see Restriction
　　Abdominal Wall 2W13X
　　Arm
　　　　Lower
　　　　　　Left 2W1DX
　　　　　　Right 2W1CX
　　　　Upper
　　　　　　Left 2W1BX
　　　　　　Right 2W1AX
　　Back 2W15X
　　Chest Wall 2W14X
　　Extremity
　　　　Lower
　　　　　　Left 2W1MX
　　　　　　Right 2W1LX
　　　　Upper
　　　　　　Left 2W19X
　　　　　　Right 2W18X
　　Face 2W11X
　　Finger
　　　　Left 2W1KX
　　　　Right 2W1JX
　　Foot
　　　　Left 2W1TX
　　　　Right 2W1SX
　　Hand
　　　　Left 2W1FX
　　　　Right 2W1EX

Compression — *continued*
  Head 2W10X
  Inguinal Region
    Left 2W17X
    Right 2W16X
  Leg
    Lower
      Left 2W1RX
      Right 2W1QX
    Upper
      Left 2W1PX
      Right 2W1NX
  Neck 2W12X
  Thumb
    Left 2W1HX
    Right 2W1GX
  Toe
    Left 2W1VX
    Right 2W1UX
Computer Assisted Procedure
  Extremity
    Lower
      No Qualifier 8E0YXBZ
      With Computerized
        Tomography 8E0YXBG
      With Fluoroscopy 8E0YXBF
      With Magnetic Resonance
        Imaging 8E0YXBH
    Upper
      No Qualifier 8E0XXBZ
      With Computerized
        Tomography 8E0XXBG
      With Fluoroscopy 8E0XXBF
      With Magnetic Resonance
        Imaging 8E0XXBH
  Head and Neck Region
    No Qualifier 8E09XBZ
    With Computerized
      Tomography 8E09XBG
    With Fluoroscopy 8E09XBF
    With Magnetic Resonance
      Imaging 8E09XBH
  Trunk Region
    No Qualifier 8E0WXBZ
    With Computerized
      Tomography 8E0WXBG
    With Fluoroscopy 8E0WXBF
    With Magnetic Resonance
      Imaging 8E0WXBH
Computerized Tomography (CT Scan)
  Abdomen BW20
    Chest and Pelvis BW25
  Abdomen and Chest BW24
  Abdomen and Pelvis BW21
  Airway, Trachea BB2F
  Ankle
    Left BQ2H
    Right BQ2G
  Aorta
    Abdominal B420
      Intravascular Optical
        Coherence B420Z2Z
    Thoracic B320
      Intravascular Optical
        Coherence B320Z2Z
  Arm
    Left BP2F
    Right BP2E
  Artery
    Celiac B421
      Intravascular Optical
        Coherence B421Z2Z
    Common Carotid
      Bilateral B325
      Intravascular Optical
        Coherence B325Z2Z

Computerized Tomography — *continued*
  Artery — *continued*
    Coronary
      Bypass Graft
        Multiple B223
          Intravascular Optical
            Coherence B223Z2Z
      Multiple B221
        Intravascular Optical
          Coherence B221Z2Z
    Internal Carotid
      Bilateral B328
      Intravascular Optical
        Coherence B328Z2Z
    Intracranial B32R
      Intravascular Optical
        Coherence B32RZ2Z
    Lower Extremity
      Bilateral B42H
        Intravascular Optical
          Coherence B42HZ2Z
      Left B42G
        Intravascular Optical
          Coherence B42GZ2Z
      Right B42F
        Intravascular Optical
          Coherence B42FZ2Z
    Pelvic B42C
      Intravascular Optical
        Coherence B42CZ2Z
    Pulmonary
      Left B32T
        Intravascular Optical
          Coherence B32TZ2Z
      Right B32S
        Intravascular Optical
          Coherence B32SZ2Z
    Renal
      Bilateral B428
        Intravascular Optical
          Coherence B428Z2Z
      Transplant B42M
        Intravascular Optical
          Coherence B42MZ2Z
    Superior Mesenteric B424
      Intravascular Optical
        Coherence B424Z2Z
    Vertebral
      Bilateral B32G
      Intravascular Optical
        Coherence B32GZ2Z
  Bladder BT20
  Bone
    Facial BN25
    Temporal BN2F
  Brain B020
  Calcaneus
    Left BQ2K
    Right BQ2J
  Cerebral Ventricle B028
  Chest, Abdomen and Pelvis BW25
  Chest and Abdomen BW24
  Cisterna B027
  Clavicle
    Left BP25
    Right BP24
  Coccyx BR2F
  Colon BD24
  Ear B920
  Elbow
    Left BP2H
    Right BP2G
  Extremity
    Lower
      Left BQ2S
      Right BQ2R

Computerized Tomography — *continued*
  Extremity — *continued*
    Upper
      Bilateral BP2V
      Left BP2U
      Right BP2T
  Eye
    Bilateral B827
    Left B826
    Right B825
  Femur
    Left BQ24
    Right BQ23
  Fibula
    Left BQ2C
    Right BQ2B
  Finger
    Left BP2S
    Right BP2R
  Foot
    Left BQ2M
    Right BQ2L
  Forearm
    Left BP2K
    Right BP2J
  Gland
    Adrenal, Bilateral BG22
    Parathyroid BG23
    Parotid, Bilateral B926
    Salivary, Bilateral B92D
    Submandibular, Bilateral B929
    Thyroid BG24
  Hand
    Left BP2P
    Right BP2N
  Hands and Wrists, Bilateral BP2Q
  Head BW28
  Head and Neck BW29
  Heart
    Right and Left B226
    Intravascular Optical
      Coherence B226Z2Z
  Hepatobiliary System, All BF2C
  Hip
    Left BQ21
    Right BQ20
  Humerus
    Left BP2B
    Right BP2A
  Intracranial Sinus B522
    Intravascular Optical
      Coherence B522Z2Z
  Joint
    Acromioclavicular, Bilateral BP23
    Finger
      Left BP2DZZZ
      Right BP2CZZZ
    Foot
      Left BQ2Y
      Right BQ2X
    Hand
      Left BP2DZZZ
      Right BP2CZZZ
    Sacroiliac BR2D
    Sternoclavicular
      Bilateral BP22
      Left BP21
      Right BP20
    Temporomandibular, Bilateral BN29
    Toe
      Left BQ2Y
      Right BQ2X
  Kidney
    Bilateral BT23
    Left BT22
    Right BT21
    Transplant BT29

Computerized Tomography — *continued*
- Knee
  - Left BQ28
  - Right BQ27
- Larynx B92J
- Leg
  - Left BQ2F
  - Right BQ2D
- Liver BF25
- Liver and Spleen BF26
- Lung, Bilateral BB24
- Mandible BN26
- Nasopharynx B92F
- Neck BW2F
- Neck and Head BW29
- Orbit, Bilateral BN23
- Oropharynx B92F
- Pancreas BF27
- Patella
  - Left BQ2W
  - Right BQ2V
- Pelvic Region BW2G
- Pelvis BR2C
  - Chest and Abdomen BW25
- Pelvis and Abdomen BW21
- Pituitary Gland B029
- Prostate BV23
- Ribs
  - Left BP2Y
  - Right BP2X
- Sacrum BR2F
- Scapula
  - Left BP27
  - Right BP26
- Sella Turcica B029
- Shoulder
  - Left BP29
  - Right BP28
- Sinus
  - Intracranial B522
    - Intravascular Optical Coherence B522Z2Z
  - Paranasal B922
- Skull BN20
- Spinal Cord B02B
- Spine
  - Cervical BR20
  - Lumbar BR29
  - Thoracic BR27
- Spleen and Liver BF26
- Thorax BP2W
- Tibia
  - Left BQ2C
  - Right BQ2B
- Toe
  - Left BQ2Q
  - Right BQ2P
- Trachea BB2F
- Tracheobronchial Tree
  - Bilateral BB29
  - Left BB28
  - Right BB27
- Vein
  - Pelvic (Iliac)
    - Left B52G
      - Intravascular Optical Coherence B52GZ2Z
    - Right B52F
      - Intravascular Optical Coherence B52FZ2Z
  - Pelvic (Iliac) Bilateral B52H
    - Intravascular Optical Coherence B52HZ2Z
  - Portal B52T
    - Intravascular Optical Coherence B52TZ2Z
  - Pulmonary

Computerized Tomography — *continued*
- Vein — *continued*
  - Bilateral B52S
    - Intravascular Optical Coherence B52SZ2Z
  - Left B52R
    - Intravascular Optical Coherence B52RZ2Z
  - Right B52Q
    - Intravascular Optical Coherence B52QZ2Z
  - Renal
    - Bilateral B52L
      - Intravascular Optical Coherence B52LZ2Z
    - Left B52K
      - Intravascular Optical Coherence B52KZ2Z
    - Right B52J
      - Intravascular Optical Coherence B52JZ2Z
  - Splanchnic B52T
    - Intravascular Optical Coherence B52TZ2Z
  - Vena Cava
    - Inferior B529
      - Intravascular Optical Coherence B529Z2Z
    - Superior B528
      - Intravascular Optical Coherence B528Z2Z
  - Ventricle, Cerebral B028
  - Wrist
    - Left BP2M
    - Right BP2L

Concentrated Bone Marrow Aspirate (CBMA) injection, intramuscular XK02303

Concerto II CRT-D
- *use* Cardiac Resynchronization Defibrillator Pulse Generator in 0JH

Condylectomy
- *see* Excision, Head and Facial Bones 0NB
- *see* Excision, Upper Bones 0PB
- *see* Excision, Lower Bones 0QB

Condyloid process
- *use* Mandible, Right
- *use* Mandible, Left

Condylotomy
- *see* Division, Head and Facial Bones 0N8
- *see* Drainage, Head and Facial Bones 0N9
- *see* Division, Upper Bones 0P8
- *see* Drainage, Upper Bones 0P9
- *see* Division, Lower Bones 0Q8
- *see* Drainage, Lower Bones 0Q9

Condylysis
- *see* Release, Head and Facial Bones 0NN
- *see* Release, Upper Bones 0PN
- *see* Release, Lower Bones 0QN

Conization, cervix
- *see* Excision, Cervix 0UBC

Conjunctivoplasty
- *see* Repair, Eye 08Q
- *see* Replacement, Eye 08R

CONSERVE® PLUS Total Resurfacing Hip System
- *use* Resurfacing Device in Lower Joints

Construction
- Auricle, ear *see* Replacement, Ear, Nose, Sinus 09R
- Ileal conduit *see* Bypass, Urinary System 0T1

Consulta CRT-D
- *use* Cardiac Resynchronization Defibrillator Pulse Generator in 0JH

Consulta CRT-P
- *use* Cardiac Resynchronization Pacemaker Pulse Generator in 0JH

Contact Radiation
- Abdomen DWY37ZZ
- Adrenal Gland DGY27ZZ
- Bile Ducts DFY27ZZ
- Bladder DTY27ZZ
- Bone, Other DPYC7ZZ
- Brain D0Y07ZZ
- Brain Stem D0Y17ZZ
- Breast
  - Left DMY07ZZ
  - Right DMY17ZZ
- Bronchus DBY17ZZ
- Cervix DUY17ZZ
- Chest DWY27ZZ
- Chest Wall DBY77ZZ
- Colon DDY57ZZ
- Diaphragm DBY87ZZ
- Duodenum DDY27ZZ
- Ear D9Y07ZZ
- Esophagus DDY07ZZ
- Eye D8Y07ZZ
- Femur DPY97ZZ
- Fibula DPYB7ZZ
- Gallbladder DFY17ZZ
- Gland
  - Adrenal DGY27ZZ
  - Parathyroid DGY47ZZ
  - Pituitary DGY07ZZ
  - Thyroid DGY57ZZ
- Glands, Salivary D9Y67ZZ
- Head and Neck DWY17ZZ
- Hemibody DWY47ZZ
- Humerus DPY67ZZ
- Hypopharynx D9Y37ZZ
- Ileum DDY47ZZ
- Jejunum DDY37ZZ
- Kidney DTY07ZZ
- Larynx D9YB7ZZ
- Liver DFY07ZZ
- Lung DBY27ZZ
- Mandible DPY37ZZ
- Maxilla DPY27ZZ
- Mediastinum DBY67ZZ
- Mouth D9Y47ZZ
- Nasopharynx D9YD7ZZ
- Neck and Head DWY17ZZ
- Nerve, Peripheral D0Y77ZZ
- Nose D9Y17ZZ
- Oropharynx D9YF7ZZ
- Ovary DUY07ZZ
- Palate
  - Hard D9Y87ZZ
  - Soft D9Y97ZZ
- Pancreas DFY37ZZ
- Parathyroid Gland DGY47ZZ
- Pelvic Bones DPY87ZZ
- Pelvic Region DWY67ZZ
- Pineal Body DGY17ZZ
- Pituitary Gland DGY07ZZ
- Pleura DBY57ZZ
- Prostate DVY07ZZ
- Radius DPY77ZZ
- Rectum DDY77ZZ
- Rib DPY57ZZ
- Sinuses D9Y77ZZ
- Skin
  - Abdomen DHY87ZZ
  - Arm DHY47ZZ
  - Back DHY77ZZ
  - Buttock DHY97ZZ
  - Chest DHY67ZZ
  - Face DHY27ZZ
  - Leg DHYB7ZZ
  - Neck DHY37ZZ
- Skull DPY07ZZ
- Spinal Cord D0Y67ZZ
- Sternum DPY47ZZ

Contact Radiation — *continued*
Stomach DDY17ZZ
Testis DVY17ZZ
Thyroid Gland DGY57ZZ
Tibia DPYB7ZZ
Tongue D9Y57ZZ
Trachea DBY07ZZ
Ulna DPY77ZZ
Ureter DTY17ZZ
Urethra DTY37ZZ
Uterus DUY27ZZ
Whole Body DWY57ZZ
ContaCT software (Measurement of intracranial arterial flow) 4A03X5D
CONTAK RENEWAL® 3 RF (HE) CRT-D
use Cardiac Resynchronization Defibrillator Pulse Generator in 0JH
Contegra Pulmonary Valved Conduit
use Zooplastic Tissue in Heart and Great Vessels
CONTEPO™
use Fosfomycin Anti-infective
Continuous Glucose Monitoring (CGM) device
use Monitoring Device
Continuous Negative Airway Pressure
24-96 Consecutive Hours, Ventilation 5A09459
Greater than 96 Consecutive Hours, Ventilation 5A09559
Less than 24 Consecutive Hours, Ventilation 5A09359
Continuous Positive Airway Pressure
24-96 Consecutive Hours, Ventilation 5A09457
Greater than 96 Consecutive Hours, Ventilation 5A09557
Less than 24 Consecutive Hours, Ventilation 5A09357
Continuous renal replacement therapy (CRRT) 5A1D90Z
Contraceptive Device
Change device in, Uterus and Cervix 0U2DXHZ
Insertion of device in
Cervix 0UHC
Subcutaneous Tissue and Fascia
Abdomen 0JH8
Chest 0JH6
Lower Arm
Left 0JHH
Right 0JHG
Lower Leg
Left 0JHP
Right 0JHN
Upper Arm
Left 0JHF
Right 0JHD
Upper Leg
Left 0JHM
Right 0JHL
Uterus 0UH9
Removal of device from
Subcutaneous Tissue and Fascia
Lower Extremity 0JPW
Trunk 0JPT
Upper Extremity 0JPV
Uterus and Cervix 0UPD
Revision of device in
Subcutaneous Tissue and Fascia
Lower Extremity 0JWW
Trunk 0JWT
Upper Extremity 0JWV
Uterus and Cervix 0UWD
Contractility Modulation Device
Abdomen 0JH8
Chest 0JH6

Control, Epistaxis
see Control bleeding in, Nasal Mucosa and Soft Tissue 093K
Control bleeding in
Abdominal Wall 0W3F
Ankle Region
Left 0Y3L
Right 0Y3K
Arm
Lower
Left 0X3F
Right 0X3D
Upper
Left 0X39
Right 0X38
Axilla
Left 0X35
Right 0X34
Back
Lower 0W3L
Upper 0W3K
Buttock
Left 0Y31
Right 0Y30
Cavity, Cranial 0W31
Chest Wall 0W38
Elbow Region
Left 0X3C
Right 0X3B
Extremity
Lower
Left 0Y3B
Right 0Y39
Upper
Left 0X37
Right 0X36
Face 0W32
Femoral Region
Left 0Y38
Right 0Y37
Foot
Left 0Y3N
Right 0Y3M
Gastrointestinal Tract 0W3P
Genitourinary Tract 0W3R
Hand
Left 0X3K
Right 0X3J
Head 0W30
Inguinal Region
Left 0Y36
Right 0Y35
Jaw
Lower 0W35
Upper 0W34
Knee Region
Left 0Y3G
Right 0Y3F
Leg
Lower
Left 0Y3J
Right 0Y3H
Upper
Left 0Y3D
Right 0Y3C
Mediastinum 0W3C
Nasal Mucosa and Soft Tissue 093K
Neck 0W36
Oral Cavity and Throat 0W33
Pelvic Cavity 0W3J
Pericardial Cavity 0W3D
Perineum
Female 0W3N
Male 0W3M
Peritoneal Cavity 0W3G
Pleural Cavity
Left 0W3B
Right 0W39

Control bleeding in — *continued*
Respiratory Tract 0W3Q
Retroperitoneum 0W3H
Shoulder Region
Left 0X33
Right 0X32
Wrist Region
Left 0X3H
Right 0X3G
Conus arteriosus
use Ventricle, Right
Conus medullaris
use Lumbar Spinal Cord
Convalescent Plasma (Nonautologous)
see New Technology, Anatomical Regions XW1
Conversion
Cardiac rhythm 5A2204Z
Gastrostomy to jejunostomy feeding device *see* Insertion of device in, Jejunum 0DHA
Cook Biodesign® Fistula Plug(s)
use Nonautologous Tissue Substitute
Cook Biodesign® Hernia Graft(s)
use Nonautologous Tissue Substitute
Cook Biodesign® Layered Graft(s)
use Nonautologous Tissue Substitute
Cook Zenapro™ Layered Graft(s)
use Nonautologous Tissue Substitute
Cook Zenith AAA Endovascular Graft
use Intraluminal Device
Cook Zenith® Fenestrated AAA Endovascular Graft
use Intraluminal Device, Branched or Fenestrated, One or Two Arteries in 04V
use Intraluminal Device, Branched or Fenestrated, Three or More Arteries in 04V
Coracoacromial ligament
use Shoulder Bursa and Ligament, Right
use Shoulder Bursa and Ligament, Left
Coracobrachialis muscle
use Upper Arm Muscle, Right
use Upper Arm Muscle, Left
Coracoclavicular ligament
use Shoulder Bursa and Ligament, Right
use Shoulder Bursa and Ligament, Left
Coracohumeral ligament
use Shoulder Bursa and Ligament, Right
use Shoulder Bursa and Ligament, Left
Coracoid process
use Scapula, Right
use Scapula, Left
Cordotomy
see Division, Central Nervous System and Cranial Nerves 008
Core needle biopsy
see Excision with qualifier Diagnostic
CoreValve transcatheter aortic valve
use Zooplastic Tissue in Heart and Great Vessels
Cormet Hip Resurfacing System
use Resurfacing Device in Lower Joints
Corniculate cartilage
use Larynx
CoRoent® XL
use Interbody Fusion Device in Lower Joints
Coronary arteriography
see Plain Radiography, Heart B20
see Fluoroscopy, Heart B21
Corox (OTW) Bipolar Lead
use Cardiac Lead, Pacemaker in 02H
use Cardiac Lead, Defibrillator in 02H
Corpus callosum
use Brain
Corpus cavernosum
use Penis
Corpus spongiosum
use Penis

Corpus striatum
 use Basal Ganglia
Corrugator supercilii muscle
 use Facial Muscle
Cortical strip neurostimulator lead
 use Neurostimulator Lead in Central
  Nervous System and Cranial Nerves
Corvia IASD®
 use Synthetic Substitute
Costatectomy
 see Excision, Upper Bones 0PB
 see Resection, Upper Bones 0PT
Costectomy
 see Excision, Upper Bones 0PB
 see Resection, Upper Bones 0PT
Costocervical trunk
 use Subclavian Artery, Right
 use Subclavian Artery, Left
Costochondrectomy
 see Excision, Upper Bones 0PB
 see Resection, Upper Bones 0PT
Costoclavicular ligament
 use Shoulder Bursa and Ligament, Right
 use Shoulder Bursa and Ligament, Left
Costosternoplasty
 see Repair, Upper Bones 0PQ
 see Replacement, Upper Bones 0PR
 see Supplement, Upper Bones 0PU
Costotomy
 see Division, Upper Bones 0P8
 see Drainage, Upper Bones 0P9
Costotransverse joint
 use Thoracic Vertebral Joint
Costotransverse ligament
 use Rib(s) Bursa and Ligament
Costovertebral joint
 use Thoracic Vertebral Joint
Costoxiphoid ligament
 use Sternum Bursa and Ligament
Counseling
 Family, for substance abuse, Other Family
  Counseling HZ63ZZZ
 Group
  12-Step HZ43ZZZ
  Behavioral HZ41ZZZ
  Cognitive HZ40ZZZ
  Cognitive-Behavioral HZ42ZZZ
  Confrontational HZ48ZZZ
  Continuing Care HZ49ZZZ
  Infectious Disease
   Post-Test HZ4CZZZ
   Pre-Test HZ4CZZZ
  Interpersonal HZ44ZZZ
  Motivational Enhancement HZ47ZZZ
  Psychoeducation HZ46ZZZ
  Spiritual HZ4BZZZ
  Vocational HZ45ZZZ
 Individual
  12-Step HZ33ZZZ
  Behavioral HZ31ZZZ
  Cognitive HZ30ZZZ
  Cognitive-Behavioral HZ32ZZZ
  Confrontational HZ38ZZZ
  Continuing Care HZ39ZZZ
  Infectious Disease
   Post-Test HZ3CZZZ
   Pre-Test HZ3CZZZ
  Interpersonal HZ34ZZZ
  Motivational Enhancement HZ37ZZZ
  Psychoeducation HZ36ZZZ
  Spiritual HZ3BZZZ
  Vocational HZ35ZZZ
 Mental Health Services
  Educational GZ60ZZZ
  Other Counseling GZ63ZZZ
  Vocational GZ61ZZZ
Countershock, cardiac 5A2204Z

COVID-19 Vaccine XW0
COVID-19 Vaccine Dose 1 XW0
COVID-19 Vaccine Dose 2 XW0
Cowper's (bulbourethral) gland
 use Urethra
CPAP (continuous positive airway pressure)
 see Assistance, Respiratory 5A09
Craniectomy
 see Excision, Head and Facial Bones 0NB
 see Resection, Head and Facial Bones 0NT
Cranioplasty
 see Repair, Head and Facial Bones 0NQ
 see Replacement, Head and Facial
  Bones 0NR
 see Supplement, Head and Facial Bones 0NU
Craniotomy
 see Drainage, Central Nervous System and
  Cranial Nerves 009
 see Division, Head and Facial Bones 0N8
 see Drainage, Head and Facial Bones 0N9
Creation
 Perineum
  Female 0W4N0
  Male 0W4M0
 Valve
  Aortic 024F0
  Mitral 024G0
  Tricuspid 024J0
Cremaster muscle
 use Perineum Muscle
Cribriform plate
 use Ethmoid Bone, Right
 use Ethmoid Bone, Left
Cricoid cartilage
 use Trachea
Cricoidectomy
 see Excision, Larynx 0CBS
Cricothyroid artery
 use Thyroid Artery, Right
 use Thyroid Artery, Left
Cricothyroid muscle
 use Neck Muscle, Right
 use Neck Muscle, Left
Crisis Intervention GZ2ZZZZ
**CRRT (Continuous renal replacement
 therapy)** 5A1D90Z
Crural fascia
 use Subcutaneous Tissue and Fascia, Right
  Upper Leg
 use Subcutaneous Tissue and Fascia, Left
  Upper Leg
Crushing, nerve
 Cranial *see* Destruction, Central Nervous
  System and Cranial Nerves 005
 Peripheral *see* Destruction, Peripheral
  Nervous System 015
Cryoablation
 see Destruction
Cryotherapy
 see Destruction
Cryptorchidectomy
 see Excision, Male Reproductive
  System 0VB
 see Resection, Male Reproductive
  System 0VT
Cryptorchiectomy
 see Excision, Male Reproductive
  System 0VB
 see Resection, Male Reproductive
  System 0VT
Cryptotomy
 see Division, Gastrointestinal System 0D8
 see Drainage, Gastrointestinal System 0D9
CT scan
 see Computerized Tomography (CT Scan)
CT sialogram
 see Computerized Tomography (CT Scan),
  Ear, Nose, Mouth and Throat B92

Cubital lymph node
 use Lymphatic, Right Upper Extremity
 use Lymphatic, Left Upper Extremity
Cubital nerve
 use Ulnar Nerve
Cuboid bone
 use Tarsal, Right
 use Tarsal, Left
Cuboideonavicular joint
 use Tarsal Joint, Right
 use Tarsal Joint, Left
Culdocentesis
 see Drainage, Cul-de-sac 0U9F
Culdoplasty
 see Repair, Cul-de-sac 0UQF
 see Supplement, Cul-de-sac 0UUF
Culdoscopy 0UJH8ZZ
Culdotomy
 see Drainage, Cul-de-sac 0U9F
Culmen
 use Cerebellum
Cultured epidermal cell autograft
 use Autologous Tissue Substitute
Cuneiform cartilage
 use Larynx
Cuneonavicular joint
 use Tarsal Joint, Right
 use Tarsal Joint, Left
Cuneonavicular ligament
 use Foot Bursa and Ligament, Right
 use Foot Bursa and Ligament, Left
Curettage
 see Excision
 see Extraction
Cutaneous (transverse) cervical nerve
 use Cervical Plexus
CVP (central venous pressure)
 see Measurement, Venous 4A04
Cyclodiathermy
 see Destruction, Eye 085
Cyclophotocoagulation
 see Destruction, Eye 085
CYPHER® Stent
 use Intraluminal Device, Drug-eluting in
  Heart and Great Vessels
Cystectomy
 see Excision, Bladder 0TBB
 see Resection, Bladder 0TTB
Cystocele repair
 see Repair, Subcutaneous Tissue and Fascia,
  Pelvic Region 0JQC
Cystography
 see Plain Radiography, Urinary
  System BT0
 see Fluoroscopy, Urinary System BT1
Cystolithotomy
 see Extirpation, Bladder 0TCB
Cystopexy
 see Repair, Bladder 0TQB
 see Reposition, Bladder 0TSB
Cystoplasty
 see Repair, Bladder 0TQB
 see Replacement, Bladder 0TRB
 see Supplement, Bladder 0TUB
Cystorrhaphy
 see Repair, Bladder 0TQB
Cystoscopy 0TJB8ZZ
Cystostomy
 see Bypass, Bladder 0T1B
Cystostomy tube
 use Drainage Device
Cystotomy
 see Drainage, Bladder 0T9B
Cystourethrography
 see Plain Radiography, Urinary System BT0
 see Fluoroscopy, Urinary System BT1

Cystourethroplasty
see Repair, Urinary System 0TQ
see Replacement, Urinary System 0TR
see Supplement, Urinary System 0TU
Cytarabine and Daunorubicin Liposome Antineoplastic XW0

D

DBS lead
use Neurostimulator Lead in Central Nervous System and Cranial Nerves
DeBakey Left Ventricular Assist Device
use Implantable Heart Assist System in Heart and Great Vessels
Debridement
Excisional see Excision
Non-excisional see Extraction
Decompression, Circulatory 6A15
Decortication, lung
see Extirpation, Respiratory System 0BC
see Release, Respiratory System 0BN
Deep brain neurostimulator lead
use Neurostimulator Lead in Central Nervous System and Cranial Nerves
Deep cervical fascia
use Subcutaneous Tissue and Fascia, Right Neck
use Subcutaneous Tissue and Fascia, Left Neck
Deep cervical vein
use Vertebral Vein, Right
use Vertebral Vein, Left
Deep circumflex iliac artery
use External Iliac Artery, Right
use External Iliac Artery, Left
Deep facial vein
use Face Vein, Right
use Face Vein, Left
Deep femoral (profunda femoris) vein
use Femoral Vein, Right
use Femoral Vein, Left
Deep femoral artery
use Femoral Artery, Right
use Femoral Artery, Left
Deep Inferior Epigastric Artery Perforator Flap
Replacement
Bilateral 0HRV077
Left 0HRU077
Right 0HRT077
Transfer
Left 0KXG
Right 0KXF
Deep palmar arch
use Hand Artery, Right
use Hand Artery, Left
Deep transverse perineal muscle
use Perineum Muscle
Deferential artery
use Internal Iliac Artery, Right
use Internal Iliac Artery, Left
Defibrillator Generator
Abdomen 0JH8
Chest 0JH6
Defibrotide Sodium Anticoagulant XW0
Defitelio
use Defibrotide Sodium Anticoagulant
Delivery
Cesarean see Extraction, Products of Conception 10D0
Forceps see Extraction, Products of Conception 10D0
Manually assisted 10E0XZZ
Products of Conception 10E0XZZ

Delivery — continued
Vacuum assisted see Extraction, Products of Conception 10D0
Delta frame external fixator
use External Fixation Device, Hybrid in 0PH
use External Fixation Device, Hybrid in 0PS
use External Fixation Device, Hybrid in 0QH
use External Fixation Device, Hybrid in 0QS
Delta III Reverse shoulder prosthesis
use Synthetic Substitute, Reverse Ball and Socket in 0RR
Deltoid fascia
use Subcutaneous Tissue and Fascia, Right Upper Arm
use Subcutaneous Tissue and Fascia, Left Upper Arm
Deltoid ligament
use Ankle Bursa and Ligament, Right
use Ankle Bursa and Ligament, Left
Deltoid muscle
use Shoulder Muscle, Right
use Shoulder Muscle, Left
Deltopectoral (infraclavicular) lymph node
use Lymphatic, Right Upper Extremity
use Lymphatic, Left Upper Extremity
Denervation
Cranial nerve see Destruction, Central Nervous System and Cranial Nerves 005
Peripheral nerve see Destruction, Peripheral Nervous System 015
Dens
use Cervical Vertebra
Densitometry
Plain Radiography
Femur
Left BQ04ZZ1
Right BQ03ZZ1
Hip
Left BQ01ZZ1
Right BQ00ZZ1
Spine
Cervical BR00ZZ1
Lumbar BR09ZZ1
Thoracic BR07ZZ1
Whole BR0GZZ1
Ultrasonography
Elbow
Left BP4HZZ1
Right BP4GZZ1
Hand
Left BP4PZZ1
Right BP4NZZ1
Shoulder
Left BP49ZZ1
Right BP48ZZ1
Wrist
Left BP4MZZ1
Right BP4LZZ1
Denticulate (dentate) ligament
use Spinal Meninges
Depressor anguli oris muscle
use Facial Muscle
Depressor labii inferioris muscle
use Facial Muscle
Depressor septi nasi muscle
use Facial Muscle
Depressor supercilii muscle
use Facial Muscle
Dermabrasion
see Extraction, Skin and Breast 0HD
Dermis
use Skin
Descending genicular artery
use Femoral Artery, Right
use Femoral Artery, Left

Destruction
Acetabulum
Left 0Q55
Right 0Q54
Adenoids 0C5Q
Ampulla of Vater 0F5C
Anal Sphincter 0D5R
Anterior Chamber
Left 08533ZZ
Right 08523ZZ
Anus 0D5Q
Aorta
Abdominal 0450
Thoracic
Ascending/Arch 025X
Descending 025W
Aortic Body 0G5D
Appendix 0D5J
Artery
Anterior Tibial
Left 045Q
Right 045P
Axillary
Left 0356
Right 0355
Brachial
Left 0358
Right 0357
Celiac 0451
Colic
Left 0457
Middle 0458
Right 0456
Common Carotid
Left 035J
Right 035H
Common Iliac
Left 045D
Right 045C
External Carotid
Left 035N
Right 035M
External Iliac
Left 045J
Right 045H
Face 035R
Femoral
Left 045L
Right 045K
Foot
Left 045W
Right 045V
Gastric 0452
Hand
Left 035F
Right 035D
Hepatic 0453
Inferior Mesenteric 045B
Innominate 0352
Internal Carotid
Left 035L
Right 035K
Internal Iliac
Left 045F
Right 045E
Internal Mammary
Left 0351
Right 0350
Intracranial 035G
Lower 045Y
Peroneal
Left 045U
Right 045T
Popliteal
Left 045N
Right 045M

Destruction — *continued*
  Artery — *continued*
    Posterior Tibial
      Left 045S
      Right 045R
    Pulmonary
      Left 025R
      Right 025Q
    Pulmonary Trunk 025P
    Radial
      Left 035C
      Right 035B
    Renal
      Left 045A
      Right 0459
    Splenic 0454
    Subclavian
      Left 0354
      Right 0353
    Superior Mesenteric 0455
    Temporal
      Left 035T
      Right 035S
    Thyroid
      Left 035V
      Right 035U
    Ulnar
      Left 035A
      Right 0359
    Upper 035Y
    Vertebral
      Left 035Q
      Right 035P
  Atrium
    Left 0257
    Right 0256
  Auditory Ossicle
    Left 095A
    Right 0959
  Basal Ganglia 0058
  Bladder 0T5B
  Bladder Neck 0T5C
  Bone
    Ethmoid
      Left 0N5G
      Right 0N5F
    Frontal 0N51
    Hyoid 0N5X
    Lacrimal
      Left 0N5J
      Right 0N5H
    Nasal 0N5B
    Occipital 0N57
    Palatine
      Left 0N5L
      Right 0N5K
    Parietal
      Left 0N54
      Right 0N53
    Pelvic
      Left 0Q53
      Right 0Q52
    Sphenoid 0N5C
    Temporal
      Left 0N56
      Right 0N55
    Zygomatic
      Left 0N5N
      Right 0N5M
  Brain 0050
  Breast
    Bilateral 0H5V
    Left 0H5U
    Right 0H5T
  Bronchus
    Lingula 0B59

Destruction — *continued*
  Bronchus — *continued*
    Lower Lobe
      Left 0B5B
      Right 0B56
    Main
      Left 0B57
      Right 0B53
    Middle Lobe, Right 0B55
    Upper Lobe
      Left 0B58
      Right 0B54
  Buccal Mucosa 0C54
  Bursa and Ligament
    Abdomen
      Left 0M5J
      Right 0M5H
    Ankle
      Left 0M5R
      Right 0M5Q
    Elbow
      Left 0M54
      Right 0M53
    Foot
      Left 0M5T
      Right 0M5S
    Hand
      Left 0M58
      Right 0M57
    Head and Neck 0M50
    Hip
      Left 0M5M
      Right 0M5L
    Knee
      Left 0M5P
      Right 0M5N
    Lower Extremity
      Left 0M5W
      Right 0M5V
    Perineum 0M5K
    Rib(s) 0M5G
    Shoulder
      Left 0M52
      Right 0M51
    Spine
      Lower 0M5D
      Upper 0M5C
    Sternum 0M5F
    Upper Extremity
      Left 0M5B
      Right 0M59
    Wrist
      Left 0M56
      Right 0M55
  Carina 0B52
  Carotid Bodies, Bilateral 0G58
  Carotid Body
    Left 0G56
    Right 0G57
  Carpal
    Left 0P5N
    Right 0P5M
  Cecum 0D5H
  Cerebellum 005C
  Cerebral Hemisphere 0057
  Cerebral Meninges 0051
  Cerebral Ventricle 0056
  Cervix 0U5C
  Chordae Tendineae 0259
  Choroid
    Left 085B
    Right 085A
  Cisterna Chyli 075L
  Clavicle
    Left 0P5B
    Right 0P59
  Clitoris 0U5J
  Coccygeal Glomus 0G5B

Destruction — *continued*
  Coccyx 0Q5S
  Colon
    Ascending 0D5K
    Descending 0D5M
    Sigmoid 0D5N
    Transverse 0D5L
  Conduction Mechanism 0258
  Conjunctiva
    Left 085TXZZ
    Right 085SXZZ
  Cord
    Bilateral 0V5H
    Left 0V5G
    Right 0V5F
  Cornea
    Left 0859XZZ
    Right 0858XZZ
  Cul-de-sac 0U5F
  Diaphragm 0B5T
  Disc
    Cervical Vertebral 0R53
    Cervicothoracic Vertebral 0R55
    Lumbar Vertebral 0S52
    Lumbosacral 0S54
    Thoracic Vertebral 0R59
    Thoracolumbar Vertebral 0R5B
  Duct
    Common Bile 0F59
    Cystic 0F58
    Hepatic
      Common 0F57
      Left 0F56
      Right 0F55
    Lacrimal
      Left 085Y
      Right 085X
    Pancreatic 0F5D
      Accessory 0F5F
    Parotid
      Left 0C5C
      Right 0C5B
  Duodenum 0D59
  Dura Mater 0052
  Ear
    External
      Left 0951
      Right 0950
    External Auditory Canal
      Left 0954
      Right 0953
    Inner
      Left 095E
      Right 095D
    Middle
      Left 0956
      Right 0955
  Endometrium 0U5B
  Epididymis
    Bilateral 0V5L
    Left 0V5K
    Right 0V5J
  Epiglottis 0C5R
  Esophagogastric Junction 0D54
  Esophagus 0D55
    Lower 0D53
    Middle 0D52
    Upper 0D51
  Eustachian Tube
    Left 095G
    Right 095F
  Eye
    Left 0851XZZ
    Right 0850XZZ
  Eyelid
    Lower
      Left 085R
      Right 085Q

Destruction — *continued*
  Eyelid — *continued*
    Upper
      Left 085P
      Right 085N
  Fallopian Tube
    Left 0U56
    Right 0U55
  Fallopian Tubes, Bilateral 0U57
  Femoral Shaft
    Left 0Q59
    Right 0Q58
  Femur
    Lower
      Left 0Q5C
      Right 0Q5B
    Upper
      Left 0Q57
      Right 0Q56
  Fibula
    Left 0Q5K
    Right 0Q5J
  Finger Nail 0H5QXZZ
  Gallbladder 0F54
  Gingiva
    Lower 0C56
    Upper 0C55
  Gland
    Adrenal
      Bilateral 0G54
      Left 0G52
      Right 0G53
    Lacrimal
      Left 085W
      Right 085V
    Minor Salivary 0C5J
    Parotid
      Left 0C59
      Right 0C58
    Pituitary 0G50
    Sublingual
      Left 0C5F
      Right 0C5D
    Submaxillary
      Left 0C5H
      Right 0C5G
    Vestibular 0U5L
  Glenoid Cavity
    Left 0P58
    Right 0P57
  Glomus Jugulare 0G5C
  Humeral Head
    Left 0P5D
    Right 0P5C
  Humeral Shaft
    Left 0P5G
    Right 0P5F
  Hymen 0U5K
  Hypothalamus 005A
  Ileocecal Valve 0D5C
  Ileum 0D5B
  Intestine
    Large 0D5E
      Left 0D5G
      Right 0D5F
    Small 0D58
  Iris
    Left 085D3ZZ
    Right 085C3ZZ
  Jejunum 0D5A
  Joint
    Acromioclavicular
      Left 0R5H
      Right 0R5G
    Ankle
      Left 0S5G
      Right 0S5F

Destruction — *continued*
  Joint — *continued*
    Carpal
      Left 0R5R
      Right 0R5Q
    Carpometacarpal
      Left 0R5T
      Right 0R5S
    Cervical Vertebral 0R51
    Cervicothoracic Vertebral 0R54
    Coccygeal 0S56
    Elbow
      Left 0R5M
      Right 0R5L
    Finger Phalangeal
      Left 0R5X
      Right 0R5W
    Hip
      Left 0S5B
      Right 0S59
    Knee
      Left 0S5D
      Right 0S5C
    Lumbar Vertebral 0S50
    Lumbosacral 0S53
    Metacarpophalangeal
      Left 0R5V
      Right 0R5U
    Metatarsal-Phalangeal
      Left 0S5N
      Right 0S5M
    Occipital-cervical 0R50
    Sacrococcygeal 0S55
    Sacroiliac
      Left 0S58
      Right 0S57
    Shoulder
      Left 0R5K
      Right 0R5J
    Sternoclavicular
      Left 0R5F
      Right 0R5E
    Tarsal
      Left 0S5J
      Right 0S5H
    Tarsometatarsal
      Left 0S5L
      Right 0S5K
    Temporomandibular
      Left 0R5D
      Right 0R5C
    Thoracic Vertebral 0R56
    Thoracolumbar Vertebral 0R5A
    Toe Phalangeal
      Left 0S5Q
      Right 0S5P
    Wrist
      Left 0R5P
      Right 0R5N
  Kidney
    Left 0T51
    Right 0T50
  Kidney Pelvis
    Left 0T54
    Right 0T53
  Larynx 0C5S
  Lens
    Left 085K3ZZ
    Right 085J3ZZ
  Lip
    Lower 0C51
    Upper 0C50
  Liver 0F50
    Left Lobe 0F52
    Right Lobe 0F51
  Lung
    Bilateral 0B5M

Destruction — *continued*
  Lung — *continued*
    Left 0B5L
    Lower Lobe
      Left 0B5J
      Right 0B5F
    Middle Lobe, Right 0B5D
    Right 0B5K
    Upper Lobe
      Left 0B5G
      Right 0B5C
  Lung Lingula 0B5H
  Lymphatic
    Aortic 075D
    Axillary
      Left 0756
      Right 0755
    Head 0750
    Inguinal
      Left 075J
      Right 075H
    Internal Mammary
      Left 0759
      Right 0758
    Lower Extremity
      Left 075G
      Right 075F
    Mesenteric 075B
    Neck
      Left 0752
      Right 0751
    Pelvis 075C
    Thoracic Duct 075K
    Thorax 0757
    Upper Extremity
      Left 0754
      Right 0753
  Mandible
    Left 0N5V
    Right 0N5T
  Maxilla 0N5R
  Medulla Oblongata 005D
  Mesentery 0D5V
  Metacarpal
    Left 0P5Q
    Right 0P5P
  Metatarsal
    Left 0Q5P
    Right 0Q5N
  Muscle
    Abdomen
      Left 0K5L
      Right 0K5K
    Extraocular
      Left 085M
      Right 085L
    Facial 0K51
    Foot
      Left 0K5W
      Right 0K5V
    Hand
      Left 0K5D
      Right 0K5C
    Head 0K50
    Hip
      Left 0K5P
      Right 0K5N
    Lower Arm and Wrist
      Left 0K5B
      Right 0K59
    Lower Leg
      Left 0K5T
      Right 0K5S
    Neck
      Left 0K53
      Right 0K52
  Papillary 025D

Destruction — *continued*
  Muscle — *continued*
    Perineum 0K5M
    Shoulder
      Left 0K56
      Right 0K55
    Thorax
      Left 0K5J
      Right 0K5H
    Tongue, Palate, Pharynx 0K54
    Trunk
      Left 0K5G
      Right 0K5F
    Upper Arm
      Left 0K58
      Right 0K57
    Upper Leg
      Left 0K5R
      Right 0K5Q
  Nasal Mucosa and Soft Tissue 095K
  Nasopharynx 095N
  Nerve
    Abdominal Sympathetic 015M
    Abducens 005L
    Accessory 005R
    Acoustic 005N
    Brachial Plexus 0153
    Cervical 0151
    Cervical Plexus 0150
    Facial 005M
    Femoral 015D
    Glossopharyngeal 005P
    Head and Neck Sympathetic 015K
    Hypoglossal 005S
    Lumbar 015B
    Lumbar Plexus 0159
    Lumbar Sympathetic 015N
    Lumbosacral Plexus 015A
    Median 0155
    Oculomotor 005H
    Olfactory 005F
    Optic 005G
    Peroneal 015H
    Phrenic 0152
    Pudendal 015C
    Radial 0156
    Sacral 015R
    Sacral Plexus 015Q
    Sacral Sympathetic 015P
    Sciatic 015F
    Thoracic 0158
    Thoracic Sympathetic 015L
    Tibial 015G
    Trigeminal 005K
    Trochlear 005J
    Ulnar 0154
    Vagus 005Q
  Nipple
    Left 0H5X
    Right 0H5W
  Omentum 0D5U
  Orbit
    Left 0N5Q
    Right 0N5P
  Ovary
    Bilateral 0U52
    Left 0U51
    Right 0U50
  Palate
    Hard 0C52
    Soft 0C53
  Pancreas 0F5G
  Para-aortic Body 0G59
  Paraganglion Extremity 0G5F
  Parathyroid Gland 0G5R
    Inferior
      Left 0G5P
      Right 0G5N

Destruction — *continued*
  Parathyroid Gland — *continued*
    Multiple 0G5Q
    Superior
      Left 0G5M
      Right 0G5L
  Patella
    Left 0Q5F
    Right 0Q5D
  Penis 0V5S
  Pericardium 025N
  Peritoneum 0D5W
  Phalanx
    Finger
      Left 0P5V
      Right 0P5T
    Thumb
      Left 0P5S
      Right 0P5R
    Toe
      Left 0Q5R
      Right 0Q5Q
  Pharynx 0C5M
  Pineal Body 0G51
  Pleura
    Left 0B5P
    Right 0B5N
  Pons 005B
  Prepuce 0V5T
  Prostate 0V50
    Robotic Waterjet Ablation XV508A4
  Radius
    Left 0P5J
    Right 0P5H
  Rectum 0D5P
  Retina
    Left 085F3ZZ
    Right 085E3ZZ
  Retinal Vessel
    Left 085H3ZZ
    Right 085G3ZZ
  Ribs
    1 to 2 0P51
    3 or More 0P52
  Sacrum 0Q51
  Scapula
    Left 0P56
    Right 0P55
  Sclera
    Left 0857XZZ
    Right 0856XZZ
  Scrotum 0V55
  Septum
    Atrial 0255
    Nasal 095M
    Ventricular 025M
  Sinus
    Accessory 095P
    Ethmoid
      Left 095V
      Right 095U
    Frontal
      Left 095T
      Right 095S
    Mastoid
      Left 095C
      Right 095B
    Maxillary
      Left 095R
      Right 095Q
    Sphenoid
      Left 095X
      Right 095W
  Skin
    Abdomen 0H57XZ
    Back 0H56XZ
    Buttock 0H58XZ

Destruction — *continued*
  Skin — *continued*
    Chest 0H55XZ
    Ear
      Left 0H53XZ
      Right 0H52XZ
    Face 0H51XZ
    Foot
      Left 0H5NXZ
      Right 0H5MXZ
    Hand
      Left 0H5GXZ
      Right 0H5FXZ
    Inguinal 0H5AXZ
    Lower Arm
      Left 0H5EXZ
      Right 0H5DXZ
    Lower Leg
      Left 0H5LXZ
      Right 0H5KXZ
    Neck 0H54XZ
    Perineum 0H59XZ
    Scalp 0H50XZ
    Upper Arm
      Left 0H5CXZ
      Right 0H5BXZ
    Upper Leg
      Left 0H5JXZ
      Right 0H5HXZ
  Skull 0N50
  Spinal Cord
    Cervical 005W
    Lumbar 005Y
    Thoracic 005X
  Spinal Meninges 005T
  Spleen 075P
  Sternum 0P50
  Stomach 0D56
    Pylorus 0D57
  Subcutaneous Tissue and Fascia
    Abdomen 0J58
    Back 0J57
    Buttock 0J59
    Chest 0J56
    Face 0J51
    Foot
      Left 0J5R
      Right 0J5Q
    Hand
      Left 0J5K
      Right 0J5J
    Lower Arm
      Left 0J5H
      Right 0J5G
    Lower Leg
      Left 0J5P
      Right 0J5N
    Neck
      Left 0J55
      Right 0J54
    Pelvic Region 0J5C
    Perineum 0J5B
    Scalp 0J50
    Upper Arm
      Left 0J5F
      Right 0J5D
    Upper Leg
      Left 0J5M
      Right 0J5L
  Tarsal
    Left 0Q5M
    Right 0Q5L
  Tendon
    Abdomen
      Left 0L5G
      Right 0L5F

Destruction — *continued*
　Tendon — *continued*
　　Ankle
　　　Left 0L5T
　　　Right 0L5S
　　Foot
　　　Left 0L5W
　　　Right 0L5V
　　Hand
　　　Left 0L58
　　　Right 0L57
　　Head and Neck 0L50
　　Hip
　　　Left 0L5K
　　　Right 0L5J
　　Knee
　　　Left 0L5R
　　　Right 0L5Q
　　Lower Arm and Wrist
　　　Left 0L56
　　　Right 0L55
　　Lower Leg
　　　Left 0L5P
　　　Right 0L5N
　　Perineum 0L5H
　　Shoulder
　　　Left 0L52
　　　Right 0L51
　　Thorax
　　　Left 0L5D
　　　Right 0L5C
　　Trunk
　　　Left 0L5B
　　　Right 0L59
　　Upper Arm
　　　Left 0L54
　　　Right 0L53
　　Upper Leg
　　　Left 0L5M
　　　Right 0L5L
　Testis
　　Bilateral 0V5C
　　Left 0V5B
　　Right 0V59
　Thalamus 0059
　Thymus 075M
　Thyroid Gland 0G5K
　　Left Lobe 0G5G
　　Right Lobe 0G5H
　Tibia
　　Left 0Q5H
　　Right 0Q5G
　Toe Nail 0H5RXZZ
　Tongue 0C57
　Tonsils 0C5P
　Tooth
　　Lower 0C5X
　　Upper 0C5W
　Trachea 0B51
　Tunica Vaginalis
　　Left 0V57
　　Right 0V56
　Turbinate, Nasal 095L
　Tympanic Membrane
　　Left 0958
　　Right 0957
　Ulna
　　Left 0P5L
　　Right 0P5K
　Ureter
　　Left 0T57
　　Right 0T56
　Urethra 0T5D
　Uterine Supporting Structure 0U54
　Uterus 0U59
　Uvula 0C5N
　Vagina 0U5G

Destruction — *continued*
　Valve
　　Aortic 025F
　　Mitral 025G
　　Pulmonary 025H
　　Tricuspid 025J
　Vas Deferens
　　Bilateral 0V5Q
　　Left 0V5P
　　Right 0V5N
　Vein
　　Axillary
　　　Left 0558
　　　Right 0557
　　Azygos 0550
　　Basilic
　　　Left 055C
　　　Right 055B
　　Brachial
　　　Left 055A
　　　Right 0559
　　Cephalic
　　　Left 055F
　　　Right 055D
　　Colic 0657
　　Common Iliac
　　　Left 065D
　　　Right 065C
　　Coronary 0254
　　Esophageal 0653
　　External Iliac
　　　Left 065G
　　　Right 065F
　　External Jugular
　　　Left 055Q
　　　Right 055P
　　Face
　　　Left 055V
　　　Right 055T
　　Femoral
　　　Left 065N
　　　Right 065M
　　Foot
　　　Left 065V
　　　Right 065T
　　Gastric 0652
　　Hand
　　　Left 055H
　　　Right 055G
　　Hemiazygos 0551
　　Hepatic 0654
　　Hypogastric
　　　Left 065J
　　　Right 065H
　　Inferior Mesenteric 0656
　　Innominate
　　　Left 0554
　　　Right 0553
　　Internal Jugular
　　　Left 055N
　　　Right 055M
　　Intracranial 055L
　　Lower 065Y
　　Portal 0658
　　Pulmonary
　　　Left 025T
　　　Right 025S
　　Renal
　　　Left 065B
　　　Right 0659
　　Saphenous
　　　Left 065Q
　　　Right 065P
　　Splenic 0651
　　Subclavian
　　　Left 0556
　　　Right 0555

Destruction — *continued*
　Vein — *continued*
　　Superior Mesenteric 0655
　　Upper 055Y
　　Vertebral
　　　Left 055S
　　　Right 055R
　Vena Cava
　　Inferior 0650
　　Superior 025V
　Ventricle
　　Left 025L
　　Right 025K
　Vertebra
　　Cervical 0P53
　　Lumbar 0Q50
　　Thoracic 0P54
　Vesicle
　　Bilateral 0V53
　　Left 0V52
　　Right 0V51
　Vitreous
　　Left 08553ZZ
　　Right 08543ZZ
　Vocal Cord
　　Left 0C5V
　　Right 0C5T
　Vulva 0U5M
Detachment
　Arm
　　Lower
　　　Left 0X6F0Z
　　　Right 0X6D0Z
　　Upper
　　　Left 0X690Z
　　　Right 0X680Z
　Elbow Region
　　Left 0X6C0ZZ
　　Right 0X6B0ZZ
　Femoral Region
　　Left 0Y680ZZ
　　Right 0Y670ZZ
　Finger
　　Index
　　　Left 0X6P0Z
　　　Right 0X6N0Z
　　Little
　　　Left 0X6W0Z
　　　Right 0X6V0Z
　　Middle
　　　Left 0X6R0Z
　　　Right 0X6Q0Z
　　Ring
　　　Left 0X6T0Z
　　　Right 0X6S0Z
　Foot
　　Left 0Y6N0Z
　　Right 0Y6M0Z
　Forequarter
　　Left 0X610ZZ
　　Right 0X600ZZ
　Hand
　　Left 0X6K0Z
　　Right 0X6J0Z
　Hindquarter
　　Bilateral 0Y640ZZ
　　Left 0Y630ZZ
　　Right 0Y620ZZ
　Knee Region
　　Left 0Y6G0ZZ
　　Right 0Y6F0ZZ
　Leg
　　Lower
　　　Left 0Y6J0Z
　　　Right 0Y6H0Z
　　Upper
　　　Left 0Y6D0Z
　　　Right 0Y6C0Z

Detachment — *continued*
Shoulder Region
Left 0X630ZZ
Right 0X620ZZ
Thumb
Left 0X6M0Z
Right 0X6L0Z
Toe
1st
Left 0Y6Q0Z
Right 0Y6P0Z
2nd
Left 0Y6S0Z
Right 0Y6R0Z
3rd
Left 0Y6U0Z
Right 0Y6T0Z
4th
Left 0Y6W0Z
Right 0Y6V0Z
5th
Left 0Y6Y0Z
Right 0Y6X0Z
Determination, Mental status GZ14ZZZ
Detorsion
see Release
see Reposition
Detoxification Services, for substance abuse HZ2ZZZZ
Device Fitting F0DZ
Diagnostic Audiology
see Audiology, Diagnostic
Diagnostic imaging
see Imaging, Diagnostic
Diagnostic radiology
see Imaging, Diagnostic
Dialysis
Hemodialysis *see* Performance, Urinary 5A1D
Peritoneal 3E1M39Z
Diaphragma sellae
use Dura Mater
Diaphragmatic pacemaker generator
use Stimulator Generator in Subcutaneous Tissue and Fascia
Diaphragmatic Pacemaker Lead
Insertion of device in, Diaphragm 0BHT
Removal of device from, Diaphragm 0BPT
Revision of device in, Diaphragm 0BWT
Digital radiography, plain
see Plain Radiography
Dilation
Ampulla of Vater 0F7C
Anus 0D7Q
Aorta
Abdominal 0470
Thoracic
Ascending/Arch 027X
Descending 027W
Artery
Anterior Tibial
Left 047Q
Sustained Release Drug-eluting Intraluminal Device X27Q385
Four or More X27Q3C5
Three X27Q3B5
Two X27Q395
Right 047P
Sustained Release Drug-eluting Intraluminal Device X27P385
Four or More X27P3C5
Three X27P3B5
Two X27P395
Axillary
Left 0376
Right 0375

Dilation — *continued*
Artery — *continued*
Brachial
Left 0378
Right 0377
Celiac 0471
Colic
Left 0477
Middle 0478
Right 0476
Common Carotid
Left 037J
Right 037H
Common Iliac
Left 047D
Right 047C
Coronary
Four or More Arteries 0273
One Artery 0270
Three Arteries 0272
Two Arteries 0271
External Carotid
Left 037N
Right 037M
External Iliac
Left 047J
Right 047H
Face 037R
Femoral
Left 047L
Sustained Release Drug-eluting Intraluminal Device X27J385
Four or More X27J3C5
Three X27J3B5
Two X27J395
Right 047K
Sustained Release Drug-eluting Intraluminal Device X27H385
Four or More X27H3C5
Three X27H3B5
Two X27H395
Foot
Left 047W
Right 047V
Gastric 0472
Hand
Left 037F
Right 037D
Hepatic 0473
Inferior Mesenteric 047B
Innominate 0372
Internal Carotid
Left 037L
Right 037K
Internal Iliac
Left 047F
Right 047E
Internal Mammary
Left 0371
Right 0370
Intracranial 037G
Lower 047Y
Peroneal
Left 047U
Sustained Release Drug-eluting Intraluminal Device X27U385
Four or More X27U3C5
Three X27U3B5
Two X27U395
Right 047T
Sustained Release Drug-eluting Intraluminal Device X27T385
Four or More X27T3C5
Three X27T3B5
Two X27T395
Popliteal
Left 047N

Dilation — *continued*
Artery — *continued*
Left Distal
Sustained Release Drug-eluting Intraluminal Device X27N385
Four or More X27N3C5
Three X27N3B5
Two X27N395
Left Proximal
Sustained Release Drug-eluting Intraluminal Device X27L385
Four or More X27L3C5
Three X27L3B5
Two X27L395
Right 047M
Right Distal
Sustained Release Drug-eluting Intraluminal Device X27M385
Four or More X27M3C5
Three X27M3B5
Two X27M395
Right Proximal
Sustained Release Drug-eluting Intraluminal Device X27K385
Four or More X27K3C5
Three X27K3B5
Two X27K395
Posterior Tibial
Left 047S
Sustained Release Drug-eluting Intraluminal Device X27S385
Four or More X27S3C5
Three X27S3B5
Two X27S395
Right 047R
Sustained Release Drug-eluting Intraluminal Device X27R385
Four or More X27R3C5
Three X27R3B5
Two X27R395
Pulmonary
Left 027R
Right 027Q
Pulmonary Trunk 027P
Radial
Left 037C
Right 037B
Renal
Left 047A
Right 0479
Splenic 0474
Subclavian
Left 0374
Right 0373
Superior Mesenteric 0475
Temporal
Left 037T
Right 037S
Thyroid
Left 037V
Right 037U
Ulnar
Left 037A
Right 0379
Upper 037Y
Vertebral
Left 037Q
Right 037P
Bladder 0T7B
Bladder Neck 0T7C
Bronchus
Lingula 0B79
Lower Lobe
Left 0B7B
Right 0B76
Main
Left 0B77
Right 0B73

Dilation — *continued*
    Bronchus — *continued*
        Middle Lobe, Right 0B75
        Upper Lobe
            Left 0B78
            Right 0B74
    Carina 0B72
    Cecum 0D7H
    Cerebral Ventricle 0076
    Cervix 0U7C
    Colon
        Ascending 0D7K
        Descending 0D7M
        Sigmoid 0D7N
        Transverse 0D7L
    Duct
        Common Bile 0F79
        Cystic 0F78
        Hepatic
            Common 0F77
            Left 0F76
            Right 0F75
        Lacrimal
            Left 087Y
            Right 087X
        Pancreatic 0F7D
            Accessory 0F7F
        Parotid
            Left 0C7C
            Right 0C7B
    Duodenum 0D79
    Esophagogastric Junction 0D74
    Esophagus 0D75
        Lower 0D73
        Middle 0D72
        Upper 0D71
    Eustachian Tube
        Left 097G
        Right 097F
    Fallopian Tube
        Left 0U76
        Right 0U75
    Fallopian Tubes, Bilateral 0U77
    Hymen 0U7K
    Ileocecal Valve 0D7C
    Ileum 0D7B
    Intestine
        Large 0D7E
            Left 0D7G
            Right 0D7F
        Small 0D78
    Jejunum 0D7A
    Kidney Pelvis
        Left 0T74
        Right 0T73
    Larynx 0C7S
    Pharynx 0C7M
    Rectum 0D7P
    Stomach 0D76
        Pylorus 0D77
    Trachea 0B71
    Ureter
        Left 0T77
        Right 0T76
    Ureters, Bilateral 0T78
    Urethra 0T7D
    Uterus 0U79
    Vagina 0U7G
    Valve
        Aortic 027F
        Mitral 027G
        Pulmonary 027H
        Tricuspid 027J
    Vas Deferens
        Bilateral 0V7Q
        Left 0V7P
        Right 0V7N

Dilation — *continued*
    Vein
        Axillary
            Left 0578
            Right 0577
        Azygos 0570
        Basilic
            Left 057C
            Right 057B
        Brachial
            Left 057A
            Right 0579
        Cephalic
            Left 057F
            Right 057D
        Colic 0677
        Common Iliac
            Left 067D
            Right 067C
        Esophageal 0673
        External Iliac
            Left 067G
            Right 067F
        External Jugular
            Left 057Q
            Right 057P
        Face
            Left 057V
            Right 057T
        Femoral
            Left 067N
            Right 067M
        Foot
            Left 067V
            Right 067T
        Gastric 0672
        Hand
            Left 057H
            Right 057G
        Hemiazygos 0571
        Hepatic 0674
        Hypogastric
            Left 067J
            Right 067H
        Inferior Mesenteric 0676
        Innominate
            Left 0574
            Right 0573
        Internal Jugular
            Left 057N
            Right 057M
        Intracranial 057L
        Lower 067Y
        Portal 0678
        Pulmonary
            Left 027T
            Right 027S
        Renal
            Left 067B
            Right 0679
        Saphenous
            Left 067Q
            Right 067P
        Splenic 0671
        Subclavian
            Left 0576
            Right 0575
        Superior Mesenteric 0675
        Upper 057Y
        Vertebral
            Left 057S
            Right 057R
    Vena Cava
        Inferior 0670
        Superior 027V
    Ventricle
        Left 027L
        Right 027K

Direct Lateral Interbody Fusion (DLIF) device
    use Interbody Fusion Device in Lower Joints
Disarticulation
    see Detachment
Discectomy, diskectomy
    see Excision, Upper Joints 0RB
    see Resection, Upper Joints 0RT
    see Excision, Lower Joints 0SB
    see Resection, Lower Joints 0ST
Discography
    see Plain Radiography, Axial Skeleton, Except Skull and Facial Bones BR0
    see Fluoroscopy, Axial Skeleton, Except Skull and Facial Bones BR1
Dismembered pyeloplasty
    see Repair, Kidney Pelvis
Distal humerus
    use Humeral Shaft, Right
    use Humeral Shaft, Left
Distal humerus, involving joint
    use Elbow Joint, Right
    use Elbow Joint, Left
Distal radioulnar joint
    use Wrist Joint, Right
    use Wrist Joint, Left
Diversion
    see Bypass
Diverticulectomy
    see Excision, Gastrointestinal System 0DB
Division
    Acetabulum
        Left 0Q85
        Right 0Q84
    Anal Sphincter 0D8R
    Basal Ganglia 0088
    Bladder Neck 0T8C
    Bone
        Ethmoid
            Left 0N8G
            Right 0N8F
        Frontal 0N81
        Hyoid 0N8X
        Lacrimal
            Left 0N8J
            Right 0N8H
        Nasal 0N8B
        Occipital 0N87
        Palatine
            Left 0N8L
            Right 0N8K
        Parietal
            Left 0N84
            Right 0N83
        Pelvic
            Left 0Q83
            Right 0Q82
        Sphenoid 0N8C
        Temporal
            Left 0N86
            Right 0N85
        Zygomatic
            Left 0N8N
            Right 0N8M
    Brain 0080
    Bursa and Ligament
        Abdomen
            Left 0M8J
            Right 0M8H
        Ankle
            Left 0M8R
            Right 0M8Q
        Elbow
            Left 0M84
            Right 0M83

Division — *continued*

Bursa and Ligament — *continued*
Foot
Left 0M8T
Right 0M8S
Hand
Left 0M88
Right 0M87
Head and Neck 0M80
Hip
Left 0M8M
Right 0M8L
Knee
Left 0M8P
Right 0M8N
Lower Extremity
Left 0M8W
Right 0M8V
Perineum 0M8K
Rib(s) 0M8G
Shoulder
Left 0M82
Right 0M81
Spine
Lower 0M8D
Upper 0M8C
Sternum 0M8F
Upper Extremity
Left 0M8B
Right 0M89
Wrist
Left 0M86
Right 0M85
Carpal
Left 0P8N
Right 0P8M
Cerebral Hemisphere 0087
Chordae Tendineae 0289
Clavicle
Left 0P8B
Right 0P89
Coccyx 0Q8S
Conduction Mechanism 0288
Esophagogastric Junction 0D84
Femoral Shaft
Left 0Q89
Right 0Q88
Femur
Lower
Left 0Q8C
Right 0Q8B
Upper
Left 0Q87
Right 0Q86
Fibula
Left 0Q8K
Right 0Q8J
Gland, Pituitary 0G80
Glenoid Cavity
Left 0P88
Right 0P87
Humeral Head
Left 0P8D
Right 0P8C
Humeral Shaft
Left 0P8G
Right 0P8F
Hymen 0U8K
Kidneys, Bilateral 0T82
Mandible
Left 0N8V
Right 0N8T
Maxilla 0N8R
Metacarpal
Left 0P8Q
Right 0P8P

Division — *continued*

Metatarsal
Left 0Q8P
Right 0Q8N
Muscle
Abdomen
Left 0K8L
Right 0K8K
Facial 0K81
Foot
Left 0K8W
Right 0K8V
Hand
Left 0K8D
Right 0K8C
Head 0K80
Hip
Left 0K8P
Right 0K8N
Lower Arm and Wrist
Left 0K8B
Right 0K89
Lower Leg
Left 0K8T
Right 0K8S
Neck
Left 0K83
Right 0K82
Papillary 028D
Perineum 0K8M
Shoulder
Left 0K86
Right 0K85
Thorax
Left 0K8J
Right 0K8H
Tongue, Palate, Pharynx 0K84
Trunk
Left 0K8G
Right 0K8F
Upper Arm
Left 0K88
Right 0K87
Upper Leg
Left 0K8R
Right 0K8Q
Nerve
Abdominal Sympathetic 018M
Abducens 008L
Accessory 008R
Acoustic 008N
Brachial Plexus 0183
Cervical 0181
Cervical Plexus 0180
Facial 008M
Femoral 018D
Glossopharyngeal 008P
Head and Neck Sympathetic 018K
Hypoglossal 008S
Lumbar 018B
Lumbar Plexus 0189
Lumbar Sympathetic 018N
Lumbosacral Plexus 018A
Median 0185
Oculomotor 008H
Olfactory 008F
Optic 008G
Peroneal 018H
Phrenic 0182
Pudendal 018C
Radial 0186
Sacral 018R
Sacral Plexus 018Q
Sacral Sympathetic 018P
Sciatic 018F
Thoracic 0188
Thoracic Sympathetic 018L

Division — *continued*

Nerve — *continued*
Tibial 018G
Trigeminal 008K
Trochlear 008J
Ulnar 0184
Vagus 008Q
Orbit
Left 0N8Q
Right 0N8P
Ovary
Bilateral 0U82
Left 0U81
Right 0U80
Pancreas 0F8G
Patella
Left 0Q8F
Right 0Q8D
Perineum, Female 0W8NXZZ
Phalanx
Finger
Left 0P8V
Right 0P8T
Thumb
Left 0P8S
Right 0P8R
Toe
Left 0Q8R
Right 0Q8Q
Radius
Left 0P8J
Right 0P8H
Ribs
1 to 2 0P81
3 or More 0P82
Sacrum 0Q81
Scapula
Left 0P86
Right 0P85
Skin
Abdomen 0H87XZZ
Back 0H86XZZ
Buttock 0H88XZZ
Chest 0H85XZZ
Ear
Left 0H83XZZ
Right 0H82XZZ
Face 0H81XZZ
Foot
Left 0H8NXZZ
Right 0H8MXZZ
Hand
Left 0H8GXZZ
Right 0H8FXZZ
Inguinal 0H8AXZZ
Lower Arm
Left 0H8EXZZ
Right 0H8DXZZ
Lower Leg
Left 0H8LXZZ
Right 0H8KXZZ
Neck 0H84XZZ
Perineum 0H89XZZ
Scalp 0H80XZZ
Upper Arm
Left 0H8CXZZ
Right 0H8BXZZ
Upper Leg
Left 0H8JXZZ
Right 0H8HXZZ
Skull 0N80
Spinal Cord
Cervical 008W
Lumbar 008Y
Thoracic 008X
Sternum 0P80
Stomach, Pylorus 0D87

Division — *continued*
  Subcutaneous Tissue and Fascia
    Abdomen 0J88
    Back 0J87
    Buttock 0J89
    Chest 0J86
    Face 0J81
    Foot
      Left 0J8R
      Right 0J8Q
    Hand
      Left 0J8K
      Right 0J8J
    Head and Neck 0J8S
    Lower Arm
      Left 0J8H
      Right 0J8G
    Lower Extremity 0J8W
    Lower Leg
      Left 0J8P
      Right 0J8N
    Neck
      Left 0J85
      Right 0J84
    Pelvic Region 0J8C
    Perineum 0J8B
    Scalp 0J80
    Trunk 0J8T
    Upper Arm
      Left 0J8F
      Right 0J8D
    Upper Extremity 0J8V
    Upper Leg
      Left 0J8M
      Right 0J8L
  Tarsal
    Left 0Q8M
    Right 0Q8L
  Tendon
    Abdomen
      Left 0L8G
      Right 0L8F
    Ankle
      Left 0L8T
      Right 0L8S
    Foot
      Left 0L8W
      Right 0L8V
    Hand
      Left 0L88
      Right 0L87
    Head and Neck 0L80
    Hip
      Left 0L8K
      Right 0L8J
    Knee
      Left 0L8R
      Right 0L8Q
    Lower Arm and Wrist
      Left 0L86
      Right 0L85
    Lower Leg
      Left 0L8P
      Right 0L8N
    Perineum 0L8H
    Shoulder
      Left 0L82
      Right 0L81
    Thorax
      Left 0L8D
      Right 0L8C
    Trunk
      Left 0L8B
      Right 0L89
    Upper Arm
      Left 0L84
      Right 0L83

Division — *continued*
  Tendon — *continued*
    Upper Leg
      Left 0L8M
      Right 0L8L
  Thyroid Gland Isthmus 0G8J
  Tibia
    Left 0Q8H
    Right 0Q8G
  Turbinate, Nasal 098L
  Ulna
    Left 0P8L
    Right 0P8K
  Uterine Supporting Structure 0U84
  Vertebra
    Cervical 0P83
    Lumbar 0Q80
    Thoracic 0P84
Doppler study
  see Ultrasonography
Dorsal digital nerve
  use Radial Nerve
Dorsal metacarpal vein
  use Hand Vein, Right
  use Hand Vein, Left
Dorsal metatarsal artery
  use Foot Artery, Right
  use Foot Artery, Left
Dorsal metatarsal vein
  use Foot Vein, Right
  use Foot Vein, Left
Dorsal scapular artery
  use Subclavian Artery, Right
  use Subclavian Artery, Left
Dorsal scapular nerve
  use Brachial Plexus
Dorsal venous arch
  use Foot Vein, Right
  use Foot Vein, Left
Dorsalis pedis artery
  use Anterior Tibial Artery, Right
  use Anterior Tibial Artery, Left
DownStream® System
  5A0512C
  5A0522C
Drainage
  Abdominal Wall 0W9F
  Acetabulum
    Left 0Q95
    Right 0Q94
  Adenoids 0C9Q
  Ampulla of Vater 0F9C
  Anal Sphincter 0D9R
  Ankle Region
    Left 0Y9L
    Right 0Y9K
  Anterior Chamber
    Left 0893
    Right 0892
  Anus 0D9Q
  Aorta, Abdominal 0490
  Aortic Body 0G9D
  Appendix 0D9J
  Arm
    Lower
      Left 0X9F
      Right 0X9D
    Upper
      Left 0X99
      Right 0X98
  Artery
    Anterior Tibial
      Left 049Q
      Right 049P
    Axillary
      Left 0396
      Right 0395

Drainage — *continued*
  Artery — *continued*
    Brachial
      Left 0398
      Right 0397
    Celiac 0491
    Colic
      Left 0497
      Middle 0498
      Right 0496
    Common Carotid
      Left 039J
      Right 039H
    Common Iliac
      Left 049D
      Right 049C
    External Carotid
      Left 039N
      Right 039M
    External Iliac
      Left 049J
      Right 049H
    Face 039R
    Femoral
      Left 049L
      Right 049K
    Foot
      Left 049W
      Right 049V
    Gastric 0492
    Hand
      Left 039F
      Right 039D
    Hepatic 0493
    Inferior Mesenteric 049B
    Innominate 0392
    Internal Carotid
      Left 039L
      Right 039K
    Internal Iliac
      Left 049F
      Right 049E
    Internal Mammary
      Left 0391
      Right 0390
    Intracranial 039G
    Lower 049Y
    Peroneal
      Left 049U
      Right 049T
    Popliteal
      Left 049N
      Right 049M
    Posterior Tibial
      Left 049S
      Right 049R
    Radial
      Left 039C
      Right 039B
    Renal
      Left 049A
      Right 0499
    Splenic 0494
    Subclavian
      Left 0394
      Right 0393
    Superior Mesenteric 0495
    Temporal
      Left 039T
      Right 039S
    Thyroid
      Left 039V
      Right 039U
    Ulnar
      Left 039A
      Right 0399
    Upper 039Y

Drainage — *continued*
  Artery — *continued*
    Vertebral
      Left 039Q
      Right 039P
  Auditory Ossicle
    Left 099A
    Right 0999
  Axilla
    Left 0X95
    Right 0X94
  Back
    Lower 0W9L
    Upper 0W9K
  Basal Ganglia 0098
  Bladder 0T9B
  Bladder Neck 0T9C
  Bone
    Ethmoid
      Left 0N9G
      Right 0N9F
    Frontal 0N91
    Hyoid 0N9X
    Lacrimal
      Left 0N9J
      Right 0N9H
    Nasal 0N9B
    Occipital 0N97
    Palatine
      Left 0N9L
      Right 0N9K
    Parietal
      Left 0N94
      Right 0N93
    Pelvic
      Left 0Q93
      Right 0Q92
    Sphenoid 0N9C
    Temporal
      Left 0N96
      Right 0N95
    Zygomatic
      Left 0N9N
      Right 0N9M
  Bone Marrow 079T
  Brain 0090
  Breast
    Bilateral 0H9V
    Left 0H9U
    Right 0H9T
  Bronchus
    Lingula 0B99
    Lower Lobe
      Left 0B9B
      Right 0B96
    Main
      Left 0B97
      Right 0B93
    Middle Lobe, Right 0B95
    Upper Lobe
      Left 0B98
      Right 0B94
  Buccal Mucosa 0C94
  Bursa and Ligament
    Abdomen
      Left 0M9J
      Right 0M9H
    Ankle
      Left 0M9R
      Right 0M9Q
    Elbow
      Left 0M94
      Right 0M93
    Foot
      Left 0M9T
      Right 0M9S

Drainage — *continued*
  Bursa and Ligament — *continued*
    Hand
      Left 0M98
      Right 0M97
    Head and Neck 0M90
    Hip
      Left 0M9M
      Right 0M9L
    Knee
      Left 0M9P
      Right 0M9N
    Lower Extremity
      Left 0M9W
      Right 0M9V
    Perineum 0M9K
    Rib(s) 0M9G
    Shoulder
      Left 0M92
      Right 0M91
    Spine
      Lower 0M9D
      Upper 0M9C
    Sternum 0M9F
    Upper Extremity
      Left 0M9B
      Right 0M99
    Wrist
      Left 0M96
      Right 0M95
  Buttock
    Left 0Y91
    Right 0Y90
  Carina 0B92
  Carotid Bodies, Bilateral 0G98
  Carotid Body
    Left 0G96
    Right 0G97
  Carpal
    Left 0P9N
    Right 0P9M
  Cavity, Cranial 0W91
  Cecum 0D9H
  Cerebellum 009C
  Cerebral Hemisphere 0097
  Cerebral Meninges 0091
  Cerebral Ventricle 0096
  Cervix 0U9C
  Chest Wall 0W98
  Choroid
    Left 089B
    Right 089A
  Cisterna Chyli 079L
  Clavicle
    Left 0P9B
    Right 0P99
  Clitoris 0U9J
  Coccygeal Glomus 0G9B
  Coccyx 0Q9S
  Colon
    Ascending 0D9K
    Descending 0D9M
    Sigmoid 0D9N
    Transverse 0D9L
  Conjunctiva
    Left 089T
    Right 089S
  Cord
    Bilateral 0V9H
    Left 0V9G
    Right 0V9F
  Cornea
    Left 0899
    Right 0898
  Cul-de-sac 0U9F
  Diaphragm 0B9T

Drainage — *continued*
  Disc
    Cervical Vertebral 0R93
    Cervicothoracic Vertebral 0R95
    Lumbar Vertebral 0S92
    Lumbosacral 0S94
    Thoracic Vertebral 0R99
    Thoracolumbar Vertebral 0R9B
  Duct
    Common Bile 0F99
    Cystic 0F98
    Hepatic
      Common 0F97
      Left 0F96
      Right 0F95
    Lacrimal
      Left 089Y
      Right 089X
    Pancreatic 0F9D
      Accessory 0F9F
    Parotid
      Left 0C9C
      Right 0C9B
  Duodenum 0D99
  Dura Mater 0092
  Ear
    External
      Left 0991
      Right 0990
    External Auditory Canal
      Left 0994
      Right 0993
    Inner
      Left 099E
      Right 099D
    Middle
      Left 0996
      Right 0995
  Elbow Region
    Left 0X9C
    Right 0X9B
  Epididymis
    Bilateral 0V9L
    Left 0V9K
    Right 0V9J
  Epidural Space, Intracranial 0093
  Epiglottis 0C9R
  Esophagogastric Junction 0D94
  Esophagus 0D95
    Lower 0D93
    Middle 0D92
    Upper 0D91
  Eustachian Tube
    Left 099G
    Right 099F
  Extremity
    Lower
      Left 0Y9B
      Right 0Y99
    Upper
      Left 0X97
      Right 0X96
  Eye
    Left 0891
    Right 0890
  Eyelid
    Lower
      Left 089R
      Right 089Q
    Upper
      Left 089P
      Right 089N
  Face 0W92
  Fallopian Tube
    Left 0U96
    Right 0U95
  Fallopian Tubes, Bilateral 0U97

Drainage — continued
  Femoral Region
    Left 0Y98
    Right 0Y97
  Femoral Shaft
    Left 0Q99
    Right 0Q98
  Femur
    Lower
      Left 0Q9C
      Right 0Q9B
    Upper
      Left 0Q97
      Right 0Q96
  Fibula
    Left 0Q9K
    Right 0Q9J
  Finger Nail 0H9Q
  Foot
    Left 0Y9N
    Right 0Y9M
  Gallbladder 0F94
  Gingiva
    Lower 0C96
    Upper 0C95
  Gland
    Adrenal
      Bilateral 0G94
      Left 0G92
      Right 0G93
    Lacrimal
      Left 089W
      Right 089V
    Minor Salivary 0C9J
    Parotid
      Left 0C99
      Right 0C98
    Pituitary 0G90
    Sublingual
      Left 0C9F
      Right 0C9D
    Submaxillary
      Left 0C9H
      Right 0C9G
    Vestibular 0U9L
  Glenoid Cavity
    Left 0P98
    Right 0P97
  Glomus Jugulare 0G9C
  Hand
    Left 0X9K
    Right 0X9J
  Head 0W90
  Humeral Head
    Left 0P9D
    Right 0P9C
  Humeral Shaft
    Left 0P9G
    Right 0P9F
  Hymen 0U9K
  Hypothalamus 009A
  Ileocecal Valve 0D9C
  Ileum 0D9B
  Inguinal Region
    Left 0Y96
    Right 0Y95
  Intestine
    Large 0D9E
      Left 0D9G
      Right 0D9F
    Small 0D98
  Iris
    Left 089D
    Right 089C
  Jaw
    Lower 0W95
    Upper 0W94

Drainage — continued
  Jejunum 0D9A
  Joint
    Acromioclavicular
      Left 0R9H
      Right 0R9G
    Ankle
      Left 0S9G
      Right 0S9F
    Carpal
      Left 0R9R
      Right 0R9Q
    Carpometacarpal
      Left 0R9T
      Right 0R9S
    Cervical Vertebral 0R91
    Cervicothoracic Vertebral 0R94
    Coccygeal 0S96
    Elbow
      Left 0R9M
      Right 0R9L
    Finger Phalangeal
      Left 0R9X
      Right 0R9W
    Hip
      Left 0S9B
      Right 0S99
    Knee
      Left 0S9D
      Right 0S9C
    Lumbar Vertebral 0S90
    Lumbosacral 0S93
    Metacarpophalangeal
      Left 0R9V
      Right 0R9U
    Metatarsal-Phalangeal
      Left 0S9N
      Right 0S9M
    Occipital-cervical 0R90
    Sacrococcygeal 0S95
    Sacroiliac
      Left 0S98
      Right 0S97
    Shoulder
      Left 0R9K
      Right 0R9J
    Sternoclavicular
      Left 0R9F
      Right 0R9E
    Tarsal
      Left 0S9J
      Right 0S9H
    Tarsometatarsal
      Left 0S9L
      Right 0S9K
    Temporomandibular
      Left 0R9D
      Right 0R9C
    Thoracic Vertebral 0R96
    Thoracolumbar Vertebral 0R9A
    Toe Phalangeal
      Left 0S9Q
      Right 0S9P
    Wrist
      Left 0R9P
      Right 0R9N
  Kidney
    Left 0T91
    Right 0T90
  Kidney Pelvis
    Left 0T94
    Right 0T93
  Knee Region
    Left 0Y9G
    Right 0Y9F
  Larynx 0C9S

Drainage — continued
  Leg
    Lower
      Left 0Y9J
      Right 0Y9H
    Upper
      Left 0Y9D
      Right 0Y9C
  Lens
    Left 089K
    Right 089J
  Lip
    Lower 0C91
    Upper 0C90
  Liver 0F90
    Left Lobe 0F92
    Right Lobe 0F91
  Lung
    Bilateral 0B9M
    Left 0B9L
    Lower Lobe
      Left 0B9J
      Right 0B9F
    Middle Lobe, Right 0B9D
    Right 0B9K
    Upper Lobe
      Left 0B9G
      Right 0B9C
  Lung Lingula 0B9H
  Lymphatic
    Aortic 079D
    Axillary
      Left 0796
      Right 0795
    Head 0790
    Inguinal
      Left 079J
      Right 079H
    Internal Mammary
      Left 0799
      Right 0798
    Lower Extremity
      Left 079G
      Right 079F
    Mesenteric 079B
    Neck
      Left 0792
      Right 0791
    Pelvis 079C
    Thoracic Duct 079K
    Thorax 0797
    Upper Extremity
      Left 0794
      Right 0793
  Mandible
    Left 0N9V
    Right 0N9T
  Maxilla 0N9R
  Mediastinum 0W9C
  Medulla Oblongata 009D
  Mesentery 0D9V
  Metacarpal
    Left 0P9Q
    Right 0P9P
  Metatarsal
    Left 0Q9P
    Right 0Q9N
  Muscle
    Abdomen
      Left 0K9L
      Right 0K9K
    Extraocular
      Left 089M
      Right 089L
    Facial 0K91
    Foot
      Left 0K9W
      Right 0K9V

Drainage — *continued*
  Muscle — *continued*
    Hand
      Left 0K9D
      Right 0K9C
    Head 0K90
    Hip
      Left 0K9P
      Right 0K9N
    Lower Arm and Wrist
      Left 0K9B
      Right 0K99
    Lower Leg
      Left 0K9T
      Right 0K9S
    Neck
      Left 0K93
      Right 0K92
    Perineum 0K9M
    Shoulder
      Left 0K96
      Right 0K95
    Thorax
      Left 0K9J
      Right 0K9H
    Tongue, Palate, Pharynx 0K94
    Trunk
      Left 0K9G
      Right 0K9F
    Upper Arm
      Left 0K98
      Right 0K97
    Upper Leg
      Left 0K9R
      Right 0K9Q
  Nasal Mucosa and Soft Tissue 099K
  Nasopharynx 099N
  Neck 0W96
  Nerve
    Abdominal Sympathetic 019M
    Abducens 009L
    Accessory 009R
    Acoustic 009N
    Brachial Plexus 0193
    Cervical 0191
    Cervical Plexus 0190
    Facial 009M
    Femoral 019D
    Glossopharyngeal 009P
    Head and Neck Sympathetic 019K
    Hypoglossal 009S
    Lumbar 019B
    Lumbar Plexus 0199
    Lumbar Sympathetic 019N
    Lumbosacral Plexus 019A
    Median 0195
    Oculomotor 009H
    Olfactory 009F
    Optic 009G
    Peroneal 019H
    Phrenic 0192
    Pudendal 019C
    Radial 0196
    Sacral 019R
    Sacral Plexus 019Q
    Sacral Sympathetic 019P
    Sciatic 019F
    Thoracic 0198
    Thoracic Sympathetic 019L
    Tibial 019G
    Trigeminal 009K
    Trochlear 009J
    Ulnar 0194
    Vagus 009Q
  Nipple
    Left 0H9X
    Right 0H9W

Drainage — *continued*
  Omentum 0D9U
  Oral Cavity and Throat 0W93
  Orbit
    Left 0N9Q
    Right 0N9P
  Ovary
    Bilateral 0U92
    Left 0U91
    Right 0U90
  Palate
    Hard 0C92
    Soft 0C93
  Pancreas 0F9G
  Para-aortic Body 0G99
  Paraganglion Extremity 0G9F
  Parathyroid Gland 0G9R
    Inferior
      Left 0G9P
      Right 0G9N
    Multiple 0G9Q
    Superior
      Left 0G9M
      Right 0G9L
  Patella
    Left 0Q9F
    Right 0Q9D
  Pelvic Cavity 0W9J
  Penis 0V9S
  Pericardial Cavity 0W9D
  Perineum
    Female 0W9N
    Male 0W9M
  Peritoneal Cavity 0W9G
  Peritoneum 0D9W
  Phalanx
    Finger
      Left 0P9V
      Right 0P9T
    Thumb
      Left 0P9S
      Right 0P9R
    Toe
      Left 0Q9R
      Right 0Q9Q
  Pharynx 0C9M
  Pineal Body 0G91
  Pleura
    Left 0B9P
    Right 0B9N
  Pleural Cavity
    Left 0W9B
    Right 0W99
  Pons 009B
  Prepuce 0V9T
  Products of Conception
    Amniotic Fluid
      Diagnostic 1090
      Therapeutic 1090
    Fetal Blood 1090
    Fetal Cerebrospinal Fluid 1090
    Fetal Fluid, Other 1090
    Fluid, Other 1090
  Prostate 0V90
  Radius
    Left 0P9J
    Right 0P9H
  Rectum 0D9P
  Retina
    Left 089F
    Right 089E
  Retinal Vessel
    Left 089H
    Right 089G
  Retroperitoneum 0W9H
  Ribs
    1 to 2 0P91
    3 or More 0P92

Drainage — *continued*
  Sacrum 0Q91
  Scapula
    Left 0P96
    Right 0P95
  Sclera
    Left 0897
    Right 0896
  Scrotum 0V95
  Septum, Nasal 099M
  Shoulder Region
    Left 0X93
    Right 0X92
  Sinus
    Accessory 099P
    Ethmoid
      Left 099V
      Right 099U
    Frontal
      Left 099T
      Right 099S
    Mastoid
      Left 099C
      Right 099B
    Maxillary
      Left 099R
      Right 099Q
    Sphenoid
      Left 099X
      Right 099W
  Skin
    Abdomen 0H97
    Back 0H96
    Buttock 0H98
    Chest 0H95
    Ear
      Left 0H93
      Right 0H92
    Face 0H91
    Foot
      Left 0H9N
      Right 0H9M
    Hand
      Left 0H9G
      Right 0H9F
    Inguinal 0H9A
    Lower Arm
      Left 0H9E
      Right 0H9D
    Lower Leg
      Left 0H9L
      Right 0H9K
    Neck 0H94
    Perineum 0H99
    Scalp 0H90
    Upper Arm
      Left 0H9C
      Right 0H9B
    Upper Leg
      Left 0H9J
      Right 0H9H
  Skull 0N90
  Spinal Canal 009U
  Spinal Cord
    Cervical 009W
    Lumbar 009Y
    Thoracic 009X
  Spinal Meninges 009T
  Spleen 079P
  Sternum 0P90
  Stomach 0D96
    Pylorus 0D97
  Subarachnoid Space, Intracranial 0095
  Subcutaneous Tissue and Fascia
    Abdomen 0J98
    Back 0J97
    Buttock 0J99

Drainage — continued

Subcutaneous Tissue and Fascia — continued
Chest 0J96
Face 0J91
Foot
  Left 0J9R
  Right 0J9Q
Hand
  Left 0J9K
  Right 0J9J
Lower Arm
  Left 0J9H
  Right 0J9G
Lower Leg
  Left 0J9P
  Right 0J9N
Neck
  Left 0J95
  Right 0J94
Pelvic Region 0J9C
Perineum 0J9B
Scalp 0J90
Upper Arm
  Left 0J9F
  Right 0J9D
Upper Leg
  Left 0J9M
  Right 0J9L
Subdural Space, Intracranial 0094
Tarsal
  Left 0Q9M
  Right 0Q9L
Tendon
  Abdomen
    Left 0L9G
    Right 0L9F
  Ankle
    Left 0L9T
    Right 0L9S
  Foot
    Left 0L9W
    Right 0L9V
  Hand
    Left 0L98
    Right 0L97
  Head and Neck 0L90
  Hip
    Left 0L9K
    Right 0L9J
  Knee
    Left 0L9R
    Right 0L9Q
  Lower Arm and Wrist
    Left 0L96
    Right 0L95
  Lower Leg
    Left 0L9P
    Right 0L9N
  Perineum 0L9H
  Shoulder
    Left 0L92
    Right 0L91
  Thorax
    Left 0L9D
    Right 0L9C
  Trunk
    Left 0L9B
    Right 0L99
  Upper Arm
    Left 0L94
    Right 0L93
  Upper Leg
    Left 0L9M
    Right 0L9L
Testis
  Bilateral 0V9C
  Left 0V9B
  Right 0V99

Drainage — continued

Thalamus 0099
Thymus 079M
Thyroid Gland 0G9K
  Left Lobe 0G9G
  Right Lobe 0G9H
Tibia
  Left 0Q9H
  Right 0Q9G
Toe Nail 0H9R
Tongue 0C97
Tonsils 0C9P
Tooth
  Lower 0C9X
  Upper 0C9W
Trachea 0B91
Tunica Vaginalis
  Left 0V97
  Right 0V96
Turbinate, Nasal 099L
Tympanic Membrane
  Left 0998
  Right 0997
Ulna
  Left 0P9L
  Right 0P9K
Ureter
  Left 0T97
  Right 0T96
Ureters, Bilateral 0T98
Urethra 0T9D
Uterine Supporting Structure 0U94
Uterus 0U99
Uvula 0C9N
Vagina 0U9G
Vas Deferens
  Bilateral 0V9Q
  Left 0V9P
  Right 0V9N
Vein
  Axillary
    Left 0598
    Right 0597
  Azygos 0590
  Basilic
    Left 059C
    Right 059B
  Brachial
    Left 059A
    Right 0599
  Cephalic
    Left 059F
    Right 059D
  Colic 0697
  Common Iliac
    Left 069D
    Right 069C
  Esophageal 0693
  External Iliac
    Left 069G
    Right 069F
  External Jugular
    Left 059Q
    Right 059P
  Face
    Left 059V
    Right 059T
  Femoral
    Left 069N
    Right 069M
  Foot
    Left 069V
    Right 069T
  Gastric 0692
  Hand
    Left 059H
    Right 059G

Drainage — continued

Vein — continued
Hemiazygos 0591
Hepatic 0694
Hypogastric
  Left 069J
  Right 069H
Inferior Mesenteric 0696
Innominate
  Left 0594
  Right 0593
Internal Jugular
  Left 059N
  Right 059M
Intracranial 059L
Lower 069Y
Portal 0698
Renal
  Left 069B
  Right 0699
Saphenous
  Left 069Q
  Right 069P
Splenic 0691
Subclavian
  Left 0596
  Right 0595
Superior Mesenteric 0695
Upper 059Y
Vertebral
  Left 059S
  Right 059R
Vena Cava, Inferior 0690
Vertebra
  Cervical 0P93
  Lumbar 0Q90
  Thoracic 0P94
Vesicle
  Bilateral 0V93
  Left 0V92
  Right 0V91
Vitreous
  Left 0895
  Right 0894
Vocal Cord
  Left 0C9V
  Right 0C9T
Vulva 0U9M
Wrist Region
  Left 0X9H
  Right 0X9G

Dressing
Abdominal Wall 2W23X4Z
Arm
  Lower
    Left 2W2DX4Z
    Right 2W2CX4Z
  Upper
    Left 2W2BX4Z
    Right 2W2AX4Z
Back 2W25X4Z
Chest Wall 2W24X4Z
Extremity
  Lower
    Left 2W2MX4Z
    Right 2W2LX4Z
  Upper
    Left 2W29X4Z
    Right 2W28X4Z
Face 2W21X4Z
Finger
  Left 2W2KX4Z
  Right 2W2JX4Z
Foot
  Left 2W2TX4Z
  Right 2W2SX4Z

Dressing — *continued*
　Hand
　　Left 2W2FX4Z
　　Right 2W2EX4Z
　Head 2W20X4Z
　Inguinal Region
　　Left 2W27X4Z
　　Right 2W26X4Z
　Leg
　　Lower
　　　Left 2W2RX4Z
　　　Right 2W2QX4Z
　　Upper
　　　Left 2W2PX4Z
　　　Right 2W2NX4Z
　Neck 2W22X4Z
　Thumb
　　Left 2W2HX4Z
　　Right 2W2GX4Z
　Toe
　　Left 2W2VX4Z
　　Right 2W2UX4Z
Driver stent (RX) (OTW)
　use Intraluminal Device
Drotrecogin alfa, infusion
　see Introduction of Recombinant Human-
　　activated Protein C
Duct of Santorini
　use Pancreatic Duct, Accessory
Duct of Wirsung
　use Pancreatic Duct
Ductogram, mammary
　see Plain Radiography, Skin, Subcutaneous
　　Tissue and Breast BH0
Ductography, mammary
　see Plain Radiography, Skin, Subcutaneous
　　Tissue and Breast BH0
Ductus deferens
　use Vas Deferens, Right
　use Vas Deferens, Left
　use Vas Deferens, Bilateral
　use Vas Deferens
Duodenal ampulla
　use Ampulla of Vater
Duodenectomy
　see Excision, Duodenum 0DB9
　see Resection, Duodenum 0DT9
Duodenocholedochotomy
　see Drainage, Gallbladder 0F94
Duodenocystostomy
　see Bypass, Gallbladder 0F14
　see Drainage, Gallbladder 0F94
Duodenoenterostomy
　see Bypass, Gastrointestinal System 0D1
　see Drainage, Gastrointestinal System 0D9
Duodenojejunal flexure
　use Jejunum
Duodenolysis
　see Release, Duodenum 0DN9
Duodenorrhaphy
　see Repair, Duodenum 0DQ9
Duodenostomy
　see Bypass, Duodenum 0D19
　see Drainage, Duodenum 0D99
Duodenotomy
　see Drainage, Duodenum 0D99
Dura mater, intracranial
　use Dura Mater
Dura mater, spinal
　use Spinal Meninges
DuraGraft® Endothelial Damage Inhibitor
　use Endothelial Damage Inhibitor
DuraHeart Left Ventricular Assist System
　use Implantable Heart Assist System in
　　Heart and Great Vessels
Dural venous sinus
　use Intracranial Vein

Durata® Defibrillation Lead
　use Cardiac Lead, Defibrillator in 02H
Durvalumab Antineoplastic XW0
DynaNail Mini®
　use Internal Fixation Device, Sustained
　　Compression in 0RG
　use Internal Fixation Device, Sustained
　　Compression in 0SG
DynaNail®
　use Internal Fixation Device, Sustained
　　Compression in 0RG
　use Internal Fixation Device, Sustained
　　Compression in 0SG
Dynesys® Dynamic Stabilization System
　use Spinal Stabilization Device, Pedicle-
　　Based in 0RH
　use Spinal Stabilization Device, Pedicle-
　　Based in 0SH

E

E-Luminexx™ (Biliary)(Vascular) Stent
　use Intraluminal Device
Earlobe
　use External Ear, Right
　use External Ear, Left
　use External Ear, Bilateral
**ECCO2R (Extracorporeal Carbon Dioxide
　Removal)** 5A0920Z
Echocardiogram
　see Ultrasonography, Heart B24
Echography
　see Ultrasonography
**EchoTip® Insight™ Portosystemic Pressure
　Gradient Measurement System** 4A044B2
ECMO
　see Performance, Circulatory 5A15
ECMO, intraoperative
　see Performance, Circulatory 5A15A
Eculizumab XW0
EDWARDS INTUITY Elite valve system
　use Zooplastic Tissue, Rapid Deployment
　　Technique in New Technology
EEG (electroencephalogram)
　see Measurement, Central Nervous 4A00
EGD (esophagogastroduodenoscopy)
　0DJ08ZZ
Eighth cranial nerve
　use Acoustic Nerve
Ejaculatory duct
　use Vas Deferens, Right
　use Vas Deferens, Left
　use Vas Deferens, Bilateral
　use Vas Deferens
EKG (electrocardiogram)
　see Measurement, Cardiac 4A02
EKOS™ EkoSonic® Endovascular System
　see Fragmentation, Artery
Eladocagene exuparvovec XW0Q316
Electrical bone growth stimulator (EBGS)
　use Bone Growth Stimulator in Head and
　　Facial Bones
　use Bone Growth Stimulator in Upper
　　Bones
　use Bone Growth Stimulator in Lower
　　Bones
Electrical muscle stimulation (EMS) lead
　use Stimulator Lead in Muscles
Electrocautery
　Destruction *see* Destruction
　Repair *see* Repair
Electroconvulsive Therapy
　Bilateral-Multiple Seizure GZB3ZZZ
　Bilateral-Single Seizure GZB2ZZZ
　Electroconvulsive Therapy, Other GZB4ZZZ

Electroconvulsive Therapy — *continued*
　Unilateral-Multiple Seizure GZB1ZZZ
　Unilateral-Single Seizure GZB0ZZZ
Electroencephalogram (EEG)
　see Measurement, Central Nervous 4A00
Electromagnetic Therapy
　Central Nervous 6A22
　Urinary 6A21
Electronic muscle stimulator lead
　use Stimulator Lead in Muscles
Electrophysiologic stimulation (EPS)
　see Measurement, Cardiac 4A02
Electroshock therapy
　see Electroconvulsive Therapy
Elevation, bone fragments, skull
　see Reposition, Head and Facial
　　Bones 0NS
Eleventh cranial nerve
　use Accessory Nerve
Ellipsys® vascular access system
　Radial Artery, Left 031C3ZF
　Radial Artery, Right 031B3ZF
　Ulnar Artery, Left 031A3ZF
　Ulnar Artery, Right 03193ZF
Eluvia™ Drug-Eluting Vascular Stent System
　use Intraluminal Device, Sustained Release
　　Drug-eluting in New Technology
　use Intraluminal Device, Sustained Release
　　Drug-eluting, Two in New Technology
　use Intraluminal Device, Sustained Release
　　Drug-eluting, Three in New Technology
　use Intraluminal Device, Sustained Release
　　Drug-eluting, Four or More in New
　　Technology
ELZONRIS™
　use Tagraxofusp-erzs Antineoplastic
Embolectomy
　see Extirpation
Embolization
　see Occlusion
　see Restriction
Embolization coil(s)
　use Intraluminal Device
EMG (electromyogram)
　see Measurement, Musculoskeletal 4A0F
Encephalon
　use Brain
Endarterectomy
　see Extirpation, Upper Arteries 03C
　see Extirpation, Lower Arteries 04C
**Endeavor® (III)(IV) (Sprint) Zotarolimus-
　eluting Coronary Stent System**
　use Intraluminal Device, Drug-eluting in
　　Heart and Great Vessels
EndoAVF procedure
　Radial Artery, Left 031C3ZF
　Radial Artery, Right 031B3ZF
　Ulnar Artery, Left 031A3ZF
　Ulnar Artery, Right 03193ZF
Endologix AFX® Endovascular AAA System
　use Intraluminal Device
EndoSure® sensor
　use Monitoring Device, Pressure Sensor
　　in 02H
**ENDOTAK RELIANCE® (G) Defibrillation
　Lead**
　use Cardiac Lead, Defibrillator in 02H
**Endothelial damage inhibitor, applied to
　vein graft** XY0VX83
Endotracheal tube (cuffed)(double-lumen)
　use Intraluminal Device, Endotracheal
　　Airway in Respiratory System
Endovascular fistula creation
　Radial Artery, Left 031C3ZF
　Radial Artery, Right 031B3ZF
　Ulnar Artery, Left 031A3ZF
　Ulnar Artery, Right 03193ZF

Endurant® Endovascular Stent Graft
   use Intraluminal Device
Endurant® II AAA stent graft system
   use Intraluminal Device
Engineered Autologous Chimeric Antigen Receptor T-cell Immunotherapy XW0
Enlargement
   see Dilation
   see Repair
EnRhythm
   use Pacemaker, Dual Chamber in 0JH
ENROUTE® Transcarotid Neuroprotection System
   see New Technology, Cardiovascular System X2A
Enterorrhaphy
   see Repair, Gastrointestinal System 0DQ
Enterra gastric neurostimulator
   use Stimulator Generator, Multiple Array in 0JH
Enucleation
   Eyeball *see* Resection, Eye 08T
   Eyeball with prosthetic implant *see* Replacement, Eye 08R
Ependyma
   use Cerebral Ventricle
Epic™ Stented Tissue Valve (aortic)
   use Zooplastic Tissue in Heart and Great Vessels
Epicel® cultured epidermal autograft
   use Autologous Tissue Substitute
Epidermis
   use Skin
Epididymectomy
   see Excision, Male Reproductive System 0VB
   see Resection, Male Reproductive System 0VT
Epididymoplasty
   see Repair, Male Reproductive System 0VQ
   see Supplement, Male Reproductive System 0VU
Epididymorrhaphy
   see Repair, Male Reproductive System 0VQ
Epididymotomy
   see Drainage, Male Reproductive System 0V9
Epidural space, spinal
   use Spinal Canal
Epiphysiodesis
   see Insertion of device in, Upper Bones 0PH
   see Repair, Upper Bones 0PQ
   see Insertion of device in, Lower Bones 0QH
   see Repair, Lower Bones 0QQ
Epiploic foramen
   use Peritoneum
Epiretinal Visual Prosthesis
   Left 08H105Z
   Right 08H005Z
Episiorrhaphy
   see Repair, Perineum, Female 0WQN
Episiotomy
   see Division, Perineum, Female 0W8N
Epithalamus
   use Thalamus
Epitrochlear lymph node
   use Lymphatic, Right Upper Extremity
   use Lymphatic, Left Upper Extremity
EPS (electrophysiologic stimulation)
   see Measurement, Cardiac 4A02
Eptifibatide, infusion
   see Introduction of Platelet Inhibitor
ERCP (endoscopic retrograde cholangiopancreatography)
   see Fluoroscopy, Hepatobiliary System and Pancreas BF1
Erdafitinib Antineoplastic XW0DXL5

Erector spinae muscle
   use Trunk Muscle, Right
   use Trunk Muscle, Left
ERLEADA™
   use Apalutamide Antineoplastic
Esketamine Hydrochloride XW097M5
Esophageal artery
   use Upper Artery
Esophageal obturator airway (EOA)
   use Intraluminal Device, Airway in Gastrointestinal System
Esophageal plexus
   use Thoracic Sympathetic Nerve
Esophagectomy
   see Excision, Gastrointestinal System 0DB
   see Resection, Gastrointestinal System 0DT
Esophagocoloplasty
   see Repair, Gastrointestinal System 0DQ
   see Supplement, Gastrointestinal System 0DU
Esophagoenterostomy
   see Bypass, Gastrointestinal System 0D1
   see Drainage, Gastrointestinal System 0D9
Esophagoesophagostomy
   see Bypass, Gastrointestinal System 0D1
   see Drainage, Gastrointestinal System 0D9
Esophagogastrectomy
   see Excision, Gastrointestinal System 0DB
   see Resection, Gastrointestinal System 0DT
Esophagogastroduodenoscopy (EGD)
   0DJ08ZZ
Esophagogastroplasty
   see Repair, Gastrointestinal System 0DQ
   see Supplement, Gastrointestinal System 0DU
Esophagogastroscopy 0DJ68ZZ
Esophagogastrostomy
   see Bypass, Gastrointestinal System 0D1
   see Drainage, Gastrointestinal System 0D9
Esophagojejunoplasty
   see Supplement, Gastrointestinal System 0DU
Esophagojejunostomy
   see Bypass, Gastrointestinal System 0D1
   see Drainage, Gastrointestinal System 0D9
Esophagomyotomy
   see Division, Esophagogastric Junction 0D84
Esophagoplasty
   see Repair, Gastrointestinal System 0DQ
   see Replacement, Esophagus 0DR5
   see Supplement, Gastrointestinal System 0DU
Esophagoplication
   see Restriction, Gastrointestinal System 0DV
Esophagorrhaphy
   see Repair, Gastrointestinal System 0DQ
Esophagoscopy 0DJ08ZZ
Esophagotomy
   see Drainage, Gastrointestinal System 0D9
Esteem® implantable hearing system
   use Hearing Device in Ear, Nose, Sinus
ESWL (extracorporeal shock wave lithotripsy)
   see Fragmentation
Etesevimab Monoclonal Antibody XW0
Ethmoidal air cell
   use Ethmoid Sinus, Right
   use Ethmoid Sinus, Left
Ethmoidectomy
   see Excision, Ear, Nose, Sinus 09B
   see Resection, Ear, Nose, Sinus 09T
   see Excision, Head and Facial Bones 0NB
   see Resection, Head and Facial Bones 0NT
Ethmoidotomy
   see Drainage, Ear, Nose, Sinus 099

Evacuation
   Hematoma *see* Extirpation
   Other Fluid *see* Drainage
Evera (XT)(S)(DR/VR)
   use Defibrillator Generator in 0JH
Everolimus-eluting coronary stent
   use Intraluminal Device, Drug-eluting in Heart and Great Vessels
Evisceration
   Eyeball *see* Resection, Eye 08T
   Eyeball with prosthetic implant *see* Replacement, Eye 08R
Ex-PRESS™ mini glaucoma shunt
   use Synthetic Substitute
Examination
   see Inspection
Exchange
   see Change device in
Excision
   Abdominal Wall 0WBF
   Acetabulum
     Left 0QB5
     Right 0QB4
   Adenoids 0CBQ
   Ampulla of Vater 0FBC
   Anal Sphincter 0DBR
   Ankle Region
     Left 0YBL
     Right 0YBK
   Anus 0DBQ
   Aorta
     Abdominal 04B0
     Thoracic
       Ascending/Arch 02BX
       Descending 02BW
   Aortic Body 0GBD
   Appendix 0DBJ
   Arm
     Lower
       Left 0XBF
       Right 0XBD
     Upper
       Left 0XB9
       Right 0XB8
   Artery
     Anterior Tibial
       Left 04BQ
       Right 04BP
     Axillary
       Left 03B6
       Right 03B5
     Brachial
       Left 03B8
       Right 03B7
     Celiac 04B1
     Colic
       Left 04B7
       Middle 04B8
       Right 04B6
     Common Carotid
       Left 03BJ
       Right 03BH
     Common Iliac
       Left 04BD
       Right 04BC
     External Carotid
       Left 03BN
       Right 03BM
     External Iliac
       Left 04BJ
       Right 04BH
     Face 03BR
     Femoral
       Left 04BL
       Right 04BK
     Foot
       Left 04BW
       Right 04BV

Excision — *continued*
  Artery — *continued*
    Gastric 04B2
    Hand
      Left 03BF
      Right 03BD
    Hepatic 04B3
    Inferior Mesenteric 04BB
    Innominate 03B2
    Internal Carotid
      Left 03BL
      Right 03BK
    Internal Iliac
      Left 04BF
      Right 04BE
    Internal Mammary
      Left 03B1
      Right 03B0
    Intracranial 03BG
    Lower 04BY
    Peroneal
      Left 04BU
      Right 04BT
    Popliteal
      Left 04BN
      Right 04BM
    Posterior Tibial
      Left 04BS
      Right 04BR
    Pulmonary
      Left 02BR
      Right 02BQ
    Pulmonary Trunk 02BP
    Radial
      Left 03BC
      Right 03BB
    Renal
      Left 04BA
      Right 04B9
    Splenic 04B4
    Subclavian
      Left 03B4
      Right 03B3
    Superior Mesenteric 04B5
    Temporal
      Left 03BT
      Right 03BS
    Thyroid
      Left 03BV
      Right 03BU
    Ulnar
      Left 03BA
      Right 03B9
    Upper 03BY
    Vertebral
      Left 03BQ
      Right 03BP
  Atrium
    Left 02B7
    Right 02B6
  Auditory Ossicle
    Left 09BA
    Right 09B9
  Axilla
    Left 0XB5
    Right 0XB4
  Back
    Lower 0WBL
    Upper 0WBK
  Basal Ganglia 00B8
  Bladder 0TBB
  Bladder Neck 0TBC
  Bone
    Ethmoid
      Left 0NBG
      Right 0NBF
    Frontal 0NB1

Excision — *continued*
  Bone — *continued*
    Hyoid 0NBX
    Lacrimal
      Left 0NBJ
      Right 0NBH
    Nasal 0NBB
    Occipital 0NB7
    Palatine
      Left 0NBL
      Right 0NBK
    Parietal
      Left 0NB4
      Right 0NB3
    Pelvic
      Left 0QB3
      Right 0QB2
    Sphenoid 0NBC
    Temporal
      Left 0NB6
      Right 0NB5
    Zygomatic
      Left 0NBN
      Right 0NBM
  Brain 00B0
  Breast
    Bilateral 0HBV
    Left 0HBU
    Right 0HBT
    Supernumerary 0HBY
  Bronchus
    Lingula 0BB9
    Lower Lobe
      Left 0BBB
      Right 0BB6
    Main
      Left 0BB7
      Right 0BB3
    Middle Lobe, Right 0BB5
    Upper Lobe
      Left 0BB8
      Right 0BB4
  Buccal Mucosa 0CB4
  Bursa and Ligament
    Abdomen
      Left 0MBJ
      Right 0MBH
    Ankle
      Left 0MBR
      Right 0MBQ
    Elbow
      Left 0MB4
      Right 0MB3
    Foot
      Left 0MBT
      Right 0MBS
    Hand
      Left 0MB8
      Right 0MB7
    Head and Neck 0MB0
    Hip
      Left 0MBM
      Right 0MBL
    Knee
      Left 0MBP
      Right 0MBN
    Lower Extremity
      Left 0MBW
      Right 0MBV
    Perineum 0MBK
    Rib(s) 0MBG
    Shoulder
      Left 0MB2
      Right 0MB1
    Spine
      Lower 0MBD
      Upper 0MBC

Excision — *continued*
  Bursa and Ligament — *continued*
    Sternum 0MBF
    Upper Extremity
      Left 0MBB
      Right 0MB9
    Wrist
      Left 0MB6
      Right 0MB5
  Buttock
    Left 0YB1
    Right 0YB0
  Carina 0BB2
  Carotid Bodies, Bilateral 0GB8
  Carotid Body
    Left 0GB6
    Right 0GB7
  Carpal
    Left 0PBN
    Right 0PBM
  Cecum 0DBH
  Cerebellum 00BC
  Cerebral Hemisphere 00B7
  Cerebral Meninges 00B1
  Cerebral Ventricle 00B6
  Cervix 0UBC
  Chest Wall 0WB8
  Chordae Tendineae 02B9
  Choroid
    Left 08BB
    Right 08BA
  Cisterna Chyli 07BL
  Clavicle
    Left 0PBB
    Right 0PB9
  Clitoris 0UBJ
  Coccygeal Glomus 0GBB
  Coccyx 0QBS
  Colon
    Ascending 0DBK
    Descending 0DBM
    Sigmoid 0DBN
    Transverse 0DBL
  Conduction Mechanism 02B8
  Conjunctiva
    Left 08BTXZ
    Right 08BSXZ
  Cord
    Bilateral 0VBH
    Left 0VBG
    Right 0VBF
  Cornea
    Left 08B9XZ
    Right 08B8XZ
  Cul-de-sac 0UBF
  Diaphragm 0BBT
  Disc
    Cervical Vertebral 0RB3
    Cervicothoracic Vertebral 0RB5
    Lumbar Vertebral 0SB2
    Lumbosacral 0SB4
    Thoracic Vertebral 0RB9
    Thoracolumbar Vertebral 0RBB
  Duct
    Common Bile 0FB9
    Cystic 0FB8
    Hepatic
      Common 0FB7
      Left 0FB6
      Right 0FB5
    Lacrimal
      Left 08BY
      Right 08BX
    Pancreatic 0FBD
      Accessory 0FBF
    Parotid
      Left 0CBC
      Right 0CBB

Excision — *continued*
  Duodenum 0DB9
  Dura Mater 00B2
  Ear
    External
      Left 09B1
      Right 09B0
    External Auditory Canal
      Left 09B4
      Right 09B3
    Inner
      Left 09BE
      Right 09BD
    Middle
      Left 09B6
      Right 09B5
  Elbow Region
    Left 0XBC
    Right 0XBB
  Epididymis
    Bilateral 0VBL
    Left 0VBK
    Right 0VBJ
  Epiglottis 0CBR
  Esophagogastric Junction 0DB4
  Esophagus 0DB5
    Lower 0DB3
    Middle 0DB2
    Upper 0DB1
  Eustachian Tube
    Left 09BG
    Right 09BF
  Extremity
    Lower
      Left 0YBB
      Right 0YB9
    Upper
      Left 0XB7
      Right 0XB6
  Eye
    Left 08B1
    Right 08B0
  Eyelid
    Lower
      Left 08BR
      Right 08BQ
    Upper
      Left 08BP
      Right 08BN
  Face 0WB2
  Fallopian Tube
    Left 0UB6
    Right 0UB5
  Fallopian Tubes, Bilateral 0UB7
  Femoral Region
    Left 0YB8
    Right 0YB7
  Femoral Shaft
    Left 0QB9
    Right 0QB8
  Femur
    Lower
      Left 0QBC
      Right 0QBB
    Upper
      Left 0QB7
      Right 0QB6
  Fibula
    Left 0QBK
    Right 0QBJ
  Finger Nail 0HBQXZ
  Floor of mouth *see* Excision, Oral Cavity and
    Throat 0WB3
  Foot
    Left 0YBN
    Right 0YBM
  Gallbladder 0FB4

Excision — *continued*
  Gingiva
    Lower 0CB6
    Upper 0CB5
  Gland
    Adrenal
      Bilateral 0GB4
      Left 0GB2
      Right 0GB3
    Lacrimal
      Left 08BW
      Right 08BV
    Minor Salivary 0CBJ
    Parotid
      Left 0CB9
      Right 0CB8
    Pituitary 0GB0
    Sublingual
      Left 0CBF
      Right 0CBD
    Submaxillary
      Left 0CBH
      Right 0CBG
    Vestibular 0UBL
  Glenoid Cavity
    Left 0PB8
    Right 0PB7
  Glomus Jugulare 0GBC
  Hand
    Left 0XBK
    Right 0XBJ
  Head 0WB0
  Humeral Head
    Left 0PBD
    Right 0PBC
  Humeral Shaft
    Left 0PBG
    Right 0PBF
  Hymen 0UBK
  Hypothalamus 00BA
  Ileocecal Valve 0DBC
  Ileum 0DBB
  Inguinal Region
    Left 0YB6
    Right 0YB5
  Intestine
    Large 0DBE
      Left 0DBG
      Right 0DBF
    Small 0DB8
  Iris
    Left 08BD3Z
    Right 08BC3Z
  Jaw
    Lower 0WB5
    Upper 0WB4
  Jejunum 0DBA
  Joint
    Acromioclavicular
      Left 0RBH
      Right 0RBG
    Ankle
      Left 0SBG
      Right 0SBF
    Carpal
      Left 0RBR
      Right 0RBQ
    Carpometacarpal
      Left 0RBT
      Right 0RBS
    Cervical Vertebral 0RB1
    Cervicothoracic Vertebral 0RB4
    Coccygeal 0SB6
    Elbow
      Left 0RBM
      Right 0RBL

Excision — *continued*
  Joint — *continued*
    Finger Phalangeal
      Left 0RBX
      Right 0RBW
    Hip
      Left 0SBB
      Right 0SB9
    Knee
      Left 0SBD
      Right 0SBC
    Lumbar Vertebral 0SB0
    Lumbosacral 0SB3
    Metacarpophalangeal
      Left 0RBV
      Right 0RBU
    Metatarsal-Phalangeal
      Left 0SBN
      Right 0SBM
    Occipital-cervical 0RB0
    Sacrococcygeal 0SB5
    Sacroiliac
      Left 0SB8
      Right 0SB7
    Shoulder
      Left 0RBK
      Right 0RBJ
    Sternoclavicular
      Left 0RBF
      Right 0RBE
    Tarsal
      Left 0SBJ
      Right 0SBH
    Tarsometatarsal
      Left 0SBL
      Right 0SBK
    Temporomandibular
      Left 0RBD
      Right 0RBC
    Thoracic Vertebral 0RB6
    Thoracolumbar Vertebral 0RBA
    Toe Phalangeal
      Left 0SBQ
      Right 0SBP
    Wrist
      Left 0RBP
      Right 0RBN
  Kidney
    Left 0TB1
    Right 0TB0
  Kidney Pelvis
    Left 0TB4
    Right 0TB3
  Knee Region
    Left 0YBG
    Right 0YBF
  Larynx 0CBS
  Leg
    Lower
      Left 0YBJ
      Right 0YBH
    Upper
      Left 0YBD
      Right 0YBC
  Lens
    Left 08BK3Z
    Right 08BJ3Z
  Lip
    Lower 0CB1
    Upper 0CB0
  Liver 0FB0
    Left Lobe 0FB2
    Right Lobe 0FB1
  Lung
    Bilateral 0BBM
    Left 0BBL

Excision — *continued*
  Lung — *continued*
    Lower Lobe
      Left 0BBJ
      Right 0BBF
    Middle Lobe, Right 0BBD
    Right 0BBK
    Upper Lobe
      Left 0BBG
      Right 0BBC
  Lung Lingula 0BBH
  Lymphatic
    Aortic 07BD
    Axillary
      Left 07B6
      Right 07B5
    Head 07B0
    Inguinal
      Left 07BJ
      Right 07BH
    Internal Mammary
      Left 07B9
      Right 07B8
    Lower Extremity
      Left 07BG
      Right 07BF
    Mesenteric 07BB
    Neck
      Left 07B2
      Right 07B1
    Pelvis 07BC
    Thoracic Duct 07BK
    Thorax 07B7
    Upper Extremity
      Left 07B4
      Right 07B3
  Mandible
    Left 0NBV
    Right 0NBT
  Maxilla 0NBR
  Mediastinum 0WBC
  Medulla Oblongata 00BD
  Mesentery 0DBV
  Metacarpal
    Left 0PBQ
    Right 0PBP
  Metatarsal
    Left 0QBP
    Right 0QBN
  Muscle
    Abdomen
      Left 0KBL
      Right 0KBK
    Extraocular
      Left 08BM
      Right 08BL
    Facial 0KB1
    Foot
      Left 0KBW
      Right 0KBV
    Hand
      Left 0KBD
      Right 0KBC
    Head 0KB0
    Hip
      Left 0KBP
      Right 0KBN
    Lower Arm and Wrist
      Left 0KBB
      Right 0KB9
    Lower Leg
      Left 0KBT
      Right 0KBS
    Neck
      Left 0KB3
      Right 0KB2
    Papillary 02BD

Excision — *continued*
  Muscle — *continued*
    Perineum 0KBM
    Shoulder
      Left 0KB6
      Right 0KB5
    Thorax
      Left 0KBJ
      Right 0KBH
    Tongue, Palate, Pharynx 0KB4
    Trunk
      Left 0KBG
      Right 0KBF
    Upper Arm
      Left 0KB8
      Right 0KB7
    Upper Leg
      Left 0KBR
      Right 0KBQ
  Nasal Mucosa and Soft Tissue 09BK
  Nasopharynx 09BN
  Neck 0WB6
  Nerve
    Abdominal Sympathetic 01BM
    Abducens 00BL
    Accessory 00BR
    Acoustic 00BN
    Brachial Plexus 01B3
    Cervical 01B1
    Cervical Plexus 01B0
    Facial 00BM
    Femoral 01BD
    Glossopharyngeal 00BP
    Head and Neck Sympathetic 01BK
    Hypoglossal 00BS
    Lumbar 01BB
    Lumbar Plexus 01B9
    Lumbar Sympathetic 01BN
    Lumbosacral Plexus 01BA
    Median 01B5
    Oculomotor 00BH
    Olfactory 00BF
    Optic 00BG
    Peroneal 01BH
    Phrenic 01B2
    Pudendal 01BC
    Radial 01B6
    Sacral 01BR
    Sacral Plexus 01BQ
    Sacral Sympathetic 01BP
    Sciatic 01BF
    Thoracic 01B8
    Thoracic Sympathetic 01BL
    Tibial 01BG
    Trigeminal 00BK
    Trochlear 00BJ
    Ulnar 01B4
    Vagus 00BQ
  Nipple
    Left 0HBX
    Right 0HBW
  Omentum 0DBU
  Oral Cavity and Throat 0WB3
  Orbit
    Left 0NBQ
    Right 0NBP
  Ovary
    Bilateral 0UB2
    Left 0UB1
    Right 0UB0
  Palate
    Hard 0CB2
    Soft 0CB3
  Pancreas 0FBG
  Para-aortic Body 0GB9
  Paraganglion Extremity 0GBF
  Parathyroid Gland 0GBR

Excision — *continued*
  Parathyroid Gland — *continued*
    Inferior
      Left 0GBP
      Right 0GBN
    Multiple 0GBQ
    Superior
      Left 0GBM
      Right 0GBL
  Patella
    Left 0QBF
    Right 0QBD
  Penis 0VBS
  Pericardium 02BN
  Perineum
    Female 0WBN
    Male 0WBM
  Peritoneum 0DBW
  Phalanx
    Finger
      Left 0PBV
      Right 0PBT
    Thumb
      Left 0PBS
      Right 0PBR
    Toe
      Left 0QBR
      Right 0QBQ
  Pharynx 0CBM
  Pineal Body 0GB1
  Pleura
    Left 0BBP
    Right 0BBN
  Pons 00BB
  Prepuce 0VBT
  Prostate 0VB0
  Radius
    Left 0PBJ
    Right 0PBH
  Rectum 0DBP
  Retina
    Left 08BF3Z
    Right 08BE3Z
  Retroperitoneum 0WBH
  Ribs
    1 to 2 0PB1
    3 or More 0PB2
  Sacrum 0QB1
  Scapula
    Left 0PB6
    Right 0PB5
  Sclera
    Left 08B7XZ
    Right 08B6XZ
  Scrotum 0VB5
  Septum
    Atrial 02B5
    Nasal 09BM
    Ventricular 02BM
  Shoulder Region
    Left 0XB3
    Right 0XB2
  Sinus
    Accessory 09BP
    Ethmoid
      Left 09BV
      Right 09BU
    Frontal
      Left 09BT
      Right 09BS
    Mastoid
      Left 09BC
      Right 09BB
    Maxillary
      Left 09BR
      Right 09BQ
    Sphenoid
      Left 09BX
      Right 09BW

Excision — *continued*

Skin
Abdomen 0HB7XZ
Back 0HB6XZ
Buttock 0HB8XZ
Chest 0HB5XZ
Ear
  Left 0HB3XZ
  Right 0HB2XZ
Face 0HB1XZ
Foot
  Left 0HBNXZ
  Right 0HBMXZ
Hand
  Left 0HBGXZ
  Right 0HBFXZ
Inguinal 0HBAXZ
Lower Arm
  Left 0HBEXZ
  Right 0HBDXZ
Lower Leg
  Left 0HBLXZ
  Right 0HBKXZ
Neck 0HB4XZ
Perineum 0HB9XZ
Scalp 0HB0XZ
Upper Arm
  Left 0HBCXZ
  Right 0HBBXZ
Upper Leg
  Left 0HBJXZ
  Right 0HBHXZ

Skull 0NB0

Spinal Cord
Cervical 00BW
Lumbar 00BY
Thoracic 00BX

Spinal Meninges 00BT
Spleen 07BP
Sternum 0PB0

Stomach 0DB6
Pylorus 0DB7

Subcutaneous Tissue and Fascia
Abdomen 0JB8
Back 0JB7
Buttock 0JB9
Chest 0JB6
Face 0JB1
Foot
  Left 0JBR
  Right 0JBQ
Hand
  Left 0JBK
  Right 0JBJ
Lower Arm
  Left 0JBH
  Right 0JBG
Lower Leg
  Left 0JBP
  Right 0JBN
Neck
  Left 0JB5
  Right 0JB4
Pelvic Region 0JBC
Perineum 0JBB
Scalp 0JB0
Upper Arm
  Left 0JBF
  Right 0JBD
Upper Leg
  Left 0JBM
  Right 0JBL

Tarsal
Left 0QBM
Right 0QBL

Tendon
Abdomen

Excision — *continued*

Tendon — *continued*
  Left 0LBG
  Right 0LBF
Ankle
  Left 0LBT
  Right 0LBS
Foot
  Left 0LBW
  Right 0LBV
Hand
  Left 0LB8
  Right 0LB7
Head and Neck 0LB0
Hip
  Left 0LBK
  Right 0LBJ
Knee
  Left 0LBR
  Right 0LBQ
Lower Arm and Wrist
  Left 0LB6
  Right 0LB5
Lower Leg
  Left 0LBP
  Right 0LBN
Perineum 0LBH
Shoulder
  Left 0LB2
  Right 0LB1
Thorax
  Left 0LBD
  Right 0LBC
Trunk
  Left 0LBB
  Right 0LB9
Upper Arm
  Left 0LB4
  Right 0LB3
Upper Leg
  Left 0LBM
  Right 0LBL

Testis
Bilateral 0VBC
Left 0VBB
Right 0VB9

Thalamus 00B9
Thymus 07BM

Thyroid Gland
Left Lobe 0GBG
Right Lobe 0GBH

Thyroid Gland Isthmus 0GBJ

Tibia
Left 0QBH
Right 0QBG

Toe Nail 0HBRXZ
Tongue 0CB7
Tonsils 0CBP

Tooth
Lower 0CBX
Upper 0CBW

Trachea 0BB1

Tunica Vaginalis
Left 0VB7
Right 0VB6

Turbinate, Nasal 09BL

Tympanic Membrane
Left 09B8
Right 09B7

Ulna
Left 0PBL
Right 0PBK

Ureter
Left 0TB7
Right 0TB6

Urethra 0TBD
Uterine Supporting Structure 0UB4

Excision — *continued*
Uterus 0UB9
Uvula 0CBN
Vagina 0UBG

Valve
Aortic 02BF
Mitral 02BG
Pulmonary 02BH
Tricuspid 02BJ

Vas Deferens
Bilateral 0VBQ
Left 0VBP
Right 0VBN

Vein
Axillary
  Left 05B8
  Right 05B7
Azygos 05B0
Basilic
  Left 05BC
  Right 05BB
Brachial
  Left 05BA
  Right 05B9
Cephalic
  Left 05BF
  Right 05BD
Colic 06B7
Common Iliac
  Left 06BD
  Right 06BC
Coronary 02B4
Esophageal 06B3
External Iliac
  Left 06BG
  Right 06BF
External Jugular
  Left 05BQ
  Right 05BP
Face
  Left 05BV
  Right 05BT
Femoral
  Left 06BN
  Right 06BM
Foot
  Left 06BV
  Right 06BT
Gastric 06B2
Hand
  Left 05BH
  Right 05BG
Hemiazygos 05B1
Hepatic 06B4
Hypogastric
  Left 06BJ
  Right 06BH
Inferior Mesenteric 06B6
Innominate
  Left 05B4
  Right 05B3
Internal Jugular
  Left 05BN
  Right 05BM
Intracranial 05BL
Lower 06BY
Portal 06B8
Pulmonary
  Left 02BT
  Right 02BS
Renal
  Left 06BB
  Right 06B9
Saphenous
  Left 06BQ
  Right 06BP
Splenic 06B1

Excision — *continued*
  Vein — *continued*
    Subclavian
      Left 05B6
      Right 05B5
    Superior Mesenteric 06B5
    Upper 05BY
    Vertebral
      Left 05BS
      Right 05BR
  Vena Cava
    Inferior 06B0
    Superior 02BV
  Ventricle
    Left 02BL
    Right 02BK
  Vertebra
    Cervical 0PB3
    Lumbar 0QB0
    Thoracic 0PB4
  Vesicle
    Bilateral 0VB3
    Left 0VB2
    Right 0VB1
  Vitreous
    Left 08B53Z
    Right 08B43Z
  Vocal Cord
    Left 0CBV
    Right 0CBT
  Vulva 0UBM
  Wrist Region
    Left 0XBH
    Right 0XBG
EXCLUDER® AAA Endoprosthesis
  use Intraluminal Device, Branched or
    Fenestrated, One or Two Arteries in 04V
  use Intraluminal Device, Branched or
    Fenestrated, Three or More Arteries in 04V
  use Intraluminal Device
EXCLUDER® IBE Endoprosthesis
  use Intraluminal Device, Branched or
    Fenestrated, One or Two Arteries in 04V
Exclusion, Left atrial appendage (LAA)
  see Occlusion, Atrium, Left 02L7
Exercise, rehabilitation
  see Motor Treatment, Rehabilitation F07
Exploration
  see Inspection
Express® (LD) Premounted Stent System
  use Intraluminal Device
**Express® Biliary SD Monorail® Premounted
Stent System**
  use Intraluminal Device
**Express® SD Renal Monorail® Premounted
Stent System**
  use Intraluminal Device
Extensor carpi radialis muscle
  use Lower Arm and Wrist Muscle, Right
  use Lower Arm and Wrist Muscle, Left
Extensor carpi ulnaris muscle
  use Lower Arm and Wrist Muscle, Right
  use Lower Arm and Wrist Muscle, Left
Extensor digitorum brevis muscle
  use Foot Muscle, Right
  use Foot Muscle, Left
Extensor digitorum longus muscle
  use Lower Leg Muscle, Right
  use Lower Leg Muscle, Left
Extensor hallucis brevis muscle
  use Foot Muscle, Right
  use Foot Muscle, Left
Extensor hallucis longus muscle
  use Lower Leg Muscle, Right
  use Lower Leg Muscle, Left
External anal sphincter
  use Anal Sphincter

External auditory meatus
  use External Auditory Canal, Right
  use External Auditory Canal, Left
External fixator
  use External Fixation Device in Head and
    Facial Bones
  use External Fixation Device in Upper
    Bones
  use External Fixation Device in Lower Bones
  use External Fixation Device in Upper Joints
  use External Fixation Device in Lower Joints
External maxillary artery
  use Face Artery
External naris
  use Nasal Mucosa and Soft Tissue
External oblique aponeurosis
  use Subcutaneous Tissue and Fascia, Trunk
External oblique muscle
  use Abdomen Muscle, Right
  use Abdomen Muscle, Left
External popliteal nerve
  use Peroneal Nerve
External pudendal artery
  use Femoral Artery, Right
  use Femoral Artery, Left
External pudendal vein
  use Saphenous Vein, Right
  use Saphenous Vein, Left
External urethral sphincter
  use Urethra
Extirpation
  Acetabulum
    Left 0QC5
    Right 0QC4
  Adenoids 0CCQ
  Ampulla of Vater 0FCC
  Anal Sphincter 0DCR
  Anterior Chamber
    Left 08C3
    Right 08C2
  Anus 0DCQ
  Aorta
    Abdominal 04C0
    Thoracic
      Ascending/Arch 02CX
      Descending 02CW
  Aortic Body 0GCD
  Appendix 0DCJ
  Artery
    Anterior Tibial
      Left 04CQ
      Right 04CP
    Axillary
      Left 03C6
      Right 03C5
    Brachial
      Left 03C8
      Right 03C7
    Celiac 04C1
    Colic
      Left 04C7
      Middle 04C8
      Right 04C6
    Common Carotid
      Left 03CJ
      Right 03CH
    Common Iliac
      Left 04CD
      Right 04CC
    Coronary
      Four or More Arteries 02C3
      One Artery 02C0
      Three Arteries 02C2
      Two Arteries 02C1
    External Carotid
      Left 03CN
      Right 03CM

Extirpation — *continued*
  Artery — *continued*
    External Iliac
      Left 04CJ
      Right 04CH
    Face 03CR
    Femoral
      Left 04CL
      Right 04CK
    Foot
      Left 04CW
      Right 04CV
    Gastric 04C2
    Hand
      Left 03CF
      Right 03CD
    Hepatic 04C3
    Inferior Mesenteric 04CB
    Innominate 03C2
    Internal Carotid
      Left 03CL
      Right 03CK
    Internal Iliac
      Left 04CF
      Right 04CE
    Internal Mammary
      Left 03C1
      Right 03C0
    Intracranial 03CG
    Lower 04CY
    Peroneal
      Left 04CU
      Right 04CT
    Popliteal
      Left 04CN
      Right 04CM
    Posterior Tibial
      Left 04CS
      Right 04CR
    Pulmonary
      Left 02CR
      Right 02CQ
    Pulmonary Trunk 02CP
    Radial
      Left 03CC
      Right 03CB
    Renal
      Left 04CA
      Right 04C9
    Splenic 04C4
    Subclavian
      Left 03C4
      Right 03C3
    Superior Mesenteric 04C5
    Temporal
      Left 03CT
      Right 03CS
    Thyroid
      Left 03CV
      Right 03CU
    Ulnar
      Left 03CA
      Right 03C9
    Upper 03CY
    Vertebral
      Left 03CQ
      Right 03CP
  Atrium
    Left 02C7
    Right 02C6
  Auditory Ossicle
    Left 09CA
    Right 09C9
  Basal Ganglia 00C8
  Bladder 0TCB
  Bladder Neck 0TCC

Extirpation — *continued*
 Bone
  Ethmoid
   Left 0NCG
   Right 0NCF
  Frontal 0NC1
  Hyoid 0NCX
  Lacrimal
   Left 0NCJ
   Right 0NCH
  Nasal 0NCB
  Occipital 0NC7
  Palatine
   Left 0NCL
   Right 0NCK
  Parietal
   Left 0NC4
   Right 0NC3
  Pelvic
   Left 0QC3
   Right 0QC2
  Sphenoid 0NCC
  Temporal
   Left 0NC6
   Right 0NC5
  Zygomatic
   Left 0NCN
   Right 0NCM
 Brain 00C0
 Breast
  Bilateral 0HCV
  Left 0HCU
  Right 0HCT
 Bronchus
  Lingula 0BC9
  Lower Lobe
   Left 0BCB
   Right 0BC6
  Main
   Left 0BC7
   Right 0BC3
  Middle Lobe, Right 0BC5
  Upper Lobe
   Left 0BC8
   Right 0BC4
 Buccal Mucosa 0CC4
 Bursa and Ligament
  Abdomen
   Left 0MCJ
   Right 0MCH
  Ankle
   Left 0MCR
   Right 0MCQ
  Elbow
   Left 0MC4
   Right 0MC3
  Foot
   Left 0MCT
   Right 0MCS
  Hand
   Left 0MC8
   Right 0MC7
  Head and Neck 0MC0
  Hip
   Left 0MCM
   Right 0MCL
  Knee
   Left 0MCP
   Right 0MCN
  Lower Extremity
   Left 0MCW
   Right 0MCV
  Perineum 0MCK
  Rib(s) 0MCG
  Shoulder
   Left 0MC2
   Right 0MC1

Extirpation — *continued*
 Bursa and Ligament — *continued*
  Spine
   Lower 0MCD
   Upper 0MCC
  Sternum 0MCF
  Upper Extremity
   Left 0MCB
   Right 0MC9
  Wrist
   Left 0MC6
   Right 0MC5
 Carina 0BC2
 Carotid Bodies, Bilateral 0GC8
 Carotid Body
  Left 0GC6
  Right 0GC7
 Carpal
  Left 0PCN
  Right 0PCM
 Cavity, Cranial 0WC1
 Cecum 0DCH
 Cerebellum 00CC
 Cerebral Hemisphere 00C7
 Cerebral Meninges 00C1
 Cerebral Ventricle 00C6
 Cervix 0UCC
 Chordae Tendineae 02C9
 Choroid
  Left 08CB
  Right 08CA
 Cisterna Chyli 07CL
 Clavicle
  Left 0PCB
  Right 0PC9
 Clitoris 0UCJ
 Coccygeal Glomus 0GCB
 Coccyx 0QCS
 Colon
  Ascending 0DCK
  Descending 0DCM
  Sigmoid 0DCN
  Transverse 0DCL
 Conduction Mechanism 02C8
 Conjunctiva
  Left 08CTXZZ
  Right 08CSXZZ
 Cord
  Bilateral 0VCH
  Left 0VCG
  Right 0VCF
 Cornea
  Left 08C9XZZ
  Right 08C8XZZ
 Cul-de-sac 0UCF
 Diaphragm 0BCT
 Disc
  Cervical Vertebral 0RC3
  Cervicothoracic Vertebral 0RC5
  Lumbar Vertebral 0SC2
  Lumbosacral 0SC4
  Thoracic Vertebral 0RC9
  Thoracolumbar Vertebral 0RCB
 Duct
  Common Bile 0FC9
  Cystic 0FC8
  Hepatic
   Common 0FC7
   Left 0FC6
   Right 0FC5
  Lacrimal
   Left 08CY
   Right 08CX
  Pancreatic 0FCD
   Accessory 0FCF
  Parotid
   Left 0CCC
   Right 0CCB

Extirpation — *continued*
 Duodenum 0DC9
 Dura Mater 00C2
 Ear
  External
   Left 09C1
   Right 09C0
  External Auditory Canal
   Left 09C4
   Right 09C3
  Inner
   Left 09CE
   Right 09CD
  Middle
   Left 09C6
   Right 09C5
 Endometrium 0UCB
 Epididymis
  Bilateral 0VCL
  Left 0VCK
  Right 0VCJ
 Epidural Space, Intracranial 00C3
 Epiglottis 0CCR
 Esophagogastric Junction 0DC4
 Esophagus 0DC5
  Lower 0DC3
  Middle 0DC2
  Upper 0DC1
 Eustachian Tube
  Left 09CG
  Right 09CF
 Eye
  Left 08C1XZZ
  Right 08C0XZZ
 Eyelid
  Lower
   Left 08CR
   Right 08CQ
  Upper
   Left 08CP
   Right 08CN
 Fallopian Tube
  Left 0UC6
  Right 0UC5
 Fallopian Tubes, Bilateral 0UC7
 Femoral Shaft
  Left 0QC9
  Right 0QC8
 Femur
  Lower
   Left 0QCC
   Right 0QCB
  Upper
   Left 0QC7
   Right 0QC6
 Fibula
  Left 0QCK
  Right 0QCJ
 Finger Nail 0HCQXZZ
 Gallbladder 0FC4
 Gastrointestinal Tract 0WCP
 Genitourinary Tract 0WCR
 Gingiva
  Lower 0CC6
  Upper 0CC5
 Gland
  Adrenal
   Bilateral 0GC4
   Left 0GC2
   Right 0GC3
  Lacrimal
   Left 08CW
   Right 08CV
  Minor Salivary 0CCJ
  Parotid
   Left 0CC9
   Right 0CC8

Extirpation — *continued*
  Gland — *continued*
    Pituitary 0GC0
    Sublingual
      Left 0CCF
      Right 0CCD
    Submaxillary
      Left 0CCH
      Right 0CCG
    Vestibular 0UCL
  Glenoid Cavity
    Left 0PC8
    Right 0PC7
  Glomus Jugulare 0GCC
  Humeral Head
    Left 0PCD
    Right 0PCC
  Humeral Shaft
    Left 0PCG
    Right 0PCF
  Hymen 0UCK
  Hypothalamus 00CA
  Ileocecal Valve 0DCC
  Ileum 0DCB
  Intestine
    Large 0DCE
      Left 0DCG
      Right 0DCF
    Small 0DC8
  Iris
    Left 08CD
    Right 08CC
  Jaw
    Lower 0WC5
    Upper 0WC4
  Jejunum 0DCA
  Joint
    Acromioclavicular
      Left 0RCH
      Right 0RCG
    Ankle
      Left 0SCG
      Right 0SCF
    Carpal
      Left 0RCR
      Right 0RCQ
    Carpometacarpal
      Left 0RCT
      Right 0RCS
    Cervical Vertebral 0RC1
    Cervicothoracic Vertebral 0RC4
    Coccygeal 0SC6
    Elbow
      Left 0RCM
      Right 0RCL
    Finger Phalangeal
      Left 0RCX
      Right 0RCW
    Hip
      Left 0SCB
      Right 0SC9
    Knee
      Left 0SCD
      Right 0SCC
    Lumbar Vertebral 0SC0
    Lumbosacral 0SC3
    Metacarpophalangeal
      Left 0RCV
      Right 0RCU
    Metatarsal-Phalangeal
      Left 0SCN
      Right 0SCM
    Occipital-cervical 0RC0
    Sacrococcygeal 0SC5
    Sacroiliac
      Left 0SC8
      Right 0SC7

Extirpation — *continued*
  Joint — *continued*
    Shoulder
      Left 0RCK
      Right 0RCJ
    Sternoclavicular
      Left 0RCF
      Right 0RCE
    Tarsal
      Left 0SCJ
      Right 0SCH
    Tarsometatarsal
      Left 0SCL
      Right 0SCK
    Temporomandibular
      Left 0RCD
      Right 0RCC
    Thoracic Vertebral 0RC6
    Thoracolumbar Vertebral 0RCA
    Toe Phalangeal
      Left 0SCQ
      Right 0SCP
    Wrist
      Left 0RCP
      Right 0RCN
  Kidney
    Left 0TC1
    Right 0TC0
  Kidney Pelvis
    Left 0TC4
    Right 0TC3
  Larynx 0CCS
  Lens
    Left 08CK
    Right 08CJ
  Lip
    Lower 0CC1
    Upper 0CC0
  Liver 0FC0
    Left Lobe 0FC2
    Right Lobe 0FC1
  Lung
    Bilateral 0BCM
    Left 0BCL
    Lower Lobe
      Left 0BCJ
      Right 0BCF
    Middle Lobe, Right 0BCD
    Right 0BCK
    Upper Lobe
      Left 0BCG
      Right 0BCC
  Lung Lingula 0BCH
  Lymphatic
    Aortic 07CD
    Axillary
      Left 07C6
      Right 07C5
    Head 07C0
    Inguinal
      Left 07CJ
      Right 07CH
    Internal Mammary
      Left 07C9
      Right 07C8
    Lower Extremity
      Left 07CG
      Right 07CF
    Mesenteric 07CB
    Neck
      Left 07C2
      Right 07C1
    Pelvis 07CC
    Thoracic Duct 07CK
    Thorax 07C7
    Upper Extremity
      Left 07C4
      Right 07C3

Extirpation — *continued*
  Mandible
    Left 0NCV
    Right 0NCT
  Maxilla 0NCR
  Mediastinum 0WCC
  Medulla Oblongata 00CD
  Mesentery 0DCV
  Metacarpal
    Left 0PCQ
    Right 0PCP
  Metatarsal
    Left 0QCP
    Right 0QCN
  Muscle
    Abdomen
      Left 0KCL
      Right 0KCK
    Extraocular
      Left 08CM
      Right 08CL
    Facial 0KC1
    Foot
      Left 0KCW
      Right 0KCV
    Hand
      Left 0KCD
      Right 0KCC
    Head 0KC0
    Hip
      Left 0KCP
      Right 0KCN
    Lower Arm and Wrist
      Left 0KCB
      Right 0KC9
    Lower Leg
      Left 0KCT
      Right 0KCS
    Neck
      Left 0KC3
      Right 0KC2
    Papillary 02CD
    Perineum 0KCM
    Shoulder
      Left 0KC6
      Right 0KC5
    Thorax
      Left 0KCJ
      Right 0KCH
    Tongue, Palate, Pharynx 0KC4
    Trunk
      Left 0KCG
      Right 0KCF
    Upper Arm
      Left 0KC8
      Right 0KC7
    Upper Leg
      Left 0KCR
      Right 0KCQ
  Nasal Mucosa and Soft Tissue 09CK
  Nasopharynx 09CN
  Nerve
    Abdominal Sympathetic 01CM
    Abducens 00CL
    Accessory 00CR
    Acoustic 00CN
    Brachial Plexus 01C3
    Cervical 01C1
    Cervical Plexus 01C0
    Facial 00CM
    Femoral 01CD
    Glossopharyngeal 00CP
    Head and Neck Sympathetic 01CK
    Hypoglossal 00CS
    Lumbar 01CB
    Lumbar Plexus 01C9
    Lumbar Sympathetic 01CN

Extirpation — *continued*
Nerve — *continued*
Lumbosacral Plexus 01CA
Median 01C5
Oculomotor 00CH
Olfactory 00CF
Optic 00CG
Peroneal 01CH
Phrenic 01C2
Pudendal 01CC
Radial 01C6
Sacral 01CR
Sacral Plexus 01CQ
Sacral Sympathetic 01CP
Sciatic 01CF
Thoracic 01C8
Thoracic Sympathetic 01CL
Tibial 01CG
Trigeminal 00CK
Trochlear 00CJ
Ulnar 01C4
Vagus 00CQ
Nipple
Left 0HCX
Right 0HCW
Omentum 0DCU
Oral Cavity and Throat 0WC3
Orbit
Left 0NCQ
Right 0NCP
Orbital Atherectomy Technology X2C
Ovary
Bilateral 0UC2
Left 0UC1
Right 0UC0
Palate
Hard 0CC2
Soft 0CC3
Pancreas 0FCG
Para-aortic Body 0GC9
Paraganglion Extremity 0GCF
Parathyroid Gland 0GCR
Inferior
Left 0GCP
Right 0GCN
Multiple 0GCQ
Superior
Left 0GCM
Right 0GCL
Patella
Left 0QCF
Right 0QCD
Pelvic Cavity 0WCJ
Penis 0VCS
Pericardial Cavity 0WCD
Pericardium 02CN
Peritoneal Cavity 0WCG
Peritoneum 0DCW
Phalanx
Finger
Left 0PCV
Right 0PCT
Thumb
Left 0PCS
Right 0PCR
Toe
Left 0QCR
Right 0QCQ
Pharynx 0CCM
Pineal Body 0GC1
Pleura
Left 0BCP
Right 0BCN
Pleural Cavity
Left 0WCB
Right 0WC9
Pons 00CB

Extirpation — *continued*
Prepuce 0VCT
Prostate 0VC0
Radius
Left 0PCJ
Right 0PCH
Rectum 0DCP
Respiratory Tract 0WCQ
Retina
Left 08CF
Right 08CE
Retinal Vessel
Left 08CH
Right 08CG
Retroperitoneum 0WCH
Ribs
1 to 2 0PC1
3 or More 0PC2
Sacrum 0QC1
Scapula
Left 0PC6
Right 0PC5
Sclera
Left 08C7XZZ
Right 08C6XZZ
Scrotum 0VC5
Septum
Atrial 02C5
Nasal 09CM
Ventricular 02CM
Sinus
Accessory 09CP
Ethmoid
Left 09CV
Right 09CU
Frontal
Left 09CT
Right 09CS
Mastoid
Left 09CC
Right 09CB
Maxillary
Left 09CR
Right 09CQ
Sphenoid
Left 09CX
Right 09CW
Skin
Abdomen 0HC7XZZ
Back 0HC6XZZ
Buttock 0HC8XZZ
Chest 0HC5XZZ
Ear
Left 0HC3XZZ
Right 0HC2XZZ
Face 0HC1XZZ
Foot
Left 0HCNXZZ
Right 0HCMXZZ
Hand
Left 0HCGXZZ
Right 0HCFXZZ
Inguinal 0HCAXZZ
Lower Arm
Left 0HCEXZZ
Right 0HCDXZZ
Lower Leg
Left 0HCLXZZ
Right 0HCKXZZ
Neck 0HC4XZZ
Perineum 0HC9XZZ
Scalp 0HC0XZZ
Upper Arm
Left 0HCCXZZ
Right 0HCBXZZ
Upper Leg
Left 0HCJXZZ
Right 0HCHXZZ

Extirpation — *continued*
Spinal Canal 00CU
Spinal Cord
Cervical 00CW
Lumbar 00CY
Thoracic 00CX
Spinal Meninges 00CT
Spleen 07CP
Sternum 0PC0
Stomach 0DC6
Pylorus 0DC7
Subarachnoid Space, Intracranial 00C5
Subcutaneous Tissue and Fascia
Abdomen 0JC8
Back 0JC7
Buttock 0JC9
Chest 0JC6
Face 0JC1
Foot
Left 0JCR
Right 0JCQ
Hand
Left 0JCK
Right 0JCJ
Lower Arm
Left 0JCH
Right 0JCG
Lower Leg
Left 0JCP
Right 0JCN
Neck
Left 0JC5
Right 0JC4
Pelvic Region 0JCC
Perineum 0JCB
Scalp 0JC0
Upper Arm
Left 0JCF
Right 0JCD
Upper Leg
Left 0JCM
Right 0JCL
Subdural Space, Intracranial 00C4
Tarsal
Left 0QCM
Right 0QCL
Tendon
Abdomen
Left 0LCG
Right 0LCF
Ankle
Left 0LCT
Right 0LCS
Foot
Left 0LCW
Right 0LCV
Hand
Left 0LC8
Right 0LC7
Head and Neck 0LC0
Hip
Left 0LCK
Right 0LCJ
Knee
Left 0LCR
Right 0LCQ
Lower Arm and Wrist
Left 0LC6
Right 0LC5
Lower Leg
Left 0LCP
Right 0LCN
Perineum 0LCH
Shoulder
Left 0LC2
Right 0LC1

Extirpation — *continued*
Tendon — *continued*
Thorax
Left 0LCD
Right 0LCC
Trunk
Left 0LCB
Right 0LC9
Upper Arm
Left 0LC4
Right 0LC3
Upper Leg
Left 0LCM
Right 0LCL
Testis
Bilateral 0VCC
Left 0VCB
Right 0VC9
Thalamus 00C9
Thymus 07CM
Thyroid Gland 0GCK
Left Lobe 0GCG
Right Lobe 0GCH
Tibia
Left 0QCH
Right 0QCG
Toe Nail 0HCRXZZ
Tongue 0CC7
Tonsils 0CCP
Tooth
Lower 0CCX
Upper 0CCW
Trachea 0BC1
Tunica Vaginalis
Left 0VC7
Right 0VC6
Turbinate, Nasal 09CL
Tympanic Membrane
Left 09C8
Right 09C7
Ulna
Left 0PCL
Right 0PCK
Ureter
Left 0TC7
Right 0TC6
Urethra 0TCD
Uterine Supporting Structure 0UC4
Uterus 0UC9
Uvula 0CCN
Vagina 0UCG
Valve
Aortic 02CF
Mitral 02CG
Pulmonary 02CH
Tricuspid 02CJ
Vas Deferens
Bilateral 0VCQ
Left 0VCP
Right 0VCN
Vein
Axillary
Left 05C8
Right 05C7
Azygos 05C0
Basilic
Left 05CC
Right 05CB
Brachial
Left 05CA
Right 05C9
Cephalic
Left 05CF
Right 05CD
Colic 06C7
Common Iliac
Left 06CD
Right 06CC

Extirpation — *continued*
Vein — *continued*
Coronary 02C4
Esophageal 06C3
External Iliac
Left 06CG
Right 06CF
External Jugular
Left 05CQ
Right 05CP
Face
Left 05CV
Right 05CT
Femoral
Left 06CN
Right 06CM
Foot
Left 06CV
Right 06CT
Gastric 06C2
Hand
Left 05CH
Right 05CG
Hemiazygos 05C1
Hepatic 06C4
Hypogastric
Left 06CJ
Right 06CH
Inferior Mesenteric 06C6
Innominate
Left 05C4
Right 05C3
Internal Jugular
Left 05CN
Right 05CM
Intracranial 05CL
Lower 06CY
Portal 06C8
Pulmonary
Left 02CT
Right 02CS
Renal
Left 06CB
Right 06C9
Saphenous
Left 06CQ
Right 06CP
Splenic 06C1
Subclavian
Left 05C6
Right 05C5
Superior Mesenteric 06C5
Upper 05CY
Vertebral
Left 05CS
Right 05CR
Vena Cava
Inferior 06C0
Superior 02CV
Ventricle
Left 02CL
Right 02CK
Vertebra
Cervical 0PC3
Lumbar 0QC0
Thoracic 0PC4
Vesicle
Bilateral 0VC3
Left 0VC2
Right 0VC1
Vitreous
Left 08C5
Right 08C4
Vocal Cord
Left 0CCV
Right 0CCT
Vulva 0UCM

Extracorporeal Carbon Dioxide Removal (ECCO2R) 5A0920Z
Extracorporeal shock wave lithotripsy
see Fragmentation
Extracranial-intracranial bypass (EC-IC)
see Bypass, Upper Arteries 031
Extraction
Acetabulum
Left 0QD50ZZ
Right 0QD40ZZ
Ampulla of Vater 0FDC
Anus 0DDQ
Appendix 0DDJ
Auditory Ossicle
Left 09DA0ZZ
Right 09D90ZZ
Bone
Ethmoid
Left 0NDG0ZZ
Right 0NDF0ZZ
Frontal 0ND10ZZ
Hyoid 0NDX0ZZ
Lacrimal
Left 0NDJ0ZZ
Right 0NDH0ZZ
Nasal 0NDB0ZZ
Occipital 0ND70ZZ
Palatine
Left 0NDL0ZZ
Right 0NDK0ZZ
Parietal
Left 0ND40ZZ
Right 0ND30ZZ
Pelvic
Left 0QD30ZZ
Right 0QD20ZZ
Sphenoid 0NDC0ZZ
Temporal
Left 0ND60ZZ
Right 0ND50ZZ
Zygomatic
Left 0NDN0ZZ
Right 0NDM0ZZ
Bone Marrow
Iliac 07DR
Sternum 07DQ
Vertebral 07DS
Breast
Bilateral 0HDV0ZZ
Left 0HDU0ZZ
Right 0HDT0ZZ
Supernumerary 0HDY0ZZ
Bronchus
Lingula 0BD9
Lower Lobe
Left 0BDB
Right 0BD6
Main
Left 0BD7
Right 0BD3
Middle Lobe, Right 0BD5
Upper Lobe
Left 0BD8
Right 0BD4
Bursa and Ligament
Abdomen
Left 0MDJ
Right 0MDH
Ankle
Left 0MDR
Right 0MDQ
Elbow
Left 0MD4
Right 0MD3
Foot
Left 0MDT
Right 0MDS

Extraction — *continued*
  Bursa and Ligament — *continued*
    Hand
      Left 0MD8
      Right 0MD7
    Head and Neck 0MD0
    Hip
      Left 0MDM
      Right 0MDL
    Knee
      Left 0MDP
      Right 0MDN
    Lower Extremity
      Left 0MDW
      Right 0MDV
    Perineum 0MDK
    Rib(s) 0MDG
    Shoulder
      Left 0MD2
      Right 0MD1
    Spine
      Lower 0MDD
      Upper 0MDC
    Sternum 0MDF
    Upper Extremity
      Left 0MDB
      Right 0MD9
    Wrist
      Left 0MD6
      Right 0MD5
  Carina 0BD2
  Carpal
    Left 0PDN0ZZ
    Right 0PDM0ZZ
  Cecum 0DDH
  Cerebral Meninges 00D1
  Cisterna Chyli 07DL
  Clavicle
    Left 0PDB0ZZ
    Right 0PD90ZZ
  Coccyx 0QDS0ZZ
  Colon
    Ascending 0DDK
    Descending 0DDM
    Sigmoid 0DDN
    Transverse 0DDL
  Cornea
    Left 08D9XZ
    Right 08D8XZ
  Duct
    Common Bile 0FD9
    Cystic 0FD8
    Hepatic
      Common 0FD7
      Left 0FD6
      Right 0FD5
    Pancreatic 0FDD
      Accessory 0FDF
  Duodenum 0DD9
  Dura Mater 00D2
  Endometrium 0UDB
  Esophagogastric Junction 0DD4
  Esophagus 0DD5
    Lower 0DD3
    Middle 0DD2
    Upper 0DD1
  Femoral Shaft
    Left 0QD90ZZ
    Right 0QD80ZZ
  Femur
    Lower
      Left 0QDC0ZZ
      Right 0QDB0ZZ
    Upper
      Left 0QD70ZZ
      Right 0QD60ZZ

Extraction — *continued*
  Fibula
    Left 0QDK0ZZ
    Right 0QDJ0ZZ
  Finger Nail 0HDQXZZ
  Gallbladder 0FD4
  Glenoid Cavity
    Left 0PD80ZZ
    Right 0PD70ZZ
  Hair 0HDSXZZ
  Humeral Head
    Left 0PDD0ZZ
    Right 0PDC0ZZ
  Humeral Shaft
    Left 0PDG0ZZ
    Right 0PDF0ZZ
  Ileocecal Valve 0DDC
  Ileum 0DDB
  Intestine
    Large 0DDE
      Left 0DDG
      Right 0DDF
    Small 0DD8
  Jejunum 0DDA
  Kidney
    Left 0TD1
    Right 0TD0
  Lens
    Left 08DK3ZZ
    Right 08DJ3ZZ
  Liver 0FD0
    Left Lobe 0FD2
    Right Lobe 0FD1
  Lung
    Bilateral 0BDM
    Left 0BDL
    Lower Lobe
      Left 0BDJ
      Right 0BDF
    Middle Lobe, Right 0BDD
    Right 0BDK
    Upper Lobe
      Left 0BDG
      Right 0BDC
  Lung Lingula 0BDH
  Lymphatic
    Aortic 07DD
    Axillary
      Left 07D6
      Right 07D5
    Head 07D0
    Inguinal
      Left 07DJ
      Right 07DH
    Internal Mammary
      Left 07D9
      Right 07D8
    Lower Extremity
      Left 07DG
      Right 07DF
    Mesenteric 07DB
    Neck
      Left 07D2
      Right 07D1
    Pelvis 07DC
    Thoracic Duct 07DK
    Thorax 07D7
    Upper Extremity
      Left 07D4
      Right 07D3
  Mandible
    Left 0NDV0ZZ
    Right 0NDT0ZZ
  Maxilla 0NDR0ZZ
  Metacarpal
    Left 0PDQ0ZZ
    Right 0PDP0ZZ

Extraction — *continued*
  Metatarsal
    Left 0QDP0ZZ
    Right 0QDN0ZZ
  Muscle
    Abdomen
      Left 0KDL0ZZ
      Right 0KDK0ZZ
    Facial 0KD10ZZ
    Foot
      Left 0KDW0ZZ
      Right 0KDV0ZZ
    Hand
      Left 0KDD0ZZ
      Right 0KDC0ZZ
    Head 0KD00ZZ
    Hip
      Left 0KDP0ZZ
      Right 0KDN0ZZ
    Lower Arm and Wrist
      Left 0KDB0ZZ
      Right 0KD90ZZ
    Lower Leg
      Left 0KDT0ZZ
      Right 0KDS0ZZ
    Neck
      Left 0KD30ZZ
      Right 0KD20ZZ
    Perineum 0KDM0ZZ
    Shoulder
      Left 0KD60ZZ
      Right 0KD50ZZ
    Thorax
      Left 0KDJ0ZZ
      Right 0KDH0ZZ
    Tongue, Palate, Pharynx 0KD40ZZ
    Trunk
      Left 0KDG0ZZ
      Right 0KDF0ZZ
    Upper Arm
      Left 0KD80ZZ
      Right 0KD70ZZ
    Upper Leg
      Left 0KDR0ZZ
      Right 0KDQ0ZZ
  Nerve
    Abdominal Sympathetic 01DM
    Abducens 00DL
    Accessory 00DR
    Acoustic 00DN
    Brachial Plexus 01D3
    Cervical 01D1
    Cervical Plexus 01D0
    Facial 00DM
    Femoral 01DD
    Glossopharyngeal 00DP
    Head and Neck Sympathetic 01DK
    Hypoglossal 00DS
    Lumbar 01DB
    Lumbar Plexus 01D9
    Lumbar Sympathetic 01DN
    Lumbosacral Plexus 01DA
    Median 01D5
    Oculomotor 00DH
    Olfactory 00DF
    Optic 00DG
    Peroneal 01DH
    Phrenic 01D2
    Pudendal 01DC
    Radial 01D6
    Sacral 01DR
    Sacral Plexus 01DQ
    Sacral Sympathetic 01DP
    Sciatic 01DF
    Thoracic 01D8
    Thoracic Sympathetic 01DL
    Tibial 01DG

Extraction — *continued*
  Nerve — *continued*
    Trigeminal 00DK
    Trochlear 00DJ
    Ulnar 01D4
    Vagus 00DQ
  Orbit
    Left 0NDQ0ZZ
    Right 0NDP0ZZ
  Ova 0UDN
  Pancreas 0FDG
  Patella
    Left 0QDF0ZZ
    Right 0QDD0ZZ
  Phalanx
    Finger
      Left 0PDV0ZZ
      Right 0PDT0ZZ
    Thumb
      Left 0PDS0ZZ
      Right 0PDR0ZZ
    Toe
      Left 0QDR0ZZ
      Right 0QDQ0ZZ
  Pleura
    Left 0BDP
    Right 0BDN
  Products of Conception
    Ectopic 10D2
    Extraperitoneal 10D00Z2
    High 10D00Z0
    High Forceps 10D07Z5
    Internal Version 10D07Z7
    Low 10D00Z1
    Low Forceps 10D07Z3
    Mid Forceps 10D07Z4
    Other 10D07Z8
    Retained 10D1
    Vacuum 10D07Z6
  Radius
    Left 0PDJ0ZZ
    Right 0PDH0ZZ
  Rectum 0DDP
  Ribs
    1 to 2 0PD10ZZ
    3 or More 0PD20ZZ
  Sacrum 0QD10ZZ
  Scapula
    Left 0PD60ZZ
    Right 0PD50ZZ
  Septum, Nasal 09DM
  Sinus
    Accessory 09DP
    Ethmoid
      Left 09DV
      Right 09DU
    Frontal
      Left 09DT
      Right 09DS
    Mastoid
      Left 09DC
      Right 09DB
    Maxillary
      Left 09DR
      Right 09DQ
    Sphenoid
      Left 09DX
      Right 09DW
  Skin
    Abdomen 0HD7XZZ
    Back 0HD6XZZ
    Buttock 0HD8XZZ
    Chest 0HD5XZZ
    Ear
      Left 0HD3XZZ
      Right 0HD2XZZ
    Face 0HD1XZZ

Extraction — *continued*
  Skin — *continued*
    Foot
      Left 0HDNXZZ
      Right 0HDMXZZ
    Hand
      Left 0HDGXZZ
      Right 0HDFXZZ
    Inguinal 0HDAXZZ
    Lower Arm
      Left 0HDEXZZ
      Right 0HDDXZZ
    Lower Leg
      Left 0HDLXZZ
      Right 0HDKXZZ
    Neck 0HD4XZZ
    Perineum 0HD9XZZ
    Scalp 0HD0XZZ
    Upper Arm
      Left 0HDCXZZ
      Right 0HDBXZZ
    Upper Leg
      Left 0HDJXZZ
      Right 0HDHXZZ
  Skull 0ND00ZZ
  Spinal Meninges 00DT
  Spleen 07DP
  Sternum 0PD00ZZ
  Stomach 0DD6
    Pylorus 0DD7
  Subcutaneous Tissue and Fascia
    Abdomen 0JD8
    Back 0JD7
    Buttock 0JD9
    Chest 0JD6
    Face 0JD1
    Foot
      Left 0JDR
      Right 0JDQ
    Hand
      Left 0JDK
      Right 0JDJ
    Lower Arm
      Left 0JDH
      Right 0JDG
    Lower Leg
      Left 0JDP
      Right 0JDN
    Neck
      Left 0JD5
      Right 0JD4
    Pelvic Region 0JDC
    Perineum 0JDB
    Scalp 0JD0
    Upper Arm
      Left 0JDF
      Right 0JDD
    Upper Leg
      Left 0JDM
      Right 0JDL
  Tarsal
    Left 0QDM0ZZ
    Right 0QDL0ZZ
  Tendon
    Abdomen
      Left 0LDG0ZZ
      Right 0LDF0ZZ
    Ankle
      Left 0LDT0ZZ
      Right 0LDS0ZZ
    Foot
      Left 0LDW0ZZ
      Right 0LDV0ZZ
    Hand
      Left 0LD80ZZ
      Right 0LD70ZZ
    Head and Neck 0LD00ZZ

Extraction — *continued*
  Tendon — *continued*
    Hip
      Left 0LDK0ZZ
      Right 0LDJ0ZZ
    Knee
      Left 0LDR0ZZ
      Right 0LDQ0ZZ
    Lower Arm and Wrist
      Left 0LD60ZZ
      Right 0LD50ZZ
    Lower Leg
      Left 0LDP0ZZ
      Right 0LDN0ZZ
    Perineum 0LDH0ZZ
    Shoulder
      Left 0LD20ZZ
      Right 0LD10ZZ
    Thorax
      Left 0LDD0ZZ
      Right 0LDC0ZZ
    Trunk
      Left 0LDB0ZZ
      Right 0LD90ZZ
    Upper Arm
      Left 0LD40ZZ
      Right 0LD30ZZ
    Upper Leg
      Left 0LDM0ZZ
      Right 0LDL0ZZ
  Thymus 07DM
  Tibia
    Left 0QDH0ZZ
    Right 0QDG0ZZ
  Toe Nail 0HDRXZZ
  Tooth
    Lower 0CDXXZ
    Upper 0CDWXZ
  Trachea 0BD1
  Turbinate, Nasal 09DL
  Tympanic Membrane
    Left 09D8
    Right 09D7
  Ulna
    Left 0PDL0ZZ
    Right 0PDK0ZZ
  Vein
    Basilic
      Left 05DC
      Right 05DB
    Brachial
      Left 05DA
      Right 05D9
    Cephalic
      Left 05DF
      Right 05DD
    Femoral
      Left 06DN
      Right 06DM
    Foot
      Left 06DV
      Right 06DT
    Hand
      Left 05DH
      Right 05DG
    Lower 06DY
    Saphenous
      Left 06DQ
      Right 06DP
    Upper 05DY
  Vertebra
    Cervical 0PD30ZZ
    Lumbar 0QD00ZZ
    Thoracic 0PD40ZZ
  Vocal Cord
    Left 0CDV
    Right 0CDT

Extradural space, intracranial
 use Epidural Space, Intracranial
Extradural space, spinal
 use Spinal Canal
EXtreme Lateral Interbody Fusion (XLIF) device
 use Interbody Fusion Device in Lower Joints

F

Face lift
 see Alteration, Face 0W02
Facet replacement spinal stabilization device
 use Spinal Stabilization Device, Facet Replacement in 0RH
 use Spinal Stabilization Device, Facet Replacement in 0SH
Facial artery
 use Face Artery
Factor Xa Inhibitor Reversal Agent, Andexanet Alfa
 use Coagulation Factor Xa, Inactivated
False vocal cord
 use Larynx
Falx cerebri
 use Dura Mater
Fascia lata
 use Subcutaneous Tissue and Fascia, Right Upper Leg
 use Subcutaneous Tissue and Fascia, Left Upper Leg
Fasciaplasty, fascioplasty
 see Repair, Subcutaneous Tissue and Fascia 0JQ
 see Replacement, Subcutaneous Tissue and Fascia 0JR
Fasciectomy
 see Excision, Subcutaneous Tissue and Fascia 0JB
Fasciorrhaphy
 see Repair, Subcutaneous Tissue and Fascia 0JQ
Fasciotomy
 see Division, Subcutaneous Tissue and Fascia 0J8
 see Drainage, Subcutaneous Tissue and Fascia 0J9
 see Release
Feeding Device
 Change device in
  Lower 0D2DXUZ
  Upper 0D20XUZ
 Insertion of device in
  Duodenum 0DH9
  Esophagus 0DH5
  Ileum 0DHB
  Intestine, Small 0DH8
  Jejunum 0DHA
  Stomach 0DH6
 Removal of device from
  Esophagus 0DP5
  Intestinal Tract
   Lower 0DPD
   Upper 0DP0
  Stomach 0DP6
 Revision of device in
  Intestinal Tract
   Lower 0DWD
   Upper 0DW0
  Stomach 0DW6
Femoral head
 use Upper Femur, Right
 use Upper Femur, Left

Femoral lymph node
 use Lymphatic, Right Lower Extremity
 use Lymphatic, Left Lower Extremity
Femoropatellar joint
 use Knee Joint, Right
 use Knee Joint, Left
 use Knee Joint, Femoral Surface, Right
 use Knee Joint, Femoral Surface, Left
Femorotibial joint
 use Knee Joint, Right
 use Knee Joint, Left
 use Knee Joint, Tibial Surface, Right
 use Knee Joint, Tibial Surface, Left
FETROJA®
 use Cefiderocol Anti-infective
FGS (fluorescence-guided surgery)
 see Fluorescence Guided Procedure
Fibular artery
 use Peroneal Artery, Right
 use Peroneal Artery, Left
Fibularis brevis muscle
 use Lower Leg Muscle, Right
 use Lower Leg Muscle, Left
Fibularis longus muscle
 use Lower Leg Muscle, Right
 use Lower Leg Muscle, Left
Fifth cranial nerve
 use Trigeminal Nerve
Filum terminale
 use Spinal Meninges
Fimbriectomy
 see Excision, Female Reproductive System 0UB
 see Resection, Female Reproductive System 0UT
Fine needle aspiration
 Fluid or gas *see* Drainage
 Tissue biopsy
  see Excision
  see Extraction
First cranial nerve
 use Olfactory Nerve
First intercostal nerve
 use Brachial Plexus
Fistulization
 see Bypass
 see Drainage
 see Repair
Fitting
 Arch bars, for fracture reduction *see* Reposition, Mouth and Throat 0CS
 Arch bars, for immobilization *see* Immobilization, Face 2W31
 Artificial limb *see* Device Fitting, Rehabilitation F0D
 Hearing aid *see* Device Fitting, Rehabilitation F0D
 Ocular prosthesis F0DZ8UZ
 Prosthesis, limb *see* Device Fitting, Rehabilitation F0D
 Prosthesis, ocular F0DZ8UZ
Fixation, bone
 External, with fracture reduction *see* Reposition
 External, without fracture reduction *see* Insertion
 Internal, with fracture reduction *see* Reposition
 Internal, without fracture reduction *see* Insertion
FLAIR® Endovascular Stent Graft
 use Intraluminal Device
Flexible Composite Mesh
 use Synthetic Substitute
Flexor carpi radialis muscle
 use Lower Arm and Wrist Muscle, Right
 use Lower Arm and Wrist Muscle, Left

Flexor carpi ulnaris muscle
 use Lower Arm and Wrist Muscle, Right
 use Lower Arm and Wrist Muscle, Left
Flexor digitorum brevis muscle
 use Foot Muscle, Right
 use Foot Muscle, Left
Flexor digitorum longus muscle
 use Lower Leg Muscle, Right
 use Lower Leg Muscle, Left
Flexor hallucis brevis muscle
 use Foot Muscle, Right
 use Foot Muscle, Left
Flexor hallucis longus muscle
 use Lower Leg Muscle, Right
 use Lower Leg Muscle, Left
Flexor pollicis longus muscle
 use Lower Arm and Wrist Muscle, Right
 use Lower Arm and Wrist Muscle, Left
Flow Diverter embolization device
 use Intraluminal Device, Flow Diverter in 03V
Fluorescence Guided Procedure
 Extremity
  Lower 8E0Y
  Upper 8E0X
 Head and Neck Region 8E09
  Aminolevulinic Acid 8E090EM
  No Qualifier 8E090EZ
 Trunk Region 8E0W
Fluorescent Pyrazine, Kidney   XT25XE5
Fluoroscopy
 Abdomen and Pelvis BW11
 Airway, Upper BB1DZZZ
 Ankle
  Left BQ1H
  Right BQ1G
 Aorta
  Abdominal B410
   Laser, Intraoperative B410
  Thoracic B310
   Laser, Intraoperative B310
  Thoraco-Abdominal B31P
   Laser, Intraoperative B31P
 Aorta and Bilateral Lower Extremity Arteries B41D
  Laser, Intraoperative B41D
 Arm
  Left BP1FZZZ
  Right BP1EZZZ
 Artery
  Brachiocephalic-Subclavian
   Right B311
    Laser, Intraoperative B311
  Bronchial B31L
   Laser, Intraoperative B31L
  Bypass Graft, Other B21F
  Cervico-Cerebral Arch B31Q
   Laser, Intraoperative B31Q
  Common Carotid
   Bilateral B315
    Laser, Intraoperative B315
   Left B314
    Laser, Intraoperative B314
   Right B313
    Laser, Intraoperative B313
  Coronary
   Bypass Graft
    Multiple B213
     Laser, Intraoperative B213
    Single B212
     Laser, Intraoperative B212
   Multiple B211
    Laser, Intraoperative B211
   Single B210
    Laser, Intraoperative B210
  External Carotid
   Bilateral B31C

Fluoroscopy — *continued*
    Artery — *continued*
        Laser, Intraoperative B31C
      Left B31B
        Laser, Intraoperative B31B
      Right B319
        Laser, Intraoperative B319
      Hepatic B412
        Laser, Intraoperative B412
      Inferior Mesenteric B415
        Laser, Intraoperative B415
      Intercostal B31L
        Laser, Intraoperative B31L
      Internal Carotid
        Bilateral B318
          Laser, Intraoperative B318
        Left B317
          Laser, Intraoperative B317
        Right B316
          Laser, Intraoperative B316
      Internal Mammary Bypass Graft
        Left B218
        Right B217
      Intra-Abdominal
        Other B41B
        Laser, Intraoperative B41B
      Intracranial B31R
        Laser, Intraoperative B31R
      Lower
        Other B41J
        Laser, Intraoperative B41J
      Lower Extremity
        Bilateral and Aorta B41D
          Laser, Intraoperative B41D
        Left B41G
          Laser, Intraoperative B41G
        Right B41F
          Laser, Intraoperative B41F
      Lumbar B419
        Laser, Intraoperative B419
      Pelvic B41C
        Laser, Intraoperative B41C
      Pulmonary
        Left B31T
          Laser, Intraoperative B31T
        Right B31S
          Laser, Intraoperative B31S
      Pulmonary Trunk B31U
        Laser, Intraoperative B31U
      Renal
        Bilateral B418
          Laser, Intraoperative B418
        Left B417
          Laser, Intraoperative B417
        Right B416
          Laser, Intraoperative B416
      Spinal B31M
        Laser, Intraoperative B31M
      Splenic B413
        Laser, Intraoperative B413
      Subclavian
        Left B312
        Laser, Intraoperative B312
      Superior Mesenteric B414
        Laser, Intraoperative B414
      Upper
        Other B31N
        Laser, Intraoperative B31N
      Upper Extremity
        Bilateral B31K
          Laser, Intraoperative B31K
        Left B31J
          Laser, Intraoperative B31J
        Right B31H
          Laser, Intraoperative B31H
      Vertebral
        Bilateral B31G

Fluoroscopy — *continued*
    Artery — *continued*
        Laser, Intraoperative B31G
      Left B31F
        Laser, Intraoperative B31F
      Right B31D
        Laser, Intraoperative B31D
    Bile Duct BF10
      Pancreatic Duct and Gallbladder BF14
    Bile Duct and Gallbladder BF13
    Biliary Duct BF11
    Bladder BT10
      Kidney and Ureter BT14
        Left BT1F
        Right BT1D
    Bladder and Urethra BT1B
    Bowel, Small BD1
    Calcaneus
      Left BQ1KZZZ
      Right BQ1JZZZ
    Clavicle
      Left BP15ZZZ
      Right BP14ZZZ
    Coccyx BR1F
    Colon BD14
    Corpora Cavernosa BV10
    Dialysis Fistula B51W
    Dialysis Shunt B51W
    Diaphragm BB16ZZZ
    Disc
      Cervical BR11
      Lumbar BR13
      Thoracic BR12
    Duodenum BD19
    Elbow
      Left BP1H
      Right BP1G
    Epiglottis B91G
    Esophagus BD11
    Extremity
      Lower BW1C
      Upper BW1J
    Facet Joint
      Cervical BR14
      Lumbar BR16
      Thoracic BR15
    Fallopian Tube
      Bilateral BU12
      Left BU11
      Right BU10
    Fallopian Tube and Uterus BU18
    Femur
      Left BQ14ZZZ
      Right BQ13ZZZ
    Finger
      Left BP1SZZZ
      Right BP1RZZZ
    Foot
      Left BQ1MZZZ
      Right BQ1LZZZ
    Forearm
      Left BP1KZZZ
      Right BP1JZZZ
    Gallbladder BF12
      Bile Duct and Pancreatic Duct BF14
    Gallbladder and Bile Duct BF13
    Gastrointestinal, Upper BD1
    Hand
      Left BP1PZZZ
      Right BP1NZZZ
    Head and Neck BW19
    Heart
      Left B215
      Right B214
      Right and Left B216
    Hip
      Left BQ11
      Right BQ10

Fluoroscopy — *continued*
    Humerus
      Left BP1BZZZ
      Right BP1AZZZ
    Ileal Diversion Loop BT1C
    Ileal Loop, Ureters and Kidney BT1G
    Intracranial Sinus B512
    Joint
      Acromioclavicular, Bilateral BP13ZZZ
      Finger
        Left BP1D
        Right BP1C
      Foot
        Left BQ1Y
        Right BQ1X
      Hand
        Left BP1D
        Right BP1C
      Lumbosacral BR1B
      Sacroiliac BR1D
      Sternoclavicular
        Bilateral BP12ZZZ
        Left BP11ZZZ
        Right BP10ZZZ
      Temporomandibular
        Bilateral BN19
        Left BN18
        Right BN17
      Thoracolumbar BR18
      Toe
        Left BQ1Y
        Right BQ1X
    Kidney
      Bilateral BT13
      Ileal Loop and Ureter BT1G
      Left BT12
      Right BT11
      Ureter and Bladder BT14
        Left BT1F
        Right BT1D
    Knee
      Left BQ18
      Right BQ17
    Larynx B91J
    Leg
      Left BQ1FZZZ
      Right BQ1DZZZ
    Lung
      Bilateral BB14ZZZ
      Left BB13ZZZ
      Right BB12ZZZ
    Mediastinum BB1CZZZ
    Mouth BD1B
    Neck and Head BW19
    Oropharynx BD1B
    Pancreatic Duct BF1
      Gallbladder and Bile Duct BF14
    Patella
      Left BQ1WZZZ
      Right BQ1VZZZ
    Pelvis BR1C
    Pelvis and Abdomen BW11
    Pharynx B91G
    Ribs
      Left BP1YZZZ
      Right BP1XZZZ
    Sacrum BR1F
    Scapula
      Left BP17ZZZ
      Right BP16ZZZ
    Shoulder
      Left BP19
      Right BP18
    Sinus, Intracranial B512
    Spinal Cord B01B
    Spine
      Cervical BR10

Fluoroscopy — *continued*
  Spine — *continued*
    Lumbar BR19
    Thoracic BR17
    Whole BR1G
  Sternum BR1H
  Stomach BD12
  Toe
    Left BQ1QZZZ
    Right BQ1PZZZ
  Tracheobronchial Tree
    Bilateral BB19YZZ
    Left BB18YZZ
    Right BB17YZZ
  Ureter
    Ileal Loop and Kidney BT1G
    Kidney and Bladder BT14
      Left BT1F
      Right BT1D
    Left BT17
    Right BT16
  Urethra BT15
  Urethra and Bladder BT1B
  Uterus BU16
  Uterus and Fallopian Tube BU18
  Vagina BU19
  Vasa Vasorum BV18
  Vein
    Cerebellar B511
    Cerebral B511
    Epidural B510
    Jugular
      Bilateral B515
      Left B514
      Right B513
    Lower Extremity
      Bilateral B51D
      Left B51C
      Right B51B
    Other B51V
    Pelvic (Iliac)
      Left B51G
      Right B51F
    Pelvic (Iliac) Bilateral B51H
    Portal B51T
    Pulmonary
      Bilateral B51S
      Left B51R
      Right B51Q
    Renal
      Bilateral B51L
      Left B51K
      Right B51J
    Splanchnic B51T
    Subclavian
      Left B517
      Right B516
    Upper Extremity
      Bilateral B51P
      Left B51N
      Right B51M
  Vena Cava
    Inferior B519
    Superior B518
  Wrist
    Left BP1M
    Right BP1L
Fluoroscopy, laser intraoperative
  see Fluoroscopy, Heart B21
  see Fluoroscopy, Upper Arteries B31
  see Fluoroscopy, Lower Arteries B41
Flushing
  see Irrigation
Foley catheter
  use Drainage Device
Fontan completion procedure Stage II
  see Bypass, Vena Cava, Inferior 0610

Foramen magnum
  use Occipital Bone
Foramen of Monro (intraventricular)
  use Cerebral Ventricle
Foreskin
  use Prepuce
Formula™ Balloon-Expandable Renal Stent System
  use Intraluminal Device
Fosfomycin Anti-infective XW0
Fosfomycin injection
  use Fosfomycin Anti-infective
Fossa of Rosenmuller
  use Nasopharynx
Fourth cranial nerve
  use Trochlear Nerve
Fourth ventricle
  use Cerebral Ventricle
Fovea
  use Retina, Right
  use Retina, Left
Fragmentation
  Ampulla of Vater 0FFC
  Anus 0DFQ
  Appendix 0DFJ
  Artery
    Anterior Tibial
      Left 04FQ3Z
      Right 04FP3Z
    Axillary
      Left 03F63Z
      Right 03F53Z
    Brachial
      Left 03F83Z
      Right 03F73Z
    Common Iliac
      Left 04FD3Z
      Right 04FC3Z
    External Iliac
      Left 04FJ3Z
      Right 04FH3Z
    Femoral
      Left 04FL3Z
      Right 04FK3Z
    Innominate 03F23Z
    Internal Iliac
      Left 04FF3Z
      Right 04FE3Z
    Lower 04FY3Z
    Peroneal
      Left 04FU3Z
      Right 04FT3Z
    Popliteal
      Left 04FN3Z
      Right 04FM3Z
    Posterior Tibial
      Left 04FS3Z
      Right 04FR3Z
    Pulmonary
      Left 02FR3Z
      Right 02FQ3Z
    Pulmonary Trunk 02FP3Z
    Radial
      Left 03FC3Z
      Right 03FB3Z
    Subclavian
      Left 03F43Z
      Right 03F33Z
    Ulnar
      Left 03FA3Z
      Right 03F93Z
    Upper 03FY3Z
  Bladder 0TFB
  Bladder Neck 0TFC
  Bronchus
    Lingula 0BF9

Fragmentation — *continued*
  Bronchus — *continued*
    Lower Lobe
      Left 0BFB
      Right 0BF6
    Main
      Left 0BF7
      Right 0BF3
    Middle Lobe, Right 0BF5
    Upper Lobe
      Left 0BF8
      Right 0BF4
  Carina 0BF2
  Cavity, Cranial 0WF1
  Cecum 0DFH
  Cerebral Ventricle 00F6
  Colon
    Ascending 0DFK
    Descending 0DFM
    Sigmoid 0DFN
    Transverse 0DFL
  Duct
    Common Bile 0FF9
    Cystic 0FF8
    Hepatic
      Common 0FF7
      Left 0FF6
      Right 0FF5
    Pancreatic 0FFD
      Accessory 0FFF
    Parotid
      Left 0CFC
      Right 0CFB
  Duodenum 0DF9
  Epidural Space, Intracranial 00F3
  Esophagus 0DF5
  Fallopian Tube
    Left 0UF6
    Right 0UF5
  Fallopian Tubes, Bilateral 0UF7
  Gallbladder 0FF4
  Gastrointestinal Tract 0WFP
  Genitourinary Tract 0WFR
  Ileum 0DFB
  Intestine
    Large 0DFE
      Left 0DFG
      Right 0DFF
    Small 0DF8
  Jejunum 0DFA
  Kidney Pelvis
    Left 0TF4
    Right 0TF3
  Mediastinum 0WFC
  Oral Cavity and Throat 0WF3
  Pelvic Cavity 0WFJ
  Pericardial Cavity 0WFD
  Pericardium 02FN
  Peritoneal Cavity 0WFG
  Pleural Cavity
    Left 0WFB
    Right 0WF9
  Rectum 0DFP
  Respiratory Tract 0WFQ
  Spinal Canal 00FU
  Stomach 0DF6
  Subarachnoid Space, Intracranial 00F5
  Subdural Space, Intracranial 00F4
  Trachea 0BF1
  Ureter
    Left 0TF7
    Right 0TF6
  Urethra 0TFD
  Uterus 0UF9
  Vein
    Axillary
      Left 05F83Z
      Right 05F73Z

Fragmentation — *continued*
  Vein — *continued*
    Basilic
      Left 05FC3Z
      Right 05FB3Z
    Brachial
      Left 05FA3Z
      Right 05F93Z
    Cephalic
      Left 05FF3Z
      Right 05FD3Z
    Common Iliac
      Left 06FD3Z
      Right 06FC3Z
    External Iliac
      Left 06FG3Z
      Right 06FF3Z
    Femoral
      Left 06FN3Z
      Right 06FM3Z
    Hypogastric
      Left 06FJ3Z
      Right 06FH3Z
    Innominate
      Left 05F43Z
      Right 05F33Z
    Lower 06FY3Z
    Pulmonary
      Left 02FT3Z
      Right 02FS3Z
    Saphenous
      Left 06FQ3Z
      Right 06FP3Z
    Subclavian
      Left 05F63Z
      Right 05F53Z
    Upper 05FY3Z
  Vitreous
    Left 08F5
    Right 08F4
Fragmentation, Ultrasonic
  see Fragmentation, Artery
Freestyle (Stentless) Aortic Root Bioprosthesis
  use Zooplastic Tissue in Heart and Great Vessels
Frenectomy
  see Excision, Mouth and Throat 0CB
  see Resection, Mouth and Throat 0CT
Frenoplasty, frenuloplasty
  see Repair, Mouth and Throat 0CQ
  see Replacement, Mouth and Throat 0CR
  see Supplement, Mouth and Throat 0CU
Frenotomy
  see Drainage, Mouth and Throat 0C9
  see Release, Mouth and Throat 0CN
Frenulotomy
  see Drainage, Mouth and Throat 0C9
  see Release, Mouth and Throat 0CN
Frenulum labii inferioris
  use Lower Lip
Frenulum labii superioris
  use Upper Lip
Frenulum linguae
  use Tongue
Frenulumectomy
  see Excision, Mouth and Throat 0CB
  see Resection, Mouth and Throat 0CT
Frontal lobe
  use Cerebral Hemisphere
Frontal vein
  use Face Vein, Right
  use Face Vein, Left
Fulguration
  see Destruction
Fundoplication, gastroesophageal
  see Restriction, Esophagogastric Junction 0DV4

Fundus uteri
  use Uterus
Fusion
  Acromioclavicular
    Left 0RGH
    Right 0RGG
  Ankle
    Left 0SGG
    Right 0SGF
  Carpal
    Left 0RGR
    Right 0RGQ
  Carpometacarpal
    Left 0RGT
    Right 0RGS
  Cervical Vertebral 0RG1
    2 or more 0RG2
      Interbody Fusion Device
        Nanotextured Surface XRG2092
        Radiolucent Porous XRG20F3
    Interbody Fusion Device
      Nanotextured Surface XRG1092
      Radiolucent Porous XRG10F3
  Cervicothoracic Vertebral 0RG4
    Interbody Fusion Device
      Nanotextured Surface XRG4092
      Radiolucent Porous XRG40F3
  Coccygeal 0SG6
  Elbow
    Left 0RGM
    Right 0RGL
  Finger Phalangeal
    Left 0RGX
    Right 0RGW
  Hip
    Left 0SGB
    Right 0SG9
  Knee
    Left 0SGD
    Right 0SGC
  Lumbar Vertebral 0SG0
    2 or more 0SG1
      Interbody Fusion Device
        Nanotextured Surface XRGC092
        Radiolucent Porous XRGC0F3
    Interbody Fusion Device
      Nanotextured Surface XRGB092
      Radiolucent Porous XRGB0F3
  Lumbosacral 0SG3
    Interbody Fusion Device
      Nanotextured Surface XRGD092
      Radiolucent Porous XRGD0F3
  Metacarpophalangeal
    Left 0RGV
    Right 0RGU
  Metatarsal-Phalangeal
    Left 0SGN
    Right 0SGM
  Occipital-cervical 0RG0
    Interbody Fusion Device
      Nanotextured Surface XRG0092
      Radiolucent Porous XRG00F3
  Sacrococcygeal 0SG5
  Sacroiliac
    Left 0SG8
    Right 0SG7
  Shoulder
    Left 0RGK
    Right 0RGJ
  Sternoclavicular
    Left 0RGF
    Right 0RGE
  Tarsal
    Left 0SGJ
    Right 0SGH

Fusion — *continued*
  Tarsometatarsal
    Left 0SGL
    Right 0SGK
  Temporomandibular
    Left 0RGD
    Right 0RGC
  Thoracic Vertebral 0RG6
    2 to 7 0RG7
      Interbody Fusion Device
        Nanotextured Surface XRG7092
        Radiolucent Porous XRG70F3
    8 or more 0RG8
      Interbody Fusion Device
        Nanotextured Surface XRG8092
        Radiolucent Porous XRG80F3
    Interbody Fusion Device
      Nanotextured Surface XRG6092
      Radiolucent Porous XRG60F3
  Thoracolumbar Vertebral 0RGA
    Interbody Fusion Device
      Nanotextured Surface XRGA092
      Radiolucent Porous XRGA0F3
  Toe Phalangeal
    Left 0SGQ
    Right 0SGP
  Wrist
    Left 0RGP
    Right 0RGN
Fusion screw (compression)(lag)(locking)
  use Internal Fixation Device in Upper Joints
  use Internal Fixation Device in Lower Joints

G

Gait training
  see Motor Treatment, Rehabilitation F07
Galea aponeurotica
  use Subcutaneous Tissue and Fascia, Scalp
GammaTile™
  use Radioactive Element, Cesium-131 Collagen Implant in 00H
Ganglion impar (ganglion of Walther)
  use Sacral Sympathetic Nerve
Ganglionectomy
  Destruction of lesion *see* Destruction
  Excision of lesion *see* Excision
Gasserian ganglion
  use Trigeminal Nerve
Gastrectomy
  Partial *see* Excision, Stomach 0DB6
  Total *see* Resection, Stomach 0DT6
  Vertical (sleeve) *see* Excision, Stomach 0DB6
Gastric electrical stimulation (GES) lead
  use Stimulator Lead in Gastrointestinal System
Gastric lymph node
  use Lymphatic, Aortic
Gastric pacemaker lead
  use Stimulator Lead in Gastrointestinal System
Gastric plexus
  use Abdominal Sympathetic Nerve
Gastrocnemius muscle
  use Lower Leg Muscle, Right
  use Lower Leg Muscle, Left
Gastrocolic ligament
  use Omentum
Gastrocolic omentum
  use Omentum
Gastrocolostomy
  see Bypass, Gastrointestinal System 0D1
  see Drainage, Gastrointestinal System 0D9
Gastroduodenal artery
  use Hepatic Artery

Gastroduodenectomy
  see Excision, Gastrointestinal System 0DB
  see Resection, Gastrointestinal System 0DT
Gastroduodenoscopy 0DJ08ZZ
Gastroenteroplasty
  see Repair, Gastrointestinal System 0DQ
  see Supplement, Gastrointestinal
    System 0DU
Gastroenterostomy
  see Bypass, Gastrointestinal System 0D1
  see Drainage, Gastrointestinal System 0D9
Gastroesophageal (GE) junction
  use Esophagogastric Junction
Gastrogastrostomy
  see Bypass, Stomach 0D16
  see Drainage, Stomach 0D96
Gastrohepatic omentum
  use Omentum
Gastrojejunostomy
  see Bypass, Stomach 0D16
  see Drainage, Stomach 0D96
Gastrolysis
  see Release, Stomach 0DN6
Gastropexy
  see Repair, Stomach 0DQ6
  see Reposition, Stomach 0DS6
Gastrophrenic ligament
  use Omentum
Gastroplasty
  see Repair, Stomach 0DQ6
  see Supplement, Stomach 0DU6
Gastroplication
  see Restriction, Stomach 0DV6
Gastropylorectomy
  see Excision, Gastrointestinal System 0DB
Gastrorrhaphy
  see Repair, Stomach 0DQ6
Gastroscopy 0DJ68ZZ
Gastrosplenic ligament
  use Omentum
Gastrostomy
  see Bypass, Stomach 0D16
  see Drainage, Stomach 0D96
Gastrotomy
  see Drainage, Stomach 0D96
Gemellus muscle
  use Hip Muscle, Right
  use Hip Muscle, Left
Geniculate ganglion
  use Facial Nerve
Geniculate nucleus
  use Thalamus
Genioglossus muscle
  use Tongue, Palate, Pharynx Muscle
Genioplasty
  see Alteration, Jaw, Lower 0W05
Genitofemoral nerve
  use Lumbar Plexus
GIAPREZA™
  use Synthetic Human Angiotensin II
Gilteritinib Antineoplastic XW0DXV5
Gingivectomy
  see Excision, Mouth and Throat 0CB
Gingivoplasty
  see Repair, Mouth and Throat 0CQ
  see Replacement, Mouth and Throat 0CR
  see Supplement, Mouth and Throat 0CU
Glans penis
  use Prepuce
Glenohumeral joint
  use Shoulder Joint, Right
  use Shoulder Joint, Left
Glenohumeral ligament
  use Shoulder Bursa and Ligament, Right
  use Shoulder Bursa and Ligament, Left
Glenoid fossa (of scapula)
  use Glenoid Cavity, Right
  use Glenoid Cavity, Left

Glenoid ligament (labrum)
  use Shoulder Joint, Right
  use Shoulder Joint, Left
Globus pallidus
  use Basal Ganglia
Glomectomy
  see Excision, Endocrine System 0GB
  see Resection, Endocrine System 0GT
Glossectomy
  see Excision, Tongue 0CB7
  see Resection, Tongue 0CT7
Glossoepiglottic fold
  use Epiglottis
Glossopexy
  see Repair, Tongue 0CQ7
  see Reposition, Tongue 0CS7
Glossoplasty
  see Repair, Tongue 0CQ7
  see Replacement, Tongue 0CR7
  see Supplement, Tongue 0CU7
Glossorrhaphy
  see Repair, Tongue 0CQ7
Glossotomy
  see Drainage, Tongue 0C97
Glottis
  use Larynx
Gluteal Artery Perforator Flap
  Replacement
    Bilateral 0HRV079
    Left 0HRU079
    Right 0HRT079
  Transfer
    Left 0KXG
    Right 0KXF
Gluteal lymph node
  use Lymphatic, Pelvis
Gluteal vein
  use Hypogastric Vein, Right
  use Hypogastric Vein, Left
Gluteus maximus muscle
  use Hip Muscle, Right
  use Hip Muscle, Left
Gluteus medius muscle
  use Hip Muscle, Right
  use Hip Muscle, Left
Gluteus minimus muscle
  use Hip Muscle, Right
  use Hip Muscle, Left
GORE EXCLUDER® AAA Endoprosthesis
  use Intraluminal Device, Branched or
    Fenestrated, One or Two Arteries in 04V
  use Intraluminal Device, Branched or
    Fenestrated, Three or More Arteries in 04V
  use Intraluminal Device
GORE EXCLUDER® IBE Endoprosthesis
  use Intraluminal Device, Branched or
    Fenestrated, One or Two Arteries in 04V
GORE TAG® Thoracic Endoprosthesis
  use Intraluminal Device
GORE® DUALMESH®
  use Synthetic Substitute
Gracilis muscle
  use Upper Leg Muscle, Right
  use Upper Leg Muscle, Left
Graft
  see Replacement
  see Supplement
Great auricular nerve
  use Cervical Plexus
Great cerebral vein
  use Intracranial Vein
Great(er) saphenous vein
  use Saphenous Vein, Right
  use Saphenous Vein, Left
Greater alar cartilage
  use Nasal Mucosa and Soft Tissue
Greater occipital nerve
  use Cervical Nerve

Greater Omentum
  use Omentum
Greater splanchnic nerve
  use Thoracic Sympathetic Nerve
Greater superficial petrosal nerve
  use Facial Nerve
Greater trochanter
  use Upper Femur, Right
  use Upper Femur, Left
Greater tuberosity
  use Humeral Head, Right
  use Humeral Head, Left
Greater vestibular (Bartholin's) gland
  use Vestibular Gland
Greater wing
  use Sphenoid Bone
GS-5734
  use Remdesivir Anti-infective
Guedel airway
  use Intraluminal Device, Airway in Mouth
    and Throat
Guidance, catheter placement
  EKG *see* Measurement, Physiological
    Systems 4A0
  Fluoroscopy *see* Fluoroscopy, Veins B51
  Ultrasound *see* Ultrasonography, Veins B54

H

Hallux
  use 1st Toe, Right
  use 1st Toe, Left
Hamate bone
  use Carpal, Right
  use Carpal, Left
Hancock Bioprosthesis (aortic) (mitral)
valve
  use Zooplastic Tissue in Heart and Great
    Vessels
Hancock Bioprosthetic Valved Conduit
  use Zooplastic Tissue in Heart and Great
    Vessels
Harvesting, stem cells
  see Pheresis, Circulatory 6A55
Head of fibula
  use Fibula, Right
  use Fibula, Left
Hearing Aid Assessment F14Z
Hearing Assessment F13Z
Hearing Device
  Bone Conduction
    Left 09HE
    Right 09HD
  Insertion of device in
    Left 0NH6
    Right 0NH5
  Multiple Channel Cochlear Prosthesis
    Left 09HE
    Right 09HD
  Removal of device from, Skull 0NP0
  Revision of device in, Skull 0NW0
  Single Channel Cochlear Prosthesis
    Left 09HE
    Right 09HD
Hearing Treatment F09Z
Heart Assist System
  Implantable
    Insertion of device in, Heart 02HA
    Removal of device from, Heart 02PA
    Revision of device in, Heart 02WA
  Short-term External
    Insertion of device in, Heart 02HA
    Removal of device from, Heart 02PA
    Revision of device in, Heart 02WA
HeartMate 3™ LVAS
  use Implantable Heart Assist System in
    Heart and Great Vessels

HeartMate II® Left Ventricular Assist Device (LVAD)
  use Implantable Heart Assist System in Heart and Great Vessels
HeartMate XVE® Left Ventricular Assist Device (LVAD)
  use Implantable Heart Assist System in Heart and Great Vessels
HeartMate® implantable heart assist system
  see Insertion of device in, Heart 02HA
Helix
  use External Ear, Right
  use External Ear, Left
  use External Ear, Bilateral
Hematopoietic cell transplant (HCT)
  see Transfusion, Circulatory 302
Hemicolectomy
  see Resection, Gastrointestinal System 0DT
Hemicystectomy
  see Excision, Urinary System 0TB
Hemigastrectomy
  see Excision, Gastrointestinal System 0DB
Hemiglossectomy
  see Excision, Mouth and Throat 0CB
Hemilaminectomy
  see Excision, Upper Bones 0PB
  see Excision, Lower Bones 0QB
Hemilaminotomy
  see Release, Central Nervous System and Cranial Nerves 00N
  see Release, Peripheral Nervous System 01N
  see Drainage, Upper Bones 0P9
  see Excision, Upper Bones 0PB
  see Release, Upper Bones 0PN
  see Drainage, Lower Bones 0Q9
  see Excision, Lower Bones 0QB
  see Release, Lower Bones 0QN
Hemilaryngectomy
  see Excision, Larynx 0CBS
Hemimandibulectomy
  see Excision, Head and Facial Bones 0NB
Hemimaxillectomy
  see Excision, Head and Facial Bones 0NB
Hemipylorectomy
  see Excision, Gastrointestinal System 0DB
Hemispherectomy
  see Excision, Central Nervous System and Cranial Nerves 00B
  see Resection, Central Nervous System and Cranial Nerves 00T
Hemithyroidectomy
  see Excision, Endocrine System 0GB
  see Resection, Endocrine System 0GT
Hemodialysis
  see Performance, Urinary 5A1D
Hemolung® Respiratory Assist System (RAS) 5A0920Z
Hemospray® Endoscopic Hemostat
  use Mineral-based Topical Hemostatic Agent
Hepatectomy
  see Excision, Hepatobiliary System and Pancreas 0FB
  see Resection, Hepatobiliary System and Pancreas 0FT
Hepatic artery proper
  use Hepatic Artery
Hepatic flexure
  use Transverse Colon
Hepatic lymph node
  use Lymphatic, Aortic
Hepatic plexus
  use Abdominal Sympathetic Nerve
Hepatic portal vein
  use Portal Vein

Hepaticoduodenostomy
  see Bypass, Hepatobiliary System and Pancreas 0F1
  see Drainage, Hepatobiliary System and Pancreas 0F9
Hepaticotomy
  see Drainage, Hepatobiliary System and Pancreas 0F9
Hepatocholedochostomy
  see Drainage, Duct, Common Bile 0F99
Hepatogastric ligament
  use Omentum
Hepatopancreatic ampulla
  use Ampulla of Vater
Hepatopexy
  see Repair, Hepatobiliary System and Pancreas 0FQ
  see Reposition, Hepatobiliary System and Pancreas 0FS
Hepatorrhaphy
  see Repair, Hepatobiliary System and Pancreas 0FQ
Hepatotomy
  see Drainage, Hepatobiliary System and Pancreas 0F9
Herculink (RX) Elite Renal Stent System
  use Intraluminal Device
Herniorrhaphy
  see Repair, Anatomical Regions, General 0WQ
  see Repair, Anatomical Regions, Lower Extremities 0YQ
  With synthetic substitute
    see Supplement, Anatomical Regions, General 0WU
    see Supplement, Anatomical Regions, Lower Extremities 0YU
Hip (joint) liner
  use Liner in Lower Joints
HIPEC (hyperthermic intraperitoneal chemotherapy) 3E0M30Y
Holter monitoring 4A12X45
Holter valve ventricular shunt
  use Synthetic Substitute
Human angiotensin II, synthetic
  use Synthetic Human Angiotensin II
Humeroradial joint
  use Elbow Joint, Right
  use Elbow Joint, Left
Humeroulnar joint
  use Elbow Joint, Right
  use Elbow Joint, Left
Humerus, distal
  use Humeral Shaft, Right
  use Humeral Shaft, Left
Hydrocelectomy
  see Excision, Male Reproductive System 0VB
Hydrotherapy
  Assisted exercise in pool see Motor Treatment, Rehabilitation F07
  Whirlpool see Activities of Daily Living Treatment, Rehabilitation F08
Hymenectomy
  see Excision, Hymen 0UBK
  see Resection, Hymen 0UTK
Hymenoplasty
  see Repair, Hymen 0UQK
  see Supplement, Hymen 0UUK
Hymenorrhaphy
  see Repair, Hymen 0UQK
Hymenotomy
  see Division, Hymen 0U8K
  see Drainage, Hymen 0U9K
Hyoglossus muscle
  use Tongue, Palate, Pharynx Muscle

Hyoid artery
  use Thyroid Artery, Right
  use Thyroid Artery, Left
Hyperalimentation
  see Introduction of substance in or on
Hyperbaric oxygenation
  Decompression sickness treatment see Decompression, Circulatory 6A15
  Wound treatment see Assistance, Circulatory 5A05
Hyperthermia
  Radiation Therapy
    Abdomen DWY38ZZ
    Adrenal Gland DGY28ZZ
    Bile Ducts DFY28ZZ
    Bladder DTY28ZZ
    Bone, Other DPYC8ZZ
    Bone Marrow D7Y08ZZ
    Brain D0Y08ZZ
    Brain Stem D0Y18ZZ
    Breast
      Left DMY08ZZ
      Right DMY18ZZ
    Bronchus DBY18ZZ
    Cervix DUY18ZZ
    Chest DWY28ZZ
    Chest Wall DBY78ZZ
    Colon DDY58ZZ
    Diaphragm DBY88ZZ
    Duodenum DDY28ZZ
    Ear D9Y08ZZ
    Esophagus DDY08ZZ
    Eye D8Y08ZZ
    Femur DPY98ZZ
    Fibula DPYB8ZZ
    Gallbladder DFY18ZZ
    Gland
      Adrenal DGY28ZZ
      Parathyroid DGY48ZZ
      Pituitary DGY08ZZ
      Thyroid DGY58ZZ
    Glands, Salivary D9Y68ZZ
    Head and Neck DWY18ZZ
    Hemibody DWY48ZZ
    Humerus DPY68ZZ
    Hypopharynx D9Y38ZZ
    Ileum DDY48ZZ
    Jejunum DDY38ZZ
    Kidney DTY08ZZ
    Larynx D9YB8ZZ
    Liver DFY08ZZ
    Lung DBY28ZZ
    Lymphatics
      Abdomen D7Y68ZZ
      Axillary D7Y48ZZ
      Inguinal D7Y88ZZ
      Neck D7Y38ZZ
      Pelvis D7Y78ZZ
      Thorax D7Y58ZZ
    Mandible DPY38ZZ
    Maxilla DPY28ZZ
    Mediastinum DBY68ZZ
    Mouth D9Y48ZZ
    Nasopharynx D9YD8ZZ
    Neck and Head DWY18ZZ
    Nerve, Peripheral D0Y78ZZ
    Nose D9Y18ZZ
    Oropharynx D9YF8ZZ
    Ovary DUY08ZZ
    Palate
      Hard D9Y88ZZ
      Soft D9Y98ZZ
    Pancreas DFY38ZZ
    Parathyroid Gland DGY48ZZ
    Pelvic Bones DPY88ZZ
    Pelvic Region DWY68ZZ

Hyperthermia — *continued*
  Radiation Therapy — *continued*
    Pineal Body DGY18ZZ
    Pituitary Gland DGY08ZZ
    Pleura DBY58ZZ
    Prostate DVY08ZZ
    Radius DPY78ZZ
    Rectum DDY78ZZ
    Rib DPY58ZZ
    Sinuses D9Y78ZZ
    Skin
      Abdomen DHY88ZZ
      Arm DHY48ZZ
      Back DHY78ZZ
      Buttock DHY98ZZ
      Chest DHY68ZZ
      Face DHY28ZZ
      Leg DHYB8ZZ
      Neck DHY38ZZ
    Skull DPY08ZZ
    Spinal Cord D0Y68ZZ
    Spleen D7Y28ZZ
    Sternum DPY48ZZ
    Stomach DDY18ZZ
    Testis DVY18ZZ
    Thymus D7Y18ZZ
    Thyroid Gland DGY58ZZ
    Tibia DPYB8ZZ
    Tongue D9Y58ZZ
    Trachea DBY08ZZ
    Ulna DPY78ZZ
    Ureter DTY18ZZ
    Urethra DTY38ZZ
    Uterus DUY28ZZ
    Whole Body DWY58ZZ
  Whole Body 6A3Z
Hyperthermic intraperitoneal chemotherapy (HIPEC) 3E0M30Y
Hypnosis GZFZZZZ
Hypogastric artery
  use Internal Iliac Artery, Right
  use Internal Iliac Artery, Left
Hypopharynx
  use Pharynx
Hypophysectomy
  see Excision, Gland, Pituitary 0GB0
  see Resection, Gland, Pituitary 0GT0
Hypophysis
  use Pituitary Gland
Hypothalamotomy
  see Destruction, Thalamus 0059
Hypothenar muscle
  use Hand Muscle, Right
  use Hand Muscle, Left
Hypothermia, Whole Body 6A4Z
Hysterectomy
  Supracervical *see* Resection, Uterus 0UT9
  Total *see* Resection, Uterus 0UT9
Hysterolysis
  see Release, Uterus 0UN9
Hysteropexy
  see Repair, Uterus 0UQ9
  see Reposition, Uterus 0US9
Hysteroplasty
  see Repair, Uterus 0UQ9
Hysterorrhaphy
  see Repair, Uterus 0UQ9
Hysteroscopy 0UJD8ZZ
Hysterotomy
  see Drainage, Uterus 0U99
Hysterotrachelectomy
  see Resection, Uterus 0UT9
  see Resection, Cervix 0UTC
Hysterotracheloplasty
  see Repair, Uterus 0UQ9
Hysterotrachelorrhaphy
  see Repair, Uterus 0UQ9

I

IABP (Intra-aortic balloon pump)
  see Assistance, Cardiac 5A02
IAEMT (Intraoperative anesthetic effect monitoring and titration)
  see Monitoring, Central Nervous 4A10
IASD® (InterAtrial Shunt Device), Corvia
  use Synthetic Substitute
Idarucizumab, Dabigatran Reversal Agent XW0
IHD (Intermittent hemodialysis) 5A1D70Z
Ileal artery
  use Superior Mesenteric Artery
Ileectomy
  see Excision, Ileum 0DBB
  see Resection, Ileum 0DTB
Ileocolic artery
  use Superior Mesenteric Artery
Ileocolic vein
  use Colic Vein
Ileopexy
  see Repair, Ileum 0DQB
  see Reposition, Ileum 0DSB
Ileorrhaphy
  see Repair, Ileum 0DQB
Ileoscopy 0DJD8ZZ
Ileostomy
  see Bypass, Ileum 0D1B
  see Drainage, Ileum 0D9B
Ileotomy
  see Drainage, Ileum 0D9B
Ileoureterostomy
  see Bypass, Urinary System 0T1
Iliac crest
  use Pelvic Bone, Right
  use Pelvic Bone, Left
Iliac fascia
  use Subcutaneous Tissue and Fascia, Right Upper Leg
  use Subcutaneous Tissue and Fascia, Left Upper Leg
Iliac lymph node
  use Lymphatic, Pelvis
Iliacus muscle
  use Hip Muscle, Right
  use Hip Muscle, Left
Iliofemoral ligament
  use Hip Bursa and Ligament, Right
  use Hip Bursa and Ligament, Left
Iliohypogastric nerve
  use Lumbar Plexus
Ilioinguinal nerve
  use Lumbar Plexus
Iliolumbar artery
  use Internal Iliac Artery, Right
  use Internal Iliac Artery, Left
Iliolumbar ligament
  use Lower Spine Bursa and Ligament
Iliotibial tract (band)
  use Subcutaneous Tissue and Fascia, Right Upper Leg
  use Subcutaneous Tissue and Fascia, Left Upper Leg
Ilium
  use Pelvic Bone, Right
  use Pelvic Bone, Left
Ilizarov external fixator
  use External Fixation Device, Ring in 0PH
  use External Fixation Device, Ring in 0PS
  use External Fixation Device, Ring in 0QH
  use External Fixation Device, Ring in 0QS
Ilizarov-Vecklich device
  use External Fixation Device, Limb Lengthening in 0PH
  use External Fixation Device, Limb Lengthening in 0QH

Imaging, diagnostic
  see Plain Radiography
  see Fluoroscopy
  see Computerized Tomography (CT Scan)
  see Magnetic Resonance Imaging (MRI)
  see Ultrasonography
IMFINZI®
  use Durvalumab Antineoplastic
IMI/REL
  use Imipenem-cilastatin-relebactam Anti-infective
Imipenem-cilastatin-relebactam Anti-infective XW0
Immobilization
  Abdominal Wall 2W33X
  Arm
    Lower
      Left 2W3DX
      Right 2W3CX
    Upper
      Left 2W3BX
      Right 2W3AX
  Back 2W35X
  Chest Wall 2W34X
  Extremity
    Lower
      Left 2W3MX
      Right 2W3LX
    Upper
      Left 2W39X
      Right 2W38X
  Face 2W31X
  Finger
    Left 2W3KX
    Right 2W3JX
  Foot
    Left 2W3TX
    Right 2W3SX
  Hand
    Left 2W3FX
    Right 2W3EX
  Head 2W30X
  Inguinal Region
    Left 2W37X
    Right 2W36X
  Leg
    Lower
      Left 2W3RX
      Right 2W3QX
    Upper
      Left 2W3PX
      Right 2W3NX
  Neck 2W32X
  Thumb
    Left 2W3HX
    Right 2W3GX
  Toe
    Left 2W3VX
    Right 2W3UX
Immunization
  see Introduction of Serum, Toxoid, and Vaccine
Immunotherapy
  see Introduction of Immunotherapeutic Substance
Immunotherapy, antineoplastic
  Interferon *see* Introduction of Low-dose Interleukin-2
  Interleukin-2, high-dose *see* Introduction of High-dose Interleukin-2
  Interleukin-2, low-dose *see* Introduction of Low dose Interleukin-2
  Monoclonal antibody *see* Introduction of Monoclonal Antibody
  Proleukin, high-dose *see* Introduction of High-dose Interleukin-2
  Proleukin, low-dose *see* Introduction of Low-dose Interleukin-2

Impella® heart pump
 use Short-term External Heart Assist System in Heart and Great Vessels
Impeller Pump
 Continuous, Output 5A0221D
 Intermittent, Output 5A0211D
Implantable cardioverter-defibrillator (ICD)
 use Defibrillator Generator in 0JH
Implantable drug infusion pump (anti-spasmodic)(chemotherapy)(pain)
 use Infusion Device, Pump in Subcutaneous Tissue and Fascia
Implantable glucose monitoring device
 use Monitoring Device
Implantable hemodynamic monitor (IHM)
 use Monitoring Device, Hemodynamic in 0JH
Implantable hemodynamic monitoring system (IHMS)
 use Monitoring Device, Hemodynamic in 0JH
Implantable Miniature Telescope™ (IMT)
 use Synthetic Substitute, Intraocular Telescope in 08R
Implantation
 see Replacement
 see Insertion
Implanted (venous)(access) port
 use Vascular Access Device, Totally Implantable in Subcutaneous Tissue and Fascia
IMV (intermittent mandatory ventilation)
 see Assistance, Respiratory 5A09
In Vitro Fertilization 8E0ZXY1
Incision, abscess
 see Drainage
Incudectomy
 see Excision, Ear, Nose, Sinus 09B
 see Resection, Ear, Nose, Sinus 09T
Incudopexy
 see Repair, Ear, Nose, Sinus 09Q
 see Reposition, Ear, Nose, Sinus 09S
Incus
 use Auditory Ossicle, Right
 use Auditory Ossicle, Left
Induction of labor
 Artificial rupture of membranes *see* Drainage, Pregnancy 109
 Oxytocin *see* Introduction of Hormone
InDura, intrathecal catheter (1P) (spinal)
 use Infusion Device
Inferior cardiac nerve
 use Thoracic Sympathetic Nerve
Inferior cerebellar vein
 use Intracranial Vein
Inferior cerebral vein
 use Intracranial Vein
Inferior epigastric artery
 use External Iliac Artery, Right
 use External Iliac Artery, Left
Inferior epigastric lymph node
 use Lymphatic, Pelvis
Inferior genicular artery
 use Popliteal Artery, Right
 use Popliteal Artery, Left
Inferior gluteal artery
 use Internal Iliac Artery, Right
 use Internal Iliac Artery, Left
Inferior gluteal nerve
 use Sacral Plexus
Inferior hypogastric plexus
 use Abdominal Sympathetic Nerve
Inferior labial artery
 use Face Artery
Inferior longitudinal muscle
 use Tongue, Palate, Pharynx Muscle

Inferior mesenteric ganglion
 use Abdominal Sympathetic Nerve
Inferior mesenteric lymph node
 use Lymphatic, Mesenteric
Inferior mesenteric plexus
 use Abdominal Sympathetic Nerve
Inferior oblique muscle
 use Extraocular Muscle, Right
 use Extraocular Muscle, Left
Inferior pancreaticoduodenal artery
 use Superior Mesenteric Artery
Inferior phrenic artery
 use Abdominal Aorta
Inferior rectus muscle
 use Extraocular Muscle, Right
 use Extraocular Muscle, Left
Inferior suprarenal artery
 use Renal Artery, Right
 use Renal Artery, Left
Inferior tarsal plate
 use Lower Eyelid, Right
 use Lower Eyelid, Left
Inferior thyroid vein
 use Innominate Vein, Right
 use Innominate Vein, Left
Inferior tibiofibular joint
 use Ankle Joint, Right
 use Ankle Joint, Left
Inferior turbinate
 use Nasal Turbinate
Inferior ulnar collateral artery
 use Brachial Artery, Right
 use Brachial Artery, Left
Inferior vesical artery
 use Internal Iliac Artery, Right
 use Internal Iliac Artery, Left
Infraauricular lymph node
 use Lymphatic, Head
Infraclavicular (deltopectoral) lymph node
 use Lymphatic, Right Upper Extremity
 use Lymphatic, Left Upper Extremity
Infrahyoid muscle
 use Neck Muscle, Right
 use Neck Muscle, Left
Infraparotid lymph node
 use Lymphatic, Head
Infraspinatus fascia
 use Subcutaneous Tissue and Fascia, Right Upper Arm
 use Subcutaneous Tissue and Fascia, Left Upper Arm
Infraspinatus muscle
 use Shoulder Muscle, Right
 use Shoulder Muscle, Left
Infundibulopelvic ligament
 use Uterine Supporting Structure
Infusion
 see Introduction of substance in or on
Infusion Device, Pump
 Insertion of device in
  Abdomen 0JH8
  Back 0JH7
  Chest 0JH6
  Lower Arm
   Left 0JHH
   Right 0JHG
  Lower Leg
   Left 0JHP
   Right 0JHN
  Trunk 0JHT
  Upper Arm
   Left 0JHF
   Right 0JHD
  Upper Leg
   Left 0JHM
   Right 0JHL

Infusion Device, Pump — *continued*
 Removal of device from
  Lower Extremity 0JPW
  Trunk 0JPT
  Upper Extremity 0JPV
 Revision of device in
  Lower Extremity 0JWW
  Trunk 0JWT
  Upper Extremity 0JWV
Infusion, glucarpidase
 Central vein 3E043GQ
 Peripheral vein 3E033GQ
Inguinal canal
 use Inguinal Region, Right
 use Inguinal Region, Left
 use Inguinal Region, Bilateral
Inguinal triangle
 use Inguinal Region, Right
 use Inguinal Region, Left
 use Inguinal Region, Bilateral
Injection
 see Introduction of substance in or on
Injection reservoir, port
 use Vascular Access Device, Totally Implantable in Subcutaneous Tissue and Fascia
Injection reservoir, pump
 use Infusion Device, Pump in Subcutaneous Tissue and Fascia
Injection, Concentrated Bone Marrow Aspirate (CBMA), intramuscular XK02303
Insemination, artificial 3E0P7LZ
Insertion
 Antimicrobial envelope *see* Introduction of Anti-infective
 Aqueous drainage shunt
  see Bypass, Eye 081
  see Drainage, Eye 089
 Products of Conception 10H0
 Spinal Stabilization Device
  see Insertion of device in, Upper Joints 0RH
  see Insertion of device in, Lower Joints 0SH
Insertion of device in
 Abdominal Wall 0WHF
 Acetabulum
  Left 0QH5
  Right 0QH4
 Anal Sphincter 0DHR
 Ankle Region
  Left 0YHL
  Right 0YHK
 Anus 0DHQ
 Aorta
  Abdominal 04H0
  Thoracic
   Ascending/Arch 02HX
   Descending 02HW
 Arm
  Lower
   Left 0XHF
   Right 0XHD
  Upper
   Left 0XH9
   Right 0XH8
 Artery
  Anterior Tibial
   Left 04HQ
   Right 04HP
  Axillary
   Left 03H6
   Right 03H5
  Brachial
   Left 03H8
   Right 03H7
  Celiac 04H1

Insertion of device in — *continued*
  Artery — *continued*
    Colic
      Left 04H7
      Middle 04H8
      Right 04H6
    Common Carotid
      Left 03HJ
      Right 03HH
    Common Iliac
      Left 04HD
      Right 04HC
    Coronary
      Four or More Arteries 02H3
      One Artery 02H0
      Three Arteries 02H2
      Two Arteries 02H1
    External Carotid
      Left 03HN
      Right 03HM
    External Iliac
      Left 04HJ
      Right 04HH
    Face 03HR
    Femoral
      Left 04HL
      Right 04HK
    Foot
      Left 04HW
      Right 04HV
    Gastric 04H2
    Hand
      Left 03HF
      Right 03HD
    Hepatic 04H3
    Inferior Mesenteric 04HB
    Innominate 03H2
    Internal Carotid
      Left 03HL
      Right 03HK
    Internal Iliac
      Left 04HF
      Right 04HE
    Internal Mammary
      Left 03H1
      Right 03H0
    Intracranial 03HG
    Lower 04HY
    Peroneal
      Left 04HU
      Right 04HT
    Popliteal
      Left 04HN
      Right 04HM
    Posterior Tibial
      Left 04HS
      Right 04HR
    Pulmonary
      Left 02HR
      Right 02HQ
    Pulmonary Trunk 02HP
    Radial
      Left 03HC
      Right 03HB
    Renal
      Left 04HA
      Right 04H9
    Splenic 04H4
    Subclavian
      Left 03H4
      Right 03H3
    Superior Mesenteric 04H5
    Temporal
      Left 03HT
      Right 03HS
    Thyroid
      Left 03HV
      Right 03HU

Insertion of device in — *continued*
  Artery — *continued*
    Ulnar
      Left 03HA
      Right 03H9
    Upper 03HY
    Vertebral
      Left 03HQ
      Right 03HP
  Atrium
    Left 02H7
    Right 02H6
  Axilla
    Left 0XH5
    Right 0XH4
  Back
    Lower 0WHL
    Upper 0WHK
  Bladder 0THB
  Bladder Neck 0THC
  Bone
    Ethmoid
      Left 0NHG
      Right 0NHF
    Facial 0NHW
    Frontal 0NH1
    Hyoid 0NHX
    Lacrimal
      Left 0NHJ
      Right 0NHH
    Lower 0QHY
    Nasal 0NHB
    Occipital 0NH7
    Palatine
      Left 0NHL
      Right 0NHK
    Parietal
      Left 0NH4
      Right 0NH3
    Pelvic
      Left 0QH3
      Right 0QH2
    Sphenoid 0NHC
    Temporal
      Left 0NH6
      Right 0NH5
    Upper 0PHY
    Zygomatic
      Left 0NHN
      Right 0NHM
  Bone Marrow 07HT
  Brain 00H0
  Breast
    Bilateral 0HHV
    Left 0HHU
    Right 0HHT
  Bronchus
    Lingula 0BH9
    Lower Lobe
      Left 0BHB
      Right 0BH6
    Main
      Left 0BH7
      Right 0BH3
    Middle Lobe, Right 0BH5
    Upper Lobe
      Left 0BH8
      Right 0BH4
  Bursa and Ligament
    Lower 0MHY
    Upper 0MHX
  Buttock
    Left 0YH1
    Right 0YH0
  Carpal
    Left 0PHN
    Right 0PHM

Insertion of device in — *continued*
  Cavity, Cranial 0WH1
  Cerebral Ventricle 00H6
  Cervix 0UHC
  Chest Wall 0WH8
  Cisterna Chyli 07HL
  Clavicle
    Left 0PHB
    Right 0PH9
  Coccyx 0QHS
  Cul-de-sac 0UHF
  Diaphragm 0BHT
  Disc
    Cervical Vertebral 0RH3
    Cervicothoracic Vertebral 0RH5
    Lumbar Vertebral 0SH2
    Lumbosacral 0SH4
    Thoracic Vertebral 0RH9
    Thoracolumbar Vertebral 0RHB
  Duct
    Hepatobiliary 0FHB
    Pancreatic 0FHD
  Duodenum 0DH9
  Ear
    Inner
      Left 09HE
      Right 09HD
    Left 09HJ
    Right 09HH
  Elbow Region
    Left 0XHC
    Right 0XHB
  Epididymis and Spermatic Cord 0VHM
  Esophagus 0DH5
  Extremity
    Lower
      Left 0YHB
      Right 0YH9
    Upper
      Left 0XH7
      Right 0XH6
  Eye
    Left 08H1
    Right 08H0
  Face 0WH2
  Fallopian Tube 0UH8
  Femoral Region
    Left 0YH8
    Right 0YH7
  Femoral Shaft
    Left 0QH9
    Right 0QH8
  Femur
    Lower
      Left 0QHC
      Right 0QHB
    Upper
      Left 0QH7
      Right 0QH6
  Fibula
    Left 0QHK
    Right 0QHJ
  Foot
    Left 0YHN
    Right 0YHM
  Gallbladder 0FH4
  Gastrointestinal Tract 0WHP
  Genitourinary Tract 0WHR
  Gland
    Endocrine 0GHS
    Salivary 0CHA
  Glenoid Cavity
    Left 0PH8
    Right 0PH7
  Hand
    Left 0XHK
    Right 0XHJ

Insertion of device in — *continued*

Head 0WH0
Heart 02HA
Humeral Head
  Left 0PHD
  Right 0PHC
Humeral Shaft
  Left 0PHG
  Right 0PHF
Ileum 0DHB
Inguinal Region
  Left 0YH6
  Right 0YH5
Intestinal Tract
  Lower 0DHD
  Upper 0DH0
Intestine
  Large 0DHE
  Small 0DH8
Jaw
  Lower 0WH5
  Upper 0WH4
Jejunum 0DHA
Joint
  Acromioclavicular
    Left 0RHH
    Right 0RHG
  Ankle
    Left 0SHG
    Right 0SHF
  Carpal
    Left 0RHR
    Right 0RHQ
  Carpometacarpal
    Left 0RHT
    Right 0RHS
  Cervical Vertebral 0RH1
  Cervicothoracic Vertebral 0RH4
  Coccygeal 0SH6
  Elbow
    Left 0RHM
    Right 0RHL
  Finger Phalangeal
    Left 0RHX
    Right 0RHW
  Hip
    Left 0SHB
    Right 0SH9
  Knee
    Left 0SHD
    Right 0SHC
  Lumbar Vertebral 0SH0
  Lumbosacral 0SH3
  Metacarpophalangeal
    Left 0RHV
    Right 0RHU
  Metatarsal-Phalangeal
    Left 0SHN
    Right 0SHM
  Occipital-cervical 0RH0
  Sacrococcygeal 0SH5
  Sacroiliac
    Left 0SH8
    Right 0SH7
  Shoulder
    Left 0RHK
    Right 0RHJ
  Sternoclavicular
    Left 0RHF
    Right 0RHE
  Tarsal
    Left 0SHJ
    Right 0SHH
  Tarsometatarsal
    Left 0SHL
    Right 0SHK

Insertion of device in — *continued*

Joint — *continued*
  Temporomandibular
    Left 0RHD
    Right 0RHC
  Thoracic Vertebral 0RH6
  Thoracolumbar Vertebral 0RHA
  Toe Phalangeal
    Left 0SHQ
    Right 0SHP
  Wrist
    Left 0RHP
    Right 0RHN
Kidney 0TH5
Knee Region
  Left 0YHG
  Right 0YHF
Larynx 0CHS
Leg
  Lower
    Left 0YHJ
    Right 0YHH
  Upper
    Left 0YHD
    Right 0YHC
Liver 0FH0
  Left Lobe 0FH2
  Right Lobe 0FH1
Lung
  Left 0BHL
  Right 0BHK
Lymphatic 07HN
  Thoracic Duct 07HK
Mandible
  Left 0NHV
  Right 0NHT
Maxilla 0NHR
Mediastinum 0WHC
Metacarpal
  Left 0PHQ
  Right 0PHP
Metatarsal
  Left 0QHP
  Right 0QHN
Mouth and Throat 0CHY
Muscle
  Lower 0KHY
  Upper 0KHX
Nasal Mucosa and Soft Tissue 09HK
Nasopharynx 09HN
Neck 0WH6
Nerve
  Cranial 00HE
  Peripheral 01HY
Nipple
  Left 0HHX
  Right 0HHW
Oral Cavity and Throat 0WH3
Orbit
  Left 0NHQ
  Right 0NHP
Ovary 0UH3
Pancreas 0FHG
Patella
  Left 0QHF
  Right 0QHD
Pelvic Cavity 0WHJ
Penis 0VHS
Pericardial Cavity 0WHD
Pericardium 02HN
Perineum
  Female 0WHN
  Male 0WHM
Peritoneal Cavity 0WHG
Phalanx
  Finger
    Left 0PHV
    Right 0PHT

Insertion of device in — *continued*

Phalanx — *continued*
  Thumb
    Left 0PHS
    Right 0PHR
  Toe
    Left 0QHR
    Right 0QHQ
Pleura 0BHQ
Pleural Cavity
  Left 0WHB
  Right 0WH9
Prostate 0VH0
Prostate and Seminal Vesicles 0VH4
Radius
  Left 0PHJ
  Right 0PHH
Rectum 0DHP
Respiratory Tract 0WHQ
Retroperitoneum 0WHH
Ribs
  1 to 2 0PH1
  3 or More 0PH2
Sacrum 0QH1
Scapula
  Left 0PH6
  Right 0PH5
Scrotum and Tunica Vaginalis 0VH8
Shoulder Region
  Left 0XH3
  Right 0XH2
Sinus 09HY
Skin 0HHPXYZ
Skull 0NH0
Spinal Canal 00HU
Spinal Cord 00HV
Spleen 07HP
Sternum 0PH0
Stomach 0DH6
Subcutaneous Tissue and Fascia
  Abdomen 0JH8
  Back 0JH7
  Buttock 0JH9
  Chest 0JH6
  Face 0JH1
  Foot
    Left 0JHR
    Right 0JHQ
  Hand
    Left 0JHK
    Right 0JHJ
  Head and Neck 0JHS
  Lower Arm
    Left 0JHH
    Right 0JHG
  Lower Extremity 0JHW
  Lower Leg
    Left 0JHP
    Right 0JHN
  Neck
    Left 0JH5
    Right 0JH4
  Pelvic Region 0JHC
  Perineum 0JHB
  Scalp 0JH0
  Trunk 0JHT
  Upper Arm
    Left 0JHF
    Right 0JHD
  Upper Extremity 0JHV
  Upper Leg
    Left 0JHM
    Right 0JHL
Tarsal
  Left 0QHM
  Right 0QHL

Insertion of device in — *continued*
Tendon
  Lower 0LHY
  Upper 0LHX
Testis 0VHD
Thymus 07HM
Tibia
  Left 0QHH
  Right 0QHG
Tongue 0CH7
Trachea 0BH1
Tracheobronchial Tree 0BH0
Ulna
  Left 0PHL
  Right 0PHK
Ureter 0TH9
Urethra 0THD
Uterus 0UH9
Uterus and Cervix 0UHD
Vagina 0UHG
Vagina and Cul-de-sac 0UHH
Vas Deferens 0VHR
Vein
  Axillary
    Left 05H8
    Right 05H7
  Azygos 05H0
  Basilic
    Left 05HC
    Right 05HB
  Brachial
    Left 05HA
    Right 05H9
  Cephalic
    Left 05HF
    Right 05HD
  Colic 06H7
  Common Iliac
    Left 06HD
    Right 06HC
  Coronary 02H4
  Esophageal 06H3
  External Iliac
    Left 06HG
    Right 06HF
  External Jugular
    Left 05HQ
    Right 05HP
  Face
    Left 05HV
    Right 05HT
  Femoral
    Left 06HN
    Right 06HM
  Foot
    Left 06HV
    Right 06HT
  Gastric 06H2
  Hand
    Left 05HH
    Right 05HG
  Hemiazygos 05H1
  Hepatic 06H4
  Hypogastric
    Left 06HJ
    Right 06HH
  Inferior Mesenteric 06H6
  Innominate
    Left 05H4
    Right 05H3
  Internal Jugular
    Left 05HN
    Right 05HM
  Intracranial 05HL
  Lower 06HY
  Portal 06H8

Insertion of device in — *continued*
Vein — *continued*
  Pulmonary
    Left 02HT
    Right 02HS
  Renal
    Left 06HB
    Right 06H9
  Saphenous
    Left 06HQ
    Right 06HP
  Splenic 06H1
  Subclavian
    Left 05H6
    Right 05H5
  Superior Mesenteric 06H5
  Upper 05HY
  Vertebral
    Left 05HS
    Right 05HR
Vena Cava
  Inferior 06H0
  Superior 02HV
Ventricle
  Left 02HL
  Right 02HK
Vertebra
  Cervical 0PH3
  Lumbar 0QH0
  Thoracic 0PH4
Wrist Region
  Left 0XHH
  Right 0XHG
Inspection
Abdominal Wall 0WJF
Ankle Region
  Left 0YJL
  Right 0YJK
Arm
  Lower
    Left 0XJF
    Right 0XJD
  Upper
    Left 0XJ9
    Right 0XJ8
Artery
  Lower 04JY
  Upper 03JY
Axilla
  Left 0XJ5
  Right 0XJ4
Back
  Lower 0WJL
  Upper 0WJK
Bladder 0TJB
Bone
  Facial 0NJW
  Lower 0QJY
  Nasal 0NJB
  Upper 0PJY
Bone Marrow 07JT
Brain 00J0
Breast
  Left 0HJU
  Right 0HJT
Bursa and Ligament
  Lower 0MJY
  Upper 0MJX
Buttock
  Left 0YJ1
  Right 0YJ0
Cavity, Cranial 0WJ1
Chest Wall 0WJ8
Cisterna Chyli 07JL
Diaphragm 0BJT
Disc
  Cervical Vertebral 0RJ3

Inspection — *continued*
Disc — *continued*
  Cervicothoracic Vertebral 0RJ5
  Lumbar Vertebral 0SJ2
  Lumbosacral 0SJ4
  Thoracic Vertebral 0RJ9
  Thoracolumbar Vertebral 0RJB
Duct
  Hepatobiliary 0FJB
  Pancreatic 0FJD
Ear
  Inner
    Left 09JE
    Right 09JD
  Left 09JJ
  Right 09JH
Elbow Region
  Left 0XJC
  Right 0XJB
Epididymis and Spermatic Cord 0VJM
Extremity
  Lower
    Left 0YJB
    Right 0YJ9
  Upper
    Left 0XJ7
    Right 0XJ6
Eye
  Left 08J1XZZ
  Right 08J0XZZ
Face 0WJ2
Fallopian Tube 0UJ8
Femoral Region
  Bilateral 0YJE
  Left 0YJ8
  Right 0YJ7
Finger Nail 0HJQXZZ
Foot
  Left 0YJN
  Right 0YJM
Gallbladder 0FJ4
Gastrointestinal Tract 0WJP
Genitourinary Tract 0WJR
Gland
  Adrenal 0GJ5
  Endocrine 0GJS
  Pituitary 0GJ0
  Salivary 0CJA
Great Vessel 02JY
Hand
  Left 0XJK
  Right 0XJJ
Head 0WJ0
Heart 02JA
Inguinal Region
  Bilateral 0YJA
  Left 0YJ6
  Right 0YJ5
Intestinal Tract
  Lower 0DJD
  Upper 0DJ0
Jaw
  Lower 0WJ5
  Upper 0WJ4
Joint
  Acromioclavicular
    Left 0RJH
    Right 0RJG
  Ankle
    Left 0SJG
    Right 0SJF
  Carpal
    Left 0RJR
    Right 0RJQ
  Carpometacarpal
    Left 0RJT
    Right 0RJS

Inspection — *continued*
  Joint — *continued*
    Cervical Vertebral 0RJ1
    Cervicothoracic Vertebral 0RJ4
    Coccygeal 0SJ6
    Elbow
      Left 0RJM
      Right 0RJL
    Finger Phalangeal
      Left 0RJX
      Right 0RJW
    Hip
      Left 0SJB
      Right 0SJ9
    Knee
      Left 0SJD
      Right 0SJC
    Lumbar Vertebral 0SJ0
    Lumbosacral 0SJ3
    Metacarpophalangeal
      Left 0RJV
      Right 0RJU
    Metatarsal-Phalangeal
      Left 0SJN
      Right 0SJM
    Occipital-cervical 0RJ0
    Sacrococcygeal 0SJ5
    Sacroiliac
      Left 0SJ8
      Right 0SJ7
    Shoulder
      Left 0RJK
      Right 0RJJ
    Sternoclavicular
      Left 0RJF
      Right 0RJE
    Tarsal
      Left 0SJJ
      Right 0SJH
    Tarsometatarsal
      Left 0SJL
      Right 0SJK
    Temporomandibular
      Left 0RJD
      Right 0RJC
    Thoracic Vertebral 0RJ6
    Thoracolumbar Vertebral 0RJA
    Toe Phalangeal
      Left 0SJQ
      Right 0SJP
    Wrist
      Left 0RJP
      Right 0RJN
  Kidney 0TJ5
  Knee Region
    Left 0YJG
    Right 0YJF
  Larynx 0CJS
  Leg
    Lower
      Left 0YJJ
      Right 0YJH
    Upper
      Left 0YJD
      Right 0YJC
  Lens
    Left 08JKXZZ
    Right 08JJXZZ
  Liver 0FJ0
  Lung
    Left 0BJL
    Right 0BJK
  Lymphatic 07JN
    Thoracic Duct 07JK
  Mediastinum 0WJC
  Mesentery 0DJV
  Mouth and Throat 0CJY

Inspection — *continued*
  Muscle
    Extraocular
      Left 08JM
      Right 08JL
    Lower 0KJY
    Upper 0KJX
  Nasal Mucosa and Soft Tissue 09JK
  Neck 0WJ6
  Nerve
    Cranial 00JE
    Peripheral 01JY
  Omentum 0DJU
  Oral Cavity and Throat 0WJ3
  Ovary 0UJ3
  Pancreas 0FJG
  Parathyroid Gland 0GJR
  Pelvic Cavity 0WJJ
  Penis 0VJS
  Pericardial Cavity 0WJD
  Perineum
    Female 0WJN
    Male 0WJM
  Peritoneal Cavity 0WJG
  Peritoneum 0DJW
  Pineal Body 0GJ1
  Pleura 0BJQ
  Pleural Cavity
    Left 0WJB
    Right 0WJ9
  Products of Conception 10J0
    Ectopic 10J2
    Retained 10J1
  Prostate and Seminal Vesicles 0VJ4
  Respiratory Tract 0WJQ
  Retroperitoneum 0WJH
  Scrotum and Tunica Vaginalis 0VJ8
  Shoulder Region
    Left 0XJ3
    Right 0XJ2
  Sinus 09JY
  Skin 0HJPXZZ
  Skull 0NJ0
  Spinal Canal 00JU
  Spinal Cord 00JV
  Spleen 07JP
  Stomach 0DJ6
  Subcutaneous Tissue and Fascia
    Head and Neck 0JJS
    Lower Extremity 0JJW
    Trunk 0JJT
    Upper Extremity 0JJV
  Tendon
    Lower 0LJY
    Upper 0LJX
  Testis 0VJD
  Thymus 07JM
  Thyroid Gland 0GJK
  Toe Nail 0HJRXZZ
  Trachea 0BJ1
  Tracheobronchial Tree 0BJ0
  Tympanic Membrane
    Left 09J8
    Right 09J7
  Ureter 0TJ9
  Urethra 0TJD
  Uterus and Cervix 0UJD
  Vagina and Cul-de-sac 0UJH
  Vas Deferens 0VJR
  Vein
    Lower 06JY
    Upper 05JY
  Vulva 0UJM
  Wrist Region
    Left 0XJH
    Right 0XJG
Instillation
  see Introduction of substance in or on

Insufflation
  see Introduction of substance in or on
Interatrial septum
  use Atrial Septum
InterAtrial Shunt Device IASD®, Corvia
  use Synthetic Substitute
Interbody fusion (spine) cage
  use Interbody Fusion Device in Upper
    Joints
  use Interbody Fusion Device in Lower
    Joints
Interbody Fusion Device
  Nanotextured Surface
    Cervical Vertebral XRG1092
      2 or more XRG2092
    Cervicothoracic Vertebral XRG4092
    Lumbar Vertebral XRGB092
      2 or more XRGC092
    Lumbosacral XRGD092
    Occipital-cervical XRG0092
    Thoracic Vertebral XRG6092
      2 to 7 XRG7092
      8 or more XRG8092
    Thoracolumbar Vertebral XRGA092
  Radiolucent Porous
    Cervical Vertebral XRG10F3
      2 or more XRG20F3
    Cervicothoracic Vertebral XRG40F3
    Lumbar Vertebral XRGB0F3
      2 or more XRGC0F3
    Lumbosacral XRGD0F3
    Occipital-cervical XRG00F3
    Thoracic Vertebral XRG60F3
      2 to 7 XRG70F3
      8 or more XRG80F3
    Thoracolumbar Vertebral XRGA0F3
Intercarpal joint
  use Carpal Joint, Right
  use Carpal Joint, Left
Intercarpal ligament
  use Hand Bursa and Ligament, Right
  use Hand Bursa and Ligament, Left
Interclavicular ligament
  use Shoulder Bursa and Ligament, Right
  use Shoulder Bursa and Ligament, Left
Intercostal lymph node
  use Lymphatic, Thorax
Intercostal muscle
  use Thorax Muscle, Right
  use Thorax Muscle, Left
Intercostal nerve
  use Thoracic Nerve
Intercostobrachial nerve
  use Thoracic Nerve
Intercuneiform joint
  use Tarsal Joint, Right
  use Tarsal Joint, Left
Intercuneiform ligament
  use Foot Bursa and Ligament, Right
  use Foot Bursa and Ligament, Left
Intermediate bronchus
  use Main Bronchus, Right
Intermediate cuneiform bone
  use Tarsal, Right
  use Tarsal, Left
Intermittent hemodialysis (IHD) 5A1D70Z
Intermittent mandatory ventilation
  see Assistance, Respiratory 5A09
Intermittent Negative Airway Pressure
  24-96 Consecutive Hours,
    Ventilation 5A0945B
  Greater than 96 Consecutive Hours,
    Ventilation 5A0955B
  Less than 24 Consecutive Hours,
    Ventilation 5A0935B

Intermittent Positive Airway Pressure
  24-96 Consecutive Hours,
    Ventilation 5A09458
  Greater than 96 Consecutive Hours,
    Ventilation 5A09558
  Less than 24 Consecutive Hours,
    Ventilation 5A09358
Intermittent positive pressure breathing
  see Assistance, Respiratory 5A09
Internal (basal) cerebral vein
  use Intracranial Vein
Internal anal sphincter
  use Anal Sphincter
Internal carotid artery, intracranial portion
  use Intracranial Artery
Internal carotid plexus
  use Head and Neck Sympathetic Nerve
Internal iliac vein
  use Hypogastric Vein, Right
  use Hypogastric Vein, Left
Internal maxillary artery
  use External Carotid Artery, Right
  use External Carotid Artery, Left
Internal naris
  use Nasal Mucosa and Soft Tissue
Internal oblique muscle
  use Abdomen Muscle, Right
  use Abdomen Muscle, Left
Internal pudendal artery
  use Internal Iliac Artery, Right
  use Internal Iliac Artery, Left
Internal pudendal vein
  use Hypogastric Vein, Right
  use Hypogastric Vein, Left
Internal thoracic artery
  use Internal Mammary Artery, Right
  use Internal Mammary Artery, Left
  use Subclavian Artery, Right
  use Subclavian Artery, Left
Internal urethral sphincter
  use Urethra
Interphalangeal (IP) joint
  use Finger Phalangeal Joint, Right
  use Finger Phalangeal Joint, Left
  use Toe Phalangeal Joint, Right
  use Toe Phalangeal Joint, Left
Interphalangeal ligament
  use Hand Bursa and Ligament, Right
  use Hand Bursa and Ligament, Left
  use Foot Bursa and Ligament, Right
  use Foot Bursa and Ligament, Left
Interrogation, cardiac rhythm related device
  Interrogation only *see* Measurement, Cardiac 4B02
  With cardiac function testing *see* Measurement, Cardiac 4A02
Interruption
  see Occlusion
Interspinalis muscle
  use Trunk Muscle, Right
  use Trunk Muscle, Left
Interspinous ligament, cervical
  use Head and Neck Bursa and Ligament
Interspinous ligament, lumbar
  use Lower Spine Bursa and Ligament
Interspinous ligament, thoracic
  use Upper Spine Bursa and Ligament
Interspinous process spinal stabilization device
  use Spinal Stabilization Device, Interspinous Process in 0RH
  use Spinal Stabilization Device, Interspinous Process in 0SH
InterStim® Therapy lead
  use Neurostimulator Lead in Peripheral Nervous System

InterStim® Therapy neurostimulator
  use Stimulator Generator, Single Array in 0JH
Intertransversarius muscle
  use Trunk Muscle, Right
  use Trunk Muscle, Left
Intertransverse ligament, cervical
  use Head and Neck Bursa and Ligament
Intertransverse ligament, lumbar
  use Lower Spine Bursa and Ligament
Intertransverse ligament, thoracic
  use Upper Spine Bursa and Ligament
Interventricular foramen (Monro)
  use Cerebral Ventricle
Interventricular septum
  use Ventricular Septum
Intestinal lymphatic trunk
  use Cisterna Chyli
Intra.OX 8E02XDZ
Intraluminal Device
  Airway
    Esophagus 0DH5
    Mouth and Throat 0CHY
    Nasopharynx 09HN
  Bioactive
    Occlusion
      Common Carotid
        Left 03LJ
        Right 03LH
      External Carotid
        Left 03LN
        Right 03LM
      Internal Carotid
        Left 03LL
        Right 03LK
      Intracranial 03LG
      Vertebral
        Left 03LQ
        Right 03LP
    Restriction
      Common Carotid
        Left 03VJ
        Right 03VH
      External Carotid
        Left 03VN
        Right 03VM
      Internal Carotid
        Left 03VL
        Right 03VK
      Intracranial 03VG
      Vertebral
        Left 03VQ
        Right 03VP
  Endobronchial Valve
    Lingula 0BH9
    Lower Lobe
      Left 0BHB
      Right 0BH6
    Main
      Left 0BH7
      Right 0BH3
    Middle Lobe, Right 0BH5
    Upper Lobe
      Left 0BH8
      Right 0BH4
  Endotracheal Airway
    Change device in, Trachea 0B21XEZ
    Insertion of device in, Trachea 0BH1
  Pessary
    Change device in, Vagina and Cul-de-sac 0U2HXGZ
    Insertion of device in
      Cul-de-sac 0UHF
      Vagina 0UHG
Intramedullary (IM) rod (nail)
  use Internal Fixation Device, Intramedullary in Upper Bones

Intramedullary (IM) rod (nail) — *continued*
  use Internal Fixation Device, Intramedullary in Lower Bones
Intramedullary skeletal kinetic distractor (ISKD)
  use Internal Fixation Device, Intramedullary in Upper Bones
  use Internal Fixation Device, Intramedullary in Lower Bones
Intraocular Telescope
  Left 08RK30Z
  Right 08RJ30Z
Intraoperative Knee Replacement Sensor XR2
Intraoperative Radiation Therapy (IORT)
  Anus DDY8CZZ
  Bile Ducts DFY2CZZ
  Bladder DTY2CZZ
  Brain D0Y0CZZ
  Brain Stem D0Y1CZZ
  Cervix DUY1CZZ
  Colon DDY5CZZ
  Duodenum DDY2CZZ
  Gallbladder DFY1CZZ
  Ileum DDY4CZZ
  Jejunum DDY3CZZ
  Kidney DTY0CZZ
  Larynx D9YBCZZ
  Liver DFY0CZZ
  Mouth D9Y4CZZ
  Nasopharynx D9YDCZZ
  Nerve, Peripheral D0Y7CZZ
  Ovary DUY0CZZ
  Pancreas DFY3CZZ
  Pharynx D9YCCZZ
  Prostate DVY0CZZ
  Rectum DDY7CZZ
  Spinal Cord D0Y6CZZ
  Stomach DDY1CZZ
  Ureter DTY1CZZ
  Urethra DTY3CZZ
  Uterus DUY2CZZ
Intrauterine device (IUD)
  use Contraceptive Device in Female Reproductive System
Intravascular fluorescence angiography (IFA)
  see Monitoring, Physiological Systems 4A1
Intravascular Lithotripsy (IVL)
  see Fragmentation
Intravascular ultrasound assisted thrombolysis
  see Fragmentation, Artery
Introduction of substance in or on
  Artery
    Central 3E06
      Analgesics 3E06
      Anesthetic, Intracirculatory 3E06
      Anti-infective 3E06
      Anti-inflammatory 3E06
      Antiarrhythmic 3E06
      Antineoplastic 3E06
      Destructive Agent 3E06
      Diagnostic Substance, Other 3E06
      Electrolytic Substance 3E06
      Hormone 3E06
      Hypnotics 3E06
      Immunotherapeutic 3E06
      Nutritional Substance 3E06
      Platelet Inhibitor 3E06
      Radioactive Substance 3E06
      Sedatives 3E06
      Serum 3E06
      Thrombolytic 3E06
      Toxoid 3E06
      Vaccine 3E06
      Vasopressor 3E06
      Water Balance Substance 3E06

Introduction of substance in or on — *continued*
  Artery — *continued*
    Coronary 3E07
      Diagnostic Substance, Other 3E07
      Platelet Inhibitor 3E07
      Thrombolytic 3E07
    Peripheral 3E05
      Analgesics 3E05
      Anesthetic, Intracirculatory 3E05
      Anti-infective 3E05
      Anti-inflammatory 3E05
      Antiarrhythmic 3E05
      Antineoplastic 3E05
      Destructive Agent 3E05
      Diagnostic Substance, Other 3E05
      Electrolytic Substance 3E05
      Hormone 3E05
      Hypnotics 3E05
      Immunotherapeutic 3E05
      Nutritional Substance 3E05
      Platelet Inhibitor 3E05
      Radioactive Substance 3E05
      Sedatives 3E05
      Serum 3E05
      Thrombolytic 3E05
      Toxoid 3E05
      Vaccine 3E05
      Vasopressor 3E05
      Water Balance Substance 3E05
  Biliary Tract 3E0J
    Analgesics 3E0J
    Anesthetic Agent 3E0J
    Anti-infective 3E0J
    Anti-inflammatory 3E0J
    Antineoplastic 3E0J
    Destructive Agent 3E0J
    Diagnostic Substance, Other 3E0J
    Electrolytic Substance 3E0J
    Gas 3E0J
    Hypnotics 3E0J
    Islet Cells, Pancreatic 3E0J
    Nutritional Substance 3E0J
    Radioactive Substance 3E0J
    Sedatives 3E0J
    Water Balance Substance 3E0J
  Bone 3E0V
    Analgesics 3E0V3NZ
    Anesthetic Agent 3E0V3BZ
    Anti-infective 3E0V32
    Anti-inflammatory 3E0V33Z
    Antineoplastic 3E0V30
    Destructive Agent 3E0V3TZ
    Diagnostic Substance, Other 3E0V3KZ
    Electrolytic Substance 3E0V37Z
    Hypnotics 3E0V3NZ
    Nutritional Substance 3E0V36Z
    Radioactive Substance 3E0V3HZ
    Sedatives 3E0V3NZ
    Water Balance Substance 3E0V37Z
  Bone Marrow 3E0A3GC
    Antineoplastic 3E0A30
  Brain 3E0Q
    Analgesics 3E0Q
    Anesthetic Agent 3E0Q
    Anti-infective 3E0Q
    Anti-inflammatory 3E0Q
    Antineoplastic 3E0Q
    Destructive Agent 3E0Q
    Diagnostic Substance, Other 3E0Q
    Electrolytic Substance 3E0Q
    Gas 3E0Q
    Hypnotics 3E0Q
    Nutritional Substance 3E0Q
    Radioactive Substance 3E0Q
    Sedatives 3E0Q
    Stem Cells
      Embryonic 3E0Q
      Somatic 3E0Q

Introduction of substance in or on — *continued*
  Brain — *continued*
    Water Balance Substance 3E0Q
  Cranial Cavity 3E0Q
    Analgesics 3E0Q
    Anesthetic Agent 3E0Q
    Anti-infective 3E0Q
    Anti-inflammatory 3E0Q
    Antineoplastic 3E0Q
    Destructive Agent 3E0Q
    Diagnostic Substance, Other 3E0Q
    Electrolytic Substance 3E0Q
    Gas 3E0Q
    Hypnotics 3E0Q
    Nutritional Substance 3E0Q
    Radioactive Substance 3E0Q
    Sedatives 3E0Q
    Stem Cells
      Embryonic 3E0Q
      Somatic 3E0Q
    Water Balance Substance 3E0Q
  Ear 3E0B
    Analgesics 3E0B
    Anesthetic Agent 3E0B
    Anti-infective 3E0B
    Anti-inflammatory 3E0B
    Antineoplastic 3E0B
    Destructive Agent 3E0B
    Diagnostic Substance, Other 3E0B
    Hypnotics 3E0B
    Radioactive Substance 3E0B
    Sedatives 3E0B
  Epidural Space 3E0S3GC
    Analgesics 3E0S3NZ
    Anesthetic Agent 3E0S3BZ
    Anti-infective 3E0S32
    Anti-inflammatory 3E0S33Z
    Antineoplastic 3E0S30
    Destructive Agent 3E0S3TZ
    Diagnostic Substance, Other 3E0S3KZ
    Electrolytic Substance 3E0S37Z
    Gas 3E0S
    Hypnotics 3E0S3NZ
    Nutritional Substance 3E0S36Z
    Radioactive Substance 3E0S3HZ
    Sedatives 3E0S3NZ
    Water Balance Substance 3E0S37Z
  Eye 3E0C
    Analgesics 3E0C
    Anesthetic Agent 3E0C
    Anti-infective 3E0C
    Anti-inflammatory 3E0C
    Antineoplastic 3E0C
    Destructive Agent 3E0C
    Diagnostic Substance, Other 3E0C
    Gas 3E0C
    Hypnotics 3E0C
    Pigment 3E0C
    Radioactive Substance 3E0C
    Sedatives 3E0C
  Gastrointestinal Tract
    Lower 3E0H
      Analgesics 3E0H
      Anesthetic Agent 3E0H
      Anti-infective 3E0H
      Anti-inflammatory 3E0H
      Antineoplastic 3E0H
      Destructive Agent 3E0H
      Diagnostic Substance, Other 3E0H
      Electrolytic Substance 3E0H
      Gas 3E0H
      Hypnotics 3E0H
      Nutritional Substance 3E0H
      Radioactive Substance 3E0H
      Sedatives 3E0H
      Water Balance Substance 3E0H

Introduction of substance in or on — *continued*
  Gastrointestinal Tract — *continued*
    Upper 3E0G
      Analgesics 3E0G
      Anesthetic Agent 3E0G
      Anti-infective 3E0G
      Anti-inflammatory 3E0G
      Antineoplastic 3E0G
      Destructive Agent 3E0G
      Diagnostic Substance, Other 3E0G
      Electrolytic Substance 3E0G
      Gas 3E0G
      Hypnotics 3E0G
      Nutritional Substance 3E0G
      Radioactive Substance 3E0G
      Sedatives 3E0G
      Water Balance Substance 3E0G
  Genitourinary Tract 3E0K
    Analgesics 3E0K
    Anesthetic Agent 3E0K
    Anti-infective 3E0K
    Anti-inflammatory 3E0K
    Antineoplastic 3E0K
    Destructive Agent 3E0K
    Diagnostic Substance, Other 3E0K
    Electrolytic Substance 3E0K
    Gas 3E0K
    Hypnotics 3E0K
    Nutritional Substance 3E0K
    Radioactive Substance 3E0K
    Sedatives 3E0K
    Water Balance Substance 3E0K
  Heart 3E08
    Diagnostic Substance, Other 3E08
    Platelet Inhibitor 3E08
    Thrombolytic 3E08
  Joint 3E0U
    Analgesics 3E0U3NZ
    Anesthetic Agent 3E0U3BZ
    Anti-infective 3E0U
    Anti-inflammatory 3E0U33Z
    Antineoplastic 3E0U30
    Destructive Agent 3E0U3TZ
    Diagnostic Substance, Other 3E0U3KZ
    Electrolytic Substance 3E0U37Z
    Gas 3E0U3SF
    Hypnotics 3E0U3NZ
    Nutritional Substance 3E0U36Z
    Radioactive Substance 3E0U3HZ
    Sedatives 3E0U3NZ
    Water Balance Substance 3E0U37Z
  Lymphatic 3E0W3GC
    Analgesics 3E0W3NZ
    Anesthetic Agent 3E0W3BZ
    Anti-infective 3E0W32
    Anti-inflammatory 3E0W33Z
    Antineoplastic 3E0W30
    Destructive Agent 3E0W3TZ
    Diagnostic Substance, Other 3E0W3KZ
    Electrolytic Substance 3E0W37Z
    Hypnotics 3E0W3NZ
    Nutritional Substance 3E0W36Z
    Radioactive Substance 3E0W3HZ
    Sedatives 3E0W3NZ
    Water Balance Substance 3E0W37Z
  Mouth 3E0D
    Analgesics 3E0D
    Anesthetic Agent 3E0D
    Anti-infective 3E0D
    Anti-inflammatory 3E0D
    Antiarrhythmic 3E0D
    Antineoplastic 3E0D
    Destructive Agent 3E0D
    Diagnostic Substance, Other 3E0D
    Electrolytic Substance 3E0D
    Hypnotics 3E0D
    Nutritional Substance 3E0D

Introduction of substance in or on — *continued*
  Mouth — *continued*
    Radioactive Substance 3E0D
    Sedatives 3E0D
    Serum 3E0D
    Toxoid 3E0D
    Vaccine 3E0D
    Water Balance Substance 3E0D
  Mucous Membrane 3E00XGC
    Analgesics 3E00XNZ
    Anesthetic Agent 3E00XBZ
    Anti-infective 3E00X2
    Anti-inflammatory 3E00X3Z
    Antineoplastic 3E00X0
    Destructive Agent 3E00XTZ
    Diagnostic Substance, Other 3E00XKZ
    Hypnotics 3E00XNZ
    Pigment 3E00XMZ
    Sedatives 3E00XNZ
    Serum 3E00X4Z
    Toxoid 3E00X4Z
    Vaccine 3E00X4Z
  Muscle 3E023GC
    Analgesics 3E023NZ
    Anesthetic Agent 3E023BZ
    Anti-infective 3E0232
    Anti-inflammatory 3E0233Z
    Antineoplastic 3E0230
    Destructive Agent 3E023TZ
    Diagnostic Substance, Other 3E023KZ
    Electrolytic Substance 3E0237Z
    Hypnotics 3E023NZ
    Nutritional Substance 3E0236Z
    Radioactive Substance 3E023HZ
    Sedatives 3E023NZ
    Serum 3E0234Z
    Toxoid 3E0234Z
    Vaccine 3E0234Z
    Water Balance Substance 3E0237Z
  Nerve
    Cranial 3E0X3GC
      Anesthetic Agent 3E0X3BZ
      Anti-inflammatory 3E0X33Z
      Destructive Agent 3E0X3TZ
    Peripheral 3E0T3GC
      Anesthetic Agent 3E0T3BZ
      Anti-inflammatory 3E0T33Z
      Destructive Agent 3E0T3TZ
    Plexus 3E0T3GC
      Anesthetic Agent 3E0T3BZ
      Anti-inflammatory 3E0T33Z
      Destructive Agent 3E0T3TZ
  Nose 3E09
    Analgesics 3E09
    Anesthetic Agent 3E09
    Anti-infective 3E09
    Anti-inflammatory 3E09
    Antineoplastic 3E09
    Destructive Agent 3E09
    Diagnostic Substance, Other 3E09
    Hypnotics 3E09
    Radioactive Substance 3E09
    Sedatives 3E09
    Serum 3E09
    Toxoid 3E09
    Vaccine 3E09
  Pancreatic Tract 3E0J
    Analgesics 3E0J
    Anesthetic Agent 3E0J
    Anti-infective 3E0J
    Anti-inflammatory 3E0J
    Antineoplastic 3E0J
    Destructive Agent 3E0J
    Diagnostic Substance, Other 3E0J
    Electrolytic Substance 3E0J
    Gas 3E0J
    Hypnotics 3E0J

Introduction of substance in or on — *continued*
  Pancreatic Tract — *continued*
    Islet Cells, Pancreatic 3E0J
    Nutritional Substance 3E0J
    Radioactive Substance 3E0J
    Sedatives 3E0J
    Water Balance Substance 3E0J
  Pericardial Cavity 3E0Y
    Analgesics 3E0Y3NZ
    Anesthetic Agent 3E0Y3BZ
    Anti-infective 3E0Y32
    Anti-inflammatory 3E0Y33Z
    Antineoplastic 3E0Y
    Destructive Agent 3E0Y3TZ
    Diagnostic Substance, Other 3E0Y3KZ
    Electrolytic Substance 3E0Y37Z
    Gas 3E0Y
    Hypnotics 3E0Y3NZ
    Nutritional Substance 3E0Y36Z
    Radioactive Substance 3E0Y3HZ
    Sedatives 3E0Y3NZ
    Water Balance Substance 3E0Y37Z
  Peritoneal Cavity 3E0M
    Adhesion Barrier 3E0M
    Analgesics 3E0M3NZ
    Anesthetic Agent 3E0M3BZ
    Anti-infective 3E0M32
    Anti-inflammatory 3E0M33Z
    Antineoplastic 3E0M
    Destructive Agent 3E0M3TZ
    Diagnostic Substance, Other 3E0M3KZ
    Electrolytic Substance 3E0M37Z
    Gas 3E0M
    Hypnotics 3E0M3NZ
    Nutritional Substance 3E0M36Z
    Radioactive Substance 3E0M3HZ
    Sedatives 3E0M3NZ
    Water Balance Substance 3E0M37Z
  Pharynx 3E0D
    Analgesics 3E0D
    Anesthetic Agent 3E0D
    Anti-infective 3E0D
    Anti-inflammatory 3E0D
    Antiarrhythmic 3E0D
    Antineoplastic 3E0D
    Destructive Agent 3E0D
    Diagnostic Substance, Other 3E0D
    Electrolytic Substance 3E0D
    Hypnotics 3E0D
    Nutritional Substance 3E0D
    Radioactive Substance 3E0D
    Sedatives 3E0D
    Serum 3E0D
    Toxoid 3E0D
    Vaccine 3E0D
    Water Balance Substance 3E0D
  Pleural Cavity 3E0L
    Adhesion Barrier 3E0L
    Analgesics 3E0L3NZ
    Anesthetic Agent 3E0L3BZ
    Anti-infective 3E0L32
    Anti-inflammatory 3E0L33Z
    Antineoplastic 3E0L
    Destructive Agent 3E0L3TZ
    Diagnostic Substance, Other 3E0L3KZ
    Electrolytic Substance 3E0L37Z
    Gas 3E0L
    Hypnotics 3E0L3NZ
    Nutritional Substance 3E0L36Z
    Radioactive Substance 3E0L3HZ
    Sedatives 3E0L3NZ
    Water Balance Substance 3E0L37Z
  Products of Conception 3E0E
    Analgesics 3E0E
    Anesthetic Agent 3E0E
    Anti-infective 3E0E
    Anti-inflammatory 3E0E

Introduction of substance in or on — *continued*
  Products of Conception — *continued*
    Antineoplastic 3E0E
    Destructive Agent 3E0E
    Diagnostic Substance, Other 3E0E
    Electrolytic Substance 3E0E
    Gas 3E0E
    Hypnotics 3E0E
    Nutritional Substance 3E0E
    Radioactive Substance 3E0E
    Sedatives 3E0E
    Water Balance Substance 3E0E
  Reproductive
    Female 3E0P
      Adhesion Barrier 3E0P
      Analgesics 3E0P
      Anesthetic Agent 3E0P
      Anti-infective 3E0P
      Anti-inflammatory 3E0P
      Antineoplastic 3E0P
      Destructive Agent 3E0P
      Diagnostic Substance, Other 3E0P
      Electrolytic Substance 3E0P
      Gas 3E0P
      Hormone 3E0P
      Hypnotics 3E0P
      Nutritional Substance 3E0P
      Ovum, Fertilized 3E0P
      Radioactive Substance 3E0P
      Sedatives 3E0P
      Sperm 3E0P
      Water Balance Substance 3E0P
    Male 3E0N
      Analgesics 3E0N
      Anesthetic Agent 3E0N
      Anti-infective 3E0N
      Anti-inflammatory 3E0N
      Antineoplastic 3E0N
      Destructive Agent 3E0N
      Diagnostic Substance, Other 3E0N
      Electrolytic Substance 3E0N
      Gas 3E0N
      Hypnotics 3E0N
      Nutritional Substance 3E0N
      Radioactive Substance 3E0N
      Sedatives 3E0N
      Water Balance Substance 3E0N
  Respiratory Tract 3E0F
    Analgesics 3E0F
    Anesthetic Agent 3E0F
    Anti-infective 3E0F
    Anti-inflammatory 3E0F
    Antineoplastic 3E0F
    Destructive Agent 3E0F
    Diagnostic Substance, Other 3E0F
    Electrolytic Substance 3E0F
    Gas 3E0F
    Hypnotics 3E0F
    Nutritional Substance 3E0F
    Radioactive Substance 3E0F
    Sedatives 3E0F
    Water Balance Substance 3E0F
  Skin 3E00XGC
    Analgesics 3E00XNZ
    Anesthetic Agent 3E00XBZ
    Anti-infective 3E00X2
    Anti-inflammatory 3E00X3Z
    Antineoplastic 3E00X0
    Destructive Agent 3E00XTZ
    Diagnostic Substance, Other 3E00XKZ
    Hypnotics 3E00XNZ
    Pigment 3E00XMZ
    Sedatives 3E00XNZ
    Serum 3E00X4Z
    Toxoid 3E00X4Z
    Vaccine 3E00X4Z

Introduction of substance in or on — *continued*
Spinal Canal 3E0R3GC
Analgesics 3E0R3NZ
Anesthetic Agent 3E0R3BZ
Anti-infective 3E0R32
Anti-inflammatory 3E0R33Z
Antineoplastic 3E0R30
Destructive Agent 3E0R3TZ
Diagnostic Substance, Other 3E0R3KZ
Electrolytic Substance 3E0R37Z
Gas 3E0R
Hypnotics 3E0R3NZ
Nutritional Substance 3E0R36Z
Radioactive Substance 3E0R3HZ
Sedatives 3E0R3NZ
Stem Cells
Embryonic 3E0R
Somatic 3E0R
Water Balance Substance 3E0R37Z
Subcutaneous Tissue 3E013GC
Analgesics 3E013NZ
Anesthetic Agent 3E013BZ
Anti-infective 3E01
Anti-inflammatory 3E0133Z
Antineoplastic 3E0130
Destructive Agent 3E013TZ
Diagnostic Substance, Other 3E013KZ
Electrolytic Substance 3E0137Z
Hormone 3E013V
Hypnotics 3E013NZ
Nutritional Substance 3E0136Z
Radioactive Substance 3E013HZ
Sedatives 3E013NZ
Serum 3E0134Z
Toxoid 3E0134Z
Vaccine 3E0134Z
Water Balance Substance 3E0137Z
Vein
Central 3E04
Analgesics 3E04
Anesthetic, Intracirculatory 3E04
Anti-infective 3E04
Anti-inflammatory 3E04
Antiarrhythmic 3E04
Antineoplastic 3E04
Destructive Agent 3E04
Diagnostic Substance, Other 3E04
Electrolytic Substance 3E04
Hormone 3E04
Hypnotics 3E04
Immunotherapeutic 3E04
Nutritional Substance 3E04
Platelet Inhibitor 3E04
Radioactive Substance 3E04
Sedatives 3E04
Serum 3E04
Thrombolytic 3E04
Toxoid 3E04
Vaccine 3E04
Vasopressor 3E04
Water Balance Substance 3E04
Peripheral 3E03
Analgesics 3E03
Anesthetic, Intracirculatory 3E03
Anti-infective 3E03
Anti-inflammatory 3E03
Antiarrhythmic 3E03
Antineoplastic 3E03
Destructive Agent 3E03
Diagnostic Substance, Other 3E03
Electrolytic Substance 3E03
Hormone 3E03
Hypnotics 3E03
Immunotherapeutic 3E03
Islet Cells, Pancreatic 3E03
Nutritional Substance 3E03
Platelet Inhibitor 3E03

Introduction of substance in or on — *continued*
Vein — *continued*
Radioactive Substance 3E03
Sedatives 3E03
Serum 3E03
Thrombolytic 3E03
Toxoid 3E03
Vaccine 3E03
Vasopressor 3E03
Water Balance Substance 3E03
Intubation
Airway
see Insertion of device in, Trachea 0BH1
see Insertion of device in, Mouth and Throat 0CHY
see Insertion of device in, Esophagus 0DH5
Drainage device *see* Drainage
Feeding Device *see* Insertion of device in, Gastrointestinal System 0DH
INTUITY Elite valve system, EDWARDS
use Zooplastic Tissue, Rapid Deployment Technique in New Technology
Iobenguane I-131 Antineoplastic XW0
Iobenguane I-131, High Specific Activity (HSA)
use Iobenguane I-131 Antineoplastic
IPPB (intermittent positive pressure breathing)
see Assistance, Respiratory 5A09
IRE (Irreversible Electroporation)
see Destruction, Hepatobiliary System and Pancreas 0F5
Iridectomy
see Excision, Eye 08B
see Resection, Eye 08T
Iridoplasty
see Repair, Eye 08Q
see Replacement, Eye 08R
see Supplement, Eye 08U
Iridotomy
see Drainage, Eye 089
Irreversible Electroporation (IRE)
see Destruction, Hepatobiliary System and Pancreas 0F5
Irrigation
Biliary Tract, Irrigating Substance 3E1J
Brain, Irrigating Substance 3E1Q38Z
Cranial Cavity, Irrigating Substance 3E1Q38Z
Ear, Irrigating Substance 3E1B
Epidural Space, Irrigating Substance 3E1S38Z
Eye, Irrigating Substance 3E1C
Gastrointestinal Tract
Lower, Irrigating Substance 3E1H
Upper, Irrigating Substance 3E1G
Genitourinary Tract, Irrigating Substance 3E1K
Irrigating Substance 3C1ZX8Z
Joint, Irrigating Substance 3E1U
Mucous Membrane, Irrigating Substance 3E10
Nose, Irrigating Substance 3E19
Pancreatic Tract, Irrigating Substance 3E1J
Pericardial Cavity, Irrigating Substance 3E1Y38Z
Peritoneal Cavity
Dialysate 3E1M39Z
Irrigating Substance 3E1M38Z
Pleural Cavity, Irrigating Substance 3E1L38Z
Reproductive
Female, Irrigating Substance 3E1P
Male, Irrigating Substance 3E1N
Respiratory Tract, Irrigating Substance 3E1F
Skin, Irrigating Substance 3E10
Spinal Canal, Irrigating Substance 3E1R38Z

Isavuconazole Anti-infective XW0
Ischiatic nerve
use Sciatic Nerve
Ischiocavernosus muscle
use Perineum Muscle
Ischiofemoral ligament
use Hip Bursa and Ligament, Right
use Hip Bursa and Ligament, Left
Ischium
use Pelvic Bone, Right
use Pelvic Bone, Left
Isolation 8E0ZXY6
Isotope Administration, Whole Body DWY5G
Itrel (3)(4) neurostimulator
use Stimulator Generator, Single Array in 0JH

J

Jakafi®
use Ruxolitinib
Jejunal artery
use Superior Mesenteric Artery
Jejunectomy
see Excision, Jejunum 0DBA
see Resection, Jejunum 0DTA
Jejunocolostomy
see Bypass, Gastrointestinal System 0D1
see Drainage, Gastrointestinal System 0D9
Jejunopexy
see Repair, Jejunum 0DQA
see Reposition, Jejunum 0DSA
Jejunostomy
see Bypass, Jejunum 0D1A
see Drainage, Jejunum 0D9A
Jejunotomy
see Drainage, Jejunum 0D9A
Joint fixation plate
use Internal Fixation Device in Upper Joints
use Internal Fixation Device in Lower Joints
Joint liner (insert)
use Liner in Lower Joints
Joint spacer (antibiotic)
use Spacer in Upper Joints
use Spacer in Lower Joints
Jugular body
use Glomus Jugulare
Jugular lymph node
use Lymphatic, Right Neck
use Lymphatic, Left Neck

K

Kappa
use Pacemaker, Dual Chamber in 0JH
Kcentra
use 4-Factor Prothrombin Complex Concentrate
Keratectomy, kerectomy
see Excision, Eye 08B
see Resection, Eye 08T
Keratocentesis
see Drainage, Eye 089
Keratoplasty
see Repair, Eye 08Q
see Replacement, Eye 08R
see Supplement, Eye 08U
Keratotomy
see Drainage, Eye 089
see Repair, Eye 08Q
KEVZARA®
use Sarilumab
Keystone Heart TriGuard 3™ CEPD (cerebral embolic protection device) X2A6325
Kirschner wire (K-wire)
use Internal Fixation Device in Head and Facial Bones

Kirschner wire (K-wire) — *continued*
  use Internal Fixation Device in Upper Bones
  use Internal Fixation Device in Lower Bones
  use Internal Fixation Device in Upper Joints
  use Internal Fixation Device in Lower Joints

Knee (implant) insert
  use Liner in Lower Joints

KUB x-ray
  see Plain Radiography, Kidney, Ureter and Bladder BT04

Kuntscher nail
  use Internal Fixation Device, Intramedullary in Upper Bones
  use Internal Fixation Device, Intramedullary in Lower Bones

KYMRIAH
  use Engineered Autologous Chimeric Antigen Receptor T-cell Immunotherapy

L

Labia majora
  use Vulva

Labia minora
  use Vulva

Labial gland
  use Upper Lip
  use Lower Lip

Labiectomy
  see Excision, Female Reproductive System 0UB
  see Resection, Female Reproductive System 0UT

Lacrimal canaliculus
  use Lacrimal Duct, Right
  use Lacrimal Duct, Left

Lacrimal punctum
  use Lacrimal Duct, Right
  use Lacrimal Duct, Left

Lacrimal sac
  use Lacrimal Duct, Right
  use Lacrimal Duct, Left

LAGB (laparoscopic adjustable gastric banding)
  Initial procedure 0DV64CZ
  Surgical correction *see* Revision of device in, Stomach 0DW6

Laminectomy
  see Release, Central Nervous System and Cranial Nerves 00N
  see Release, Peripheral Nervous System 01N
  see Excision, Upper Bones 0PB
  see Excision, Lower Bones 0QB

Laminotomy
  see Release, Central Nervous System and Cranial Nerves 00N
  see Release, Peripheral Nervous System 01N
  see Drainage, Upper Bones 0P9
  see Excision, Upper Bones 0PB
  see Release, Upper Bones 0PN
  see Drainage, Lower Bones 0Q9
  see Excision, Lower Bones 0QB
  see Release, Lower Bones 0QN

LAP-BAND® adjustable gastric banding system
  use Extraluminal Device

Laparoscopic-assisted transanal pull-through
  see Excision, Gastrointestinal System 0DB
  see Resection, Gastrointestinal System 0DT

Laparoscopy
  see Inspection

Laparotomy
  Drainage *see* Drainage, Peritoneal Cavity 0W9G
  Exploratory *see* Inspection, Peritoneal Cavity 0WJG

Laryngectomy
  see Excision, Larynx 0CBS
  see Resection, Larynx 0CTS

Laryngocentesis
  see Drainage, Larynx 0C9S

Laryngogram
  see Fluoroscopy, Larynx B91J

Laryngopexy
  see Repair, Larynx 0CQS

Laryngopharynx
  use Pharynx

Laryngoplasty
  see Repair, Larynx 0CQS
  see Replacement, Larynx 0CRS
  see Supplement, Larynx 0CUS

Laryngorrhaphy
  see Repair, Larynx 0CQS

Laryngoscopy 0CJS8ZZ

Laryngotomy
  see Drainage, Larynx 0C9S

Laser Interstitial Thermal Therapy
  Adrenal Gland DGY2KZZ
  Anus DDY8KZZ
  Bile Ducts DFY2KZZ
  Brain D0Y0KZZ
  Brain Stem D0Y1KZZ
  Breast
    Left DMY0KZZ
    Right DMY1KZZ
  Bronchus DBY1KZZ
  Chest Wall DBY7KZZ
  Colon DDY5KZZ
  Diaphragm DBY8KZZ
  Duodenum DDY2KZZ
  Esophagus DDY0KZZ
  Gallbladder DFY1KZZ
  Gland
    Adrenal DGY2KZZ
    Parathyroid DGY4KZZ
    Pituitary DGY0KZZ
    Thyroid DGY5KZZ
  Ileum DDY4KZZ
  Jejunum DDY3KZZ
  Liver DFY0KZZ
  Lung DBY2KZZ
  Mediastinum DBY6KZZ
  Nerve, Peripheral D0Y7KZZ
  Pancreas DFY3KZZ
  Parathyroid Gland DGY4KZZ
  Pineal Body DGY1KZZ
  Pituitary Gland DGY0KZZ
  Pleura DBY5KZZ
  Prostate DVY0KZZ
  Rectum DDY7KZZ
  Spinal Cord D0Y6KZZ
  Stomach DDY1KZZ
  Thyroid Gland DGY5KZZ
  Trachea DBY0KZZ

Lateral (brachial) lymph node
  use Lymphatic, Right Axillary
  use Lymphatic, Left Axillary

Lateral canthus
  use Upper Eyelid, Right
  use Upper Eyelid, Left

Lateral collateral ligament (LCL)
  use Knee Bursa and Ligament, Right
  use Knee Bursa and Ligament, Left

Lateral condyle of femur
  use Lower Femur, Right
  use Lower Femur, Left

Lateral condyle of tibia
  use Tibia, Right
  use Tibia, Left

Lateral cuneiform bone
  use Tarsal, Right
  use Tarsal, Left

Lateral epicondyle of femur
  use Lower Femur, Right
  use Lower Femur, Left

Lateral epicondyle of humerus
  use Humeral Shaft, Right
  use Humeral Shaft, Left

Lateral femoral cutaneous nerve
  use Lumbar Plexus

Lateral malleolus
  use Fibula, Right
  use Fibula, Left

Lateral meniscus
  use Knee Joint, Right
  use Knee Joint, Left

Lateral nasal cartilage
  use Nasal Mucosa and Soft Tissue

Lateral plantar artery
  use Foot Artery, Right
  use Foot Artery, Left

Lateral plantar nerve
  use Tibial Nerve

Lateral rectus muscle
  use Extraocular Muscle, Right
  use Extraocular Muscle, Left

Lateral sacral artery
  use Internal Iliac Artery, Right
  use Internal Iliac Artery, Left

Lateral sacral vein
  use Hypogastric Vein, Right
  use Hypogastric Vein, Left

Lateral sural cutaneous nerve
  use Peroneal Nerve

Lateral tarsal artery
  use Foot Artery, Right
  use Foot Artery, Left

Lateral temporomandibular ligament
  use Head and Neck Bursa and Ligament

Lateral thoracic artery
  use Axillary Artery, Right
  use Axillary Artery, Left

Latissimus dorsi muscle
  use Trunk Muscle, Right
  use Trunk Muscle, Left

Latissimus Dorsi Myocutaneous Flap
  Replacement
    Bilateral 0HRV075
    Left 0HRU075
    Right 0HRT075
  Transfer
    Left 0KXG
    Right 0KXF

Lavage
  see Irrigation
  Bronchial alveolar, diagnostic *see* Drainage, Respiratory System 0B9

Least splanchnic nerve
  use Thoracic Sympathetic Nerve

Lefamulin Anti-infective XW0

Left ascending lumbar vein
  use Hemiazygos Vein

Left atrioventricular valve
  use Mitral Valve

Left auricular appendix
  use Atrium, Left

Left colic vein
  use Colic Vein

Left coronary sulcus
  use Heart, Left

Left gastric artery
  use Gastric Artery

Left gastroepiploic artery
  use Splenic Artery

Left gastroepiploic vein
  use Splenic Vein

Left inferior phrenic vein
  use Renal Vein, Left
Left inferior pulmonary vein
  use Pulmonary Vein, Left
Left jugular trunk
  use Thoracic Duct
Left lateral ventricle
  use Cerebral Ventricle
Left ovarian vein
  use Renal Vein, Left
Left second lumbar vein
  use Renal Vein, Left
Left subclavian trunk
  use Thoracic Duct
Left subcostal vein
  use Hemiazygos Vein
Left superior pulmonary vein
  use Pulmonary Vein, Left
Left suprarenal vein
  use Renal Vein, Left
Left testicular vein
  use Renal Vein, Left
Lengthening
  Bone, with device *see* Insertion of Limb
    Lengthening Device
  Muscle, by incision *see* Division,
    Muscles 0K8
  Tendon, by incision *see* Division,
    Tendons 0L8
Leptomeninges, intracranial
  use Cerebral Meninges
Leptomeninges, spinal
  use Spinal Meninges
Leronlimab Monoclonal Antibody XW013K6
Lesser alar cartilage
  use Nasal Mucosa and Soft Tissue
Lesser occipital nerve
  use Cervical Plexus
Lesser Omentum
  use Omentum
Lesser saphenous vein
  use Saphenous Vein, Right
  use Saphenous Vein, Left
Lesser splanchnic nerve
  use Thoracic Sympathetic Nerve
Lesser trochanter
  use Upper Femur, Right
  use Upper Femur, Left
Lesser tuberosity
  use Humeral Head, Right
  use Humeral Head, Left
Lesser wing
  use Sphenoid Bone
Leukopheresis, therapeutic
  see Pheresis, Circulatory 6A55
Levator anguli oris muscle
  use Facial Muscle
Levator ani muscle
  use Perineum Muscle
Levator labii superioris alaeque nasi muscle
  use Facial Muscle
Levator labii superioris muscle
  use Facial Muscle
Levator palpebrae superioris muscle
  use Upper Eyelid, Right
  use Upper Eyelid, Left
Levator scapulae muscle
  use Neck Muscle, Right
  use Neck Muscle, Left
Levator veli palatini muscle
  use Tongue, Palate, Pharynx Muscle
Levatores costarum muscle
  use Thorax Muscle, Right
  use Thorax Muscle, Left
**LifeStent® (Flexstar)(XL) Vascular Stent
System**
  use Intraluminal Device

Ligament of head of fibula
  use Knee Bursa and Ligament, Right
  use Knee Bursa and Ligament, Left
Ligament of the lateral malleolus
  use Ankle Bursa and Ligament, Right
  use Ankle Bursa and Ligament, Left
Ligamentum flavum, cervical
  use Head and Neck Bursa and Ligament
Ligamentum flavum, lumbar
  use Lower Spine Bursa and Ligament
Ligamentum flavum, thoracic
  use Upper Spine Bursa and Ligament
Ligation
  see Occlusion
Ligation, hemorrhoid
  see Occlusion, Lower Veins, Hemorrhoidal
  Plexus
Light Therapy GZJZZZZ
Liner
  Removal of device from
    Hip
      Left 0SPB09Z
      Right 0SP909Z
    Knee
      Left 0SPD09Z
      Right 0SPC09Z
  Revision of device in
    Hip
      Left 0SWB09Z
      Right 0SW909Z
    Knee
      Left 0SWD09Z
      Right 0SWC09Z
  Supplement
    Hip
      Left 0SUB09Z
        Acetabular Surface 0SUE09Z
        Femoral Surface 0SUS09Z
      Right 0SU909Z
        Acetabular Surface 0SUA09Z
        Femoral Surface 0SUR09Z
    Knee
      Left 0SUD09
        Femoral Surface 0SUU09Z
        Tibial Surface 0SUW09Z
      Right 0SUC09
        Femoral Surface 0SUT09Z
        Tibial Surface 0SUV09Z
Lingual artery
  use External Carotid Artery, Right
  use External Carotid Artery, Left
Lingual tonsil
  use Pharynx
Lingulectomy, lung
  see Excision, Lung Lingula 0BBH
  see Resection, Lung Lingula 0BTH
Lisocabtagene Maraleucel
  use Lisocabtagene Maraleucel
    Immunotherapy
**Lisocabtagene Maraleucel
Immunotherapy** XW2
Lithoplasty
  see Fragmentation
Lithotripsy
  see Fragmentation
  With removal of fragments *see* Extirpation
LITT (laser interstitial thermal therapy)
  see Laser Interstitial Thermal Therapy
LIVIAN™ CRT-D
  use Cardiac Resynchronization Defibrillator
    Pulse Generator in 0JH
Lobectomy
  see Excision, Central Nervous System and
    Cranial Nerves 00B
  see Excision, Respiratory System 0BB
  see Resection, Respiratory System 0BT

Lobectomy — *continued*
  see Excision, Hepatobiliary System and
    Pancreas 0FB
  see Resection, Hepatobiliary System and
    Pancreas 0FT
  see Excision, Endocrine System 0GB
  see Resection, Endocrine System 0GT
Lobotomy
  see Division, Brain 0080
Localization
  see Map
  see Imaging
Locus ceruleus
  use Pons
Long thoracic nerve
  use Brachial Plexus
Loop ileostomy
  see Bypass, Ileum 0D1B
Loop recorder, implantable
  use Monitoring Device
Lower GI series
  see Fluoroscopy, Colon BD14
**Lower Respiratory Fluid Nucleic Acid-base
Microbial Detection** XXEBXQ6
Lumbar artery
  use Abdominal Aorta
Lumbar facet joint
  use Lumbar Vertebral Joint
Lumbar ganglion
  use Lumbar Sympathetic Nerve
Lumbar lymph node
  use Lymphatic, Aortic
Lumbar lymphatic trunk
  use Cisterna Chyli
Lumbar splanchnic nerve
  use Lumbar Sympathetic Nerve
Lumbosacral facet joint
  use Lumbosacral Joint
Lumbosacral trunk
  use Lumbar Nerve
Lumpectomy
  see Excision
Lunate bone
  use Carpal, Right
  use Carpal, Left
Lunotriquetral ligament
  use Hand Bursa and Ligament, Right
  use Hand Bursa and Ligament, Left
Lymphadenectomy
  see Excision, Lymphatic and Hemic
    Systems 07B
  see Resection, Lymphatic and Hemic
    Systems 07T
Lymphadenotomy
  see Drainage, Lymphatic and Hemic
    Systems 079
Lymphangiectomy
  see Excision, Lymphatic and Hemic
    Systems 07B
  see Resection, Lymphatic and Hemic
    Systems 07T
Lymphangiogram
  see Plain Radiography, Lymphatic
    System B70
Lymphangioplasty
  see Repair, Lymphatic and Hemic
    Systems 07Q
  see Supplement, Lymphatic and Hemic
    Systems 07U
Lymphangiorrhaphy
  see Repair, Lymphatic and Hemic
    Systems 07Q
Lymphangiotomy
  see Drainage, Lymphatic and Hemic
    Systems 079
Lysis
  see Release

M

Macula
use Retina, Right
use Retina, Left
MAGEC® Spinal Bracing and Distraction System
use Magnetically Controlled Growth Rod(s) in New Technology
Magnet extraction, ocular foreign body
see Extirpation, Eye 08C
Magnetic Resonance Imaging (MRI)
Abdomen BW30
Ankle
   Left BQ3H
   Right BQ3G
Aorta
   Abdominal B430
   Thoracic B330
Arm
   Left BP3F
   Right BP3E
Artery
   Celiac B431
   Cervico-Cerebral Arch B33Q
   Common Carotid, Bilateral B335
   Coronary
      Bypass Graft, Multiple B233
      Multiple B231
   Internal Carotid, Bilateral B338
   Intracranial B33R
   Lower Extremity
      Bilateral B43H
      Left B43G
      Right B43F
   Pelvic B43C
   Renal, Bilateral B438
   Spinal B33M
   Superior Mesenteric B434
   Upper Extremity
      Bilateral B33K
      Left B33J
      Right B33H
   Vertebral, Bilateral B33G
Bladder BT30
Brachial Plexus BW3P
Brain B030
Breast
   Bilateral BH32
   Left BH31
   Right BH30
Calcaneus
   Left BQ3K
   Right BQ3J
Chest BW33Y
Coccyx BR3F
Connective Tissue
   Lower Extremity BL31
   Upper Extremity BL30
Corpora Cavernosa BV30
Disc
   Cervical BR31
   Lumbar BR33
   Thoracic BR32
Ear B930
Elbow
   Left BP3H
   Right BP3G
Eye
   Bilateral B837
   Left B836
   Right B835
Femur
   Left BQ34
   Right BQ33
Fetal Abdomen BY33

Magnetic Resonance Imaging — *continued*
Fetal Extremity BY35
Fetal Head BY30
Fetal Heart BY31
Fetal Spine BY34
Fetal Thorax BY32
Fetus, Whole BY36
Foot
   Left BQ3M
   Right BQ3L
Forearm
   Left BP3K
   Right BP3J
Gland
   Adrenal, Bilateral BG32
   Parathyroid BG33
   Parotid, Bilateral B936
   Salivary, Bilateral B93D
   Submandibular, Bilateral B939
   Thyroid BG34
Head BW38
Heart, Right and Left B236
Hip
   Left BQ31
   Right BQ30
Intracranial Sinus B532
Joint
   Finger
      Left BP3D
      Right BP3C
   Hand
      Left BP3D
      Right BP3C
   Temporomandibular, Bilateral BN39
Kidney
   Bilateral BT33
   Left BT32
   Right BT31
   Transplant BT39
Knee
   Left BQ38
   Right BQ37
Larynx B93J
Leg
   Left BQ3F
   Right BQ3D
Liver BF35
Liver and Spleen BF36
Lung Apices BB3G
Nasopharynx B93F
Neck BW3F
Nerve
   Acoustic B03C
   Brachial Plexus BW3P
Oropharynx B93F
Ovary
   Bilateral BU35
   Left BU34
   Right BU33
Ovary and Uterus BU3C
Pancreas BF37
Patella
   Left BQ3W
   Right BQ3V
Pelvic Region BW3G
Pelvis BR3C
Pituitary Gland B039
Plexus, Brachial BW3P
Prostate BV33
Retroperitoneum BW3H
Sacrum BR3F
Scrotum BV34
Sella Turcica B039
Shoulder
   Left BP39
   Right BP38

Magnetic Resonance Imaging — *continued*
Sinus
   Intracranial B532
   Paranasal B932
Spinal Cord B03B
Spine
   Cervical BR30
   Lumbar BR39
   Thoracic BR37
Spleen and Liver BF36
Subcutaneous Tissue
   Abdomen BH3H
   Extremity
      Lower BH3J
      Upper BH3F
   Head BH3D
   Neck BH3D
   Pelvis BH3H
   Thorax BH3G
Tendon
   Lower Extremity BL33
   Upper Extremity BL32
Testicle
   Bilateral BV37
   Left BV36
   Right BV35
Toe
   Left BQ3Q
   Right BQ3P
Uterus BU36
   Pregnant BU3B
Uterus and Ovary BU3C
Vagina BU39
Vein
   Cerebellar B531
   Cerebral B531
   Jugular, Bilateral B535
   Lower Extremity
      Bilateral B53D
      Left B53C
      Right B53B
   Other B53V
   Pelvic (Iliac) Bilateral B53H
   Portal B53T
   Pulmonary, Bilateral B53S
   Renal, Bilateral B53L
   Splanchnic B53T
   Upper Extremity
      Bilateral B53P
      Left B53N
      Right B53M
Vena Cava
   Inferior B539
   Superior B538
Wrist
   Left BP3M
   Right BP3L
Magnetic-guided radiofrequency endovascular fistula
Radial Artery, Left 031C3ZF
Radial Artery, Right 031B3ZF
Ulnar Artery, Left 031A3ZF
Ulnar Artery, Right 03193ZF
Magnetically Controlled Growth Rod(s)
Cervical XNS3
Lumbar XNS0
Thoracic XNS4
Malleotomy
see Drainage, Ear, Nose, Sinus 099
Malleus
use Auditory Ossicle, Right
use Auditory Ossicle, Left
Mammaplasty, mammoplasty
see Alteration, Skin and Breast 0H0
see Repair, Skin and Breast 0HQ
see Replacement, Skin and Breast 0HR
see Supplement, Skin and Breast 0HU

Mammary duct
use Breast, Right
use Breast, Left
use Breast, Bilateral
Mammary gland
use Breast, Right
use Breast, Left
use Breast, Bilateral
Mammectomy
see Excision, Skin and Breast 0HB
see Resection, Skin and Breast 0HT
Mammillary body
use Hypothalamus
Mammography
see Plain Radiography, Skin, Subcutaneous Tissue and Breast BH0
Mammotomy
see Drainage, Skin and Breast 0H9
Mandibular nerve
use Trigeminal Nerve
Mandibular notch
use Mandible, Right
use Mandible, Left
Mandibulectomy
see Excision, Head and Facial Bones 0NB
see Resection, Head and Facial Bones 0NT
Manipulation
Adhesions see Release
Chiropractic see Chiropractic Manipulation
Manual removal, retained placenta
see Extraction, Products of Conception, Retained 10D1
Manubrium
use Sternum
Map
Basal Ganglia 00K8
Brain 00K0
Cerebellum 00KC
Cerebral Hemisphere 00K7
Conduction Mechanism 02K8
Hypothalamus 00KA
Medulla Oblongata 00KD
Pons 00KB
Thalamus 00K9
Mapping
Doppler ultrasound see Ultrasonography
Electrocardiogram only see Measurement, Cardiac 4A02
Mark IV Breathing Pacemaker System
use Stimulator Generator in Subcutaneous Tissue and Fascia
Marsupialization
see Drainage
see Excision
Massage, cardiac
External 5A12012
Open 02QA0ZZ
Masseter muscle
use Head Muscle
Masseteric fascia
use Subcutaneous Tissue and Fascia, Face
Mastectomy
see Excision, Skin and Breast 0HB
see Resection, Skin and Breast 0HT
Mastoid (postauricular) lymph node
use Lymphatic, Right Neck
use Lymphatic, Left Neck
Mastoid air cells
use Mastoid Sinus, Right
use Mastoid Sinus, Left
Mastoid process
use Temporal Bone, Right
use Temporal Bone, Left
Mastoidectomy
see Excision, Ear, Nose, Sinus 09B
see Resection, Ear, Nose, Sinus 09T

Mastoidotomy
see Drainage, Ear, Nose, Sinus 099
Mastopexy
see Repair, Skin and Breast 0HQ
see Reposition, Skin and Breast 0HS
Mastorrhaphy
see Repair, Skin and Breast 0HQ
Mastotomy
see Drainage, Skin and Breast 0H9
Maxillary artery
use External Carotid Artery, Right
use External Carotid Artery, Left
Maxillary nerve
use Trigeminal Nerve
Maximo II DR (VR)
use Defibrillator Generator in 0JH
Maximo II DR CRT-D
use Cardiac Resynchronization Defibrillator Pulse Generator in 0JH
Measurement
Arterial
Flow
Coronary 4A03
Intracranial 4A03X5D
Peripheral 4A03
Pulmonary 4A03
Pressure
Coronary 4A03
Peripheral 4A03
Pulmonary 4A03
Thoracic, Other 4A03
Pulse
Coronary 4A03
Peripheral 4A03
Pulmonary 4A03
Saturation, Peripheral 4A03
Sound, Peripheral 4A03
Biliary
Flow 4A0C
Pressure 4A0C
Cardiac
Action Currents 4A02
Defibrillator 4B02XTZ
Electrical Activity 4A02
Guidance 4A02X4A
No Qualifier 4A02X4Z
Output 4A02
Pacemaker 4B02XSZ
Rate 4A02
Rhythm 4A02
Sampling and Pressure
Bilateral 4A02
Left Heart 4A02
Right Heart 4A02
Sound 4A02
Total Activity, Stress 4A02XM4
Central Nervous
Conductivity 4A00
Electrical Activity 4A00
Pressure 4A000BZ
Intracranial 4A00
Saturation, Intracranial 4A00
Stimulator 4B00XVZ
Temperature, Intracranial 4A00
Circulatory, Volume 4A05XLZ
Gastrointestinal
Motility 4A0B
Pressure 4A0B
Secretion 4A0B
Lower Respiratory Fluid Nucleic Acid-base Microbial Detection XXEBXQ6
Lymphatic
Flow 4A06
Pressure 4A06
Metabolism 4A0Z

Measurement — continued
Musculoskeletal
Contractility 4A0F
Pressure 4A0F3BE
Stimulator 4B0FXVZ
Olfactory, Acuity 4A08X0Z
Peripheral Nervous
Conductivity
Motor 4A01
Sensory 4A01
Electrical Activity 4A01
Stimulator 4B01XVZ
Positive Blood Culture Fluorescence Hybridization for Organism Identification, Concentration and Susceptibility XXE5XN6
Products of Conception
Cardiac
Electrical Activity 4A0H
Rate 4A0H
Rhythm 4A0H
Sound 4A0H
Nervous
Conductivity 4A0J
Electrical Activity 4A0J
Pressure 4A0J
Respiratory
Capacity 4A09
Flow 4A09
Pacemaker 4B09XSZ
Rate 4A09
Resistance 4A09
Total Activity 4A09
Volume 4A09
Sleep 4A0ZXQZ
Temperature 4A0Z
Urinary
Contractility 4A0D
Flow 4A0D
Pressure 4A0D
Resistance 4A0D
Volume 4A0D
Venous
Flow
Central 4A04
Peripheral 4A04
Portal 4A04
Pulmonary 4A04
Pressure
Central 4A04
Peripheral 4A04
Portal 4A04
Pulmonary 4A04
Pulse
Central 4A04
Peripheral 4A04
Portal 4A04
Pulmonary 4A04
Saturation, Peripheral 4A04
Visual
Acuity 4A07X0Z
Mobility 4A07X7Z
Pressure 4A07XBZ
Whole Blood Nucleic Acid-base Microbial Detection XXE5XM5
Meatoplasty, urethra
see Repair, Urethra 0TQD
Meatotomy
see Drainage, Urinary System 0T9
Mechanical ventilation
see Performance, Respiratory 5A19
Medial canthus
use Lower Eyelid, Right
use Lower Eyelid, Left
Medial collateral ligament (MCL)
use Knee Bursa and Ligament, Right
use Knee Bursa and Ligament, Left

Medial condyle of femur
  use Lower Femur, Right
  use Lower Femur, Left
Medial condyle of tibia
  use Tibia, Right
  use Tibia, Left
Medial cuneiform bone
  use Tarsal, Right
  use Tarsal, Left
Medial epicondyle of femur
  use Lower Femur, Right
  use Lower Femur, Left
Medial epicondyle of humerus
  use Humeral Shaft, Right
  use Humeral Shaft, Left
Medial malleolus
  use Tibia, Right
  use Tibia, Left
Medial meniscus
  use Knee Joint, Right
  use Knee Joint, Left
Medial plantar artery
  use Foot Artery, Right
  use Foot Artery, Left
Medial plantar nerve
  use Tibial Nerve
Medial popliteal nerve
  use Tibial Nerve
Medial rectus muscle
  use Extraocular Muscle, Right
  use Extraocular Muscle, Left
Medial sural cutaneous nerve
  use Tibial Nerve
Median antebrachial vein
  use Basilic Vein, Right
  use Basilic Vein, Left
Median cubital vein
  use Basilic Vein, Right
  use Basilic Vein, Left
Median sacral artery
  use Abdominal Aorta
Mediastinal cavity
  use Mediastinum
Mediastinal lymph node
  use Lymphatic, Thorax
Mediastinal space
  use Mediastinum
Mediastinoscopy 0WJC4ZZ
Medication Management GZ3ZZZZ
  for substance abuse
    Antabuse HZ83ZZZ
    Bupropion HZ87ZZZ
    Clonidine HZ86ZZZ
    Levo-alpha-acetyl-methadol
      (LAAM) HZ82ZZZ
    Methadone Maintenance HZ81ZZZ
    Naloxone HZ85ZZZ
    Naltrexone HZ84ZZZ
    Nicotine Replacement HZ80ZZZ
    Other Replacement
      Medication HZ89ZZZ
    Psychiatric Medication HZ88ZZZ
Meditation 8E0ZXY5
Medtronic Endurant® II AAA stent graft system
  use Intraluminal Device
Meissner's (submucous) plexus
  use Abdominal Sympathetic Nerve
Melody® transcatheter pulmonary valve
  use Zooplastic Tissue in Heart and Great Vessels
Membranous urethra
  use Urethra
Meningeorrhaphy
  see Repair, Cerebral Meninges 00Q1
  see Repair, Spinal Meninges 00QT

Meniscectomy, knee
  see Excision, Joint, Knee, Right 0SBC
  see Excision, Joint, Knee, Left 0SBD
Mental foramen
  use Mandible, Right
  use Mandible, Left
Mentalis muscle
  use Facial Muscle
Mentoplasty
  see Alteration, Jaw, Lower 0W05
Meropenem-vaborbactam Anti-infective XW0
Mesenterectomy
  see Excision, Mesentery 0DBV
Mesenteriorrhaphy, mesenterorrhaphy
  see Repair, Mesentery 0DQV
Mesenteriplication
  see Repair, Mesentery 0DQV
Mesoappendix
  use Mesentery
Mesocolon
  use Mesentery
Metacarpal ligament
  use Hand Bursa and Ligament, Right
  use Hand Bursa and Ligament, Left
Metacarpophalangeal ligament
  use Hand Bursa and Ligament, Right
  use Hand Bursa and Ligament, Left
Metal on metal bearing surface
  use Synthetic Substitute, Metal in 0SR
Metatarsal ligament
  use Foot Bursa and Ligament, Right
  use Foot Bursa and Ligament, Left
Metatarsectomy
  see Excision, Lower Bones 0QB
  see Resection, Lower Bones 0QT
Metatarsophalangeal (MTP) joint
  use Metatarsal-Phalangeal Joint, Right
  use Metatarsal-Phalangeal Joint, Left
Metatarsophalangeal ligament
  use Foot Bursa and Ligament, Right
  use Foot Bursa and Ligament, Left
Metathalamus
  use Thalamus
Micro-Driver stent (RX) (OTW)
  use Intraluminal Device
MicroMed HeartAssist
  use Implantable Heart Assist System in Heart and Great Vessels
Micrus CERECYTE microcoil
  use Intraluminal Device, Bioactive in Upper Arteries
Midcarpal joint
  use Carpal Joint, Right
  use Carpal Joint, Left
Middle cardiac nerve
  use Thoracic Sympathetic Nerve
Middle cerebral artery
  use Intracranial Artery
Middle cerebral vein
  use Intracranial Vein
Middle colic vein
  use Colic Vein
Middle genicular artery
  use Popliteal Artery, Right
  use Popliteal Artery, Left
Middle hemorrhoidal vein
  use Hypogastric Vein, Right
  use Hypogastric Vein, Left
Middle rectal artery
  use Internal Iliac Artery, Right
  use Internal Iliac Artery, Left
Middle suprarenal artery
  use Abdominal Aorta
Middle temporal artery
  use Temporal Artery, Right
  use Temporal Artery, Left

Middle turbinate
  use Nasal Turbinate
Mineral-based Topical Hemostatic Agent XW0
MIRODERM™ Biologic Wound Matrix
  use Skin Substitute, Porcine Liver Derived in New Technology
MitraClip valve repair system
  use Synthetic Substitute
Mitral annulus
  use Mitral Valve
Mitroflow® Aortic Pericardial Heart Valve
  use Zooplastic Tissue in Heart and Great Vessels
Mobilization, adhesions
  see Release
Molar gland
  use Buccal Mucosa
MolecuLight i:X® wound imaging
  see Other Imaging, Anatomical Regions BW5
Monitoring
  Arterial
    Flow
      Coronary 4A13
      Peripheral 4A13
      Pulmonary 4A13
    Pressure
      Coronary 4A13
      Peripheral 4A13
      Pulmonary 4A13
    Pulse
      Coronary 4A13
      Peripheral 4A13
      Pulmonary 4A13
    Saturation, Peripheral 4A13
    Sound, Peripheral 4A13
  Cardiac
    Electrical Activity 4A12
      Ambulatory 4A12X45
      No Qualifier 4A12X4Z
    Output 4A12
    Rate 4A12
    Rhythm 4A12
    Sound 4A12
    Total Activity, Stress 4A12XM4
    Vascular Perfusion, Indocyanine Green Dye 4A12XSH
  Central Nervous
    Conductivity 4A10
    Electrical Activity
      Intraoperative 4A10
      No Qualifier 4A10
    Pressure 4A100BZ
      Intracranial 4A10
    Saturation, Intracranial 4A10
    Temperature, Intracranial 4A10
  Gastrointestinal
    Motility 4A1B
    Pressure 4A1B
    Secretion 4A1B
    Vascular Perfusion, Indocyanine Green Dye 4A1BXSH
  Intraoperative Knee Replacement Sensor XR2
  Kidney, Fluorescent Pyrazine XT25XE5
  Lymphatic
    Flow
      Indocyanine Green Dye 4A16
      No Qualifier 4A16
    Pressure 4A16
  Peripheral Nervous
    Conductivity
      Motor 4A11
      Sensory 4A11
    Electrical Activity
      Intraoperative 4A11
      No Qualifier 4A11

Monitoring — *continued*
  Products of Conception
    Cardiac
      Electrical Activity 4A1H
      Rate 4A1H
      Rhythm 4A1H
      Sound 4A1H
    Nervous
      Conductivity 4A1J
      Electrical Activity 4A1J
      Pressure 4A1J
    Respiratory
      Capacity 4A19
      Flow 4A19
      Rate 4A19
      Resistance 4A19
      Volume 4A19
  Skin and Breast, Vascular Perfusion,
    Indocyanine Green Dye 4A1GXSH
  Sleep 4A1ZXQZ
  Temperature 4A1Z
  Urinary
    Contractility 4A1D
    Flow 4A1D
    Pressure 4A1D
    Resistance 4A1D
    Volume 4A1D
  Venous
    Flow
      Central 4A14
      Peripheral 4A14
      Portal 4A14
      Pulmonary 4A14
    Pressure
      Central 4A14
      Peripheral 4A14
      Portal 4A14
      Pulmonary 4A14
    Pulse
      Central 4A14
      Peripheral 4A14
      Portal 4A14
      Pulmonary 4A14
    Saturation
      Central 4A14
      Portal 4A14
      Pulmonary 4A14
Monitoring Device, Hemodynamic
  Abdomen 0JH8
  Chest 0JH6
Mosaic Bioprosthesis (aortic) (mitral) valve
  use Zooplastic Tissue in Heart and Great
    Vessels
Motor Function Assessment F01
Motor Treatment F07
MR Angiography
  see Magnetic Resonance Imaging (MRI),
    Heart B23
  see Magnetic Resonance Imaging (MRI),
    Upper Arteries B33
  see Magnetic Resonance Imaging (MRI),
    Lower Arteries B43
**MULTI-LINK (VISION)(MINI-VISION)(ULTRA)
  Coronary Stent System**
  use Intraluminal Device
Multiple sleep latency test 4A0ZXQZ
Musculocutaneous nerve
  use Brachial Plexus
Musculopexy
  see Repair, Muscles 0KQ
  see Reposition, Muscles 0KS
Musculophrenic artery
  use Internal Mammary Artery, Right
  use Internal Mammary Artery, Left
Musculoplasty
  see Repair, Muscles 0KQ
  see Supplement, Muscles 0KU

Musculorrhaphy
  see Repair, Muscles 0KQ
Musculospiral nerve
  use Radial Nerve
Myectomy
  see Excision, Muscles 0KB
  see Resection, Muscles 0KT
Myelencephalon
  use Medulla Oblongata
Myelogram
  CT *see* Computerized Tomography (CT
    Scan), Central Nervous System B02
  MRI *see* Magnetic Resonance Imaging
    (MRI), Central Nervous System B03
Myenteric (Auerbach's) plexus
  use Abdominal Sympathetic Nerve
Myocardial Bridge Release
  see Release, Artery, Coronary
Myomectomy
  see Excision, Female Reproductive
    System 0UB
Myometrium
  use Uterus
Myopexy
  see Repair, Muscles 0KQ
  see Reposition, Muscles 0KS
Myoplasty
  see Repair, Muscles 0KQ
  see Supplement, Muscles 0KU
Myorrhaphy
  see Repair, Muscles 0KQ
Myoscopy
  see Inspection, Muscles 0KJ
Myotomy
  see Division, Muscles 0K8
  see Drainage, Muscles 0K9
Myringectomy
  see Excision, Ear, Nose, Sinus 09B
  see Resection, Ear, Nose, Sinus 09T
Myringoplasty
  see Repair, Ear, Nose, Sinus 09Q
  see Replacement, Ear, Nose, Sinus 09R
  see Supplement, Ear, Nose, Sinus 09U
Myringostomy
  see Drainage, Ear, Nose, Sinus 099
Myringotomy
  see Drainage, Ear, Nose, Sinus 099

N

NA-1 (Nerinitide)
  use Nerinitide
Nail bed
  use Finger Nail
  use Toe Nail
Nail plate
  use Finger Nail
  use Toe Nail
nanoLOCK™ interbody fusion device
  use Interbody Fusion Device, Nanotextured
    Surface in New Technology
Narcosynthesis GZGZZZZ
Nasal cavity
  use Nasal Mucosa and Soft Tissue
Nasal concha
  use Nasal Turbinate
Nasalis muscle
  use Facial Muscle
Nasolacrimal duct
  use Lacrimal Duct, Right
  use Lacrimal Duct, Left
Nasopharyngeal airway (NPA)
  use Intraluminal Device, Airway in Ear,
    Nose, Sinus

Navicular bone
  use Tarsal, Right
  use Tarsal, Left
**Near Infrared Spectroscopy, Circulatory
  System** 8E02
Neck of femur
  use Upper Femur, Right
  use Upper Femur, Left
Neck of humerus (anatomical)(surgical)
  use Humeral Head, Right
  use Humeral Head, Left
Nephrectomy
  see Excision, Urinary System 0TB
  see Resection, Urinary System 0TT
Nephrolithotomy
  see Extirpation, Urinary System 0TC
Nephrolysis
  see Release, Urinary System 0TN
Nephropexy
  see Repair, Urinary System 0TQ
  see Reposition, Urinary System 0TS
Nephroplasty
  see Repair, Urinary System 0TQ
  see Supplement, Urinary System 0TU
Nephropyeloureterostomy
  see Bypass, Urinary System 0T1
  see Drainage, Urinary System 0T9
Nephrorrhaphy
  see Repair, Urinary System 0TQ
Nephroscopy, transurethral 0TJ58ZZ
Nephrostomy
  see Bypass, Urinary System 0T1
  see Drainage, Urinary System 0T9
Nephrotomography
  see Plain Radiography, Urinary System BT0
  see Fluoroscopy, Urinary System BT1
Nephrotomy
  see Division, Urinary System 0T8
  see Drainage, Urinary System 0T9
Nerinitide XW0
Nerve conduction study
  see Measurement, Central Nervous 4A00
  see Measurement, Peripheral Nervous 4A01
Nerve Function Assessment F01
Nerve to the stapedius
  use Facial Nerve
Nesiritide
  use Human B-type Natriuretic Peptide
Neurectomy
  see Excision, Central Nervous System and
    Cranial Nerves 00B
  see Excision, Peripheral Nervous
    System 01B
Neurexeresis
  see Extraction, Central Nervous System and
    Cranial Nerves 00D
  see Extraction, Peripheral Nervous
    System 01D
Neurohypophysis
  use Pituitary Gland
Neurolysis
  see Release, Central Nervous System and
    Cranial Nerves 00N
  see Release, Peripheral Nervous
    System 01N
**Neuromuscular electrical stimulation
  (NEMS) lead**
  use Stimulator Lead in Muscles
Neurophysiologic monitoring
  see Monitoring, Central Nervous 4A10
Neuroplasty
  see Repair, Central Nervous System and
    Cranial Nerves 00Q
  see Supplement, Central Nervous System
    and Cranial Nerves 00U
  see Repair, Peripheral Nervous System 01Q

Neurorrhaphy
   see Repair, Central Nervous System and
      Cranial Nerves 00Q
   see Repair, Peripheral Nervous
      System 01Q

Neurostimulator Generator
   Insertion of device in, Skull 0NH00NZ
   Removal of device from, Skull 0NP00NZ
   Revision of device in, Skull 0NW00NZ

Neurostimulator generator, multiple channel
   use Stimulator Generator, Multiple Array
      in 0JH

Neurostimulator generator, multiple channel rechargeable
   use Stimulator Generator, Multiple Array
      Rechargeable in 0JH

Neurostimulator generator, single channel
   use Stimulator Generator, Single Array
      in 0JH

Neurostimulator generator, single channel rechargeable
   use Stimulator Generator, Single Array
      Rechargeable in 0JH

Neurostimulator Lead
   Insertion of device in
      Brain 00H0
      Cerebral Ventricle 00H6
      Nerve
         Cranial 00HE
         Peripheral 01HY
      Spinal Canal 00HU
      Spinal Cord 00HV
      Vein
         Azygos 05H0
         Innominate
            Left 05H4
            Right 05H3
   Removal of device from
      Brain 00P0
      Cerebral Ventricle 00P6
      Nerve
         Cranial 00PE
         Peripheral 01PY
      Spinal Canal 00PU
      Spinal Cord 00PV
      Vein
         Azygos 05P0
         Innominate
            Left 05P4
            Right 05P3
   Revision of device in
      Brain 00W0
      Cerebral Ventricle 00W6
      Nerve
         Cranial 00WE
         Peripheral 01WY
      Spinal Canal 00WU
      Spinal Cord 00WV
      Vein
         Azygos 05W0
         Innominate
            Left 05W4
            Right 05W3

Neurotomy
   see Division, Central Nervous System and
      Cranial Nerves 008
   see Division, Peripheral Nervous
      System 018

Neurotripsy
   see Destruction, Central Nervous System
      and Cranial Nerves 005
   see Destruction, Peripheral Nervous
      System 015

Neutralization plate
   use Internal Fixation Device in Head and
      Facial Bones
   use Internal Fixation Device in Upper Bones
   use Internal Fixation Device in Lower Bones

New Technology
   Apalutamide Antineoplastic XW0DXJ5
   Atezolizumab Antineoplastic XW0
   Bamlanivimab Monoclonal Antibody XW0
   Baricitinib XW0
   Bezlotoxumab Monoclonal Antibody XW0
   Blinatumomab Antineoplastic
      Immunotherapy XW0
   Brexanolone XW0
   Brexucabtagene Autoleucel
      Immunotherapy XW2
   Caplacizumab XW0
   CD24Fc Immunomodulator XW0
   Cefiderocol Anti-infective XW0
   Ceftazidime-Avibactam Anti-infective XW0
   Ceftolozane/Tazobactam Anti-
      infective XW0
   Cerebral Embolic Filtration
      Dual Filter X2A5312
      Extracorporeal Flow Reversal Circuit X2A
      Single Deflection Filter X2A6325
   Coagulation Factor Xa, Inactivated XW0
   Concentrated Bone Marrow
      Aspirate XK02303
   COVID-19 Vaccine XW0
   COVID-19 Vaccine Dose 1 XW0
   COVID-19 Vaccine Dose 2 XW0
   Cytarabine and Daunorubicin Liposome
      Antineoplastic XW0
   Defibrotide Sodium Anticoagulant XW0
   Destruction, Prostate, Robotic Waterjet
      Ablation XV508A4
   Dilation
      Anterior Tibial
         Left
            Sustained Release Drug-eluting
               Intraluminal Device X27Q385
            Four or More X27Q3C5
            Three X27Q3B5
            Two X27Q395
         Right
            Sustained Release Drug-eluting
               Intraluminal Device X27P385
            Four or More X27P3C5
            Three X27P3B5
            Two X27P395
      Femoral
         Left
            Sustained Release Drug-eluting
               Intraluminal Device X27J385
            Four or More X27J3C5
            Three X27J3B5
            Two X27J395
         Right
            Sustained Release Drug-eluting
               Intraluminal Device X27H385
            Four or More X27H3C5
            Three X27H3B5
            Two X27H395
      Peroneal
         Left
            Sustained Release Drug-eluting
               Intraluminal Device X27U385
            Four or More X27U3C5
            Three X27U3B5
            Two X27U395
         Right
            Sustained Release Drug-eluting
               Intraluminal Device X27T385
            Four or More X27T3C5
            Three X27T3B5
            Two X27T395
      Popliteal
         Left Distal
            Sustained Release Drug-eluting
               Intraluminal Device X27N385
            Four or More X27N3C5
            Three X27N3B5

New Technology — *continued*
   Dilation — *continued*
            Two X27N395
         Left Proximal
            Sustained Release Drug-eluting
               Intraluminal Device X27L385
            Four or More X27L3C5
            Three X27L3B5
            Two X27L395
         Right Distal
            Sustained Release Drug-eluting
               Intraluminal Device X27M385
            Four or More X27M3C5
            Three X27M3B5
            Two X27M395
         Right Proximal
            Sustained Release Drug-eluting
               Intraluminal Device X27K385
            Four or More X27K3C5
            Three X27K3B5
            Two X27K395
      Posterior Tibial
         Left
            Sustained Release Drug-eluting
               Intraluminal Device X27S385
            Four or More X27S3C5
            Three X27S3B5
            Two X27S395
         Right
            Sustained Release Drug-eluting
               Intraluminal Device X27R385
            Four or More X27R3C5
            Three X27R3B5
            Two X27R395
   Durvalumab Antineoplastic XW0
   Eculizumab XW0
   Eladocagene exuparvovec XW0Q316
   Endothelial Damage Inhibitor XY0VX83
   Engineered Autologous Chimeric Antigen
      Receptor T-cell Immunotherapy XW0
   Erdafitinib Antineoplastic XW0DXL5
   Esketamine Hydrochloride XW097M5
   Etesevimab Monoclonal Antibody XW0
   Fosfomycin Anti-infective XW0
   Fusion
      Cervical Vertebral
         2 or more
            Nanotextured Surface XRG2092
            Radiolucent Porous XRG20F3
            Interbody Fusion Device
               Nanotextured Surface XRG1092
               Radiolucent Porous XRG10F3
      Cervicothoracic Vertebral
         Nanotextured Surface XRG4092
         Radiolucent Porous XRG40F3
      Lumbar Vertebral
         2 or more
            Nanotextured Surface XRGC092
            Radiolucent Porous XRGC0F3
         Interbody Fusion Device
            Nanotextured Surface XRGB092
            Radiolucent Porous XRGB0F3
      Lumbosacral
         Nanotextured Surface XRGD092
         Radiolucent Porous XRGD0F3
      Occipital-cervical
         Nanotextured Surface XRG0092
         Radiolucent Porous XRG00F3
      Thoracic Vertebral
         2 to 7
            Nanotextured Surface XRG7092
            Radiolucent Porous XRG70F3
         8 or more
            Nanotextured Surface XRG8092
            Radiolucent Porous XRG80F3
         Interbody Fusion Device
            Nanotextured Surface XRG6092
            Radiolucent Porous XRG60F3

Etesevimab Monoclonal — *continued*
  Fusion — *continued*
    Thoracolumbar Vertebral
      Nanotextured Surface XRGA092
      Radiolucent Porous XRGA0F3
  Gilteritinib Antineoplastic XW0DXV5
  Idarucizumab, Dabigatran Reversal
    Agent XW0
  Imipenem-cilastatin-relebactam Anti-
    infective XW0
  Intraoperative Knee Replacement
    Sensor XR2
  Iobenguane I-131 Antineoplastic XW0
  Isavuconazole Anti-infective XW0
  Kidney, Fluorescent Pyrazine XT25XE5
  Lefamulin Anti-infective XW0
  Leronlimab Monoclonal Antibody
    XW013K6
  Lisocabtagene Maraleucel
    Immunotherapy XW2
  Lower Respiratory Fluid Nucleic Acid-base
    Microbial Detection XXEBXQ6
  Meropenem-vaborbactam Anti-
    infective XW0
  Mineral-based Topical Hemostatic
    Agent XW0K
  Nerinitide XW0
  Omadacycline Anti-infective XW0
  Orbital Atherectomy Technology X2C
  Other New Technology Monoclonal
    Antibody XW0
  Other New Technology Therapeutic
    Substance XW0
  Plasma, Convalescent (Nonautologous) XW1
  Plazomicin Anti-infective XW0
  Positive Blood Culture Fluorescence
    Hybridization for Organism
    Identification, Concentration and
    Susceptibility XXE5XN6
  REGN-COV2 Monoclonal Antibody XW0
  Remdesivir Anti-infective XW0
  Replacement
    Skin Substitute, Porcine Liver
      Derived XHRPXL2
    Zooplastic Tissue, Rapid Deployment
      Technique X2RF
  Reposition
    Cervical, Magnetically Controlled Growth
      Rod(s) XNS3
    Lumbar, Magnetically Controlled Growth
      Rod(s) XNS0
    Thoracic, Magnetically Controlled
      Growth Rod(s) XNS4
  Ruxolitinib XW0DXT5
  Sarilumab XW0
  Supplement
    Lumbar, Mechanically Expandable
      (Paired) Synthetic Substitute XNU0356
    Thoracic, Mechanically Expandable
      (Paired) Synthetic Substitute XNU4356
  Synthetic Human Angiotensin II XW0
  Tagraxofusp-erzs Antineoplastic XW0
  Tocilizumab XW0
  Uridine Triacetate XW0DX82
  Venetoclax Antineoplastic XW0DXR5
  Whole Blood Nucleic Acid-base Microbial
    Detection XXE5XM5
Ninth cranial nerve
  use Glossopharyngeal Nerve
NIRS (Near Infrared Spectroscopy)
  see Physiological Systems and Anatomical
    Regions 8E0
Nitinol framed polymer mesh
  use Synthetic Substitute
Non-tunneled central venous catheter
  use Infusion Device
Nonimaging Nuclear Medicine Assay
  Bladder, Kidneys and Ureters CT63
  Blood C763
  Kidneys, Ureters and Bladder CT63

Nonimaging Nuclear Medicine Assay
  — *continued*
  Lymphatics and Hematologic
    System C76YYZZ
  Ureters, Kidneys and Bladder CT63
  Urinary System CT6YYZZ
Nonimaging Nuclear Medicine Probe
  Abdomen CW50
  Abdomen and Chest CW54
  Abdomen and Pelvis CW51
  Brain C050
  Central Nervous System C05YYZZ
  Chest CW53
  Chest and Abdomen CW54
  Chest and Neck CW56
  Extremity
    Lower CP5PZZZ
    Upper CP5NZZZ
  Head and Neck CW5B
  Heart C25YYZZ
    Right and Left C256
  Lymphatics
    Head C75J
    Head and Neck C755
    Lower Extremity C75P
    Neck C75K
    Pelvic C75D
    Trunk C75M
    Upper Chest C75L
    Upper Extremity C75N
  Lymphatics and Hematologic
    System C75YYZZ
  Musculoskeletal System, Other CP5YYZZ
  Neck and Chest CW56
  Neck and Head CW5B
  Pelvic Region CW5J
  Pelvis and Abdomen CW51
  Spine CP55ZZZ
Nonimaging Nuclear Medicine Uptake
  Endocrine System CG4YYZZ
  Gland, Thyroid CG42
Nostril
  use Nasal Mucosa and Soft Tissue
Novacor Left Ventricular Assist Device
  use Implantable Heart Assist System in
    Heart and Great Vessels
**Novation® Ceramic AHS® (Articulation Hip
System)**
  use Synthetic Substitute, Ceramic in 0SR
Nuclear medicine
  see Planar Nuclear Medicine Imaging
  see Tomographic (Tomo) Nuclear Medicine
    Imaging
  see Positron Emission Tomographic (PET)
    Imaging
  see Nonimaging Nuclear Medicine Uptake
  see Nonimaging Nuclear Medicine Probe
  see Nonimaging Nuclear Medicine Assay
  see Systemic Nuclear Medicine Therapy
Nuclear scintigraphy
  see Nuclear Medicine
Nutrition, concentrated substances
  Enteral infusion 3E0G36Z
  Parenteral (peripheral) infusion *see*
    Introduction of Nutritional Substance
NUZYRA™
  use Omadacycline Anti-infective

O

Obliteration
  see Destruction
Obturator artery
  use Internal Iliac Artery, Right
  use Internal Iliac Artery, Left
Obturator lymph node
  use Lymphatic, Pelvis
Obturator muscle
  use Hip Muscle, Right
  use Hip Muscle, Left

Obturator nerve
  use Lumbar Plexus
Obturator vein
  use Hypogastric Vein, Right
  use Hypogastric Vein, Left
Obtuse margin
  use Heart, Left
Occipital artery
  use External Carotid Artery, Right
  use External Carotid Artery, Left
Occipital lobe
  use Cerebral Hemisphere
Occipital lymph node
  use Lymphatic, Right Neck
  use Lymphatic, Left Neck
Occipitofrontalis muscle
  use Facial Muscle
Occlusion
  Ampulla of Vater 0FLC
  Anus 0DLQ
  Aorta
    Abdominal 04L0
    Thoracic, Descending 02LW3DJ
  Artery
    Anterior Tibial
      Left 04LQ
      Right 04LP
    Axillary
      Left 03L6
      Right 03L5
    Brachial
      Left 03L8
      Right 03L7
    Celiac 04L1
    Colic
      Left 04L7
      Middle 04L8
      Right 04L6
    Common Carotid
      Left 03LJ
      Right 03LH
    Common Iliac
      Left 04LD
      Right 04LC
    External Carotid
      Left 03LN
      Right 03LM
    External Iliac
      Left 04LJ
      Right 04LH
    Face 03LR
    Femoral
      Left 04LL
      Right 04LK
    Foot
      Left 04LW
      Right 04LV
    Gastric 04L2
    Hand
      Left 03LF
      Right 03LD
    Hepatic 04L3
    Inferior Mesenteric 04LB
    Innominate 03L2
    Internal Carotid
      Left 03LL
      Right 03LK
    Internal Iliac
      Left 04LF
      Right 04LE
    Internal Mammary
      Left 03L1
      Right 03L0
    Intracranial 03LG
    Lower 04LY
    Peroneal
      Left 04LU
      Right 04LT

Occlusion — *continued*
  Artery — *continued*
    Popliteal
      Left 04LN
      Right 04LM
    Posterior Tibial
      Left 04LS
      Right 04LR
    Pulmonary
      Left 02LR
      Right 02LQ
    Pulmonary Trunk 02LP
    Radial
      Left 03LC
      Right 03LB
    Renal
      Left 04LA
      Right 04L9
    Splenic 04L4
    Subclavian
      Left 03L4
      Right 03L3
    Superior Mesenteric 04L5
    Temporal
      Left 03LT
      Right 03LS
    Thyroid
      Left 03LV
      Right 03LU
    Ulnar
      Left 03LA
      Right 03L9
    Upper 03LY
    Vertebral
      Left 03LQ
      Right 03LP
  Atrium, Left 02L7
  Bladder 0TLB
  Bladder Neck 0TLC
  Bronchus
    Lingula 0BL9
    Lower Lobe
      Left 0BLB
      Right 0BL6
    Main
      Left 0BL7
      Right 0BL3
    Middle Lobe, Right 0BL5
    Upper Lobe
      Left 0BL8
      Right 0BL4
  Carina 0BL2
  Cecum 0DLH
  Cisterna Chyli 07LL
  Colon
    Ascending 0DLK
    Descending 0DLM
    Sigmoid 0DLN
    Transverse 0DLL
  Cord
    Bilateral 0VLH
    Left 0VLG
    Right 0VLF
  Cul-de-sac 0ULF
  Duct
    Common Bile 0FL9
    Cystic 0FL8
    Hepatic
      Common 0FL7
      Left 0FL6
      Right 0FL5
    Lacrimal
      Left 08LY
      Right 08LX
    Pancreatic 0FLD
      Accessory 0FLF

Occlusion — *continued*
  Duct — *continued*
    Parotid
      Left 0CLC
      Right 0CLB
  Duodenum 0DL9
  Esophagogastric Junction 0DL4
  Esophagus 0DL5
    Lower 0DL3
    Middle 0DL2
    Upper 0DL1
  Fallopian Tube
    Left 0UL6
    Right 0UL5
  Fallopian Tubes, Bilateral 0UL7
  Ileocecal Valve 0DLC
  Ileum 0DLB
  Intestine
    Large 0DLE
      Left 0DLG
      Right 0DLF
    Small 0DL8
  Jejunum 0DLA
  Kidney Pelvis
    Left 0TL4
    Right 0TL3
  Left atrial appendage (LAA) *see* Occlusion,
    Atrium, Left 02L7
  Lymphatic
    Aortic 07LD
    Axillary
      Left 07L6
      Right 07L5
    Head 07L0
    Inguinal
      Left 07LJ
      Right 07LH
    Internal Mammary
      Left 07L9
      Right 07L8
    Lower Extremity
      Left 07LG
      Right 07LF
    Mesenteric 07LB
    Neck
      Left 07L2
      Right 07L1
    Pelvis 07LC
    Thoracic Duct 07LK
    Thorax 07L7
    Upper Extremity
      Left 07L4
      Right 07L3
  Rectum 0DLP
  Stomach 0DL6
    Pylorus 0DL7
  Trachea 0BL1
  Ureter
    Left 0TL7
    Right 0TL6
  Urethra 0TLD
  Vagina 0ULG
  Valve, Pulmonary 02LH
  Vas Deferens
    Bilateral 0VLQ
    Left 0VLP
    Right 0VLN
  Vein
    Axillary
      Left 05L8
      Right 05L7
    Azygos 05L0
    Basilic
      Left 05LC
      Right 05LB
    Brachial
      Left 05LA
      Right 05L9

Occlusion — *continued*
  Vein — *continued*
    Cephalic
      Left 05LF
      Right 05LD
    Colic 06L7
    Common Iliac
      Left 06LD
      Right 06LC
    Esophageal 06L3
    External Iliac
      Left 06LG
      Right 06LF
    External Jugular
      Left 05LQ
      Right 05LP
    Face
      Left 05LV
      Right 05LT
    Femoral
      Left 06LN
      Right 06LM
    Foot
      Left 06LV
      Right 06LT
    Gastric 06L2
    Hand
      Left 05LH
      Right 05LG
    Hemiazygos 05L1
    Hepatic 06L4
    Hypogastric
      Left 06LJ
      Right 06LH
    Inferior Mesenteric 06L6
    Innominate
      Left 05L4
      Right 05L3
    Internal Jugular
      Left 05LN
      Right 05LM
    Intracranial 05LL
    Lower 06LY
    Portal 06L8
    Pulmonary
      Left 02LT
      Right 02LS
    Renal
      Left 06LB
      Right 06L9
    Saphenous
      Left 06LQ
      Right 06LP
    Splenic 06L1
    Subclavian
      Left 05L6
      Right 05L5
    Superior Mesenteric 06L5
    Upper 05LY
    Vertebral
      Left 05LS
      Right 05LR
  Vena Cava
    Inferior 06L0
    Superior 02LV
**Occlusion, REBOA (resuscitative
endovascular balloon occlusion of the
aorta)**
  02LW3DJ
  04L03DJ
Occupational therapy
  see Activities of Daily Living Treatment,
    Rehabilitation F08
Odentectomy
  see Excision, Mouth and Throat 0CB
  see Resection, Mouth and Throat 0CT

Odontoid process
  use Cervical Vertebra
Olecranon bursa
  use Elbow Bursa and Ligament, Right
  use Elbow Bursa and Ligament, Left
Olecranon process
  use Ulna, Right
  use Ulna, Left
Olfactory bulb
  use Olfactory Nerve
Olumiant® *use* Baricitinib
Omadacycline Anti-infective XW0
Omentectomy, omentumectomy
  see Excision, Gastrointestinal System 0DB
  see Resection, Gastrointestinal System 0DT
Omentofixation
  see Repair, Gastrointestinal System 0DQ
Omentoplasty
  see Repair, Gastrointestinal System 0DQ
  see Replacement, Gastrointestinal
    System 0DR
  see Supplement, Gastrointestinal
    System 0DU
Omentorrhaphy
  see Repair, Gastrointestinal System 0DQ
Omentotomy
  see Drainage, Gastrointestinal System 0D9
Omnilink Elite Vascular Balloon
  Expandable Stent System
  use Intraluminal Device
Onychectomy
  see Excision, Skin and Breast 0HB
  see Resection, Skin and Breast 0HT
Onychoplasty
  see Repair, Skin and Breast 0HQ
  see Replacement, Skin and Breast 0HR
Onychotomy
  see Drainage, Skin and Breast 0H9
Oophorectomy
  see Excision, Female Reproductive
    System 0UB
  see Resection, Female Reproductive
    System 0UT
Oophoropexy
  see Repair, Female Reproductive
    System 0UQ
  see Reposition, Female Reproductive
    System 0US
Oophoroplasty
  see Repair, Female Reproductive
    System 0UQ
  see Supplement, Female Reproductive
    System 0UU
Oophororrhaphy
  see Repair, Female Reproductive
    System 0UQ
Oophorostomy
  see Drainage, Female Reproductive
    System 0U9
Oophorotomy
  see Division, Female Reproductive
    System 0U8
  see Drainage, Female Reproductive
    System 0U9
Oophorrhaphy
  see Repair, Female Reproductive
    System 0UQ
Open Pivot (mechanical) valve
  use Synthetic Substitute
Open Pivot Aortic Valve Graft (AVG)
  use Synthetic Substitute
Ophthalmic artery
  use Intracranial Artery
Ophthalmic nerve
  use Trigeminal Nerve
Ophthalmic vein
  use Intracranial Vein

Opponensplasty
  Tendon replacement *see* Replacement,
    Tendons 0LR
  Tendon transfer *see* Transfer, Tendons 0LX
Optic chiasma
  use Optic Nerve
Optic disc
  use Retina, Right
  use Retina, Left
Optic foramen
  use Sphenoid Bone
Optical coherence tomography,
  intravascular
  see Computerized Tomography (CT Scan)
Optimizer™ III implantable pulse generator
  use Contractility Modulation Device in 0JH
Orbicularis oculi muscle
  use Upper Eyelid, Right
  use Upper Eyelid, Left
Orbicularis oris muscle
  use Facial Muscle
Orbital Atherectomy Technology X2C
Orbital fascia
  use Subcutaneous Tissue and Fascia, Face
Orbital portion of ethmoid bone
  use Orbit, Right
  use Orbit, Left
Orbital portion of frontal bone
  use Orbit, Right
  use Orbit, Left
Orbital portion of lacrimal bone
  use Orbit, Right
  use Orbit, Left
Orbital portion of maxilla
  use Orbit, Right
  use Orbit, Left
Orbital portion of palatine bone
  use Orbit, Right
  use Orbit, Left
Orbital portion of sphenoid bone
  use Orbit, Right
  use Orbit, Left
Orbital portion of zygomatic bone
  use Orbit, Right
  use Orbit, Left
Orchectomy, orchidectomy, orchiectomy
  see Excision, Male Reproductive
    System 0VB
  see Resection, Male Reproductive
    System 0VT
Orchidoplasty, orchioplasty
  see Repair, Male Reproductive
    System 0VQ
  see Replacement, Male Reproductive
    System 0VR
  see Supplement, Male Reproductive
    System 0VU
Orchidorrhaphy, orchiorrhaphy
  see Repair, Male Reproductive System 0VQ
Orchidotomy, orchiotomy, orchotomy
  see Drainage, Male Reproductive
    System 0V9
Orchiopexy
  see Repair, Male Reproductive System 0VQ
  see Reposition, Male Reproductive
    System 0VS
Oropharyngeal airway (OPA)
  use Intraluminal Device, Airway in Mouth
    and Throat
Oropharynx
  use Pharynx
Ossiculectomy
  see Excision, Ear, Nose, Sinus 09B
  see Resection, Ear, Nose, Sinus 09T
Ossiculotomy
  see Drainage, Ear, Nose, Sinus 099

Ostectomy
  see Excision, Head and Facial Bones 0NB
  see Resection, Head and Facial Bones 0NT
  see Excision, Upper Bones 0PB
  see Resection, Upper Bones 0PT
  see Excision, Lower Bones 0QB
  see Resection, Lower Bones 0QT
Osteoclasis
  see Division, Head and Facial Bones 0N8
  see Division, Upper Bones 0P8
  see Division, Lower Bones 0Q8
Osteolysis
  see Release, Head and Facial Bones 0NN
  see Release, Upper Bones 0PN
  see Release, Lower Bones 0QN
Osteopathic Treatment
  Abdomen 7W09X
  Cervical 7W01X
  Extremity
    Lower 7W06X
    Upper 7W07X
  Head 7W00X
  Lumbar 7W03X
  Pelvis 7W05X
  Rib Cage 7W08X
  Sacrum 7W04X
  Thoracic 7W02X
Osteopexy
  see Repair, Head and Facial Bones 0NQ
  see Reposition, Head and Facial Bones 0NS
  see Repair, Upper Bones 0PQ
  see Reposition, Upper Bones 0PS
  see Repair, Lower Bones 0QQ
  see Reposition, Lower Bones 0QS
Osteoplasty
  see Repair, Head and Facial Bones 0NQ
  see Replacement, Head and Facial
    Bones 0NR
  see Supplement, Head and Facial
    Bones 0NU
  see Repair, Upper Bones 0PQ
  see Replacement, Upper Bones 0PR
  see Supplement, Upper Bones 0PU
  see Repair, Lower Bones 0QQ
  see Replacement, Lower Bones 0QR
  see Supplement, Lower Bones 0QU
Osteorrhaphy
  see Repair, Head and Facial Bones 0NQ
  see Repair, Upper Bones 0PQ
  see Repair, Lower Bones 0QQ
Osteotomy, ostotomy
  see Division, Head and Facial Bones 0N8
  see Drainage, Head and Facial Bones 0N9
  see Division, Upper Bones 0P8
  see Drainage, Upper Bones 0P9
  see Division, Lower Bones 0Q8
  see Drainage, Lower Bones 0Q9
Other Imaging
  Bile Duct, Indocyanine Green Dye,
    Intraoperative BF50200
  Bile Duct and Gallbladder, Indocyanine
    Green Dye, Intraoperative BF53200
  Extremity
    Lower BW5CZ1Z
    Upper BW5JZ1Z
  Gallbladder, Indocyanine Green Dye,
    Intraoperative BF52200
  Gallbladder and Bile Duct, Indocyanine
    Green Dye, Intraoperative BF53200
  Head and Neck BW59Z1Z
  Hepatobiliary System, All, Indocyanine
    Green Dye, Intraoperative BF5C200
  Liver, Indocyanine Green Dye,
    Intraoperative BF55200
  Liver and Spleen, Indocyanine Green Dye,
    Intraoperative BF56200
  Neck and Head BW59Z1Z

Other Imaging — *continued*
    Pancreas, Indocyanine Green Dye,
      Intraoperative BF57200
    Spleen and Liver, Indocyanine Green Dye,
      Intraoperative BF56200
    Trunk BW52Z1Z
Other New Technology Monoclonal
   Antibody XW0
Other New Technology Therapeutic
   Substance XW0
Otic ganglion
   use Head and Neck Sympathetic Nerve
OTL-101
   use Hematopoietic Stem/Progenitor Cells,
     Genetically Modified
Otoplasty
   see Repair, Ear, Nose, Sinus 09Q
   see Replacement, Ear, Nose, Sinus 09R
   see Supplement, Ear, Nose, Sinus 09U
Otoscopy
   see Inspection, Ear, Nose, Sinus 09J
Oval window
   use Middle Ear, Right
   use Middle Ear, Left
Ovarian artery
   use Abdominal Aorta
Ovarian ligament
   use Uterine Supporting Structure
Ovariectomy
   see Excision, Female Reproductive
     System 0UB
   see Resection, Female Reproductive
     System 0UT
Ovariocentesis
   see Drainage, Female Reproductive
     System 0U9
Ovariopexy
   see Repair, Female Reproductive
     System 0UQ
   see Reposition, Female Reproductive
     System 0US
Ovariotomy
   see Division, Female Reproductive
     System 0U8
   see Drainage, Female Reproductive
     System 0U9
Ovatio™ CRT-D
   use Cardiac Resynchronization Defibrillator
     Pulse Generator in 0JH
Oversewing
   Gastrointestinal ulcer *see* Repair,
     Gastrointestinal System 0DQ
   Pleural bleb *see* Repair, Respiratory
     System 0BQ
Oviduct
   use Fallopian Tube, Right
   use Fallopian Tube, Left
Oximetry, Fetal pulse 10H073Z
OXINIUM
   use Synthetic Substitute, Oxidized
     Zirconium on Polyethylene in 0SR
Oxygenation
   Extracorporeal membrane (ECMO) *see*
     Performance, Circulatory 5A15
   Hyperbaric *see* Assistance,
     Circulatory 5A05
   Supersaturated *see* Assistance,
     Circulatory 5A05

P

Pacemaker
   Dual Chamber
     Abdomen 0JH8
     Chest 0JH6
   Intracardiac
     Insertion of device in

Pacemaker — *continued*
   Intracardiac — *continued*
     Atrium
       Left 02H7
       Right 02H6
     Vein, Coronary 02H4
     Ventricle
       Left 02HL
       Right 02HK
     Removal of device from, Heart 02PA
     Revision of device in, Heart 02WA
   Single Chamber
     Abdomen 0JH8
     Chest 0JH6
   Single Chamber Rate Responsive
     Abdomen 0JH8
     Chest 0JH6
Packing
   Abdominal Wall 2W43X5Z
   Anorectal 2Y43X5Z
   Arm
     Lower
       Left 2W4DX5Z
       Right 2W4CX5Z
     Upper
       Left 2W4BX5Z
       Right 2W4AX5Z
   Back 2W45X5Z
   Chest Wall 2W44X5Z
   Ear 2Y42X5Z
   Extremity
     Lower
       Left 2W4MX5Z
       Right 2W4LX5Z
     Upper
       Left 2W49X5Z
       Right 2W48X5Z
   Face 2W41X5Z
   Finger
     Left 2W4KX5Z
     Right 2W4JX5Z
   Foot
     Left 2W4TX5Z
     Right 2W4SX5Z
   Genital Tract, Female 2Y44X5Z
   Hand
     Left 2W4FX5Z
     Right 2W4EX5Z
   Head 2W40X5Z
   Inguinal Region
     Left 2W47X5Z
     Right 2W46X5Z
   Leg
     Lower
       Left 2W4RX5Z
       Right 2W4QX5Z
     Upper
       Left 2W4PX5Z
       Right 2W4NX5Z
   Mouth and Pharynx 2Y40X5Z
   Nasal 2Y41X5Z
   Neck 2W42X5Z
   Thumb
     Left 2W4HX5Z
     Right 2W4GX5Z
   Toe
     Left 2W4VX5Z
     Right 2W4UX5Z
   Urethra 2Y45X5Z
Paclitaxel-eluting coronary stent
   use Intraluminal Device, Drug-eluting in
     Heart and Great Vessels
Paclitaxel-eluting peripheral stent
   use Intraluminal Device, Drug-eluting in
     Upper Arteries
   use Intraluminal Device, Drug-eluting in
     Lower Arteries

Palatine gland
   use Buccal Mucosa
Palatine tonsil
   use Tonsils
Palatine uvula
   use Uvula
Palatoglossal muscle
   use Tongue, Palate, Pharynx Muscle
Palatopharyngeal muscle
   use Tongue, Palate, Pharynx Muscle
Palatoplasty
   see Repair, Mouth and Throat 0CQ
   see Replacement, Mouth and Throat 0CR
   see Supplement, Mouth and Throat 0CU
Palatorrhaphy
   see Repair, Mouth and Throat 0CQ
Palmar (volar) digital vein
   use Hand Vein, Right
   use Hand Vein, Left
Palmar (volar) metacarpal vein
   use Hand Vein, Right
   use Hand Vein, Left
Palmar cutaneous nerve
   use Median Nerve
   use Radial Nerve
Palmar fascia (aponeurosis)
   use Subcutaneous Tissue and Fascia, Right
     Hand
   use Subcutaneous Tissue and Fascia, Left
     Hand
Palmar interosseous muscle
   use Hand Muscle, Right
   use Hand Muscle, Left
Palmar ulnocarpal ligament
   use Wrist Bursa and Ligament, Right
   use Wrist Bursa and Ligament, Left
Palmaris longus muscle
   use Lower Arm and Wrist Muscle, Right
   use Lower Arm and Wrist Muscle, Left
Pancreatectomy
   see Excision, Pancreas 0FBG
   see Resection, Pancreas 0FTG
Pancreatic artery
   use Splenic Artery
Pancreatic plexus
   use Abdominal Sympathetic Nerve
Pancreatic vein
   use Splenic Vein
Pancreaticoduodenostomy
   see Bypass, Hepatobiliary System and
     Pancreas 0F1
Pancreaticosplenic lymph node
   use Lymphatic, Aortic
Pancreatogram, endoscopic retrograde
   see Fluoroscopy, Pancreatic Duct BF18
Pancreatolithotomy
   see Extirpation, Pancreas 0FCG
Pancreatotomy
   see Division, Pancreas 0F8G
   see Drainage, Pancreas 0F9G
Panniculectomy
   see Excision, Skin, Abdomen 0HB7
   see Excision, Subcutaneous Tissue and
     Fascia, Abdomen 0JB8
Paraaortic lymph node
   use Lymphatic, Aortic
Paracentesis
   Eye *see* Drainage, Eye 089
   Peritoneal Cavity *see* Drainage, Peritoneal
     Cavity 0W9G
   Tympanum *see* Drainage, Ear, Nose,
     Sinus 099
Pararectal lymph node
   use Lymphatic, Mesenteric
Parasternal lymph node
   use Lymphatic, Thorax

Parathyroidectomy
  see Excision, Endocrine System 0GB
  see Resection, Endocrine System 0GT
Paratracheal lymph node
  use Lymphatic, Thorax
Paraurethral (Skene's) gland
  use Vestibular Gland
Parenteral nutrition, total
  see Introduction of Nutritional Substance
Parietal lobe
  use Cerebral Hemisphere
Parotid lymph node
  use Lymphatic, Head
Parotid plexus
  use Facial Nerve
Parotidectomy
  see Excision, Mouth and Throat 0CB
  see Resection, Mouth and Throat 0CT
Pars flaccida
  use Tympanic Membrane, Right
  use Tympanic Membrane, Left
Partial joint replacement
  Hip see Replacement, Lower Joints 0SR
  Knee see Replacement, Lower Joints 0SR
  Shoulder see Replacement, Upper
    Joints 0RR
Partially absorbable mesh
  use Synthetic Substitute
Patch, blood, spinal 3E0R3GC
Patellapexy
  see Repair, Lower Bones 0QQ
  see Reposition, Lower Bones 0QS
Patellaplasty
  see Repair, Lower Bones 0QQ
  see Replacement, Lower Bones 0QR
  see Supplement, Lower Bones 0QU
Patellar ligament
  use Knee Bursa and Ligament, Right
  use Knee Bursa and Ligament, Left
Patellar tendon
  use Knee Tendon, Right
  use Knee Tendon, Left
Patellectomy
  see Excision, Lower Bones 0QB
  see Resection, Lower Bones 0QT
Patellofemoral joint
  use Knee Joint, Right
  use Knee Joint, Left
  use Knee Joint, Femoral Surface, Right
  use Knee Joint, Femoral Surface, Left
Pectineus muscle
  use Upper Leg Muscle, Right
  use Upper Leg Muscle, Left
Pectoral (anterior) lymph node
  use Lymphatic, Right Axillary
  use Lymphatic, Left Axillary
Pectoral fascia
  use Subcutaneous Tissue and Fascia, Chest
Pectoralis major muscle
  use Thorax Muscle, Right
  use Thorax Muscle, Left
Pectoralis minor muscle
  use Thorax Muscle, Right
  use Thorax Muscle, Left
**Pedicle-based dynamic stabilization
  device**
  use Spinal Stabilization Device, Pedicle-
    Based in 0RH
  use Spinal Stabilization Device, Pedicle-
    Based in 0SH
PEEP (positive end expiratory pressure)
  see Assistance, Respiratory 5A09
**PEG (percutaneous endoscopic
  gastrostomy)** 0DH63UZ
**PEJ (percutaneous endoscopic
  jejunostomy)** 0DHA3UZ

Pelvic splanchnic nerve
  use Abdominal Sympathetic Nerve
  use Sacral Sympathetic Nerve
Penectomy
  see Excision, Male Reproductive System 0VB
  see Resection, Male Reproductive
    System 0VT
Penile urethra
  use Urethra
Perceval sutureless valve
  use Zooplastic Tissue, Rapid Deployment
    Technique in New Technology
**Percutaneous endoscopic
  gastrojejunostomy (PEG/J) tube**
  use Feeding Device in Gastrointestinal
    System
**Percutaneous endoscopic gastrostomy
  (PEG) tube**
  use Feeding Device in Gastrointestinal
    System
Percutaneous nephrostomy catheter
  use Drainage Device
**Percutaneous transluminal coronary
  angioplasty (PTCA)**
  see Dilation, Heart and Great Vessels 027
Performance
  Biliary
    Multiple, Filtration 5A1C60Z
    Single, Filtration 5A1C00Z
  Cardiac
    Continuous
      Output 5A1221Z
      Pacing 5A1223Z
    Intermittent, Pacing 5A1213Z
    Single, Output, Manual 5A12012
  Circulatory
    Continuous
      Central Membrane 5A1522F
      Peripheral Veno-arterial
        Membrane 5A1522G
      Peripheral Veno-venous
        Membrane 5A1522H
    Intraoperative
      Central Membrane 5A15A2F
      Peripheral Veno-arterial
        Membrane 5A15A2G
      Peripheral Veno-venous
        Membrane 5A15A2H
  Respiratory
    24-96 Consecutive Hours,
      Ventilation 5A1945Z
    Greater than 96 Consecutive Hours,
      Ventilation 5A1955Z
    Less than 24 Consecutive Hours,
      Ventilation 5A1935Z
    Single, Ventilation,
      Nonmechanical 5A19054
  Urinary
    Continuous, Greater than 18 hours per
      day, Filtration 5A1D90Z
    Intermittent, Less than 6 Hours Per Day,
      Filtration 5A1D70Z
    Prolonged Intermittent, 6-18 hours per
      day, Filtration 5A1D80Z
Perfusion
  see Introduction of substance in or on
Perfusion, donor organ
  Heart 6AB50BZ
  Kidney(s) 6ABT0BZ
  Liver 6ABF0BZ
  Lung(s) 6ABB0BZ
Pericardiectomy
  see Excision, Pericardium 02BN
  see Resection, Pericardium 02TN
Pericardiocentesis
  see Drainage, Pericardial Cavity 0W9D

Pericardiolysis
  see Release, Pericardium 02NN
Pericardiophrenic artery
  use Internal Mammary Artery, Right
  use Internal Mammary Artery, Left
Pericardioplasty
  see Repair, Pericardium 02QN
  see Replacement, Pericardium 02RN
  see Supplement, Pericardium 02UN
Pericardiorrhaphy
  see Repair, Pericardium 02QN
Pericardiostomy
  see Drainage, Pericardial Cavity 0W9D
Pericardiotomy
  see Drainage, Pericardial Cavity 0W9D
Perimetrium
  use Uterus
**Peripheral Intravascular Lithotripsy
  (Peripheral IVL)**
  see Fragmentation
Peripheral parenteral nutrition
  see Introduction of Nutritional Substance
**Peripherally inserted central catheter
  (PICC)**
  use Infusion Device
Peritoneal dialysis 3E1M39Z
Peritoneocentesis
  see Drainage, Peritoneum 0D9W
  see Drainage, Peritoneal Cavity 0W9G
Peritoneoplasty
  see Repair, Peritoneum 0DQW
  see Replacement, Peritoneum 0DRW
  see Supplement, Peritoneum 0DUW
Peritoneoscopy 0DJW4ZZ
Peritoneotomy
  see Drainage, Peritoneum 0D9W
Peritoneumectomy
  see Excision, Peritoneum 0DBW
Peroneus brevis muscle
  use Lower Leg Muscle, Right
  use Lower Leg Muscle, Left
Peroneus longus muscle
  use Lower Leg Muscle, Right
  use Lower Leg Muscle, Left
Pessary ring
  use Intraluminal Device, Pessary in Female
    Reproductive System
PET scan
  see Positron Emission Tomographic (PET)
    Imaging
Petrous part of temporal bone
  use Temporal Bone, Right
  use Temporal Bone, Left
Phacoemulsification, lens
  With IOL implant see Replacement, Eye 08R
  Without IOL implant see Extraction,
    Eye 08D
Phalangectomy
  see Excision, Upper Bones 0PB
  see Resection, Upper Bones 0PT
  see Excision, Lower Bones 0QB
  see Resection, Lower Bones 0QT
Phallectomy
  see Excision, Penis 0VBS
  see Resection, Penis 0VTS
Phalloplasty
  see Repair, Penis 0VQS
  see Supplement, Penis 0VUS
Phallotomy
  see Drainage, Penis 0V9S
Pharmacotherapy, for substance abuse
  Antabuse HZ93ZZZ
  Bupropion HZ97ZZZ
  Clonidine HZ96ZZZ
  Levo-alpha-acetyl-methadol
    (LAAM) HZ92ZZZ

Pharmacotherapy, for substance abuse
— *continued*
  Methadone Maintenance HZ91ZZZ
  Naloxone HZ95ZZZ
  Naltrexone HZ94ZZZ
  Nicotine Replacement HZ90ZZZ
  Psychiatric Medication HZ98ZZZ
  Replacement Medication, Other HZ99ZZZ
Pharyngeal constrictor muscle
  use Tongue, Palate, Pharynx Muscle
Pharyngeal plexus
  use Vagus Nerve
Pharyngeal recess
  use Nasopharynx
Pharyngeal tonsil
  use Adenoids
Pharyngogram
  see Fluoroscopy, Pharynix B91G
Pharyngoplasty
  see Repair, Mouth and Throat 0CQ
  see Replacement, Mouth and Throat 0CR
  see Supplement, Mouth and Throat 0CU
Pharyngorrhaphy
  see Repair, Mouth and Throat 0CQ
Pharyngotomy
  see Drainage, Mouth and Throat 0C9
Pharyngotympanic tube
  use Eustachian Tube, Right
  use Eustachian Tube, Left
Pheresis
  Erythrocytes 6A55
  Leukocytes 6A55
  Plasma 6A55
  Platelets 6A55
  Stem Cells
    Cord Blood 6A55
    Hematopoietic 6A55
Phlebectomy
  see Excision, Upper Veins 05B
  see Extraction, Upper Veins 05D
  see Excision, Lower Veins 06B
  see Extraction, Lower Veins 06D
Phlebography
  see Plain Radiography, Veins B50
  Impedance 4A04X51
Phleborrhaphy
  see Repair, Upper Veins 05Q
  see Repair, Lower Veins 06Q
Phlebotomy
  see Drainage, Upper Veins 059
  see Drainage, Lower Veins 069
Photocoagulation
  For Destruction *see* Destruction
  For Repair *see* Repair
Photopheresis, therapeutic
  see Phototherapy, Circulatory 6A65
Phototherapy
  Circulatory 6A65
  Skin 6A60
  Ultraviolet light *see* Ultraviolet Light
    Therapy, Physiological Systems 6A8
Phrenectomy, phrenoneurectomy
  see Excision, Nerve, Phrenic 01B2
Phrenemphraxis
  see Destruction, Nerve, Phrenic 0152
Phrenic nerve stimulator generator
  use Stimulator Generator in Subcutaneous
    Tissue and Fascia
Phrenic nerve stimulator lead
  use Diaphragmatic Pacemaker Lead in
    Respiratory System
Phreniclasis
  see Destruction, Nerve, Phrenic 0152
Phrenicoexeresis
  see Extraction, Nerve, Phrenic 01D2
Phrenicotomy
  see Division, Nerve, Phrenic 0182

Phrenicotripsy
  see Destruction, Nerve, Phrenic 0152
Phrenoplasty
  see Repair, Respiratory System 0BQ
  see Supplement, Respiratory System 0BU
Phrenotomy
  see Drainage, Respiratory System 0B9
Physiatry
  see Motor Treatment, Rehabilitation F07
Physical medicine
  see Motor Treatment, Rehabilitation F07
Physical therapy
  see Motor Treatment, Rehabilitation F07
PHYSIOMESH™ Flexible Composite Mesh
  use Synthetic Substitute
Pia mater, intracranial
  use Cerebral Meninges
Pia mater, spinal
  use Spinal Meninges
Pinealectomy
  see Excision, Pineal Body 0GB1
  see Resection, Pineal Body 0GT1
Pinealoscopy 0GJ14ZZ
Pinealotomy
  see Drainage, Pineal Body 0G91
Pinna
  use External Ear, Right
  use External Ear, Left
  use External Ear, Bilateral
Pipeline™ (Flex) embolization device
  use Intraluminal Device, Flow Diverter
    in 03V
Piriform recess (sinus)
  use Pharynx
Piriformis muscle
  use Hip Muscle, Right
  use Hip Muscle, Left
PIRRT (Prolonged intermittent renal
  replacement therapy) 5A1D80Z
Pisiform bone
  use Carpal, Right
  use Carpal, Left
Pisohamate ligament
  use Hand Bursa and Ligament, Right
  use Hand Bursa and Ligament, Left
Pisometacarpal ligament
  use Hand Bursa and Ligament, Right
  use Hand Bursa and Ligament, Left
Pituitectomy
  see Excision, Gland, Pituitary 0GB0
  see Resection, Gland, Pituitary 0GT0
Plain film radiology
  see Plain Radiography
Plain Radiography
  Abdomen BW00ZZZ
  Abdomen and Pelvis BW01ZZZ
  Abdominal Lymphatic
    Bilateral B701
    Unilateral B700
  Airway, Upper BB0DZZZ
  Ankle
    Left BQ0H
    Right BQ0G
  Aorta
    Abdominal B400
    Thoracic B300
    Thoraco-Abdominal B30P
  Aorta and Bilateral Lower Extremity
    Arteries B40D
  Arch
    Bilateral BN0DZZZ
    Left BN0CZZZ
    Right BN0BZZZ
  Arm
    Left BP0FZZZ
    Right BP0EZZZ

Plain Radiography — *continued*
  Artery
    Brachiocephalic-Subclavian, Right B301
    Bronchial B30L
    Bypass Graft, Other B20F
    Cervico-Cerebral Arch B30Q
    Common Carotid
      Bilateral B305
      Left B304
      Right B303
    Coronary
      Bypass Graft
        Multiple B203
        Single B202
      Multiple B201
      Single B200
    External Carotid
      Bilateral B30C
      Left B30B
      Right B309
    Hepatic B402
    Inferior Mesenteric B405
    Intercostal B30L
    Internal Carotid
      Bilateral B308
      Left B307
      Right B306
    Internal Mammary Bypass Graft
      Left B208
      Right B207
    Intra-Abdominal, Other B40B
    Intracranial B30R
    Lower, Other B40J
    Lower Extremity
      Bilateral and Aorta B40D
      Left B40G
      Right B40F
    Lumbar B409
    Pelvic B40C
    Pulmonary
      Left B30T
      Right B30S
    Renal
      Bilateral B408
      Left B407
      Right B406
      Transplant B40M
    Spinal B30M
    Splenic B403
    Subclavian, Left B302
    Superior Mesenteric B404
    Upper, Other B30N
    Upper Extremity
      Bilateral B30K
      Left B30J
      Right B30H
    Vertebral
      Bilateral B30G
      Left B30F
      Right B30D
  Bile Duct BF00
  Bile Duct and Gallbladder BF03
  Bladder BT00
    Kidney and Ureter BT04
  Bladder and Urethra BT0B
  Bone
    Facial BN05ZZZ
    Nasal BN04ZZZ
  Bones, Long, All BW0BZZZ
  Breast
    Bilateral BH02ZZZ
    Left BH01ZZZ
    Right BH00ZZZ
  Calcaneus
    Left BQ0KZZZ
    Right BQ0JZZZ
  Chest BW03ZZZ

Plain Radiography — *continued*
  Clavicle
    Left BP05ZZZ
    Right BP04ZZZ
  Coccyx BR0FZZZ
  Corpora Cavernosa BV00
  Dialysis Fistula B50W
  Dialysis Shunt B50W
  Disc
    Cervical BR01
    Lumbar BR03
    Thoracic BR02
  Duct
    Lacrimal
      Bilateral B802
      Left B801
      Right B800
    Mammary
      Multiple
        Left BH06
        Right BH05
      Single
        Left BH04
        Right BH03
  Elbow
    Left BP0H
    Right BP0G
  Epididymis
    Left BV02
    Right BV01
  Extremity
    Lower BW0CZZZ
    Upper BW0JZZZ
  Eye
    Bilateral B807ZZZ
    Left B806ZZZ
    Right B805ZZZ
  Facet Joint
    Cervical BR04
    Lumbar BR06
    Thoracic BR05
  Fallopian Tube
    Bilateral BU02
    Left BU01
    Right BU00
  Fallopian Tube and Uterus BU08
  Femur
    Left, Densitometry BQ04ZZ1
    Right, Densitometry BQ03ZZ1
  Finger
    Left BP0SZZZ
    Right BP0RZZZ
  Foot
    Left BQ0MZZZ
    Right BQ0LZZZ
  Forearm
    Left BP0KZZZ
    Right BP0JZZZ
  Gallbladder and Bile Duct BF03
  Gland
    Parotid
      Bilateral B906
      Left B905
      Right B904
    Salivary
      Bilateral B90D
      Left B90C
      Right B90B
    Submandibular
      Bilateral B909
      Left B908
      Right B907
  Hand
    Left BP0PZZZ
    Right BP0NZZZ
  Heart
    Left B205

Plain Radiography — *continued*
  Heart — *continued*
    Right B204
    Right and Left B206
  Hepatobiliary System, All BF0C
  Hip
    Left BQ01
      Densitometry BQ01ZZ1
    Right BQ00
      Densitometry BQ00ZZ1
  Humerus
    Left BP0BZZZ
    Right BP0AZZZ
  Ileal Diversion Loop BT0C
  Intracranial Sinus B502
  Joint
    Acromioclavicular, Bilateral BP03ZZZ
    Finger
      Left BP0D
      Right BP0C
    Foot
      Left BQ0Y
      Right BQ0X
    Hand
      Left BP0D
      Right BP0C
    Lumbosacral BR0BZZZ
    Sacroiliac BR0D
    Sternoclavicular
      Bilateral BP02ZZZ
      Left BP01ZZZ
      Right BP00ZZZ
    Temporomandibular
      Bilateral BN09
      Left BN08
      Right BN07
    Thoracolumbar BR08ZZZ
    Toe
      Left BQ0Y
      Right BQ0X
  Kidney
    Bilateral BT03
    Left BT02
    Right BT01
    Ureter and Bladder BT04
  Knee
    Left BQ08
    Right BQ07
  Leg
    Left BQ0FZZZ
    Right BQ0DZZZ
  Lymphatic
    Head B704
    Lower Extremity
      Bilateral B70B
      Left B709
      Right B708
    Neck B704
    Pelvic B70C
    Upper Extremity
      Bilateral B707
      Left B706
      Right B705
  Mandible BN06ZZZ
  Mastoid B90HZZZ
  Nasopharynx B90FZZZ
  Optic Foramina
    Left B804ZZZ
    Right B803ZZZ
  Orbit
    Bilateral BN03ZZZ
    Left BN02ZZZ
    Right BN01ZZZ
  Oropharynx B90FZZZ
  Patella
    Left BQ0WZZZ
    Right BQ0VZZZ

Plain Radiography — *continued*
  Pelvis BR0CZZZ
  Pelvis and Abdomen BW01ZZZ
  Prostate BV03
  Retroperitoneal Lymphatic
    Bilateral B701
    Unilateral B700
  Ribs
    Left BP0YZZZ
    Right BP0XZZZ
  Sacrum BR0FZZZ
  Scapula
    Left BP07ZZZ
    Right BP06ZZZ
  Shoulder
    Left BP09
    Right BP08
  Sinus
    Intracranial B502
    Paranasal B902ZZZ
  Skull BN00ZZZ
  Spinal Cord B00B
  Spine
    Cervical, Densitometry BR00ZZ1
    Lumbar, Densitometry BR09ZZ1
    Thoracic, Densitometry BR07ZZ1
    Whole, Densitometry BR0GZZ1
  Sternum BR0HZZZ
  Teeth
    All BN0JZZZ
    Multiple BN0HZZZ
  Testicle
    Left BV06
    Right BV05
  Toe
    Left BQ0QZZZ
    Right BQ0PZZZ
  Tooth, Single BN0GZZZ
  Tracheobronchial Tree
    Bilateral BB09YZZ
    Left BB08YZZ
    Right BB07YZZ
  Ureter
    Bilateral BT08
    Kidney and Bladder BT04
    Left BT07
    Right BT06
  Urethra BT05
  Urethra and Bladder BT0B
  Uterus BU06
  Uterus and Fallopian Tube BU08
  Vagina BU09
  Vasa Vasorum BV08
  Vein
    Cerebellar B501
    Cerebral B501
    Epidural B500
    Jugular
      Bilateral B505
      Left B504
      Right B503
    Lower Extremity
      Bilateral B50D
      Left B50C
      Right B50B
    Other B50V
    Pelvic (Iliac)
      Left B50G
      Right B50F
    Pelvic (Iliac) Bilateral B50H
    Portal B50T
    Pulmonary
      Bilateral B50S
      Left B50R
      Right B50Q
    Renal
      Bilateral B50L

Plain Radiography — *continued*
Vein — *continued*
　　Left B50K
　　Right B50J
　　Splanchnic B50T
　　Subclavian
　　　Left B507
　　　Right B506
　　Upper Extremity
　　　Bilateral B50P
　　　Left B50N
　　　Right B50M
　Vena Cava
　　Inferior B509
　　Superior B508
　Whole Body BW0KZZZ
　　Infant BW0MZZZ
　Whole Skeleton BW0LZZZ
　Wrist
　　Left BP0M
　　Right BP0L
Planar Nuclear Medicine Imaging
Abdomen CW10
Abdomen and Chest CW14
Abdomen and Pelvis CW11
Anatomical Region, Other CW1ZZZZ
Anatomical Regions, Multiple CW1YYZZ
Bladder, Kidneys and Ureters CT13
Bladder and Ureters CT1H
Blood C713
Bone Marrow C710
Brain C010
Breast CH1YYZZ
　Bilateral CH12
　Left CH11
　Right CH10
Bronchi and Lungs CB12
Central Nervous System C01YYZZ
Cerebrospinal Fluid C015
Chest CW13
Chest and Abdomen CW14
Chest and Neck CW16
Digestive System CD1YYZZ
Ducts, Lacrimal, Bilateral C819
Ear, Nose, Mouth and Throat C91YYZZ
Endocrine System CG1YYZZ
Extremity
　Lower CW1D
　　Bilateral CP1F
　　Left CP1D
　　Right CP1C
　Upper CW1M
　　Bilateral CP1B
　　Left CP19
　　Right CP18
Eye C81YYZZ
Gallbladder CF14
Gastrointestinal Tract CD17
　Upper CD15
Gland
　Adrenal, Bilateral CG14
　Parathyroid CG11
　Thyroid CG12
Glands, Salivary, Bilateral C91B
Head and Neck CW1B
Heart C21YYZZ
　Right and Left C216
Hepatobiliary System, All CF1C
Hepatobiliary System and
　Pancreas CF1YYZZ
Kidneys, Ureters and Bladder CT13
Liver CF15
Liver and Spleen CF16
Lungs and Bronchi CB12
Lymphatics
　Head C71J
　Head and Neck C715

Planar Nuclear Medicine Imaging — *continued*
Lymphatics — *continued*
　Lower Extremity C71P
　Neck C71K
　Pelvic C71D
　Trunk C71M
　Upper Chest C71L
　Upper Extremity C71N
Lymphatics and Hematologic
　System C71YYZZ
Musculoskeletal System
　All CP1Z
　Other CP1YYZZ
Myocardium C21G
Neck and Chest CW16
Neck and Head CW1B
Pancreas and Hepatobiliary
　System CF1YYZZ
Pelvic Region CW1J
Pelvis CP16
Pelvis and Abdomen CW11
Pelvis and Spine CP17
Reproductive System, Male CV1YYZZ
Respiratory System CB1YYZZ
Skin CH1YYZZ
Skull CP11
Spine CP15
Spine and Pelvis CP17
Spleen C712
Spleen and Liver CF16
Subcutaneous Tissue CH1YYZZ
Testicles, Bilateral CV19
Thorax CP14
Ureters, Kidneys and Bladder CT13
Ureters and Bladder CT1H
Urinary System CT1YYZZ
Veins C51YYZZ
　Central C51R
　Lower Extremity
　　Bilateral C51D
　　Left C51C
　　Right C51B
　Upper Extremity
　　Bilateral C51Q
　　Left C51P
　　Right C51N
Whole Body CW1N
Plantar digital vein
　use Foot Vein, Right
　use Foot Vein, Left
Plantar fascia (aponeurosis)
　use Subcutaneous Tissue and Fascia, Right
　　Foot
　use Subcutaneous Tissue and Fascia, Left
　　Foot
Plantar metatarsal vein
　use Foot Vein, Right
　use Foot Vein, Left
Plantar venous arch
　use Foot Vein, Right
　use Foot Vein, Left
Plaque Radiation
Abdomen DWY3FZZ
Adrenal Gland DGY2FZZ
Anus DDY8FZZ
Bile Ducts DFY2FZZ
Bladder DTY2FZZ
Bone, Other DPYCFZZ
Bone Marrow D7Y0FZZ
Brain D0Y0FZZ
Brain Stem D0Y1FZZ
Breast
　Left DMY0FZZ
　Right DMY1FZZ
Bronchus DBY1FZZ
Cervix DUY1FZZ
Chest DWY2FZZ

Plaque Radiation — *continued*
Chest Wall DBY7FZZ
Colon DDY5FZZ
Diaphragm DBY8FZZ
Duodenum DDY2FZZ
Ear D9Y0FZZ
Esophagus DDY0FZZ
Eye D8Y0FZZ
Femur DPY9FZZ
Fibula DPYBFZZ
Gallbladder DFY1FZZ
Gland
　Adrenal DGY2FZZ
　Parathyroid DGY4FZZ
　Pituitary DGY0FZZ
　Thyroid DGY5FZZ
Glands, Salivary D9Y6FZZ
Head and Neck DWY1FZZ
Hemibody DWY4FZZ
Humerus DPY6FZZ
Ileum DDY4FZZ
Jejunum DDY3FZZ
Kidney DTY0FZZ
Larynx D9YBFZZ
Liver DFY0FZZ
Lung DBY2FZZ
Lymphatics
　Abdomen D7Y6FZZ
　Axillary D7Y4FZZ
　Inguinal D7Y8FZZ
　Neck D7Y3FZZ
　Pelvis D7Y7FZZ
　Thorax D7Y5FZZ
Mandible DPY3FZZ
Maxilla DPY2FZZ
Mediastinum DBY6FZZ
Mouth D9Y4FZZ
Nasopharynx D9YDFZZ
Neck and Head DWY1FZZ
Nerve, Peripheral D0Y7FZZ
Nose D9Y1FZZ
Ovary DUY0FZZ
Palate
　Hard D9Y8FZZ
　Soft D9Y9FZZ
Pancreas DFY3FZZ
Parathyroid Gland DGY4FZZ
Pelvic Bones DPY8FZZ
Pelvic Region DWY6FZZ
Pharynx D9YCFZZ
Pineal Body DGY1FZZ
Pituitary Gland DGY0FZZ
Pleura DBY5FZZ
Prostate DVY0FZZ
Radius DPY7FZZ
Rectum DDY7FZZ
Rib DPY5FZZ
Sinuses D9Y7FZZ
Skin
　Abdomen DHY8FZZ
　Arm DHY4FZZ
　Back DHY7FZZ
　Buttock DHY9FZZ
　Chest DHY6FZZ
　Face DHY2FZZ
　Foot DHYCFZZ
　Hand DHY5FZZ
　Leg DHYBFZZ
　Neck DHY3FZZ
Skull DPY0FZZ
Spinal Cord D0Y6FZZ
Spleen D7Y2FZZ
Sternum DPY4FZZ
Stomach DDY1FZZ
Testis DVY1FZZ
Thymus D7Y1FZZ
Thyroid Gland DGY5FZZ

Plaque Radiation — *continued*
- Tibia DPYBFZZ
- Tongue D9Y5FZZ
- Trachea DBY0FZZ
- Ulna DPY7FZZ
- Ureter DTY1FZZ
- Urethra DTY3FZZ
- Uterus DUY2FZZ
- Whole Body DWY5FZZ

Plasma, Convalescent (Nonautologous) XW1

Plasmapheresis, therapeutic
see Pheresis, Physiological Systems 6A5

Plateletpheresis, therapeutic
see Pheresis, Physiological Systems 6A5

Platysma muscle
use Neck Muscle, Right
use Neck Muscle, Left

Plazomicin Anti-infective XW0

Pleurectomy
see Excision, Respiratory System 0BB
see Resection, Respiratory System 0BT

Pleurocentesis
see Drainage, Anatomical Regions, General 0W9

Pleurodesis, pleurosclerosis
Chemical injection *see* Introduction of substance in or on, Pleural Cavity 3E0L
Surgical *see* Destruction, Respiratory System 0B5

Pleurolysis
see Release, Respiratory System 0BN

Pleuroscopy 0BJQ4ZZ

Pleurotomy
see Drainage, Respiratory System 0B9

Plica semilunaris
use Conjunctiva, Right
use Conjunctiva, Left

Plication
see Restriction

Pneumectomy
see Excision, Respiratory System 0BB
see Resection, Respiratory System 0BT

Pneumocentesis
see Drainage, Respiratory System 0B9

Pneumogastric nerve
use Vagus Nerve

Pneumolysis
see Release, Respiratory System 0BN

Pneumonectomy
see Resection, Respiratory System 0BT

Pneumonolysis
see Release, Respiratory System 0BN

Pneumonopexy
see Repair, Respiratory System 0BQ
see Reposition, Respiratory System 0BS

Pneumonorrhaphy
see Repair, Respiratory System 0BQ

Pneumonotomy
see Drainage, Respiratory System 0B9

Pneumotaxic center
use Pons

Pneumotomy
see Drainage, Respiratory System 0B9

Pollicization
see Transfer, Anatomical Regions, Upper Extremities 0XX

Polyethylene socket
use Synthetic Substitute, Polyethylene in 0SR

Polymethylmethacrylate (PMMA)
use Synthetic Substitute

Polypectomy, gastrointestinal
see Excision, Gastrointestinal System 0DB

Polypropylene mesh
use Synthetic Substitute

Polysomnogram 4A1ZXQZ

Pontine tegmentum
use Pons

Popliteal ligament
use Knee Bursa and Ligament, Right
use Knee Bursa and Ligament, Left

Popliteal lymph node
use Lymphatic, Right Lower Extremity
use Lymphatic, Left Lower Extremity

Popliteal vein
use Femoral Vein, Right
use Femoral Vein, Left

Popliteus muscle
use Lower Leg Muscle, Right
use Lower Leg Muscle, Left

Porcine (bioprosthetic) valve
use Zooplastic Tissue in Heart and Great Vessels

Positive Blood Culture Fluorescence Hybridization for Organism Identification, Concentration and Susceptibility XXE5XN6

Positive end expiratory pressure
see Performance, Respiratory 5A19

Positron Emission Tomographic (PET) Imaging
- Brain C030
- Bronchi and Lungs CB32
- Central Nervous System C03YYZZ
- Heart C23YYZZ
- Lungs and Bronchi CB32
- Myocardium C23G
- Respiratory System CB3YYZZ
- Whole Body CW3NYZZ

Positron emission tomography
see Positron Emission Tomographic (PET) Imaging

Postauricular (mastoid) lymph node
use Lymphatic, Right Neck
use Lymphatic, Left Neck

Postcava
use Inferior Vena Cava

Posterior (subscapular) lymph node
use Lymphatic, Right Axillary
use Lymphatic, Left Axillary

Posterior auricular artery
use External Carotid Artery, Right
use External Carotid Artery, Left

Posterior auricular nerve
use Facial Nerve

Posterior auricular vein
use External Jugular Vein, Right
use External Jugular Vein, Left

Posterior cerebral artery
use Intracranial Artery

Posterior chamber
use Eye, Right
use Eye, Left

Posterior circumflex humeral artery
use Axillary Artery, Right
use Axillary Artery, Left

Posterior communicating artery
use Intracranial Artery

Posterior cruciate ligament (PCL)
use Knee Bursa and Ligament, Right
use Knee Bursa and Ligament, Left

Posterior facial (retromandibular) vein
use Face Vein, Right
use Face Vein, Left

Posterior femoral cutaneous nerve
use Sacral Plexus

Posterior inferior cerebellar artery (PICA)
use Intracranial Artery

Posterior interosseous nerve
use Radial Nerve

Posterior labial nerve
use Pudendal Nerve

Posterior scrotal nerve
use Pudendal Nerve

Posterior spinal artery
use Vertebral Artery, Right
use Vertebral Artery, Left

Posterior tibial recurrent artery
use Anterior Tibial Artery, Right
use Anterior Tibial Artery, Left

Posterior ulnar recurrent artery
use Ulnar Artery, Right
use Ulnar Artery, Left

Posterior vagal trunk
use Vagus Nerve

PPN (peripheral parenteral nutrition)
see Introduction of Nutritional Substance

Preauricular lymph node
use Lymphatic, Head

Precava
use Superior Vena Cava

PRECICE intramedullary limb lengthening system
use Internal Fixation Device, Intramedullary Limb Lengthening in 0PH
use Internal Fixation Device, Intramedullary Limb Lengthening in 0QH

Prepatellar bursa
use Knee Bursa and Ligament, Right
use Knee Bursa and Ligament, Left

Preputiotomy
see Drainage, Male Reproductive System 0V9

Pressure support ventilation
see Performance, Respiratory 5A19

PRESTIGE® Cervical Disc
use Synthetic Substitute

Pretracheal fascia
use Subcutaneous Tissue and Fascia, Right Neck
use Subcutaneous Tissue and Fascia, Left Neck

Prevertebral fascia
use Subcutaneous Tissue and Fascia, Right Neck
use Subcutaneous Tissue and Fascia, Left Neck

PrimeAdvanced neurostimulator (SureScan)(MRI Safe)
use Stimulator Generator, Multiple Array in 0JH

Princeps pollicis artery
use Hand Artery, Right
use Hand Artery, Left

Probing, duct
Diagnostic *see* Inspection
Dilation *see* Dilation

PROCEED™ Ventral Patch
use Synthetic Substitute

Procerus muscle
use Facial Muscle

Proctectomy
see Excision, Rectum 0DBP
see Resection, Rectum 0DTP

Proctoclysis
see Introduction of substance in or on, Gastrointestinal Tract, Lower 3E0H

Proctocolectomy
see Excision, Gastrointestinal System 0DB
see Resection, Gastrointestinal System 0DT

Proctocolpoplasty
see Repair, Gastrointestinal System 0DQ
see Supplement, Gastrointestinal System 0DU

Proctoperineoplasty
see Repair, Gastrointestinal System 0DQ
see Supplement, Gastrointestinal System 0DU

Proctoperineorrhaphy
see Repair, Gastrointestinal System 0DQ

Proctopexy
see Repair, Rectum 0DQP
see Reposition, Rectum 0DSP
Proctoplasty
see Repair, Rectum 0DQP
see Supplement, Rectum 0DUP
Proctorrhaphy
see Repair, Rectum 0DQP
Proctoscopy 0DJD8ZZ
Proctosigmoidectomy
see Excision, Gastrointestinal System 0DB
see Resection, Gastrointestinal System 0DT
Proctosigmoidoscopy 0DJD8ZZ
Proctostomy
see Drainage, Rectum 0D9P
Proctotomy
see Drainage, Rectum 0D9P
Prodisc-C
use Synthetic Substitute
Prodisc-L
use Synthetic Substitute
Production, atrial septal defect
see Excision, Septum, Atrial 02B5
Profunda brachii
use Brachial Artery, Right
use Brachial Artery, Left
Profunda femoris (deep femoral) vein
use Femoral Vein, Right
use Femoral Vein, Left
PROLENE Polypropylene Hernia System (PHS)
use Synthetic Substitute
Prolonged intermittent renal replacement therapy (PIRRT) 5A1D80Z
Pronator quadratus muscle
use Lower Arm and Wrist Muscle, Right
use Lower Arm and Wrist Muscle, Left
Pronator teres muscle
use Lower Arm and Wrist Muscle, Right
use Lower Arm and Wrist Muscle, Left
Prostatectomy
see Excision, Prostate 0VB0
see Resection, Prostate 0VT0
Prostatic urethra
use Urethra
Prostatomy, prostatotomy
see Drainage, Prostate 0V90
Protecta XT CRT-D
use Cardiac Resynchronization Defibrillator Pulse Generator in 0JH
Protecta XT DR (XT VR)
use Defibrillator Generator in 0JH
Protege® RX Carotid Stent System
use Intraluminal Device
Proximal radioulnar joint
use Elbow Joint, Right
use Elbow Joint, Left
Psoas muscle
use Hip Muscle, Right
use Hip Muscle, Left
PSV (pressure support ventilation)
see Performance, Respiratory 5A19
Psychoanalysis GZ54ZZZ
Psychological Tests
Cognitive Status GZ14ZZZ
Developmental GZ10ZZZ
Intellectual and Psychoeducational GZ12ZZZ
Neurobehavioral Status GZ14ZZZ
Neuropsychological GZ13ZZZ
Personality and Behavioral GZ11ZZZ
Psychotherapy
Family, Mental Health Services GZ72ZZZ
Group
GZHZZZZ
Mental Health Services GZHZZZZ

Psychotherapy — continued
Individual
see Psychotherapy, Individual, Mental Health Services
for substance abuse
12-Step HZ53ZZZ
Behavioral HZ51ZZZ
Cognitive HZ50ZZZ
Cognitive-Behavioral HZ52ZZZ
Confrontational HZ58ZZZ
Interactive HZ55ZZZ
Interpersonal HZ54ZZZ
Motivational Enhancement HZ57ZZZ
Psychoanalysis HZ5BZZZ
Psychodynamic HZ5CZZZ
Psychoeducation HZ56ZZZ
Psychophysiological HZ5DZZZ
Supportive HZ59ZZZ
Mental Health Services
Behavioral GZ51ZZZ
Cognitive GZ52ZZZ
Cognitive-Behavioral GZ58ZZZ
Interactive GZ50ZZZ
Interpersonal GZ53ZZZ
Psychoanalysis GZ54ZZZ
Psychodynamic GZ55ZZZ
Psychophysiological GZ59ZZZ
Supportive GZ56ZZZ
PTCA (percutaneous transluminal coronary angioplasty)
see Dilation, Heart and Great Vessels 027
Pterygoid muscle
use Head Muscle
Pterygoid process
use Sphenoid Bone
Pterygopalatine (sphenopalatine) ganglion
use Head and Neck Sympathetic Nerve
Pubis
use Pelvic Bone, Right
use Pelvic Bone, Left
Pubofemoral ligament
use Hip Bursa and Ligament, Right
use Hip Bursa and Ligament, Left
Pudendal nerve
use Sacral Plexus
Pull-through, laparoscopic-assisted transanal
see Excision, Gastrointestinal System 0DB
see Resection, Gastrointestinal System 0DT
Pull-through, rectal
see Resection, Rectum 0DTP
Pulmoaortic canal
use Pulmonary Artery, Left
Pulmonary annulus
use Pulmonary Valve
Pulmonary artery wedge monitoring
see Monitoring, Arterial 4A13
Pulmonary plexus
use Vagus Nerve
use Thoracic Sympathetic Nerve
Pulmonic valve
use Pulmonary Valve
Pulpectomy
see Excision, Mouth and Throat 0CB
Pulverization
see Fragmentation
Pulvinar
use Thalamus
Pump reservoir
use Infusion Device, Pump in Subcutaneous Tissue and Fascia
Punch biopsy
see Excision with qualifier Diagnostic
Puncture
see Drainage
Puncture, lumbar
see Drainage, Spinal Canal 009U

Pyelography
see Plain Radiography, Urinary System BT0
see Fluoroscopy, Urinary System BT1
Pyeloileostomy, urinary diversion
see Bypass, Urinary System 0T1
Pyeloplasty
see Repair, Urinary System 0TQ
see Replacement, Urinary System 0TR
see Supplement, Urinary System 0TU
Pyeloplasty, dismembered
see Repair, Kidney Pelvis
Pyelorrhaphy
see Repair, Urinary System 0TQ
Pyeloscopy 0TJ58ZZ
Pyelostomy
see Bypass, Urinary System 0T1
see Drainage, Urinary System 0T9
Pyelotomy
see Drainage, Urinary System 0T9
Pylorectomy
see Excision, Stomach, Pylorus 0DB7
see Resection, Stomach, Pylorus 0DT7
Pyloric antrum
use Stomach, Pylorus
Pyloric canal
use Stomach, Pylorus
Pyloric sphincter
use Stomach, Pylorus
Pylorodiosis
see Dilation, Stomach, Pylorus 0D77
Pylorogastrectomy
see Excision, Gastrointestinal System 0DB
see Resection, Gastrointestinal System 0DT
Pyloroplasty
see Repair, Stomach, Pylorus 0DQ7
see Supplement, Stomach, Pylorus 0DU7
Pyloroscopy 0DJ68ZZ
Pylorotomy
see Drainage, Stomach, Pylorus 0D97
Pyramidalis muscle
use Abdomen Muscle, Right
use Abdomen Muscle, Left

Q

Quadrangular cartilage
use Nasal Septum
Quadrant resection of breast
see Excision, Skin and Breast 0HB
Quadrate lobe
use Liver
Quadratus femoris muscle
use Hip Muscle, Right
use Hip Muscle, Left
Quadratus lumborum muscle
use Trunk Muscle, Right
use Trunk Muscle, Left
Quadratus plantae muscle
use Foot Muscle, Right
use Foot Muscle, Left
Quadriceps (femoris)
use Upper Leg Muscle, Right
use Upper Leg Muscle, Left
Quarantine 8E0ZXY6

R

Radial collateral carpal ligament
use Wrist Bursa and Ligament, Right
use Wrist Bursa and Ligament, Left
Radial collateral ligament
use Elbow Bursa and Ligament, Right
use Elbow Bursa and Ligament, Left
Radial notch
use Ulna, Right
use Ulna, Left

Radial recurrent artery
  use Radial Artery, Right
  use Radial Artery, Left
Radial vein
  use Brachial Vein, Right
  use Brachial Vein, Left
Radialis indicis
  use Hand Artery, Right
  use Hand Artery, Left
Radiation Therapy
  see Beam Radiation
  see Brachytherapy
  see Stereotactic Radiosurgery
Radiation treatment
  see Radiation Therapy
Radiocarpal joint
  use Wrist Joint, Right
  use Wrist Joint, Left
Radiocarpal ligament
  use Wrist Bursa and Ligament, Right
  use Wrist Bursa and Ligament, Left
Radiography
  see Plain Radiography
Radiology, analog
  see Plain Radiography
Radiology, diagnostic
  see Imaging, Diagnostic
Radioulnar ligament
  use Wrist Bursa and Ligament, Right
  use Wrist Bursa and Ligament, Left
Range of motion testing
  see Motor Function Assessment, Rehabilitation F01
REALIZE® Adjustable Gastric Band
  use Extraluminal Device
Reattachment
  Abdominal Wall 0WMF0ZZ
  Ampulla of Vater 0FMC
  Ankle Region
    Left 0YML0ZZ
    Right 0YMK0ZZ
  Arm
    Lower
      Left 0XMF0ZZ
      Right 0XMD0ZZ
    Upper
      Left 0XM90ZZ
      Right 0XM80ZZ
  Axilla
    Left 0XM50ZZ
    Right 0XM40ZZ
  Back
    Lower 0WML0ZZ
    Upper 0WMK0ZZ
  Bladder 0TMB
  Bladder Neck 0TMC
  Breast
    Bilateral 0HMVXZZ
    Left 0HMUXZZ
    Right 0HMTXZZ
  Bronchus
    Lingula 0BM90ZZ
    Lower Lobe
      Left 0BMB0ZZ
      Right 0BM60ZZ
    Main
      Left 0BM70ZZ
      Right 0BM30ZZ
    Middle Lobe, Right 0BM50ZZ
    Upper Lobe
      Left 0BM80ZZ
      Right 0BM40ZZ
  Bursa and Ligament
    Abdomen
      Left 0MMJ
      Right 0MMH

Reattachment — *continued*
  Bursa and Ligament — *continued*
    Ankle
      Left 0MMR
      Right 0MMQ
    Elbow
      Left 0MM4
      Right 0MM3
    Foot
      Left 0MMT
      Right 0MMS
    Hand
      Left 0MM8
      Right 0MM7
    Head and Neck 0MM0
    Hip
      Left 0MMM
      Right 0MML
    Knee
      Left 0MMP
      Right 0MMN
    Lower Extremity
      Left 0MMW
      Right 0MMV
    Perineum 0MMK
    Rib(s) 0MMG
    Shoulder
      Left 0MM2
      Right 0MM1
    Spine
      Lower 0MMD
      Upper 0MMC
    Sternum 0MMF
    Upper Extremity
      Left 0MMB
      Right 0MM9
    Wrist
      Left 0MM6
      Right 0MM5
  Buttock
    Left 0YM10ZZ
    Right 0YM00ZZ
  Carina 0BM20ZZ
  Cecum 0DMH
  Cervix 0UMC
  Chest Wall 0WM80ZZ
  Clitoris 0UMJXZZ
  Colon
    Ascending 0DMK
    Descending 0DMM
    Sigmoid 0DMN
    Transverse 0DML
  Cord
    Bilateral 0VMH
    Left 0VMG
    Right 0VMF
  Cul-de-sac 0UMF
  Diaphragm 0BMT0ZZ
  Duct
    Common Bile 0FM9
    Cystic 0FM8
    Hepatic
      Common 0FM7
      Left 0FM6
      Right 0FM5
    Pancreatic 0FMD
      Accessory 0FMF
  Duodenum 0DM9
  Ear
    Left 09M1XZZ
    Right 09M0XZZ
  Elbow Region
    Left 0XMC0ZZ
    Right 0XMB0ZZ
  Esophagus 0DM5
  Extremity
    Lower

Reattachment — *continued*
  Extremity — *continued*
      Left 0YMB0ZZ
      Right 0YM90ZZ
    Upper
      Left 0XM70ZZ
      Right 0XM60ZZ
  Eyelid
    Lower
      Left 08MRXZZ
      Right 08MQXZZ
    Upper
      Left 08MPXZZ
      Right 08MNXZZ
  Face 0WM20ZZ
  Fallopian Tube
    Left 0UM6
    Right 0UM5
  Fallopian Tubes, Bilateral 0UM7
  Femoral Region
    Left 0YM80ZZ
    Right 0YM70ZZ
  Finger
    Index
      Left 0XMP0ZZ
      Right 0XMN0ZZ
    Little
      Left 0XMW0ZZ
      Right 0XMV0ZZ
    Middle
      Left 0XMR0ZZ
      Right 0XMQ0ZZ
    Ring
      Left 0XMT0ZZ
      Right 0XMS0ZZ
  Foot
    Left 0YMN0ZZ
    Right 0YMM0ZZ
  Forequarter
    Left 0XM10ZZ
    Right 0XM00ZZ
  Gallbladder 0FM4
  Gland
    Left 0GM2
    Right 0GM3
  Hand
    Left 0XMK0ZZ
    Right 0XMJ0ZZ
  Hindquarter
    Bilateral 0YM40ZZ
    Left 0YM30ZZ
    Right 0YM20ZZ
  Hymen 0UMK
  Ileum 0DMB
  Inguinal Region
    Left 0YM60ZZ
    Right 0YM50ZZ
  Intestine
    Large 0DME
      Left 0DMG
      Right 0DMF
    Small 0DM8
  Jaw
    Lower 0WM50ZZ
    Upper 0WM40ZZ
  Jejunum 0DMA
  Kidney
    Left 0TM1
    Right 0TM0
  Kidney Pelvis
    Left 0TM4
    Right 0TM3
  Kidneys, Bilateral 0TM2
  Knee Region
    Left 0YMG0ZZ
    Right 0YMF0ZZ

Reattachment — *continued*
Leg
  Lower
    Left 0YMJ0ZZ
    Right 0YMH0ZZ
  Upper
    Left 0YMD0ZZ
    Right 0YMC0ZZ
Lip
  Lower 0CM10ZZ
  Upper 0CM00ZZ
Liver 0FM0
  Left Lobe 0FM2
  Right Lobe 0FM1
Lung
  Left 0BML0ZZ
  Lower Lobe
    Left 0BMJ0ZZ
    Right 0BMF0ZZ
  Middle Lobe, Right 0BMD0ZZ
  Right 0BMK0ZZ
  Upper Lobe
    Left 0BMG0ZZ
    Right 0BMC0ZZ
Lung Lingula 0BMH0ZZ
Muscle
  Abdomen
    Left 0KML
    Right 0KMK
  Facial 0KM1
  Foot
    Left 0KMW
    Right 0KMV
  Hand
    Left 0KMD
    Right 0KMC
  Head 0KM0
  Hip
    Left 0KMP
    Right 0KMN
  Lower Arm and Wrist
    Left 0KMB
    Right 0KM9
  Lower Leg
    Left 0KMT
    Right 0KMS
  Neck
    Left 0KM3
    Right 0KM2
  Perineum 0KMM
  Shoulder
    Left 0KM6
    Right 0KM5
  Thorax
    Left 0KMJ
    Right 0KMH
  Tongue, Palate, Pharynx 0KM4
  Trunk
    Left 0KMG
    Right 0KMF
  Upper Arm
    Left 0KM8
    Right 0KM7
  Upper Leg
    Left 0KMR
    Right 0KMQ
Nasal Mucosa and Soft Tissue 09MKXZZ
Neck 0WM60ZZ
Nipple
  Left 0HMXXZZ
  Right 0HMWXZZ
Ovary
  Bilateral 0UM2
  Left 0UM1
  Right 0UM0
Palate, Soft 0CM30ZZ
Pancreas 0FMG

Reattachment — *continued*
Parathyroid Gland 0GMR
  Inferior
    Left 0GMP
    Right 0GMN
  Multiple 0GMQ
  Superior
    Left 0GMM
    Right 0GML
Penis 0VMSXZZ
Perineum
  Female 0WMN0ZZ
  Male 0WMM0ZZ
Rectum 0DMP
Scrotum 0VM5XZZ
Shoulder Region
  Left 0XM30ZZ
  Right 0XM20ZZ
Skin
  Abdomen 0HM7XZZ
  Back 0HM6XZZ
  Buttock 0HM8XZZ
  Chest 0HM5XZZ
  Ear
    Left 0HM3XZZ
    Right 0HM2XZZ
  Face 0HM1XZZ
  Foot
    Left 0HMNXZZ
    Right 0HMMXZZ
  Hand
    Left 0HMGXZZ
    Right 0HMFXZZ
  Inguinal 0HMAXZZ
  Lower Arm
    Left 0HMEXZZ
    Right 0HMDXZZ
  Lower Leg
    Left 0HMLXZZ
    Right 0HMKXZZ
  Neck 0HM4XZZ
  Perineum 0HM9XZZ
  Scalp 0HM0XZZ
  Upper Arm
    Left 0HMCXZZ
    Right 0HMBXZZ
  Upper Leg
    Left 0HMJXZZ
    Right 0HMHXZZ
Stomach 0DM6
Tendon
  Abdomen
    Left 0LMG
    Right 0LMF
  Ankle
    Left 0LMT
    Right 0LMS
  Foot
    Left 0LMW
    Right 0LMV
  Hand
    Left 0LM8
    Right 0LM7
  Head and Neck 0LM0
  Hip
    Left 0LMK
    Right 0LMJ
  Knee
    Left 0LMR
    Right 0LMQ
  Lower Arm and Wrist
    Left 0LM6
    Right 0LM5
  Lower Leg
    Left 0LMP
    Right 0LMN
  Perineum 0LMH

Reattachment — *continued*
Tendon — *continued*
  Shoulder
    Left 0LM2
    Right 0LM1
  Thorax
    Left 0LMD
    Right 0LMC
  Trunk
    Left 0LMB
    Right 0LM9
  Upper Arm
    Left 0LM4
    Right 0LM3
  Upper Leg
    Left 0LMM
    Right 0LML
Testis
  Bilateral 0VMC
  Left 0VMB
  Right 0VM9
Thumb
  Left 0XMM0ZZ
  Right 0XML0ZZ
Thyroid Gland
  Left Lobe 0GMG
  Right Lobe 0GMH
Toe
  1st
    Left 0YMQ0ZZ
    Right 0YMP0ZZ
  2nd
    Left 0YMS0ZZ
    Right 0YMR0ZZ
  3rd
    Left 0YMU0ZZ
    Right 0YMT0ZZ
  4th
    Left 0YMW0ZZ
    Right 0YMV0ZZ
  5th
    Left 0YMY0ZZ
    Right 0YMX0ZZ
Tongue 0CM70ZZ
Tooth
  Lower 0CMX
  Upper 0CMW
Trachea 0BM10ZZ
Tunica Vaginalis
  Left 0VM7
  Right 0VM6
Ureter
  Left 0TM7
  Right 0TM6
Ureters, Bilateral 0TM8
Urethra 0TMD
Uterine Supporting Structure 0UM4
Uterus 0UM9
Uvula 0CMN0ZZ
Vagina 0UMG
Vulva 0UMMXZZ
Wrist Region
  Left 0XMH0ZZ
  Right 0XMG0ZZ
REBOA (resuscitative endovascular balloon occlusion of the aorta)
  02LW3DJ
  04L03DJ
Rebound HRD® (Hernia Repair Device)
  use Synthetic Substitute
RECELL® cell suspension autograft
  see Replacement, Skin and Breast 0HR
Recession
  see Repair
  see Reposition
Reclosure, disrupted abdominal wall
  0WQFXZZ

Reconstruction - Release

ICD-10-PCS INDEX

Reconstruction
 see Repair
 see Replacement
 see Supplement
Rectectomy
 see Excision, Rectum 0DBP
 see Resection, Rectum 0DTP
Rectocele repair
 see Repair, Subcutaneous Tissue and Fascia, Pelvic Region 0JQC
Rectopexy
 see Repair, Gastrointestinal System 0DQ
 see Reposition, Gastrointestinal System 0DS
Rectoplasty
 see Repair, Gastrointestinal System 0DQ
 see Supplement, Gastrointestinal System 0DU
Rectorrhaphy
 see Repair, Gastrointestinal System 0DQ
Rectoscopy 0DJD8ZZ
Rectosigmoid junction
 use Sigmoid Colon
Rectosigmoidectomy
 see Excision, Gastrointestinal System 0DB
 see Resection, Gastrointestinal System 0DT
Rectostomy
 see Drainage, Rectum 0D9P
Rectotomy
 see Drainage, Rectum 0D9P
Rectus abdominis muscle
 use Abdomen Muscle, Right
 use Abdomen Muscle, Left
Rectus femoris muscle
 use Upper Leg Muscle, Right
 use Upper Leg Muscle, Left
Recurrent laryngeal nerve
 use Vagus Nerve
Reduction
 Dislocation *see* Reposition
 Fracture *see* Reposition
 Intussusception, intestinal *see* Reposition, Gastrointestinal System 0DS
 Mammoplasty *see* Excision, Skin and Breast 0HB
 Prolapse *see* Reposition
 Torsion *see* Reposition
 Volvulus, gastrointestinal *see* Reposition, Gastrointestinal System 0DS
Refusion
 see Fusion
REGN-COV2 Monoclonal Antibody XW0
Rehabilitation
 see Speech Assessment, Rehabilitation F00
 see Motor Function Assessment, Rehabilitation F01
 see Activities of Daily Living Assessment, Rehabilitation F02
 see Speech Treatment, Rehabilitation F06
 see Motor Treatment, Rehabilitation F07
 see Activities of Daily Living Treatment, Rehabilitation F08
 see Hearing Treatment, Rehabilitation F09
 see Cochlear Implant Treatment, Rehabilitation F0B
 see Vestibular Treatment, Rehabilitation F0C
 see Device Fitting, Rehabilitation F0D
 see Caregiver Training, Rehabilitation F0F
Reimplantation
 see Reattachment
 see Reposition
 see Transfer
Reinforcement
 see Repair
 see Supplement
Relaxation, scar tissue
 see Release

Release
 Acetabulum
  Left 0QN5
  Right 0QN4
 Adenoids 0CNQ
 Ampulla of Vater 0FNC
 Anal Sphincter 0DNR
 Anterior Chamber
  Left 08N33ZZ
  Right 08N23ZZ
 Anus 0DNQ
 Aorta
  Abdominal 04N0
  Thoracic
   Ascending/Arch 02NX
   Descending 02NW
 Aortic Body 0GND
 Appendix 0DNJ
 Artery
  Anterior Tibial
   Left 04NQ
   Right 04NP
  Axillary
   Left 03N6
   Right 03N5
  Brachial
   Left 03N8
   Right 03N7
  Celiac 04N1
  Colic
   Left 04N7
   Middle 04N8
   Right 04N6
  Common Carotid
   Left 03NJ
   Right 03NH
  Common Iliac
   Left 04ND
   Right 04NC
  Coronary
   Four or More Arteries 02N3
   One Artery 02N0
   Three Arteries 02N2
   Two Arteries 02N1
  External Carotid
   Left 03NN
   Right 03NM
  External Iliac
   Left 04NJ
   Right 04NH
  Face 03NR
  Femoral
   Left 04NL
   Right 04NK
  Foot
   Left 04NW
   Right 04NV
  Gastric 04N2
  Hand
   Left 03NF
   Right 03ND
  Hepatic 04N3
  Inferior Mesenteric 04NB
  Innominate 03N2
  Internal Carotid
   Left 03NL
   Right 03NK
  Internal Iliac
   Left 04NF
   Right 04NE
  Internal Mammary
   Left 03N1
   Right 03N0
  Intracranial 03NG
  Lower 04NY
  Peroneal

Release — *continued*
 Artery — *continued*
   Left 04NU
   Right 04NT
  Popliteal
   Left 04NN
   Right 04NM
  Posterior Tibial
   Left 04NS
   Right 04NR
  Pulmonary
   Left 02NR
   Right 02NQ
  Pulmonary Trunk 02NP
  Radial
   Left 03NC
   Right 03NB
  Renal
   Left 04NA
   Right 04N9
  Splenic 04N4
  Subclavian
   Left 03N4
   Right 03N3
  Superior Mesenteric 04N5
  Temporal
   Left 03NT
   Right 03NS
  Thyroid
   Left 03NV
   Right 03NU
  Ulnar
   Left 03NA
   Right 03N9
  Upper 03NY
  Vertebral
   Left 03NQ
   Right 03NP
 Atrium
  Left 02N7
  Right 02N6
 Auditory Ossicle
  Left 09NA
  Right 09N9
 Basal Ganglia 00N8
 Bladder 0TNB
 Bladder Neck 0TNC
 Bone
  Ethmoid
   Left 0NNG
   Right 0NNF
  Frontal 0NN1
  Hyoid 0NNX
  Lacrimal
   Left 0NNJ
   Right 0NNH
  Nasal 0NNB
  Occipital 0NN7
  Palatine
   Left 0NNL
   Right 0NNK
  Parietal
   Left 0NN4
   Right 0NN3
  Pelvic
   Left 0QN3
   Right 0QN2
  Sphenoid 0NNC
  Temporal
   Left 0NN6
   Right 0NN5
  Zygomatic
   Left 0NNN
   Right 0NNM
 Brain 00N0
 Breast
  Bilateral 0HNV

Release — *continued*
  Breast — *continued*
    Left 0HNU
    Right 0HNT
  Bronchus
    Lingula 0BN9
    Lower Lobe
      Left 0BNB
      Right 0BN6
    Main
      Left 0BN7
      Right 0BN3
    Middle Lobe, Right 0BN5
    Upper Lobe
      Left 0BN8
      Right 0BN4
  Buccal Mucosa 0CN4
  Bursa and Ligament
    Abdomen
      Left 0MNJ
      Right 0MNH
    Ankle
      Left 0MNR
      Right 0MNQ
    Elbow
      Left 0MN4
      Right 0MN3
    Foot
      Left 0MNT
      Right 0MNS
    Hand
      Left 0MN8
      Right 0MN7
    Head and Neck 0MN0
    Hip
      Left 0MNM
      Right 0MNL
    Knee
      Left 0MNP
      Right 0MNN
    Lower Extremity
      Left 0MNW
      Right 0MNV
    Perineum 0MNK
    Rib(s) 0MNG
    Shoulder
      Left 0MN2
      Right 0MN1
    Spine
      Lower 0MND
      Upper 0MNC
    Sternum 0MNF
    Upper Extremity
      Left 0MNB
      Right 0MN9
    Wrist
      Left 0MN6
      Right 0MN5
  Carina 0BN2
  Carotid Bodies, Bilateral 0GN8
  Carotid Body
    Left 0GN6
    Right 0GN7
  Carpal
    Left 0PNN
    Right 0PNM
  Cecum 0DNH
  Cerebellum 00NC
  Cerebral Hemisphere 00N7
  Cerebral Meninges 00N1
  Cerebral Ventricle 00N6
  Cervix 0UNC
  Chordae Tendineae 02N9
  Choroid
    Left 08NB
    Right 08NA
  Cisterna Chyli 07NL

Release — *continued*
  Clavicle
    Left 0PNB
    Right 0PN9
  Clitoris 0UNJ
  Coccygeal Glomus 0GNB
  Coccyx 0QNS
  Colon
    Ascending 0DNK
    Descending 0DNM
    Sigmoid 0DNN
    Transverse 0DNL
  Conduction Mechanism 02N8
  Conjunctiva
    Left 08NTXZZ
    Right 08NSXZZ
  Cord
    Bilateral 0VNH
    Left 0VNG
    Right 0VNF
  Cornea
    Left 08N9XZZ
    Right 08N8XZZ
  Cul-de-sac 0UNF
  Diaphragm 0BNT
  Disc
    Cervical Vertebral 0RN3
    Cervicothoracic Vertebral 0RN5
    Lumbar Vertebral 0SN2
    Lumbosacral 0SN4
    Thoracic Vertebral 0RN9
    Thoracolumbar Vertebral 0RNB
  Duct
    Common Bile 0FN9
    Cystic 0FN8
    Hepatic
      Common 0FN7
      Left 0FN6
      Right 0FN5
    Lacrimal
      Left 08NY
      Right 08NX
    Pancreatic 0FND
      Accessory 0FNF
    Parotid
      Left 0CNC
      Right 0CNB
  Duodenum 0DN9
  Dura Mater 00N2
  Ear
    External
      Left 09N1
      Right 09N0
    External Auditory Canal
      Left 09N4
      Right 09N3
    Inner
      Left 09NE
      Right 09ND
    Middle
      Left 09N6
      Right 09N5
  Epididymis
    Bilateral 0VNL
    Left 0VNK
    Right 0VNJ
  Epiglottis 0CNR
  Esophagogastric Junction 0DN4
  Esophagus 0DN5
    Lower 0DN3
    Middle 0DN2
    Upper 0DN1
  Eustachian Tube
    Left 09NG
    Right 09NF
  Eye
    Left 08N1XZZ
    Right 08N0XZZ

Release — *continued*
  Eyelid
    Lower
      Left 08NR
      Right 08NQ
    Upper
      Left 08NP
      Right 08NN
  Fallopian Tube
    Left 0UN6
    Right 0UN5
  Fallopian Tubes, Bilateral 0UN7
  Femoral Shaft
    Left 0QN9
    Right 0QN8
  Femur
    Lower
      Left 0QNC
      Right 0QNB
    Upper
      Left 0QN7
      Right 0QN6
  Fibula
    Left 0QNK
    Right 0QNJ
  Finger Nail 0HNQXZZ
  Gallbladder 0FN4
  Gingiva
    Lower 0CN6
    Upper 0CN5
  Gland
    Adrenal
      Bilateral 0GN4
      Left 0GN2
      Right 0GN3
    Lacrimal
      Left 08NW
      Right 08NV
    Minor Salivary 0CNJ
    Parotid
      Left 0CN9
      Right 0CN8
    Pituitary 0GN0
    Sublingual
      Left 0CNF
      Right 0CND
    Submaxillary
      Left 0CNH
      Right 0CNG
    Vestibular 0UNL
  Glenoid Cavity
    Left 0PN8
    Right 0PN7
  Glomus Jugulare 0GNC
  Humeral Head
    Left 0PND
    Right 0PNC
  Humeral Shaft
    Left 0PNG
    Right 0PNF
  Hymen 0UNK
  Hypothalamus 00NA
  Ileocecal Valve 0DNC
  Ileum 0DNB
  Intestine
    Large 0DNE
      Left 0DNG
      Right 0DNF
    Small 0DN8
  Iris
    Left 08ND3ZZ
    Right 08NC3ZZ
  Jejunum 0DNA
  Joint
    Acromioclavicular
      Left 0RNH
      Right 0RNG

Release — *continued*
  Joint — *continued*
    Ankle
      Left 0SNG
      Right 0SNF
    Carpal
      Left 0RNR
      Right 0RNQ
    Carpometacarpal
      Left 0RNT
      Right 0RNS
    Cervical Vertebral 0RN1
    Cervicothoracic Vertebral 0RN4
    Coccygeal 0SN6
    Elbow
      Left 0RNM
      Right 0RNL
    Finger Phalangeal
      Left 0RNX
      Right 0RNW
    Hip
      Left 0SNB
      Right 0SN9
    Knee
      Left 0SND
      Right 0SNC
    Lumbar Vertebral 0SN0
    Lumbosacral 0SN3
    Metacarpophalangeal
      Left 0RNV
      Right 0RNU
    Metatarsal-Phalangeal
      Left 0SNN
      Right 0SNM
    Occipital-cervical 0RN0
    Sacrococcygeal 0SN5
    Sacroiliac
      Left 0SN8
      Right 0SN7
    Shoulder
      Left 0RNK
      Right 0RNJ
    Sternoclavicular
      Left 0RNF
      Right 0RNE
    Tarsal
      Left 0SNJ
      Right 0SNH
    Tarsometatarsal
      Left 0SNL
      Right 0SNK
    Temporomandibular
      Left 0RND
      Right 0RNC
    Thoracic Vertebral 0RN6
    Thoracolumbar Vertebral 0RNA
    Toe Phalangeal
      Left 0SNQ
      Right 0SNP
    Wrist
      Left 0RNP
      Right 0RNN
  Kidney
    Left 0TN1
    Right 0TN0
  Kidney Pelvis
    Left 0TN4
    Right 0TN3
  Larynx 0CNS
  Lens
    Left 08NK3ZZ
    Right 08NJ3ZZ
  Lip
    Lower 0CN1
    Upper 0CN0
  Liver 0FN0
    Left Lobe 0FN2
    Right Lobe 0FN1

Release — *continued*
  Lung
    Bilateral 0BNM
    Left 0BNL
    Lower Lobe
      Left 0BNJ
      Right 0BNF
    Middle Lobe, Right 0BND
    Right 0BNK
    Upper Lobe
      Left 0BNG
      Right 0BNC
  Lung Lingula 0BNH
  Lymphatic
    Aortic 07ND
    Axillary
      Left 07N6
      Right 07N5
    Head 07N0
    Inguinal
      Left 07NJ
      Right 07NH
    Internal Mammary
      Left 07N9
      Right 07N8
    Lower Extremity
      Left 07NG
      Right 07NF
    Mesenteric 07NB
    Neck
      Left 07N2
      Right 07N1
    Pelvis 07NC
    Thoracic Duct 07NK
    Thorax 07N7
    Upper Extremity
      Left 07N4
      Right 07N3
  Mandible
    Left 0NNV
    Right 0NNT
  Maxilla 0NNR
  Medulla Oblongata 00ND
  Mesentery 0DNV
  Metacarpal
    Left 0PNQ
    Right 0PNP
  Metatarsal
    Left 0QNP
    Right 0QNN
  Muscle
    Abdomen
      Left 0KNL
      Right 0KNK
    Extraocular
      Left 08NM
      Right 08NL
    Facial 0KN1
    Foot
      Left 0KNW
      Right 0KNV
    Hand
      Left 0KND
      Right 0KNC
    Head 0KN0
    Hip
      Left 0KNP
      Right 0KNN
    Lower Arm and Wrist
      Left 0KNB
      Right 0KN9
    Lower Leg
      Left 0KNT
      Right 0KNS
    Neck
      Left 0KN3
      Right 0KN2

Release — *continued*
  Muscle — *continued*
    Papillary 02ND
    Perineum 0KNM
    Shoulder
      Left 0KN6
      Right 0KN5
    Thorax
      Left 0KNJ
      Right 0KNH
    Tongue, Palate, Pharynx 0KN4
    Trunk
      Left 0KNG
      Right 0KNF
    Upper Arm
      Left 0KN8
      Right 0KN7
    Upper Leg
      Left 0KNR
      Right 0KNQ
  Myocardial Bridge *see* Release, Artery, Coronary
  Nasal Mucosa and Soft Tissue 09NK
  Nasopharynx 09NN
  Nerve
    Abdominal Sympathetic 01NM
    Abducens 00NL
    Accessory 00NR
    Acoustic 00NN
    Brachial Plexus 01N3
    Cervical 01N1
    Cervical Plexus 01N0
    Facial 00NM
    Femoral 01ND
    Glossopharyngeal 00NP
    Head and Neck Sympathetic 01NK
    Hypoglossal 00NS
    Lumbar 01NB
    Lumbar Plexus 01N9
    Lumbar Sympathetic 01NN
    Lumbosacral Plexus 01NA
    Median 01N5
    Oculomotor 00NH
    Olfactory 00NF
    Optic 00NG
    Peroneal 01NH
    Phrenic 01N2
    Pudendal 01NC
    Radial 01N6
    Sacral 01NR
    Sacral Plexus 01NQ
    Sacral Sympathetic 01NP
    Sciatic 01NF
    Thoracic 01N8
    Thoracic Sympathetic 01NL
    Tibial 01NG
    Trigeminal 00NK
    Trochlear 00NJ
    Ulnar 01N4
    Vagus 00NQ
  Nipple
    Left 0HNX
    Right 0HNW
  Omentum 0DNU
  Orbit
    Left 0NNQ
    Right 0NNP
  Ovary
    Bilateral 0UN2
    Left 0UN1
    Right 0UN0
  Palate
    Hard 0CN2
    Soft 0CN3
  Pancreas 0FNG
  Para-aortic Body 0GN9
  Paraganglion Extremity 0GNF

Release — *continued*
  Parathyroid Gland 0GNR
    Inferior
      Left 0GNP
      Right 0GNN
    Multiple 0GNQ
    Superior
      Left 0GNM
      Right 0GNL
  Patella
    Left 0QNF
    Right 0QND
  Penis 0VNS
  Pericardium 02NN
  Peritoneum 0DNW
  Phalanx
    Finger
      Left 0PNV
      Right 0PNT
    Thumb
      Left 0PNS
      Right 0PNR
    Toe
      Left 0QNR
      Right 0QNQ
  Pharynx 0CNM
  Pineal Body 0GN1
  Pleura
    Left 0BNP
    Right 0BNN
  Pons 00NB
  Prepuce 0VNT
  Prostate 0VN0
  Radius
    Left 0PNJ
    Right 0PNH
  Rectum 0DNP
  Retina
    Left 08NF3ZZ
    Right 08NE3ZZ
  Retinal Vessel
    Left 08NH3ZZ
    Right 08NG3ZZ
  Ribs
    1 to 2 0PN1
    3 or More 0PN2
  Sacrum 0QN1
  Scapula
    Left 0PN6
    Right 0PN5
  Sclera
    Left 08N7XZZ
    Right 08N6XZZ
  Scrotum 0VN5
  Septum
    Atrial 02N5
    Nasal 09NM
    Ventricular 02NM
  Sinus
    Accessory 09NP
    Ethmoid
      Left 09NV
      Right 09NU
    Frontal
      Left 09NT
      Right 09NS
    Mastoid
      Left 09NC
      Right 09NB
    Maxillary
      Left 09NR
      Right 09NQ
    Sphenoid
      Left 09NX
      Right 09NW
  Skin
    Abdomen 0HN7XZZ

Release — *continued*
  Skin — *continued*
    Back 0HN6XZZ
    Buttock 0HN8XZZ
    Chest 0HN5XZZ
    Ear
      Left 0HN3XZZ
      Right 0HN2XZZ
    Face 0HN1XZZ
    Foot
      Left 0HNNXZZ
      Right 0HNMXZZ
    Hand
      Left 0HNGXZZ
      Right 0HNFXZZ
    Inguinal 0HNAXZZ
    Lower Arm
      Left 0HNEXZZ
      Right 0HNDXZZ
    Lower Leg
      Left 0HNLXZZ
      Right 0HNKXZZ
    Neck 0HN4XZZ
    Perineum 0HN9XZZ
    Scalp 0HN0XZZ
    Upper Arm
      Left 0HNCXZZ
      Right 0HNBXZZ
    Upper Leg
      Left 0HNJXZZ
      Right 0HNHXZZ
  Spinal Cord
    Cervical 00NW
    Lumbar 00NY
    Thoracic 00NX
  Spinal Meninges 00NT
  Spleen 07NP
  Sternum 0PN0
  Stomach 0DN6
    Pylorus 0DN7
  Subcutaneous Tissue and Fascia
    Abdomen 0JN8
    Back 0JN7
    Buttock 0JN9
    Chest 0JN6
    Face 0JN1
    Foot
      Left 0JNR
      Right 0JNQ
    Hand
      Left 0JNK
      Right 0JNJ
    Lower Arm
      Left 0JNH
      Right 0JNG
    Lower Leg
      Left 0JNP
      Right 0JNN
    Neck
      Left 0JN5
      Right 0JN4
    Pelvic Region 0JNC
    Perineum 0JNB
    Scalp 0JN0
    Upper Arm
      Left 0JNF
      Right 0JND
    Upper Leg
      Left 0JNM
      Right 0JNL
  Tarsal
    Left 0QNM
    Right 0QNL
  Tendon
    Abdomen
      Left 0LNG
      Right 0LNF

Release — *continued*
  Tendon — *continued*
    Ankle
      Left 0LNT
      Right 0LNS
    Foot
      Left 0LNW
      Right 0LNV
    Hand
      Left 0LN8
      Right 0LN7
    Head and Neck 0LN0
    Hip
      Left 0LNK
      Right 0LNJ
    Knee
      Left 0LNR
      Right 0LNQ
    Lower Arm and Wrist
      Left 0LN6
      Right 0LN5
    Lower Leg
      Left 0LNP
      Right 0LNN
    Perineum 0LNH
    Shoulder
      Left 0LN2
      Right 0LN1
    Thorax
      Left 0LND
      Right 0LNC
    Trunk
      Left 0LNB
      Right 0LN9
    Upper Arm
      Left 0LN4
      Right 0LN3
    Upper Leg
      Left 0LNM
      Right 0LNL
  Testis
    Bilateral 0VNC
    Left 0VNB
    Right 0VN9
  Thalamus 00N9
  Thymus 07NM
  Thyroid Gland 0GNK
    Left Lobe 0GNG
    Right Lobe 0GNH
  Tibia
    Left 0QNH
    Right 0QNG
  Toe Nail 0HNRXZZ
  Tongue 0CN7
  Tonsils 0CNP
  Tooth
    Lower 0CNX
    Upper 0CNW
  Trachea 0BN1
  Tunica Vaginalis
    Left 0VN7
    Right 0VN6
  Turbinate, Nasal 09NL
  Tympanic Membrane
    Left 09N8
    Right 09N7
  Ulna
    Left 0PNL
    Right 0PNK
  Ureter
    Left 0TN7
    Right 0TN6
  Urethra 0TND
  Uterine Supporting Structure 0UN4
  Uterus 0UN9
  Uvula 0CNN
  Vagina 0UNG

Release — continued
Valve
Aortic 02NF
Mitral 02NG
Pulmonary 02NH
Tricuspid 02NJ
Vas Deferens
Bilateral 0VNQ
Left 0VNP
Right 0VNN
Vein
Axillary
Left 05N8
Right 05N7
Azygos 05N0
Basilic
Left 05NC
Right 05NB
Brachial
Left 05NA
Right 05N9
Cephalic
Left 05NF
Right 05ND
Colic 06N7
Common Iliac
Left 06ND
Right 06NC
Coronary 02N4
Esophageal 06N3
External Iliac
Left 06NG
Right 06NF
External Jugular
Left 05NQ
Right 05NP
Face
Left 05NV
Right 05NT
Femoral
Left 06NN
Right 06NM
Foot
Left 06NV
Right 06NT
Gastric 06N2
Hand
Left 05NH
Right 05NG
Hemiazygos 05N1
Hepatic 06N4
Hypogastric
Left 06NJ
Right 06NH
Inferior Mesenteric 06N6
Innominate
Left 05N4
Right 05N3
Internal Jugular
Left 05NN
Right 05NM
Intracranial 05NL
Lower 06NY
Portal 06N8
Pulmonary
Left 02NT
Right 02NS
Renal
Left 06NB
Right 06N9
Saphenous
Left 06NQ
Right 06NP
Splenic 06N1
Subclavian
Left 05N6
Right 05N5

Release — continued
Vein — continued
Superior Mesenteric 06N5
Upper 05NY
Vertebral
Left 05NS
Right 05NR
Vena Cava
Inferior 06N0
Superior 02NV
Ventricle
Left 02NL
Right 02NK
Vertebra
Cervical 0PN3
Lumbar 0QN0
Thoracic 0PN4
Vesicle
Bilateral 0VN3
Left 0VN2
Right 0VN1
Vitreous
Left 08N53ZZ
Right 08N43ZZ
Vocal Cord
Left 0CNV
Right 0CNT
Vulva 0UNM
Relocation
see Reposition
Remdesivir Anti-infective XW0
Removal
Abdominal Wall 2W53X
Anorectal 2Y53X5Z
Arm
Lower
Left 2W5DX
Right 2W5CX
Upper
Left 2W5BX
Right 2W5AX
Back 2W55X
Chest Wall 2W54X
Ear 2Y52X5Z
Extremity
Lower
Left 2W5MX
Right 2W5LX
Upper
Left 2W59X
Right 2W58X
Face 2W51X
Finger
Left 2W5KX
Right 2W5JX
Foot
Left 2W5TX
Right 2W5SX
Genital Tract, Female 2Y54X5Z
Hand
Left 2W5FX
Right 2W5EX
Head 2W50X
Inguinal Region
Left 2W57X
Right 2W56X
Leg
Lower
Left 2W5RX
Right 2W5QX
Upper
Left 2W5PX
Right 2W5NX
Mouth and Pharynx 2Y50X5Z
Nasal 2Y51X5Z
Neck 2W52X
Thumb
Left 2W5HX
Right 2W5GX

Removal — continued
Toe
Left 2W5VX
Right 2W5UX
Urethra 2Y55X5Z
Removal of device from
Abdominal Wall 0WPF
Acetabulum
Left 0QP5
Right 0QP4
Anal Sphincter 0DPR
Anus 0DPQ
Artery
Lower 04PY
Upper 03PY
Back
Lower 0WPL
Upper 0WPK
Bladder 0TPB
Bone
Facial 0NPW
Lower 0QPY
Nasal 0NPB
Pelvic
Left 0QP3
Right 0QP2
Upper 0PPY
Bone Marrow 07PT
Brain 00P0
Breast
Left 0HPU
Right 0HPT
Bursa and Ligament
Lower 0MPY
Upper 0MPX
Carpal
Left 0PPN
Right 0PPM
Cavity, Cranial 0WP1
Cerebral Ventricle 00P6
Chest Wall 0WP8
Cisterna Chyli 07PL
Clavicle
Left 0PPB
Right 0PP9
Coccyx 0QPS
Diaphragm 0BPT
Disc
Cervical Vertebral 0RP3
Cervicothoracic Vertebral 0RP5
Lumbar Vertebral 0SP2
Lumbosacral 0SP4
Thoracic Vertebral 0RP9
Thoracolumbar Vertebral 0RPB
Duct
Hepatobiliary 0FPB
Pancreatic 0FPD
Ear
Inner
Left 09PE
Right 09PD
Left 09PJ
Right 09PH
Epididymis and Spermatic Cord 0VPM
Esophagus 0DP5
Extremity
Lower
Left 0YPB
Right 0YP9
Upper
Left 0XP7
Right 0XP6
Eye
Left 08P1
Right 08P0
Face 0WP2
Fallopian Tube 0UP8

Removal of device from — *continued*
Femoral Shaft
    Left 0QP9
    Right 0QP8
Femur
    Lower
        Left 0QPC
        Right 0QPB
    Upper
        Left 0QP7
        Right 0QP6
Fibula
    Left 0QPK
    Right 0QPJ
Finger Nail 0HPQX
Gallbladder 0FP4
Gastrointestinal Tract 0WPP
Genitourinary Tract 0WPR
Gland
    Adrenal 0GP5
    Endocrine 0GPS
    Pituitary 0GP0
    Salivary 0CPA
Glenoid Cavity
    Left 0PP8
    Right 0PP7
Great Vessel 02PY
Hair 0HPSX
Head 0WP0
Heart 02PA
Humeral Head
    Left 0PPD
    Right 0PPC
Humeral Shaft
    Left 0PPG
    Right 0PPF
Intestinal Tract
    Lower 0DPD
    Upper 0DP0
Jaw
    Lower 0WP5
    Upper 0WP4
Joint
    Acromioclavicular
        Left 0RPH
        Right 0RPG
    Ankle
        Left 0SPG
        Right 0SPF
    Carpal
        Left 0RPR
        Right 0RPQ
    Carpometacarpal
        Left 0RPT
        Right 0RPS
    Cervical Vertebral 0RP1
    Cervicothoracic Vertebral 0RP4
    Coccygeal 0SP6
    Elbow
        Left 0RPM
        Right 0RPL
    Finger Phalangeal
        Left 0RPX
        Right 0RPW
    Hip
        Left 0SPB
            Acetabular Surface 0SPE
            Femoral Surface 0SPS
        Right 0SP9
            Acetabular Surface 0SPA
            Femoral Surface 0SPR
    Knee
        Left 0SPD
            Femoral Surface 0SPU
            Tibial Surface 0SPW
        Right 0SPC
            Femoral Surface 0SPT
            Tibial Surface 0SPV

Removal of device from — *continued*
Joint — *continued*
    Lumbar Vertebral 0SP0
    Lumbosacral 0SP3
    Metacarpophalangeal
        Left 0RPV
        Right 0RPU
    Metatarsal-Phalangeal
        Left 0SPN
        Right 0SPM
    Occipital-cervical 0RP0
    Sacrococcygeal 0SP5
    Sacroiliac
        Left 0SP8
        Right 0SP7
    Shoulder
        Left 0RPK
        Right 0RPJ
    Sternoclavicular
        Left 0RPF
        Right 0RPE
    Tarsal
        Left 0SPJ
        Right 0SPH
    Tarsometatarsal
        Left 0SPL
        Right 0SPK
    Temporomandibular
        Left 0RPD
        Right 0RPC
    Thoracic Vertebral 0RP6
    Thoracolumbar Vertebral 0RPA
    Toe Phalangeal
        Left 0SPQ
        Right 0SPP
    Wrist
        Left 0RPP
        Right 0RPN
Kidney 0TP5
Larynx 0CPS
Lens
    Left 08PK3
    Right 08PJ3
Liver 0FP0
Lung
    Left 0BPL
    Right 0BPK
Lymphatic 07PN
    Thoracic Duct 07PK
Mediastinum 0WPC
Mesentery 0DPV
Metacarpal
    Left 0PPQ
    Right 0PPP
Metatarsal
    Left 0QPP
    Right 0QPN
Mouth and Throat 0CPY
Muscle
    Extraocular
        Left 08PM
        Right 08PL
    Lower 0KPY
    Upper 0KPX
Nasal Mucosa and Soft Tissue 09PK
Neck 0WP6
Nerve
    Cranial 00PE
    Peripheral 01PY
Omentum 0DPU
Ovary 0UP3
Pancreas 0FPG
Parathyroid Gland 0GPR
Patella
    Left 0QPF
    Right 0QPD

Removal of device from — *continued*
Pelvic Cavity 0WPJ
Penis 0VPS
Pericardial Cavity 0WPD
Perineum
    Female 0WPN
    Male 0WPM
Peritoneal Cavity 0WPG
Peritoneum 0DPW
Phalanx
    Finger
        Left 0PPV
        Right 0PPT
    Thumb
        Left 0PPS
        Right 0PPR
    Toe
        Left 0QPR
        Right 0QPQ
Pineal Body 0GP1
Pleura 0BPQ
Pleural Cavity
    Left 0WPB
    Right 0WP9
Products of Conception 10P0
Prostate and Seminal Vesicles 0VP4
Radius
    Left 0PPJ
    Right 0PPH
Rectum 0DPP
Respiratory Tract 0WPQ
Retroperitoneum 0WPH
Ribs
    1 to 2 0PP1
    3 or More 0PP2
Sacrum 0QP1
Scapula
    Left 0PP6
    Right 0PP5
Scrotum and Tunica Vaginalis 0VP8
Sinus 09PY
Skin 0HPPX
Skull 0NP0
Spinal Canal 00PU
Spinal Cord 00PV
Spleen 07PP
Sternum 0PP0
Stomach 0DP6
Subcutaneous Tissue and Fascia
    Head and Neck 0JPS
    Lower Extremity 0JPW
    Trunk 0JPT
    Upper Extremity 0JPV
Tarsal
    Left 0QPM
    Right 0QPL
Tendon
    Lower 0LPY
    Upper 0LPX
Testis 0VPD
Thymus 07PM
Thyroid Gland 0GPK
Tibia
    Left 0QPH
    Right 0QPG
Toe Nail 0HPRX
Trachea 0BP1
Tracheobronchial Tree 0BP0
Tympanic Membrane
    Left 09P8
    Right 09P7
Ulna
    Left 0PPL
    Right 0PPK
Ureter 0TP9
Urethra 0TPD
Uterus and Cervix 0UPD

Removal of device from — *continued*
Vagina and Cul-de-sac 0UPH
Vas Deferens 0VPR
Vein
　Azygos 05P0
　Innominate
　　Left 05P4
　　Right 05P3
　Lower 06PY
　Upper 05PY
Vertebra
　Cervical 0PP3
　Lumbar 0QP0
　Thoracic 0PP4
Vulva 0UPM
Renal calyx
use Kidney, Right
use Kidney, Left
use Kidneys, Bilateral
use Kidney
Renal capsule
use Kidney, Right
use Kidney, Left
use Kidneys, Bilateral
use Kidney
Renal cortex
use Kidney, Right
use Kidney, Left
use Kidneys, Bilateral
use Kidney
Renal dialysis
see Performance, Urinary 5A1D
Renal nerve
use Abdominal Sympathetic Nerve
Renal plexus
use Abdominal Sympathetic Nerve
Renal segment
use Kidney, Right
use Kidney, Left
use Kidneys, Bilateral
use Kidney
Renal segmental artery
use Renal Artery, Right
use Renal Artery, Left
Reopening, operative site
Control of bleeding *see* Control bleeding in
Inspection only *see* Inspection
Repair
Abdominal Wall 0WQF
Acetabulum
　Left 0QQ5
　Right 0QQ4
Adenoids 0CQQ
Ampulla of Vater 0FQC
Anal Sphincter 0DQR
Ankle Region
　Left 0YQL
　Right 0YQK
Anterior Chamber
　Left 08Q33ZZ
　Right 08Q23ZZ
Anus 0DQQ
Aorta
　Abdominal 04Q0
　Thoracic
　　Ascending/Arch 02QX
　　Descending 02QW
Aortic Body 0GQD
Appendix 0DQJ
Arm
　Lower
　　Left 0XQF
　　Right 0XQD
　Upper
　　Left 0XQ9
　　Right 0XQ8

Repair — *continued*
Artery
　Anterior Tibial
　　Left 04QQ
　　Right 04QP
　Axillary
　　Left 03Q6
　　Right 03Q5
　Brachial
　　Left 03Q8
　　Right 03Q7
　Celiac 04Q1
　Colic
　　Left 04Q7
　　Middle 04Q8
　　Right 04Q6
　Common Carotid
　　Left 03QJ
　　Right 03QH
　Common Iliac
　　Left 04QD
　　Right 04QC
　Coronary
　　Four or More Arteries 02Q3
　　One Artery 02Q0
　　Three Arteries 02Q2
　　Two Arteries 02Q1
　External Carotid
　　Left 03QN
　　Right 03QM
　External Iliac
　　Left 04QJ
　　Right 04QH
　Face 03QR
　Femoral
　　Left 04QL
　　Right 04QK
　Foot
　　Left 04QW
　　Right 04QV
　Gastric 04Q2
　Hand
　　Left 03QF
　　Right 03QD
　Hepatic 04Q3
　Inferior Mesenteric 04QB
　Innominate 03Q2
　Internal Carotid
　　Left 03QL
　　Right 03QK
　Internal Iliac
　　Left 04QF
　　Right 04QE
　Internal Mammary
　　Left 03Q1
　　Right 03Q0
　Intracranial 03QG
　Lower 04QY
　Peroneal
　　Left 04QU
　　Right 04QT
　Popliteal
　　Left 04QN
　　Right 04QM
　Posterior Tibial
　　Left 04QS
　　Right 04QR
　Pulmonary
　　Left 02QR
　　Right 02QQ
　Pulmonary Trunk 02QP
　Radial
　　Left 03QC
　　Right 03QB
　Renal
　　Left 04QA
　　Right 04Q9

Repair — *continued*
Artery — *continued*
　Splenic 04Q4
　Subclavian
　　Left 03Q4
　　Right 03Q3
　Superior Mesenteric 04Q5
　Temporal
　　Left 03QT
　　Right 03QS
　Thyroid
　　Left 03QV
　　Right 03QU
　Ulnar
　　Left 03QA
　　Right 03Q9
　Upper 03QY
　Vertebral
　　Left 03QQ
　　Right 03QP
Atrium
　Left 02Q7
　Right 02Q6
Auditory Ossicle
　Left 09QA
　Right 09Q9
Axilla
　Left 0XQ5
　Right 0XQ4
Back
　Lower 0WQL
　Upper 0WQK
Basal Ganglia 00Q8
Bladder 0TQB
Bladder Neck 0TQC
Bone
　Ethmoid
　　Left 0NQG
　　Right 0NQF
　Frontal 0NQ1
　Hyoid 0NQX
　Lacrimal
　　Left 0NQJ
　　Right 0NQH
　Nasal 0NQB
　Occipital 0NQ7
　Palatine
　　Left 0NQL
　　Right 0NQK
　Parietal
　　Left 0NQ4
　　Right 0NQ3
　Pelvic
　　Left 0QQ3
　　Right 0QQ2
　Sphenoid 0NQC
　Temporal
　　Left 0NQ6
　　Right 0NQ5
　Zygomatic
　　Left 0NQN
　　Right 0NQM
Brain 00Q0
Breast
　Bilateral 0HQV
　Left 0HQU
　Right 0HQT
　Supernumerary 0HQY
Bronchus
　Lingula 0BQ9
　Lower Lobe
　　Left 0BQB
　　Right 0BQ6
　Main
　　Left 0BQ7
　　Right 0BQ3
　Middle Lobe, Right 0BQ5

Repair — *continued*
  Bronchus — *continued*
    Upper Lobe
      Left 0BQ8
      Right 0BQ4
  Buccal Mucosa 0CQ4
  Bursa and Ligament
    Abdomen
      Left 0MQJ
      Right 0MQH
    Ankle
      Left 0MQR
      Right 0MQQ
    Elbow
      Left 0MQ4
      Right 0MQ3
    Foot
      Left 0MQT
      Right 0MQS
    Hand
      Left 0MQ8
      Right 0MQ7
    Head and Neck 0MQ0
    Hip
      Left 0MQM
      Right 0MQL
    Knee
      Left 0MQP
      Right 0MQN
    Lower Extremity
      Left 0MQW
      Right 0MQV
    Perineum 0MQK
    Rib(s) 0MQG
    Shoulder
      Left 0MQ2
      Right 0MQ1
    Spine
      Lower 0MQD
      Upper 0MQC
    Sternum 0MQF
    Upper Extremity
      Left 0MQB
      Right 0MQ9
    Wrist
      Left 0MQ6
      Right 0MQ5
  Buttock
    Left 0YQ1
    Right 0YQ0
  Carina 0BQ2
  Carotid Bodies, Bilateral 0GQ8
  Carotid Body
    Left 0GQ6
    Right 0GQ7
  Carpal
    Left 0PQN
    Right 0PQM
  Cecum 0DQH
  Cerebellum 00QC
  Cerebral Hemisphere 00Q7
  Cerebral Meninges 00Q1
  Cerebral Ventricle 00Q6
  Cervix 0UQC
  Chest Wall 0WQ8
  Chordae Tendineae 02Q9
  Choroid
    Left 08QB
    Right 08QA
  Cisterna Chyli 07QL
  Clavicle
    Left 0PQB
    Right 0PQ9
  Clitoris 0UQJ
  Coccygeal Glomus 0GQB
  Coccyx 0QQS

Repair — *continued*
  Colon
    Ascending 0DQK
    Descending 0DQM
    Sigmoid 0DQN
    Transverse 0DQL
  Conduction Mechanism 02Q8
  Conjunctiva
    Left 08QTXZZ
    Right 08QSXZZ
  Cord
    Bilateral 0VQH
    Left 0VQG
    Right 0VQF
  Cornea
    Left 08Q9XZZ
    Right 08Q8XZZ
  Cul-de-sac 0UQF
  Diaphragm 0BQT
  Disc
    Cervical Vertebral 0RQ3
    Cervicothoracic Vertebral 0RQ5
    Lumbar Vertebral 0SQ2
    Lumbosacral 0SQ4
    Thoracic Vertebral 0RQ9
    Thoracolumbar Vertebral 0RQB
  Duct
    Common Bile 0FQ9
    Cystic 0FQ8
    Hepatic
      Common 0FQ7
      Left 0FQ6
      Right 0FQ5
    Lacrimal
      Left 08QY
      Right 08QX
    Pancreatic 0FQD
      Accessory 0FQF
    Parotid
      Left 0CQC
      Right 0CQB
  Duodenum 0DQ9
  Dura Mater 00Q2
  Ear
    External
      Bilateral 09Q2
      Left 09Q1
      Right 09Q0
    External Auditory Canal
      Left 09Q4
      Right 09Q3
    Inner
      Left 09QE
      Right 09QD
    Middle
      Left 09Q6
      Right 09Q5
  Elbow Region
    Left 0XQC
    Right 0XQB
  Epididymis
    Bilateral 0VQL
    Left 0VQK
    Right 0VQJ
  Epiglottis 0CQR
  Esophagogastric Junction 0DQ4
  Esophagus 0DQ5
    Lower 0DQ3
    Middle 0DQ2
    Upper 0DQ1
  Eustachian Tube
    Left 09QG
    Right 09QF
  Extremity
    Lower
      Left 0YQB
      Right 0YQ9

Repair — *continued*
  Extremity — *continued*
    Upper
      Left 0XQ7
      Right 0XQ6
  Eye
    Left 08Q1XZZ
    Right 08Q0XZZ
  Eyelid
    Lower
      Left 08QR
      Right 08QQ
    Upper
      Left 08QP
      Right 08QN
  Face 0WQ2
  Fallopian Tube
    Left 0UQ6
    Right 0UQ5
  Fallopian Tubes, Bilateral 0UQ7
  Femoral Region
    Bilateral 0YQE
    Left 0YQ8
    Right 0YQ7
  Femoral Shaft
    Left 0QQ9
    Right 0QQ8
  Femur
    Lower
      Left 0QQC
      Right 0QQB
    Upper
      Left 0QQ7
      Right 0QQ6
  Fibula
    Left 0QQK
    Right 0QQJ
  Finger
    Index
      Left 0XQP
      Right 0XQN
    Little
      Left 0XQW
      Right 0XQV
    Middle
      Left 0XQR
      Right 0XQQ
    Ring
      Left 0XQT
      Right 0XQS
  Finger Nail 0HQQXZZ
  Floor of mouth *see* Repair, Oral Cavity and
    Throat 0WQ3
  Foot
    Left 0YQN
    Right 0YQM
  Gallbladder 0FQ4
  Gingiva
    Lower 0CQ6
    Upper 0CQ5
  Gland
    Adrenal
      Bilateral 0GQ4
      Left 0GQ2
      Right 0GQ3
    Lacrimal
      Left 08QW
      Right 08QV
    Minor Salivary 0CQJ
    Parotid
      Left 0CQ9
      Right 0CQ8
    Pituitary 0GQ0
    Sublingual
      Left 0CQF
      Right 0CQD

Repair — continued
  Gland — continued
    Submaxillary
      Left 0CQH
      Right 0CQG
    Vestibular 0UQL
  Glenoid Cavity
    Left 0PQ8
    Right 0PQ7
  Glomus Jugulare 0GQC
  Hand
    Left 0XQK
    Right 0XQJ
  Head 0WQ0
  Heart 02QA
    Left 02QC
    Right 02QB
  Humeral Head
    Left 0PQD
    Right 0PQC
  Humeral Shaft
    Left 0PQG
    Right 0PQF
  Hymen 0UQK
  Hypothalamus 00QA
  Ileocecal Valve 0DQC
  Ileum 0DQB
  Inguinal Region
    Bilateral 0YQA
    Left 0YQ6
    Right 0YQ5
  Intestine
    Large 0DQE
      Left 0DQG
      Right 0DQF
    Small 0DQ8
  Iris
    Left 08QD3ZZ
    Right 08QC3ZZ
  Jaw
    Lower 0WQ5
    Upper 0WQ4
  Jejunum 0DQA
  Joint
    Acromioclavicular
      Left 0RQH
      Right 0RQG
    Ankle
      Left 0SQG
      Right 0SQF
    Carpal
      Left 0RQR
      Right 0RQQ
    Carpometacarpal
      Left 0RQT
      Right 0RQS
    Cervical Vertebral 0RQ1
    Cervicothoracic Vertebral 0RQ4
    Coccygeal 0SQ6
    Elbow
      Left 0RQM
      Right 0RQL
    Finger Phalangeal
      Left 0RQX
      Right 0RQW
    Hip
      Left 0SQB
      Right 0SQ9
    Knee
      Left 0SQD
      Right 0SQC
    Lumbar Vertebral 0SQ0
    Lumbosacral 0SQ3
    Metacarpophalangeal
      Left 0RQV
      Right 0RQU

Repair — continued
  Joint — continued
    Metatarsal-Phalangeal
      Left 0SQN
      Right 0SQM
    Occipital-cervical 0RQ0
    Sacrococcygeal 0SQ5
    Sacroiliac
      Left 0SQ8
      Right 0SQ7
    Shoulder
      Left 0RQK
      Right 0RQJ
    Sternoclavicular
      Left 0RQF
      Right 0RQE
    Tarsal
      Left 0SQJ
      Right 0SQH
    Tarsometatarsal
      Left 0SQL
      Right 0SQK
    Temporomandibular
      Left 0RQD
      Right 0RQC
    Thoracic Vertebral 0RQ6
    Thoracolumbar Vertebral 0RQA
    Toe Phalangeal
      Left 0SQQ
      Right 0SQP
    Wrist
      Left 0RQP
      Right 0RQN
  Kidney
    Left 0TQ1
    Right 0TQ0
  Kidney Pelvis
    Left 0TQ4
    Right 0TQ3
  Knee Region
    Left 0YQG
    Right 0YQF
  Larynx 0CQS
  Leg
    Lower
      Left 0YQJ
      Right 0YQH
    Upper
      Left 0YQD
      Right 0YQC
  Lens
    Left 08QK3ZZ
    Right 08QJ3ZZ
  Lip
    Lower 0CQ1
    Upper 0CQ0
  Liver 0FQ0
    Left Lobe 0FQ2
    Right Lobe 0FQ1
  Lung
    Bilateral 0BQM
    Left 0BQL
    Lower Lobe
      Left 0BQJ
      Right 0BQF
    Middle Lobe, Right 0BQD
    Right 0BQK
    Upper Lobe
      Left 0BQG
      Right 0BQC
  Lung Lingula 0BQH
  Lymphatic
    Aortic 07QD
    Axillary
      Left 07Q6
      Right 07Q5
    Head 07Q0

Repair — continued
  Lymphatic — continued
    Inguinal
      Left 07QJ
      Right 07QH
    Internal Mammary
      Left 07Q9
      Right 07Q8
    Lower Extremity
      Left 07QG
      Right 07QF
    Mesenteric 07QB
    Neck
      Left 07Q2
      Right 07Q1
    Pelvis 07QC
    Thoracic Duct 07QK
    Thorax 07Q7
    Upper Extremity
      Left 07Q4
      Right 07Q3
  Mandible
    Left 0NQV
    Right 0NQT
  Maxilla 0NQR
  Mediastinum 0WQC
  Medulla Oblongata 00QD
  Mesentery 0DQV
  Metacarpal
    Left 0PQQ
    Right 0PQP
  Metatarsal
    Left 0QQP
    Right 0QQN
  Muscle
    Abdomen
      Left 0KQL
      Right 0KQK
    Extraocular
      Left 08QM
      Right 08QL
    Facial 0KQ1
    Foot
      Left 0KQW
      Right 0KQV
    Hand
      Left 0KQD
      Right 0KQC
    Head 0KQ0
    Hip
      Left 0KQP
      Right 0KQN
    Lower Arm and Wrist
      Left 0KQB
      Right 0KQ9
    Lower Leg
      Left 0KQT
      Right 0KQS
    Neck
      Left 0KQ3
      Right 0KQ2
    Papillary 02QD
    Perineum 0KQM
    Shoulder
      Left 0KQ6
      Right 0KQ5
    Thorax
      Left 0KQJ
      Right 0KQH
    Tongue, Palate, Pharynx 0KQ4
    Trunk
      Left 0KQG
      Right 0KQF
    Upper Arm
      Left 0KQ8
      Right 0KQ7

Repair — *continued*
  Muscle — *continued*
    Upper Leg
      Left 0KQR
      Right 0KQQ
  Nasal Mucosa and Soft Tissue 09QK
  Nasopharynx 09QN
  Neck 0WQ6
  Nerve
    Abdominal Sympathetic 01QM
    Abducens 00QL
    Accessory 00QR
    Acoustic 00QN
    Brachial Plexus 01Q3
    Cervical 01Q1
    Cervical Plexus 01Q0
    Facial 00QM
    Femoral 01QD
    Glossopharyngeal 00QP
    Head and Neck Sympathetic 01QK
    Hypoglossal 00QS
    Lumbar 01QB
    Lumbar Plexus 01Q9
    Lumbar Sympathetic 01QN
    Lumbosacral Plexus 01QA
    Median 01Q5
    Oculomotor 00QH
    Olfactory 00QF
    Optic 00QG
    Peroneal 01QH
    Phrenic 01Q2
    Pudendal 01QC
    Radial 01Q6
    Sacral 01QR
    Sacral Plexus 01QQ
    Sacral Sympathetic 01QP
    Sciatic 01QF
    Thoracic 01Q8
    Thoracic Sympathetic 01QL
    Tibial 01QG
    Trigeminal 00QK
    Trochlear 00QJ
    Ulnar 01Q4
    Vagus 00QQ
  Nipple
    Left 0HQX
    Right 0HQW
  Omentum 0DQU
  Oral Cavity and Throat 0WQ3
  Orbit
    Left 0NQQ
    Right 0NQP
  Ovary
    Bilateral 0UQ2
    Left 0UQ1
    Right 0UQ0
  Palate
    Hard 0CQ2
    Soft 0CQ3
  Pancreas 0FQG
  Para-aortic Body 0GQ9
  Paraganglion Extremity 0GQF
  Parathyroid Gland 0GQR
    Inferior
      Left 0GQP
      Right 0GQN
    Multiple 0GQQ
    Superior
      Left 0GQM
      Right 0GQL
  Patella
    Left 0QQF
    Right 0QQD
  Penis 0VQS
  Pericardium 02QN
  Perineum
    Female 0WQN
    Male 0WQM

Repair — *continued*
  Peritoneum 0DQW
  Phalanx
    Finger
      Left 0PQV
      Right 0PQT
    Thumb
      Left 0PQS
      Right 0PQR
    Toe
      Left 0QQR
      Right 0QQQ
  Pharynx 0CQM
  Pineal Body 0GQ1
  Pleura
    Left 0BQP
    Right 0BQN
  Pons 00QB
  Prepuce 0VQT
  Products of Conception 10Q0
  Prostate 0VQ0
  Radius
    Left 0PQJ
    Right 0PQH
  Rectum 0DQP
  Retina
    Left 08QF3ZZ
    Right 08QE3ZZ
  Retinal Vessel
    Left 08QH3ZZ
    Right 08QG3ZZ
  Ribs
    1 to 2 0PQ1
    3 or More 0PQ2
  Sacrum 0QQ1
  Scapula
    Left 0PQ6
    Right 0PQ5
  Sclera
    Left 08Q7XZZ
    Right 08Q6XZZ
  Scrotum 0VQ5
  Septum
    Atrial 02Q5
    Nasal 09QM
    Ventricular 02QM
  Shoulder Region
    Left 0XQ3
    Right 0XQ2
  Sinus
    Accessory 09QP
    Ethmoid
      Left 09QV
      Right 09QU
    Frontal
      Left 09QT
      Right 09QS
    Mastoid
      Left 09QC
      Right 09QB
    Maxillary
      Left 09QR
      Right 09QQ
    Sphenoid
      Left 09QX
      Right 09QW
  Skin
    Abdomen 0HQ7XZZ
    Back 0HQ6XZZ
    Buttock 0HQ8XZZ
    Chest 0HQ5XZZ
    Ear
      Left 0HQ3XZZ
      Right 0HQ2XZZ
    Face 0HQ1XZZ
    Foot
      Left 0HQNXZZ
      Right 0HQMXZZ

Repair — *continued*
  Skin — *continued*
    Hand
      Left 0HQGXZZ
      Right 0HQFXZZ
    Inguinal 0HQAXZZ
    Lower Arm
      Left 0HQEXZZ
      Right 0HQDXZZ
    Lower Leg
      Left 0HQLXZZ
      Right 0HQKXZZ
    Neck 0HQ4XZZ
    Perineum 0HQ9XZZ
    Scalp 0HQ0XZZ
    Upper Arm
      Left 0HQCXZZ
      Right 0HQBXZZ
    Upper Leg
      Left 0HQJXZZ
      Right 0HQHXZZ
  Skull 0NQ0
  Spinal Cord
    Cervical 00QW
    Lumbar 00QY
    Thoracic 00QX
  Spinal Meninges 00QT
  Spleen 07QP
  Sternum 0PQ0
  Stomach 0DQ6
    Pylorus 0DQ7
  Subcutaneous Tissue and Fascia
    Abdomen 0JQ8
    Back 0JQ7
    Buttock 0JQ9
    Chest 0JQ6
    Face 0JQ1
    Foot
      Left 0JQR
      Right 0JQQ
    Hand
      Left 0JQK
      Right 0JQJ
    Lower Arm
      Left 0JQH
      Right 0JQG
    Lower Leg
      Left 0JQP
      Right 0JQN
    Neck
      Left 0JQ5
      Right 0JQ4
    Pelvic Region 0JQC
    Perineum 0JQB
    Scalp 0JQ0
    Upper Arm
      Left 0JQF
      Right 0JQD
    Upper Leg
      Left 0JQM
      Right 0JQL
  Tarsal
    Left 0QQM
    Right 0QQL
  Tendon
    Abdomen
      Left 0LQG
      Right 0LQF
    Ankle
      Left 0LQT
      Right 0LQS
    Foot
      Left 0LQW
      Right 0LQV
    Hand
      Left 0LQ8
      Right 0LQ7

Repair — *continued*
Tendon — *continued*
Head and Neck 0LQ0
Hip
Left 0LQK
Right 0LQJ
Knee
Left 0LQR
Right 0LQQ
Lower Arm and Wrist
Left 0LQ6
Right 0LQ5
Lower Leg
Left 0LQP
Right 0LQN
Perineum 0LQH
Shoulder
Left 0LQ2
Right 0LQ1
Thorax
Left 0LQD
Right 0LQC
Trunk
Left 0LQB
Right 0LQ9
Upper Arm
Left 0LQ4
Right 0LQ3
Upper Leg
Left 0LQM
Right 0LQL
Testis
Bilateral 0VQC
Left 0VQB
Right 0VQ9
Thalamus 00Q9
Thumb
Left 0XQM
Right 0XQL
Thymus 07QM
Thyroid Gland 0GQK
Left Lobe 0GQG
Right Lobe 0GQH
Thyroid Gland Isthmus 0GQJ
Tibia
Left 0QQH
Right 0QQG
Toe
1st
Left 0YQQ
Right 0YQP
2nd
Left 0YQS
Right 0YQR
3rd
Left 0YQU
Right 0YQT
4th
Left 0YQW
Right 0YQV
5th
Left 0YQY
Right 0YQX
Toe Nail 0HQRXZZ
Tongue 0CQ7
Tonsils 0CQP
Tooth
Lower 0CQX
Upper 0CQW
Trachea 0BQ1
Tunica Vaginalis
Left 0VQ7
Right 0VQ6
Turbinate, Nasal 09QL
Tympanic Membrane
Left 09Q8
Right 09Q7

Repair — *continued*
Ulna
Left 0PQL
Right 0PQK
Ureter
Left 0TQ7
Right 0TQ6
Urethra 0TQD
Uterine Supporting Structure 0UQ4
Uterus 0UQ9
Uvula 0CQN
Vagina 0UQG
Valve
Aortic 02QF
Mitral 02QG
Pulmonary 02QH
Tricuspid 02QJ
Vas Deferens
Bilateral 0VQQ
Left 0VQP
Right 0VQN
Vein
Axillary
Left 05Q8
Right 05Q7
Azygos 05Q0
Basilic
Left 05QC
Right 05QB
Brachial
Left 05QA
Right 05Q9
Cephalic
Left 05QF
Right 05QD
Colic 06Q7
Common Iliac
Left 06QD
Right 06QC
Coronary 02Q4
Esophageal 06Q3
External Iliac
Left 06QG
Right 06QF
External Jugular
Left 05QQ
Right 05QP
Face
Left 05QV
Right 05QT
Femoral
Left 06QN
Right 06QM
Foot
Left 06QV
Right 06QT
Gastric 06Q2
Hand
Left 05QH
Right 05QG
Hemiazygos 05Q1
Hepatic 06Q4
Hypogastric
Left 06QJ
Right 06QH
Inferior Mesenteric 06Q6
Innominate
Left 05Q4
Right 05Q3
Internal Jugular
Left 05QN
Right 05QM
Intracranial 05QL
Lower 06QY
Portal 06Q8
Pulmonary
Left 02QT
Right 02QS

Repair — *continued*
Vein — *continued*
Renal
Left 06QB
Right 06Q9
Saphenous
Left 06QQ
Right 06QP
Splenic 06Q1
Subclavian
Left 05Q6
Right 05Q5
Superior Mesenteric 06Q5
Upper 05QY
Vertebral
Left 05QS
Right 05QR
Vena Cava
Inferior 06Q0
Superior 02QV
Ventricle
Left 02QL
Right 02QK
Vertebra
Cervical 0PQ3
Lumbar 0QQ0
Thoracic 0PQ4
Vesicle
Bilateral 0VQ3
Left 0VQ2
Right 0VQ1
Vitreous
Left 08Q53ZZ
Right 08Q43ZZ
Vocal Cord
Left 0CQV
Right 0CQT
Vulva 0UQM
Wrist Region
Left 0XQH
Right 0XQG
Repair, obstetric laceration, periurethral
0UQMXZZ
Replacement
Acetabulum
Left 0QR5
Right 0QR4
Ampulla of Vater 0FRC
Anal Sphincter 0DRR
Aorta
Abdominal 04R0
Thoracic
Ascending/Arch 02RX
Descending 02RW
Artery
Anterior Tibial
Left 04RQ
Right 04RP
Axillary
Left 03R6
Right 03R5
Brachial
Left 03R8
Right 03R7
Celiac 04R1
Colic
Left 04R7
Middle 04R8
Right 04R6
Common Carotid
Left 03RJ
Right 03RH
Common Iliac
Left 04RD
Right 04RC
External Carotid
Left 03RN
Right 03RM

Replacement — *continued*
  Artery — *continued*
    External Iliac
      Left 04RJ
      Right 04RH
    Face 03RR
    Femoral
      Left 04RL
      Right 04RK
    Foot
      Left 04RW
      Right 04RV
    Gastric 04R2
    Hand
      Left 03RF
      Right 03RD
    Hepatic 04R3
    Inferior Mesenteric 04RB
    Innominate 03R2
    Internal Carotid
      Left 03RL
      Right 03RK
    Internal Iliac
      Left 04RF
      Right 04RE
    Internal Mammary
      Left 03R1
      Right 03R0
    Intracranial 03RG
    Lower 04RY
    Peroneal
      Left 04RU
      Right 04RT
    Popliteal
      Left 04RN
      Right 04RM
    Posterior Tibial
      Left 04RS
      Right 04RR
    Pulmonary
      Left 02RR
      Right 02RQ
    Pulmonary Trunk 02RP
    Radial
      Left 03RC
      Right 03RB
    Renal
      Left 04RA
      Right 04R9
    Splenic 04R4
    Subclavian
      Left 03R4
      Right 03R3
    Superior Mesenteric 04R5
    Temporal
      Left 03RT
      Right 03RS
    Thyroid
      Left 03RV
      Right 03RU
    Ulnar
      Left 03RA
      Right 03R9
    Upper 03RY
    Vertebral
      Left 03RQ
      Right 03RP
  Atrium
    Left 02R7
    Right 02R6
  Auditory Ossicle
    Left 09RA0
    Right 09R90
  Bladder 0TRB
  Bladder Neck 0TRC
  Bone
    Ethmoid

Replacement — *continued*
  Bone — *continued*
      Left 0NRG
      Right 0NRF
    Frontal 0NR1
    Hyoid 0NRX
    Lacrimal
      Left 0NRJ
      Right 0NRH
    Nasal 0NRB
    Occipital 0NR7
    Palatine
      Left 0NRL
      Right 0NRK
    Parietal
      Left 0NR4
      Right 0NR3
    Pelvic
      Left 0QR3
      Right 0QR2
    Sphenoid 0NRC
    Temporal
      Left 0NR6
      Right 0NR5
    Zygomatic
      Left 0NRN
      Right 0NRM
  Breast
    Bilateral 0HRV
    Left 0HRU
    Right 0HRT
  Bronchus
    Lingula 0BR9
    Lower Lobe
      Left 0BRB
      Right 0BR6
    Main
      Left 0BR7
      Right 0BR3
    Middle Lobe, Right 0BR5
    Upper Lobe
      Left 0BR8
      Right 0BR4
  Buccal Mucosa 0CR4
  Bursa and Ligament
    Abdomen
      Left 0MRJ
      Right 0MRH
    Ankle
      Left 0MRR
      Right 0MRQ
    Elbow
      Left 0MR4
      Right 0MR3
    Foot
      Left 0MRT
      Right 0MRS
    Hand
      Left 0MR8
      Right 0MR7
    Head and Neck 0MR0
    Hip
      Left 0MRM
      Right 0MRL
    Knee
      Left 0MRP
      Right 0MRN
    Lower Extremity
      Left 0MRW
      Right 0MRV
    Perineum 0MRK
    Rib(s) 0MRG
    Shoulder
      Left 0MR2
      Right 0MR1
    Spine
      Lower 0MRD
      Upper 0MRC

Replacement — *continued*
  Bursa and Ligament — *continued*
    Sternum 0MRF
    Upper Extremity
      Left 0MRB
      Right 0MR9
    Wrist
      Left 0MR6
      Right 0MR5
  Carina 0BR2
  Carpal
    Left 0PRN
    Right 0PRM
  Cerebral Meninges 00R1
  Cerebral Ventricle 00R6
  Chordae Tendineae 02R9
  Choroid
    Left 08RB
    Right 08RA
  Clavicle
    Left 0PRB
    Right 0PR9
  Coccyx 0QRS
  Conjunctiva
    Left 08RTX
    Right 08RSX
  Cornea
    Left 08R9
    Right 08R8
  Diaphragm 0BRT
  Disc
    Cervical Vertebral 0RR30
    Cervicothoracic Vertebral 0RR50
    Lumbar Vertebral 0SR20
    Lumbosacral 0SR40
    Thoracic Vertebral 0RR90
    Thoracolumbar Vertebral 0RRB0
  Duct
    Common Bile 0FR9
    Cystic 0FR8
    Hepatic
      Common 0FR7
      Left 0FR6
      Right 0FR5
    Lacrimal
      Left 08RY
      Right 08RX
    Pancreatic 0FRD
      Accessory 0FRF
    Parotid
      Left 0CRC
      Right 0CRB
  Dura Mater 00R2
  Ear
    External
      Bilateral 09R2
      Left 09R1
      Right 09R0
    Inner
      Left 09RE0
      Right 09RD0
    Middle
      Left 09R60
      Right 09R50
  Epiglottis 0CRR
  Esophagus 0DR5
  Eye
    Left 08R1
    Right 08R0
  Eyelid
    Lower
      Left 08RR
      Right 08RQ
    Upper
      Left 08RP
      Right 08RN

Replacement — *continued*
  Femoral Shaft
    Left 0QR9
    Right 0QR8
  Femur
    Lower
      Left 0QRC
      Right 0QRB
    Upper
      Left 0QR7
      Right 0QR6
  Fibula
    Left 0QRK
    Right 0QRJ
  Finger Nail 0HRQX
  Gingiva
    Lower 0CR6
    Upper 0CR5
  Glenoid Cavity
    Left 0PR8
    Right 0PR7
  Hair 0HRSX
  Humeral Head
    Left 0PRD
    Right 0PRC
  Humeral Shaft
    Left 0PRG
    Right 0PRF
  Iris
    Left 08RD3
    Right 08RC3
  Joint
    Acromioclavicular
      Left 0RRH0
      Right 0RRG0
    Ankle
      Left 0SRG
      Right 0SRF
    Carpal
      Left 0RRR0
      Right 0RRQ0
    Carpometacarpal
      Left 0RRT0
      Right 0RRS0
    Cervical Vertebral 0RR10
    Cervicothoracic Vertebral 0RR40
    Coccygeal 0SR60
    Elbow
      Left 0RRM0
      Right 0RRL0
    Finger Phalangeal
      Left 0RRX0
      Right 0RRW0
    Hip
      Left 0SRB
        Acetabular Surface 0SRE
        Femoral Surface 0SRS
      Right 0SR9
        Acetabular Surface 0SRA
        Femoral Surface 0SRR
    Knee
      Left 0SRD
        Femoral Surface 0SRU
        Tibial Surface 0SRW
      Right 0SRC
        Femoral Surface 0SRT
        Tibial Surface 0SRV
    Lumbar Vertebral 0SR00
    Lumbosacral 0SR30
    Metacarpophalangeal
      Left 0RRV0
      Right 0RRU0
    Metatarsal-Phalangeal
      Left 0SRN0
      Right 0SRM0
    Occipital-cervical 0RR00
    Sacrococcygeal 0SR50

Replacement — *continued*
  Joint — *continued*
    Sacroiliac
      Left 0SR80
      Right 0SR70
    Shoulder
      Left 0RRK
      Right 0RRJ
    Sternoclavicular
      Left 0RRF0
      Right 0RRE0
    Tarsal
      Left 0SRJ0
      Right 0SRH0
    Tarsometatarsal
      Left 0SRL0
      Right 0SRK0
    Temporomandibular
      Left 0RRD0
      Right 0RRC0
    Thoracic Vertebral 0RR60
    Thoracolumbar Vertebral 0RRA0
    Toe Phalangeal
      Left 0SRQ0
      Right 0SRP0
    Wrist
      Left 0RRP0
      Right 0RRN0
  Kidney Pelvis
    Left 0TR4
    Right 0TR3
  Larynx 0CRS
  Lens
    Left 08RK30Z
    Right 08RJ30Z
  Lip
    Lower 0CR1
    Upper 0CR0
  Mandible
    Left 0NRV
    Right 0NRT
  Maxilla 0NRR
  Mesentery 0DRV
  Metacarpal
    Left 0PRQ
    Right 0PRP
  Metatarsal
    Left 0QRP
    Right 0QRN
  Muscle
    Abdomen
      Left 0KRL
      Right 0KRK
    Facial 0KR1
    Foot
      Left 0KRW
      Right 0KRV
    Hand
      Left 0KRD
      Right 0KRC
    Head 0KR0
    Hip
      Left 0KRP
      Right 0KRN
    Lower Arm and Wrist
      Left 0KRB
      Right 0KR9
    Lower Leg
      Left 0KRT
      Right 0KRS
    Neck
      Left 0KR3
      Right 0KR2
    Papillary 02RD
    Perineum 0KRM
    Shoulder
      Left 0KR6
      Right 0KR5

Replacement — *continued*
  Muscle — *continued*
    Thorax
      Left 0KRJ
      Right 0KRH
    Tongue, Palate, Pharynx 0KR4
    Trunk
      Left 0KRG
      Right 0KRF
    Upper Arm
      Left 0KR8
      Right 0KR7
    Upper Leg
      Left 0KRR
      Right 0KRQ
  Nasal Mucosa and Soft Tissue 09RK
  Nasopharynx 09RN
  Nerve
    Abducens 00RL
    Accessory 00RR
    Acoustic 00RN
    Cervical 01R1
    Facial 00RM
    Femoral 01RD
    Glossopharyngeal 00RP
    Hypoglossal 00RS
    Lumbar 01RB
    Median 01R5
    Oculomotor 00RH
    Olfactory 00RF
    Optic 00RG
    Peroneal 01RH
    Phrenic 01R2
    Pudendal 01RC
    Radial 01R6
    Sacral 01RR
    Sciatic 01RF
    Thoracic 01R8
    Tibial 01RG
    Trigeminal 00RK
    Trochlear 00RJ
    Ulnar 01R4
    Vagus 00RQ
  Nipple
    Left 0HRX
    Right 0HRW
  Omentum 0DRU
  Orbit
    Left 0NRQ
    Right 0NRP
  Palate
    Hard 0CR2
    Soft 0CR3
  Patella
    Left 0QRF
    Right 0QRD
  Pericardium 02RN
  Peritoneum 0DRW
  Phalanx
    Finger
      Left 0PRV
      Right 0PRT
    Thumb
      Left 0PRS
      Right 0PRR
    Toe
      Left 0QRR
      Right 0QRQ
  Pharynx 0CRM
  Radius
    Left 0PRJ
    Right 0PRH
  Retinal Vessel
    Left 08RH3
    Right 08RG3
  Ribs
    1 to 2 0PR1
    3 or More 0PR2

Replacement — *continued*
  Sacrum 0QR1
  Scapula
    Left 0PR6
    Right 0PR5
  Sclera
    Left 08R7X
    Right 08R6X
  Septum
    Atrial 02R5
    Nasal 09RM
    Ventricular 02RM
  Skin
    Abdomen 0HR7
    Back 0HR6
    Buttock 0HR8
    Chest 0HR5
    Ear
      Left 0HR3
      Right 0HR2
    Face 0HR1
    Foot
      Left 0HRN
      Right 0HRM
    Hand
      Left 0HRG
      Right 0HRF
    Inguinal 0HRA
    Lower Arm
      Left 0HRE
      Right 0HRD
    Lower Leg
      Left 0HRL
      Right 0HRK
    Neck 0HR4
    Perineum 0HR9
    Scalp 0HR0
    Upper Arm
      Left 0HRC
      Right 0HRB
    Upper Leg
      Left 0HRJ
      Right 0HRH
  Skin Substitute, Porcine Liver
    Derived XHRPXL2
  Skull 0NR0
  Spinal Meninges 00RT
  Sternum 0PR0
  Subcutaneous Tissue and Fascia
    Abdomen 0JR8
    Back 0JR7
    Buttock 0JR9
    Chest 0JR6
    Face 0JR1
    Foot
      Left 0JRR
      Right 0JRQ
    Hand
      Left 0JRK
      Right 0JRJ
    Lower Arm
      Left 0JRH
      Right 0JRG
    Lower Leg
      Left 0JRP
      Right 0JRN
    Neck
      Left 0JR5
      Right 0JR4
    Pelvic Region 0JRC
    Perineum 0JRB
    Scalp 0JR0
    Upper Arm
      Left 0JRF
      Right 0JRD
    Upper Leg
      Left 0JRM
      Right 0JRL

Replacement — *continued*
  Tarsal
    Left 0QRM
    Right 0QRL
  Tendon
    Abdomen
      Left 0LRG
      Right 0LRF
    Ankle
      Left 0LRT
      Right 0LRS
    Foot
      Left 0LRW
      Right 0LRV
    Hand
      Left 0LR8
      Right 0LR7
    Head and Neck 0LR0
    Hip
      Left 0LRK
      Right 0LRJ
    Knee
      Left 0LRR
      Right 0LRQ
    Lower Arm and Wrist
      Left 0LR6
      Right 0LR5
    Lower Leg
      Left 0LRP
      Right 0LRN
    Perineum 0LRH
    Shoulder
      Left 0LR2
      Right 0LR1
    Thorax
      Left 0LRD
      Right 0LRC
    Trunk
      Left 0LRB
      Right 0LR9
    Upper Arm
      Left 0LR4
      Right 0LR3
    Upper Leg
      Left 0LRM
      Right 0LRL
  Testis
    Bilateral 0VRC0JZ
    Left 0VRB0JZ
    Right 0VR90JZ
  Thumb
    Left 0XRM
    Right 0XRL
  Tibia
    Left 0QRH
    Right 0QRG
  Toe Nail 0HRRX
  Tongue 0CR7
  Tooth
    Lower 0CRX
    Upper 0CRW
  Trachea 0BR1
  Turbinate, Nasal 09RL
  Tympanic Membrane
    Left 09R8
    Right 09R7
  Ulna
    Left 0PRL
    Right 0PRK
  Ureter
    Left 0TR7
    Right 0TR6
  Urethra 0TRD
  Uvula 0CRN
  Valve
    Aortic 02RF
    Mitral 02RG

Replacement — *continued*
  Valve — *continued*
    Pulmonary 02RH
    Tricuspid 02RJ
  Vein
    Axillary
      Left 05R8
      Right 05R7
    Azygos 05R0
    Basilic
      Left 05RC
      Right 05RB
    Brachial
      Left 05RA
      Right 05R9
    Cephalic
      Left 05RF
      Right 05RD
    Colic 06R7
    Common Iliac
      Left 06RD
      Right 06RC
    Esophageal 06R3
    External Iliac
      Left 06RG
      Right 06RF
    External Jugular
      Left 05RQ
      Right 05RP
    Face
      Left 05RV
      Right 05RT
    Femoral
      Left 06RN
      Right 06RM
    Foot
      Left 06RV
      Right 06RT
    Gastric 06R2
    Hand
      Left 05RH
      Right 05RG
    Hemiazygos 05R1
    Hepatic 06R4
    Hypogastric
      Left 06RJ
      Right 06RH
    Inferior Mesenteric 06R6
    Innominate
      Left 05R4
      Right 05R3
    Internal Jugular
      Left 05RN
      Right 05RM
    Intracranial 05RL
    Lower 06RY
    Portal 06R8
    Pulmonary
      Left 02RT
      Right 02RS
    Renal
      Left 06RB
      Right 06R9
    Saphenous
      Left 06RQ
      Right 06RP
    Splenic 06R1
    Subclavian
      Left 05R6
      Right 05R5
    Superior Mesenteric 06R5
    Upper 05RY
    Vertebral
      Left 05RS
      Right 05RR
  Vena Cava
    Inferior 06R0
    Superior 02RV

Replacement — *continued*
Ventricle
Left 02RL
Right 02RK
Vertebra
Cervical 0PR3
Lumbar 0QR0
Thoracic 0PR4
Vitreous
Left 08R53
Right 08R43
Vocal Cord
Left 0CRV
Right 0CRT
Zooplastic Tissue, Rapid Deployment
Technique X2RF
Replacement, hip
Partial or total *see* Replacement, Lower
Joints 0SR
Resurfacing only *see* Supplement, Lower
Joints 0SU
Replantation
see Reposition
Replantation, scalp
see Reattachment, Skin, Scalp 0HM0
Reposition
Acetabulum
Left 0QS5
Right 0QS4
Ampulla of Vater 0FSC
Anus 0DSQ
Aorta
Abdominal 04S0
Thoracic
Ascending/Arch 02SX0ZZ
Descending 02SW0ZZ
Artery
Anterior Tibial
Left 04SQ
Right 04SP
Axillary
Left 03S6
Right 03S5
Brachial
Left 03S8
Right 03S7
Celiac 04S1
Colic
Left 04S7
Middle 04S8
Right 04S6
Common Carotid
Left 03SJ
Right 03SH
Common Iliac
Left 04SD
Right 04SC
Coronary
One Artery 02S00ZZ
Two Arteries 02S10ZZ
External Carotid
Left 03SN
Right 03SM
External Iliac
Left 04SJ
Right 04SH
Face 03SR
Femoral
Left 04SL
Right 04SK
Foot
Left 04SW
Right 04SV
Gastric 04S2
Hand
Left 03SF
Right 03SD

Reposition — *continued*
Artery — *continued*
Hepatic 04S3
Inferior Mesenteric 04SB
Innominate 03S2
Internal Carotid
Left 03SL
Right 03SK
Internal Iliac
Left 04SF
Right 04SE
Internal Mammary
Left 03S1
Right 03S0
Intracranial 03SG
Lower 04SY
Peroneal
Left 04SU
Right 04ST
Popliteal
Left 04SN
Right 04SM
Posterior Tibial
Left 04SS
Right 04SR
Pulmonary
Left 02SR0ZZ
Right 02SQ0ZZ
Pulmonary Trunk 02SP0ZZ
Radial
Left 03SC
Right 03SB
Renal
Left 04SA
Right 04S9
Splenic 04S4
Subclavian
Left 03S4
Right 03S3
Superior Mesenteric 04S5
Temporal
Left 03ST
Right 03SS
Thyroid
Left 03SV
Right 03SU
Ulnar
Left 03SA
Right 03S9
Upper 03SY
Vertebral
Left 03SQ
Right 03SP
Auditory Ossicle
Left 09SA
Right 09S9
Bladder 0TSB
Bladder Neck 0TSC
Bone
Ethmoid
Left 0NSG
Right 0NSF
Frontal 0NS1
Hyoid 0NSX
Lacrimal
Left 0NSJ
Right 0NSH
Nasal 0NSB
Occipital 0NS7
Palatine
Left 0NSL
Right 0NSK
Parietal
Left 0NS4
Right 0NS3
Pelvic
Left 0QS3
Right 0QS2

Reposition — *continued*
Bone — *continued*
Sphenoid 0NSC
Temporal
Left 0NS6
Right 0NS5
Zygomatic
Left 0NSN
Right 0NSM
Breast
Bilateral 0HSV0ZZ
Left 0HSU0ZZ
Right 0HST0ZZ
Bronchus
Lingula 0BS90ZZ
Lower Lobe
Left 0BSB0ZZ
Right 0BS60ZZ
Main
Left 0BS70ZZ
Right 0BS30ZZ
Middle Lobe, Right 0BS50ZZ
Upper Lobe
Left 0BS80ZZ
Right 0BS40ZZ
Bursa and Ligament
Abdomen
Left 0MSJ
Right 0MSH
Ankle
Left 0MSR
Right 0MSQ
Elbow
Left 0MS4
Right 0MS3
Foot
Left 0MST
Right 0MSS
Hand
Left 0MS8
Right 0MS7
Head and Neck 0MS0
Hip
Left 0MSM
Right 0MSL
Knee
Left 0MSP
Right 0MSN
Lower Extremity
Left 0MSW
Right 0MSV
Perineum 0MSK
Rib(s) 0MSG
Shoulder
Left 0MS2
Right 0MS1
Spine
Lower 0MSD
Upper 0MSC
Sternum 0MSF
Upper Extremity
Left 0MSB
Right 0MS9
Wrist
Left 0MS6
Right 0MS5
Carina 0BS20ZZ
Carpal
Left 0PSN
Right 0PSM
Cecum 0DSH
Cervix 0USC
Clavicle
Left 0PSB
Right 0PS9
Coccyx 0QSS

Reposition — *continued*
- Colon
  - Ascending 0DSK
  - Descending 0DSM
  - Sigmoid 0DSN
  - Transverse 0DSL
- Cord
  - Bilateral 0VSH
  - Left 0VSG
  - Right 0VSF
- Cul-de-sac 0USF
- Diaphragm 0BST0ZZ
- Duct
  - Common Bile 0FS9
  - Cystic 0FS8
  - Hepatic
    - Common 0FS7
    - Left 0FS6
    - Right 0FS5
  - Lacrimal
    - Left 08SY
    - Right 08SX
  - Pancreatic 0FSD
    - Accessory 0FSF
  - Parotid
    - Left 0CSC
    - Right 0CSB
- Duodenum 0DS9
- Ear
  - Bilateral 09S2
  - Left 09S1
  - Right 09S0
- Epiglottis 0CSR
- Esophagus 0DS5
- Eustachian Tube
  - Left 09SG
  - Right 09SF
- Eyelid
  - Lower
    - Left 08SR
    - Right 08SQ
  - Upper
    - Left 08SP
    - Right 08SN
- Fallopian Tube
  - Left 0US6
  - Right 0US5
- Fallopian Tubes, Bilateral 0US7
- Femoral Shaft
  - Left 0QS9
  - Right 0QS8
- Femur
  - Lower
    - Left 0QSC
    - Right 0QSB
  - Upper
    - Left 0QS7
    - Right 0QS6
- Fibula
  - Left 0QSK
  - Right 0QSJ
- Gallbladder 0FS4
- Gland
  - Adrenal
    - Left 0GS2
    - Right 0GS3
  - Lacrimal
    - Left 08SW
    - Right 08SV
- Glenoid Cavity
  - Left 0PS8
  - Right 0PS7
- Hair 0HSSXZZ
- Humeral Head
  - Left 0PSD
  - Right 0PSC

Reposition — *continued*
- Humeral Shaft
  - Left 0PSG
  - Right 0PSF
- Ileum 0DSB
- Intestine
  - Large 0DSE
  - Small 0DS8
- Iris
  - Left 08SD3ZZ
  - Right 08SC3ZZ
- Jejunum 0DSA
- Joint
  - Acromioclavicular
    - Left 0RSH
    - Right 0RSG
  - Ankle
    - Left 0SSG
    - Right 0SSF
  - Carpal
    - Left 0RSR
    - Right 0RSQ
  - Carpometacarpal
    - Left 0RST
    - Right 0RSS
  - Cervical Vertebral 0RS1
  - Cervicothoracic Vertebral 0RS4
  - Coccygeal 0SS6
  - Elbow
    - Left 0RSM
    - Right 0RSL
  - Finger Phalangeal
    - Left 0RSX
    - Right 0RSW
  - Hip
    - Left 0SSB
    - Right 0SS9
  - Knee
    - Left 0SSD
    - Right 0SSC
  - Lumbar Vertebral 0SS0
  - Lumbosacral 0SS3
  - Metacarpophalangeal
    - Left 0RSV
    - Right 0RSU
  - Metatarsal-Phalangeal
    - Left 0SSN
    - Right 0SSM
  - Occipital-cervical 0RS0
  - Sacrococcygeal 0SS5
  - Sacroiliac
    - Left 0SS8
    - Right 0SS7
  - Shoulder
    - Left 0RSK
    - Right 0RSJ
  - Sternoclavicular
    - Left 0RSF
    - Right 0RSE
  - Tarsal
    - Left 0SSJ
    - Right 0SSH
  - Tarsometatarsal
    - Left 0SSL
    - Right 0SSK
  - Temporomandibular
    - Left 0RSD
    - Right 0RSC
  - Thoracic Vertebral 0RS6
  - Thoracolumbar Vertebral 0RSA
  - Toe Phalangeal
    - Left 0SSQ
    - Right 0SSP
  - Wrist
    - Left 0RSP
    - Right 0RSN

Reposition — *continued*
- Kidney
  - Left 0TS1
  - Right 0TS0
- Kidney Pelvis
  - Left 0TS4
  - Right 0TS3
- Kidneys, Bilateral 0TS2
- Lens
  - Left 08SK3ZZ
  - Right 08SJ3ZZ
- Lip
  - Lower 0CS1
  - Upper 0CS0
- Liver 0FS0
- Lung
  - Left 0BSL0ZZ
  - Lower Lobe
    - Left 0BSJ0ZZ
    - Right 0BSF0ZZ
  - Middle Lobe, Right 0BSD0ZZ
  - Right 0BSK0ZZ
  - Upper Lobe
    - Left 0BSG0ZZ
    - Right 0BSC0ZZ
- Lung Lingula 0BSH0ZZ
- Mandible
  - Left 0NSV
  - Right 0NST
- Maxilla 0NSR
- Metacarpal
  - Left 0PSQ
  - Right 0PSP
- Metatarsal
  - Left 0QSP
  - Right 0QSN
- Muscle
  - Abdomen
    - Left 0KSL
    - Right 0KSK
  - Extraocular
    - Left 08SM
    - Right 08SL
  - Facial 0KS1
  - Foot
    - Left 0KSW
    - Right 0KSV
  - Hand
    - Left 0KSD
    - Right 0KSC
  - Head 0KS0
  - Hip
    - Left 0KSP
    - Right 0KSN
  - Lower Arm and Wrist
    - Left 0KSB
    - Right 0KS9
  - Lower Leg
    - Left 0KST
    - Right 0KSS
  - Neck
    - Left 0KS3
    - Right 0KS2
  - Perineum 0KSM
  - Shoulder
    - Left 0KS6
    - Right 0KS5
  - Thorax
    - Left 0KSJ
    - Right 0KSH
  - Tongue, Palate, Pharynx 0KS4
  - Trunk
    - Left 0KSG
    - Right 0KSF
  - Upper Arm
    - Left 0KS8
    - Right 0KS7

Reposition — *continued*
- Muscle — *continued*
  - Upper Leg
    - Left 0KSR
    - Right 0KSQ
- Nasal Mucosa and Soft Tissue 09SK
- Nerve
  - Abducens 00SL
  - Accessory 00SR
  - Acoustic 00SN
  - Brachial Plexus 01S3
  - Cervical 01S1
  - Cervical Plexus 01S0
  - Facial 00SM
  - Femoral 01SD
  - Glossopharyngeal 00SP
  - Hypoglossal 00SS
  - Lumbar 01SB
  - Lumbar Plexus 01S9
  - Lumbosacral Plexus 01SA
  - Median 01S5
  - Oculomotor 00SH
  - Olfactory 00SF
  - Optic 00SG
  - Peroneal 01SH
  - Phrenic 01S2
  - Pudendal 01SC
  - Radial 01S6
  - Sacral 01SR
  - Sacral Plexus 01SQ
  - Sciatic 01SF
  - Thoracic 01S8
  - Tibial 01SG
  - Trigeminal 00SK
  - Trochlear 00SJ
  - Ulnar 01S4
  - Vagus 00SQ
- Nipple
  - Left 0HSXXZZ
  - Right 0HSWXZZ
- Orbit
  - Left 0NSQ
  - Right 0NSP
- Ovary
  - Bilateral 0US2
  - Left 0US1
  - Right 0US0
- Palate
  - Hard 0CS2
  - Soft 0CS3
- Pancreas 0FSG
- Parathyroid Gland 0GSR
  - Inferior
    - Left 0GSP
    - Right 0GSN
  - Multiple 0GSQ
  - Superior
    - Left 0GSM
    - Right 0GSL
- Patella
  - Left 0QSF
  - Right 0QSD
- Phalanx
  - Finger
    - Left 0PSV
    - Right 0PST
  - Thumb
    - Left 0PSS
    - Right 0PSR
  - Toe
    - Left 0QSR
    - Right 0QSQ
- Products of Conception 10S0
  - Ectopic 10S2
- Radius
  - Left 0PSJ
  - Right 0PSH

Reposition — *continued*
- Rectum 0DSP
- Retinal Vessel
  - Left 08SH3ZZ
  - Right 08SG3ZZ
- Ribs
  - 1 to 2 0PS1
  - 3 or More 0PS2
- Sacrum 0QS1
- Scapula
  - Left 0PS6
  - Right 0PS5
- Septum, Nasal 09SM
- Sesamoid Bone(s) 1st Toe
  - *see* Reposition, Metatarsal, Right 0QSN
  - *see* Reposition, Metatarsal, Left 0QSP
- Skull 0NS0
- Spinal Cord
  - Cervical 00SW
  - Lumbar 00SY
  - Thoracic 00SX
- Spleen 07SP0ZZ
- Sternum 0PS0
- Stomach 0DS6
- Tarsal
  - Left 0QSM
  - Right 0QSL
- Tendon
  - Abdomen
    - Left 0LSG
    - Right 0LSF
  - Ankle
    - Left 0LST
    - Right 0LSS
  - Foot
    - Left 0LSW
    - Right 0LSV
  - Hand
    - Left 0LS8
    - Right 0LS7
  - Head and Neck 0LS0
  - Hip
    - Left 0LSK
    - Right 0LSJ
  - Knee
    - Left 0LSR
    - Right 0LSQ
  - Lower Arm and Wrist
    - Left 0LS6
    - Right 0LS5
  - Lower Leg
    - Left 0LSP
    - Right 0LSN
  - Perineum 0LSH
  - Shoulder
    - Left 0LS2
    - Right 0LS1
  - Thorax
    - Left 0LSD
    - Right 0LSC
  - Trunk
    - Left 0LSB
    - Right 0LS9
  - Upper Arm
    - Left 0LS4
    - Right 0LS3
  - Upper Leg
    - Left 0LSM
    - Right 0LSL
- Testis
  - Bilateral 0VSC
  - Left 0VSB
  - Right 0VS9
- Thymus 07SM0ZZ
- Thyroid Gland
  - Left Lobe 0GSG
  - Right Lobe 0GSH

Reposition — *continued*
- Tibia
  - Left 0QSH
  - Right 0QSG
- Tongue 0CS7
- Tooth
  - Lower 0CSX
  - Upper 0CSW
- Trachea 0BS10ZZ
- Turbinate, Nasal 09SL
- Tympanic Membrane
  - Left 09S8
  - Right 09S7
- Ulna
  - Left 0PSL
  - Right 0PSK
- Ureter
  - Left 0TS7
  - Right 0TS6
- Ureters, Bilateral 0TS8
- Urethra 0TSD
- Uterine Supporting Structure 0US4
- Uterus 0US9
- Uvula 0CSN
- Vagina 0USG
- Vein
  - Axillary
    - Left 05S8
    - Right 05S7
  - Azygos 05S0
  - Basilic
    - Left 05SC
    - Right 05SB
  - Brachial
    - Left 05SA
    - Right 05S9
  - Cephalic
    - Left 05SF
    - Right 05SD
  - Colic 06S7
  - Common Iliac
    - Left 06SD
    - Right 06SC
  - Esophageal 06S3
  - External Iliac
    - Left 06SG
    - Right 06SF
  - External Jugular
    - Left 05SQ
    - Right 05SP
  - Face
    - Left 05SV
    - Right 05ST
  - Femoral
    - Left 06SN
    - Right 06SM
  - Foot
    - Left 06SV
    - Right 06ST
  - Gastric 06S2
  - Hand
    - Left 05SH
    - Right 05SG
  - Hemiazygos 05S1
  - Hepatic 06S4
  - Hypogastric
    - Left 06SJ
    - Right 06SH
  - Inferior Mesenteric 06S6
  - Innominate
    - Left 05S4
    - Right 05S3
  - Internal Jugular
    - Left 05SN
    - Right 05SM
  - Intracranial 05SL
  - Lower 06SY

Reposition — *continued*
    Vein — *continued*
        Portal 06S8
        Pulmonary
            Left 02ST0ZZ
            Right 02SS0ZZ
        Renal
            Left 06SB
            Right 06S9
        Saphenous
            Left 06SQ
            Right 06SP
        Splenic 06S1
        Subclavian
            Left 05S6
            Right 05S5
        Superior Mesenteric 06S5
        Upper 05SY
        Vertebral
            Left 05SS
            Right 05SR
    Vena Cava
        Inferior 06S0
        Superior 02SV0ZZ
    Vertebra
        Cervical 0PS3
            Magnetically Controlled Growth
                Rod(s) XNS3
        Lumbar 0QS0
            Magnetically Controlled Growth
                Rod(s) XNS0
        Thoracic 0PS4
            Magnetically Controlled Growth
                Rod(s) XNS4
    Vocal Cord
        Left 0CSV
        Right 0CST
Resection
    Acetabulum
        Left 0QT50ZZ
        Right 0QT40ZZ
    Adenoids 0CTQ
    Ampulla of Vater 0FTC
    Anal Sphincter 0DTR
    Anus 0DTQ
    Aortic Body 0GTD
    Appendix 0DTJ
    Auditory Ossicle
        Left 09TA
        Right 09T9
    Bladder 0TTB
    Bladder Neck 0TTC
    Bone
        Ethmoid
            Left 0NTG0ZZ
            Right 0NTF0ZZ
        Frontal 0NT10ZZ
        Hyoid 0NTX0ZZ
        Lacrimal
            Left 0NTJ0ZZ
            Right 0NTH0ZZ
        Nasal 0NTB0ZZ
        Occipital 0NT70ZZ
        Palatine
            Left 0NTL0ZZ
            Right 0NTK0ZZ
        Parietal
            Left 0NT40ZZ
            Right 0NT30ZZ
        Pelvic
            Left 0QT30ZZ
            Right 0QT20ZZ
        Sphenoid 0NTC0ZZ
        Temporal
            Left 0NT60ZZ
            Right 0NT50ZZ

Resection — *continued*
    Bone — *continued*
        Zygomatic
            Left 0NTN0ZZ
            Right 0NTM0ZZ
    Breast
        Bilateral 0HTV0ZZ
        Left 0HTU0ZZ
        Right 0HTT0ZZ
        Supernumerary 0HTY0ZZ
    Bronchus
        Lingula 0BT9
        Lower Lobe
            Left 0BTB
            Right 0BT6
        Main
            Left 0BT7
            Right 0BT3
        Middle Lobe, Right 0BT5
        Upper Lobe
            Left 0BT8
            Right 0BT4
    Bursa and Ligament
        Abdomen
            Left 0MTJ
            Right 0MTH
        Ankle
            Left 0MTR
            Right 0MTQ
        Elbow
            Left 0MT4
            Right 0MT3
        Foot
            Left 0MTT
            Right 0MTS
        Hand
            Left 0MT8
            Right 0MT7
        Head and Neck 0MT0
        Hip
            Left 0MTM
            Right 0MTL
        Knee
            Left 0MTP
            Right 0MTN
        Lower Extremity
            Left 0MTW
            Right 0MTV
        Perineum 0MTK
        Rib(s) 0MTG
        Shoulder
            Left 0MT2
            Right 0MT1
        Spine
            Lower 0MTD
            Upper 0MTC
        Sternum 0MTF
        Upper Extremity
            Left 0MTB
            Right 0MT9
        Wrist
            Left 0MT6
            Right 0MT5
    Carina 0BT2
    Carotid Bodies, Bilateral 0GT8
    Carotid Body
        Left 0GT6
        Right 0GT7
    Carpal
        Left 0PTN0ZZ
        Right 0PTM0ZZ
    Cecum 0DTH
    Cerebral Hemisphere 00T7
    Cervix 0UTC
    Chordae Tendineae 02T9
    Cisterna Chyli 07TL

Resection — *continued*
    Clavicle
        Left 0PTB0ZZ
        Right 0PT90ZZ
    Clitoris 0UTJ
    Coccygeal Glomus 0GTB
    Coccyx 0QTS0ZZ
    Colon
        Ascending 0DTK
        Descending 0DTM
        Sigmoid 0DTN
        Transverse 0DTL
    Conduction Mechanism 02T8
    Cord
        Bilateral 0VTH
        Left 0VTG
        Right 0VTF
    Cornea
        Left 08T9XZZ
        Right 08T8XZZ
    Cul-de-sac 0UTF
    Diaphragm 0BTT
    Disc
        Cervical Vertebral 0RT30ZZ
        Cervicothoracic Vertebral 0RT50ZZ
        Lumbar Vertebral 0ST20ZZ
        Lumbosacral 0ST40ZZ
        Thoracic Vertebral 0RT90ZZ
        Thoracolumbar Vertebral 0RTB0ZZ
    Duct
        Common Bile 0FT9
        Cystic 0FT8
        Hepatic
            Common 0FT7
            Left 0FT6
            Right 0FT5
        Lacrimal
            Left 08TY
            Right 08TX
        Pancreatic 0FTD
            Accessory 0FTF
        Parotid
            Left 0CTC0ZZ
            Right 0CTB0ZZ
    Duodenum 0DT9
    Ear
        External
            Left 09T1
            Right 09T0
        Inner
            Left 09TE
            Right 09TD
        Middle
            Left 09T6
            Right 09T5
    Epididymis
        Bilateral 0VTL
        Left 0VTK
        Right 0VTJ
    Epiglottis 0CTR
    Esophagogastric Junction 0DT4
    Esophagus 0DT5
        Lower 0DT3
        Middle 0DT2
        Upper 0DT1
    Eustachian Tube
        Left 09TG
        Right 09TF
    Eye
        Left 08T1XZZ
        Right 08T0XZZ
    Eyelid
        Lower
            Left 08TR
            Right 08TQ
        Upper
            Left 08TP
            Right 08TN

Resection — *continued*
Fallopian Tube
Left 0UT6
Right 0UT5
Fallopian Tubes, Bilateral 0UT7
Femoral Shaft
Left 0QT90ZZ
Right 0QT80ZZ
Femur
Lower
Left 0QTC0ZZ
Right 0QTB0ZZ
Upper
Left 0QT70ZZ
Right 0QT60ZZ
Fibula
Left 0QTK0ZZ
Right 0QTJ0ZZ
Finger Nail 0HTQXZZ
Gallbladder 0FT4
Gland
Adrenal
Bilateral 0GT4
Left 0GT2
Right 0GT3
Lacrimal
Left 08TW
Right 08TV
Minor Salivary 0CTJ0ZZ
Parotid
Left 0CT90ZZ
Right 0CT80ZZ
Pituitary 0GT0
Sublingual
Left 0CTF0ZZ
Right 0CTD0ZZ
Submaxillary
Left 0CTH0ZZ
Right 0CTG0ZZ
Vestibular 0UTL
Glenoid Cavity
Left 0PT80ZZ
Right 0PT70ZZ
Glomus Jugulare 0GTC
Humeral Head
Left 0PTD0ZZ
Right 0PTC0ZZ
Humeral Shaft
Left 0PTG0ZZ
Right 0PTF0ZZ
Hymen 0UTK
Ileocecal Valve 0DTC
Ileum 0DTB
Intestine
Large 0DTE
Left 0DTG
Right 0DTF
Small 0DT8
Iris
Left 08TD3ZZ
Right 08TC3ZZ
Jejunum 0DTA
Joint
Acromioclavicular
Left 0RTH0ZZ
Right 0RTG0ZZ
Ankle
Left 0STG0ZZ
Right 0STF0ZZ
Carpal
Left 0RTR0ZZ
Right 0RTQ0ZZ
Carpometacarpal
Left 0RTT0ZZ
Right 0RTS0ZZ
Cervicothoracic Vertebral 0RT40ZZ
Coccygeal 0ST60ZZ

Resection — *continued*
Joint — *continued*
Elbow
Left 0RTM0ZZ
Right 0RTL0ZZ
Finger Phalangeal
Left 0RTX0ZZ
Right 0RTW0ZZ
Hip
Left 0STB0ZZ
Right 0ST90ZZ
Knee
Left 0STD0ZZ
Right 0STC0ZZ
Metacarpophalangeal
Left 0RTV0ZZ
Right 0RTU0ZZ
Metatarsal-Phalangeal
Left 0STN0ZZ
Right 0STM0ZZ
Sacrococcygeal 0ST50ZZ
Sacroiliac
Left 0ST80ZZ
Right 0ST70ZZ
Shoulder
Left 0RTK0ZZ
Right 0RTJ0ZZ
Sternoclavicular
Left 0RTF0ZZ
Right 0RTE0ZZ
Tarsal
Left 0STJ0ZZ
Right 0STH0ZZ
Tarsometatarsal
Left 0STL0ZZ
Right 0STK0ZZ
Temporomandibular
Left 0RTD0ZZ
Right 0RTC0ZZ
Toe Phalangeal
Left 0STQ0ZZ
Right 0STP0ZZ
Wrist
Left 0RTP0ZZ
Right 0RTN0ZZ
Kidney
Left 0TT1
Right 0TT0
Kidney Pelvis
Left 0TT4
Right 0TT3
Kidneys, Bilateral 0TT2
Larynx 0CTS
Lens
Left 08TK3ZZ
Right 08TJ3ZZ
Lip
Lower 0CT1
Upper 0CT0
Liver 0FT0
Left Lobe 0FT2
Right Lobe 0FT1
Lung
Bilateral 0BTM
Left 0BTL
Lower Lobe
Left 0BTJ
Right 0BTF
Middle Lobe, Right 0BTD
Right 0BTK
Upper Lobe
Left 0BTG
Right 0BTC
Lung Lingula 0BTH
Lymphatic
Aortic 07TD

Resection — *continued*
Lymphatic — *continued*
Axillary
Left 07T6
Right 07T5
Head 07T0
Inguinal
Left 07TJ
Right 07TH
Internal Mammary
Left 07T9
Right 07T8
Lower Extremity
Left 07TG
Right 07TF
Mesenteric 07TB
Neck
Left 07T2
Right 07T1
Pelvis 07TC
Thoracic Duct 07TK
Thorax 07T7
Upper Extremity
Left 07T4
Right 07T3
Mandible
Left 0NTV0ZZ
Right 0NTT0ZZ
Maxilla 0NTR0ZZ
Metacarpal
Left 0PTQ0ZZ
Right 0PTP0ZZ
Metatarsal
Left 0QTP0ZZ
Right 0QTN0ZZ
Muscle
Abdomen
Left 0KTL
Right 0KTK
Extraocular
Left 08TM
Right 08TL
Facial 0KT1
Foot
Left 0KTW
Right 0KTV
Hand
Left 0KTD
Right 0KTC
Head 0KT0
Hip
Left 0KTP
Right 0KTN
Lower Arm and Wrist
Left 0KTB
Right 0KT9
Lower Leg
Left 0KTT
Right 0KTS
Neck
Left 0KT3
Right 0KT2
Papillary 02TD
Perineum 0KTM
Shoulder
Left 0KT6
Right 0KT5
Thorax
Left 0KTJ
Right 0KTH
Tongue, Palate, Pharynx 0KT4
Trunk
Left 0KTG
Right 0KTF
Upper Arm
Left 0KT8
Right 0KT7

Resection — *continued*
  Muscle — *continued*
    Upper Leg
      Left 0KTR
      Right 0KTQ
  Nasal Mucosa and Soft Tissue 09TK
  Nasopharynx 09TN
  Nipple
    Left 0HTXXZZ
    Right 0HTWXZZ
  Omentum 0DTU
  Orbit
    Left 0NTQ0ZZ
    Right 0NTP0ZZ
  Ovary
    Bilateral 0UT2
    Left 0UT1
    Right 0UT0
  Palate
    Hard 0CT2
    Soft 0CT3
  Pancreas 0FTG
  Para-aortic Body 0GT9
  Paraganglion Extremity 0GTF
  Parathyroid Gland 0GTR
    Inferior
      Left 0GTP
      Right 0GTN
    Multiple 0GTQ
    Superior
      Left 0GTM
      Right 0GTL
  Patella
    Left 0QTF0ZZ
    Right 0QTD0ZZ
  Penis 0VTS
  Pericardium 02TN
  Phalanx
    Finger
      Left 0PTV0ZZ
      Right 0PTT0ZZ
    Thumb
      Left 0PTS0ZZ
      Right 0PTR0ZZ
    Toe
      Left 0QTR0ZZ
      Right 0QTQ0ZZ
  Pharynx 0CTM
  Pineal Body 0GT1
  Prepuce 0VTT
  Products of Conception, Ectopic 10T2
  Prostate 0VT0
  Radius
    Left 0PTJ0ZZ
    Right 0PTH0ZZ
  Rectum 0DTP
  Ribs
    1 to 2 0PT10ZZ
    3 or More 0PT20ZZ
  Scapula
    Left 0PT60ZZ
    Right 0PT50ZZ
  Scrotum 0VT5
  Septum
    Atrial 02T5
    Nasal 09TM
    Ventricular 02TM
  Sinus
    Accessory 09TP
    Ethmoid
      Left 09TV
      Right 09TU
    Frontal
      Left 09TT
      Right 09TS
    Mastoid
      Left 09TC
      Right 09TB

Resection — *continued*
  Sinus — *continued*
    Maxillary
      Left 09TR
      Right 09TQ
    Sphenoid
      Left 09TX
      Right 09TW
  Spleen 07TP
  Sternum 0PT00ZZ
  Stomach 0DT6
    Pylorus 0DT7
  Tarsal
    Left 0QTM0ZZ
    Right 0QTL0ZZ
  Tendon
    Abdomen
      Left 0LTG
      Right 0LTF
    Ankle
      Left 0LTT
      Right 0LTS
    Foot
      Left 0LTW
      Right 0LTV
    Hand
      Left 0LT8
      Right 0LT7
    Head and Neck 0LT0
    Hip
      Left 0LTK
      Right 0LTJ
    Knee
      Left 0LTR
      Right 0LTQ
    Lower Arm and Wrist
      Left 0LT6
      Right 0LT5
    Lower Leg
      Left 0LTP
      Right 0LTN
    Perineum 0LTH
    Shoulder
      Left 0LT2
      Right 0LT1
    Thorax
      Left 0LTD
      Right 0LTC
    Trunk
      Left 0LTB
      Right 0LT9
    Upper Arm
      Left 0LT4
      Right 0LT3
    Upper Leg
      Left 0LTM
      Right 0LTL
  Testis
    Bilateral 0VTC
    Left 0VTB
    Right 0VT9
  Thymus 07TM
  Thyroid Gland 0GTK
    Left Lobe 0GTG
    Right Lobe 0GTH
  Thyroid Gland Isthmus 0GTJ
  Tibia
    Left 0QTH0ZZ
    Right 0QTG0ZZ
  Toe Nail 0HTRXZZ
  Tongue 0CT7
  Tonsils 0CTP
  Tooth
    Lower 0CTX0Z
    Upper 0CTW0Z
  Trachea 0BT1

Resection — *continued*
  Tunica Vaginalis
    Left 0VT7
    Right 0VT6
  Turbinate, Nasal 09TL
  Tympanic Membrane
    Left 09T8
    Right 09T7
  Ulna
    Left 0PTL0ZZ
    Right 0PTK0ZZ
  Ureter
    Left 0TT7
    Right 0TT6
  Urethra 0TTD
  Uterine Supporting Structure 0UT4
  Uterus 0UT9
  Uvula 0CTN
  Vagina 0UTG
  Valve, Pulmonary 02TH
  Vas Deferens
    Bilateral 0VTQ
    Left 0VTP
    Right 0VTN
  Vesicle
    Bilateral 0VT3
    Left 0VT2
    Right 0VT1
  Vitreous
    Left 08T53ZZ
    Right 08T43ZZ
  Vocal Cord
    Left 0CTV
    Right 0CTT
  Vulva 0UTM
Resection, Left ventricular outflow tract obstruction (LVOT)
  see Dilation, Ventricle, Left 027L
Resection, Subaortic membrane (Left ventricular outflow tract obstruction)
  see Dilation, Ventricle, Left 027L
Restoration, Cardiac, Single, Rhythm 5A2204Z
RestoreAdvanced neurostimulator (SureScan)(MRI Safe)
  use Stimulator Generator, Multiple Array Rechargeable in 0JH
RestoreSensor neurostimulator (SureScan) (MRI Safe)
  use Stimulator Generator, Multiple Array Rechargeable in 0JH
RestoreUltra neurostimulator (SureScan) (MRI Safe)
  use Stimulator Generator, Multiple Array Rechargeable in 0JH
Restriction
  Ampulla of Vater 0FVC
  Anus 0DVQ
  Aorta
    Abdominal 04V0
      Intraluminal Device, Branched or Fenestrated 04V0
    Thoracic
      Ascending/Arch, Intraluminal Device, Branched or Fenestrated 02VX
      Descending, Intraluminal Device, Branched or Fenestrated 02VW
  Artery
    Anterior Tibial
      Left 04VQ
      Right 04VP
    Axillary
      Left 03V6
      Right 03V5
    Brachial
      Left 03V8
      Right 03V7

Restriction — *continued*
Artery — *continued*
Celiac 04V1
Colic
Left 04V7
Middle 04V8
Right 04V6
Common Carotid
Left 03VJ
Right 03VH
Common Iliac
Left 04VD
Right 04VC
External Carotid
Left 03VN
Right 03VM
External Iliac
Left 04VJ
Right 04VH
Face 03VR
Femoral
Left 04VL
Right 04VK
Foot
Left 04VW
Right 04VV
Gastric 04V2
Hand
Left 03VF
Right 03VD
Hepatic 04V3
Inferior Mesenteric 04VB
Innominate 03V2
Internal Carotid
Left 03VL
Right 03VK
Internal Iliac
Left 04VF
Right 04VE
Internal Mammary
Left 03V1
Right 03V0
Intracranial 03VG
Lower 04VY
Peroneal
Left 04VU
Right 04VT
Popliteal
Left 04VN
Right 04VM
Posterior Tibial
Left 04VS
Right 04VR
Pulmonary
Left 02VR
Right 02VQ
Pulmonary Trunk 02VP
Radial
Left 03VC
Right 03VB
Renal
Left 04VA
Right 04V9
Splenic 04V4
Subclavian
Left 03V4
Right 03V3
Superior Mesenteric 04V5
Temporal
Left 03VT
Right 03VS
Thyroid
Left 03VV
Right 03VU
Ulnar
Left 03VA
Right 03V9

Restriction — *continued*
Artery — *continued*
Upper 03VY
Vertebral
Left 03VQ
Right 03VP
Bladder 0TVB
Bladder Neck 0TVC
Bronchus
Lingula 0BV9
Lower Lobe
Left 0BVB
Right 0BV6
Main
Left 0BV7
Right 0BV3
Middle Lobe, Right 0BV5
Upper Lobe
Left 0BV8
Right 0BV4
Carina 0BV2
Cecum 0DVH
Cervix 0UVC
Cisterna Chyli 07VL
Colon
Ascending 0DVK
Descending 0DVM
Sigmoid 0DVN
Transverse 0DVL
Duct
Common Bile 0FV9
Cystic 0FV8
Hepatic
Common 0FV7
Left 0FV6
Right 0FV5
Lacrimal
Left 08VY
Right 08VX
Pancreatic 0FVD
Accessory 0FVF
Parotid
Left 0CVC
Right 0CVB
Duodenum 0DV9
Esophagogastric Junction 0DV4
Esophagus 0DV5
Lower 0DV3
Middle 0DV2
Upper 0DV1
Heart 02VA
Ileocecal Valve 0DVC
Ileum 0DVB
Intestine
Large 0DVE
Left 0DVG
Right 0DVF
Small 0DV8
Jejunum 0DVA
Kidney Pelvis
Left 0TV4
Right 0TV3
Lymphatic
Aortic 07VD
Axillary
Left 07V6
Right 07V5
Head 07V0
Inguinal
Left 07VJ
Right 07VH
Internal Mammary
Left 07V9
Right 07V8
Lower Extremity
Left 07VG
Right 07VF

Restriction — *continued*
Lymphatic — *continued*
Mesenteric 07VB
Neck
Left 07V2
Right 07V1
Pelvis 07VC
Thoracic Duct 07VK
Thorax 07V7
Upper Extremity
Left 07V4
Right 07V3
Rectum 0DVP
Stomach 0DV6
Pylorus 0DV7
Trachea 0BV1
Ureter
Left 0TV7
Right 0TV6
Urethra 0TVD
Valve, Mitral 02VG
Vein
Axillary
Left 05V8
Right 05V7
Azygos 05V0
Basilic
Left 05VC
Right 05VB
Brachial
Left 05VA
Right 05V9
Cephalic
Left 05VF
Right 05VD
Colic 06V7
Common Iliac
Left 06VD
Right 06VC
Esophageal 06V3
External Iliac
Left 06VG
Right 06VF
External Jugular
Left 05VQ
Right 05VP
Face
Left 05VV
Right 05VT
Femoral
Left 06VN
Right 06VM
Foot
Left 06VV
Right 06VT
Gastric 06V2
Hand
Left 05VH
Right 05VG
Hemiazygos 05V1
Hepatic 06V4
Hypogastric
Left 06VJ
Right 06VH
Inferior Mesenteric 06V6
Innominate
Left 05V4
Right 05V3
Internal Jugular
Left 05VN
Right 05VM
Intracranial 05VL
Lower 06VY
Portal 06V8
Pulmonary
Left 02VT
Right 02VS

Restriction — *continued*
  Vein — *continued*
    Renal
      Left 06VB
      Right 06V9
    Saphenous
      Left 06VQ
      Right 06VP
    Splenic 06V1
    Subclavian
      Left 05V6
      Right 05V5
    Superior Mesenteric 06V5
    Upper 05VY
    Vertebral
      Left 05VS
      Right 05VR
  Vena Cava
    Inferior 06V0
    Superior 02VV
Resurfacing Device
  Removal of device from
    Left 0SPB0BZ
    Right 0SP90BZ
  Revision of device in
    Left 0SWB0BZ
    Right 0SW90BZ
  Supplement
    Left 0SUB0BZ
      Acetabular Surface 0SUE0BZ
      Femoral Surface 0SUS0BZ
    Right 0SU90BZ
      Acetabular Surface 0SUA0BZ
      Femoral Surface 0SUR0BZ
Resuscitation
  Cardiopulmonary *see* Assistance,
    Cardiac 5A02
  Cardioversion 5A2204Z
  Defibrillation 5A2204Z
  Endotracheal intubation *see* Insertion of
    device in, Trachea 0BH1
  External chest compression 5A12012
  Pulmonary 5A19054
Resuscitative endovascular balloon
  occlusion of the aorta (REBOA)
    02LW3DJ
    04L03DJ
Resuture, Heart valve prosthesis
  see Revision of device in, Heart and Great
    Vessels 02W
Retained placenta, manual removal
  see Extraction, Products of Conception,
    Retained 10D1
Retraining
  Cardiac *see* Motor Treatment,
    Rehabilitation F07
  Vocational *see* Activities of Daily Living
    Treatment, Rehabilitation F08
Retrogasserian rhizotomy
  see Division, Nerve, Trigeminal 008K
Retroperitoneal cavity
  use Retroperitoneum
Retroperitoneal lymph node
  use Lymphatic, Aortic
Retroperitoneal space
  use Retroperitoneum
Retropharyngeal lymph node
  use Lymphatic, Right Neck
  use Lymphatic, Left Neck
Retropubic space
  use Pelvic Cavity
Reveal (LINQ)(DX)(XT)
  use Monitoring Device
Reverse total shoulder replacement
  see Replacement, Upper Joints 0RR

Reverse® Shoulder Prosthesis
  use Synthetic Substitute, Reverse Ball and
    Socket in 0RR
Revision
  Correcting a portion of existing device *see*
    Revision of device in
  Removal of device without replacement
    see Removal of device from
  Replacement of existing device
    see Removal of device from
    see Root operation to place new
      device, e.g., Insertion, Replacement,
      Supplement
Revision of device in
  Abdominal Wall 0WWF
  Acetabulum
    Left 0QW5
    Right 0QW4
  Anal Sphincter 0DWR
  Anus 0DWQ
  Artery
    Lower 04WY
    Upper 03WY
  Auditory Ossicle
    Left 09WA
    Right 09W9
  Back
    Lower 0WWL
    Upper 0WWK
  Bladder 0TWB
  Bone
    Facial 0NWW
    Lower 0QWY
    Nasal 0NWB
    Pelvic
      Left 0QW3
      Right 0QW2
    Upper 0PWY
  Bone Marrow 07WT
  Brain 00W0
  Breast
    Left 0HWU
    Right 0HWT
  Bursa and Ligament
    Lower 0MWY
    Upper 0MWX
  Carpal
    Left 0PWN
    Right 0PWM
  Cavity, Cranial 0WW1
  Cerebral Ventricle 00W6
  Chest Wall 0WW8
  Cisterna Chyli 07WL
  Clavicle
    Left 0PWB
    Right 0PW9
  Coccyx 0QWS
  Diaphragm 0BWT
  Disc
    Cervical Vertebral 0RW3
    Cervicothoracic Vertebral 0RW5
    Lumbar Vertebral 0SW2
    Lumbosacral 0SW4
    Thoracic Vertebral 0RW9
    Thoracolumbar Vertebral 0RWB
  Duct
    Hepatobiliary 0FWB
    Pancreatic 0FWD
  Ear
    Inner
      Left 09WE
      Right 09WD
    Left 09WJ
    Right 09WH
  Epididymis and Spermatic Cord 0VWM
  Esophagus 0DW5

Revision of device in — *continued*
  Extremity
    Lower
      Left 0YWB
      Right 0YW9
    Upper
      Left 0XW7
      Right 0XW6
  Eye
    Left 08W1
    Right 08W0
  Face 0WW2
  Fallopian Tube 0UW8
  Femoral Shaft
    Left 0QW9
    Right 0QW8
  Femur
    Lower
      Left 0QWC
      Right 0QWB
    Upper
      Left 0QW7
      Right 0QW6
  Fibula
    Left 0QWK
    Right 0QWJ
  Finger Nail 0HWQX
  Gallbladder 0FW4
  Gastrointestinal Tract 0WWP
  Genitourinary Tract 0WWR
  Gland
    Adrenal 0GW5
    Endocrine 0GWS
    Pituitary 0GW0
    Salivary 0CWA
  Glenoid Cavity
    Left 0PW8
    Right 0PW7
  Great Vessel 02WY
  Hair 0HWSX
  Head 0WW0
  Heart 02WA
  Humeral Head
    Left 0PWD
    Right 0PWC
  Humeral Shaft
    Left 0PWG
    Right 0PWF
  Intestinal Tract
    Lower 0DWD
    Upper 0DW0
  Intestine
    Large 0DWE
    Small 0DW8
  Jaw
    Lower 0WW5
    Upper 0WW4
  Joint
    Acromioclavicular
      Left 0RWH
      Right 0RWG
    Ankle
      Left 0SWG
      Right 0SWF
    Carpal
      Left 0RWR
      Right 0RWQ
    Carpometacarpal
      Left 0RWT
      Right 0RWS
    Cervical Vertebral 0RW1
    Cervicothoracic Vertebral 0RW4
    Coccygeal 0SW6
    Elbow
      Left 0RWM
      Right 0RWL

Revision of device in — *continued*
  Joint — *continued*
    Finger Phalangeal
      Left 0RWX
      Right 0RWW
    Hip
      Left 0SWB
        Acetabular Surface 0SWE
        Femoral Surface 0SWS
      Right 0SW9
        Acetabular Surface 0SWA
        Femoral Surface 0SWR
    Knee
      Left 0SWD
        Femoral Surface 0SWU
        Tibial Surface 0SWW
      Right 0SWC
        Femoral Surface 0SWT
        Tibial Surface 0SWV
    Lumbar Vertebral 0SW0
    Lumbosacral 0SW3
    Metacarpophalangeal
      Left 0RWV
      Right 0RWU
    Metatarsal-Phalangeal
      Left 0SWN
      Right 0SWM
    Occipital-cervical 0RW0
    Sacrococcygeal 0SW5
    Sacroiliac
      Left 0SW8
      Right 0SW7
    Shoulder
      Left 0RWK
      Right 0RWJ
    Sternoclavicular
      Left 0RWF
      Right 0RWE
    Tarsal
      Left 0SWJ
      Right 0SWH
    Tarsometatarsal
      Left 0SWL
      Right 0SWK
    Temporomandibular
      Left 0RWD
      Right 0RWC
    Thoracic Vertebral 0RW6
    Thoracolumbar Vertebral 0RWA
    Toe Phalangeal
      Left 0SWQ
      Right 0SWP
    Wrist
      Left 0RWP
      Right 0RWN
  Kidney 0TW5
  Larynx 0CWS
  Lens
    Left 08WK
    Right 08WJ
  Liver 0FW0
  Lung
    Left 0BWL
    Right 0BWK
  Lymphatic 07WN
    Thoracic Duct 07WK
  Mediastinum 0WWC
  Mesentery 0DWV
  Metacarpal
    Left 0PWQ
    Right 0PWP
  Metatarsal
    Left 0QWP
    Right 0QWN
  Mouth and Throat 0CWY
  Muscle
    Extraocular

Revision of device in — *continued*
  Muscle — *continued*
      Left 08WM
      Right 08WL
    Lower 0KWY
    Upper 0KWX
  Nasal Mucosa and Soft Tissue 09WK
  Neck 0WW6
  Nerve
    Cranial 00WE
    Peripheral 01WY
  Omentum 0DWU
  Ovary 0UW3
  Pancreas 0FWG
  Parathyroid Gland 0GWR
  Patella
    Left 0QWF
    Right 0QWD
  Pelvic Cavity 0WWJ
  Penis 0VWS
  Pericardial Cavity 0WWD
  Perineum
    Female 0WWN
    Male 0WWM
  Peritoneal Cavity 0WWG
  Peritoneum 0DWW
  Phalanx
    Finger
      Left 0PWV
      Right 0PWT
    Thumb
      Left 0PWS
      Right 0PWR
    Toe
      Left 0QWR
      Right 0QWQ
  Pineal Body 0GW1
  Pleura 0BWQ
  Pleural Cavity
    Left 0WWB
    Right 0WW9
  Prostate and Seminal Vesicles 0VW4
  Radius
    Left 0PWJ
    Right 0PWH
  Respiratory Tract 0WWQ
  Retroperitoneum 0WWH
  Ribs
    1 to 2 0PW1
    3 or More 0PW2
  Sacrum 0QW1
  Scapula
    Left 0PW6
    Right 0PW5
  Scrotum and Tunica Vaginalis 0VW8
  Septum
    Atrial 02W5
    Ventricular 02WM
  Sinus 09WY
  Skin 0HWPX
  Skull 0NW0
  Spinal Canal 00WU
  Spinal Cord 00WV
  Spleen 07WP
  Sternum 0PW0
  Stomach 0DW6
  Subcutaneous Tissue and Fascia
    Head and Neck 0JWS
    Lower Extremity 0JWW
    Trunk 0JWT
    Upper Extremity 0JWV
  Tarsal
    Left 0QWM
    Right 0QWL
  Tendon
    Lower 0LWY
    Upper 0LWX

Revision of device in — *continued*
  Testis 0VWD
  Thymus 07WM
  Thyroid Gland 0GWK
  Tibia
    Left 0QWH
    Right 0QWG
  Toe Nail 0HWRX
  Trachea 0BW1
  Tracheobronchial Tree 0BW0
  Tympanic Membrane
    Left 09W8
    Right 09W7
  Ulna
    Left 0PWL
    Right 0PWK
  Ureter 0TW9
  Urethra 0TWD
  Uterus and Cervix 0UWD
  Vagina and Cul-de-sac 0UWH
  Valve
    Aortic 02WF
    Mitral 02WG
    Pulmonary 02WH
    Tricuspid 02WJ
  Vas Deferens 0VWR
  Vein
    Azygos 05W0
    Innominate
      Left 05W4
      Right 05W3
    Lower 06WY
    Upper 05WY
  Vertebra
    Cervical 0PW3
    Lumbar 0QW0
    Thoracic 0PW4
  Vulva 0UWM
Revo MRI™ SureScan® pacemaker
  use Pacemaker, Dual Chamber in 0JH
rhBMP-2
  use Recombinant Bone Morphogenetic
    Protein
Rheos® System device
  use Stimulator Generator in Subcutaneous
    Tissue and Fascia
Rheos® System lead
  use Stimulator Lead in Upper Arteries
Rhinopharynx
  use Nasopharynx
Rhinoplasty
  see Alteration, Nasal Mucosa and Soft
    Tissue 090K
  see Repair, Nasal Mucosa and Soft
    Tissue 09QK
  see Replacement, Nasal Mucosa and Soft
    Tissue 09RK
  see Supplement, Nasal Mucosa and Soft
    Tissue 09UK
Rhinorrhaphy
  see Repair, Nasal Mucosa and Soft
    Tissue 09QK
Rhinoscopy 09JKXZZ
Rhizotomy
  see Division, Central Nervous System and
    Cranial Nerves 008
  see Division, Peripheral Nervous System 018
Rhomboid major muscle
  use Trunk Muscle, Right
  use Trunk Muscle, Left
Rhomboid minor muscle
  use Trunk Muscle, Right
  use Trunk Muscle, Left
Rhythm electrocardiogram
  see Measurement, Cardiac 4A02

Rhytidectomy
see Alteration, Face 0W02
Right ascending lumbar vein
use Azygos Vein
Right atrioventricular valve
use Tricuspid Valve
Right auricular appendix
use Atrium, Right
Right colic vein
use Colic Vein
Right coronary sulcus
use Heart, Right
Right gastric artery
use Gastric Artery
Right gastroepiploic vein
use Superior Mesenteric Vein
Right inferior phrenic vein
use Inferior Vena Cava
Right inferior pulmonary vein
use Pulmonary Vein, Right
Right jugular trunk
use Lymphatic, Right Neck
Right lateral ventricle
use Cerebral Ventricle
Right lymphatic duct
use Lymphatic, Right Neck
Right ovarian vein
use Inferior Vena Cava
Right second lumbar vein
use Inferior Vena Cava
Right subclavian trunk
use Lymphatic, Right Neck
Right subcostal vein
use Azygos Vein
Right superior pulmonary vein
use Pulmonary Vein, Right
Right suprarenal vein
use Inferior Vena Cava
Right testicular vein
use Inferior Vena Cava
Rima glottidis
use Larynx
Risorius muscle
use Facial Muscle
RNS System lead
use Neurostimulator Lead in Central
Nervous System and Cranial Nerves
RNS system neurostimulator generator
use Neurostimulator Generator in Head
and Facial Bones
Robotic Assisted Procedure
Extremity
Lower 8E0Y
Upper 8E0X
Head and Neck Region 8E09
Trunk Region 8E0W
**Robotic Waterjet Ablation, Destruction,
Prostate** XV508A4
Rotation of fetal head
Forceps 10S07ZZ
Manual 10S0XZZ
Round ligament of uterus
use Uterine Supporting Structure
Round window
use Inner Ear, Right
use Inner Ear, Left
Roux-en-Y operation
see Bypass, Gastrointestinal System 0D1
see Bypass, Hepatobiliary System and
Pancreas 0F1
Rupture
Adhesions *see* Release
Fluid collection *see* Drainage
Ruxolitinib XW0DXT5

S

S-ICD™ lead
use Subcutaneous Defibrillator Lead in
Subcutaneous Tissue and Fascia
Sacral ganglion
use Sacral Sympathetic Nerve
Sacral lymph node
use Lymphatic, Pelvis
Sacral nerve modulation (SNM) lead
use Stimulator Lead in Urinary System
Sacral neuromodulation lead
use Stimulator Lead in Urinary System
Sacral splanchnic nerve
use Sacral Sympathetic Nerve
Sacrectomy
see Excision, Lower Bones 0QB
Sacrococcygeal ligament
use Lower Spine Bursa and Ligament
Sacrococcygeal symphysis
use Sacrococcygeal Joint
Sacroiliac ligament
use Lower Spine Bursa and Ligament
Sacrospinous ligament
use Lower Spine Bursa and Ligament
Sacrotuberous ligament
use Lower Spine Bursa and Ligament
Salpingectomy
see Excision, Female Reproductive
System 0UB
see Resection, Female Reproductive
System 0UT
Salpingolysis
see Release, Female Reproductive
System 0UN
Salpingopexy
see Repair, Female Reproductive
System 0UQ
see Reposition, Female Reproductive
System 0US
Salpingopharyngeus muscle
use Tongue, Palate, Pharynx Muscle
Salpingoplasty
see Repair, Female Reproductive
System 0UQ
see Supplement, Female Reproductive
System 0UU
Salpingorrhaphy
see Repair, Female Reproductive
System 0UQ
Salpingoscopy 0UJ88ZZ
Salpingostomy
see Drainage, Female Reproductive
System 0U9
Salpingotomy
see Drainage, Female Reproductive
System 0U9
Salpinx
use Fallopian Tube, Right
use Fallopian Tube, Left
Saphenous nerve
use Femoral Nerve
SAPIEN transcatheter aortic valve
use Zooplastic Tissue in Heart and Great
Vessels
Sarilumab XW0
Sartorius muscle
use Upper Leg Muscle, Right
use Upper Leg Muscle, Left
**SAVAL below-the-knee (BTK) drug-eluting
stent system**
use Intraluminal Device, Sustained Release
Drug-eluting in New Technology
use Intraluminal Device, Sustained Release
Drug-eluting, Two in New Technology
use Intraluminal Device, Sustained Release
Drug-eluting, Three in New Technology

**SAVAL below-the-knee (BTK) drug-eluting
stent system** — *continued*
use Intraluminal Device, Sustained Release
Drug-eluting, Four or More in New
Technology
Scalene muscle
use Neck Muscle, Right
use Neck Muscle, Left
Scan
Computerized Tomography (CT) *see*
Computerized Tomography (CT Scan)
Radioisotope *see* Planar Nuclear Medicine
Imaging
Scaphoid bone
use Carpal, Right
use Carpal, Left
Scapholunate ligament
use Wrist Bursa and Ligament, Right
use Wrist Bursa and Ligament, Left
Scaphotrapezium ligament
use Hand Bursa and Ligament, Right
use Hand Bursa and Ligament, Left
Scapulectomy
see Excision, Upper Bones 0PB
see Resection, Upper Bones 0PT
Scapulopexy
see Repair, Upper Bones 0PQ
see Reposition, Upper Bones 0PS
Scarpa's (vestibular) ganglion
use Acoustic Nerve
Sclerectomy
see Excision, Eye 08B
Sclerotherapy, mechanical
see Destruction
**Sclerotherapy, via injection of sclerosing
agent**
see Introduction, Destructive Agent
Sclerotomy
see Drainage, Eye 089
Scrotectomy
see Excision, Male Reproductive
System 0VB
see Resection, Male Reproductive
System 0VT
Scrotoplasty
see Repair, Male Reproductive
System 0VQ
see Supplement, Male Reproductive
System 0VU
Scrotorrhaphy
see Repair, Male Reproductive System 0VQ
Scrototomy
see Drainage, Male Reproductive
System 0V9
Sebaceous gland
use Skin
Second cranial nerve
use Optic Nerve
Section, cesarean
see Extraction, Pregnancy 10D
Secura (DR) (VR)
use Defibrillator Generator in 0JH
Sella turcica
use Sphenoid Bone
Semicircular canal
use Inner Ear, Right
use Inner Ear, Left
Semimembranosus muscle
use Upper Leg Muscle, Right
use Upper Leg Muscle, Left
Semitendinosus muscle
use Upper Leg Muscle, Right
use Upper Leg Muscle, Left
**Sentinel ™ Cerebral Protection System
(CPS)** X2A5312
Seprafilm
use Adhesion Barrier

Septal cartilage
  use Nasal Septum
Septectomy
  see Excision, Heart and Great Vessels 02B
  see Resection, Heart and Great Vessels 02T
  see Excision, Ear, Nose, Sinus 09B
  see Resection, Ear, Nose, Sinus 09T
Septoplasty
  see Repair, Heart and Great Vessels 02Q
  see Replacement, Heart and Great Vessels 02R
  see Supplement, Heart and Great Vessels 02U
  see Repair, Ear, Nose, Sinus 09Q
  see Replacement, Ear, Nose, Sinus 09R
  see Reposition, Ear, Nose, Sinus 09S
  see Supplement, Ear, Nose, Sinus 09U
Septostomy, balloon atrial 02163Z7
Septotomy
  see Drainage, Ear, Nose, Sinus 099
Sequestrectomy, bone
  see Extirpation
Serratus anterior muscle
  use Thorax Muscle, Right
  use Thorax Muscle, Left
Serratus posterior muscle
  use Trunk Muscle, Right
  use Trunk Muscle, Left
Seventh cranial nerve
  use Facial Nerve
Sheffield hybrid external fixator
  use External Fixation Device, Hybrid in 0PH
  use External Fixation Device, Hybrid in 0PS
  use External Fixation Device, Hybrid in 0QH
  use External Fixation Device, Hybrid in 0QS
Sheffield ring external fixator
  use External Fixation Device, Ring in 0PH
  use External Fixation Device, Ring in 0PS
  use External Fixation Device, Ring in 0QH
  use External Fixation Device, Ring in 0QS
Shirodkar cervical cerclage 0UVC7ZZ
Shock Wave Therapy, Musculoskeletal 6A93
Shockwave Intravascular Lithotripsy (Shockwave IVL)
  see Fragmentation
Short gastric artery
  use Splenic Artery
Shortening
  see Excision
  see Repair
  see Reposition
Shunt creation
  see Bypass
Sialoadenectomy
  Complete *see* Resection, Mouth and Throat 0CT
  Partial *see* Excision, Mouth and Throat 0CB
Sialodochoplasty
  see Repair, Mouth and Throat 0CQ
  see Replacement, Mouth and Throat 0CR
  see Supplement, Mouth and Throat 0CU
Sialoectomy
  see Excision, Mouth and Throat 0CB
  see Resection, Mouth and Throat 0CT
Sialography
  see Plain Radiography, Ear, Nose, Mouth and Throat B90
Sialolithotomy
  see Extirpation, Mouth and Throat 0CC
Sigmoid artery
  use Inferior Mesenteric Artery
Sigmoid flexure
  use Sigmoid Colon
Sigmoid vein
  use Inferior Mesenteric Vein

Sigmoidectomy
  see Excision, Gastrointestinal System 0DB
  see Resection, Gastrointestinal System 0DT
Sigmoidorrhaphy
  see Repair, Gastrointestinal System 0DQ
Sigmoidoscopy 0DJD8ZZ
Sigmoidotomy
  see Drainage, Gastrointestinal System 0D9
Single lead pacemaker (atrium)(ventricle)
  use Pacemaker, Single Chamber in 0JH
Single lead rate responsive pacemaker (atrium)(ventricle)
  use Pacemaker, Single Chamber Rate Responsive in 0JH
Sinoatrial node
  use Conduction Mechanism
Sinogram
  Abdominal Wall *see* Fluoroscopy, Abdomen and Pelvis BW11
  Chest Wall *see* Plain Radiography, Chest BW03
  Retroperitoneum *see* Fluoroscopy, Abdomen and Pelvis BW11
Sinus venosus
  use Atrium, Right
Sinusectomy
  see Excision, Ear, Nose, Sinus 09B
  see Resection, Ear, Nose, Sinus 09T
Sinusoscopy 09JY4ZZ
Sinusotomy
  see Drainage, Ear, Nose, Sinus 099
Sirolimus-eluting coronary stent
  use Intraluminal Device, Drug-eluting in Heart and Great Vessels
Sixth cranial nerve
  use Abducens Nerve
Size reduction, breast
  see Excision, Skin and Breast 0HB
SJM Biocor® Stented Valve System
  use Zooplastic Tissue in Heart and Great Vessels
Skene's (paraurethral) gland
  use Vestibular Gland
Skin Substitute, Porcine Liver Derived, Replacement XHRPXL2
Sling
  Fascial, orbicularis muscle (mouth) *see* Supplement, Muscle, Facial 0KU1
  Levator muscle, for urethral suspension *see* Reposition, Bladder Neck 0TSC
  Pubococcygeal, for urethral suspension *see* Reposition, Bladder Neck 0TSC
  Rectum *see* Reposition, Rectum 0DSP
Small bowel series
  see Fluoroscopy, Bowel, Small BD13
Small saphenous vein
  use Saphenous Vein, Right
  use Saphenous Vein, Left
Snapshot_NIR 8E02XDZ
Snaring, polyp, colon
  see Excision, Gastrointestinal System 0DB
Solar (celiac) plexus
  use Abdominal Sympathetic Nerve
Soleus muscle
  use Lower Leg Muscle, Right
  use Lower Leg Muscle, Left
Soliris®
  use Eculizumab
Spacer
  Insertion of device in
    Disc
      Lumbar Vertebral 0SH2
      Lumbosacral 0SH4
    Joint
      Acromioclavicular
        Left 0RHH
        Right 0RHG

Spacer — *continued*
  Insertion of device in — *continued*
    Ankle
      Left 0SHG
      Right 0SHF
    Carpal
      Left 0RHR
      Right 0RHQ
    Carpometacarpal
      Left 0RHT
      Right 0RHS
    Cervical Vertebral 0RH1
    Cervicothoracic Vertebral 0RH4
    Coccygeal 0SH6
    Elbow
      Left 0RHM
      Right 0RHL
    Finger Phalangeal
      Left 0RHX
      Right 0RHW
    Hip
      Left 0SHB
      Right 0SH9
    Knee
      Left 0SHD
      Right 0SHC
    Lumbar Vertebral 0SH0
    Lumbosacral 0SH3
    Metacarpophalangeal
      Left 0RHV
      Right 0RHU
    Metatarsal-Phalangeal
      Left 0SHN
      Right 0SHM
    Occipital-cervical 0RH0
    Sacrococcygeal 0SH5
    Sacroiliac
      Left 0SH8
      Right 0SH7
    Shoulder
      Left 0RHK
      Right 0RHJ
    Sternoclavicular
      Left 0RHF
      Right 0RHE
    Tarsal
      Left 0SHJ
      Right 0SHH
    Tarsometatarsal
      Left 0SHL
      Right 0SHK
    Temporomandibular
      Left 0RHD
      Right 0RHC
    Thoracic Vertebral 0RH6
    Thoracolumbar Vertebral 0RHA
    Toe Phalangeal
      Left 0SHQ
      Right 0SHP
    Wrist
      Left 0RHP
      Right 0RHN
  Removal of device from
    Acromioclavicular
      Left 0RPH
      Right 0RPG
    Ankle
      Left 0SPG
      Right 0SPF
    Carpal
      Left 0RPR
      Right 0RPQ
    Carpometacarpal
      Left 0RPT
      Right 0RPS
    Cervical Vertebral 0RP1
    Cervicothoracic Vertebral 0RP4

Spacer — *continued*
Removal of device from — *continued*
Coccygeal 0SP6
Elbow
Left 0RPM
Right 0RPL
Finger Phalangeal
Left 0RPX
Right 0RPW
Hip
Left 0SPB
Right 0SP9
Knee
Left 0SPD
Right 0SPC
Lumbar Vertebral 0SP0
Lumbosacral 0SP3
Metacarpophalangeal
Left 0RPV
Right 0RPU
Metatarsal-Phalangeal
Left 0SPN
Right 0SPM
Occipital-cervical 0RP0
Sacrococcygeal 0SP5
Sacroiliac
Left 0SP8
Right 0SP7
Shoulder
Left 0RPK
Right 0RPJ
Sternoclavicular
Left 0RPF
Right 0RPE
Tarsal
Left 0SPJ
Right 0SPH
Tarsometatarsal
Left 0SPL
Right 0SPK
Temporomandibular
Left 0RPD
Right 0RPC
Thoracic Vertebral 0RP6
Thoracolumbar Vertebral 0RPA
Toe Phalangeal
Left 0SPQ
Right 0SPP
Wrist
Left 0RPP
Right 0RPN
Revision of device in
Acromioclavicular
Left 0RWH
Right 0RWG
Ankle
Left 0SWG
Right 0SWF
Carpal
Left 0RWR
Right 0RWQ
Carpometacarpal
Left 0RWT
Right 0RWS
Cervical Vertebral 0RW1
Cervicothoracic Vertebral 0RW4
Coccygeal 0SW6
Elbow
Left 0RWM
Right 0RWL
Finger Phalangeal
Left 0RWX
Right 0RWW
Hip
Left 0SWB
Right 0SW9

Spacer — *continued*
Revision of device in — *continued*
Knee
Left 0SWD
Right 0SWC
Lumbar Vertebral 0SW0
Lumbosacral 0SW3
Metacarpophalangeal
Left 0RWV
Right 0RWU
Metatarsal-Phalangeal
Left 0SWN
Right 0SWM
Occipital-cervical 0RW0
Sacrococcygeal 0SW5
Sacroiliac
Left 0SW8
Right 0SW7
Shoulder
Left 0RWK
Right 0RWJ
Sternoclavicular
Left 0RWF
Right 0RWE
Tarsal
Left 0SWJ
Right 0SWH
Tarsometatarsal
Left 0SWL
Right 0SWK
Temporomandibular
Left 0RWD
Right 0RWC
Thoracic Vertebral 0RW6
Thoracolumbar Vertebral 0RWA
Toe Phalangeal
Left 0SWQ
Right 0SWP
Wrist
Left 0RWP
Right 0RWN
Spacer, Articulating (Antibiotic)
use Articulating Spacer in Lower Joints
Spacer, Static (Antibiotic)
use Spacer in Lower Joints
Spectroscopy
Intravascular Near Infrared 8E023DZ
Near Infrared *see* Physiological Systems and Anatomical Regions 8E0
Speech Assessment F00
Speech therapy
see Speech Treatment, Rehabilitation F06
Speech Treatment F06
Sphenoidectomy
see Excision, Ear, Nose, Sinus 09B
see Resection, Ear, Nose, Sinus 09T
see Excision, Head and Facial Bones 0NB
see Resection, Head and Facial Bones 0NT
Sphenoidotomy
see Drainage, Ear, Nose, Sinus 099
Sphenomandibular ligament
use Head and Neck Bursa and Ligament
Sphenopalatine (pterygopalatine) ganglion
use Head and Neck Sympathetic Nerve
Sphincterorrhaphy, anal
see Repair, Anal Sphincter 0DQR
Sphincterotomy, anal
see Division, Anal Sphincter 0D8R
see Drainage, Anal Sphincter 0D9R
Spinal cord neurostimulator lead
use Neurostimulator Lead in Central Nervous System and Cranial Nerves
Spinal growth rods, magnetically controlled
use Magnetically Controlled Growth Rod(s) in New Technology

Spinal nerve, cervical
use Cervical Nerve
Spinal nerve, lumbar
use Lumbar Nerve
Spinal nerve, sacral
use Sacral Nerve
Spinal nerve, thoracic
use Thoracic Nerve
Spinal Stabilization Device
Facet Replacement
Cervical Vertebral 0RH1
Cervicothoracic Vertebral 0RH4
Lumbar Vertebral 0SH0
Lumbosacral 0SH3
Occipital-cervical 0RH0
Thoracic Vertebral 0RH6
Thoracolumbar Vertebral 0RHA
Interspinous Process
Cervical Vertebral 0RH1
Cervicothoracic Vertebral 0RH4
Lumbar Vertebral 0SH0
Lumbosacral 0SH3
Occipital-cervical 0RH0
Thoracic Vertebral 0RH6
Thoracolumbar Vertebral 0RHA
Pedicle-Based
Cervical Vertebral 0RH1
Cervicothoracic Vertebral 0RH4
Lumbar Vertebral 0SH0
Lumbosacral 0SH3
Occipital-cervical 0RH0
Thoracic Vertebral 0RH6
Thoracolumbar Vertebral 0RHA
SpineJack® system
use Synthetic Substitute, Mechanically Expandable (Paired) in New Technology
Spinous process
use Cervical Vertebra
use Thoracic Vertebra
use Lumbar Vertebra
Spiral ganglion
use Acoustic Nerve
Spiration IBV™ Valve System
use Intraluminal Device, Endobronchial Valve in Respiratory System
Splenectomy
see Excision, Lymphatic and Hemic Systems 07B
see Resection, Lymphatic and Hemic Systems 07T
Splenic flexure
use Transverse Colon
Splenic plexus
use Abdominal Sympathetic Nerve
Splenius capitis muscle
use Head Muscle
Splenius cervicis muscle
use Neck Muscle, Right
use Neck Muscle, Left
Splenolysis
see Release, Lymphatic and Hemic Systems 07N
Splenopexy
see Repair, Lymphatic and Hemic Systems 07Q
see Reposition, Lymphatic and Hemic Systems 07S
Splenoplasty
see Repair, Lymphatic and Hemic Systems 07Q
Splenorrhaphy
see Repair, Lymphatic and Hemic Systems 07Q
Splenotomy
see Drainage, Lymphatic and Hemic Systems 079

Splinting, musculoskeletal
see Immobilization, Anatomical Regions 2W3

SPRAVATO™
use Esketamine Hydrochloride

SPY PINPOINT fluorescence imaging system
see Monitoring, Physiological Systems 4A1
see Other Imaging, Hepatobiliary System and Pancreas BF5

SPY system intraoperative fluorescence cholangiography
see Other Imaging, Hepatobiliary System and Pancreas BF5

SPY system intravascular fluorescence angiography
see Monitoring, Physiological Systems 4A1

Stapedectomy
see Excision, Ear, Nose, Sinus 09B
see Resection, Ear, Nose, Sinus 09T

Stapediolysis
see Release, Ear, Nose, Sinus 09N

Stapedioplasty
see Repair, Ear, Nose, Sinus 09Q
see Replacement, Ear, Nose, Sinus 09R
see Supplement, Ear, Nose, Sinus 09U

Stapedotomy
see Drainage, Ear, Nose, Sinus 099

Stapes
use Auditory Ossicle, Right
use Auditory Ossicle, Left

Static Spacer (Antibiotic)
use Spacer in Lower Joints

STELARA®
use Other New Technology Therapeutic Substance

Stellate ganglion
use Head and Neck Sympathetic Nerve

Stem cell transplant
see Transfusion, Circulatory 302

Stensen's duct
use Parotid Duct, Right
use Parotid Duct, Left

Stent retriever thrombectomy
see Extirpation, Upper Arteries 03C

Stent, intraluminal (cardiovascular) (gastrointestinal)(hepatobiliary)(urinary)
use Intraluminal Device

Stented tissue valve
use Zooplastic Tissue in Heart and Great Vessels

Stereotactic Radiosurgery
Abdomen DW23
Adrenal Gland DG22
Bile Ducts DF22
Bladder DT22
Bone Marrow D720
Brain D020
Brain Stem D021
Breast
  Left DM20
  Right DM21
Bronchus DB21
Cervix DU21
Chest DW22
Chest Wall DB27
Colon DD25
Diaphragm DB28
Duodenum DD22
Ear D920
Esophagus DD20
Eye D820
Gallbladder DF21
Gamma Beam
  Abdomen DW23JZZ
  Adrenal Gland DG22JZZ

Stereotactic Radiosurgery — continued
Gamma Beam — continued
  Bile Ducts DF22JZZ
  Bladder DT22JZZ
  Bone Marrow D720JZZ
  Brain D020JZZ
  Brain Stem D021JZZ
  Breast
    Left DM20JZZ
    Right DM21JZZ
  Bronchus DB21JZZ
  Cervix DU21JZZ
  Chest DW22JZZ
  Chest Wall DB27JZZ
  Colon DD25JZZ
  Diaphragm DB28JZZ
  Duodenum DD22JZZ
  Ear D920JZZ
  Esophagus DD20JZZ
  Eye D820JZZ
  Gallbladder DF21JZZ
  Gland
    Adrenal DG22JZZ
    Parathyroid DG24JZZ
    Pituitary DG20JZZ
    Thyroid DG25JZZ
  Glands, Salivary D926JZZ
  Head and Neck DW21JZZ
  Ileum DD24JZZ
  Jejunum DD23JZZ
  Kidney DT20JZZ
  Larynx D92BJZZ
  Liver DF20JZZ
  Lung DB22JZZ
  Lymphatics
    Abdomen D726JZZ
    Axillary D724JZZ
    Inguinal D728JZZ
    Neck D723JZZ
    Pelvis D727JZZ
    Thorax D725JZZ
  Mediastinum DB26JZZ
  Mouth D924JZZ
  Nasopharynx D92DJZZ
  Neck and Head DW21JZZ
  Nerve, Peripheral D027JZZ
  Nose D921JZZ
  Ovary DU20JZZ
  Palate
    Hard D928JZZ
    Soft D929JZZ
  Pancreas DF23JZZ
  Parathyroid Gland DG24JZZ
  Pelvic Region DW26JZZ
  Pharynx D92CJZZ
  Pineal Body DG21JZZ
  Pituitary Gland DG20JZZ
  Pleura DB25JZZ
  Prostate DV20JZZ
  Rectum DD27JZZ
  Sinuses D927JZZ
  Spinal Cord D026JZZ
  Spleen D722JZZ
  Stomach DD21JZZ
  Testis DV21JZZ
  Thymus D721JZZ
  Thyroid Gland DG25JZZ
  Tongue D925JZZ
  Trachea DB20JZZ
  Ureter DT21JZZ
  Urethra DT23JZZ
  Uterus DU22JZZ
Gland
  Adrenal DG22
  Parathyroid DG24
  Pituitary DG20
  Thyroid DG25

Stereotactic Radiosurgery — continued
Glands, Salivary D926
Head and Neck DW21
Ileum DD24
Jejunum DD23
Kidney DT20
Larynx D92B
Liver DF20
Lung DB22
Lymphatics
  Abdomen D726
  Axillary D724
  Inguinal D728
  Neck D723
  Pelvis D727
  Thorax D725
Mediastinum DB26
Mouth D924
Nasopharynx D92D
Neck and Head DW21
Nerve, Peripheral D027
Nose D921
Other Photon
  Abdomen DW23DZZ
  Adrenal Gland DG22DZZ
  Bile Ducts DF22DZZ
  Bladder DT22DZZ
  Bone Marrow D720DZZ
  Brain D020DZZ
  Brain Stem D021DZZ
  Breast
    Left DM20DZZ
    Right DM21DZZ
  Bronchus DB21DZZ
  Cervix DU21DZZ
  Chest DW22DZZ
  Chest Wall DB27DZZ
  Colon DD25DZZ
  Diaphragm DB28DZZ
  Duodenum DD22DZZ
  Ear D920DZZ
  Esophagus DD20DZZ
  Eye D820DZZ
  Gallbladder DF21DZZ
  Gland
    Adrenal DG22DZZ
    Parathyroid DG24DZZ
    Pituitary DG20DZZ
    Thyroid DG25DZZ
  Glands, Salivary D926DZZ
  Head and Neck DW21DZZ
  Ileum DD24DZZ
  Jejunum DD23DZZ
  Kidney DT20DZZ
  Larynx D92BDZZ
  Liver DF20DZZ
  Lung DB22DZZ
  Lymphatics
    Abdomen D726DZZ
    Axillary D724DZZ
    Inguinal D728DZZ
    Neck D723DZZ
    Pelvis D727DZZ
    Thorax D725DZZ
  Mediastinum DB26DZZ
  Mouth D924DZZ
  Nasopharynx D92DDZZ
  Neck and Head DW21DZZ
  Nerve, Peripheral D027DZZ
  Nose D921DZZ
  Ovary DU20DZZ
  Palate
    Hard D928DZZ
    Soft D929DZZ
  Pancreas DF23DZZ
  Parathyroid Gland DG24DZZ
  Pelvic Region DW26DZZ

Stereotactic Radiosurgery — *continued*
　Other Photon — *continued*
　　Pharynx D92CDZZ
　　Pineal Body DG21DZZ
　　Pituitary Gland DG20DZZ
　　Pleura DB25DZZ
　　Prostate DV20DZZ
　　Rectum DD27DZZ
　　Sinuses D927DZZ
　　Spinal Cord D026DZZ
　　Spleen D722DZZ
　　Stomach DD21DZZ
　　Testis DV21DZZ
　　Thymus D721DZZ
　　Thyroid Gland DG25DZZ
　　Tongue D925DZZ
　　Trachea DB20DZZ
　　Ureter DT21DZZ
　　Urethra DT23DZZ
　　Uterus DU22DZZ
　Ovary DU20
　Palate
　　Hard D928
　　Soft D929
　Pancreas DF23
　Parathyroid Gland DG24
　Particulate
　　Abdomen DW23HZZ
　　Adrenal Gland DG22HZZ
　　Bile Ducts DF22HZZ
　　Bladder DT22HZZ
　　Bone Marrow D720HZZ
　　Brain D020HZZ
　　Brain Stem D021HZZ
　　Breast
　　　Left DM20HZZ
　　　Right DM21HZZ
　　Bronchus DB21HZZ
　　Cervix DU21HZZ
　　Chest DW22HZZ
　　Chest Wall DB27HZZ
　　Colon DD25HZZ
　　Diaphragm DB28HZZ
　　Duodenum DD22HZZ
　　Ear D920HZZ
　　Esophagus DD20HZZ
　　Eye D820HZZ
　　Gallbladder DF21HZZ
　　Gland
　　　Adrenal DG22HZZ
　　　Parathyroid DG24HZZ
　　　Pituitary DG20HZZ
　　　Thyroid DG25HZZ
　　Glands, Salivary D926HZZ
　　Head and Neck DW21HZZ
　　Ileum DD24HZZ
　　Jejunum DD23HZZ
　　Kidney DT20HZZ
　　Larynx D92BHZZ
　　Liver DF20HZZ
　　Lung DB22HZZ
　　Lymphatics
　　　Abdomen D726HZZ
　　　Axillary D724HZZ
　　　Inguinal D728HZZ
　　　Neck D723HZZ
　　　Pelvis D727HZZ
　　　Thorax D725HZZ
　　Mediastinum DB26HZZ
　　Mouth D924HZZ
　　Nasopharynx D92DHZZ
　　Neck and Head DW21HZZ
　　Nerve, Peripheral D027HZZ
　　Nose D921HZZ
　　Ovary DU20HZZ
　　Palate
　　　Hard D928HZZ
　　　Soft D929HZZ

Stereotactic Radiosurgery — *continued*
　Particulate — *continued*
　　Pancreas DF23HZZ
　　Parathyroid Gland DG24HZZ
　　Pelvic Region DW26HZZ
　　Pharynx D92CHZZ
　　Pineal Body DG21HZZ
　　Pituitary Gland DG20HZZ
　　Pleura DB25HZZ
　　Prostate DV20HZZ
　　Rectum DD27HZZ
　　Sinuses D927HZZ
　　Spinal Cord D026HZZ
　　Spleen D722HZZ
　　Stomach DD21HZZ
　　Testis DV21HZZ
　　Thymus D721HZZ
　　Thyroid Gland DG25HZZ
　　Tongue D925HZZ
　　Trachea DB20HZZ
　　Ureter DT21HZZ
　　Urethra DT23HZZ
　　Uterus DU22HZZ
　Pelvic Region DW26
　Pharynx D92C
　Pineal Body DG21
　Pituitary Gland DG20
　Pleura DB25
　Prostate DV20
　Rectum DD27
　Sinuses D927
　Spinal Cord D026
　Spleen D722
　Stomach DD21
　Testis DV21
　Thymus D721
　Thyroid Gland DG25
　Tongue D925
　Trachea DB20
　Ureter DT21
　Urethra DT23
　Uterus DU22
Sternoclavicular ligament
　use Shoulder Bursa and Ligament, Right
　use Shoulder Bursa and Ligament, Left
Sternocleidomastoid artery
　use Thyroid Artery, Right
　use Thyroid Artery, Left
Sternocleidomastoid muscle
　use Neck Muscle, Right
　use Neck Muscle, Left
Sternocostal ligament
　use Sternum Bursa and Ligament
Sternotomy
　see Division, Sternum 0P80
　see Drainage, Sternum 0P90
Stimulation, cardiac
　Cardioversion 5A2204Z
　Electrophysiologic testing *see*
　　Measurement, Cardiac 4A02
Stimulator Generator
　Insertion of device in
　　Abdomen 0JH8
　　Back 0JH7
　　Chest 0JH6
　　Multiple Array
　　　Abdomen 0JH8
　　　Back 0JH7
　　　Chest 0JH6
　　Multiple Array Rechargeable
　　　Abdomen 0JH8
　　　Back 0JH7
　　　Chest 0JH6
　Removal of device from, Subcutaneous
　　Tissue and Fascia, Trunk 0JPT
　Revision of device in, Subcutaneous Tissue
　　and Fascia, Trunk 0JWT

Stimulator Generator — *continued*
　Single Array
　　Abdomen 0JH8
　　Back 0JH7
　　Chest 0JH6
　Single Array Rechargeable
　　Abdomen 0JH8
　　Back 0JH7
　　Chest 0JH6
Stimulator Lead
　Insertion of device in
　　Anal Sphincter 0DHR
　　Artery
　　　Left 03HL
　　　Right 03HK
　　Bladder 0THB
　　Muscle
　　　Lower 0KHY
　　　Upper 0KHX
　　Stomach 0DH6
　　Ureter 0TH9
　Removal of device from
　　Anal Sphincter 0DPR
　　Artery, Upper 03PY
　　Bladder 0TPB
　　Muscle
　　　Lower 0KPY
　　　Upper 0KPX
　　Stomach 0DP6
　　Ureter 0TP9
　Revision of device in
　　Anal Sphincter 0DWR
　　Artery, Upper 03WY
　　Bladder 0TWB
　　Muscle
　　　Lower 0KWY
　　　Upper 0KWX
　　Stomach 0DW6
　　Ureter 0TW9
Stoma
　Excision
　　Abdominal Wall 0WBFXZ2
　　Neck 0WB6XZ2
　Repair
　　Abdominal Wall 0WQFXZ2
　　Neck 0WQ6XZ2
Stomatoplasty
　see Repair, Mouth and Throat 0CQ
　see Replacement, Mouth and Throat 0CR
　see Supplement, Mouth and Throat 0CU
Stomatorrhaphy
　see Repair, Mouth and Throat 0CQ
Stratos LV
　use Cardiac Resynchronization Pacemaker
　　Pulse Generator in 0JH
Stress test
　4A02XM4
　4A12XM4
Stripping
　see Extraction
Study
　Electrophysiologic stimulation, cardiac *see*
　　Measurement, Cardiac 4A02
　Ocular motility 4A07X7Z
　Pulmonary airway flow measurement *see*
　　Measurement, Respiratory 4A09
　Visual acuity 4A07X0Z
Styloglossus muscle
　use Tongue, Palate, Pharynx Muscle
Stylomandibular ligament
　use Head and Neck Bursa and Ligament
Stylopharyngeus muscle
　use Tongue, Palate, Pharynx Muscle
Subacromial bursa
　use Shoulder Bursa and Ligament, Right
　use Shoulder Bursa and Ligament, Left

Subaortic (common iliac) lymph node
use Lymphatic, Pelvis
Subarachnoid space, spinal
use Spinal Canal
Subclavicular (apical) lymph node
use Lymphatic, Right Axillary
use Lymphatic, Left Axillary
Subclavius muscle
use Thorax Muscle, Right
use Thorax Muscle, Left
Subclavius nerve
use Brachial Plexus
Subcostal artery
use Upper Artery
Subcostal muscle
use Thorax Muscle, Right
use Thorax Muscle, Left
Subcostal nerve
use Thoracic Nerve
Subcutaneous Defibrillator Lead
Insertion of device in, Subcutaneous Tissue and Fascia, Chest 0JH6
Removal of device from, Subcutaneous Tissue and Fascia, Trunk 0JPT
Revision of device in, Subcutaneous Tissue and Fascia, Trunk 0JWT
Subcutaneous injection reservoir, port
use Vascular Access Device, Totally Implantable in Subcutaneous Tissue and Fascia
Subcutaneous injection reservoir, pump
use Infusion Device, Pump in Subcutaneous Tissue and Fascia
Subdermal progesterone implant
use Contraceptive Device in Subcutaneous Tissue and Fascia
Subdural space, spinal
use Spinal Canal
Submandibular ganglion
use Facial Nerve
use Head and Neck Sympathetic Nerve
Submandibular gland
use Submaxillary Gland, Right
use Submaxillary Gland, Left
Submandibular lymph node
use Lymphatic, Head
Submandibular space
use Subcutaneous Tissue and Fascia, Face
Submaxillary ganglion
use Head and Neck Sympathetic Nerve
Submaxillary lymph node
use Lymphatic, Head
Submental artery
use Face Artery
Submental lymph node
use Lymphatic, Head
Submucous (Meissner's) plexus
use Abdominal Sympathetic Nerve
Suboccipital nerve
use Cervical Nerve
Suboccipital venous plexus
use Vertebral Vein, Right
use Vertebral Vein, Left
Subparotid lymph node
use Lymphatic, Head
Subscapular (posterior) lymph node
use Lymphatic, Right Axillary
use Lymphatic, Left Axillary
Subscapular aponeurosis
use Subcutaneous Tissue and Fascia, Right Upper Arm
use Subcutaneous Tissue and Fascia, Left Upper Arm
Subscapular artery
use Axillary Artery, Right
use Axillary Artery, Left

Subscapularis muscle
use Shoulder Muscle, Right
use Shoulder Muscle, Left
Substance Abuse Treatment
Counseling
Family, for substance abuse, Other Family Counseling HZ63ZZZ
Group
12-Step HZ43ZZZ
Behavioral HZ41ZZZ
Cognitive HZ40ZZZ
Cognitive-Behavioral HZ42ZZZ
Confrontational HZ48ZZZ
Continuing Care HZ49ZZZ
Infectious Disease
Post-Test HZ4CZZZ
Pre-Test HZ4CZZZ
Interpersonal HZ44ZZZ
Motivational Enhancement HZ47ZZZ
Psychoeducation HZ46ZZZ
Spiritual HZ4BZZZ
Vocational HZ45ZZZ
Individual
12-Step HZ33ZZZ
Behavioral HZ31ZZZ
Cognitive HZ30ZZZ
Cognitive-Behavioral HZ32ZZZ
Confrontational HZ38ZZZ
Continuing Care HZ39ZZZ
Infectious Disease
Post-Test HZ3CZZZ
Pre-Test HZ3CZZZ
Interpersonal HZ34ZZZ
Motivational Enhancement HZ37ZZZ
Psychoeducation HZ36ZZZ
Spiritual HZ3BZZZ
Vocational HZ35ZZZ
Detoxification Services, for substance abuse HZ2ZZZZ
Medication Management
Antabuse HZ83ZZZ
Bupropion HZ87ZZZ
Clonidine HZ86ZZZ
Levo-alpha-acetyl-methadol (LAAM) HZ82ZZZ
Methadone Maintenance HZ81ZZZ
Naloxone HZ85ZZZ
Naltrexone HZ84ZZZ
Nicotine Replacement HZ80ZZZ
Other Replacement Medication HZ89ZZZ
Psychiatric Medication HZ88ZZZ
Pharmacotherapy
Antabuse HZ93ZZZ
Bupropion HZ97ZZZ
Clonidine HZ96ZZZ
Levo-alpha-acetyl-methadol (LAAM) HZ92ZZZ
Methadone Maintenance HZ91ZZZ
Naloxone HZ95ZZZ
Naltrexone HZ94ZZZ
Nicotine Replacement HZ90ZZZ
Psychiatric Medication HZ98ZZZ
Replacement Medication, Other HZ99ZZZ
Psychotherapy
12-Step HZ53ZZZ
Behavioral HZ51ZZZ
Cognitive HZ50ZZZ
Cognitive-Behavioral HZ52ZZZ
Confrontational HZ58ZZZ
Interactive HZ55ZZZ
Interpersonal HZ54ZZZ
Motivational Enhancement HZ57ZZZ
Psychoanalysis HZ5BZZZ
Psychodynamic HZ5CZZZ

Substance Abuse Treatment — continued
Psychotherapy — continued
Psychoeducation HZ56ZZZ
Psychophysiological HZ5DZZZ
Supportive HZ59ZZZ
Substantia nigra
use Basal Ganglia
Subtalar (talocalcaneal) joint
use Tarsal Joint, Right
use Tarsal Joint, Left
Subtalar ligament
use Foot Bursa and Ligament, Right
use Foot Bursa and Ligament, Left
Subthalamic nucleus
use Basal Ganglia
Suction curettage (D&C), nonobstetric
see Extraction, Endometrium 0UDB
Suction curettage, obstetric post-delivery
see Extraction, Products of Conception, Retained 10D1
Superficial circumflex iliac vein
use Saphenous Vein, Right
use Saphenous Vein, Left
Superficial epigastric artery
use Femoral Artery, Right
use Femoral Artery, Left
Superficial epigastric vein
use Saphenous Vein, Right
use Saphenous Vein, Left
Superficial Inferior Epigastric Artery Flap
Replacement
Bilateral 0HRV078
Left 0HRU078
Right 0HRT078
Transfer
Left 0KXG
Right 0KXF
Superficial palmar arch
use Hand Artery, Right
use Hand Artery, Left
Superficial palmar venous arch
use Hand Vein, Right
use Hand Vein, Left
Superficial temporal artery
use Temporal Artery, Right
use Temporal Artery, Left
Superficial transverse perineal muscle
use Perineum Muscle
Superior cardiac nerve
use Thoracic Sympathetic Nerve
Superior cerebellar vein
use Intracranial Vein
Superior cerebral vein
use Intracranial Vein
Superior clunic (cluneal) nerve
use Lumbar Nerve
Superior epigastric artery
use Internal Mammary Artery, Right
use Internal Mammary Artery, Left
Superior genicular artery
use Popliteal Artery, Right
use Popliteal Artery, Left
Superior gluteal artery
use Internal Iliac Artery, Right
use Internal Iliac Artery, Left
Superior gluteal nerve
use Lumbar Plexus
Superior hypogastric plexus
use Abdominal Sympathetic Nerve
Superior labial artery
use Face Artery
Superior laryngeal artery
use Thyroid Artery, Right
use Thyroid Artery, Left
Superior laryngeal nerve
use Vagus Nerve

Superior longitudinal muscle
   use Tongue, Palate, Pharynx Muscle
Superior mesenteric ganglion
   use Abdominal Sympathetic Nerve
Superior mesenteric lymph node
   use Lymphatic, Mesenteric
Superior mesenteric plexus
   use Abdominal Sympathetic Nerve
Superior oblique muscle
   use Extraocular Muscle, Right
   use Extraocular Muscle, Left
Superior olivary nucleus
   use Pons
Superior rectal artery
   use Inferior Mesenteric Artery
Superior rectal vein
   use Inferior Mesenteric Vein
Superior rectus muscle
   use Extraocular Muscle, Right
   use Extraocular Muscle, Left
Superior tarsal plate
   use Upper Eyelid, Right
   use Upper Eyelid, Left
Superior thoracic artery
   use Axillary Artery, Right
   use Axillary Artery, Left
Superior thyroid artery
   use External Carotid Artery, Right
   use External Carotid Artery, Left
   use Thyroid Artery, Right
   use Thyroid Artery, Left
Superior turbinate
   use Nasal Turbinate
Superior ulnar collateral artery
   use Brachial Artery, Right
   use Brachial Artery, Left
Supersaturated Oxygen therapy
   5A0512C
   5A0522C
Supplement
   Abdominal Wall 0WUF
   Acetabulum
      Left 0QU5
      Right 0QU4
   Ampulla of Vater 0FUC
   Anal Sphincter 0DUR
   Ankle Region
      Left 0YUL
      Right 0YUK
   Anus 0DUQ
   Aorta
      Abdominal 04U0
      Thoracic
         Ascending/Arch 02UX
         Descending 02UW
   Arm
      Lower
         Left 0XUF
         Right 0XUD
      Upper
         Left 0XU9
         Right 0XU8
   Artery
      Anterior Tibial
         Left 04UQ
         Right 04UP
      Axillary
         Left 03U6
         Right 03U5
      Brachial
         Left 03U8
         Right 03U7
      Celiac 04U1
      Colic
         Left 04U7
         Middle 04U8
         Right 04U6

Supplement — *continued*
   Artery — *continued*
      Common Carotid
         Left 03UJ
         Right 03UH
      Common Iliac
         Left 04UD
         Right 04UC
      Coronary
         Four or More Arteries 02U3
         One Artery 02U0
         Three Arteries 02U2
         Two Arteries 02U1
      External Carotid
         Left 03UN
         Right 03UM
      External Iliac
         Left 04UJ
         Right 04UH
      Face 03UR
      Femoral
         Left 04UL
         Right 04UK
      Foot
         Left 04UW
         Right 04UV
      Gastric 04U2
      Hand
         Left 03UF
         Right 03UD
      Hepatic 04U3
      Inferior Mesenteric 04UB
      Innominate 03U2
      Internal Carotid
         Left 03UL
         Right 03UK
      Internal Iliac
         Left 04UF
         Right 04UE
      Internal Mammary
         Left 03U1
         Right 03U0
      Intracranial 03UG
      Lower 04UY
      Peroneal
         Left 04UU
         Right 04UT
      Popliteal
         Left 04UN
         Right 04UM
      Posterior Tibial
         Left 04US
         Right 04UR
      Pulmonary
         Left 02UR
         Right 02UQ
      Pulmonary Trunk 02UP
      Radial
         Left 03UC
         Right 03UB
      Renal
         Left 04UA
         Right 04U9
      Splenic 04U4
      Subclavian
         Left 03U4
         Right 03U3
      Superior Mesenteric 04U5
      Temporal
         Left 03UT
         Right 03US
      Thyroid
         Left 03UV
         Right 03UU
      Ulnar
         Left 03UA
         Right 03U9

Supplement — *continued*
   Artery — *continued*
      Upper 03UY
      Vertebral
         Left 03UQ
         Right 03UP
   Atrium
      Left 02U7
      Right 02U6
   Auditory Ossicle
      Left 09UA
      Right 09U9
   Axilla
      Left 0XU5
      Right 0XU4
   Back
      Lower 0WUL
      Upper 0WUK
   Bladder 0TUB
   Bladder Neck 0TUC
   Bone
      Ethmoid
         Left 0NUG
         Right 0NUF
      Frontal 0NU1
      Hyoid 0NUX
      Lacrimal
         Left 0NUJ
         Right 0NUH
      Nasal 0NUB
      Occipital 0NU7
      Palatine
         Left 0NUL
         Right 0NUK
      Parietal
         Left 0NU4
         Right 0NU3
      Pelvic
         Left 0QU3
         Right 0QU2
      Sphenoid 0NUC
      Temporal
         Left 0NU6
         Right 0NU5
      Zygomatic
         Left 0NUN
         Right 0NUM
   Breast
      Bilateral 0HUV
      Left 0HUU
      Right 0HUT
   Bronchus
      Lingula 0BU9
      Lower Lobe
         Left 0BUB
         Right 0BU6
      Main
         Left 0BU7
         Right 0BU3
      Middle Lobe, Right 0BU5
      Upper Lobe
         Left 0BU8
         Right 0BU4
   Buccal Mucosa 0CU4
   Bursa and Ligament
      Abdomen
         Left 0MUJ
         Right 0MUH
      Ankle
         Left 0MUR
         Right 0MUQ
      Elbow
         Left 0MU4
         Right 0MU3
      Foot
         Left 0MUT
         Right 0MUS

Supplement — *continued*
  Bursa and Ligament — *continued*
    Hand
      Left 0MU8
      Right 0MU7
    Head and Neck 0MU0
    Hip
      Left 0MUM
      Right 0MUL
    Knee
      Left 0MUP
      Right 0MUN
    Lower Extremity
      Left 0MUW
      Right 0MUV
    Perineum 0MUK
    Rib(s) 0MUG
    Shoulder
      Left 0MU2
      Right 0MU1
    Spine
      Lower 0MUD
      Upper 0MUC
    Sternum 0MUF
    Upper Extremity
      Left 0MUB
      Right 0MU9
    Wrist
      Left 0MU6
      Right 0MU5
  Buttock
    Left 0YU1
    Right 0YU0
  Carina 0BU2
  Carpal
    Left 0PUN
    Right 0PUM
  Cecum 0DUH
  Cerebral Meninges 00U1
  Cerebral Ventricle 00U6
  Chest Wall 0WU8
  Chordae Tendineae 02U9
  Cisterna Chyli 07UL
  Clavicle
    Left 0PUB
    Right 0PU9
  Clitoris 0UUJ
  Coccyx 0QUS
  Colon
    Ascending 0DUK
    Descending 0DUM
    Sigmoid 0DUN
    Transverse 0DUL
  Cord
    Bilateral 0VUH
    Left 0VUG
    Right 0VUF
  Cornea
    Left 08U9
    Right 08U8
  Cul-de-sac 0UUF
  Diaphragm 0BUT
  Disc
    Cervical Vertebral 0RU3
    Cervicothoracic Vertebral 0RU5
    Lumbar Vertebral 0SU2
    Lumbosacral 0SU4
    Thoracic Vertebral 0RU9
    Thoracolumbar Vertebral 0RUB
  Duct
    Common Bile 0FU9
    Cystic 0FU8
    Hepatic
      Common 0FU7
      Left 0FU6
      Right 0FU5

Supplement — *continued*
  Duct — *continued*
    Lacrimal
      Left 08UY
      Right 08UX
    Pancreatic 0FUD
      Accessory 0FUF
  Duodenum 0DU9
  Dura Mater 00U2
  Ear
    External
      Bilateral 09U2
      Left 09U1
      Right 09U0
    Inner
      Left 09UE
      Right 09UD
    Middle
      Left 09U6
      Right 09U5
  Elbow Region
    Left 0XUC
    Right 0XUB
  Epididymis
    Bilateral 0VUL
    Left 0VUK
    Right 0VUJ
  Epiglottis 0CUR
  Esophagogastric Junction 0DU4
  Esophagus 0DU5
    Lower 0DU3
    Middle 0DU2
    Upper 0DU1
  Extremity
    Lower
      Left 0YUB
      Right 0YU9
    Upper
      Left 0XU7
      Right 0XU6
  Eye
    Left 08U1
    Right 08U0
  Eyelid
    Lower
      Left 08UR
      Right 08UQ
    Upper
      Left 08UP
      Right 08UN
  Face 0WU2
  Fallopian Tube
    Left 0UU6
    Right 0UU5
  Fallopian Tubes, Bilateral 0UU7
  Femoral Region
    Bilateral 0YUE
    Left 0YU8
    Right 0YU7
  Femoral Shaft
    Left 0QU9
    Right 0QU8
  Femur
    Lower
      Left 0QUC
      Right 0QUB
    Upper
      Left 0QU7
      Right 0QU6
  Fibula
    Left 0QUK
    Right 0QUJ
  Finger
    Index
      Left 0XUP
      Right 0XUN

Supplement — *continued*
  Finger — *continued*
    Little
      Left 0XUW
      Right 0XUV
    Middle
      Left 0XUR
      Right 0XUQ
    Ring
      Left 0XUT
      Right 0XUS
  Foot
    Left 0YUN
    Right 0YUM
  Gingiva
    Lower 0CU6
    Upper 0CU5
  Glenoid Cavity
    Left 0PU8
    Right 0PU7
  Hand
    Left 0XUK
    Right 0XUJ
  Head 0WU0
  Heart 02UA
  Humeral Head
    Left 0PUD
    Right 0PUC
  Humeral Shaft
    Left 0PUG
    Right 0PUF
  Hymen 0UUK
  Ileocecal Valve 0DUC
  Ileum 0DUB
  Inguinal Region
    Bilateral 0YUA
    Left 0YU6
    Right 0YU5
  Intestine
    Large 0DUE
      Left 0DUG
      Right 0DUF
    Small 0DU8
  Iris
    Left 08UD
    Right 08UC
  Jaw
    Lower 0WU5
    Upper 0WU4
  Jejunum 0DUA
  Joint
    Acromioclavicular
      Left 0RUH
      Right 0RUG
    Ankle
      Left 0SUG
      Right 0SUF
    Carpal
      Left 0RUR
      Right 0RUQ
    Carpometacarpal
      Left 0RUT
      Right 0RUS
    Cervical Vertebral 0RU1
    Cervicothoracic Vertebral 0RU4
    Coccygeal 0SU6
    Elbow
      Left 0RUM
      Right 0RUL
    Finger Phalangeal
      Left 0RUX
      Right 0RUW
    Hip
      Left 0SUB
        Acetabular Surface 0SUE
        Femoral Surface 0SUS
      Right 0SU9
        Acetabular Surface 0SUA
        Femoral Surface 0SUR

Supplement — *continued*
  Joint — *continued*
    Knee
      Left 0SUD
        Femoral Surface 0SUU09Z
        Tibial Surface 0SUW09Z
      Right 0SUC
        Femoral Surface 0SUT09Z
        Tibial Surface 0SUV09Z
    Lumbar Vertebral 0SU0
    Lumbosacral 0SU3
    Metacarpophalangeal
      Left 0RUV
      Right 0RUU
    Metatarsal-Phalangeal
      Left 0SUN
      Right 0SUM
    Occipital-cervical 0RU0
    Sacrococcygeal 0SU5
    Sacroiliac
      Left 0SU8
      Right 0SU7
    Shoulder
      Left 0RUK
      Right 0RUJ
    Sternoclavicular
      Left 0RUF
      Right 0RUE
    Tarsal
      Left 0SUJ
      Right 0SUH
    Tarsometatarsal
      Left 0SUL
      Right 0SUK
    Temporomandibular
      Left 0RUD
      Right 0RUC
    Thoracic Vertebral 0RU6
    Thoracolumbar Vertebral 0RUA
    Toe Phalangeal
      Left 0SUQ
      Right 0SUP
    Wrist
      Left 0RUP
      Right 0RUN
  Kidney Pelvis
    Left 0TU4
    Right 0TU3
  Knee Region
    Left 0YUG
    Right 0YUF
  Larynx 0CUS
  Leg
    Lower
      Left 0YUJ
      Right 0YUH
    Upper
      Left 0YUD
      Right 0YUC
  Lip
    Lower 0CU1
    Upper 0CU0
  Lymphatic
    Aortic 07UD
    Axillary
      Left 07U6
      Right 07U5
    Head 07U0
    Inguinal
      Left 07UJ
      Right 07UH
    Internal Mammary
      Left 07U9
      Right 07U8
    Lower Extremity
      Left 07UG
      Right 07UF

Supplement — *continued*
  Lymphatic — *continued*
    Mesenteric 07UB
    Neck
      Left 07U2
      Right 07U1
    Pelvis 07UC
    Thoracic Duct 07UK
    Thorax 07U7
    Upper Extremity
      Left 07U4
      Right 07U3
  Mandible
    Left 0NUV
    Right 0NUT
  Maxilla 0NUR
  Mediastinum 0WUC
  Mesentery 0DUV
  Metacarpal
    Left 0PUQ
    Right 0PUP
  Metatarsal
    Left 0QUP
    Right 0QUN
  Muscle
    Abdomen
      Left 0KUL
      Right 0KUK
    Extraocular
      Left 08UM
      Right 08UL
    Facial 0KU1
    Foot
      Left 0KUW
      Right 0KUV
    Hand
      Left 0KUD
      Right 0KUC
    Head 0KU0
    Hip
      Left 0KUP
      Right 0KUN
    Lower Arm and Wrist
      Left 0KUB
      Right 0KU9
    Lower Leg
      Left 0KUT
      Right 0KUS
    Neck
      Left 0KU3
      Right 0KU2
    Papillary 02UD
    Perineum 0KUM
    Shoulder
      Left 0KU6
      Right 0KU5
    Thorax
      Left 0KUJ
      Right 0KUH
    Tongue, Palate, Pharynx 0KU4
    Trunk
      Left 0KUG
      Right 0KUF
    Upper Arm
      Left 0KU8
      Right 0KU7
    Upper Leg
      Left 0KUR
      Right 0KUQ
  Nasal Mucosa and Soft Tissue 09UK
  Nasopharynx 09UN
  Neck 0WU6
  Nerve
    Abducens 00UL
    Accessory 00UR
    Acoustic 00UN
    Cervical 01U1

Supplement — *continued*
  Nerve — *continued*
    Facial 00UM
    Femoral 01UD
    Glossopharyngeal 00UP
    Hypoglossal 00US
    Lumbar 01UB
    Median 01U5
    Oculomotor 00UH
    Olfactory 00UF
    Optic 00UG
    Peroneal 01UH
    Phrenic 01U2
    Pudendal 01UC
    Radial 01U6
    Sacral 01UR
    Sciatic 01UF
    Thoracic 01U8
    Tibial 01UG
    Trigeminal 00UK
    Trochlear 00UJ
    Ulnar 01U4
    Vagus 00UQ
  Nipple
    Left 0HUX
    Right 0HUW
  Omentum 0DUU
  Orbit
    Left 0NUQ
    Right 0NUP
  Palate
    Hard 0CU2
    Soft 0CU3
  Patella
    Left 0QUF
    Right 0QUD
  Penis 0VUS
  Pericardium 02UN
  Perineum
    Female 0WUN
    Male 0WUM
  Peritoneum 0DUW
  Phalanx
    Finger
      Left 0PUV
      Right 0PUT
    Thumb
      Left 0PUS
      Right 0PUR
    Toe
      Left 0QUR
      Right 0QUQ
  Pharynx 0CUM
  Prepuce 0VUT
  Radius
    Left 0PUJ
    Right 0PUH
  Rectum 0DUP
  Retina
    Left 08UF
    Right 08UE
  Retinal Vessel
    Left 08UH
    Right 08UG
  Ribs
    1 to 2 0PU1
    3 or More 0PU2
  Sacrum 0QU1
  Scapula
    Left 0PU6
    Right 0PU5
  Scrotum 0VU5
  Septum
    Atrial 02U5
    Nasal 09UM
    Ventricular 02UM

Supplement — *continued*
  Shoulder Region
    Left 0XU3
    Right 0XU2
  Sinus
    Accessory 09UP
    Ethmoid
      Left 09UV
      Right 09UU
    Frontal
      Left 09UT
      Right 09US
    Mastoid
      Left 09UC
      Right 09UB
    Maxillary
      Left 09UR
      Right 09UQ
    Sphenoid
      Left 09UX
      Right 09UW
  Skull 0NU0
  Spinal Meninges 00UT
  Sternum 0PU0
  Stomach 0DU6
    Pylorus 0DU7
  Subcutaneous Tissue and Fascia
    Abdomen 0JU8
    Back 0JU7
    Buttock 0JU9
    Chest 0JU6
    Face 0JU1
    Foot
      Left 0JUR
      Right 0JUQ
    Hand
      Left 0JUK
      Right 0JUJ
    Lower Arm
      Left 0JUH
      Right 0JUG
    Lower Leg
      Left 0JUP
      Right 0JUN
    Neck
      Left 0JU5
      Right 0JU4
    Pelvic Region 0JUC
    Perineum 0JUB
    Scalp 0JU0
    Upper Arm
      Left 0JUF
      Right 0JUD
    Upper Leg
      Left 0JUM
      Right 0JUL
  Tarsal
    Left 0QUM
    Right 0QUL
  Tendon
    Abdomen
      Left 0LUG
      Right 0LUF
    Ankle
      Left 0LUT
      Right 0LUS
    Foot
      Left 0LUW
      Right 0LUV
    Hand
      Left 0LU8
      Right 0LU7
    Head and Neck 0LU0
    Hip
      Left 0LUK
      Right 0LUJ

Supplement — *continued*
  Tendon — *continued*
    Knee
      Left 0LUR
      Right 0LUQ
    Lower Arm and Wrist
      Left 0LU6
      Right 0LU5
    Lower Leg
      Left 0LUP
      Right 0LUN
    Perineum 0LUH
    Shoulder
      Left 0LU2
      Right 0LU1
    Thorax
      Left 0LUD
      Right 0LUC
    Trunk
      Left 0LUB
      Right 0LU9
    Upper Arm
      Left 0LU4
      Right 0LU3
    Upper Leg
      Left 0LUM
      Right 0LUL
  Testis
    Bilateral 0VUC0
    Left 0VUB0
    Right 0VU90
  Thumb
    Left 0XUM
    Right 0XUL
  Tibia
    Left 0QUH
    Right 0QUG
  Toe
    1st
      Left 0YUQ
      Right 0YUP
    2nd
      Left 0YUS
      Right 0YUR
    3rd
      Left 0YUU
      Right 0YUT
    4th
      Left 0YUW
      Right 0YUV
    5th
      Left 0YUY
      Right 0YUX
  Tongue 0CU7
  Trachea 0BU1
  Tunica Vaginalis
    Left 0VU7
    Right 0VU6
  Turbinate, Nasal 09UL
  Tympanic Membrane
    Left 09U8
    Right 09U7
  Ulna
    Left 0PUL
    Right 0PUK
  Ureter
    Left 0TU7
    Right 0TU6
  Urethra 0TUD
  Uterine Supporting Structure 0UU4
  Uvula 0CUN
  Vagina 0UUG
  Valve
    Aortic 02UF
    Mitral 02UG
    Pulmonary 02UH
    Tricuspid 02UJ

Supplement — *continued*
  Vas Deferens
    Bilateral 0VUQ
    Left 0VUP
    Right 0VUN
  Vein
    Axillary
      Left 05U8
      Right 05U7
    Azygos 05U0
    Basilic
      Left 05UC
      Right 05UB
    Brachial
      Left 05UA
      Right 05U9
    Cephalic
      Left 05UF
      Right 05UD
    Colic 06U7
    Common Iliac
      Left 06UD
      Right 06UC
    Esophageal 06U3
    External Iliac
      Left 06UG
      Right 06UF
    External Jugular
      Left 05UQ
      Right 05UP
    Face
      Left 05UV
      Right 05UT
    Femoral
      Left 06UN
      Right 06UM
    Foot
      Left 06UV
      Right 06UT
    Gastric 06U2
    Hand
      Left 05UH
      Right 05UG
    Hemiazygos 05U1
    Hepatic 06U4
    Hypogastric
      Left 06UJ
      Right 06UH
    Inferior Mesenteric 06U6
    Innominate
      Left 05U4
      Right 05U3
    Internal Jugular
      Left 05UN
      Right 05UM
    Intracranial 05UL
    Lower 06UY
    Portal 06U8
    Pulmonary
      Left 02UT
      Right 02US
    Renal
      Left 06UB
      Right 06U9
    Saphenous
      Left 06UQ
      Right 06UP
    Splenic 06U1
    Subclavian
      Left 05U6
      Right 05U5
    Superior Mesenteric 06U5
    Upper 05UY
    Vertebral
      Left 05US
      Right 05UR

Supplement — *continued*
  Vena Cava
    Inferior 06U0
    Superior 02UV
  Ventricle
    Left 02UL
    Right 02UK
  Vertebra
    Cervical 0PU3
    Lumbar 0QU0
      Mechanically Expandable (Paired)
        Synthetic Substitute XNU0356
    Thoracic 0PU4
      Mechanically Expandable (Paired)
        Synthetic Substitute XNU4356
  Vesicle
    Bilateral 0VU3
    Left 0VU2
    Right 0VU1
  Vocal Cord
    Left 0CUV
    Right 0CUT
  Vulva 0UUM
  Wrist Region
    Left 0XUH
    Right 0XUG
Supraclavicular (Virchow's) lymph node
  use Lymphatic, Right Neck
  use Lymphatic, Left Neck
Supraclavicular nerve
  use Cervical Plexus
Suprahyoid lymph node
  use Lymphatic, Head
Suprahyoid muscle
  use Neck Muscle, Right
  use Neck Muscle, Left
Suprainguinal lymph node
  use Lymphatic, Pelvis
Supraorbital vein
  use Face Vein, Right
  use Face Vein, Left
Suprarenal gland
  use Adrenal Gland, Left
  use Adrenal Gland, Right
  use Adrenal Glands, Bilateral
  use Adrenal Gland
Suprarenal plexus
  use Abdominal Sympathetic Nerve
Suprascapular nerve
  use Brachial Plexus
Supraspinatus fascia
  use Subcutaneous Tissue and Fascia, Right Upper Arm
  use Subcutaneous Tissue and Fascia, Left Upper Arm
Supraspinatus muscle
  use Shoulder Muscle, Right
  use Shoulder Muscle, Left
Supraspinous ligament
  use Upper Spine Bursa and Ligament
  use Lower Spine Bursa and Ligament
Suprasternal notch
  use Sternum
Supratrochlear lymph node
  use Lymphatic, Right Upper Extremity
  use Lymphatic, Left Upper Extremity
Sural artery
  use Popliteal Artery, Right
  use Popliteal Artery, Left
Surpass Streamline™ Flow Diverter
  use Intraluminal Device, Flow Diverter in 03V
Suspension
  Bladder Neck *see* Reposition, Bladder Neck 0TSC
  Kidney *see* Reposition, Urinary System 0TS
  Urethra *see* Reposition, Urinary System 0TS

Suspension — *continued*
  Urethrovesical *see* Reposition, Bladder Neck 0TSC
  Uterus *see* Reposition, Uterus 0US9
  Vagina *see* Reposition, Vagina 0USG
Sustained Release Drug-eluting Intraluminal Device
  Dilation
    Anterior Tibial
      Left X27Q385
      Right X27P385
    Femoral
      Left X27J385
      Right X27H385
    Peroneal
      Left X27U385
      Right X27T385
    Popliteal
      Left Distal X27N385
      Left Proximal X27L385
      Right Distal X27M385
      Right Proximal X27K385
    Posterior Tibial
      Left X27S385
      Right X27R385
  Four or More
    Anterior Tibial
      Left X27Q3C5
      Right X27P3C5
    Femoral
      Left X27J3C5
      Right X27H3C5
    Peroneal
      Left X27U3C5
      Right X27T3C5
    Popliteal
      Left Distal X27N3C5
      Left Proximal X27L3C5
      Right Distal X27M3C5
      Right Proximal X27K3C5
    Posterior Tibial
      Left X27S3C5
      Right X27R3C5
  Three
    Anterior Tibial
      Left X27Q3B5
      Right X27P3B5
    Femoral
      Left X27J3B5
      Right X27H3B5
    Peroneal
      Left X27U3B5
      Right X27T3B5
    Popliteal
      Left Distal X27N3B5
      Left Proximal X27L3B5
      Right Distal X27M3B5
      Right Proximal X27K3B5
    Posterior Tibial
      Left X27S3B5
      Right X27R3B5
  Two
    Anterior Tibial
      Left X27Q395
      Right X27P395
    Femoral
      Left X27J395
      Right X27H395
    Peroneal
      Left X27U395
      Right X27T395
    Popliteal
      Left Distal X27N395
      Left Proximal X27L395
      Right Distal X27M395
      Right Proximal X27K395

Sustained Release Drug-eluting Intraluminal Device — *continued*
  Two — *continued*
    Posterior Tibial
      Left X27S395
      Right X27R395
Suture
  Laceration repair *see* Repair
  Ligation *see* Occlusion
Suture Removal
  Extremity
    Lower 8E0YXY8
    Upper 8E0XXY8
  Head and Neck Region 8E09XY8
  Trunk Region 8E0WXY8
Sutureless valve, Perceval
  use Zooplastic Tissue, Rapid Deployment Technique in New Technology
Sweat gland
  use Skin
Sympathectomy
  see Excision, Peripheral Nervous System 01B
SynCardia Total Artificial Heart
  use Synthetic Substitute
Synchra CRT-P
  use Cardiac Resynchronization Pacemaker Pulse Generator in 0JH
SynchroMed pump
  use Infusion Device, Pump in Subcutaneous Tissue and Fascia
Synechiotomy, iris
  see Release, Eye 08N
Synovectomy
  Lower joint *see* Excision, Lower Joints 0SB
  Upper joint *see* Excision, Upper Joints 0RB
Synthetic Human Angiotensin II XW0
Systemic Nuclear Medicine Therapy
  Abdomen CW70
  Anatomical Regions, Multiple CW7YYZZ
  Chest CW73
  Thyroid CW7G
  Whole Body CW7N

T

Tagraxofusp-erzs Antineoplastic XW0
Takedown
  Arteriovenous shunt *see* Removal of device from, Upper Arteries 03P
  Arteriovenous shunt, with creation of new shunt *see* Bypass, Upper Arteries 031
  Stoma
    see Excision
    see Reposition
Talent® Converter
  use Intraluminal Device
Talent® Occluder
  use Intraluminal Device
Talent® Stent Graft (abdominal)(thoracic)
  use Intraluminal Device
Talocalcaneal (subtalar) joint
  use Tarsal Joint, Right
  use Tarsal Joint, Left
Talocalcaneal ligament
  use Foot Bursa and Ligament, Right
  use Foot Bursa and Ligament, Left
Talocalcaneonavicular joint
  use Tarsal Joint, Right
  use Tarsal Joint, Left
Talocalcaneonavicular ligament
  use Foot Bursa and Ligament, Right
  use Foot Bursa and Ligament, Left
Talocrural joint
  use Ankle Joint, Right
  use Ankle Joint, Left

Talofibular ligament
use Ankle Bursa and Ligament, Right
use Ankle Bursa and Ligament, Left
Talus bone
use Tarsal, Right
use Tarsal, Left
TandemHeart® System
use Short-term External Heart Assist System in Heart and Great Vessels
Tarsectomy
see Excision, Lower Bones 0QB
see Resection, Lower Bones 0QT
Tarsometatarsal ligament
use Foot Bursa and Ligament, Right
use Foot Bursa and Ligament, Left
Tarsorrhaphy
see Repair, Eye 08Q
Tattooing
Cornea 3E0CXMZ
Skin *see* Introduction of substance in or on, Skin 3E00
TAXUS® Liberte® Paclitaxel-eluting Coronary Stent System
use Intraluminal Device, Drug-eluting in Heart and Great Vessels
TBNA (transbronchial needle aspiration)
Fluid or gas *see* Drainage, Respiratory System 0B9
Tissue biopsy *see* Extraction, Respiratory System 0BD
TECENTRIQ®
use Atezolizumab Antineoplastic
Telemetry
4A12X4Z
Ambulatory 4A12X45
Temperature gradient study 4A0ZXKZ
Temporal lobe
use Cerebral Hemisphere
Temporalis muscle
use Head Muscle
Temporoparietalis muscle
use Head Muscle
Tendolysis
see Release, Tendons 0LN
Tendonectomy
see Excision, Tendons 0LB
see Resection, Tendons 0LT
Tendonoplasty, tenoplasty
see Repair, Tendons 0LQ
see Replacement, Tendons 0LR
see Supplement, Tendons 0LU
Tendorrhaphy
see Repair, Tendons 0LQ
Tendototomy
see Division, Tendons 0L8
see Drainage, Tendons 0L9
Tenectomy, tenonectomy
see Excision, Tendons 0LB
see Resection, Tendons 0LT
Tenolysis
see Release, Tendons 0LN
Tenontorrhaphy
see Repair, Tendons 0LQ
Tenontotomy
see Division, Tendons 0L8
see Drainage, Tendons 0L9
Tenorrhaphy
see Repair, Tendons 0LQ
Tenosynovectomy
see Excision, Tendons 0LB
see Resection, Tendons 0LT
Tenotomy
see Division, Tendons 0L8
see Drainage, Tendons 0L9
Tensor fasciae latae muscle
use Hip Muscle, Right
use Hip Muscle, Left

Tensor veli palatini muscle
use Tongue, Palate, Pharynx Muscle
Tenth cranial nerve
use Vagus Nerve
Tentorium cerebelli
use Dura Mater
Teres major muscle
use Shoulder Muscle, Right
use Shoulder Muscle, Left
Teres minor muscle
use Shoulder Muscle, Right
use Shoulder Muscle, Left
Termination of pregnancy
Aspiration curettage 10A07ZZ
Dilation and curettage 10A07ZZ
Hysterotomy 10A00ZZ
Intra-amniotic injection 10A03ZZ
Laminaria 10A07ZW
Vacuum 10A07Z6
Testectomy
see Excision, Male Reproductive System 0VB
see Resection, Male Reproductive System 0VT
Testicular artery
use Abdominal Aorta
Testing
Glaucoma 4A07XBZ
Hearing *see* Hearing Assessment, Diagnostic Audiology F13
Mental health *see* Psychological Tests
Muscle function, electromyography (EMG) *see* Measurement, Musculoskeletal 4A0F
Muscle function, manual *see* Motor Function Assessment, Rehabilitation F01
Neurophysiologic monitoring, intra-operative *see* Monitoring, Physiological Systems 4A1
Range of motion *see* Motor Function Assessment, Rehabilitation F01
Vestibular function *see* Vestibular Assessment, Diagnostic Audiology F15
Thalamectomy
see Excision, Thalamus 00B9
Thalamotomy
see Drainage, Thalamus 0099
Thenar muscle
use Hand Muscle, Right
use Hand Muscle, Left
Therapeutic Massage
Musculoskeletal System 8E0KX1Z
Reproductive System
Prostate 8E0VX1C
Rectum 8E0VX1D
Therapeutic occlusion coil(s)
use Intraluminal Device
Thermography 4A0ZXKZ
Thermotherapy, prostate
see Destruction, Prostate 0V50
Third cranial nerve
use Oculomotor Nerve
Third occipital nerve
use Cervical Nerve
Third ventricle
use Cerebral Ventricle
Thoracectomy
see Excision, Anatomical Regions, General 0WB
Thoracentesis
see Drainage, Anatomical Regions, General 0W9
Thoracic aortic plexus
use Thoracic Sympathetic Nerve
Thoracic esophagus
use Esophagus, Middle
Thoracic facet joint
use Thoracic Vertebral Joint

Thoracic ganglion
use Thoracic Sympathetic Nerve
Thoracoacromial artery
use Axillary Artery, Right
use Axillary Artery, Left
Thoracocentesis
see Drainage, Anatomical Regions, General 0W9
Thoracolumbar facet joint
use Thoracolumbar Vertebral Joint
Thoracoplasty
see Repair, Anatomical Regions, General 0WQ
see Supplement, Anatomical Regions, General 0WU
Thoracostomy tube
use Drainage Device
Thoracostomy, for lung collapse
see Drainage, Respiratory System 0B9
Thoracotomy
see Drainage, Anatomical Regions, General 0W9
Thoratec IVAD (Implantable Ventricular Assist Device)
use Implantable Heart Assist System in Heart and Great Vessels
Thoratec Paracorporeal Ventricular Assist Device
use Short-term External Heart Assist System in Heart and Great Vessels
Thrombectomy
see Extirpation
Thrombolysis, Ultrasound assisted
see Fragmentation, Artery
Thymectomy
see Excision, Lymphatic and Hemic Systems 07B
see Resection, Lymphatic and Hemic Systems 07T
Thymopexy
see Repair, Lymphatic and Hemic Systems 07Q
see Reposition, Lymphatic and Hemic Systems 07S
Thymus gland
use Thymus
Thyroarytenoid muscle
use Neck Muscle, Right
use Neck Muscle, Left
Thyrocervical trunk
use Thyroid Artery, Right
use Thyroid Artery, Left
Thyroid cartilage
use Larynx
Thyroidectomy
see Excision, Endocrine System 0GB
see Resection, Endocrine System 0GT
Thyroidorrhaphy
see Repair, Endocrine System 0GQ
Thyroidoscopy 0GJK4ZZ
Thyroidotomy
see Drainage, Endocrine System 0G9
Tibial insert
use Liner in Lower Joints
Tibialis anterior muscle
use Lower Leg Muscle, Right
use Lower Leg Muscle, Left
Tibialis posterior muscle
use Lower Leg Muscle, Right
use Lower Leg Muscle, Left
Tibiofemoral joint
use Knee Joint, Right
use Knee Joint, Left
use Knee Joint, Tibial Surface, Right
use Knee Joint, Tibial Surface, Left

Tibioperoneal trunk
  use Popliteal Artery, Right
  use Popliteal Artery, Left
Tisagenlecleucel
  use Engineered Autologous Chimeric
    Antigen Receptor T-cell Immunotherapy
Tissue bank graft
  use Nonautologous Tissue Substitute
Tissue Expander
  Insertion of device in
    Breast
      Bilateral 0HHV
      Left 0HHU
      Right 0HHT
    Nipple
      Left 0HHX
      Right 0HHW
    Subcutaneous Tissue and Fascia
      Abdomen 0JH8
      Back 0JH7
      Buttock 0JH9
      Chest 0JH6
      Face 0JH1
      Foot
        Left 0JHR
        Right 0JHQ
      Hand
        Left 0JHK
        Right 0JHJ
      Lower Arm
        Left 0JHH
        Right 0JHG
      Lower Leg
        Left 0JHP
        Right 0JHN
      Neck
        Left 0JH5
        Right 0JH4
      Pelvic Region 0JHC
      Perineum 0JHB
      Scalp 0JH0
      Upper Arm
        Left 0JHF
        Right 0JHD
      Upper Leg
        Left 0JHM
        Right 0JHL
  Removal of device from
    Breast
      Left 0HPU
      Right 0HPT
    Subcutaneous Tissue and Fascia
      Head and Neck 0JPS
      Lower Extremity 0JPW
      Trunk 0JPT
      Upper Extremity 0JPV
  Revision of device in
    Breast
      Left 0HWU
      Right 0HWT
    Subcutaneous Tissue and Fascia
      Head and Neck 0JWS
      Lower Extremity 0JWW
      Trunk 0JWT
      Upper Extremity 0JWV
Tissue expander (inflatable)(injectable)
  use Tissue Expander in Skin and Breast
  use Tissue Expander in Subcutaneous
    Tissue and Fascia
Tissue Plasminogen Activator (tPA)(r-tPA)
  use Other Thrombolytic
Titanium Sternal Fixation System (TSFS)
  use Internal Fixation Device, Rigid Plate
    in 0PH
  use Internal Fixation Device, Rigid Plate
    in 0PS
Tocilizumab XW0

Tomographic (Tomo) Nuclear Medicine Imaging
  Abdomen CW20
  Abdomen and Chest CW24
  Abdomen and Pelvis CW21
  Anatomical Regions, Multiple CW2YYZZ
  Bladder, Kidneys and Ureters CT23
  Brain C020
  Breast CH2YYZZ
    Bilateral CH22
    Left CH21
    Right CH20
  Bronchi and Lungs CB22
  Central Nervous System C02YYZZ
  Cerebrospinal Fluid C025
  Chest CW23
  Chest and Abdomen CW24
  Chest and Neck CW26
  Digestive System CD2YYZZ
  Endocrine System CG2YYZZ
  Extremity
    Lower CW2D
      Bilateral CP2F
      Left CP2D
      Right CP2C
    Upper CW2M
      Bilateral CP2B
      Left CP29
      Right CP28
  Gallbladder CF24
  Gastrointestinal Tract CD27
  Gland, Parathyroid CG21
  Head and Neck CW2B
  Heart C22YYZZ
    Right and Left C226
  Hepatobiliary System and
    Pancreas CF2YYZZ
  Kidneys, Ureters and Bladder CT23
  Liver CF25
  Liver and Spleen CF26
  Lungs and Bronchi CB22
  Lymphatics and Hematologic
    System C72YYZZ
  Musculoskeletal System, Other CP2YYZZ
  Myocardium C22G
  Neck and Chest CW26
  Neck and Head CW2B
  Pancreas and Hepatobiliary
    System CF2YYZZ
  Pelvic Region CW2J
  Pelvis CP26
  Pelvis and Abdomen CW21
  Pelvis and Spine CP27
  Respiratory System CB2YYZZ
  Skin CH2YYZZ
  Skull CP21
  Skull and Cervical Spine CP23
  Spine
    Cervical CP22
    Cervical and Skull CP23
    Lumbar CP2H
    Thoracic CP2G
    Thoracolumbar CP2J
  Spine and Pelvis CP27
  Spleen C722
  Spleen and Liver CF26
  Subcutaneous Tissue CH2YYZZ
  Thorax CP24
  Ureters, Kidneys and Bladder CT23
  Urinary System CT2YYZZ
Tomography, computerized
  see Computerized Tomography (CT Scan)
Tongue, base of
  use Pharynx
Tonometry 4A07XBZ
Tonsillectomy
  see Excision, Mouth and Throat 0CB
  see Resection, Mouth and Throat 0CT

Tonsillotomy
  see Drainage, Mouth and Throat 0C9
Total Anomalous Pulmonary Venous
  Return (TAPVR) repair
  see Bypass, Atrium, Left 0217
  see Bypass, Vena Cava, Superior 021V
Total artificial (replacement) heart
  use Synthetic Substitute
Total parenteral nutrition (TPN)
  see Introduction of Nutritional Substance
Trachectomy
  see Excision, Trachea 0BB1
  see Resection, Trachea 0BT1
Trachelectomy
  see Excision, Cervix 0UBC
  see Resection, Cervix 0UTC
Trachelopexy
  see Repair, Cervix 0UQC
  see Reposition, Cervix 0USC
Tracheloplasty
  see Repair, Cervix 0UQC
Trachelorrhaphy
  see Repair, Cervix 0UQC
Trachelotomy
  see Drainage, Cervix 0U9C
Tracheobronchial lymph node
  use Lymphatic, Thorax
Tracheoesophageal fistulization 0B110D6
Tracheolysis
  see Release, Respiratory System 0BN
Tracheoplasty
  see Repair, Respiratory System 0BQ
  see Supplement, Respiratory System 0BU
Tracheorrhaphy
  see Repair, Respiratory System 0BQ
Tracheoscopy 0BJ18ZZ
Tracheostomy
  see Bypass, Respiratory System 0B1
Tracheostomy Device
  Bypass, Trachea 0B11
  Change device in, Trachea 0B21XFZ
  Removal of device from, Trachea 0BP1
  Revision of device in, Trachea 0BW1
Tracheostomy tube
  use Tracheostomy Device in Respiratory
    System
Tracheotomy
  see Drainage, Respiratory System 0B9
Traction
  Abdominal Wall 2W63X
  Arm
    Lower
      Left 2W6DX
      Right 2W6CX
    Upper
      Left 2W6BX
      Right 2W6AX
  Back 2W65X
  Chest Wall 2W64X
  Extremity
    Lower
      Left 2W6MX
      Right 2W6LX
    Upper
      Left 2W69X
      Right 2W68X
  Face 2W61X
  Finger
    Left 2W6KX
    Right 2W6JX
  Foot
    Left 2W6TX
    Right 2W6SX
  Hand
    Left 2W6FX
    Right 2W6EX
  Head 2W60X

Traction — *continued*
Inguinal Region
Left 2W67X
Right 2W66X
Leg
Lower
Left 2W6RX
Right 2W6QX
Upper
Left 2W6PX
Right 2W6NX
Neck 2W62X
Thumb
Left 2W6HX
Right 2W6GX
Toe
Left 2W6VX
Right 2W6UX
Tractotomy
see Division, Central Nervous System and Cranial Nerves 008
Tragus
use External Ear, Right
use External Ear, Left
use External Ear, Bilateral
Training, caregiver
see Caregiver Training
TRAM (transverse rectus abdominis myocutaneous) flap reconstruction
Free *see* Replacement, Skin and Breast 0HR
Pedicled *see* Transfer, Muscles 0KX
Transdermal Glomerular Filtration Rate (GFR) Measurement System XT25XE5
Transection
see Division
Transfer
Buccal Mucosa 0CX4
Bursa and Ligament
Abdomen
Left 0MXJ
Right 0MXH
Ankle
Left 0MXR
Right 0MXQ
Elbow
Left 0MX4
Right 0MX3
Foot
Left 0MXT
Right 0MXS
Hand
Left 0MX8
Right 0MX7
Head and Neck 0MX0
Hip
Left 0MXM
Right 0MXL
Knee
Left 0MXP
Right 0MXN
Lower Extremity
Left 0MXW
Right 0MXV
Perineum 0MXK
Rib(s) 0MXG
Shoulder
Left 0MX2
Right 0MX1
Spine
Lower 0MXD
Upper 0MXC
Sternum 0MXF
Upper Extremity
Left 0MXB
Right 0MX9
Wrist
Left 0MX6
Right 0MX5

Transfer — *continued*
Finger
Left 0XXP0ZM
Right 0XXN0ZL
Gingiva
Lower 0CX6
Upper 0CX5
Intestine
Large 0DXE
Small 0DX8
Lip
Lower 0CX1
Upper 0CX0
Muscle
Abdomen
Left 0KXL
Right 0KXK
Extraocular
Left 08XM
Right 08XL
Facial 0KX1
Foot
Left 0KXW
Right 0KXV
Hand
Left 0KXD
Right 0KXC
Head 0KX0
Hip
Left 0KXP
Right 0KXN
Lower Arm and Wrist
Left 0KXB
Right 0KX9
Lower Leg
Left 0KXT
Right 0KXS
Neck
Left 0KX3
Right 0KX2
Perineum 0KXM
Shoulder
Left 0KX6
Right 0KX5
Thorax
Left 0KXJ
Right 0KXH
Tongue, Palate, Pharynx 0KX4
Trunk
Left 0KXG
Right 0KXF
Upper Arm
Left 0KX8
Right 0KX7
Upper Leg
Left 0KXR
Right 0KXQ
Nerve
Abducens 00XL
Accessory 00XR
Acoustic 00XN
Cervical 01X1
Facial 00XM
Femoral 01XD
Glossopharyngeal 00XP
Hypoglossal 00XS
Lumbar 01XB
Median 01X5
Oculomotor 00XH
Olfactory 00XF
Optic 00XG
Peroneal 01XH
Phrenic 01X2
Pudendal 01XC
Radial 01X6
Sciatic 01XF
Thoracic 01X8

Transfer — *continued*
Nerve — *continued*
Tibial 01XG
Trigeminal 00XK
Trochlear 00XJ
Ulnar 01X4
Vagus 00XQ
Palate, Soft 0CX3
Prepuce 0VXT
Skin
Abdomen 0HX7XZZ
Back 0HX6XZZ
Buttock 0HX8XZZ
Chest 0HX5XZZ
Ear
Left 0HX3XZZ
Right 0HX2XZZ
Face 0HX1XZZ
Foot
Left 0HXNXZZ
Right 0HXMXZZ
Hand
Left 0HXGXZZ
Right 0HXFXZZ
Inguinal 0HXAXZZ
Lower Arm
Left 0HXEXZZ
Right 0HXDXZZ
Lower Leg
Left 0HXLXZZ
Right 0HXKXZZ
Neck 0HX4XZZ
Perineum 0HX9XZZ
Scalp 0HX0XZZ
Upper Arm
Left 0HXCXZZ
Right 0HXBXZZ
Upper Leg
Left 0HXJXZZ
Right 0HXHXZZ
Stomach 0DX6
Subcutaneous Tissue and Fascia
Abdomen 0JX8
Back 0JX7
Buttock 0JX9
Chest 0JX6
Face 0JX1
Foot
Left 0JXR
Right 0JXQ
Hand
Left 0JXK
Right 0JXJ
Lower Arm
Left 0JXH
Right 0JXG
Lower Leg
Left 0JXP
Right 0JXN
Neck
Left 0JX5
Right 0JX4
Pelvic Region 0JXC
Perineum 0JXB
Scalp 0JX0
Upper Arm
Left 0JXF
Right 0JXD
Upper Leg
Left 0JXM
Right 0JXL
Tendon
Abdomen
Left 0LXG
Right 0LXF
Ankle
Left 0LXT
Right 0LXS

Transfer — *continued*
  Tendon — *continued*
    Foot
      Left 0LXW
      Right 0LXV
    Hand
      Left 0LX8
      Right 0LX7
    Head and Neck 0LX0
    Hip
      Left 0LXK
      Right 0LXJ
    Knee
      Left 0LXR
      Right 0LXQ
    Lower Arm and Wrist
      Left 0LX6
      Right 0LX5
    Lower Leg
      Left 0LXP
      Right 0LXN
    Perineum 0LXH
    Shoulder
      Left 0LX2
      Right 0LX1
    Thorax
      Left 0LXD
      Right 0LXC
    Trunk
      Left 0LXB
      Right 0LX9
    Upper Arm
      Left 0LX4
      Right 0LX3
    Upper Leg
      Left 0LXM
      Right 0LXL
  Tongue 0CX7
Transfusion
  Immunotherapy *see* New Technology,
    Anatomical Regions XW2
  Products of Conception
    Antihemophilic Factors 3027
    Blood
      Platelets 3027
      Red Cells 3027
        Frozen 3027
      White Cells 3027
      Whole 3027
    Factor IX 3027
    Fibrinogen 3027
    Globulin 3027
    Plasma
      Fresh 3027
      Frozen 3027
    Plasma Cryoprecipitate 3027
    Serum Albumin 3027
  Vein
    4-Factor Prothrombin Complex
      Concentrate 3028
    Central
      Antihemophilic Factors 3024
      Blood
        Platelets 3024
        Red Cells 3024
          Frozen 3024
        White Cells 3024
        Whole 3024
      Bone Marrow 3024
      Factor IX 3024
      Fibrinogen 3024
      Globulin 3024
      Hematopoietic Stem/Progenitor Cells
        (HSPC), Genetically Modified 3024
      Plasma
        Fresh 3024
        Frozen 3024

Transfusion — *continued*
  Vein — *continued*
    Plasma Cryoprecipitate 3024
    Serum Albumin 3024
    Stem Cells
      Cord Blood 3024
      Embryonic 3024
      Hematopoietic 3024
      T-cell Depleted Hematopoietic 3024
  Peripheral
    Antihemophilic Factors 3023
    Blood
      Platelets 3023
      Red Cells 3023
        Frozen 3023
      White Cells 3023
      Whole 3023
    Bone Marrow 3023
    Factor IX 3023
    Fibrinogen 3023
    Globulin 3023
    Hematopoietic Stem/Progenitor Cells
      (HSPC), Genetically Modified 3023
    Plasma
      Fresh 3023
      Frozen 3023
    Plasma Cryoprecipitate 3023
    Serum Albumin 3023
    Stem Cells
      Cord Blood 3023
      Embryonic 3023
      Hematopoietic 3023
      T-cell Depleted Hematopoietic 3023
Transplant
  see Transplantation
Transplantation
  Bone marrow *see* Transfusion,
    Circulatory 302
  Esophagus 0DY50Z
  Face 0WY20Z
  Hand
    Left 0XYK0Z
    Right 0XYJ0Z
  Heart 02YA0Z
  Hematopoietic cell *see* Transfusion,
    Circulatory 302
  Intestine
    Large 0DYE0Z
    Small 0DY80Z
  Kidney
    Left 0TY10Z
    Right 0TY00Z
  Liver 0FY00Z
  Lung
    Bilateral 0BYM0Z
    Left 0BYL0Z
    Lower Lobe
      Left 0BYJ0Z
      Right 0BYF0Z
    Middle Lobe, Right 0BYD0Z
    Right 0BYK0Z
    Upper Lobe
      Left 0BYG0Z
      Right 0BYC0Z
  Lung Lingula 0BYH0Z
  Ovary
    Left 0UY10Z
    Right 0UY00Z
  Pancreas 0FYG0Z
  Penis 0VYS0Z
  Products of Conception 10Y0
  Scrotum 0VY50Z
  Spleen 07YP0Z
  Stem cell *see* Transfusion, Circulatory 302
  Stomach 0DY60Z
  Thymus 07YM0Z
  Uterus 0UY90Z

Transposition
  see Bypass
  see Reposition
  see Transfer
Transversalis fascia
  use Subcutaneous Tissue and Fascia, Trunk
Transverse (cutaneous) cervical nerve
  use Cervical Plexus
Transverse acetabular ligament
  use Hip Bursa and Ligament, Right
  use Hip Bursa and Ligament, Left
Transverse facial artery
  use Temporal Artery, Right
  use Temporal Artery, Left
Transverse foramen
  use Cervical Vertebra
Transverse humeral ligament
  use Shoulder Bursa and Ligament, Right
  use Shoulder Bursa and Ligament, Left
Transverse ligament of atlas
  use Head and Neck Bursa and Ligament
Transverse process
  use Cervical Vertebra
  use Thoracic Vertebra
  use Lumbar Vertebra
Transverse Rectus Abdominis
  Myocutaneous Flap
  Replacement
    Bilateral 0HRV076
    Left 0HRU076
    Right 0HRT076
  Transfer
    Left 0KXL
    Right 0KXK
Transverse scapular ligament
  use Shoulder Bursa and Ligament, Right
  use Shoulder Bursa and Ligament, Left
Transverse thoracis muscle
  use Thorax Muscle, Right
  use Thorax Muscle, Left
Transversospinalis muscle
  use Trunk Muscle, Right
  use Trunk Muscle, Left
Transversus abdominis muscle
  use Abdomen Muscle, Right
  use Abdomen Muscle, Left
Trapezium bone
  use Carpal, Right
  use Carpal, Left
Trapezius muscle
  use Trunk Muscle, Right
  use Trunk Muscle, Left
Trapezoid bone
  use Carpal, Right
  use Carpal, Left
Triceps brachii muscle
  use Upper Arm Muscle, Right
  use Upper Arm Muscle, Left
Tricuspid annulus
  use Tricuspid Valve
Trifacial nerve
  use Trigeminal Nerve
Trifecta™ Valve (aortic)
  use Zooplastic Tissue in Heart and Great
    Vessels
Trigone of bladder
  use Bladder
**TriGuard 3™ CEPD (cerebral embolic
  protection device)** X2A6325
Trimming, excisional
  see Excision
Triquetral bone
  use Carpal, Right
  use Carpal, Left
Trochanteric bursa
  use Hip Bursa and Ligament, Right
  use Hip Bursa and Ligament, Left

TUMT (Transurethral microwave thermotherapy of prostate) 0V507ZZ

TUNA (transurethral needle ablation of prostate) 0V507ZZ

Tunneled central venous catheter
use Vascular Access Device, Tunneled in Subcutaneous Tissue and Fascia

Tunneled spinal (intrathecal) catheter
use Infusion Device

Turbinectomy
see Excision, Ear, Nose, Sinus 09B
see Resection, Ear, Nose, Sinus 09T

Turbinoplasty
see Repair, Ear, Nose, Sinus 09Q
see Replacement, Ear, Nose, Sinus 09R
see Supplement, Ear, Nose, Sinus 09U

Turbinotomy
see Division, Ear, Nose, Sinus 098
see Drainage, Ear, Nose, Sinus 099

TURP (transurethral resection of prostate)
see Excision, Prostate 0VB0
see Resection, Prostate 0VT0

Twelfth cranial nerve
use Hypoglossal Nerve

Two lead pacemaker
use Pacemaker, Dual Chamber in 0JH

Tympanic cavity
use Middle Ear, Right
use Middle Ear, Left

Tympanic nerve
use Glossopharyngeal Nerve

Tympanic part of temporal bone
use Temporal Bone, Right
use Temporal Bone, Left

Tympanogram
see Hearing Assessment, Diagnostic Audiology F13

Tympanoplasty
see Repair, Ear, Nose, Sinus 09Q
see Replacement, Ear, Nose, Sinus 09R
see Supplement, Ear, Nose, Sinus 09U

Tympanosympathectomy
see Excision, Nerve, Head and Neck Sympathetic 01BK

Tympanotomy
see Drainage, Ear, Nose, Sinus 099

TYRX Antibacterial Envelope
use Anti-Infective Envelope

U

Ulnar collateral carpal ligament
use Wrist Bursa and Ligament, Right
use Wrist Bursa and Ligament, Left

Ulnar collateral ligament
use Elbow Bursa and Ligament, Right
use Elbow Bursa and Ligament, Left

Ulnar notch
use Radius, Right
use Radius, Left

Ulnar vein
use Brachial Vein, Right
use Brachial Vein, Left

Ultrafiltration
Hemodialysis *see* Performance, Urinary 5A1D
Therapeutic plasmapheresis *see* Pheresis, Circulatory 6A55

Ultraflex™ Precision Colonic Stent System
use Intraluminal Device

ULTRAPRO Hernia System (UHS)
use Synthetic Substitute

ULTRAPRO Partially Absorbable Lightweight Mesh
use Synthetic Substitute

ULTRAPRO Plug
use Synthetic Substitute

Ultrasonic osteogenic stimulator
use Bone Growth Stimulator in Head and Facial Bones
use Bone Growth Stimulator in Upper Bones
use Bone Growth Stimulator in Lower Bones

Ultrasonography
Abdomen BW40ZZZ
Abdomen and Pelvis BW41ZZZ
Abdominal Wall BH49ZZZ
Aorta
  Abdominal, Intravascular B440ZZ3
  Thoracic, Intravascular B340ZZ3
Appendix BD48ZZZ
Artery
  Brachiocephalic-Subclavian, Right, Intravascular B341ZZ3
  Celiac and Mesenteric, Intravascular B44KZZ3
  Common Carotid
    Bilateral, Intravascular B345ZZ3
    Left, Intravascular B344ZZ3
    Right, Intravascular B343ZZ3
  Coronary
    Multiple B241YZZ
      Intravascular B241ZZ3
      Transesophageal B241ZZ4
    Single B240YZZ
      Intravascular B240ZZ3
      Transesophageal B240ZZ4
  Femoral, Intravascular B44LZZ3
  Inferior Mesenteric, Intravascular B445ZZ3
  Internal Carotid
    Bilateral, Intravascular B348ZZ3
    Left, Intravascular B347ZZ3
    Right, Intravascular B346ZZ3
  Intra-Abdominal, Other, Intravascular B44BZZ3
  Intracranial, Intravascular B34RZZ3
  Lower Extremity
    Bilateral, Intravascular B44HZZ3
    Left, Intravascular B44GZZ3
    Right, Intravascular B44FZZ3
  Mesenteric and Celiac, Intravascular B44KZZ3
  Ophthalmic, Intravascular B34VZZ3
  Penile, Intravascular B44NZZ3
  Pulmonary
    Left, Intravascular B34TZZ3
    Right, Intravascular B34SZZ3
  Renal
    Bilateral, Intravascular B448ZZ3
    Left, Intravascular B447ZZ3
    Right, Intravascular B446ZZ3
  Subclavian, Left, Intravascular B342ZZ3
  Superior Mesenteric, Intravascular B444ZZ3
  Upper Extremity
    Bilateral, Intravascular B34KZZ3
    Left, Intravascular B34JZZ3
    Right, Intravascular B34HZZ3
Bile Duct BF40ZZZ
Bile Duct and Gallbladder BF43ZZZ
Bladder BT40ZZZ
  and Kidney BT4JZZZ
Brain B040ZZZ
Breast
  Bilateral BH42ZZZ
  Left BH41ZZZ
  Right BH40ZZZ
Chest Wall BH4BZZZ
Coccyx BR4FZZZ

Ultrasonography — *continued*
Connective Tissue
  Lower Extremity BL41ZZZ
  Upper Extremity BL40ZZZ
Duodenum BD49ZZZ
Elbow
  Left, Densitometry BP4HZZ1
  Right, Densitometry BP4GZZ1
Esophagus BD41ZZZ
Extremity
  Lower BH48ZZZ
  Upper BH47ZZZ
Eye
  Bilateral B847ZZZ
  Left B846ZZZ
  Right B845ZZZ
Fallopian Tube
  Bilateral BU42
  Left BU41
  Right BU40
Fetal Umbilical Cord BY47ZZZ
Fetus
  First Trimester, Multiple Gestation BY4BZZZ
  Second Trimester, Multiple Gestation BY4DZZZ
  Single
    First Trimester BY49ZZZ
    Second Trimester BY4CZZZ
    Third Trimester BY4FZZZ
  Third Trimester, Multiple Gestation BY4GZZZ
Gallbladder BF42ZZZ
Gallbladder and Bile Duct BF43ZZZ
Gastrointestinal Tract BD47ZZZ
Gland
  Adrenal
    Bilateral BG42ZZZ
    Left BG41ZZZ
    Right BG40ZZZ
  Parathyroid BG43ZZZ
  Thyroid BG44ZZZ
Hand
  Left, Densitometry BP4PZZ1
  Right, Densitometry BP4NZZ1
Head and Neck BH4CZZZ
Heart
  Left B245YZZ
    Intravascular B245ZZ3
    Transesophageal B245ZZ4
  Pediatric B24DYZZ
    Intravascular B24DZZ3
    Transesophageal B24DZZ4
  Right B244YZZ
    Intravascular B244ZZ3
    Transesophageal B244ZZ4
  Right and Left B246YZZ
    Intravascular B246ZZ3
    Transesophageal B246ZZ4
Heart with Aorta B24BYZZ
  Intravascular B24BZZ3
  Transesophageal B24BZZ4
Hepatobiliary System, All BF4CZZZ
Hip
  Bilateral BQ42ZZZ
  Left BQ41ZZZ
  Right BQ40ZZZ
Kidney
  and Bladder BT4JZZZ
  Bilateral BT43ZZZ
  Left BT42ZZZ
  Right BT41ZZZ
  Transplant BT49ZZZ
Knee
  Bilateral BQ49ZZZ
  Left BQ48ZZZ
  Right BQ47ZZZ

Ultrasonography — *continued*
  Liver BF45ZZZ
  Liver and Spleen BF46ZZZ
  Mediastinum BB4CZZZ
  Neck BW4FZZZ
  Ovary
    Bilateral BU45
    Left BU44
    Right BU43
  Ovary and Uterus BU4C
  Pancreas BF47ZZZ
  Pelvic Region BW4GZZZ
  Pelvis and Abdomen BW41ZZZ
  Penis BV4BZZZ
  Pericardium B24CYZZ
    Intravascular B24CZZ3
    Transesophageal B24CZZ4
  Placenta BY48ZZZ
  Pleura BB4BZZZ
  Prostate and Seminal Vesicle BV49ZZZ
  Rectum BD4CZZZ
  Sacrum BR4FZZZ
  Scrotum BV44ZZZ
  Seminal Vesicle and Prostate BV49ZZZ
  Shoulder
    Left, Densitometry BP49ZZ1
    Right, Densitometry BP48ZZ1
  Spinal Cord B04BZZZ
  Spine
    Cervical BR40ZZZ
    Lumbar BR49ZZZ
    Thoracic BR47ZZZ
  Spleen and Liver BF46ZZZ
  Stomach BD42ZZZ
  Tendon
    Lower Extremity BL43ZZZ
    Upper Extremity BL42ZZZ
  Ureter
    Bilateral BT48ZZZ
    Left BT47ZZZ
    Right BT46ZZZ
  Urethra BT45ZZZ
  Uterus BU46
  Uterus and Ovary BU4C
  Vein
    Jugular
      Left, Intravascular B544ZZ3
      Right, Intravascular B543ZZ3
    Lower Extremity
      Bilateral, Intravascular B54DZZ3
      Left, Intravascular B54CZZ3
      Right, Intravascular B54BZZ3
    Portal, Intravascular B54TZZ3
    Renal
      Bilateral, Intravascular B54LZZ3
      Left, Intravascular B54KZZ3
      Right, Intravascular B54JZZ3
    Splanchnic, Intravascular B54TZZ3
    Subclavian
      Left, Intravascular B547ZZ3
      Right, Intravascular B546ZZ3
    Upper Extremity
      Bilateral, Intravascular B54PZZ3
      Left, Intravascular B54NZZ3
      Right, Intravascular B54MZZ3
  Vena Cava
    Inferior, Intravascular B549ZZ3
    Superior, Intravascular B548ZZ3
  Wrist
    Left, Densitometry BP4MZZ1
    Right, Densitometry BP4LZZ1
Ultrasound bone healing system
  use Bone Growth Stimulator in Head and Facial Bones
  use Bone Growth Stimulator in Upper Bones
  use Bone Growth Stimulator in Lower Bones

Ultrasound Therapy
  Heart 6A75
  No Qualifier 6A75
  Vessels
    Head and Neck 6A75
    Other 6A75
    Peripheral 6A75
Ultraviolet Light Therapy, Skin 6A80
Umbilical artery
  use Internal Iliac Artery, Right
  use Internal Iliac Artery, Left
  use Lower Artery
Uniplanar external fixator
  use External Fixation Device, Monoplanar in 0PH
  use External Fixation Device, Monoplanar in 0PS
  use External Fixation Device, Monoplanar in 0QH
  use External Fixation Device, Monoplanar in 0QS
Upper GI series
  see Fluoroscopy, Gastrointestinal, Upper BD15
Ureteral orifice
  use Ureter, Right
  use Ureter, Left
  use Ureters, Bilateral
  use Ureter
Ureterectomy
  see Excision, Urinary System 0TB
  see Resection, Urinary System 0TT
Ureterocolostomy
  see Bypass, Urinary System 0T1
Ureterocystostomy
  see Bypass, Urinary System 0T1
Ureteroenterostomy
  see Bypass, Urinary System 0T1
Ureteroileostomy
  see Bypass, Urinary System 0T1
Ureterolithotomy
  see Extirpation, Urinary System 0TC
Ureterolysis
  see Release, Urinary System 0TN
Ureteroneocystostomy
  see Bypass, Urinary System 0T1
  see Reposition, Urinary System 0TS
Ureteropelvic junction (UPJ)
  use Kidney Pelvis, Right
  use Kidney Pelvis, Left
Ureteropexy
  see Repair, Urinary System 0TQ
  see Reposition, Urinary System 0TS
Ureteroplasty
  see Repair, Urinary System 0TQ
  see Replacement, Urinary System 0TR
  see Supplement, Urinary System 0TU
Ureteroplication
  see Restriction, Urinary System 0TV
Ureteropyelography
  see Fluoroscopy, Urinary System BT1
Ureterorrhaphy
  see Repair, Urinary System 0TQ
Ureteroscopy 0TJ98ZZ
Ureterostomy
  see Bypass, Urinary System 0T1
  see Drainage, Urinary System 0T9
Ureterotomy
  see Drainage, Urinary System 0T9
Ureteroureterostomy
  see Bypass, Urinary System 0T1
Ureterovesical orifice
  use Ureter, Right
  use Ureter, Left
  use Ureters, Bilateral
  use Ureter

Urethral catheterization, indwelling 0T9B70Z
Urethrectomy
  see Excision, Urethra 0TBD
  see Resection, Urethra 0TTD
Urethrolithotomy
  see Extirpation, Urethra 0TCD
Urethrolysis
  see Release, Urethra 0TND
Urethropexy
  see Repair, Urethra 0TQD
  see Reposition, Urethra 0TSD
Urethroplasty
  see Repair, Urethra 0TQD
  see Replacement, Urethra 0TRD
  see Supplement, Urethra 0TUD
Urethrorrhaphy
  see Repair, Urethra 0TQD
Urethroscopy 0TJD8ZZ
Urethrotomy
  see Drainage, Urethra 0T9D
Uridine Triacetate XW0DX82
Urinary incontinence stimulator lead
  use Stimulator Lead in Urinary System
Urography
  see Fluoroscopy, Urinary System BT1
Ustekinumab
  use Other New Technology Therapeutic Substance
Uterine Artery
  use Internal Iliac Artery, Right
  use Internal Iliac Artery, Left
Uterine artery embolization (UAE)
  see Occlusion, Lower Arteries 04L
Uterine cornu
  use Uterus
Uterine tube
  use Fallopian Tube, Right
  use Fallopian Tube, Left
Uterine vein
  use Hypogastric Vein, Right
  use Hypogastric Vein, Left
Uvulectomy
  see Excision, Uvula 0CBN
  see Resection, Uvula 0CTN
Uvulorrhaphy
  see Repair, Uvula 0CQN
Uvulotomy
  see Drainage, Uvula 0C9N

V

V-Wave Interatrial Shunt System
  use Synthetic Substitute
Vabomere™
  use Meropenem-vaborbactam Anti-infective
Vaccination
  see Introduction of Serum, Toxoid, and Vaccine
Vacuum extraction, obstetric 10D07Z6
Vaginal artery
  use Internal Iliac Artery, Right
  use Internal Iliac Artery, Left
Vaginal pessary
  use Intraluminal Device, Pessary in Female Reproductive System
Vaginal vein
  use Hypogastric Vein, Right
  use Hypogastric Vein, Left
Vaginectomy
  see Excision, Vagina 0UBG
  see Resection, Vagina 0UTG
Vaginofixation
  see Repair, Vagina 0UQG
  see Reposition, Vagina 0USG

Vaginoplasty
see Repair, Vagina 0UQG
see Supplement, Vagina 0UUG
Vaginorrhaphy
see Repair, Vagina 0UQG
Vaginoscopy 0UJH8ZZ
Vaginotomy
see Drainage, Female Reproductive System 0U9
Vagotomy
see Division, Nerve, Vagus 008Q
Valiant Thoracic Stent Graft
use Intraluminal Device
Valvotomy, valvulotomy
see Division, Heart and Great Vessels 028
see Release, Heart and Great Vessels 02N
Valvuloplasty
see Repair, Heart and Great Vessels 02Q
see Replacement, Heart and Great Vessels 02R
see Supplement, Heart and Great Vessels 02U
Valvuloplasty, Alfieri Stitch
see Restriction, Valve, Mitral 02VG
Vascular Access Device
Totally Implantable
Insertion of device in
Abdomen 0JH8
Chest 0JH6
Lower Arm
Left 0JHH
Right 0JHG
Lower Leg
Left 0JHP
Right 0JHN
Upper Arm
Left 0JHF
Right 0JHD
Upper Leg
Left 0JHM
Right 0JHL
Removal of device from
Lower Extremity 0JPW
Trunk 0JPT
Upper Extremity 0JPV
Revision of device in
Lower Extremity 0JWW
Trunk 0JWT
Upper Extremity 0JWV
Tunneled
Insertion of device in
Abdomen 0JH8
Chest 0JH6
Lower Arm
Left 0JHH
Right 0JHG
Lower Leg
Left 0JHP
Right 0JHN
Upper Arm
Left 0JHF
Right 0JHD
Upper Leg
Left 0JHM
Right 0JHL
Removal of device from
Lower Extremity 0JPW
Trunk 0JPT
Upper Extremity 0JPV
Revision of device in
Lower Extremity 0JWW
Trunk 0JWT
Upper Extremity 0JWV
Vasectomy
see Excision, Male Reproductive System 0VB

Vasography
see Plain Radiography, Male Reproductive System BV0
see Fluoroscopy, Male Reproductive System BV1
Vasoligation
see Occlusion, Male Reproductive System 0VL
Vasorrhaphy
see Repair, Male Reproductive System 0VQ
Vasostomy
see Bypass, Male Reproductive System 0V1
Vasotomy
Drainage see Drainage, Male Reproductive System 0V9
With ligation see Occlusion, Male Reproductive System 0VL
Vasovasostomy
see Repair, Male Reproductive System 0VQ
Vastus intermedius muscle
use Upper Leg Muscle, Right
use Upper Leg Muscle, Left
Vastus lateralis muscle
use Upper Leg Muscle, Right
use Upper Leg Muscle, Left
Vastus medialis muscle
use Upper Leg Muscle, Right
use Upper Leg Muscle, Left
VCG (vectorcardiogram)
see Measurement, Cardiac 4A02
Vectra® Vascular Access Graft
use Vascular Access Device, Tunneled in Subcutaneous Tissue and Fascia
Veklury use Remdesivir Anti-infective
Venclexta®
use Venetoclax Antineoplastic
Venectomy
see Excision, Upper Veins 05B
see Excision, Lower Veins 06B
Venetoclax Antineoplastic XW0DXR5
Venography
see Plain Radiography, Veins B50
see Fluoroscopy, Veins B51
Venorrhaphy
see Repair, Upper Veins 05Q
see Repair, Lower Veins 06Q
Venotripsy
see Occlusion, Upper Veins 05L
see Occlusion, Lower Veins 06L
Ventricular fold
use Larynx
Ventriculoatriostomy
see Bypass, Central Nervous System and Cranial Nerves 001
Ventriculocisternostomy
see Bypass, Central Nervous System and Cranial Nerves 001
Ventriculogram, cardiac
Combined left and right heart see Fluoroscopy, Heart, Right and Left B216
Left ventricle see Fluoroscopy, Heart, Left B215
Right ventricle see Fluoroscopy, Heart, Right B214
Ventriculopuncture, through previously implanted catheter 8C01X6J
Ventriculoscopy 00J04ZZ
Ventriculostomy
External drainage see Drainage, Cerebral Ventricle 0096
Internal shunt see Bypass, Cerebral Ventricle 0016
Ventriculovenostomy
see Bypass, Cerebral Ventricle 0016
Ventrio™ Hernia Patch
use Synthetic Substitute
VEP (visual evoked potential) 4A07X0Z

Vermiform appendix
use Appendix
Vermilion border
use Upper Lip
use Lower Lip
Versa
use Pacemaker, Dual Chamber in 0JH
Version, obstetric
External 10S0XZZ
Internal 10S07ZZ
Vertebral arch
use Cervical Vertebra
use Thoracic Vertebra
use Lumbar Vertebra
Vertebral body
use Cervical Vertebra
use Thoracic Vertebra
use Lumbar Vertebra
Vertebral canal
use Spinal Canal
Vertebral foramen
use Cervical Vertebra
use Thoracic Vertebra
use Lumbar Vertebra
Vertebral lamina
use Cervical Vertebra
use Thoracic Vertebra
use Lumbar Vertebra
Vertebral pedicle
use Cervical Vertebra
use Thoracic Vertebra
use Lumbar Vertebra
Vesical vein
use Hypogastric Vein, Right
use Hypogastric Vein, Left
Vesicotomy
see Drainage, Urinary System 0T9
Vesiculectomy
see Excision, Male Reproductive System 0VB
see Resection, Male Reproductive System 0VT
Vesiculogram, seminal
see Plain Radiography, Male Reproductive System BV0
Vesiculotomy
see Drainage, Male Reproductive System 0V9
Vestibular (Scarpa's) ganglion
use Acoustic Nerve
Vestibular Assessment F15Z
Vestibular nerve
use Acoustic Nerve
Vestibular Treatment F0C
Vestibulocochlear nerve
use Acoustic Nerve
VH-IVUS (virtual histology intravascular ultrasound)
see Ultrasonography, Heart B24
Virchow's (supraclavicular) lymph node
use Lymphatic, Right Neck
use Lymphatic, Left Neck
Virtuoso (II) (DR) (VR)
use Defibrillator Generator in 0JH
Vistogard®
use Uridine Triacetate
Vitrectomy
see Excision, Eye 08B
see Resection, Eye 08T
Vitreous body
use Vitreous, Right
use Vitreous, Left
Viva (XT)(S)
use Cardiac Resynchronization Defibrillator Pulse Generator in 0JH

Vocal fold
　　use Vocal Cord, Right
　　use Vocal Cord, Left
Vocational
　　Assessment *see* Activities of Daily Living
　　　Assessment, Rehabilitation F02
　　Retraining *see* Activities of Daily Living
　　　Treatment, Rehabilitation F08
Volar (palmar) digital vein
　　use Hand Vein, Right
　　use Hand Vein, Left
Volar (palmar) metacarpal vein
　　use Hand Vein, Right
　　use Hand Vein, Left
Vomer bone
　　use Nasal Septum
Vomer of nasal septum
　　use Nasal Bone
Voraxaze
　　use Glucarpidase
Vulvectomy
　　see Excision, Female Reproductive
　　　System 0UB
　　see Resection, Female Reproductive
　　　System 0UT
VYXEOS™
　　use Cytarabine and Daunorubicin
　　　Liposome Antineoplastic

W

WALLSTENT® Endoprosthesis
　　use Intraluminal Device
Washing
　　see Irrigation
WavelinQ EndoAVF system
　　Radial Artery, Left 031C3ZF
　　Radial Artery, Right 031B3ZF
　　Ulnar Artery, Left 031A3ZF
　　Ulnar Artery, Right 03193ZF
Wedge resection, pulmonary
　　see Excision, Respiratory System 0BB
Whole Blood Nucleic Acid-base Microbial
　　Detection XXE5XM5
Window
　　see Drainage
Wiring, dental 2W31X9Z

X

X-ray
　　see Plain Radiography
X-STOP® Spacer
　　use Spinal Stabilization Device,
　　　Interspinous Process in 0RH
　　use Spinal Stabilization Device,
　　　Interspinous Process in 0SH
Xact Carotid Stent System
　　use Intraluminal Device
XENLETA™
　　use Lefamulin Anti-infective
Xenograft
　　use Zooplastic Tissue in Heart and Great
　　　Vessels
XIENCE Everolimus Eluting Coronary Stent
　　System
　　use Intraluminal Device, Drug-eluting in
　　　Heart and Great Vessels
Xiphoid process
　　use Sternum
XLIF® System
　　use Interbody Fusion Device in Lower
　　　Joints
XOSPATA®
　　use Gilteritinib Antineoplastic

Y

Yoga Therapy 8E0ZXY4

Z

Z-plasty, skin for scar contracture
　　see Release, Skin and Breast 0HN
Zenith AAA Endovascular Graft
　　use Intraluminal Device
Zenith Flex® AAA Endovascular Graft
　　use Intraluminal Device
Zenith TX2® TAA Endovascular Graft
　　use Intraluminal Device
Zenith® Fenestrated AAA Endovascular
　　Graft
　　use Intraluminal Device, Branched or
　　　Fenestrated, One or Two Arteries in 04V
　　use Intraluminal Device, Branched or
　　　Fenestrated, Three or More Arteries in 04V
Zenith® Renu™ AAA Ancillary Graft
　　use Intraluminal Device
ZERBAXA®
　　use Ceftolozane/Tazobactam Anti-infective
Zilver® PTX® (paclitaxel) Drug-Eluting
　　Peripheral Stent
　　use Intraluminal Device, Drug-eluting in
　　　Upper Arteries
　　use Intraluminal Device, Drug-eluting in
　　　Lower Arteries
Zimmer® NexGen® LPS Mobile Bearing
　　Knee
　　use Synthetic Substitute
Zimmer® NexGen® LPS-Flex Mobile Knee
　　use Synthetic Substitute
ZINPLAVA™
　　use Bezlotoxumab Monoclonal Antibody
Zonule of Zinn
　　use Lens, Right
　　use Lens, Left
Zooplastic Tissue, Rapid Deployment
　　Technique, Replacement X2RF
Zotarolimus-eluting coronary stent
　　use Intraluminal Device, Drug-eluting in
　　　Heart and Great Vessels
ZULRESSO™
　　use Brexanolone
Zygomatic process of frontal bone
　　use Frontal Bone
Zygomatic process of temporal bone
　　use Temporal Bone, Right
　　use Temporal Bone, Left
Zygomaticus muscle
　　use Facial Muscle
Zyvox
　　use Oxazolidinones

This page intentionally left blank

Medical and Surgical 001-0YW

Central Nervous System and Cranial Nerves 001-00X

0 **Medical and Surgical**
0 **Central Nervous System and Cranial Nerves**
1 **Bypass:** Altering the route of passage of the contents of a tubular body part

Body Part	Approach	Device	Qualifier
Character 4	Character 5	Character 6	Character 7
6 Cerebral Ventricle	0 Open 3 Percutaneous 4 Percutaneous Endoscopic	7 Autologous Tissue Substitute J Synthetic Substitute K Nonautologous Tissue Substitute	0 Nasopharynx 1 Mastoid Sinus 2 Atrium 3 Blood Vessel 4 Pleural Cavity 5 Intestine 6 Peritoneal Cavity 7 Urinary Tract 8 Bone Marrow A Subgaleal Space B Cerebral Cisterns
6 Cerebral Ventricle	0 Open 3 Percutaneous 4 Percutaneous Endoscopic	Z No Device	B Cerebral Cisterns
U Spinal Canal	0 Open 3 Percutaneous 4 Percutaneous Endoscopic	7 Autologous Tissue Substitute J Synthetic Substitute K Nonautologous Tissue Substitute	2 Atrium 4 Pleural Cavity 6 Peritoneal Cavity 7 Urinary Tract 9 Fallopian Tube

0 **Medical and Surgical**
0 **Central Nervous System and Cranial Nerves**
2 **Change:** Taking out or off a device from a body part and putting back an identical or similar device in or on the same body part without cutting or puncturing the skin or a mucous membrane

Body Part	Approach	Device	Qualifier
Character 4	Character 5	Character 6	Character 7
0 Brain E Cranial Nerve U Spinal Canal	X External	0 Drainage Device Y Other Device	Z No Qualifier

0 Medical and Surgical
0 Central Nervous System and Cranial Nerves
5 Destruction: Physical eradication of all or a portion of a body part by the direct use of energy, force, or a destructive agent

Body Part	Approach	Device	Qualifier
Character 4	Character 5	Character 6	Character 7
0 Brain 1 Cerebral Meninges 2 Dura Mater 6 Cerebral Ventricle 7 Cerebral Hemisphere 8 Basal Ganglia 9 Thalamus A Hypothalamus B Pons C Cerebellum D Medulla Oblongata F Olfactory Nerve G Optic Nerve H Oculomotor Nerve J Trochlear Nerve K Trigeminal Nerve L Abducens Nerve M Facial Nerve N Acoustic Nerve P Glossopharyngeal Nerve Q Vagus Nerve R Accessory Nerve S Hypoglossal Nerve T Spinal Meninges W Cervical Spinal Cord X Thoracic Spinal Cord Y Lumbar Spinal Cord	0 Open 3 Percutaneous 4 Percutaneous Endoscopic	Z No Device	Z No Qualifier

0 Medical and Surgical
0 Central Nervous System and Cranial Nerves
7 Dilation: Expanding an orifice or the lumen of a tubular body part

Body Part	Approach	Device	Qualifier
Character 4	Character 5	Character 6	Character 7
6 Cerebral Ventricle	0 Open 3 Percutaneous 4 Percutaneous Endoscopic	Z No Device	Z No Qualifier

0 Medical and Surgical
0 Central Nervous System and Cranial Nerves
8 Division: Cutting into a body part, without draining fluids and/or gases from the body part, in order to separate or transect a body part

Body Part	Approach	Device	Qualifier
Character 4	Character 5	Character 6	Character 7
0 Brain 7 Cerebral Hemisphere 8 Basal Ganglia F Olfactory Nerve G Optic Nerve H Oculomotor Nerve J Trochlear Nerve K Trigeminal Nerve L Abducens Nerve M Facial Nerve N Acoustic Nerve P Glossopharyngeal Nerve Q Vagus Nerve R Accessory Nerve S Hypoglossal Nerve W Cervical Spinal Cord X Thoracic Spinal Cord Y Lumbar Spinal Cord	0 Open 3 Percutaneous 4 Percutaneous Endoscopic	Z No Device	Z No Qualifier

LC Limited Coverage   NC Noncovered   HAC HAC-associated Procedure   CC Combination Cluster - See Appendix G for code lists
DRG Non-OR-Affecting MS-DRG Assignment   New/Revised Text in Orange   ♂ Male   ♀ Female

174   2021 ICD-10-PCS

0   Medical and Surgical
0   Central Nervous System and Cranial Nerves
9   Drainage: Taking or letting out fluids and/or gases from a body part

Body Part	Approach	Device	Qualifier
Character 4	Character 5	Character 6	Character 7
0 Brain 1 Cerebral Meninges 2 Dura Mater 3 Epidural Space, Intracranial 4 Subdural Space, Intracranial 5 Subarachnoid Space, Intracranial 6 Cerebral Ventricle 7 Cerebral Hemisphere 8 Basal Ganglia 9 Thalamus A Hypothalamus B Pons C Cerebellum D Medulla Oblongata F Olfactory Nerve G Optic Nerve H Oculomotor Nerve J Trochlear Nerve K Trigeminal Nerve L Abducens Nerve M Facial Nerve N Acoustic Nerve P Glossopharyngeal Nerve Q Vagus Nerve R Accessory Nerve S Hypoglossal Nerve T Spinal Meninges U Spinal Canal W Cervical Spinal Cord X Thoracic Spinal Cord Y Lumbar Spinal Cord	0 Open 3 Percutaneous 4 Percutaneous Endoscopic	0 Drainage Device	Z No Qualifier
0 Brain 1 Cerebral Meninges 2 Dura Mater 3 Epidural Space, Intracranial 4 Subdural Space, Intracranial 5 Subarachnoid Space, Intracranial 6 Cerebral Ventricle 7 Cerebral Hemisphere 8 Basal Ganglia 9 Thalamus A Hypothalamus B Pons C Cerebellum D Medulla Oblongata F Olfactory Nerve G Optic Nerve H Oculomotor Nerve J Trochlear Nerve K Trigeminal Nerve L Abducens Nerve M Facial Nerve N Acoustic Nerve P Glossopharyngeal Nerve Q Vagus Nerve R Accessory Nerve S Hypoglossal Nerve T Spinal Meninges U Spinal Canal W Cervical Spinal Cord X Thoracic Spinal Cord Y Lumbar Spinal Cord	0 Open 3 Percutaneous 4 Percutaneous Endoscopic	Z No Device	X Diagnostic Z No Qualifier

0 Medical and Surgical
0 Central Nervous System and Cranial Nerves
B Excision: Cutting out or off, without replacement, a portion of a body part

Body Part	Approach	Device	Qualifier
Character 4	Character 5	Character 6	Character 7
0 Brain	0 Open	Z No Device	X Diagnostic
1 Cerebral Meninges	3 Percutaneous		Z No Qualifier
2 Dura Mater	4 Percutaneous Endoscopic		
6 Cerebral Ventricle			
7 Cerebral Hemisphere			
8 Basal Ganglia			
9 Thalamus			
A Hypothalamus			
B Pons			
C Cerebellum			
D Medulla Oblongata			
F Olfactory Nerve			
G Optic Nerve			
H Oculomotor Nerve			
J Trochlear Nerve			
K Trigeminal Nerve			
L Abducens Nerve			
M Facial Nerve			
N Acoustic Nerve			
P Glossopharyngeal Nerve			
Q Vagus Nerve			
R Accessory Nerve			
S Hypoglossal Nerve			
T Spinal Meninges			
W Cervical Spinal Cord			
X Thoracic Spinal Cord			
Y Lumbar Spinal Cord			

0   **Medical and Surgical**
0   **Central Nervous System and Cranial Nerves**
C   **Extirpation:** Taking or cutting out solid matter from a body part

Body Part	Approach	Device	Qualifier
Character 4	Character 5	Character 6	Character 7
0 Brain 1 Cerebral Meninges 2 Dura Mater 3 Epidural Space, Intracranial 4 Subdural Space, Intracranial 5 Subarachnoid Space, Intracranial 6 Cerebral Ventricle 7 Cerebral Hemisphere 8 Basal Ganglia 9 Thalamus A Hypothalamus B Pons C Cerebellum D Medulla Oblongata F Olfactory Nerve G Optic Nerve H Oculomotor Nerve J Trochlear Nerve K Trigeminal Nerve L Abducens Nerve M Facial Nerve N Acoustic Nerve P Glossopharyngeal Nerve Q Vagus Nerve R Accessory Nerve S Hypoglossal Nerve T Spinal Meninges U Spinal Canal W Cervical Spinal Cord X Thoracic Spinal Cord Y Lumbar Spinal Cord	0 Open 3 Percutaneous 4 Percutaneous Endoscopic	Z No Device	Z No Qualifier

0   **Medical and Surgical**
0   **Central Nervous System and Cranial Nerves**
D   **Extraction:** Pulling or stripping out or off all or a portion of a body part by the use of force

Body Part	Approach	Device	Qualifier
Character 4	Character 5	Character 6	Character 7
1 Cerebral Meninges 2 Dura Mater F Olfactory Nerve G Optic Nerve H Oculomotor Nerve J Trochlear Nerve K Trigeminal Nerve L Abducens Nerve M Facial Nerve N Acoustic Nerve P Glossopharyngeal Nerve Q Vagus Nerve R Accessory Nerve S Hypoglossal Nerve T Spinal Meninges	0 Open 3 Percutaneous 4 Percutaneous Endoscopic	Z No Device	Z No Qualifier

LC Limited Coverage   NC Noncovered   HAC HAC-associated Procedure   CC Combination Cluster - See Appendix G for code lists
DRG Non-OR-Affecting MS-DRG Assignment   New/Revised Text in **Orange**   ♂ Male   ♀ Female

0 Medical and Surgical
0 Central Nervous System and Cranial Nerves
F Fragmentation: Breaking solid matter in a body part into pieces

Body Part	Approach	Device	Qualifier
Character 4	Character 5	Character 6	Character 7
3 Epidural Space, Intracranial NC 4 Subdural Space, Intracranial NC 5 Subarachnoid Space, Intracranial NC 6 Cerebral Ventricle NC U Spinal Canal	0 Open 3 Percutaneous 4 Percutaneous Endoscopic X External	Z No Device	Z No Qualifier

NC 00F3XZZ 00F4XZZ 00F5XZZ 00F6XZZ

0 Medical and Surgical
0 Central Nervous System and Cranial Nerves
H Insertion: Putting in a nonbiological appliance that monitors, assists, performs, or prevents a physiological function but does not physically take the place of a body part

Body Part	Approach	Device	Qualifier
Character 4	Character 5	Character 6	Character 7
0 Brain CC DRG	0 Open	1 Radioactive Element 2 Monitoring Device 3 Infusion Device 4 Radioactive Element, Cesium-131 Collagen Implant M Neurostimulator Lead Y Other Device	Z No Qualifier
0 Brain CC	3 Percutaneous 4 Percutaneous Endoscopic	1 Radioactive Element 2 Monitoring Device 3 Infusion Device M Neurostimulator Lead Y Other Device	Z No Qualifier
6 Cerebral Ventricle CC E Cranial Nerve CC U Spinal Canal CC V Spinal Cord CC	0 Open 3 Percutaneous 4 Percutaneous Endoscopic	1 Radioactive Element 2 Monitoring Device 3 Infusion Device M Neurostimulator Lead Y Other Device	Z No Qualifier

CC 00H00MZ 00H03MZ 00H04MZ 00H60MZ 00H63MZ 00H64MZ 00HE0MZ 00HE3MZ 00HE4MZ 00HU0MZ 00HU3MZ 00HU4MZ 00HV0MZ
00HV3MZ 00HV4MZ
DRG 00H004Z

0 Medical and Surgical
0 Central Nervous System and Cranial Nerves
J Inspection: Visually and/or manually exploring a body part

Body Part	Approach	Device	Qualifier
Character 4	Character 5	Character 6	Character 7
0 Brain E Cranial Nerve U Spinal Canal V Spinal Cord	0 Open 3 Percutaneous 4 Percutaneous Endoscopic	Z No Device	Z No Qualifier

LC Limited Coverage   NC Noncovered   HAC HAC-associated Procedure   CC Combination Cluster - See Appendix G for code lists
DRG Non-OR-Affecting MS-DRG Assignment   New/Revised Text in Orange   ♂ Male   ♀ Female

178

2021 ICD-10-PCS

0   **Medical and Surgical**

0   **Central Nervous System and Cranial Nerves**

K   **Map:** Locating the route of passage of electrical impulses and/or locating functional areas in a body part

Body Part	Approach	Device	Qualifier
Character 4	Character 5	Character 6	Character 7
0 Brain **7** Cerebral Hemisphere **8** Basal Ganglia **9** Thalamus **A** Hypothalamus **B** Pons **C** Cerebellum **D** Medulla Oblongata	**0** Open **3** Percutaneous **4** Percutaneous Endoscopic	**Z** No Device	**Z** No Qualifier

0   **Medical and Surgical**

0   **Central Nervous System and Cranial Nerves**

N   **Release:** Freeing a body part from an abnormal physical constraint by cutting or by the use of force

Body Part	Approach	Device	Qualifier
Character 4	Character 5	Character 6	Character 7
0 Brain **1** Cerebral Meninges **2** Dura Mater **6** Cerebral Ventricle **7** Cerebral Hemisphere **8** Basal Ganglia **9** Thalamus **A** Hypothalamus **B** Pons **C** Cerebellum **D** Medulla Oblongata **F** Olfactory Nerve **G** Optic Nerve **H** Oculomotor Nerve **J** Trochlear Nerve **K** Trigeminal Nerve **L** Abducens Nerve **M** Facial Nerve **N** Acoustic Nerve **P** Glossopharyngeal Nerve **Q** Vagus Nerve **R** Accessory Nerve **S** Hypoglossal Nerve **T** Spinal Meninges **W** Cervical Spinal Cord **X** Thoracic Spinal Cord **Y** Lumbar Spinal Cord	**0** Open **3** Percutaneous **4** Percutaneous Endoscopic	**Z** No Device	**Z** No Qualifier

LC Limited Coverage   **NC** Noncovered   **HAC** HAC-associated Procedure   **CC** Combination Cluster - See Appendix G for code lists

DRG Non-OR-Affecting MS-DRG Assignment   New/Revised Text in **Orange**   ♂ Male   ♀ Female

2021 ICD-10-PCS

179

0 **Medical and Surgical**
0 **Central Nervous System and Cranial Nerves**
P **Removal:** Taking out or off a device from a body part

Body Part	Approach	Device	Qualifier
Character 4	Character 5	Character 6	Character 7
0 Brain V Spinal Cord	0 Open 3 Percutaneous 4 Percutaneous Endoscopic	0 Drainage Device 2 Monitoring Device 3 Infusion Device 7 Autologous Tissue Substitute J Synthetic Substitute K Nonautologous Tissue Substitute M Neurostimulator Lead Y Other Device	Z No Qualifier
0 Brain V Spinal Cord	X External	0 Drainage Device 2 Monitoring Device 3 Infusion Device M Neurostimulator Lead	Z No Qualifier
6 Cerebral Ventricle U Spinal Canal	0 Open 3 Percutaneous 4 Percutaneous Endoscopic	0 Drainage Device 2 Monitoring Device 3 Infusion Device J Synthetic Substitute M Neurostimulator Lead Y Other Device	Z No Qualifier
6 Cerebral Ventricle U Spinal Canal	X External	0 Drainage Device 2 Monitoring Device 3 Infusion Device M Neurostimulator Lead	Z No Qualifier
E Cranial Nerve	0 Open 3 Percutaneous 4 Percutaneous Endoscopic	0 Drainage Device 2 Monitoring Device 3 Infusion Device 7 Autologous Tissue Substitute M Neurostimulator Lead Y Other Device	Z No Qualifier
E Cranial Nerve	X External	0 Drainage Device 2 Monitoring Device 3 Infusion Device M Neurostimulator Lead	Z No Qualifier

LC Limited Coverage   NC Noncovered   HAC HAC-associated Procedure   CC Combination Cluster - See Appendix G for code lists
DRG Non-OR-Affecting MS-DRG Assignment   New/Revised Text in Orange   ♂ Male   ♀ Female

180

2021 ICD-10-PCS

0 **Medical and Surgical**
0 **Central Nervous System and Cranial Nerves**
Q **Repair:** Restoring, to the extent possible, a body part to its normal anatomic structure and function

Body Part	Approach	Device	Qualifier
Character 4	Character 5	Character 6	Character 7
0 Brain	0 Open	Z No Device	Z No Qualifier
1 Cerebral Meninges	3 Percutaneous		
2 Dura Mater	4 Percutaneous Endoscopic		
6 Cerebral Ventricle			
7 Cerebral Hemisphere			
8 Basal Ganglia			
9 Thalamus			
A Hypothalamus			
B Pons			
C Cerebellum			
D Medulla Oblongata			
F Olfactory Nerve			
G Optic Nerve			
H Oculomotor Nerve			
J Trochlear Nerve			
K Trigeminal Nerve			
L Abducens Nerve			
M Facial Nerve			
N Acoustic Nerve			
P Glossopharyngeal Nerve			
Q Vagus Nerve			
R Accessory Nerve			
S Hypoglossal Nerve			
T Spinal Meninges			
W Cervical Spinal Cord			
X Thoracic Spinal Cord			
Y Lumbar Spinal Cord			

0 **Medical and Surgical**
0 **Central Nervous System and Cranial Nerves**
R **Replacement:** Putting in or on biological or synthetic material that physically takes the place and/or function of all or a portion of a body part

Body Part	Approach	Device	Qualifier
Character 4	Character 5	Character 6	Character 7
1 Cerebral Meninges	0 Open	7 Autologous Tissue Substitute	Z No Qualifier
2 Dura Mater	4 Percutaneous Endoscopic	J Synthetic Substitute	
6 Cerebral Ventricle		K Nonautologous Tissue Substitute	
F Olfactory Nerve			
G Optic Nerve			
H Oculomotor Nerve			
J Trochlear Nerve			
K Trigeminal Nerve			
L Abducens Nerve			
M Facial Nerve			
N Acoustic Nerve			
P Glossopharyngeal Nerve			
Q Vagus Nerve			
R Accessory Nerve			
S Hypoglossal Nerve			
T Spinal Meninges			

0   Medical and Surgical
0   Central Nervous System and Cranial Nerves
S   Reposition: Moving to its normal location, or other suitable location, all or a portion of a body part

Body Part	Approach	Device	Qualifier
Character 4	Character 5	Character 6	Character 7
F Olfactory Nerve **G** Optic Nerve **H** Oculomotor Nerve **J** Trochlear Nerve **K** Trigeminal Nerve **L** Abducens Nerve **M** Facial Nerve **N** Acoustic Nerve **P** Glossopharyngeal Nerve **Q** Vagus Nerve **R** Accessory Nerve **S** Hypoglossal Nerve **W** Cervical Spinal Cord **X** Thoracic Spinal Cord **Y** Lumbar Spinal Cord	**0** Open **3** Percutaneous **4** Percutaneous Endoscopic	**Z** No Device	**Z** No Qualifier

0   Medical and Surgical
0   Central Nervous System and Cranial Nerves
T   Resection: Cutting out or off, without replacement, all of a body part

Body Part	Approach	Device	Qualifier
Character 4	Character 5	Character 6	Character 7
7 Cerebral Hemisphere	**0** Open **3** Percutaneous **4** Percutaneous Endoscopic	**Z** No Device	**Z** No Qualifier

0   Medical and Surgical
0   Central Nervous System and Cranial Nerves
U   Supplement: Putting in or on biological or synthetic material that physically reinforces and/or augments the function of a portion of a body part

Body Part	Approach	Device	Qualifier
Character 4	Character 5	Character 6	Character 7
1 Cerebral Meninges **2** Dura Mater **6** Cerebral Ventricle **F** Olfactory Nerve **G** Optic Nerve **H** Oculomotor Nerve **J** Trochlear Nerve **K** Trigeminal Nerve **L** Abducens Nerve **M** Facial Nerve **N** Acoustic Nerve **P** Glossopharyngeal Nerve **Q** Vagus Nerve **R** Accessory Nerve **S** Hypoglossal Nerve **T** Spinal Meninges	**0** Open **3** Percutaneous **4** Percutaneous Endoscopic	**7** Autologous Tissue Substitute **J** Synthetic Substitute **K** Nonautologous Tissue Substitute	**Z** No Qualifier

LC Limited Coverage   **NC** Noncovered   **HAC** HAC-associated Procedure   **CC** Combination Cluster - See Appendix G for code lists
DRG Non-OR-Affecting MS-DRG Assignment   New/Revised Text in **Orange**   ♂ Male   ♀ Female

182

2021 ICD-10-PCS

0 Medical and Surgical
0 Central Nervous System and Cranial Nerves
W Revision: Correcting, to the extent possible, a portion of a malfunctioning device or the position of a displaced device

Body Part	Approach	Device	Qualifier
Character 4	Character 5	Character 6	Character 7
0 Brain **V** Spinal Cord	**0** Open **3** Percutaneous **4** Percutaneous Endoscopic	**0** Drainage Device **2** Monitoring Device **3** Infusion Device **7** Autologous Tissue Substitute **J** Synthetic Substitute **K** Nonautologous Tissue Substitute **M** Neurostimulator Lead **Y** Other Device	**Z** No Qualifier
0 Brain **V** Spinal Cord	**X** External	**0** Drainage Device **2** Monitoring Device **3** Infusion Device **7** Autologous Tissue Substitute **J** Synthetic Substitute **K** Nonautologous Tissue Substitute **M** Neurostimulator Lead	**Z** No Qualifier
6 Cerebral Ventricle **U** Spinal Canal	**0** Open **3** Percutaneous **4** Percutaneous Endoscopic	**0** Drainage Device **2** Monitoring Device **3** Infusion Device **J** Synthetic Substitute **M** Neurostimulator Lead **Y** Other Device	**Z** No Qualifier
6 Cerebral Ventricle **U** Spinal Canal	**X** External	**0** Drainage Device **2** Monitoring Device **3** Infusion Device **J** Synthetic Substitute **M** Neurostimulator Lead	**Z** No Qualifier
E Cranial Nerve	**0** Open **3** Percutaneous **4** Percutaneous Endoscopic	**0** Drainage Device **2** Monitoring Device **3** Infusion Device **7** Autologous Tissue Substitute **M** Neurostimulator Lead **Y** Other Device	**Z** No Qualifier
E Cranial Nerve	**X** External	**0** Drainage Device **2** Monitoring Device **3** Infusion Device **7** Autologous Tissue Substitute **M** Neurostimulator Lead	**Z** No Qualifier

0 Medical and Surgical
0 Central Nervous System and Cranial Nerves
X Transfer: Moving, without taking out, all or a portion of a body part to another location to take over the function of all or a portion of a body part

Body Part	Approach	Device	Qualifier
Character 4	Character 5	Character 6	Character 7
F Olfactory Nerve **G** Optic Nerve **H** Oculomotor Nerve **J** Trochlear Nerve **K** Trigeminal Nerve **L** Abducens Nerve **M** Facial Nerve **N** Acoustic Nerve **P** Glossopharyngeal Nerve **Q** Vagus Nerve **R** Accessory Nerve **S** Hypoglossal Nerve	**0** Open **4** Percutaneous Endoscopic	**Z** No Device	**F** Olfactory Nerve **G** Optic Nerve **H** Oculomotor Nerve **J** Trochlear Nerve **K** Trigeminal Nerve **L** Abducens Nerve **M** Facial Nerve **N** Acoustic Nerve **P** Glossopharyngeal Nerve **Q** Vagus Nerve **R** Accessory Nerve **S** Hypoglossal Nerve

NOTES

Peripheral Nervous System 012-01X

0 Medical and Surgical
1 Peripheral Nervous System
2 **Change:** Taking out or off a device from a body part and putting back an identical or similar device in or on the same body part without cutting or puncturing the skin or a mucous membrane

Body Part	Approach	Device	Qualifier
Character 4	Character 5	Character 6	Character 7
Y Peripheral Nerve	**X** External	**0** Drainage Device **Y** Other Device	**Z** No Qualifier

0 Medical and Surgical
1 Peripheral Nervous System
5 **Destruction:** Physical eradication of all or a portion of a body part by the direct use of energy, force, or a destructive agent

Body Part	Approach	Device	Qualifier
Character 4	Character 5	Character 6	Character 7
0 Cervical Plexus **1** Cervical Nerve **2** Phrenic Nerve **3** Brachial Plexus **4** Ulnar Nerve **5** Median Nerve **6** Radial Nerve **8** Thoracic Nerve **9** Lumbar Plexus **A** Lumbosacral Plexus **B** Lumbar Nerve **C** Pudendal Nerve **D** Femoral Nerve **F** Sciatic Nerve **G** Tibial Nerve **H** Peroneal Nerve **K** Head and Neck Sympathetic Nerve **L** Thoracic Sympathetic Nerve **M** Abdominal Sympathetic Nerve **N** Lumbar Sympathetic Nerve **P** Sacral Sympathetic Nerve **Q** Sacral Plexus **R** Sacral Nerve	**0** Open **3** Percutaneous **4** Percutaneous Endoscopic	**Z** No Device	**Z** No Qualifier

---

IC Limited Coverage   **NC** Noncovered   **HAC** HAC-associated Procedure   **CC** Combination Cluster - See Appendix G for code lists

DRG Non-OR-Affecting MS-DRG Assignment   New/Revised Text in Orange   ♂ Male   ♀ Female

2021 ICD-10-PCS

185

PERIPHERAL NERVOUS SYSTEM 012-01X

018-019

0 Medical and Surgical
1 Peripheral Nervous System
8 Division: Cutting into a body part, without draining fluids and/or gases from the body part, in order to separate or transect a body part

Body Part	Approach	Device	Qualifier
Character 4	Character 5	Character 6	Character 7
0 Cervical Plexus 1 Cervical Nerve 2 Phrenic Nerve 3 Brachial Plexus 4 Ulnar Nerve 5 Median Nerve 6 Radial Nerve 8 Thoracic Nerve 9 Lumbar Plexus A Lumbosacral Plexus B Lumbar Nerve C Pudendal Nerve D Femoral Nerve F Sciatic Nerve G Tibial Nerve H Peroneal Nerve K Head and Neck Sympathetic Nerve L Thoracic Sympathetic Nerve M Abdominal Sympathetic Nerve N Lumbar Sympathetic Nerve P Sacral Sympathetic Nerve Q Sacral Plexus R Sacral Nerve	0 Open 3 Percutaneous 4 Percutaneous Endoscopic	Z No Device	Z No Qualifier

0 Medical and Surgical
1 Peripheral Nervous System
9 Drainage: Taking or letting out fluids and/or gases from a body part

Body Part	Approach	Device	Qualifier
Character 4	Character 5	Character 6	Character 7
0 Cervical Plexus 1 Cervical Nerve 2 Phrenic Nerve 3 Brachial Plexus 4 Ulnar Nerve 5 Median Nerve 6 Radial Nerve 8 Thoracic Nerve 9 Lumbar Plexus A Lumbosacral Plexus B Lumbar Nerve C Pudendal Nerve D Femoral Nerve F Sciatic Nerve G Tibial Nerve H Peroneal Nerve K Head and Neck Sympathetic Nerve L Thoracic Sympathetic Nerve M Abdominal Sympathetic Nerve N Lumbar Sympathetic Nerve P Sacral Sympathetic Nerve Q Sacral Plexus R Sacral Nerve	0 Open 3 Percutaneous 4 Percutaneous Endoscopic	0 Drainage Device	Z No Qualifier

019 continued on next page

0   Medical and Surgical
1   Peripheral Nervous System
9   **Drainage:** Taking or letting out fluids and/or gases from a body part

019 continued from previous page

Body Part	Approach	Device	Qualifier
Character 4	Character 5	Character 6	Character 7
0 Cervical Plexus 1 Cervical Nerve 2 Phrenic Nerve 3 Brachial Plexus 4 Ulnar Nerve 5 Median Nerve 6 Radial Nerve 8 Thoracic Nerve 9 Lumbar Plexus A Lumbosacral Plexus B Lumbar Nerve C Pudendal Nerve D Femoral Nerve F Sciatic Nerve G Tibial Nerve H Peroneal Nerve K Head and Neck Sympathetic Nerve L Thoracic Sympathetic Nerve M Abdominal Sympathetic Nerve N Lumbar Sympathetic Nerve P Sacral Sympathetic Nerve Q Sacral Plexus R Sacral Nerve	0 Open 3 Percutaneous 4 Percutaneous Endoscopic	Z No Device	X Diagnostic Z No Qualifier

0   Medical and Surgical
1   Peripheral Nervous System
B   **Excision:** Cutting out or off, without replacement, a portion of a body part

Body Part	Approach	Device	Qualifier
Character 4	Character 5	Character 6	Character 7
0 Cervical Plexus 1 Cervical Nerve 2 Phrenic Nerve 3 Brachial Plexus 4 Ulnar Nerve 5 Median Nerve 6 Radial Nerve 8 Thoracic Nerve 9 Lumbar Plexus A Lumbosacral Plexus B Lumbar Nerve C Pudendal Nerve D Femoral Nerve F Sciatic Nerve G Tibial Nerve H Peroneal Nerve K Head and Neck Sympathetic Nerve L Thoracic Sympathetic Nerve M Abdominal Sympathetic Nerve N Lumbar Sympathetic Nerve P Sacral Sympathetic Nerve Q Sacral Plexus R Sacral Nerve	0 Open 3 Percutaneous 4 Percutaneous Endoscopic	Z No Device	X Diagnostic Z No Qualifier

0 **Medical and Surgical**
1 **Peripheral Nervous System**
C **Extirpation:** Taking or cutting out solid matter from a body part

Body Part	Approach	Device	Qualifier
Character 4	Character 5	Character 6	Character 7
0 Cervical Plexus	0 Open	Z No Device	Z No Qualifier
1 Cervical Nerve	3 Percutaneous		
2 Phrenic Nerve	4 Percutaneous Endoscopic		
3 Brachial Plexus			
4 Ulnar Nerve			
5 Median Nerve			
6 Radial Nerve			
8 Thoracic Nerve			
9 Lumbar Plexus			
A Lumbosacral Plexus			
B Lumbar Nerve			
C Pudendal Nerve			
D Femoral Nerve			
F Sciatic Nerve			
G Tibial Nerve			
H Peroneal Nerve			
K Head and Neck Sympathetic Nerve			
L Thoracic Sympathetic Nerve			
M Abdominal Sympathetic Nerve			
N Lumbar Sympathetic Nerve			
P Sacral Sympathetic Nerve			
Q Sacral Plexus			
R Sacral Nerve			

0 **Medical and Surgical**
1 **Peripheral Nervous System**
D **Extraction:** Pulling or stripping out or off all or a portion of a body part by the use of force

Body Part	Approach	Device	Qualifier
Character 4	Character 5	Character 6	Character 7
0 Cervical Plexus	0 Open	Z No Device	Z No Qualifier
1 Cervical Nerve	3 Percutaneous		
2 Phrenic Nerve	4 Percutaneous Endoscopic		
3 Brachial Plexus			
4 Ulnar Nerve			
5 Median Nerve			
6 Radial Nerve			
8 Thoracic Nerve			
9 Lumbar Plexus			
A Lumbosacral Plexus			
B Lumbar Nerve			
C Pudendal Nerve			
D Femoral Nerve			
F Sciatic Nerve			
G Tibial Nerve			
H Peroneal Nerve			
K Head and Neck Sympathetic Nerve			
L Thoracic Sympathetic Nerve			
M Abdominal Sympathetic Nerve			
N Lumbar Sympathetic Nerve			
P Sacral Sympathetic Nerve			
Q Sacral Plexus			
R Sacral Nerve			

LC Limited Coverage   NC Noncovered   HAC HAC-associated Procedure   CC Combination Cluster - See Appendix G for code lists
Non-OR-Affecting MS-DRG Assignment   New/Revised Text in **Orange**   ♂ Male   ♀ Female

PERIPHERAL NERVOUS SYSTEM 012-01X

188   2021 ICD-10-PCS

0 **Medical and Surgical**
1 **Peripheral Nervous System**
H **Insertion:** Putting in a nonbiological appliance that monitors, assists, performs, or prevents a physiological function but does not physically take the place of a body part

Body Part	Approach	Device	Qualifier
Character 4	Character 5	Character 6	Character 7
Y Peripheral Nerve ᴄᴄ	**0** Open **3** Percutaneous **4** Percutaneous Endoscopic	**1** Radioactive Element **2** Monitoring Device **M** Neurostimulator Lead **Y** Other Device	**Z** No Qualifier

ᴄᴄ   01HY0MZ   01HY3MZ   01HY4MZ

0 **Medical and Surgical**
1 **Peripheral Nervous System**
J **Inspection:** Visually and/or manually exploring a body part

Body Part	Approach	Device	Qualifier
Character 4	Character 5	Character 6	Character 7
Y Peripheral Nerve	**0** Open **3** Percutaneous **4** Percutaneous Endoscopic	**Z** No Device	**Z** No Qualifier

0 **Medical and Surgical**
1 **Peripheral Nervous System**
N **Release:** Freeing a body part from an abnormal physical constraint by cutting or by the use of force

Body Part	Approach	Device	Qualifier
Character 4	Character 5	Character 6	Character 7
0 Cervical Plexus **1** Cervical Nerve **2** Phrenic Nerve **3** Brachial Plexus **4** Ulnar Nerve **5** Median Nerve **6** Radial Nerve **8** Thoracic Nerve **9** Lumbar Plexus **A** Lumbosacral Plexus **B** Lumbar Nerve **C** Pudendal Nerve **D** Femoral Nerve **F** Sciatic Nerve **G** Tibial Nerve **H** Peroneal Nerve **K** Head and Neck Sympathetic Nerve **L** Thoracic Sympathetic Nerve **M** Abdominal Sympathetic Nerve **N** Lumbar Sympathetic Nerve **P** Sacral Sympathetic Nerve **Q** Sacral Plexus **R** Sacral Nerve	**0** Open **3** Percutaneous **4** Percutaneous Endoscopic	**Z** No Device	**Z** No Qualifier

ʟᴄ Limited Coverage   ɴᴄ Noncovered   ʜᴀᴄ HAC-associated Procedure   ᴄᴄ Combination Cluster - See Appendix G for code lists
🚫 Non-OR-Affecting MS-DRG Assignment   New/Revised Text in **Orange**   ♂ Male   ♀ Female

2021 ICD-10-PCS

189

PERIPHERAL NERVOUS SYSTEM 012-01X

01H-01N

0   Medical and Surgical
1   Peripheral Nervous System
P   Removal: Taking out or off a device from a body part

Body Part	Approach	Device	Qualifier
Character 4	Character 5	Character 6	Character 7
Y Peripheral Nerve	**0** Open **3** Percutaneous **4** Percutaneous Endoscopic	**0** Drainage Device **2** Monitoring Device **7** Autologous Tissue Substitute **M** Neurostimulator Lead **Y** Other Device	**Z** No Qualifier
Y Peripheral Nerve	**X** External	**0** Drainage Device **2** Monitoring Device **M** Neurostimulator Lead	**Z** No Qualifier

0   Medical and Surgical
1   Peripheral Nervous System
Q   Repair: Restoring, to the extent possible, a body part to its normal anatomic structure and function

Body Part	Approach	Device	Qualifier
Character 4	Character 5	Character 6	Character 7
0 Cervical Plexus **1** Cervical Nerve **2** Phrenic Nerve **3** Brachial Plexus **4** Ulnar Nerve **5** Median Nerve **6** Radial Nerve **8** Thoracic Nerve **9** Lumbar Plexus **A** Lumbosacral Plexus **B** Lumbar Nerve **C** Pudendal Nerve **D** Femoral Nerve **F** Sciatic Nerve **G** Tibial Nerve **H** Peroneal Nerve **K** Head and Neck Sympathetic Nerve **L** Thoracic Sympathetic Nerve **M** Abdominal Sympathetic Nerve **N** Lumbar Sympathetic Nerve **P** Sacral Sympathetic Nerve **Q** Sacral Plexus **R** Sacral Nerve	**0** Open **3** Percutaneous **4** Percutaneous Endoscopic	**Z** No Device	**Z** No Qualifier

0   Medical and Surgical
1   Peripheral Nervous System
R   Replacement: Putting in or on biological or synthetic material that physically takes the place and/or function of all or a portion of a body part

Body Part	Approach	Device	Qualifier
Character 4	Character 5	Character 6	Character 7
1 Cervical Nerve **2** Phrenic Nerve **4** Ulnar Nerve **5** Median Nerve **6** Radial Nerve **8** Thoracic Nerve **B** Lumbar Nerve **C** Pudendal Nerve **D** Femoral Nerve **F** Sciatic Nerve **G** Tibial Nerve **H** Peroneal Nerve **R** Sacral Nerve	**0** Open **4** Percutaneous Endoscopic	**7** Autologous Tissue Substitute **J** Synthetic Substitute **K** Nonautologous Tissue Substitute	**Z** No Qualifier

LC Limited Coverage   **NC** Noncovered   **HAC** HAC-associated Procedure   **CC** Combination Cluster - See Appendix G for code lists
DRG Non-OR-Affecting MS-DRG Assignment   New/Revised Text in **Orange**   ♂ Male   ♀ Female

190

2021 ICD-10-PCS

0   **Medical and Surgical**
1   **Peripheral Nervous System**
S   **Reposition:** Moving to its normal location, or other suitable location, all or a portion of a body part

Body Part	Approach	Device	Qualifier
Character 4	Character 5	Character 6	Character 7
0 Cervical Plexus 1 Cervical Nerve 2 Phrenic Nerve 3 Brachial Plexus 4 Ulnar Nerve 5 Median Nerve 6 Radial Nerve 8 Thoracic Nerve 9 Lumbar Plexus A Lumbosacral Plexus B Lumbar Nerve C Pudendal Nerve D Femoral Nerve F Sciatic Nerve G Tibial Nerve H Peroneal Nerve Q Sacral Plexus R Sacral Nerve	0 Open 3 Percutaneous 4 Percutaneous Endoscopic	Z No Device	Z No Qualifier

0   **Medical and Surgical**
1   **Peripheral Nervous System**
U   **Supplement:** Putting in or on biological or synthetic material that physically reinforces and/or augments the function of a portion of a body part

Body Part	Approach	Device	Qualifier
Character 4	Character 5	Character 6	Character 7
1 Cervical Nerve 2 Phrenic Nerve 4 Ulnar Nerve 5 Median Nerve 6 Radial Nerve 8 Thoracic Nerve B Lumbar Nerve C Pudendal Nerve D Femoral Nerve F Sciatic Nerve G Tibial Nerve H Peroneal Nerve R Sacral Nerve	0 Open 3 Percutaneous 4 Percutaneous Endoscopic	7 Autologous Tissue Substitute J Synthetic Substitute K Nonautologous Tissue Substitute	Z No Qualifier

0   **Medical and Surgical**
1   **Peripheral Nervous System**
W   **Revision:** Correcting, to the extent possible, a portion of a malfunctioning device or the position of a displaced device

Body Part	Approach	Device	Qualifier
Character 4	Character 5	Character 6	Character 7
Y Peripheral Nerve	0 Open 3 Percutaneous 4 Percutaneous Endoscopic	0 Drainage Device 2 Monitoring Device 7 Autologous Tissue Substitute M Neurostimulator Lead Y Other Device	Z No Qualifier
Y Peripheral Nerve	X External	0 Drainage Device 2 Monitoring Device 7 Autologous Tissue Substitute M Neurostimulator Lead	Z No Qualifier

LC Limited Coverage   NC Noncovered   HAC HAC-associated Procedure   CC Combination Cluster - See Appendix G for code lists
DRG Non-OR-Affecting MS-DRG Assignment   New/Revised Text in Orange   ♂ Male   ♀ Female

2021 ICD-10-PCS

191

0   Medical and Surgical
1   Peripheral Nervous System
X   Transfer: Moving, without taking out, all or a portion of a body part to another location to take over the function of all or a portion of a body part

Body Part		Approach		Device		Qualifier	
Character 4		**Character 5**		**Character 6**		**Character 7**	
1	Cervical Nerve	0	Open	Z	No Device	1	Cervical Nerve
2	Phrenic Nerve	4	Percutaneous Endoscopic			2	Phrenic Nerve
4	Ulnar Nerve	0	Open	Z	No Device	4	Ulnar Nerve
5	Median Nerve	4	Percutaneous Endoscopic			5	Median Nerve
6	Radial Nerve					6	Radial Nerve
8	Thoracic Nerve	0	Open	Z	No Device	8	Thoracic Nerve
		4	Percutaneous Endoscopic				
B	Lumbar Nerve	0	Open	Z	No Device	B	Lumbar Nerve
C	Pudendal Nerve	4	Percutaneous Endoscopic			C	Perineal Nerve
D	Femoral Nerve	0	Open	Z	No Device	D	Femoral Nerve
F	Sciatic Nerve	4	Percutaneous Endoscopic			F	Sciatic Nerve
G	Tibial Nerve					G	Tibial Nerve
H	Peroneal Nerve					H	Peroneal Nerve

IC Limited Coverage   NC Noncovered   HAC HAC-associated Procedure   CC Combination Cluster - See Appendix G for code lists
DRG Non-OR-Affecting MS-DRG Assignment   New/Revised Text in **Orange**   ♂ Male   ♀ Female

192

2021 ICD-10-PCS

NOTES

NOTES

Heart and Great Vessels 021-02Y

0 Medical and Surgical
2 Heart and Great Vessels
1 Bypass: Altering the route of passage of the contents of a tubular body part

Body Part	Approach	Device	Qualifier
Character 4	Character 5	Character 6	Character 7
0 Coronary Artery, One Artery HAC 1 Coronary Artery, Two Arteries HAC 2 Coronary Artery, Three Arteries HAC 3 Coronary Artery, Four or More Arteries HAC	0 Open	8 Zooplastic Tissue 9 Autologous Venous Tissue A Autologous Arterial Tissue J Synthetic Substitute K Nonautologous Tissue Substitute	3 Coronary Artery 8 Internal Mammary, Right 9 Internal Mammary, Left C Thoracic Artery F Abdominal Artery W Aorta
0 Coronary Artery, One Artery HAC 1 Coronary Artery, Two Arteries HAC 2 Coronary Artery, Three Arteries HAC 3 Coronary Artery, Four or More Arteries HAC	0 Open	Z No Device	3 Coronary Artery 8 Internal Mammary, Right 9 Internal Mammary, Left C Thoracic Artery F Abdominal Artery
0 Coronary Artery, One Artery 1 Coronary Artery, Two Arteries 2 Coronary Artery, Three Arteries 3 Coronary Artery, Four or More Arteries	3 Percutaneous	4 Intraluminal Device, Drug-eluting D Intraluminal Device	4 Coronary Vein
0 Coronary Artery, One Artery 1 Coronary Artery, Two Arteries 2 Coronary Artery, Three Arteries 3 Coronary Artery, Four or More Arteries	4 Percutaneous Endoscopic	4 Intraluminal Device, Drug-eluting D Intraluminal Device	4 Coronary Vein
0 Coronary Artery, One Artery HAC 1 Coronary Artery, Two Arteries HAC 2 Coronary Artery, Three Arteries HAC 3 Coronary Artery, Four or More Arteries HAC	4 Percutaneous Endoscopic	8 Zooplastic Tissue 9 Autologous Venous Tissue A Autologous Arterial Tissue J Synthetic Substitute K Nonautologous Tissue Substitute	3 Coronary Artery 8 Internal Mammary, Right 9 Internal Mammary, Left C Thoracic Artery F Abdominal Artery W Aorta
0 Coronary Artery, One Artery HAC 1 Coronary Artery, Two Arteries HAC 2 Coronary Artery, Three Arteries HAC 3 Coronary Artery, Four or More Arteries HAC	4 Percutaneous Endoscopic	Z No Device	3 Coronary Artery 8 Internal Mammary, Right 9 Internal Mammary, Left C Thoracic Artery F Abdominal Artery
6 Atrium, Right	0 Open 4 Percutaneous Endoscopic	8 Zooplastic Tissue 9 Autologous Venous Tissue A Autologous Arterial Tissue J Synthetic Substitute K Nonautologous Tissue Substitute	P Pulmonary Trunk Q Pulmonary Artery, Right R Pulmonary Artery, Left
6 Atrium, Right	0 Open 4 Percutaneous Endoscopic	Z No Device	7 Atrium, Left P Pulmonary Trunk Q Pulmonary Artery, Right R Pulmonary Artery, Left

021 continued on next page

LC Limited Coverage   NC Noncovered   HAC HAC-associated Procedure   CC Combination Cluster - See Appendix G for code lists
DRG Non-OR-Affecting MS-DRG Assignment   New/Revised Text in Orange   ♂ Male   ♀ Female

0 Medical and Surgical
2 Heart and Great Vessels
1 Bypass: Altering the route of passage of the contents of a tubular body part

021 continued from previous page

Body Part	Approach	Device	Qualifier
Character 4	Character 5	Character 6	Character 7
6 Atrium, Right	**3** Percutaneous	**Z** No Device	**7** Atrium, Left
7 Atrium, Left	**0** Open **4** Percutaneous Endoscopic	**8** Zooplastic Tissue **9** Autologous Venous Tissue **A** Autologous Arterial Tissue **J** Synthetic Substitute **K** Nonautologous Tissue Substitute **Z** No Device	**P** Pulmonary Trunk **Q** Pulmonary Artery, Right **R** Pulmonary Artery, Left **S** Pulmonary Vein, Right **T** Pulmonary Vein, Left **U** Pulmonary Vein, Confluence
7 Atrium, Left	**3** Percutaneous	**J** Synthetic Substitute	**6** Atrium, Right
K Ventricle, Right **L** Ventricle, Left	**0** Open **4** Percutaneous Endoscopic	**8** Zooplastic Tissue **9** Autologous Venous Tissue **A** Autologous Arterial Tissue **J** Synthetic Substitute **K** Nonautologous Tissue Substitute	**P** Pulmonary Trunk **Q** Pulmonary Artery, Right **R** Pulmonary Artery, Left
K Ventricle, Right **L** Ventricle, Left	**0** Open **4** Percutaneous Endoscopic	**Z** No Device	**5** Coronary Circulation **8** Internal Mammary, Right **9** Internal Mammary, Left **C** Thoracic Artery **F** Abdominal Artery **P** Pulmonary Trunk **Q** Pulmonary Artery, Right **R** Pulmonary Artery, Left **W** Aorta
P Pulmonary Trunk **Q** Pulmonary Artery, Right **R** Pulmonary Artery, Left	**0** Open **4** Percutaneous Endoscopic	**8** Zooplastic Tissue **9** Autologous Venous Tissue **A** Autologous Arterial Tissue **J** Synthetic Substitute **K** Nonautologous Tissue Substitute **Z** No Device	**A** Innominate Artery **B** Subclavian **D** Carotid
V Superior Vena Cava	**0** Open **4** Percutaneous Endoscopic	**8** Zooplastic Tissue **9** Autologous Venous Tissue **A** Autologous Arterial Tissue **J** Synthetic Substitute **K** Nonautologous Tissue Substitute **Z** No Device	**P** Pulmonary Trunk **Q** Pulmonary Artery, Right **R** Pulmonary Artery, Left **S** Pulmonary Vein, Right **T** Pulmonary Vein, Left **U** Pulmonary Vein, Confluence
W Thoracic Aorta, Descending	**0** Open	**8** Zooplastic Tissue **9** Autologous Venous Tissue **A** Autologous Arterial Tissue **J** Synthetic Substitute **K** Nonautologous Tissue Substitute	**A** Innominate Artery **B** Subclavian **D** Carotid **F** Abdominal Artery **G** Axillary Artery **H** Brachial Artery **P** Pulmonary Trunk **Q** Pulmonary Artery, Right **R** Pulmonary Artery, Left **V** Lower Extremity Artery
W Thoracic Aorta, Descending	**0** Open	**Z** No Device	**A** Innominate Artery **B** Subclavian **D** Carotid **P** Pulmonary Trunk **Q** Pulmonary Artery, Right **R** Pulmonary Artery, Left

021 continued on next page

LC Limited Coverage   NC Noncovered   HAC HAC-associated Procedure   CC Combination Cluster - See Appendix G for code lists
⬛ Non-OR-Affecting MS-DRG Assignment   New/Revised Text in **Orange**   ♂ Male   ♀ Female

0 **Medical and Surgical**

021 continued from previous page

2 **Heart and Great Vessels**
1 **Bypass:** Altering the route of passage of the contents of a tubular body part

Body Part	Approach	Device	Qualifier
Character 4	Character 5	Character 6	Character 7
W Thoracic Aorta, Descending	**4** Percutaneous Endoscopic	**8** Zooplastic Tissue **9** Autologous Venous Tissue **A** Autologous Arterial Tissue **J** Synthetic Substitute **K** Nonautologous Tissue Substitute **Z** No Device	**A** Innominate Artery **B** Subclavian **D** Carotid **P** Pulmonary Trunk **Q** Pulmonary Artery, Right **R** Pulmonary Artery, Left
X Thoracic Aorta, Ascending/Arch	**0** Open **4** Percutaneous Endoscopic	**8** Zooplastic Tissue **9** Autologous Venous Tissue **A** Autologous Arterial Tissue **J** Synthetic Substitute **K** Nonautologous Tissue Substitute **Z** No Device	**A** Innominate Artery **B** Subclavian **D** Carotid **P** Pulmonary Trunk **Q** Pulmonary Artery, Right **R** Pulmonary Artery, Left

HAC

0210083	0210088	0210089	021008C	021008F	021008W	0210093	0210098	0210099	021009C	021009F	021009W	02100A3
02100A8	02100A9	02100AC	02100AF	02100AW	02100J3	02100J8	02100J9	02100JC	02100JF	02100JW	02100K3	02100K8
02100K9	02100KC	02100KF	02100KW	02100Z3	02100Z8	02100Z9	02100ZC	02100ZF	0210483	0210488	0210489	021048C
021048F	021048W	0210493	0210498	0210499	021049C	021049F	021049W	02104A3	02104A8	02104A9	02104AC	02104AF
02104AW	02104J3	02104J8	02104J9	02104JC	02104JF	02104JW	02104K3	02104K8	02104K9	02104KC	02104KF	02104KW
02104Z3	02104Z8	02104Z9	02104ZC	02104ZF	0211083	0211088	0211089	021108C	021108F	021108W	0211093	0211098
0211099	021109C	021109F	021109W	02110A3	02110A8	02110A9	02110AC	02110AF	02110AW	02110J3	02110J8	02110J9
02110JC	02110JF	02110JW	02110K3	02110K8	02110K9	02110KC	02110KF	02110KW	02110Z3	02110Z8	02110Z9	02110ZC
02110ZF	0211483	0211488	0211489	021148C	021148F	021148W	0211493	0211498	0211499	021149C	021149F	021149W
02114A3	02114A8	02114A9	02114AC	02114AF	02114AW	02114J3	02114J8	02114J9	02114JC	02114JF	02114JW	02114K3
02114K8	02114K9	02114KC	02114KF	02114KW	02114Z3	02114Z8	02114Z9	02114ZC	02114ZF	0212083	0212088	0212089
021208C	021208F	021208W	0212093	0212098	0212099	021209C	021209F	021209W	02120A3	02120A8	02120A9	02120AC
02120AF	02120AW	02120J3	02120J8	02120J9	02120JC	02120JF	02120JW	02120K3	02120K8	02120K9	02120KC	02120KF
02120KW	02120Z3	02120Z8	02120Z9	02120ZC	02120ZF	0212483	0212488	0212489	021248C	021248F	021248W	0212493
0212498	0212499	021249C	021249F	021249W	02124A3	02124A8	02124A9	02124AC	02124AF	02124AW	02124J3	02124J8
02124J9	02124JC	02124JF	02124JW	02124K3	02124K8	02124K9	02124KC	02124KF	02124KW	02124Z3	02124Z8	02124Z9
02124ZC	02124ZF	0213083	0213088	0213089	021308C	021308F	0213088	0213093	0213098	0213099	021309C	021309F
021309W	02130A3	02130A8	02130A9	02130AC	02130AF	02130AW	02130J3	02130J8	02130J9	02130JC	02130JF	02130JW
02130K3	02130K8	02130K9	02130KC	02130KF	02130KW	02130Z3	02130Z8	02130Z9	02130ZC	02130ZF	0213483	0213488
0213489	021348C	021348F	021348W	0213493	0213498	0213499	021349C	021349F	021349W	02134A3	02134A8	02134A9
02134AC	02134AF	02134AW	02134J3	02134J8	02134J9	02134JC	02134JF	02134JW	02134K3	02134K8	02134K9	02134KC
02134KF	02134KW	02134Z3	02134Z8	02134Z9	02134ZC	02134ZF						

Surgical site infection-mediastinitis after coronary bypass graft (CABG) and secondary diagnosis J98.51, J98.59.

0 **Medical and Surgical**

2 **Heart and Great Vessels**

4 **Creation:** Putting in or on biological or synthetic material to form a new body part that to the extent possible replicates the anatomic structure or function of an absent body part

Body Part	Approach	Device	Qualifier
Character 4	Character 5	Character 6	Character 7
F Aortic Valve	**0** Open	**7** Autologous Tissue Substitute **8** Zooplastic Tissue **J** Synthetic Substitute **K** Nonautologous Tissue Substitute	**J** Truncal Valve
G Mitral Valve **J** Tricuspid Valve	**0** Open	**7** Autologous Tissue Substitute **8** Zooplastic Tissue **J** Synthetic Substitute **K** Nonautologous Tissue Substitute	**2** Common Atrioventricular Valve

LC Limited Coverage   **NC** Noncovered   **HAC** HAC-associated Procedure   **CC** Combination Cluster - See Appendix G for code lists
DRG Non-OR-Affecting MS-DRG Assignment   New/Revised Text in **Orange**   ♂ Male   ♀ Female

0   Medical and Surgical
2   Heart and Great Vessels
5   Destruction: Physical eradication of all or a portion of a body part by the direct use of energy, force, or a destructive agent

Body Part	Approach	Device	Qualifier
Character 4	Character 5	Character 6	Character 7
4 Coronary Vein 5 Atrial Septum 6 Atrium, Right 8 Conduction Mechanism 9 Chordae Tendineae D Papillary Muscle F Aortic Valve G Mitral Valve H Pulmonary Valve J Tricuspid Valve K Ventricle, Right L Ventricle, Left M Ventricular Septum N Pericardium P Pulmonary Trunk Q Pulmonary Artery, Right R Pulmonary Artery, Left S Pulmonary Vein, Right T Pulmonary Vein, Left V Superior Vena Cava W Thoracic Aorta, Descending X Thoracic Aorta, Ascending/Arch	0 Open 3 Percutaneous 4 Percutaneous Endoscopic	Z No Device	Z No Qualifier
7 Atrium, Left ᴰᴿᴳ	0 Open 3 Percutaneous 4 Percutaneous Endoscopic	Z No Device	K Left Atrial Appendage Z No Qualifier

ᴰᴿᴳ   02570ZK   02573ZK   02574ZK

ᴸᶜ Limited Coverage   ᴺᶜ Noncovered   ᴴᴬᶜ HAC-associated Procedure   ᶜᶜ Combination Cluster - See Appendix G for code lists
ᴰᴿᴳ Non-OR-Affecting MS-DRG Assignment   New/Revised Text in **Orange**   ♂ Male   ♀ Female

198

2021 ICD-10-PCS

0 **Medical and Surgical**
2 **Heart and Great Vessels**
7 **Dilation:** Expanding an orifice or the lumen of a tubular body part

Body Part	Approach	Device	Qualifier
Character 4	Character 5	Character 6	Character 7
0 Coronary Artery, One Artery **1** Coronary Artery, Two Arteries **2** Coronary Artery, Three Arteries **3** Coronary Artery, Four or More Arteries	**0** Open **3** Percutaneous **4** Percutaneous Endoscopic	**4** Intraluminal Device, Drug-eluting **5** Intraluminal Device, Drug-eluting, Two **6** Intraluminal Device, Drug-eluting, Three **7** Intraluminal Device, Drug-eluting, Four or More **D** Intraluminal Device **E** Intraluminal Device, Two **F** Intraluminal Device, Three **G** Intraluminal Device, Four or More **T** Intraluminal Device, Radioactive **Z** No Device	**6** Bifurcation **Z** No Qualifier
F Aortic Valve **G** Mitral Valve **H** Pulmonary Valve **J** Tricuspid Valve **K** Ventricle, Right **L** Ventricle, Left **P** Pulmonary Trunk **Q** Pulmonary Artery, Right **S** Pulmonary Vein, Right **T** Pulmonary Vein, Left **V** Superior Vena Cava **W** Thoracic Aorta, Descending **X** Thoracic Aorta, Ascending/Arch	**0** Open **3** Percutaneous **4** Percutaneous Endoscopic	**4** Intraluminal Device, Drug-eluting **D** Intraluminal Device **Z** No Device	**Z** No Qualifier
R Pulmonary Artery, Left	**0** Open **3** Percutaneous **4** Percutaneous Endoscopic	**4** Intraluminal Device, Drug-eluting **D** Intraluminal Device **Z** No Device	**T** Ductus Arteriosus **Z** No Qualifier

LC Limited Coverage **NC** Noncovered **HAC** HAC-associated Procedure **CC** Combination Cluster - See Appendix G for code lists
non Non-OR-Affecting MS-DRG Assignment New/Revised Text in **Orange** ♂ Male ♀ Female

2021 ICD-10-PCS 199

0 **Medical and Surgical**
2 **Heart and Great Vessels**
8 **Division:** Cutting into a body part, without draining fluids and/or gases from the body part, in order to separate or transect a body part

Body Part	Approach	Device	Qualifier
Character 4	Character 5	Character 6	Character 7
8 Conduction Mechanism **9** Chordae Tendineae **D** Papillary Muscle	**0** Open **3** Percutaneous **4** Percutaneous Endoscopic	**Z** No Device	**Z** No Qualifier

0 **Medical and Surgical**
2 **Heart and Great Vessels**
B **Excision:** Cutting out or off, without replacement, a portion of a body part

Body Part	Approach	Device	Qualifier
Character 4	Character 5	Character 6	Character 7
4 Coronary Vein **5** Atrial Septum **6** Atrium, Right **8** Conduction Mechanism **9** Chordae Tendineae **D** Papillary Muscle **F** Aortic Valve **G** Mitral Valve **H** Pulmonary Valve **J** Tricuspid Valve **K** Ventricle, Right **NC** **L** Ventricle, Left **NC** **M** Ventricular Septum **N** Pericardium **P** Pulmonary Trunk **Q** Pulmonary Artery, Right **R** Pulmonary Artery, Left **S** Pulmonary Vein, Right **T** Pulmonary Vein, Left **V** Superior Vena Cava **W** Thoracic Aorta, Descending **X** Thoracic Aorta, Ascending/Arch	**0** Open **3** Percutaneous **4** Percutaneous Endoscopic	**Z** No Device	**X** Diagnostic **Z** No Qualifier
7 Atrium, Left **DRG**	**0** Open **3** Percutaneous **4** Percutaneous Endoscopic	**Z** No Device	**K** Left Atrial Appendage **X** Diagnostic **Z** No Qualifier

NC 02BK0ZZ   02BK3ZZ   02BK4ZZ   02BL0ZZ   02BL3ZZ   02BL4ZZ
DRG 02B70ZK   02B73ZK   02B74ZK

LC Limited Coverage   **NC** Noncovered   **HAC** HAC-associated Procedure   **CC** Combination Cluster - See Appendix G for code lists
DRG Non-OR-Affecting MS-DRG Assignment   New/Revised Text in **Orange**   ♂ Male   ♀ Female

200

2021 ICD-10-PCS

0 **Medical and Surgical**
2 **Heart and Great Vessels**
C **Extirpation:** Taking or cutting out solid matter from a body part

Body Part	Approach	Device	Qualifier
Character 4	Character 5	Character 6	Character 7
0 Coronary Artery, One Artery **1** Coronary Artery, Two Arteries **2** Coronary Artery, Three Arteries **3** Coronary Artery, Four or More Arteries	**0** Open **3** Percutaneous **4** Percutaneous Endoscopic	**Z** No Device	**6** Bifurcation **Z** No Qualifier
4 Coronary Vein **5** Atrial Septum **6** Atrium, Right **7** Atrium, Left **8** Conduction Mechanism **9** Chordae Tendineae **D** Papillary Muscle **F** Aortic Valve **G** Mitral Valve **H** Pulmonary Valve **J** Tricuspid Valve **K** Ventricle, Right **L** Ventricle, Left **M** Ventricular Septum **N** Pericardium **P** Pulmonary Trunk **Q** Pulmonary Artery, Right **R** Pulmonary Artery, Left **S** Pulmonary Vein, Right **T** Pulmonary Vein, Left **V** Superior Vena Cava **W** Thoracic Aorta, Descending **X** Thoracic Aorta, Ascending/Arch	**0** Open **3** Percutaneous **4** Percutaneous Endoscopic	**Z** No Device	**Z** No Qualifier

0 **Medical and Surgical**
2 **Heart and Great Vessels**
F **Fragmentation:** Breaking solid matter in a body part into pieces

Body Part	Approach	Device	Qualifier
Character 4	Character 5	Character 6	Character 7
N Pericardium 🅝🅒	**0** Open **3** Percutaneous **4** Percutaneous Endoscopic **X** External	**Z** No Device	**Z** No Qualifier
P Pulmonary Trunk **Q** Pulmonary Artery, Right **R** Pulmonary Artery, Left **S** Pulmonary Vein, Right **T** Pulmonary Vein, Left	**3** Percutaneous	**Z** No Device	**0** Ultrasonic **Z** No Qualifier

🅝🅒 02FNXZZ

0 Medical and Surgical
2 Heart and Great Vessels
H Insertion: Putting in a nonbiological appliance that monitors, assists, performs, or prevents a physiological function but does not physically take the place of a body part

Body Part	Approach	Device	Qualifier
Character 4	**Character 5**	**Character 6**	**Character 7**
0 Coronary Artery, One Artery 1 Coronary Artery, Two Arteries 2 Coronary Artery, Three Arteries 3 Coronary Artery, Four or More Arteries	0 Open 3 Percutaneous 4 Percutaneous Endoscopic	D Intraluminal Device Y Other Device	Z No Qualifier
4 Coronary Vein ᴴᴬᶜ ᶜᶜ ᴰᴿᴳ 6 Atrium, Right ᴴᴬᶜ ᶜᶜ ᴰᴿᴳ 7 Atrium, Left ᴴᴬᶜ ᶜᶜ ᴰᴿᴳ K Ventricle, Right ᴴᴬᶜ ᶜᶜ ᴰᴿᴳ L Ventricle, Left ᴴᴬᶜ ᶜᶜ ᴰᴿᴳ	0 Open 3 Percutaneous 4 Percutaneous Endoscopic	0 Monitoring Device, Pressure Sensor 2 Monitoring Device 3 Infusion Device D Intraluminal Device J Cardiac Lead, Pacemaker K Cardiac Lead, Defibrillator M Cardiac Lead N Intracardiac Pacemaker Y Other Device	Z No Qualifier
A Heart ᴸᶜ ᴺᶜ	0 Open 3 Percutaneous 4 Percutaneous Endoscopic	Q Implantable Heart Assist System Y Other Device	Z No Qualifier
A Heart ᶜᶜ	0 Open 3 Percutaneous 4 Percutaneous Endoscopic	R Short term External Heart Assist System	J Intraoperative S Biventricular Z No Qualifier
N Pericardium ᴴᴬᶜ ᶜᶜ ᴰᴿᴳ	0 Open 3 Percutaneous 4 Percutaneous Endoscopic	0 Monitoring Device, Pressure Sensor 2 Monitoring Device J Cardiac Lead, Pacemaker K Cardiac Lead, Defibrillator M Cardiac Lead Y Other Device	Z No Qualifier
P Pulmonary Trunk Q Pulmonary Artery, Right R Pulmonary Artery, Left S Pulmonary Vein, Right ᴴᴬᶜ T Pulmonary Vein, Left ᴴᴬᶜ V Superior Vena Cava ᴴᴬᶜ W Thoracic Aorta, Descending	0 Open 3 Percutaneous 4 Percutaneous Endoscopic	0 Monitoring Device, Pressure Sensor 2 Monitoring Device 3 Infusion Device D Intraluminal Device Y Other Device	Z No Qualifier
X Thoracic Aorta, Ascending/Arch	0 Open 3 Percutaneous 4 Percutaneous Endoscopic	0 Monitoring Device, Pressure Sensor 2 Monitoring Device 3 Infusion Device D Intraluminal Device	Z No Qualifier

ᴸᶜ 02HA0QZ

ᴺᶜ 02HA3QZ   02HA4QZ

ᴴᴬᶜ 02H43JZ   02H43KZ   02H43MZ   02H633Z   02H63JZ   02H63MZ   02H73JZ   02H73MZ   02HK33Z   02HK3JZ   02HL3JZ   02HN0JZ   02HN0MZ
02HN3JZ   02HN3MZ   02HN4JZ   02HN4MZ

Surgical site infection (SSI) following cardiac implantable electronic device (CIED) procedures and secondary diagnosis K68.11, T81.40XA, T81.41XA, T81.42XA, T81.43XA, T81.44XA, T81.49XA, T82.6XXA, T82.7XXA.

ᴴᴬᶜ 02HS33Z   02HS43Z   02HT33Z   02HT43Z   02HV33Z   02HV43Z

Iatrogenic pneumothorax w/ venous catheterization procedures and secondary diagnosis J95.811.

ᶜᶜ 02H40JZ   02H40KZ   02H40MZ   02H43JZ   02H43KZ   02H43MZ   02H44JZ   02H44KZ   02H44MZ   02H60JZ   02H60KZ   02H60MZ   02H63JZ
02H63KZ   02H63MZ   02H64JZ   02H64KZ   02H64MZ   02H70JZ   02H70KZ   02H70MZ   02H73JZ   02H73KZ   02H73MZ   02H74JZ   02H74KZ
02H74MZ   02HA0RS   02HA0RZ   02HA3RS   02HA4RS   02HA4RZ   02HK0JZ   02HK0KZ   02HK0MZ   02HK3JZ   02HK3KZ   02HK3MZ   02HK4JZ
02HK4KZ   02HK4MZ   02HL0JZ   02HL0KZ   02HL0MZ   02HL3JZ   02HL3KZ   02HL3MZ   02HL4JZ   02HL4KZ   02HL4MZ   02HN0JZ   02HN0KZ
02HN0MZ   02HN3JZ   02HN3KZ   02HN3MZ   02HN4JZ   02HN4KZ   02HN4MZ

ᴰᴿᴳ 02H40JZ   02H40MZ   02H43JZ   02H43MZ   02H44JZ   02H44MZ   02H60JZ   02H60MZ   02H63JZ   02H63MZ   02H64JZ   02H64MZ   02H70JZ
02H70MZ   02H73JZ   02H73MZ   02H74JZ   02H74MZ   02HK0JZ   02HK0MZ   02HK32Z   02HK3JZ   02HK3MZ   02HK4JZ   02HK4MZ   02HL0JZ
02HL0MZ   02HL3JZ   02HL3MZ   02HL4JZ   02HL4MZ   02HN0JZ   02HN0MZ   02HN3JZ   02HN3MZ   02HN4JZ   02HN4MZ

ᴸᶜ Limited Coverage   ᴺᶜ Noncovered   ᴴᴬᶜ HAC-associated Procedure   ᶜᶜ Combination Cluster - See Appendix G for code lists
ᴰᴿᴳ Non-OR-Affecting MS-DRG Assignment   New/Revised Text in Orange   ♂ Male   ♀ Female

202   **2021 ICD-10-PCS**

0 Medical and Surgical
2 Heart and Great Vessels
J Inspection: Visually and/or manually exploring a body part

Body Part	Approach	Device	Qualifier
Character 4	Character 5	Character 6	Character 7
A Heart Y Great Vessel	0 Open 3 Percutaneous 4 Percutaneous Endoscopic	Z No Device	Z No Qualifier

0 Medical and Surgical
2 Heart and Great Vessels
K Map: Locating the route of passage of electrical impulses and/or locating functional areas in a body part

Body Part	Approach	Device	Qualifier
Character 4	Character 5	Character 6	Character 7
8 Conduction Mechanism ᴅᴿᴳ	0 Open 3 Percutaneous 4 Percutaneous Endoscopic	Z No Device	Z No Qualifier

ᴅᴿᴳ 02K80ZZ   02K83ZZ   02K84ZZ

0 Medical and Surgical
2 Heart and Great Vessels
L Occlusion: Completely closing an orifice or the lumen of a tubular body part

Body Part	Approach	Device	Qualifier
Character 4	Character 5	Character 6	Character 7
7 Atrium, Left ᴅᴿᴳ	0 Open 3 Percutaneous 4 Percutaneous Endoscopic	C Extraluminal Device D Intraluminal Device Z No Device	K Left Atrial Appendage
H Pulmonary Valve P Pulmonary Trunk Q Pulmonary Artery, Right S Pulmonary Vein, Right T Pulmonary Vein, Left V Superior Vena Cava	0 Open 3 Percutaneous 4 Percutaneous Endoscopic	C Extraluminal Device D Intraluminal Device Z No Device	Z No Qualifier
R Pulmonary Artery, Left	0 Open 3 Percutaneous 4 Percutaneous Endoscopic	C Extraluminal Device D Intraluminal Device Z No Device	T Ductus Arteriosus Z No Qualifier
W Thoracic Aorta, Descending	3 Percutaneous	D Intraluminal Device	J Temporary

ᴅᴿᴳ 02L70CK   02L70DK   02L70ZK   02L73CK   02L73DK   02L73ZK   02L74CK   02L74DK   02L74ZK

ᴸᶜ Limited Coverage   ᴺᶜ Noncovered   ᴴᴬᶜ HAC-associated Procedure   ᶜᶜ Combination Cluster - See Appendix G for code lists
ᴅᴿᴳ Non-OR-Affecting MS-DRG Assignment   New/Revised Text in **Orange**   ♂ Male   ♀ Female

2021 ICD-10-PCS

203

HEART AND GREAT VESSELS 021-02Y

0 **Medical and Surgical**
2 **Heart and Great Vessels**
N **Release:** Freeing a body part from an abnormal physical constraint by cutting or by the use of force

Body Part	Approach	Device	Qualifier
Character 4	**Character 5**	**Character 6**	**Character 7**
0 Coronary Artery, One Artery	0 Open	Z No Device	Z No Qualifier
1 Coronary Artery, Two Arteries	3 Percutaneous		
2 Coronary Artery, Three Arteries	4 Percutaneous Endoscopic		
3 Coronary Artery, Four or More Arteries			
4 Coronary Vein			
5 Atrial Septum			
6 Atrium, Right			
7 Atrium, Left			
8 Conduction Mechanism			
9 Chordae Tendineae			
D Papillary Muscle			
F Aortic Valve			
G Mitral Valve			
H Pulmonary Valve			
J Tricuspid Valve			
K Ventricle, Right			
L Ventricle, Left			
M Ventricular Septum			
N Pericardium			
P Pulmonary Trunk			
Q Pulmonary Artery, Right			
R Pulmonary Artery, Left			
S Pulmonary Vein, Right			
T Pulmonary Vein, Left			
V Superior Vena Cava			
W Thoracic Aorta, Descending			
X Thoracic Aorta, Ascending/Arch			

LC Limited Coverage   **NC** Noncovered   **HAC** HAC-associated Procedure   **CC** Combination Cluster - See Appendix G for code lists
DRG Non-OR-Affecting MS-DRG Assignment   New/Revised Text in **Orange**   ♂ Male   ♀ Female

204   **2021 ICD-10-PCS**

0 Medical and Surgical
2 Heart and Great Vessels
P Removal: Taking out or off a device from a body part

Body Part	Approach	Device	Qualifier
Character 4	Character 5	Character 6	Character 7
A Heart HAC	0 Open 3 Percutaneous 4 Percutaneous Endoscopic	2 Monitoring Device 3 Infusion Device 7 Autologous Tissue Substitute 8 Zooplastic Tissue C Extraluminal Device D Intraluminal Device J Synthetic Substitute K Nonautologous Tissue Substitute M Cardiac Lead N Intracardiac Pacemaker Q Implantable Heart Assist System Y Other Device	Z No Qualifier
A Heart CC	0 Open 3 Percutaneous 4 Percutaneous Endoscopic	R Short-term External Heart Assist System	S Biventricular Z No Qualifier
A Heart	X External	2 Monitoring Device 3 Infusion Device D Intraluminal Device M Cardiac Lead	Z No Qualifier
Y Great Vessel	0 Open 3 Percutaneous 4 Percutaneous Endoscopic	2 Monitoring Device 3 Infusion Device 7 Autologous Tissue Substitute 8 Zooplastic Tissue C Extraluminal Device D Intraluminal Device J Synthetic Substitute K Nonautologous Tissue Substitute Y Other Device	Z No Qualifier
Y Great Vessel	X External	2 Monitoring Device 3 Infusion Device D Intraluminal Device	Z No Qualifier

HAC 02PA0MZ   02PA3MZ   02PA4MZ   02PAXMZ

Surgical site infection (SSI) following cardiac implantable electronic device (CIED) procedures and secondary diagnosis K68.11, T81.40XA, T81.41XA, T81.42XA, T81.43XA, T81.44XA, T81.49XA, T82.6XXA, T82.7XXA.

CC 02PA0RZ   02PA3RZ   02PA4RZ

02Q

0 Medical and Surgical
2 Heart and Great Vessels
Q Repair: Restoring, to the extent possible, a body part to its normal anatomic structure and function

Body Part	Approach	Device	Qualifier
Character 4	**Character 5**	**Character 6**	**Character 7**

0 Coronary Artery, One Artery
1 Coronary Artery, Two Arteries
2 Coronary Artery, Three Arteries
3 Coronary Artery, Four or More
    Arteries
4 Coronary Vein
5 Atrial Septum
6 Atrium, Right
7 Atrium, Left
8 Conduction Mechanism
9 Chordae Tendineae
A Heart
B Heart, Right
C Heart, Left
D Papillary Muscle
H Pulmonary Valve
K Ventricle, Right
L Ventricle, Left
M Ventricular Septum
N Pericardium
P Pulmonary Trunk
Q Pulmonary Artery, Right
R Pulmonary Artery, Left
S Pulmonary Vein, Right
T Pulmonary Vein, Left
V Superior Vena Cava
W Thoracic Aorta, Descending
X Thoracic Aorta,
    Ascending/Arch
	0 Open
	3 Percutaneous
	4 Percutaneous Endoscopic
		Z No Device	**Z** No Qualifier

F Aortic Valve	**0** Open **3** Percutaneous **4** Percutaneous Endoscopic	**Z** No Device	**J** Truncal Valve **Z** No Qualifier
G Mitral Valve	**0** Open **3** Percutaneous **4** Percutaneous Endoscopic	**Z** No Device	**E** Atrioventricular Valve, Left **Z** No Qualifier
J Tricuspid Valve	**0** Open **3** Percutaneous **4** Percutaneous Endoscopic	**Z** No Device	**G** Atrioventricular Valve, Right **Z** No Qualifier

LC Limited Coverage **NC** Noncovered **HAC** HAC-associated Procedure **CC** Combination Cluster - See Appendix G for code lists

Non-OR-Affecting MS-DRG Assignment New/Revised Text in Orange ♂ Male ♀ Female

206

2021 ICD-10-PCS

0 Medical and Surgical

2 Heart and Great Vessels

R Replacement: Putting in or on biological or synthetic material that physically takes the place and/or function of all or a portion of a body part

Body Part	Approach	Device	Qualifier
Character 4	Character 5	Character 6	Character 7
5 Atrial Septum **6** Atrium, Right **7** Atrium, Left **9** Chordae Tendineae **D** Papillary Muscle **K** Ventricle, Right LC NC CC **L** Ventricle, Left LC NC CC **M** Ventricular Septum **N** Pericardium **P** Pulmonary Trunk **Q** Pulmonary Artery, Right **R** Pulmonary Artery, Left **S** Pulmonary Vein, Right **T** Pulmonary Vein, Left **V** Superior Vena Cava **W** Thoracic Aorta, Descending **X** Thoracic Aorta, Ascending/Arch	**0** Open **4** Percutaneous Endoscopic	**7** Autologous Tissue Substitute **8** Zooplastic Tissue **J** Synthetic Substitute **K** Nonautologous Tissue Substitute	**Z** No Qualifier
F Aortic Valve **G** Mitral Valve **H** Pulmonary Valve **J** Tricuspid Valve	**0** Open **4** Percutaneous Endoscopic	**7** Autologous Tissue Substitute **8** Zooplastic Tissue **J** Synthetic Substitute **K** Nonautologous Tissue Substitute	**Z** No Qualifier
F Aortic Valve **G** Mitral Valve **H** Pulmonary Valve **J** Tricuspid Valve	**3** Percutaneous	**7** Autologous Tissue Substitute **8** Zooplastic Tissue **J** Synthetic Substitute **K** Nonautologous Tissue Substitute	**H** Transapical **Z** No Qualifier

LC 02RK0JZ with 02RL0JZ

The procedures shown below are identified as limited coverage procedures when combined with diagnosis code Z00.6

NC 02RK0JZ   02RL0JZ

Noncovered except when combined with diagnosis code Z00.6.

CC 02RK0JZ   02RL0JZ

0 Medical and Surgical

2 Heart and Great Vessels

S Reposition: Moving to its normal location, or other suitable location, all or a portion of a body part

Body Part	Approach	Device	Qualifier
Character 4	Character 5	Character 6	Character 7
0 Coronary Artery, One Artery **1** Coronary Artery, Two Arteries **P** Pulmonary Trunk **Q** Pulmonary Artery, Right **R** Pulmonary Artery, Left **S** Pulmonary Vein, Right **T** Pulmonary Vein, Left **V** Superior Vena Cava **W** Thoracic Aorta, Descending **X** Thoracic Aorta, Ascending/Arch	**0** Open	**Z** No Device	**Z** No Qualifier

02T-02U

HEART AND GREAT VESSELS 021-02Y

0   Medical and Surgical
2   Heart and Great Vessels
T   Resection: Cutting out or off, without replacement, all of a body part

Body Part	Approach	Device	Qualifier
Character 4	Character 5	Character 6	Character 7
5 Atrial Septum 8 Conduction Mechanism 9 Chordae Tendineae D Papillary Muscle H Pulmonary Valve M Ventricular Septum N Pericardium	0 Open 3 Percutaneous 4 Percutaneous Endoscopic	Z No Device	Z No Qualifier

0   Medical and Surgical
2   Heart and Great Vessels
U   Supplement: Putting in or on biological or synthetic material that physically reinforces and/or augments the function of a portion of a body part

Body Part	Approach	Device	Qualifier
Character 4	Character 5	Character 6	Character 7
0 Coronary Artery, One Artery 1 Coronary Artery, Two Arteries 2 Coronary Artery, Three Arteries 3 Coronary Artery, Four or More Arteries 5 Atrial Septum 6 Atrium, Right 7 Atrium, Left ᴰᴿᴳ 9 Chordae Tendineae A Heart D Papillary Muscle H Pulmonary Valve K Ventricle, Right L Ventricle, Left M Ventricular Septum N Pericardium P Pulmonary Trunk Q Pulmonary Artery, Right R Pulmonary Artery, Left S Pulmonary Vein, Right T Pulmonary Vein, Left V Superior Vena Cava W Thoracic Aorta, Descending X Thoracic Aorta, Ascending/Arch	0 Open 3 Percutaneous 4 Percutaneous Endoscopic	7 Autologous Tissue Substitute 8 Zooplastic Tissue J Synthetic Substitute K Nonautologous Tissue Substitute	Z No Qualifier
F Aortic Valve	0 Open 3 Percutaneous 4 Percutaneous Endoscopic	7 Autologous Tissue Substitute 8 Zooplastic Tissue J Synthetic Substitute K Nonautologous Tissue Substitute	J Truncal Valve Z No Qualifier
G Mitral Valve	0 Open 4 Percutaneous Endoscopic	7 Autologous Tissue Substitute 8 Zooplastic Tissue J Synthetic Substitute K Nonautologous Tissue Substitute	E Atrioventricular Valve, Left Z No Qualifier
G Mitral Valve	3 Percutaneous	7 Autologous Tissue Substitute 8 Zooplastic Tissue K Nonautologous Tissue Substitute	E Atrioventricular Valve, Left Z No Qualifier
G Mitral Valve	3 Percutaneous	J Synthetic Substitute	E Atrioventricular Valve, Left H Transapical Z No Qualifier
J Tricuspid Valve	0 Open 3 Percutaneous 4 Percutaneous Endoscopic	7 Autologous Tissue Substitute 8 Zooplastic Tissue J Synthetic Substitute K Nonautologous Tissue Substitute	G Atrioventricular Valve, Right Z No Qualifier

ᴰᴿᴳ   02U73JZ   02U74JZ

0   **Medical and Surgical**
2   **Heart and Great Vessels**
V   **Restriction:** Partially closing an orifice or the lumen of a tubular body part

Body Part	Approach	Device	Qualifier
Character 4	Character 5	Character 6	Character 7
A Heart	**0** Open **3** Percutaneous **4** Percutaneous Endoscopic	**C** Extraluminal Device **Z** No Device	**Z** No Qualifier
G Mitral Valve	**0** Open **3** Percutaneous **4** Percutaneous Endoscopic	**Z** No Device	**Z** No Qualifier
P Pulmonary Trunk **Q** Pulmonary Artery, Right **S** Pulmonary Vein, Right **T** Pulmonary Vein, Left **V** Superior Vena Cava	**0** Open **3** Percutaneous **4** Percutaneous Endoscopic	**C** Extraluminal Device **D** Intraluminal Device **Z** No Device	**Z** No Qualifier
R Pulmonary Artery, Left	**0** Open **3** Percutaneous **4** Percutaneous Endoscopic	**C** Extraluminal Device **D** Intraluminal Device **Z** No Device	**T** Ductus Arteriosus **Z** No Qualifier
W Thoracic Aorta, Descending **X** Thoracic Aorta, Ascending/Arch	**0** Open **3** Percutaneous **4** Percutaneous Endoscopic	**C** Extraluminal Device **D** Intraluminal Device **E** Intraluminal Device, Branched or Fenestrated, One or Two Arteries **F** Intraluminal Device, Branched or Fenestrated, Three or More Arteries **Z** No Device	**Z** No Qualifier

0   **Medical and Surgical**
2   **Heart and Great Vessels**
W   **Revision:** Correcting, to the extent possible, a portion of a malfunctioning device or the position of a displaced device

Body Part	Approach	Device	Qualifier
Character 4	Character 5	Character 6	Character 7
5 Atrial Septum **M** Ventricular Septum	**0** Open **4** Percutaneous Endoscopic	**J** Synthetic Substitute	**Z** No Qualifier
A Heart LC NC HAC CC	**0** Open **3** Percutaneous **4** Percutaneous Endoscopic	**2** Monitoring Device **3** Infusion Device **7** Autologous Tissue Substitute **8** Zooplastic Tissue **C** Extraluminal Device **D** Intraluminal Device **J** Synthetic Substitute **K** Nonautologous Tissue Substitute **M** Cardiac Lead **N** Intracardiac Pacemaker **Q** Implantable Heart Assist System **Y** Other Device	**Z** No Qualifier
A Heart CC	**0** Open **3** Percutaneous **4** Percutaneous Endoscopic	**R** Short-term External Heart Assist System	**S** Biventricular **Z** No Qualifier
A Heart	**X** External	**2** Monitoring Device **3** Infusion Device **7** Autologous Tissue Substitute **8** Zooplastic Tissue **C** Extraluminal Device **D** Intraluminal Device **J** Synthetic Substitute **K** Nonautologous Tissue Substitute **M** Cardiac Lead **N** Intracardiac Pacemaker **Q** Implantable Heart Assist System	**Z** No Qualifier
A Heart	**X** External	**R** Short-term External Heart Assist System	**S** Biventricular **Z** No Qualifier

02W continued on next page

LC Limited Coverage   NC Noncovered   HAC HAC-associated Procedure   CC Combination Cluster - See Appendix G for code lists
DRG Non-OR-Affecting MS-DRG Assignment   New/Revised Text in Orange   ♂ Male   ♀ Female

0   Medical and Surgical   02W continued from previous page
2   Heart and Great Vessels
W   Revision: Correcting, to the extent possible, a portion of a malfunctioning device or the position of a displaced device

Body Part	Approach	Device	Qualifier
Character 4	Character 5	Character 6	Character 7
F Aortic Valve G Mitral Valve H Pulmonary Valve J Tricuspid Valve	0 Open 3 Percutaneous 4 Percutaneous Endoscopic	7 Autologous Tissue Substitute 8 Zooplastic Tissue J Synthetic Substitute K Nonautologous Tissue Substitute	Z No Qualifier
Y Great Vessel	0 Open 3 Percutaneous 4 Percutaneous Endoscopic	2 Monitoring Device 3 Infusion Device 7 Autologous Tissue Substitute 8 Zooplastic Tissue C Extraluminal Device D Intraluminal Device J Synthetic Substitute K Nonautologous Tissue Substitute Y Other Device	Z No Qualifier
Y Great Vessel	X External	2 Monitoring Device 3 Infusion Device 7 Autologous Tissue Substitute 8 Zooplastic Tissue C Extraluminal Device D Intraluminal Device J Synthetic Substitute K Nonautologous Tissue Substitute	Z No Qualifier

LC   02WA0JZ   02WA0QZ
NC   02WA3QZ   02WA4QZ
HAC   02WA0MZ   02WA3MZ   02WA4MZ
Surgical site infection (SSI) following cardiac implantable electronic device (CIED) procedures and secondary diagnosis K68.11, T81.40XA, T81.41XA, T81.42XA, T81.43XA, T81.44XA, T81.49XA, T82.6XXA, T82.7XXA.
CC   02WA0QZ   02WA0RZ   02WA3QZ   02WA3RZ   02WA4QZ   02WA4RZ

0   Medical and Surgical
2   Heart and Great Vessels
Y   Transplantation: Putting in or on all or a portion of a living body part taken from another individual or animal to physically take the place and/or function of all or a portion of a similar body part

Body Part	Approach	Device	Qualifier
Character 4	Character 5	Character 6	Character 7
A Heart **LC**	0 Open	Z No Device	0 Allogeneic 1 Syngeneic 2 Zooplastic

LC   02YA0Z0   02YA0Z1   02YA0Z2

LC Limited Coverage   **NC** Noncovered   **HAC** HAC-associated Procedure   **CC** Combination Cluster - See Appendix G for code lists
DRG Non-OR-Affecting MS-DRG Assignment   New/Revised Text in Orange   ♂ Male   ♀ Female

210   2021 ICD-10-PCS

NOTES

NOTES

Upper Arteries 031-03W

0 **Medical and Surgical**
3 **Upper Arteries**
1 **Bypass:** Altering the route of passage of the contents of a tubular body part

Body Part	Approach	Device	Qualifier
Character 4	Character 5	Character 6	Character 7
2 Innominate Artery	**0** Open	**9** Autologous Venous Tissue **A** Autologous Arterial Tissue **J** Synthetic Substitute **K** Nonautologous Tissue Substitute **Z** No Device	**0** Upper Arm Artery, Right **1** Upper Arm Artery, Left **2** Upper Arm Artery, Bilateral **3** Lower Arm Artery, Right **4** Lower Arm Artery, Left **5** Lower Arm Artery, Bilateral **6** Upper Leg Artery, Right **7** Upper Leg Artery, Left **8** Upper Leg Artery, Bilateral **9** Lower Leg Artery, Right **B** Lower Leg Artery, Left **C** Lower Leg Artery, Bilateral **D** Upper Arm Vein **F** Lower Arm Vein **J** Extracranial Artery, Right **K** Extracranial Artery, Left **W** Lower Extremity Vein
3 Subclavian Artery, Right **4** Subclavian Artery, Left	**0** Open	**9** Autologous Venous Tissue **A** Autologous Arterial Tissue **J** Synthetic Substitute **K** Nonautologous Tissue Substitute **Z** No Device	**0** Upper Arm Artery, Right **1** Upper Arm Artery, Left **2** Upper Arm Artery, Bilateral **3** Lower Arm Artery, Right **4** Lower Arm Artery, Left **5** Lower Arm Artery, Bilateral **6** Upper Leg Artery, Right **7** Upper Leg Artery, Left **8** Upper Leg Artery, Bilateral **9** Lower Leg Artery, Right **B** Lower Leg Artery, Left **C** Lower Leg Artery, Bilateral **D** Upper Arm Vein **F** Lower Arm Vein **J** Extracranial Artery, Right **K** Extracranial Artery, Left **M** Pulmonary Artery, Right **N** Pulmonary Artery, Left **W** Lower Extremity Vein
5 Axillary Artery, Right **6** Axillary Artery, Left	**0** Open	**9** Autologous Venous Tissue **A** Autologous Arterial Tissue **J** Synthetic Substitute **K** Nonautologous Tissue Substitute **Z** No Device	**0** Upper Arm Artery, Right **1** Upper Arm Artery, Left **2** Upper Arm Artery, Bilateral **3** Lower Arm Artery, Right **4** Lower Arm Artery, Left **5** Lower Arm Artery, Bilateral **6** Upper Leg Artery, Right **7** Upper Leg Artery, Left **8** Upper Leg Artery, Bilateral **9** Lower Leg Artery, Right **B** Lower Leg Artery, Left **C** Lower Leg Artery, Bilateral **D** Upper Arm Vein **F** Lower Arm Vein **J** Extracranial Artery, Right **K** Extracranial Artery, Left **T** Abdominal Artery **V** Superior Vena Cava **W** Lower Extremity Vein

031 continued on next page

LC Limited Coverage   NC Noncovered   HAC HAC-associated Procedure   CC Combination Cluster - See Appendix G for code lists
DRG Non-OR-Affecting MS-DRG Assignment   New/Revised Text in **Orange**   ♂ Male   ♀ Female

0 Medical and Surgical
3 Upper Arteries
1 Bypass: Altering the route of passage of the contents of a tubular body part

031 continued from previous page

Body Part		Approach		Device		Qualifier	
Character 4		**Character 5**		**Character 6**		**Character 7**	
7	Brachial Artery, Right	**0**	Open	**9** **A** **J** **K** **Z**	Autologous Venous Tissue Autologous Arterial Tissue Synthetic Substitute Nonautologous Tissue Substitute No Device	**0** **3** **D** **F** **V** **W**	Upper Arm Artery, Right Lower Arm Artery, Right Upper Arm Vein Lower Arm Vein Superior Vena Cava Lower Extremity Vein
8	Brachial Artery, Left	**0**	Open	**9** **A** **J** **K** **Z**	Autologous Venous Tissue Autologous Arterial Tissue Synthetic Substitute Nonautologous Tissue Substitute No Device	**1** **4** **D** **F** **V** **W**	Upper Arm Artery, Left Lower Arm Artery, Left Upper Arm Vein Lower Arm Vein Superior Vena Cava Lower Extremity Vein
9 **B**	Ulnar Artery, Right Radial Artery, Right	**0**	Open	**9** **A** **J** **K** **Z**	Autologous Venous Tissue Autologous Arterial Tissue Synthetic Substitute Nonautologous Tissue Substitute No Device	**3** **F**	Lower Arm Artery, Right Lower Arm Vein
9 **B**	Ulnar Artery, Right Radial Artery, Right	**3**	Percutaneous	**Z**	No Device	**F**	Lower Arm Vein
A **C**	Ulnar Artery, Left Radial Artery, Left	**0**	Open	**9** **A** **J** **K** **Z**	Autologous Venous Tissue Autologous Arterial Tissue Synthetic Substitute Nonautologous Tissue Substitute No Device	**4** **F**	Lower Arm Artery, Left Lower Arm Vein
A **C**	Ulnar Artery, Left Radial Artery, Left	**3**	Percutaneous	**Z**	No Device	**F**	Lower Arm Vein
G **S** **T**	Intracranial Artery Temporal Artery, Right Temporal Artery, Left	**0**	Open	**9** **A** **J** **K** **Z**	Autologous Venous Tissue Autologous Arterial Tissue Synthetic Substitute Nonautologous Tissue Substitute No Device	**G**	Intracranial Artery
H **J**	Common Carotid Artery, Right Common Carotid Artery, Left	**0**	Open	**9** **A** **J** **K** **Z**	Autologous Venous Tissue Autologous Arterial Tissue Synthetic Substitute Nonautologous Tissue Substitute No Device	**G** **J** **K** **Y**	Intracranial Artery Extracranial Artery, Right Extracranial Artery, Left Upper Artery
K **L** **M** **N**	Internal Carotid Artery, Right Internal Carotid Artery, Left External Carotid Artery, Right External Carotid Artery, Left	**0**	Open	**9** **A** **J** **K** **Z**	Autologous Venous Tissue Autologous Arterial Tissue Synthetic Substitute Nonautologous Tissue Substitute No Device	**J** **K**	Extracranial Artery, Right Extracranial Artery, Left

LC Limited Coverage **NC** Noncovered **HAC** HAC-associated Procedure **CC** Combination Cluster - See Appendix G for code lists
DRG Non-OR-Affecting MS-DRG Assignment New/Revised Text in **Orange** ♂ Male ♀ Female

214

2021 ICD-10-PCS

0 **Medical and Surgical**
3 **Upper Arteries**
5 **Destruction:** Physical eradication of all or a portion of a body part by the direct use of energy, force, or a destructive agent

Body Part	Approach	Device	Qualifier
Character 4	**Character 5**	**Character 6**	**Character 7**
0 Internal Mammary Artery, Right 1 Internal Mammary Artery, Left 2 Innominate Artery 3 Subclavian Artery, Right 4 Subclavian Artery, Left 5 Axillary Artery, Right 6 Axillary Artery, Left 7 Brachial Artery, Right 8 Brachial Artery, Left 9 Ulnar Artery, Right A Ulnar Artery, Left B Radial Artery, Right C Radial Artery, Left D Hand Artery, Right F Hand Artery, Left G Intracranial Artery H Common Carotid Artery, Right J Common Carotid Artery, Left K Internal Carotid Artery, Right L Internal Carotid Artery, Left M External Carotid Artery, Right N External Carotid Artery, Left P Vertebral Artery, Right Q Vertebral Artery, Left R Face Artery S Temporal Artery, Right T Temporal Artery, Left U Thyroid Artery, Right V Thyroid Artery, Left Y Upper Artery	0 Open 3 Percutaneous 4 Percutaneous Endoscopic	Z No Device	Z No Qualifier

LC Limited Coverage   **NC** Noncovered   **HAC** HAC-associated Procedure   **CC** Combination Cluster - See Appendix G for code lists
⊕ Non-OR-Affecting MS-DRG Assignment   New/Revised Text in **Orange**   ♂ Male   ♀ Female

2021 ICD-10-PCS   215

0   **Medical and Surgical**
3   **Upper Arteries**
7   **Dilation:** Expanding an orifice or the lumen of a tubular body part

Body Part	Approach	Device	Qualifier
Character 4	Character 5	Character 6	Character 7
0 Internal Mammary Artery, Right 1 Internal Mammary Artery, Left 2 Innominate Artery 3 Subclavian Artery, Right 4 Subclavian Artery, Left 5 Axillary Artery, Right 6 Axillary Artery, Left 7 Brachial Artery, Right 8 Brachial Artery, Left 9 Ulnar Artery, Right A Ulnar Artery, Left B Radial Artery, Right C Radial Artery, Left	0 Open 3 Percutaneous 4 Percutaneous Endoscopic	4 Intraluminal Device, Drug-eluting 5 Intraluminal Device, Drug-eluting, Two 6 Intraluminal Device, Drug-eluting, Three 7 Intraluminal Device, Drug-eluting, Four or More E Intraluminal Device, Two F Intraluminal Device, Three G Intraluminal Device, Four or More	Z No Qualifier
0 Internal Mammary Artery, Right 1 Internal Mammary Artery, Left 2 Innominate Artery 3 Subclavian Artery, Right 4 Subclavian Artery, Left 5 Axillary Artery, Right 6 Axillary Artery, Left 7 Brachial Artery, Right 8 Brachial Artery, Left 9 Ulnar Artery, Right A Ulnar Artery, Left B Radial Artery, Right C Radial Artery, Left	0 Open 3 Percutaneous 4 Percutaneous Endoscopic	D Intraluminal Device Z No Device	1 Drug-Coated Balloon Z No Qualifier
D Hand Artery, Right F Hand Artery, Left G Intracranial Artery 🅽🅲 H Common Carotid Artery, Right J Common Carotid Artery, Left K Internal Carotid Artery, Right L Internal Carotid Artery, Left M External Carotid Artery, Right N External Carotid Artery, Left P Vertebral Artery, Right Q Vertebral Artery, Left R Face Artery S Temporal Artery, Right T Temporal Artery, Left U Thyroid Artery, Right V Thyroid Artery, Left Y Upper Artery	0 Open 3 Percutaneous 4 Percutaneous Endoscopic	4 Intraluminal Device, Drug-eluting 5 Intraluminal Device, Drug-eluting, Two 6 Intraluminal Device, Drug-eluting, Three 7 Intraluminal Device, Drug-eluting, Four or More D Intraluminal Device E Intraluminal Device, Two F Intraluminal Device, Three G Intraluminal Device, Four or More Z No Device	Z No Qualifier

🅽🅲   037G3ZZ   037G4ZZ

🅻🅲 Limited Coverage   🅽🅲 Noncovered   🅷🅰🅲 HAC-associated Procedure   🅲🅲 Combination Cluster - See Appendix G for code lists
🔵 Non-OR-Affecting MS-DRG Assignment   New/Revised Text in Orange   ♂ Male   ♀ Female

216

2021 ICD-10-PCS

0 **Medical and Surgical**
3 **Upper Arteries**
9 **Drainage:** Taking or letting out fluids and/or gases from a body part

Body Part	Approach	Device	Qualifier
Character 4	Character 5	Character 6	Character 7
0 Internal Mammary Artery, Right 1 Internal Mammary Artery, Left 2 Innominate Artery 3 Subclavian Artery, Right 4 Subclavian Artery, Left 5 Axillary Artery, Right 6 Axillary Artery, Left 7 Brachial Artery, Right 8 Brachial Artery, Left 9 Ulnar Artery, Right A Ulnar Artery, Left B Radial Artery, Right C Radial Artery, Left D Hand Artery, Right F Hand Artery, Left G Intracranial Artery H Common Carotid Artery, Right J Common Carotid Artery, Left K Internal Carotid Artery, Right L Internal Carotid Artery, Left M External Carotid Artery, Right N External Carotid Artery, Left P Vertebral Artery, Right Q Vertebral Artery, Left R Face Artery S Temporal Artery, Right T Temporal Artery, Left U Thyroid Artery, Right V Thyroid Artery, Left Y Upper Artery	0 Open 3 Percutaneous 4 Percutaneous Endoscopic	0 Drainage Device	Z No Qualifier
0 Internal Mammary Artery, Right 1 Internal Mammary Artery, Left 2 Innominate Artery 3 Subclavian Artery, Right 4 Subclavian Artery, Left 5 Axillary Artery, Right 6 Axillary Artery, Left 7 Brachial Artery, Right 8 Brachial Artery, Left 9 Ulnar Artery, Right A Ulnar Artery, Left B Radial Artery, Right C Radial Artery, Left D Hand Artery, Right F Hand Artery, Left G Intracranial Artery H Common Carotid Artery, Right J Common Carotid Artery, Left K Internal Carotid Artery, Right L Internal Carotid Artery, Left M External Carotid Artery, Right N External Carotid Artery, Left P Vertebral Artery, Right Q Vertebral Artery, Left R Face Artery S Temporal Artery, Right T Temporal Artery, Left U Thyroid Artery, Right V Thyroid Artery, Left Y Upper Artery	0 Open 3 Percutaneous 4 Percutaneous Endoscopic	Z No Device	X Diagnostic Z No Qualifier

LC Limited Coverage   NC Noncovered   HAC HAC-associated Procedure   CC Combination Cluster - See Appendix G for code lists
DRG Non-OR-Affecting MS-DRG Assignment   New/Revised Text in Orange   ♂ Male   ♀ Female

2021 ICD-10-PCS

217

0 **Medical and Surgical**
3 **Upper Arteries**
B **Excision:** Cutting out or off, without replacement, a portion of a body part

Body Part	Approach	Device	Qualifier
Character 4	Character 5	Character 6	Character 7
0 Internal Mammary Artery, Right	0 Open	Z No Device	X Diagnostic
1 Internal Mammary Artery, Left	3 Percutaneous		Z No Qualifier
2 Innominate Artery	4 Percutaneous Endoscopic		
3 Subclavian Artery, Right			
4 Subclavian Artery, Left			
5 Axillary Artery, Right			
6 Axillary Artery, Left			
7 Brachial Artery, Right			
8 Brachial Artery, Left			
9 Ulnar Artery, Right			
A Ulnar Artery, Left			
B Radial Artery, Right			
C Radial Artery, Left			
D Hand Artery, Right			
F Hand Artery, Left			
G Intracranial Artery			
H Common Carotid Artery, Right			
J Common Carotid Artery, Left			
K Internal Carotid Artery, Right			
L Internal Carotid Artery, Left			
M External Carotid Artery, Right			
N External Carotid Artery, Left			
P Vertebral Artery, Right			
Q Vertebral Artery, Left			
R Face Artery			
S Temporal Artery, Right			
T Temporal Artery, Left			
U Thyroid Artery, Right			
V Thyroid Artery, Left			
Y Upper Artery			

LC Limited Coverage   **NC** Noncovered   **HAC** HAC-associated Procedure   **CC** Combination Cluster - See Appendix G for code lists
DRG Non-OR-Affecting MS-DRG Assignment   New/Revised Text in **Orange**   ♂ Male   ♀ Female

218

2021 ICD-10-PCS

0 Medical and Surgical
3 Upper Arteries
C Extirpation: Taking or cutting out solid matter from a body part

Body Part	Approach	Device	Qualifier
Character 4	Character 5	Character 6	Character 7
0 Internal Mammary Artery, Right **1** Internal Mammary Artery, Left **2** Innominate Artery **3** Subclavian Artery, Right **4** Subclavian Artery, Left **5** Axillary Artery, Right **6** Axillary Artery, Left **7** Brachial Artery, Right **8** Brachial Artery, Left **9** Ulnar Artery, Right **A** Ulnar Artery, Left **B** Radial Artery, Right **C** Radial Artery, Left **D** Hand Artery, Right **F** Hand Artery, Left **R** Face Artery **S** Temporal Artery, Right **T** Temporal Artery, Left **U** Thyroid Artery, Right **V** Thyroid Artery, Left **Y** Upper Artery	**0** Open **3** Percutaneous **4** Percutaneous Endoscopic	**Z** No Device	**Z** No Qualifier
G Intracranial Artery **H** Common Carotid Artery, Right **J** Common Carotid Artery, Left **K** Internal Carotid Artery, Right **L** Internal Carotid Artery, Left **M** External Carotid Artery, Right **N** External Carotid Artery, Left **P** Vertebral Artery, Right **Q** Vertebral Artery, Left	**0** Open **4** Percutaneous Endoscopic	**Z** No Device	**Z** No Qualifier
G Intracranial Artery **H** Common Carotid Artery, Right **J** Common Carotid Artery, Left **K** Internal Carotid Artery, Right **L** Internal Carotid Artery, Left **M** External Carotid Artery, Right **N** External Carotid Artery, Left **P** Vertebral Artery, Right **Q** Vertebral Artery, Left	**3** Percutaneous	**Z** No Device	**7** Stent Retriever **Z** No Qualifier

0 Medical and Surgical
3 Upper Arteries
F Fragmentation: Breaking solid matter in a body part into pieces

Body Part	Approach	Device	Qualifier
Character 4	Character 5	Character 6	Character 7
2 Innominate Artery **3** Subclavian Artery, Right **4** Subclavian Artery, Left **5** Axillary Artery, Right **6** Axillary Artery, Left **7** Brachial Artery, Right **8** Brachial Artery, Left **9** Ulnar Artery, Right **A** Ulnar Artery, Left **B** Radial Artery, Right **C** Radial Artery, Left **Y** Upper Artery	**3** Percutaneous	**Z** No Device	**0** Ultrasonic **Z** No Qualifier

0 **Medical and Surgical**
3 **Upper Arteries**
H **Insertion:** Putting in a nonbiological appliance that monitors, assists, performs, or prevents a physiological function but does not physically take the place of a body part

Body Part	Approach	Device	Qualifier
Character 4	Character 5	Character 6	Character 7
0 Internal Mammary Artery, Right **1** Internal Mammary Artery, Left **2** Innominate Artery **3** Subclavian Artery, Right **4** Subclavian Artery, Left **5** Axillary Artery, Right **6** Axillary Artery, Left **7** Brachial Artery, Right **8** Brachial Artery, Left **9** Ulnar Artery, Right **A** Ulnar Artery, Left **B** Radial Artery, Right **C** Radial Artery, Left **D** Hand Artery, Right **F** Hand Artery, Left **G** Intracranial Artery **H** Common Carotid Artery, Right **J** Common Carotid Artery, Left **M** External Carotid Artery, Right **N** External Carotid Artery, Left **P** Vertebral Artery, Right **Q** Vertebral Artery, Left **R** Face Artery **S** Temporal Artery, Right **T** Temporal Artery, Left **U** Thyroid Artery, Right **V** Thyroid Artery, Left	**0** Open **3** Percutaneous **4** Percutaneous Endoscopic	**3** Infusion Device **D** Intraluminal Device	**Z** No Qualifier
K Internal Carotid Artery, Right **L** Internal Carotid Artery, Left	**0** Open **3** Percutaneous **4** Percutaneous Endoscopic	**3** Infusion Device **D** Intraluminal Device **M** Stimulator Lead	**Z** No Qualifier
Y Upper Artery	**0** Open **3** Percutaneous **4** Percutaneous Endoscopic	**2** Monitoring Device **3** Infusion Device **D** Intraluminal Device **Y** Other Device	**Z** No Qualifier

0 **Medical and Surgical**
3 **Upper Arteries**
J **Inspection:** Visually and/or manually exploring a body part

Body Part	Approach	Device	Qualifier
Character 4	Character 5	Character 6	Character 7
Y Upper Artery	**0** Open **3** Percutaneous **4** Percutaneous Endoscopic **X** External	**Z** No Device	**Z** No Qualifier

0 **Medical and Surgical**
3 **Upper Arteries**
L **Occlusion:** Completely closing an orifice or the lumen of a tubular body part

Body Part	Approach	Device	Qualifier
Character 4	Character 5	Character 6	Character 7
0 Internal Mammary Artery, Right 1 Internal Mammary Artery, Left 2 Innominate Artery 3 Subclavian Artery, Right 4 Subclavian Artery, Left 5 Axillary Artery, Right 6 Axillary Artery, Left 7 Brachial Artery, Right 8 Brachial Artery, Left 9 Ulnar Artery, Right A Ulnar Artery, Left B Radial Artery, Right C Radial Artery, Left D Hand Artery, Right F Hand Artery, Left R Face Artery S Temporal Artery, Right T Temporal Artery, Left U Thyroid Artery, Right V Thyroid Artery, Left Y Upper Artery	0 Open 3 Percutaneous 4 Percutaneous Endoscopic	C Extraluminal Device D Intraluminal Device Z No Device	Z No Qualifier
G Intracranial Artery H Common Carotid Artery, Right J Common Carotid Artery, Left K Internal Carotid Artery, Right L Internal Carotid Artery, Left M External Carotid Artery, Right N External Carotid Artery, Left P Vertebral Artery, Right Q Vertebral Artery, Left	0 Open 3 Percutaneous 4 Percutaneous Endoscopic	B Intraluminal Device, Bioactive C Extraluminal Device D Intraluminal Device Z No Device	Z No Qualifier

IC Limited Coverage   **NC** Noncovered   **HAC** HAC-associated Procedure   **CC** Combination Cluster - See Appendix G for code lists

DRG Non-OR-Affecting MS-DRG Assignment   New/Revised Text in **Orange**   ♂ Male   ♀ Female

2021 ICD-10-PCS

UPPER ARTERIES 031-03W

221

0 **Medical and Surgical**
3 **Upper Arteries**
N **Release:** Freeing a body part from an abnormal physical constraint by cutting or by the use of force

Body Part	Approach	Device	Qualifier
Character 4	Character 5	Character 6	Character 7
0 Internal Mammary Artery, Right **1** Internal Mammary Artery, Left **2** Innominate Artery **3** Subclavian Artery, Right **4** Subclavian Artery, Left **5** Axillary Artery, Right **6** Axillary Artery, Left **7** Brachial Artery, Right **8** Brachial Artery, Left **9** Ulnar Artery, Right **A** Ulnar Artery, Left **B** Radial Artery, Right **C** Radial Artery, Left **D** Hand Artery, Right **F** Hand Artery, Left **G** Intracranial Artery **H** Common Carotid Artery, Right **J** Common Carotid Artery, Left **K** Internal Carotid Artery, Right **L** Internal Carotid Artery, Left **M** External Carotid Artery, Right **N** External Carotid Artery, Left **P** Vertebral Artery, Right **Q** Vertebral Artery, Left **R** Face Artery **S** Temporal Artery, Right **T** Temporal Artery, Left **U** Thyroid Artery, Right **V** Thyroid Artery, Left **Y** Upper Artery	**0** Open **3** Percutaneous **4** Percutaneous Endoscopic	**Z** No Device	**Z** No Qualifier

0 **Medical and Surgical**
3 **Upper Arteries**
P **Removal:** Taking out or off a device from a body part

Body Part	Approach	Device	Qualifier
Character 4	Character 5	Character 6	Character 7
Y Upper Artery	**0** Open **3** Percutaneous **4** Percutaneous Endoscopic	**0** Drainage Device **2** Monitoring Device **3** Infusion Device **7** Autologous Tissue Substitute **C** Extraluminal Device **D** Intraluminal Device **J** Synthetic Substitute **K** Nonautologous Tissue Substitute **M** Stimulator Lead **Y** Other Device	**Z** No Qualifier
Y Upper Artery	**X** External	**0** Drainage Device **2** Monitoring Device **3** Infusion Device **D** Intraluminal Device **M** Stimulator Lead	**Z** No Qualifier

LC Limited Coverage   **NC** Noncovered   **HAC** HAC-associated Procedure   **CC** Combination Cluster - See Appendix G for code lists
DRG Non-OR-Affecting MS-DRG Assignment   New/Revised Text in **Orange**   ♂ Male ♀ Female

222

2021 ICD-10-PCS

0 Medical and Surgical
3 Upper Arteries
Q **Repair:** Restoring, to the extent possible, a body part to its normal anatomic structure and function

Body Part	Approach	Device	Qualifier
Character 4	Character 5	Character 6	Character 7
0 Internal Mammary Artery, Right	**0** Open	**Z** No Device	**Z** No Qualifier
1 Internal Mammary Artery, Left	**3** Percutaneous		
2 Innominate Artery	**4** Percutaneous Endoscopic		
3 Subclavian Artery, Right			
4 Subclavian Artery, Left			
5 Axillary Artery, Right			
6 Axillary Artery, Left			
7 Brachial Artery, Right			
8 Brachial Artery, Left			
9 Ulnar Artery, Right			
A Ulnar Artery, Left			
B Radial Artery, Right			
C Radial Artery, Left			
D Hand Artery, Right			
F Hand Artery, Left			
G Intracranial Artery			
H Common Carotid Artery, Right			
J Common Carotid Artery, Left			
K Internal Carotid Artery, Right			
L Internal Carotid Artery, Left			
M External Carotid Artery, Right			
N External Carotid Artery, Left			
P Vertebral Artery, Right			
Q Vertebral Artery, Left			
R Face Artery			
S Temporal Artery, Right			
T Temporal Artery, Left			
U Thyroid Artery, Right			
V Thyroid Artery, Left			
Y Upper Artery			

03R

UPPER ARTERIES 031-03W

0 **Medical and Surgical**
3 **Upper Arteries**
R **Replacement:** Putting in or on biological or synthetic material that physically takes the place and/or function of all or a portion of a body part

Body Part	Approach	Device	Qualifier
Character 4	Character 5	Character 6	Character 7
0 Internal Mammary Artery, Right **1** Internal Mammary Artery, Left **2** Innominate Artery **3** Subclavian Artery, Right **4** Subclavian Artery, Left **5** Axillary Artery, Right **6** Axillary Artery, Left **7** Brachial Artery, Right **8** Brachial Artery, Left **9** Ulnar Artery, Right **A** Ulnar Artery, Left **B** Radial Artery, Right **C** Radial Artery, Left **D** Hand Artery, Right **F** Hand Artery, Left **G** Intracranial Artery **H** Common Carotid Artery, Right **J** Common Carotid Artery, Left **K** Internal Carotid Artery, Right **L** Internal Carotid Artery, Left **M** External Carotid Artery, Right **N** External Carotid Artery, Left **P** Vertebral Artery, Right **Q** Vertebral Artery, Left **R** Face Artery **S** Temporal Artery, Right **T** Temporal Artery, Left **U** Thyroid Artery, Right **V** Thyroid Artery, Left **Y** Upper Artery	**0** Open **4** Percutaneous Endoscopic	**7** Autologous Tissue Substitute **J** Synthetic Substitute **K** Nonautologous Tissue Substitute	**Z** No Qualifier

LC Limited Coverage   **NC** Noncovered   **HAC** HAC-associated Procedure   **CC** Combination Cluster - See Appendix G for code lists
DRG Non-OR-Affecting MS-DRG Assignment   New/Revised Text in **Orange**   ♂ Male   ♀ Female

224   **2021 ICD-10-PCS**

0 **Medical and Surgical**
3 **Upper Arteries**
S **Reposition:** Moving to its normal location, or other suitable location, all or a portion of a body part

Body Part	Approach	Device	Qualifier
Character 4	Character 5	Character 6	Character 7
0 Internal Mammary Artery, Right	**0** Open	**Z** No Device	**Z** No Qualifier
1 Internal Mammary Artery, Left	**3** Percutaneous		
2 Innominate Artery	**4** Percutaneous Endoscopic		
3 Subclavian Artery, Right			
4 Subclavian Artery, Left			
5 Axillary Artery, Right			
6 Axillary Artery, Left			
7 Brachial Artery, Right			
8 Brachial Artery, Left			
9 Ulnar Artery, Right			
A Ulnar Artery, Left			
B Radial Artery, Right			
C Radial Artery, Left			
D Hand Artery, Right			
F Hand Artery, Left			
G Intracranial Artery			
H Common Carotid Artery, Right			
J Common Carotid Artery, Left			
K Internal Carotid Artery, Right			
L Internal Carotid Artery, Left			
M External Carotid Artery, Right			
N External Carotid Artery, Left			
P Vertebral Artery, Right			
Q Vertebral Artery, Left			
R Face Artery			
S Temporal Artery, Right			
T Temporal Artery, Left			
U Thyroid Artery, Right			
V Thyroid Artery, Left			
Y Upper Artery			

0 **Medical and Surgical**
3 **Upper Arteries**
U **Supplement:** Putting in or on biological or synthetic material that physically reinforces and/or augments the function of a portion of a body part

Body Part	Approach	Device	Qualifier
Character 4	Character 5	Character 6	Character 7
0 Internal Mammary Artery, Right **1** Internal Mammary Artery, Left **2** Innominate Artery **3** Subclavian Artery, Right **4** Subclavian Artery, Left **5** Axillary Artery, Right **6** Axillary Artery, Left **7** Brachial Artery, Right **8** Brachial Artery, Left **9** Ulnar Artery, Right **A** Ulnar Artery, Left **B** Radial Artery, Right **C** Radial Artery, Left **D** Hand Artery, Right **F** Hand Artery, Left **G** Intracranial Artery **H** Common Carotid Artery, Right **J** Common Carotid Artery, Left **K** Internal Carotid Artery, Right **L** Internal Carotid Artery, Left **M** External Carotid Artery, Right **N** External Carotid Artery, Left **P** Vertebral Artery, Right **Q** Vertebral Artery, Left **R** Face Artery **S** Temporal Artery, Right **T** Temporal Artery, Left **U** Thyroid Artery, Right **V** Thyroid Artery, Left **Y** Upper Artery	**0** Open **3** Percutaneous **4** Percutaneous Endoscopic	**7** Autologous Tissue Substitute **J** Synthetic Substitute **K** Nonautologous Tissue Substitute	**Z** No Qualifier

LC Limited Coverage   NC Noncovered   HAC HAC-associated Procedure   CC Combination Cluster - See Appendix G for code lists
Non-OR-Affecting MS-DRG Assignment   New/Revised Text in **Orange**   ♂ Male   ♀ Female

226

2021 ICD-10-PCS

0 **Medical and Surgical**
3 **Upper Arteries**
V **Restriction:** Partially closing an orifice or the lumen of a tubular body part

Body Part	Approach	Device	Qualifier
Character 4	**Character 5**	**Character 6**	**Character 7**
0 Internal Mammary Artery, Right 1 Internal Mammary Artery, Left 2 Innominate Artery 3 Subclavian Artery, Right 4 Subclavian Artery, Left 5 Axillary Artery, Right 6 Axillary Artery, Left 7 Brachial Artery, Right 8 Brachial Artery, Left 9 Ulnar Artery, Right A Ulnar Artery, Left B Radial Artery, Right C Radial Artery, Left D Hand Artery, Right F Hand Artery, Left R Face Artery S Temporal Artery, Right T Temporal Artery, Left U Thyroid Artery, Right V Thyroid Artery, Left Y Upper Artery	0 Open 3 Percutaneous 4 Percutaneous Endoscopic	C Extraluminal Device D Intraluminal Device Z No Device	Z No Qualifier
G Intracranial Artery H Common Carotid Artery, Right J Common Carotid Artery, Left K Internal Carotid Artery, Right L Internal Carotid Artery, Left M External Carotid Artery, Right N External Carotid Artery, Left P Vertebral Artery, Right Q Vertebral Artery, Left	0 Open 3 Percutaneous 4 Percutaneous Endoscopic	B Intraluminal Device, Bioactive C Extraluminal Device D Intraluminal Device H Intraluminal Device, Flow Diverter Z No Device	Z No Qualifier

0 **Medical and Surgical**
3 **Upper Arteries**
W **Revision:** Correcting, to the extent possible, a portion of a malfunctioning device or the position of a displaced device

Body Part	Approach	Device	Qualifier
Character 4	**Character 5**	**Character 6**	**Character 7**
Y Upper Artery	0 Open 3 Percutaneous 4 Percutaneous Endoscopic	0 Drainage Device 2 Monitoring Device 3 Infusion Device 7 Autologous Tissue Substitute C Extraluminal Device D Intraluminal Device J Synthetic Substitute K Nonautologous Tissue Substitute M Stimulator Lead Y Other Device	Z No Qualifier
Y Upper Artery	X External	0 Drainage Device 2 Monitoring Device 3 Infusion Device 7 Autologous Tissue Substitute C Extraluminal Device D Intraluminal Device J Synthetic Substitute K Nonautologous Tissue Substitute M Stimulator Lead	Z No Qualifier

NOTES

Lower Arteries 041-04W

0 **Medical and Surgical**
4 **Lower Arteries**
1 **Bypass:** Altering the route of passage of the contents of a tubular body part

Body Part	Approach	Device	Qualifier
Character 4	**Character 5**	**Character 6**	**Character 7**
0 Abdominal Aorta C Common Iliac Artery, Right D Common Iliac Artery, Left	0 Open 4 Percutaneous Endoscopic	9 Autologous Venous Tissue A Autologous Arterial Tissue J Synthetic Substitute K Nonautologous Tissue Substitute Z No Device	0 Abdominal Aorta 1 Celiac Artery 2 Mesenteric Artery 3 Renal Artery, Right 4 Renal Artery, Left 5 Renal Artery, Bilateral 6 Common Iliac Artery, Right 7 Common Iliac Artery, Left 8 Common Iliac Arteries, Bilateral 9 Internal Iliac Artery, Right B Internal Iliac Artery, Left C Internal Iliac Arteries, Bilateral D External Iliac Artery, Right F External Iliac Artery, Left G External Iliac Arteries, Bilateral H Femoral Artery, Right J Femoral Artery, Left K Femoral Arteries, Bilateral Q Lower Extremity Artery R Lower Artery
3 Hepatic Artery 4 Splenic Artery	0 Open 4 Percutaneous Endoscopic	9 Autologous Venous Tissue A Autologous Arterial Tissue J Synthetic Substitute K Nonautologous Tissue Substitute Z No Device	3 Renal Artery, Right 4 Renal Artery, Left 5 Renal Artery, Bilateral
E Internal Iliac Artery, Right F Internal Iliac Artery, Left H External Iliac Artery, Right J External Iliac Artery, Left	0 Open 4 Percutaneous Endoscopic	9 Autologous Venous Tissue A Autologous Arterial Tissue J Synthetic Substitute K Nonautologous Tissue Substitute Z No Device	9 Internal Iliac Artery, Right B Internal Iliac Artery, Left C Internal Iliac Arteries, Bilateral D External Iliac Artery, Right F External Iliac Artery, Left G External Iliac Arteries, Bilateral H Femoral Artery, Right J Femoral Artery, Left K Femoral Arteries, Bilateral P Foot Artery Q Lower Extremity Artery
K Femoral Artery, Right L Femoral Artery, Left	0 Open 4 Percutaneous Endoscopic	9 Autologous Venous Tissue A Autologous Arterial Tissue J Synthetic Substitute K Nonautologous Tissue Substitute Z No Device	H Femoral Artery, Right J Femoral Artery, Left K Femoral Arteries, Bilateral L Popliteal Artery M Peroneal Artery N Posterior Tibial Artery P Foot Artery Q Lower Extremity Artery S Lower Extremity Vein
K Femoral Artery, Right L Femoral Artery, Left	3 Percutaneous	J Synthetic Substitute	Q Lower Extremity Artery S Lower Extremity Vein
M Popliteal Artery, Right N Popliteal Artery, Left	0 Open 4 Percutaneous Endoscopic	9 Autologous Venous Tissue A Autologous Arterial Tissue J Synthetic Substitute K Nonautologous Tissue Substitute Z No Device	L Popliteal Artery M Peroneal Artery P Foot Artery Q Lower Extremity Artery S Lower Extremity Vein

041 continued on next page

IC Limited Coverage   **NC** Noncovered   **HAC** HAC-associated Procedure   **CC** Combination Cluster - See Appendix G for code lists   **DRG** Non-OR-Affecting MS-DRG Assignment   New/Revised Text in **Orange**   ♂ Male   ♀ Female

2021 ICD-10-PCS   **229**

0   Medical and Surgical   041 continued from previous page
4   Lower Arteries
1   Bypass: Altering the route of passage of the contents of a tubular body part

Body Part	Approach	Device	Qualifier
Character 4	**Character 5**	**Character 6**	**Character 7**
M Popliteal Artery, Right N Popliteal Artery, Left	3 Percutaneous	J Synthetic Substitute	Q Lower Extremity Artery S Lower Extremity Vein
P Anterior Tibial Artery, Right Q Anterior Tibial Artery, Left R Posterior Tibial Artery, Right S Posterior Tibial Artery	0 Open 3 Percutaneous 4 Percutaneous Endoscopic	J Synthetic Substitute	Q Lower Extremity Artery S Lower Extremity Vein
T Peroneal Artery, Right U Peroneal Artery, Left V Foot Artery, Right W Foot Artery, Left	0 Open 4 Percutaneous Endoscopic	9 Autologous Venous Tissue A Autologous Arterial Tissue J Synthetic Substitute K Nonautologous Tissue Substitute Z No Device	P Foot Artery Q Lower Extremity Artery S Lower Extremity Vein
T Peroneal Artery, Right U Peroneal Artery, Left V Foot Artery, Right W Foot Artery, Left	3 Percutaneous	J Synthetic Substitute	Q Lower Extremity Artery S Lower Extremity Vein

0   Medical and Surgical
4   Lower Arteries
5   Destruction: Physical eradication of all or a portion of a body part by the direct use of energy, force, or a destructive agent

Body Part	Approach	Device	Qualifier
Character 4	**Character 5**	**Character 6**	**Character 7**
0 Abdominal Aorta 1 Celiac Artery 2 Gastric Artery 3 Hepatic Artery 4 Splenic Artery 5 Superior Mesenteric Artery 6 Colic Artery, Right 7 Colic Artery, Left 8 Colic Artery, Middle 9 Renal Artery, Right A Renal Artery, Left B Inferior Mesenteric Artery C Common Iliac Artery, Right D Common Iliac Artery, Left E Internal Iliac Artery, Right F Internal Iliac Artery, Left H External Iliac Artery, Right J External Iliac Artery, Left K Femoral Artery, Right L Femoral Artery, Left M Popliteal Artery, Right N Popliteal Artery, Left P Anterior Tibial Artery, Right Q Anterior Tibial Artery, Left R Posterior Tibial Artery, Right S Posterior Tibial Artery, Left T Peroneal Artery, Right U Peroneal Artery, Left V Foot Artery, Right W Foot Artery, Left Y Lower Artery	0 Open 3 Percutaneous 4 Percutaneous Endoscopic	Z No Device	Z No Qualifier

0   **Medical and Surgical**
4   **Lower Arteries**
7   **Dilation:** Expanding an orifice or the lumen of a tubular body part

Body Part	Approach	Device	Qualifier
Character 4	**Character 5**	**Character 6**	**Character 7**
0 Abdominal Aorta **1** Celiac Artery **2** Gastric Artery **3** Hepatic Artery **4** Splenic Artery **5** Superior Mesenteric Artery **6** Colic Artery, Right **7** Colic Artery, Left **8** Colic Artery, Middle **9** Renal Artery, Right **A** Renal Artery, Left **B** Inferior Mesenteric Artery **C** Common Iliac Artery, Right **D** Common Iliac Artery, Left **E** Internal Iliac Artery, Right **F** Internal Iliac Artery, Left **H** External Iliac Artery, Right **J** External Iliac Artery, Left **K** Femoral Artery, Right **L** Femoral Artery, Left **M** Popliteal Artery, Right **N** Popliteal Artery, Left **P** Anterior Tibial Artery, Right **Q** Anterior Tibial Artery, Left **R** Posterior Tibial Artery, Right **S** Posterior Tibial Artery, Left **T** Peroneal Artery, Right **U** Peroneal Artery, Left **V** Foot Artery, Right **W** Foot Artery, Left **Y** Lower Artery	**0** Open **3** Percutaneous **4** Percutaneous Endoscopic	**4** Intraluminal Device, Drug-eluting **D** Intraluminal Device **Z** No Device	**1** Drug-Coated Balloon **Z** No Qualifier
0 Abdominal Aorta **1** Celiac Artery **2** Gastric Artery **3** Hepatic Artery **4** Splenic Artery **5** Superior Mesenteric Artery **6** Colic Artery, Right **7** Colic Artery, Left **8** Colic Artery, Middle **9** Renal Artery, Right **A** Renal Artery, Left **B** Inferior Mesenteric Artery **C** Common Iliac Artery, Right **D** Common Iliac Artery, Left **E** Internal Iliac Artery, Right **F** Internal Iliac Artery, Left **H** External Iliac Artery, Right **J** External Iliac Artery, Left **K** Femoral Artery, Right **L** Femoral Artery, Left **M** Popliteal Artery, Right **N** Popliteal Artery, Left **P** Anterior Tibial Artery, Right **Q** Anterior Tibial Artery, Left **R** Posterior Tibial Artery, Right **S** Posterior Tibial Artery, Left **T** Peroneal Artery, Right **U** Peroneal Artery, Left **V** Foot Artery, Right **W** Foot Artery, Left **Y** Lower Artery	**0** Open **3** Percutaneous **4** Percutaneous Endoscopic	**5** Intraluminal Device, Drug-eluting, Two **6** Intraluminal Device, Drug-eluting, Three **7** Intraluminal Device, Drug-eluting, Four or More **E** Intraluminal Device, Two **F** Intraluminal Device, Three **G** Intraluminal Device, Four or More	**Z** No Qualifier

LC Limited Coverage   **NC** Noncovered   **HAC** HAC-associated Procedure   **CC** Combination Cluster - See Appendix G for code lists
DRG Non-OR-Affecting MS-DRG Assignment   New/Revised Text in **Orange**   ♂ Male   ♀ Female

2021 ICD-10-PCS   231

0 **Medical and Surgical**
4 **Lower Arteries**
9 **Drainage:** Taking or letting out fluids and/or gases from a body part

Body Part	Approach	Device	Qualifier
Character 4	**Character 5**	**Character 6**	**Character 7**
0 Abdominal Aorta	0 Open	0 Drainage Device	Z No Qualifier
1 Celiac Artery	3 Percutaneous		
2 Gastric Artery	4 Percutaneous Endoscopic		
3 Hepatic Artery			
4 Splenic Artery			
5 Superior Mesenteric Artery			
6 Colic Artery, Right			
7 Colic Artery, Left			
8 Colic Artery, Middle			
9 Renal Artery, Right			
A Renal Artery, Left			
B Inferior Mesenteric Artery			
C Common Iliac Artery, Right			
D Common Iliac Artery, Left			
E Internal Iliac Artery, Right			
F Internal Iliac Artery, Left			
H External Iliac Artery, Right			
J External Iliac Artery, Left			
K Femoral Artery, Right			
L Femoral Artery, Left			
M Popliteal Artery, Right			
N Popliteal Artery, Left			
P Anterior Tibial Artery, Right			
Q Anterior Tibial Artery, Left			
R Posterior Tibial Artery, Right			
S Posterior Tibial Artery, Left			
T Peroneal Artery, Right			
U Peroneal Artery, Left			
V Foot Artery, Right			
W Foot Artery, Left			
Y Lower Artery			
0 Abdominal Aorta	0 Open	Z No Device	X Diagnostic
1 Celiac Artery	3 Percutaneous		Z No Qualifier
2 Gastric Artery	4 Percutaneous Endoscopic		
3 Hepatic Artery			
4 Splenic Artery			
5 Superior Mesenteric Artery			
6 Colic Artery, Right			
7 Colic Artery, Left			
8 Colic Artery, Middle			
9 Renal Artery, Right			
A Renal Artery, Left			
B Inferior Mesenteric Artery			
C Common Iliac Artery, Right			
D Common Iliac Artery, Left			
E Internal Iliac Artery, Right			
F Internal Iliac Artery, Left			
H External Iliac Artery, Right			
J External Iliac Artery, Left			
K Femoral Artery, Right			
L Femoral Artery, Left			
M Popliteal Artery, Right			
N Popliteal Artery, Left			
P Anterior Tibial Artery, Right			
Q Anterior Tibial Artery, Left			
R Posterior Tibial Artery, Right			
S Posterior Tibial Artery, Left			
T Peroneal Artery, Right			
U Peroneal Artery, Left			
V Foot Artery, Right			
W Foot Artery, Left			
Y Lower Artery			

0 Medical and Surgical
4 Lower Arteries
B Excision: Cutting out or off, without replacement, a portion of a body part

Body Part	Approach	Device	Qualifier
Character 4	Character 5	Character 6	Character 7
0 Abdominal Aorta	0 Open	Z No Device	X Diagnostic
1 Celiac Artery	3 Percutaneous		Z No Qualifier
2 Gastric Artery	4 Percutaneous Endoscopic		
3 Hepatic Artery			
4 Splenic Artery			
5 Superior Mesenteric Artery			
6 Colic Artery, Right			
7 Colic Artery, Left			
8 Colic Artery, Middle			
9 Renal Artery, Right			
A Renal Artery, Left			
B Inferior Mesenteric Artery			
C Common Iliac Artery, Right			
D Common Iliac Artery, Left			
E Internal Iliac Artery, Right			
F Internal Iliac Artery, Left			
H External Iliac Artery, Right			
J External Iliac Artery, Left			
K Femoral Artery, Right			
L Femoral Artery, Left			
M Popliteal Artery, Right			
N Popliteal Artery, Left			
P Anterior Tibial Artery, Right			
Q Anterior Tibial Artery, Left			
R Posterior Tibial Artery, Right			
S Posterior Tibial Artery, Left			
T Peroneal Artery, Right			
U Peroneal Artery, Left			
V Foot Artery, Right			
W Foot Artery, Left			
Y Lower Artery			

LC Limited Coverage   NC Noncovered   HAC HAC-associated Procedure   CC Combination Cluster - See Appendix G for code lists
DRG Non-OR-Affecting MS-DRG Assignment   New/Revised Text in Orange   ♂ Male   ♀ Female

2021 ICD-10-PCS 233

0 Medical and Surgical
4 Lower Arteries
C Extirpation: Taking or cutting out solid matter from a body part

Body Part	Approach	Device	Qualifier
Character 4	Character 5	Character 6	Character 7
0 Abdominal Aorta **1** Celiac Artery **2** Gastric Artery **3** Hepatic Artery **4** Splenic Artery **5** Superior Mesenteric Artery **6** Colic Artery, Right **7** Colic Artery, Left **8** Colic Artery, Middle **9** Renal Artery, Right **A** Renal Artery, Left **B** Inferior Mesenteric Artery **C** Common Iliac Artery, Right **D** Common Iliac Artery, Left **E** Internal Iliac Artery, Right **F** Internal Iliac Artery, Left **H** External Iliac Artery, Right **J** External Iliac Artery, Left **K** Femoral Artery, Right **L** Femoral Artery, Left **M** Popliteal Artery, Right **N** Popliteal Artery, Left **P** Anterior Tibial Artery, Right **Q** Anterior Tibial Artery, Left **R** Posterior Tibial Artery, Right **S** Posterior Tibial Artery, Left **T** Peroneal Artery, Right **U** Peroneal Artery, Left **V** Foot Artery, Right **W** Foot Artery, Left **Y** Lower Artery	**0** Open **3** Percutaneous **4** Percutaneous Endoscopic	**Z** No Device	**Z** No Qualifier

0 Medical and Surgical
4 Lower Arteries
F Fragmentation: Breaking solid matter in a body part into pieces

Body Part	Approach	Device	Qualifier
Character 4	Character 5	Character 6	Character 7
C Common Iliac Artery, Right **D** Common Iliac Artery, Left **E** Internal Iliac Artery, Right **F** Internal Iliac Artery, Left **H** External Iliac Artery, Right **J** External Iliac Artery, Left **K** Femoral Artery, Right **L** Femoral Artery, Left **M** Popliteal Artery, Right **N** Popliteal Artery, Left **P** Anterior Tibial Artery, Right **Q** Anterior Tibial Artery, Left **R** Posterior Tibial Artery, Right **S** Posterior Tibial Artery, Left **T** Peroneal Artery, Right **U** Peroneal Artery, Left **Y** Lower Artery	**3** Percutaneous	**Z** No Device	**0** Ultrasonic **Z** No Qualifier

0 **Medical and Surgical**
4 **Lower Arteries**
H **Insertion:** Putting in a nonbiological appliance that monitors, assists, performs, or prevents a physiological function but does not physically take the place of a body part

Body Part	Approach	Device	Qualifier
Character 4	**Character 5**	**Character 6**	**Character 7**
0 Abdominal Aorta	**0** Open **3** Percutaneous **4** Percutaneous Endoscopic	**2** Monitoring Device **3** Infusion Device **D** Intraluminal Device	**Z** No Qualifier
1 Celiac Artery **2** Gastric Artery **3** Hepatic Artery **4** Splenic Artery **5** Superior Mesenteric Artery **6** Colic Artery, Right **7** Colic Artery, Left **8** Colic Artery, Middle **9** Renal Artery, Right **A** Renal Artery, Left **B** Inferior Mesenteric Artery **C** Common Iliac Artery, Right **D** Common Iliac Artery, Left **E** Internal Iliac Artery, Right **F** Internal Iliac Artery, Left **H** External Iliac Artery, Right **J** External Iliac Artery, Left **K** Femoral Artery, Right **L** Femoral Artery, Left **M** Popliteal Artery, Right **N** Popliteal Artery, Left **P** Anterior Tibial Artery, Right **Q** Anterior Tibial Artery, Left **R** Posterior Tibial Artery, Right **S** Posterior Tibial Artery, Left **T** Peroneal Artery, Right **U** Peroneal Artery, Left **V** Foot Artery, Right **W** Foot Artery, Left	**0** Open **3** Percutaneous **4** Percutaneous Endoscopic	**3** Infusion Device **D** Intraluminal Device	**Z** No Qualifier
Y Lower Artery	**0** Open **3** Percutaneous **4** Percutaneous Endoscopic	**2** Monitoring Device **3** Infusion Device **D** Intraluminal Device **Y** Other Device	**Z** No Qualifier

0 **Medical and Surgical**
4 **Lower Arteries**
J **Inspection:** Visually and/or manually exploring a body part

Body Part	Approach	Device	Qualifier
Character 4	**Character 5**	**Character 6**	**Character 7**
Y Lower Artery	**0** Open **3** Percutaneous **4** Percutaneous Endoscopic **X** External	**Z** No Device	**Z** No Qualifier

LC Limited Coverage   NC Noncovered   HAC HAC-associated Procedure   CC Combination Cluster - See Appendix G for code lists
DRG Non-OR-Affecting MS-DRG Assignment   New/Revised Text in Orange   ♂ Male   ♀ Female

2021 ICD-10-PCS   235

0   **Medical and Surgical**
4   **Lower Arteries**
L   **Occlusion:** Completely closing an orifice or the lumen of a tubular body part

Body Part	Approach	Device	Qualifier
Character 4	Character 5	Character 6	Character 7
0 Abdominal Aorta	**0** Open **4** Percutaneous Endoscopic	**C** Extraluminal Device **D** Intraluminal Device **Z** No Device	**Z** No Qualifier
0 Abdominal Aorta	**3** Percutaneous	**C** Extraluminal Device **Z** No Device	**Z** No Qualifier
0 Abdominal Aorta	**3** Percutaneous	**D** Intraluminal Device	**J** Temporary **Z** No Qualifier
1 Celiac Artery **2** Gastric Artery **3** Hepatic Artery **4** Splenic Artery **5** Superior Mesenteric Artery **6** Colic Artery, Right **7** Colic Artery, Left **8** Colic Artery, Middle **9** Renal Artery, Right **A** Renal Artery, Left **B** Inferior Mesenteric Artery **C** Common Iliac Artery, Right **D** Common Iliac Artery, Left **H** External Iliac Artery, Right **J** External Iliac Artery, Left **K** Femoral Artery, Right **L** Femoral Artery, Left **M** Popliteal Artery, Right **N** Popliteal Artery, Left **P** Anterior Tibial Artery, Right **Q** Anterior Tibial Artery, Left **R** Posterior Tibial Artery, Right **S** Posterior Tibial Artery, Left **T** Peroneal Artery, Right **U** Peroneal Artery, Left **V** Foot Artery, Right **W** Foot Artery, Left **Y** Lower Artery	**0** Open **3** Percutaneous **4** Percutaneous Endoscopic	**C** Extraluminal Device **D** Intraluminal Device **Z** No Device	**Z** No Qualifier
E Internal Iliac Artery, Right ♀	**0** Open **3** Percutaneous **4** Percutaneous Endoscopic	**C** Extraluminal Device **D** Intraluminal Device **Z** No Device	**T** Uterine Artery, Right **Z** No Qualifier
F Internal Iliac Artery, Left ♀	**0** Open **3** Percutaneous **4** Percutaneous Endoscopic	**C** Extraluminal Device **D** Intraluminal Device **Z** No Device	**U** Uterine Artery, Left **Z** No Qualifier

♀   04LE0CT   04LE0DT   04LE0ZT   04LE3CT   04LE3DT   04LE3ZT   04LE4CT   04LE4DT   04LE4ZT   04LF0CU   04LF0DU   04LF0ZU   04LF3CU
    04LF3DU   04LF3ZU   04LF4CU   04LF4DU   04LF4ZU

LC Limited Coverage   NC Noncovered   HAC HAC-associated Procedure   CC Combination Cluster - See Appendix G for code lists
DRG Non-OR-Affecting MS-DRG Assignment   New/Revised Text in Orange   ♂ Male   ♀ Female

236

2021 ICD-10-PCS

0 Medical and Surgical
4 Lower Arteries
N Release: Freeing a body part from an abnormal physical constraint by cutting or by the use of force

Body Part	Approach	Device	Qualifier
Character 4	Character 5	Character 6	Character 7
0 Abdominal Aorta	**0** Open	**Z** No Device	**Z** No Qualifier
1 Celiac Artery	**3** Percutaneous		
2 Gastric Artery	**4** Percutaneous Endoscopic		
3 Hepatic Artery			
4 Splenic Artery			
5 Superior Mesenteric Artery			
6 Colic Artery, Right			
7 Colic Artery, Left			
8 Colic Artery, Middle			
9 Renal Artery, Right			
A Renal Artery, Left			
B Inferior Mesenteric Artery			
C Common Iliac Artery, Right			
D Common Iliac Artery, Left			
E Internal Iliac Artery, Right			
F Internal Iliac Artery, Left			
H External Iliac Artery, Right			
J External Iliac Artery, Left			
K Femoral Artery, Right			
L Femoral Artery, Left			
M Popliteal Artery, Right			
N Popliteal Artery, Left			
P Anterior Tibial Artery, Right			
Q Anterior Tibial Artery, Left			
R Posterior Tibial Artery, Right			
S Posterior Tibial Artery, Left			
T Peroneal Artery, Right			
U Peroneal Artery, Left			
V Foot Artery, Right			
W Foot Artery, Left			
Y Lower Artery			

0 Medical and Surgical
4 Lower Arteries
P Removal: Taking out or off a device from a body part

Body Part	Approach	Device	Qualifier
Character 4	Character 5	Character 6	Character 7
Y Lower Artery	**0** Open	**0** Drainage Device	**Z** No Qualifier
	3 Percutaneous	**2** Monitoring Device	
	4 Percutaneous Endoscopic	**3** Infusion Device	
		7 Autologous Tissue Substitute	
		C Extraluminal Device	
		D Intraluminal Device	
		J Synthetic Substitute	
		K Nonautologous Tissue Substitute	
		Y Other Device	
Y Lower Artery	**X** External	**0** Drainage Device	**Z** No Qualifier
		1 Radioactive Element	
		2 Monitoring Device	
		3 Infusion Device	
		D Intraluminal Device	

0 **Medical and Surgical**
4 **Lower Arteries**
Q **Repair:** Restoring, to the extent possible, a body part to its normal anatomic structure and function

Body Part	Approach	Device	Qualifier
Character 4	Character 5	Character 6	Character 7
0 Abdominal Aorta	**0** Open	**Z** No Device	**Z** No Qualifier
1 Celiac Artery	**3** Percutaneous		
2 Gastric Artery	**4** Percutaneous Endoscopic		
3 Hepatic Artery			
4 Splenic Artery			
5 Superior Mesenteric Artery			
6 Colic Artery, Right			
7 Colic Artery, Left			
8 Colic Artery, Middle			
9 Renal Artery, Right			
A Renal Artery, Left			
B Inferior Mesenteric Artery			
C Common Iliac Artery, Right			
D Common Iliac Artery, Left			
E Internal Iliac Artery, Right			
F Internal Iliac Artery, Left			
H External Iliac Artery, Right			
J External Iliac Artery, Left			
K Femoral Artery, Right			
L Femoral Artery, Left			
M Popliteal Artery, Right			
N Popliteal Artery, Left			
P Anterior Tibial Artery, Right			
Q Anterior Tibial Artery, Left			
R Posterior Tibial Artery, Right			
S Posterior Tibial Artery, Left			
T Peroneal Artery, Right			
U Peroneal Artery, Left			
V Foot Artery, Right			
W Foot Artery, Left			
Y Lower Artery			

LC Limited Coverage   NC Noncovered   HAC HAC-associated Procedure   CC Combination Cluster - See Appendix G for code lists
DRG Non-OR-Affecting MS-DRG Assignment   New/Revised Text in **Orange**   ♂ Male   ♀ Female

238   **2021 ICD-10-PCS**

0   Medical and Surgical
4   Lower Arteries
R   Replacement: Putting in or on biological or synthetic material that physically takes the place and/or function of all or a portion of a body part

Body Part	Approach	Device	Qualifier
Character 4	**Character 5**	**Character 6**	**Character 7**
0 Abdominal Aorta	**0** Open	**7** Autologous Tissue Substitute	**Z** No Qualifier
1 Celiac Artery	**4** Percutaneous Endoscopic	**J** Synthetic Substitute	
2 Gastric Artery		**K** Nonautologous Tissue	
3 Hepatic Artery		Substitute	
4 Splenic Artery			
5 Superior Mesenteric Artery			
6 Colic Artery, Right			
7 Colic Artery, Left			
8 Colic Artery, Middle			
9 Renal Artery, Right			
A Renal Artery, Left			
B Inferior Mesenteric Artery			
C Common Iliac Artery, Right			
D Common Iliac Artery, Left			
E Internal Iliac Artery, Right			
F Internal Iliac Artery, Left			
H External Iliac Artery, Right			
J External Iliac Artery, Left			
K Femoral Artery, Right			
L Femoral Artery, Left			
M Popliteal Artery, Right			
N Popliteal Artery, Left			
P Anterior Tibial Artery, Right			
Q Anterior Tibial Artery, Left			
R Posterior Tibial Artery, Right			
S Posterior Tibial Artery, Left			
T Peroneal Artery, Right			
U Peroneal Artery, Left			
V Foot Artery, Right			
W Foot Artery, Left			
Y Lower Artery			

LC Limited Coverage   NC Noncovered   HAC HAC-associated Procedure   CC Combination Cluster - See Appendix G for code lists
DRG Non-OR-Affecting MS-DRG Assignment   New/Revised Text in Orange   ♂ Male   ♀ Female

2021 ICD-10-PCS   239

0   **Medical and Surgical**
4   **Lower Arteries**
S   **Reposition:** Moving to its normal location, or other suitable location, all or a portion of a body part

Body Part	Approach	Device	Qualifier
Character 4	Character 5	Character 6	Character 7
0 Abdominal Aorta	**0** Open	**Z** No Device	**Z** No Qualifier
1 Celiac Artery	**3** Percutaneous		
2 Gastric Artery	**4** Percutaneous Endoscopic		
3 Hepatic Artery			
4 Splenic Artery			
5 Superior Mesenteric Artery			
6 Colic Artery, Right			
7 Colic Artery, Left			
8 Colic Artery, Middle			
9 Renal Artery, Right			
A Renal Artery, Left			
B Inferior Mesenteric Artery			
C Common Iliac Artery, Right			
D Common Iliac Artery, Left			
E Internal Iliac Artery, Right			
F Internal Iliac Artery, Left			
H External Iliac Artery, Right			
J External Iliac Artery, Left			
K Femoral Artery, Right			
L Femoral Artery, Left			
M Popliteal Artery, Right			
N Popliteal Artery, Left			
P Anterior Tibial Artery, Right			
Q Anterior Tibial Artery, Left			
R Posterior Tibial Artery, Right			
S Posterior Tibial Artery, Left			
T Peroneal Artery, Right			
U Peroneal Artery, Left			
V Foot Artery, Right			
W Foot Artery, Left			
Y Lower Artery			

LC Limited Coverage   **NC** Noncovered   **HAC** HAC-associated Procedure   **CC** Combination Cluster - See Appendix G for code lists
DRG Non-OR-Affecting MS-DRG Assignment   New/Revised Text in **Orange**   ♂ Male   ♀ Female

240

2021 ICD-10-PCS

0 **Medical and Surgical**
4 **Lower Arteries**
U **Supplement:** Putting in or on biological or synthetic material that physically reinforces and/or augments the function of a portion of a body part

Body Part	Approach	Device	Qualifier
Character 4	Character 5	Character 6	Character 7
0 Abdominal Aorta **1** Celiac Artery **2** Gastric Artery **3** Hepatic Artery **4** Splenic Artery **5** Superior Mesenteric Artery **6** Colic Artery, Right **7** Colic Artery, Left **8** Colic Artery, Middle **9** Renal Artery, Right **A** Renal Artery, Left **B** Inferior Mesenteric Artery **C** Common Iliac Artery, Right **D** Common Iliac Artery, Left **E** Internal Iliac Artery, Right **F** Internal Iliac Artery, Left **H** External Iliac Artery, Right **J** External Iliac Artery, Left **K** Femoral Artery, Right **L** Femoral Artery, Left **M** Popliteal Artery, Right **N** Popliteal Artery, Left **P** Anterior Tibial Artery, Right **Q** Anterior Tibial Artery, Left **R** Posterior Tibial Artery, Right **S** Posterior Tibial Artery, Left **T** Peroneal Artery, Right **U** Peroneal Artery, Left **V** Foot Artery, Right **W** Foot Artery, Left **Y** Lower Artery	**0** Open **3** Percutaneous **4** Percutaneous Endoscopic	**7** Autologous Tissue Substitute **J** Synthetic Substitute **K** Nonautologous Tissue Substitute	**Z** No Qualifier

LC Limited Coverage   NC Noncovered   HAC HAC-associated Procedure   CC Combination Cluster - See Appendix G for code lists
Non-OR-Affecting MS-DRG Assignment   New/Revised Text in **Orange**   ♂ Male   ♀ Female

2021 ICD-10-PCS

241

0 Medical and Surgical
4 Lower Arteries
V Restriction: Partially closing an orifice or the lumen of a tubular body part

Body Part	Approach	Device	Qualifier
Character 4	**Character 5**	**Character 6**	**Character 7**
0 Abdominal Aorta	**0** Open **3** Percutaneous **4** Percutaneous Endoscopic	**C** Extraluminal Device **E** Intraluminal Device, Branched or Fenestrated, One or Two Arteries **F** Intraluminal Device, Branched or Fenestrated, Three or More Arteries **Z** No Device	**Z** No Qualifier
0 Abdominal Aorta	**0** Open **3** Percutaneous **4** Percutaneous Endoscopic	**D** Intraluminal Device	**J** Temporary **Z** No Qualifier
1 Celiac Artery **2** Gastric Artery **3** Hepatic Artery **4** Splenic Artery **5** Superior Mesenteric Artery **6** Colic Artery, Right **7** Colic Artery, Left **8** Colic Artery, Middle **9** Renal Artery, Right **A** Renal Artery, Left **B** Inferior Mesenteric Artery **E** Internal Iliac Artery, Right **F** Internal Iliac Artery, Left **H** External Iliac Artery, Right **J** External Iliac Artery, Left **K** Femoral Artery, Right **L** Femoral Artery, Left **M** Popliteal Artery, Right **N** Popliteal Artery, Left **P** Anterior Tibial Artery, Right **Q** Anterior Tibial Artery, Left **R** Posterior Tibial Artery, Right **S** Posterior Tibial Artery, Left **T** Peroneal Artery, Right **U** Peroneal Artery, Left **V** Foot Artery, Right **W** Foot Artery, Left **Y** Lower Artery	**0** Open **3** Percutaneous **4** Percutaneous Endoscopic	**C** Extraluminal Device **D** Intraluminal Device **Z** No Device	**Z** No Qualifier
C Common Iliac Artery, Right **D** Common Iliac Artery, Left	**0** Open **3** Percutaneous **4** Percutaneous Endoscopic	**C** Extraluminal Device **D** Intraluminal Device **E** Intraluminal Device, Branched or Fenestrated, One or Two Arteries **Z** No Device	**Z** No Qualifier

LC Limited Coverage   **NC** Noncovered   **HAC** HAC-associated Procedure   **CC** Combination Cluster - See Appendix G for code lists
DRG Non-OR-Affecting MS-DRG Assignment   New/Revised Text in **Orange**   ♂ Male   ♀ Female

242   **2021 ICD-10-PCS**

0   Medical and Surgical
4   Lower Arteries
W Revision: Correcting, to the extent possible, a portion of a malfunctioning device or the position of a displaced device

Body Part	Approach	Device	Qualifier
Character 4	Character 5	Character 6	Character 7
Y Lower Artery	**0** Open **3** Percutaneous **4** Percutaneous Endoscopic	**0** Drainage Device **2** Monitoring Device **3** Infusion Device **7** Autologous Tissue Substitute **C** Extraluminal Device **D** Intraluminal Device **J** Synthetic Substitute **K** Nonautologous Tissue Substitute **Y** Other Device	**Z** No Qualifier
Y Lower Artery	**X** External	**0** Drainage Device **2** Monitoring Device **3** Infusion Device **7** Autologous Tissue Substitute **C** Extraluminal Device **D** Intraluminal Device **J** Synthetic Substitute **K** Nonautologous Tissue Substitute	**Z** No Qualifier

LC Limited Coverage   **NC** Noncovered   **HAC** HAC-associated Procedure   **CC** Combination Cluster - See Appendix G for code lists
DRG Non-OR-Affecting MS-DRG Assignment   New/Revised Text in **Orange**   ♂ Male   ♀ Female

2021 ICD-10-PCS

243

NOTES

Upper Veins 051-05W

0   **Medical and Surgical**
5   **Upper Veins**
1   **Bypass:** Altering the route of passage of the contents of a tubular body part

Body Part	Approach	Device	Qualifier
Character 4	**Character 5**	**Character 6**	**Character 7**
0 Azygos Vein	0 Open	7 Autologous Tissue Substitute	Y Upper Vein
1 Hemiazygos Vein	4 Percutaneous Endoscopic	9 Autologous Venous Tissue	
3 Innominate Vein, Right		A Autologous Arterial Tissue	
4 Innominate Vein, Left		J Synthetic Substitute	
5 Subclavian Vein, Right		K Nonautologous Tissue	
6 Subclavian Vein, Left		Substitute	
7 Axillary Vein, Right		Z No Device	
8 Axillary Vein, Left			
9 Brachial Vein, Right			
A Brachial Vein, Left			
B Basilic Vein, Right			
C Basilic Vein, Left			
D Cephalic Vein, Right			
F Cephalic Vein, Left			
G Hand Vein, Right			
H Hand Vein, Left			
L Intracranial Vein			
M Internal Jugular Vein, Right			
N Internal Jugular Vein, Left			
P External Jugular Vein, Right			
Q External Jugular Vein, Left			
R Vertebral Vein, Right			
S Vertebral Vein, Left			
T Face Vein, Right			
V Face Vein, Left			

LC Limited Coverage   **NC** Noncovered   **HAC** HAC-associated Procedure   **CC** Combination Cluster - See Appendix G for code lists

DRG Non-OR-Affecting MS-DRG Assignment   New/Revised Text in **Orange**   ♂ Male   ♀ Female

0 Medical and Surgical
5 Upper Veins
5 Destruction: Physical eradication of all or a portion of a body part by the direct use of energy, force, or a destructive agent

Body Part	Approach	Device	Qualifier
Character 4	Character 5	Character 6	Character 7
0 Azygos Vein	0 Open	Z No Device	Z No Qualifier
1 Hemiazygos Vein	3 Percutaneous		
3 Innominate Vein, Right	4 Percutaneous Endoscopic		
4 Innominate Vein, Left			
5 Subclavian Vein, Right			
6 Subclavian Vein, Left			
7 Axillary Vein, Right			
8 Axillary Vein, Left			
9 Brachial Vein, Right			
A Brachial Vein, Left			
B Basilic Vein, Right			
C Basilic Vein, Left			
D Cephalic Vein, Right			
F Cephalic Vein, Left			
G Hand Vein, Right			
H Hand Vein, Left			
L Intracranial Vein			
M Internal Jugular Vein, Right			
N Internal Jugular Vein, Left			
P External Jugular Vein, Right			
Q External Jugular Vein, Left			
R Vertebral Vein, Right			
S Vertebral Vein, Left			
T Face Vein, Right			
V Face Vein, Left			
Y Upper Vein			

0 Medical and Surgical
5 Upper Veins
7 Dilation: Expanding an orifice or the lumen of a tubular body part

Body Part	Approach	Device	Qualifier
Character 4	Character 5	Character 6	Character 7
0 Azygos Vein	0 Open	D Intraluminal Device	Z No Qualifier
1 Hemiazygos Vein	3 Percutaneous	Z No Device	
G Hand Vein, Right	4 Percutaneous Endoscopic		
H Hand Vein, Left			
L Intracranial Vein NC			
M Internal Jugular Vein, Right			
N Internal Jugular Vein, Left			
P External Jugular Vein, Right			
Q External Jugular Vein, Left			
R Vertebral Vein, Right			
S Vertebral Vein, Left			
T Face Vein, Right			
V Face Vein, Left			
Y Upper Vein			
3 Innominate Vein, Right	0 Open	D Intraluminal Device	1 Drug-Coated Balloon
4 Innominate Vein, Left	3 Percutaneous	Z No Device	Z No Qualifier
5 Subclavian Vein, Right	4 Percutaneous Endoscopic		
6 Subclavian Vein, Left			
7 Axillary Vein, Right			
8 Axillary Vein, Left			
9 Brachial Vein, Right			
A Brachial Vein, Left			
B Basilic Vein, Right			
C Basilic Vein, Left			
D Cephalic Vein, Right			
F Cephalic Vein, Left			

NC 057L3ZZ   057L4ZZ

LC Limited Coverage NC Noncovered HAC HAC-associated Procedure CC Combination Cluster - See Appendix G for code lists
DRG Non-OR-Affecting MS-DRG Assignment   New/Revised Text in Orange   ♂ Male   ♀ Female

0   **Medical and Surgical**
5   **Upper Veins**
9   **Drainage:** Taking or letting out fluids and/or gases from a body part

Body Part	Approach	Device	Qualifier
Character 4	Character 5	Character 6	Character 7
0 Azygos Vein 1 Hemiazygos Vein 3 Innominate Vein, Right 4 Innominate Vein, Left 5 Subclavian Vein, Right 6 Subclavian Vein, Left 7 Axillary Vein, Right 8 Axillary Vein, Left 9 Brachial Vein, Right A Brachial Vein, Left B Basilic Vein, Right C Basilic Vein, Left D Cephalic Vein, Right F Cephalic Vein, Left G Hand Vein, Right H Hand Vein, Left L Intracranial Vein M Internal Jugular Vein, Right N Internal Jugular Vein, Left P External Jugular Vein, Right Q External Jugular Vein, Left R Vertebral Vein, Right S Vertebral Vein, Left T Face Vein, Right V Face Vein, Left Y Upper Vein	0 Open 3 Percutaneous 4 Percutaneous Endoscopic	0 Drainage Device	Z No Qualifier
0 Azygos Vein 1 Hemiazygos Vein 3 Innominate Vein, Right 4 Innominate Vein, Left 5 Subclavian Vein, Right 6 Subclavian Vein, Left 7 Axillary Vein, Right 8 Axillary Vein, Left 9 Brachial Vein, Right A Brachial Vein, Left B Basilic Vein, Right C Basilic Vein, Left D Cephalic Vein, Right F Cephalic Vein, Left G Hand Vein, Right H Hand Vein, Left L Intracranial Vein M Internal Jugular Vein, Right N Internal Jugular Vein, Left P External Jugular Vein, Right Q External Jugular Vein, Left R Vertebral Vein, Right S Vertebral Vein, Left T Face Vein, Right V Face Vein, Left Y Upper Vein	0 Open 3 Percutaneous 4 Percutaneous Endoscopic	Z No Device	X Diagnostic Z No Qualifier

0 **Medical and Surgical**
5 **Upper Veins**
B **Excision:** Cutting out or off, without replacement, a portion of a body part

Body Part	Approach	Device	Qualifier
Character 4	Character 5	Character 6	Character 7
0 Azygos Vein	**0** Open	**Z** No Device	**X** Diagnostic
1 Hemiazygos Vein	**3** Percutaneous		**Z** No Qualifier
3 Innominate Vein, Right	**4** Percutaneous Endoscopic		
4 Innominate Vein, Left			
5 Subclavian Vein, Right			
6 Subclavian Vein, Left			
7 Axillary Vein, Right			
8 Axillary Vein, Left			
9 Brachial Vein, Right			
A Brachial Vein, Left			
B Basilic Vein, Right			
C Basilic Vein, Left			
D Cephalic Vein, Right			
F Cephalic Vein, Left			
G Hand Vein, Right			
H Hand Vein, Left			
L Intracranial Vein			
M Internal Jugular Vein, Right			
N Internal Jugular Vein, Left			
P External Jugular Vein, Right			
Q External Jugular Vein, Left			
R Vertebral Vein, Right			
S Vertebral Vein, Left			
T Face Vein, Right			
V Face Vein, Left			
Y Upper Vein			

0 **Medical and Surgical**
5 **Upper Veins**
C **Extirpation:** Taking or cutting out solid matter from a body part

Body Part	Approach	Device	Qualifier
Character 4	Character 5	Character 6	Character 7
0 Azygos Vein	**0** Open	**Z** No Device	**Z** No Qualifier
1 Hemiazygos Vein	**3** Percutaneous		
3 Innominate Vein, Right	**4** Percutaneous Endoscopic		
4 Innominate Vein, Left			
5 Subclavian Vein, Right			
6 Subclavian Vein, Left			
7 Axillary Vein, Right			
8 Axillary Vein, Left			
9 Brachial Vein, Right			
A Brachial Vein, Left			
B Basilic Vein, Right			
C Basilic Vein, Left			
D Cephalic Vein, Right			
F Cephalic Vein, Left			
G Hand Vein, Right			
H Hand Vein, Left			
L Intracranial Vein			
M Internal Jugular Vein, Right			
N Internal Jugular Vein, Left			
P External Jugular Vein, Right			
Q External Jugular Vein, Left			
R Vertebral Vein, Right			
S Vertebral Vein, Left			
T Face Vein, Right			
V Face Vein, Left			
Y Upper Vein			

0 **Medical and Surgical**
5 **Upper Veins**
D **Extraction:** Pulling or stripping out or off all or a portion of a body part by the use of force

Body Part	Approach	Device	Qualifier
Character 4	Character 5	Character 6	Character 7
9 Brachial Vein, Right	**0** Open	**Z** No Device	**Z** No Qualifier
A Brachial Vein, Left	**3** Percutaneous		
B Basilic Vein, Right			
C Basilic Vein, Left			
D Cephalic Vein, Right			
F Cephalic Vein, Left			
G Hand Vein, Right			
H Hand Vein, Left			
Y Upper Vein			

0 **Medical and Surgical**
5 **Lower Arteries**
F **Fragmentation:** Breaking solid matter in a body part into pieces

Body Part	Approach	Device	Qualifier
Character 4	Character 5	Character 6	Character 7
3 Innominate Vein, Right	**3** Percutaneous	**Z** No Device	**0** Ultrasonic
4 Innominate Vein, Left			**Z** No Qualifier
5 Subclavian Vein, Right			
6 Subclavian Vein, Left			
7 Axillary Vein, Right			
8 Axillary Vein, Left			
9 Brachial Vein, Right			
A Brachial Vein, Left			
B Basilic Vein, Right			
C Basilic Vein, Left			
D Cephalic Vein, Right			
F Cephalic Vein, Left			
Y Upper Vein			

0   Medical and Surgical
5   Upper Veins
H   Insertion: Putting in a nonbiological appliance that monitors, assists, performs, or prevents a physiological function but does not physically take the place of a body part

Body Part	Approach	Device	Qualifier
Character 4	Character 5	Character 6	Character 7
0 Azygos Vein `HAC` `CC`	**0** Open **3** Percutaneous **4** Percutaneous Endoscopic	**2** Monitoring Device **3** Infusion Device **D** Intraluminal Device **M** Neurostimulator Lead	**Z** No Qualifier
1 Hemiazygos Vein `HAC` **5** Subclavian Vein, Right `HAC` **6** Subclavian Vein, Left `HAC` **7** Axillary Vein, Right **8** Axillary Vein, Left **9** Brachial Vein, Right **A** Brachial Vein, Left **B** Basilic Vein, Right **C** Basilic Vein, Left **D** Cephalic Vein, Right **F** Cephalic Vein, Left **G** Hand Vein, Right **H** Hand Vein, Left **L** Intracranial Vein **M** Internal Jugular Vein, Right `HAC` **N** Internal Jugular Vein, Left `HAC` **P** External Jugular Vein, Right `HAC` **Q** External Jugular Vein, Left `HAC` **R** Vertebral Vein, Right **S** Vertebral Vein, Left **T** Face Vein, Right **V** Face Vein, Left	**0** Open **3** Percutaneous **4** Percutaneous Endoscopic	**3** Infusion Device **D** Intraluminal Device	**Z** No Qualifier
3 Innominate Vein, Right `HAC` `CC` **4** Innominate Vein, Left `HAC` `CC`	**0** Open **3** Percutaneous **4** Percutaneous Endoscopic	**3** Infusion Device **D** Intraluminal Device **M** Neurostimulator Lead	**Z** No Qualifier
Y Upper Vein	**0** Open **3** Percutaneous **4** Percutaneous Endoscopic	**2** Monitoring Device **3** Infusion Device **D** Intraluminal Device **Y** Other Device	**Z** No Qualifier

`HAC` 05H033Z   05H043Z   05H133Z   05H143Z   05H333Z   05H343Z   05H433Z   05H443Z   05H533Z   05H543Z   05H633Z   05H643Z   05HM33Z
05HN33Z   05HP33Z   05HQ33Z

Iatrogenic pneumothorax w/ venous catheterization procedures and secondary diagnosis J95.811.

`CC` 05H00MZ   05H03MZ   05H04MZ   05H30MZ   05H33MZ   05H34MZ   05H40MZ   05H43MZ   05H44MZ

LC Limited Coverage   **NC** Noncovered   **HAC** HAC-associated Procedure   **CC** Combination Cluster - See Appendix G for code lists
NG Non-OR-Affecting MS-DRG Assignment   New/Revised Text in **Orange**   ♂ Male   ♀ Female

250

2021 ICD-10-PCS

0   **Medical and Surgical**
5   **Upper Veins**
J   **Inspection:** Visually and/or manually exploring a body part

Body Part	Approach	Device	Qualifier
Character 4	Character 5	Character 6	Character 7
Y Upper Vein	**0** Open **3** Percutaneous **4** Percutaneous Endoscopic **X** External	**Z** No Device	**Z** No Qualifier

0   **Medical and Surgical**
5   **Upper Veins**
L   **Occlusion:** Completely closing an orifice or the lumen of a tubular body part

Body Part	Approach	Device	Qualifier
Character 4	Character 5	Character 6	Character 7
0 Azygos Vein **1** Hemiazygos Vein **3** Innominate Vein, Right **4** Innominate Vein, Left **5** Subclavian Vein, Right **6** Subclavian Vein, Left **7** Axillary Vein, Right **8** Axillary Vein, Left **9** Brachial Vein, Right **A** Brachial Vein, Left **B** Basilic Vein, Right **C** Basilic Vein, Left **D** Cephalic Vein, Right **F** Cephalic Vein, Left **G** Hand Vein, Right **H** Hand Vein, Left **L** Intracranial Vein **M** Internal Jugular Vein, Right **N** Internal Jugular Vein, Left **P** External Jugular Vein, Right **Q** External Jugular Vein, Left **R** Vertebral Vein, Right **S** Vertebral Vein, Left **T** Face Vein, Right **V** Face Vein, Left **Y** Upper Vein	**0** Open **3** Percutaneous **4** Percutaneous Endoscopic	**C** Extraluminal Device **D** Intraluminal Device **Z** No Device	**Z** No Qualifier

0 Medical and Surgical
5 Upper Veins
N Release: Freeing a body part from an abnormal physical constraint by cutting or by the use of force

Body Part	Approach	Device	Qualifier
Character 4	Character 5	Character 6	Character 7
0 Azygos Vein **1** Hemiazygos Vein **3** Innominate Vein, Right **4** Innominate Vein, Left **5** Subclavian Vein, Right **6** Subclavian Vein, Left **7** Axillary Vein, Right **8** Axillary Vein, Left **9** Brachial Vein, Right **A** Brachial Vein, Left **B** Basilic Vein, Right **C** Basilic Vein, Left **D** Cephalic Vein, Right **F** Cephalic Vein, Left **G** Hand Vein, Right **H** Hand Vein, Left **L** Intracranial Vein **M** Internal Jugular Vein, Right **N** Internal Jugular Vein, Left **P** External Jugular Vein, Right **Q** External Jugular Vein, Left **R** Vertebral Vein, Right **S** Vertebral Vein, Left **T** Face Vein, Right **V** Face Vein, Left **Y** Upper Vein	**0** Open **3** Percutaneous **4** Percutaneous Endoscopic	**Z** No Device	**Z** No Qualifier

0 Medical and Surgical
5 Upper Veins
P Removal: Taking out or off a device from a body part

Body Part	Approach	Device	Qualifier
Character 4	Character 5	Character 6	Character 7
0 Azygos Vein	**0** Open **3** Percutaneous **4** Percutaneous Endoscopic **X** External	**2** Monitoring Device **M** Neurostimulator Lead	**Z** No Qualifier
3 Innominate Vein, Right **4** Innominate Vein, Left	**0** Open **3** Percutaneous **4** Percutaneous Endoscopic **X** External	**M** Neurostimulator Lead	**Z** No Qualifier
Y Upper Vein	**0** Open **3** Percutaneous **4** Percutaneous Endoscopic	**0** Drainage Device **2** Monitoring Device **3** Infusion Device **7** Autologous Tissue Substitute **C** Extraluminal Device **D** Intraluminal Device **J** Synthetic Substitute **K** Nonautologous Tissue Substitute **Y** Other Device	**Z** No Qualifier
Y Upper Vein	**X** External	**0** Drainage Device **2** Monitoring Device **3** Infusion Device **D** Intraluminal Device	**Z** No Qualifier

LC Limited Coverage   **NC** Noncovered   **HAC** HAC-associated Procedure   **CC** Combination Cluster - See Appendix G for code lists
DRG Non-OR-Affecting MS-DRG Assignment   New/Revised Text in **Orange**   ♂ Male   ♀ Female

252

2021 ICD-10-PCS

0 Medical and Surgical
5 Upper Veins
Q Repair: Restoring, to the extent possible, a body part to its normal anatomic structure and function

Body Part	Approach	Device	Qualifier
Character 4	Character 5	Character 6	Character 7
0 Azygos Vein	0 Open	Z No Device	Z No Qualifier
1 Hemiazygos Vein	3 Percutaneous		
3 Innominate Vein, Right	4 Percutaneous Endoscopic		
4 Innominate Vein, Left			
5 Subclavian Vein, Right			
6 Subclavian Vein, Left			
7 Axillary Vein, Right			
8 Axillary Vein, Left			
9 Brachial Vein, Right			
A Brachial Vein, Left			
B Basilic Vein, Right			
C Basilic Vein, Left			
D Cephalic Vein, Right			
F Cephalic Vein, Left			
G Hand Vein, Right			
H Hand Vein, Left			
L Intracranial Vein			
M Internal Jugular Vein, Right			
N Internal Jugular Vein, Left			
P External Jugular Vein, Right			
Q External Jugular Vein, Left			
R Vertebral Vein, Right			
S Vertebral Vein, Left			
T Face Vein, Right			
V Face Vein, Left			
Y Upper Vein			

0 Medical and Surgical
5 Upper Veins
R Replacement: Putting in or on biological or synthetic material that physically takes the place and/or function of all or a portion of a body part

Body Part	Approach	Device	Qualifier
Character 4	Character 5	Character 6	Character 7
0 Azygos Vein	0 Open	7 Autologous Tissue Substitute	Z No Qualifier
1 Hemiazygos Vein	4 Percutaneous Endoscopic	J Synthetic Substitute	
3 Innominate Vein, Right		K Nonautologous Tissue Substitute	
4 Innominate Vein, Left			
5 Subclavian Vein, Right			
6 Subclavian Vein, Left			
7 Axillary Vein, Right			
8 Axillary Vein, Left			
9 Brachial Vein, Right			
A Brachial Vein, Left			
B Basilic Vein, Right			
C Basilic Vein, Left			
D Cephalic Vein, Right			
F Cephalic Vein, Left			
G Hand Vein, Right			
H Hand Vein, Left			
L Intracranial Vein			
M Internal Jugular Vein, Right			
N Internal Jugular Vein, Left			
P External Jugular Vein, Right			
Q External Jugular Vein, Left			
R Vertebral Vein, Right			
S Vertebral Vein, Left			
T Face Vein, Right			
V Face Vein, Left			
Y Upper Vein			

0 Medical and Surgical
5 Upper Veins
S Reposition: Moving to its normal location, or other suitable location, all or a portion of a body part

Body Part	Approach	Device	Qualifier
Character 4	Character 5	Character 6	Character 7
0 Azygos Vein	0 Open	Z No Device	Z No Qualifier
1 Hemiazygos Vein	3 Percutaneous		
3 Innominate Vein, Right	4 Percutaneous Endoscopic		
4 Innominate Vein, Left			
5 Subclavian Vein, Right			
6 Subclavian Vein, Left			
7 Axillary Vein, Right			
8 Axillary Vein, Left			
9 Brachial Vein, Right			
A Brachial Vein, Left			
B Basilic Vein, Right			
C Basilic Vein, Left			
D Cephalic Vein, Right			
F Cephalic Vein, Left			
G Hand Vein, Right			
H Hand Vein, Left			
L Intracranial Vein			
M Internal Jugular Vein, Right			
N Internal Jugular Vein, Left			
P External Jugular Vein, Right			
Q External Jugular Vein, Left			
R Vertebral Vein, Right			
S Vertebral Vein, Left			
T Face Vein, Right			
V Face Vein, Left			
Y Upper Vein			

0 Medical and Surgical
5 Upper Veins
U Supplement: Putting in or on biological or synthetic material that physically reinforces and/or augments the function of a portion of a body part

Body Part	Approach	Device	Qualifier
Character 4	Character 5	Character 6	Character 7
0 Azygos Vein	0 Open	7 Autologous Tissue Substitute	Z No Qualifier
1 Hemiazygos Vein	3 Percutaneous	J Synthetic Substitute	
3 Innominate Vein, Right	4 Percutaneous Endoscopic	K Nonautologous Tissue Substitute	
4 Innominate Vein, Left			
5 Subclavian Vein, Right			
6 Subclavian Vein, Left			
7 Axillary Vein, Right			
8 Axillary Vein, Left			
9 Brachial Vein, Right			
A Brachial Vein, Left			
B Basilic Vein, Right			
C Basilic Vein, Left			
D Cephalic Vein, Right			
F Cephalic Vein, Left			
G Hand Vein, Right			
H Hand Vein, Left			
L Intracranial Vein			
M Internal Jugular Vein, Right			
N Internal Jugular Vein, Left			
P External Jugular Vein, Right			
Q External Jugular Vein, Left			
R Vertebral Vein, Right			
S Vertebral Vein, Left			
T Face Vein, Right			
V Face Vein, Left			
Y Upper Vein			

LC Limited Coverage   NC Noncovered   HAC HAC-associated Procedure   CC Combination Cluster - See Appendix G for code lists
DRG Non-OR-Affecting MS-DRG Assignment   New/Revised Text in Orange   ♂ Male   ♀ Female

254

2021 ICD-10-PCS

0 Medical and Surgical

5 Upper Veins

V Restriction: Partially closing an orifice or the lumen of a tubular body part

Body Part	Approach	Device	Qualifier
Character 4	Character 5	Character 6	Character 7
0 Azygos Vein	0 Open	C Extraluminal Device	Z No Qualifier
1 Hemiazygos Vein	3 Percutaneous	D Intraluminal Device	
3 Innominate Vein, Right	4 Percutaneous Endoscopic	Z No Device	
4 Innominate Vein, Left			
5 Subclavian Vein, Right			
6 Subclavian Vein, Left			
7 Axillary Vein, Right			
8 Axillary Vein, Left			
9 Brachial Vein, Right			
A Brachial Vein, Left			
B Basilic Vein, Right			
C Basilic Vein, Left			
D Cephalic Vein, Right			
F Cephalic Vein, Left			
G Hand Vein, Right			
H Hand Vein, Left			
L Intracranial Vein			
M Internal Jugular Vein, Right			
N Internal Jugular Vein, Left			
P External Jugular Vein, Right			
Q External Jugular Vein, Left			
R Vertebral Vein, Right			
S Vertebral Vein, Left			
T Face Vein, Right			
V Face Vein, Left			
Y Upper Vein			

0 Medical and Surgical

5 Upper Veins

W Revision: Correcting, to the extent possible, a portion of a malfunctioning device or the position of a displaced device

Body Part	Approach	Device	Qualifier
Character 4	Character 5	Character 6	Character 7
0 Azygos Vein	0 Open 3 Percutaneous 4 Percutaneous Endoscopic X External	2 Monitoring Device M Neurostimulator Lead	Z No Qualifier
3 Innominate Vein, Right 4 Innominate Vein, Left	0 Open 3 Percutaneous 4 Percutaneous Endoscopic X External	M Neurostimulator Lead	Z No Qualifier
Y Upper Vein	0 Open 3 Percutaneous 4 Percutaneous Endoscopic	0 Drainage Device 2 Monitoring Device 3 Infusion Device 7 Autologous Tissue Substitute C Extraluminal Device D Intraluminal Device J Synthetic Substitute K Nonautologous Tissue Substitute Y Other Device	Z No Qualifier
Y Upper Vein	X External	0 Drainage Device 2 Monitoring Device 3 Infusion Device 7 Autologous Tissue Substitute C Extraluminal Device D Intraluminal Device J Synthetic Substitute K Nonautologous Tissue Substitute	Z No Qualifier

LC Limited Coverage   **NC** Noncovered   **HAC** HAC-associated Procedure   **CC** Combination Cluster - See Appendix G for code lists

DRG Non-OR-Affecting MS-DRG Assignment   New/Revised Text in **Orange**   ♂ Male   ♀ Female

NOTES

Lower Veins 061-06W

0 Medical and Surgical
6 Lower Veins
1 Bypass: Altering the route of passage of the contents of a tubular body part

Body Part	Approach	Device	Qualifier
Character 4	Character 5	Character 6	Character 7
0 Inferior Vena Cava	**0** Open **4** Percutaneous Endoscopic	**7** Autologous Tissue Substitute **9** Autologous Venous Tissue **A** Autologous Arterial Tissue **J** Synthetic Substitute **K** Nonautologous Tissue Substitute **Z** No Device	**5** Superior Mesenteric Vein **6** Inferior Mesenteric Vein **P** Pulmonary Trunk **Q** Pulmonary Artery, Right **R** Pulmonary Artery, Left **Y** Lower Vein
1 Splenic Vein	**0** Open **4** Percutaneous Endoscopic	**7** Autologous Tissue Substitute **9** Autologous Venous Tissue **A** Autologous Arterial Tissue **J** Synthetic Substitute **K** Nonautologous Tissue Substitute **Z** No Device	**9** Renal Vein, Right **B** Renal Vein, Left **Y** Lower Vein
2 Gastric Vein **3** Esophageal Vein **4** Hepatic Vein **5** Superior Mesenteric Vein **6** Inferior Mesenteric Vein **7** Colic Vein **9** Renal Vein, Right **B** Renal Vein, Left **C** Common Iliac Vein, Right **D** Common Iliac Vein, Left **F** External Iliac Vein, Right **G** External Iliac Vein, Left **H** Hypogastric Vein, Right **J** Hypogastric Vein, Left **M** Femoral Vein, Right **N** Femoral Vein, Left **P** Saphenous Vein, Right **Q** Saphenous Vein, Left **T** Foot Vein, Right **V** Foot Vein, Left	**0** Open **4** Percutaneous Endoscopic	**7** Autologous Tissue Substitute **9** Autologous Venous Tissue **A** Autologous Arterial Tissue **J** Synthetic Substitute **K** Nonautologous Tissue Substitute **Z** No Device	**Y** Lower Vein
8 Portal Vein	**0** Open	**7** Autologous Tissue Substitute **9** Autologous Venous Tissue **A** Autologous Arterial Tissue **J** Synthetic Substitute **K** Nonautologous Tissue Substitute **Z** No Device	**9** Renal Vein, Right **B** Renal Vein, Left **Y** Lower Vein
8 Portal Vein	**3** Percutaneous	**J** Synthetic Substitute	**4** Hepatic Vein **Y** Lower Vein
8 Portal Vein	**4** Percutaneous Endoscopic	**7** Autologous Tissue Substitute **9** Autologous Venous Tissue **A** Autologous Arterial Tissue **K** Nonautologous Tissue Substitute **Z** No Device	**9** Renal Vein, Right **B** Renal Vein, Left **Y** Lower Vein
8 Portal Vein	**4** Percutaneous Endoscopic	**J** Synthetic Substitute	**4** Hepatic Vein **9** Renal Vein, Right **B** Renal Vein, Left **Y** Lower Vein

LC Limited Coverage   **NC** Noncovered   **HAC** HAC-associated Procedure   **CC** Combination Cluster - See Appendix G for code lists
DRG Non-OR-Affecting MS-DRG Assignment   New/Revised Text in **Orange**   ♂ Male ♀ Female

0 Medical and Surgical
6 Lower Veins
5 Destruction: Physical eradication of all or a portion of a body part by the direct use of energy, force, or a destructive agent

Body Part	Approach	Device	Qualifier
Character 4	Character 5	Character 6	Character 7
0 Inferior Vena Cava **1** Splenic Vein **2** Gastric Vein **3** Esophageal Vein **4** Hepatic Vein **5** Superior Mesenteric Vein **6** Inferior Mesenteric Vein **7** Colic Vein **8** Portal Vein **9** Renal Vein, Right **B** Renal Vein, Left **C** Common Iliac Vein, Right **D** Common Iliac Vein, Left **F** External Iliac Vein, Right **G** External Iliac Vein, Left **H** Hypogastric Vein, Right **J** Hypogastric Vein, Left **M** Femoral Vein, Right **N** Femoral Vein, Left **P** Saphenous Vein, Right **Q** Saphenous Vein, Left **T** Foot Vein, Right **V** Foot Vein, Left	**0** Open **3** Percutaneous **4** Percutaneous Endoscopic	**Z** No Device	**Z** No Qualifier
Y Lower Vein	**0** Open **3** Percutaneous **4** Percutaneous Endoscopic	**Z** No Device	**C** Hemorrhoidal Plexus **Z** No Qualifier

0 Medical and Surgical
6 Lower Veins
7 Dilation: Expanding an orifice or the lumen of a tubular body part

Body Part	Approach	Device	Qualifier
Character 4	Character 5	Character 6	Character 7
0 Inferior Vena Cava **1** Splenic Vein **2** Gastric Vein **3** Esophageal Vein **4** Hepatic Vein **5** Superior Mesenteric Vein **6** Inferior Mesenteric Vein **7** Colic Vein **8** Portal Vein **9** Renal Vein, Right **B** Renal Vein, Left **C** Common Iliac Vein, Right **D** Common Iliac Vein, Left **F** External Iliac Vein, Right **G** External Iliac Vein, Left **H** Hypogastric Vein, Right **J** Hypogastric Vein, Left **M** Femoral Vein, Right **N** Femoral Vein, Left **P** Saphenous Vein, Right **Q** Saphenous Vein, Left **T** Foot Vein, Right **V** Foot Vein, Left **Y** Lower Vein	**0** Open **3** Percutaneous **4** Percutaneous Endoscopic	**D** Intraluminal Device **Z** No Device	**Z** No Qualifier

0 Medical and Surgical
6 Lower Veins
9 Drainage: Taking or letting out fluids and/or gases from a body part

Body Part	Approach	Device	Qualifier
Character 4	Character 5	Character 6	Character 7
0 Inferior Vena Cava **1** Splenic Vein **2** Gastric Vein **3** Esophageal Vein **4** Hepatic Vein **5** Superior Mesenteric Vein **6** Inferior Mesenteric Vein **7** Colic Vein **8** Portal Vein **9** Renal Vein, Right **B** Renal Vein, Left **C** Common Iliac Vein, Right **D** Common Iliac Vein, Left **F** External Iliac Vein, Right **G** External Iliac Vein, Left **H** Hypogastric Vein, Right **J** Hypogastric Vein, Left **M** Femoral Vein, Right **N** Femoral Vein, Left **P** Saphenous Vein, Right **Q** Saphenous Vein, Left **T** Foot Vein, Right **V** Foot Vein, Left **Y** Lower Vein	**0** Open **3** Percutaneous **4** Percutaneous Endoscopic	**0** Drainage Device	**Z** No Qualifier
0 Inferior Vena Cava **1** Splenic Vein **2** Gastric Vein **3** Esophageal Vein **4** Hepatic Vein **5** Superior Mesenteric Vein **6** Inferior Mesenteric Vein **7** Colic Vein **8** Portal Vein **9** Renal Vein, Right **B** Renal Vein, Left **C** Common Iliac Vein, Right **D** Common Iliac Vein, Left **F** External Iliac Vein, Right **G** External Iliac Vein, Left **H** Hypogastric Vein, Right **J** Hypogastric Vein, Left **M** Femoral Vein, Right **N** Femoral Vein, Left **P** Saphenous Vein, Right **Q** Saphenous Vein, Left **T** Foot Vein, Right **V** Foot Vein, Left **Y** Lower Vein	**0** Open **3** Percutaneous **4** Percutaneous Endoscopic	**Z** No Device	**X** Diagnostic **Z** No Qualifier

LC Limited Coverage NC Noncovered HAC HAC-associated Procedure CC Combination Cluster - See Appendix G for code lists
DRG Non-OR-Affecting MS-DRG Assignment New/Revised Text in Orange ♂ Male ♀ Female

2021 ICD-10-PCS 259

0   Medical and Surgical
6   Lower Veins
B   Excision: Cutting out or off, without replacement, a portion of a body part

Body Part	Approach	Device	Qualifier
Character 4	Character 5	Character 6	Character 7
0 Inferior Vena Cava 1 Splenic Vein 2 Gastric Vein 3 Esophageal Vein 4 Hepatic Vein 5 Superior Mesenteric Vein 6 Inferior Mesenteric Vein 7 Colic Vein 8 Portal Vein 9 Renal Vein, Right B Renal Vein, Left C Common Iliac Vein, Right D Common Iliac Vein, Left F External Iliac Vein, Right G External Iliac Vein, Left H Hypogastric Vein, Right J Hypogastric Vein, Left M Femoral Vein, Right N Femoral Vein, Left P Saphenous Vein, Right Q Saphenous Vein, Left T Foot Vein, Right V Foot Vein, Left	0 Open 3 Percutaneous 4 Percutaneous Endoscopic	Z No Device	X Diagnostic Z No Qualifier
Y Lower Vein	0 Open 3 Percutaneous 4 Percutaneous Endoscopic	Z No Device	C Hemorrhoidal Plexus X Diagnostic Z No Qualifier

0   Medical and Surgical
6   Lower Veins
C   Extirpation: Taking or cutting out solid matter from a body part

Body Part	Approach	Device	Qualifier
Character 4	Character 5	Character 6	Character 7
0 Inferior Vena Cava 1 Splenic Vein 2 Gastric Vein 3 Esophageal Vein 4 Hepatic Vein 5 Superior Mesenteric Vein 6 Inferior Mesenteric Vein 7 Colic Vein 8 Portal Vein 9 Renal Vein, Right B Renal Vein, Left C Common Iliac Vein, Right D Common Iliac Vein, Left F External Iliac Vein, Right G External Iliac Vein, Left H Hypogastric Vein, Right J Hypogastric Vein, Left M Femoral Vein, Right N Femoral Vein, Left P Saphenous Vein, Right Q Saphenous Vein, Left T Foot Vein, Right V Foot Vein, Left Y Lower Vein	0 Open 3 Percutaneous 4 Percutaneous Endoscopic	Z No Device	Z No Qualifier

LC Limited Coverage   NC Noncovered   HAC HAC-associated Procedure   CC Combination Cluster - See Appendix G for code lists
DRG Non-OR-Affecting MS-DRG Assignment   New/Revised Text in **Orange**   ♂ Male   ♀ Female

260   2021 ICD-10-PCS

0   Medical and Surgical
6   Lower Veins
D   Extraction: Pulling or stripping out or off all or a portion of a body part by the use of force

Body Part	Approach	Device	Qualifier
Character 4	Character 5	Character 6	Character 7
M Femoral Vein, Right **N** Femoral Vein, Left **P** Saphenous Vein, Right **Q** Saphenous Vein, Left **T** Foot Vein, Right **V** Foot Vein, Left **Y** Lower Vein	**0** Open **3** Percutaneous **4** Percutaneous Endoscopic	**Z** No Device	**Z** No Qualifier

0   Medical and Surgical
6   Lower Arteries
F   Fragmentation: Breaking solid matter in a body part into pieces

Body Part	Approach	Device	Qualifier
Character 4	Character 5	Character 6	Character 7
C Common Iliac Vein, Right **D** Common Iliac Vein, Left **F** External Iliac Vein, Right **G** External Iliac Vein, Left **H** Hypogastric Vein, Right **J** Hypogastric Vein, Left **M** Femoral Vein, Right **N** Femoral Vein, Left **P** Saphenous Vein, Right **Q** Saphenous Vein, Left **Y** Lower Vein	**3** Percutaneous	**Z** No Device	**0** Ultrasonic **Z** No Qualifier

0 Medical and Surgical
6 Lower Veins
H **Insertion:** Putting in a nonbiological appliance that monitors, assists, performs, or prevents a physiological function but does not physically take the place of a body part

Body Part	Approach	Device	Qualifier
Character 4	Character 5	Character 6	Character 7
0 Inferior Vena Cava	**0** Open **3** Percutaneous	**3** Infusion Device	**T** Via Umbilical Vein **Z** No Qualifier
0 Inferior Vena Cava	**0** Open **3** Percutaneous	**D** Intraluminal Device	**Z** No Qualifier
0 Inferior Vena Cava	**4** Percutaneous Endoscopic	**3** Infusion Device **D** Intraluminal Device	**Z** No Qualifier
1 Splenic Vein **2** Gastric Vein **3** Esophageal Vein **4** Hepatic Vein **5** Superior Mesenteric Vein **6** Inferior Mesenteric Vein **7** Colic Vein **8** Portal Vein **9** Renal Vein, Right **B** Renal Vein, Left **C** Common Iliac Vein, Right **D** Common Iliac Vein, Left **F** External Iliac Vein, Right **G** External Iliac Vein, Left **H** Hypogastric Vein, Right **J** Hypogastric Vein, Left **M** Femoral Vein, Right **N** Femoral Vein, Left **P** Saphenous Vein, Right **Q** Saphenous Vein, Left **T** Foot Vein, Right **V** Foot Vein, Left	**0** Open **3** Percutaneous **4** Percutaneous Endoscopic	**3** Infusion Device **D** Intraluminal Device	**Z** No Qualifier
Y Lower Vein	**0** Open **3** Percutaneous **4** Percutaneous Endoscopic	**2** Monitoring Device **3** Infusion Device **D** Intraluminal Device **Y** Other Device	**Z** No Qualifier

0 Medical and Surgical
6 Lower Veins
J **Inspection:** Visually and/or manually exploring a body part

Body Part	Approach	Device	Qualifier
Character 4	Character 5	Character 6	Character 7
Y Lower Vein	**0** Open **3** Percutaneous **4** Percutaneous Endoscopic **X** External	**Z** No Device	**Z** No Qualifier

0   **Medical and Surgical**
6   **Lower Veins**
L   **Occlusion:** Completely closing an orifice or the lumen of a tubular body part

Body Part	Approach	Device	Qualifier
Character 4	Character 5	Character 6	Character 7
0 Inferior Vena Cava 1 Splenic Vein 4 Hepatic Vein 5 Superior Mesenteric Vein 6 Inferior Mesenteric Vein 7 Colic Vein 8 Portal Vein 9 Renal Vein, Right B Renal Vein, Left C Common Iliac Vein, Right D Common Iliac Vein, Left F External Iliac Vein, Right G External Iliac Vein, Left H Hypogastric Vein, Right J Hypogastric Vein, Left M Femoral Vein, Right N Femoral Vein, Left P Saphenous Vein, Right Q Saphenous Vein, Left T Foot Vein, Right V Foot Vein, Left	0 Open 3 Percutaneous 4 Percutaneous Endoscopic	C Extraluminal Device D Intraluminal Device Z No Device	Z No Qualifier
2 Gastric Vein 3 Esophageal Vein	0 Open 3 Percutaneous 4 Percutaneous Endoscopic 7 Via Natural or Artificial Opening 8 Via Natural or Artificial Opening Endoscopic	C Extraluminal Device D Intraluminal Device Z No Device	Z No Qualifier
Y Lower Vein	0 Open 3 Percutaneous 4 Percutaneous Endoscopic	C Extraluminal Device D Intraluminal Device Z No Device	C Hemorrhoidal Plexus Z No Qualifier

0 Medical and Surgical
6 Lower Veins
N Release: Freeing a body part from an abnormal physical constraint by cutting or by the use of force

Body Part	Approach	Device	Qualifier
Character 4	Character 5	Character 6	Character 7
0 Inferior Vena Cava 1 Splenic Vein 2 Gastric Vein 3 Esophageal Vein 4 Hepatic Vein 5 Superior Mesenteric Vein 6 Inferior Mesenteric Vein 7 Colic Vein 8 Portal Vein 9 Renal Vein, Right B Renal Vein, Left C Common Iliac Vein, Right D Common Iliac Vein, Left F External Iliac Vein, Right G External Iliac Vein, Left H Hypogastric Vein, Right J Hypogastric Vein, Left M Femoral Vein, Right N Femoral Vein, Left P Saphenous Vein, Right Q Saphenous Vein, Left T Foot Vein, Right V Foot Vein, Left Y Lower Vein	0 Open 3 Percutaneous 4 Percutaneous Endoscopic	Z No Device	Z No Qualifier

0 Medical and Surgical
6 Lower Veins
P Removal: Taking out or off a device from a body part

Body Part	Approach	Device	Qualifier
Character 4	Character 5	Character 6	Character 7
Y Lower Vein	0 Open 3 Percutaneous 4 Percutaneous Endoscopic	0 Drainage Device 2 Monitoring Device 3 Infusion Device 7 Autologous Tissue Substitute C Extraluminal Device D Intraluminal Device J Synthetic Substitute K Nonautologous Tissue Substitute Y Other Device	Z No Qualifier
Y Lower Vein	X External	0 Drainage Device 2 Monitoring Device 3 Infusion Device D Intraluminal Device	Z No Qualifier

LC Limited Coverage   NC Noncovered   HAC HAC-associated Procedure   CC Combination Cluster - See Appendix G for code lists
Non-OR-Affecting MS-DRG Assignment   New/Revised Text in Orange   ♂ Male   ♀ Female

264   2021 ICD-10-PCS

0 Medical and Surgical
6 Lower Veins
Q Repair: Restoring, to the extent possible, a body part to its normal anatomic structure and function

Body Part	Approach	Device	Qualifier
Character 4	Character 5	Character 6	Character 7
0 Inferior Vena Cava **1** Splenic Vein **2** Gastric Vein **3** Esophageal Vein **4** Hepatic Vein **5** Superior Mesenteric Vein **6** Inferior Mesenteric Vein **7** Colic Vein **8** Portal Vein **9** Renal Vein, Right **B** Renal Vein, Left **C** Common Iliac Vein, Right **D** Common Iliac Vein, Left **F** External Iliac Vein, Right **G** External Iliac Vein, Left **H** Hypogastric Vein, Right **J** Hypogastric Vein, Left **M** Femoral Vein, Right **N** Femoral Vein, Left **P** Saphenous Vein, Right **Q** Saphenous Vein, Left **T** Foot Vein, Right **V** Foot Vein, Left **Y** Lower Vein	**0** Open **3** Percutaneous **4** Percutaneous Endoscopic	**Z** No Device	**Z** No Qualifier

0 Medical and Surgical
6 Lower Veins
R Replacement: Putting in or on biological or synthetic material that physically takes the place and/or function of all or a portion of a body part

Body Part	Approach	Device	Qualifier
Character 4	Character 5	Character 6	Character 7
0 Inferior Vena Cava **1** Splenic Vein **2** Gastric Vein **3** Esophageal Vein **4** Hepatic Vein **5** Superior Mesenteric Vein **6** Inferior Mesenteric Vein **7** Colic Vein **8** Portal Vein **9** Renal Vein, Right **B** Renal Vein, Left **C** Common Iliac Vein, Right **D** Common Iliac Vein, Left **F** External Iliac Vein, Right **G** External Iliac Vein, Left **H** Hypogastric Vein, Right **J** Hypogastric Vein, Left **M** Femoral Vein, Right **N** Femoral Vein, Left **P** Saphenous Vein, Right **Q** Saphenous Vein, Left **T** Foot Vein, Right **V** Foot Vein, Left **Y** Lower Vein	**0** Open **4** Percutaneous Endoscopic	**7** Autologous Tissue Substitute **J** Synthetic Substitute **K** Nonautologous Tissue Substitute	**Z** No Qualifier

0 Medical and Surgical
6 Lower Veins
S Reposition: Moving to its normal location, or other suitable location, all or a portion of a body part

Body Part		Approach		Device		Qualifier	
Character 4		**Character 5**		**Character 6**		**Character 7**	
0	Inferior Vena Cava	0	Open	Z	No Device	Z	No Qualifier
1	Splenic Vein	3	Percutaneous				
2	Gastric Vein	4	Percutaneous Endoscopic				
3	Esophageal Vein						
4	Hepatic Vein						
5	Superior Mesenteric Vein						
6	Inferior Mesenteric Vein						
7	Colic Vein						
8	Portal Vein						
9	Renal Vein, Right						
B	Renal Vein, Left						
C	Common Iliac Vein, Right						
D	Common Iliac Vein, Left						
F	External Iliac Vein, Right						
G	External Iliac Vein, Left						
H	Hypogastric Vein, Right						
J	Hypogastric Vein, Left						
M	Femoral Vein, Right						
N	Femoral Vein, Left						
P	Saphenous Vein, Right						
Q	Saphenous Vein, Left						
T	Foot Vein, Right						
V	Foot Vein, Left						
Y	Lower Vein						

0 Medical and Surgical
6 Lower Veins
U Supplement: Putting in or on biological or synthetic material that physically reinforces and/or augments the function of a portion of a body part

Body Part		Approach		Device		Qualifier	
Character 4		**Character 5**		**Character 6**		**Character 7**	
0	Inferior Vena Cava	0	Open	7	Autologous Tissue Substitute	Z	No Qualifier
1	Splenic Vein	3	Percutaneous	J	Synthetic Substitute		
2	Gastric Vein	4	Percutaneous Endoscopic	K	Nonautologous Tissue Substitute		
3	Esophageal Vein						
4	Hepatic Vein						
5	Superior Mesenteric Vein						
6	Inferior Mesenteric Vein						
7	Colic Vein						
8	Portal Vein						
9	Renal Vein, Right						
B	Renal Vein, Left						
C	Common Iliac Vein, Right						
D	Common Iliac Vein, Left						
F	External Iliac Vein, Right						
G	External Iliac Vein, Left						
H	Hypogastric Vein, Right						
J	Hypogastric Vein, Left						
M	Femoral Vein, Right						
N	Femoral Vein, Left						
P	Saphenous Vein, Right						
Q	Saphenous Vein, Left						
T	Foot Vein, Right						
V	Foot Vein, Left						
Y	Lower Vein						

LC Limited Coverage   NC Noncovered   HAC HAC-associated Procedure   CC Combination Cluster - See Appendix G for code lists
DRG Non-OR-Affecting MS-DRG Assignment   New/Revised Text in Orange   ♂ Male   ♀ Female

266

2021 ICD-10-PCS

0   **Medical and Surgical**
6   **Lower Veins**
V   **Restriction:** Partially closing an orifice or the lumen of a tubular body part

Body Part	Approach	Device	Qualifier
Character 4	Character 5	Character 6	Character 7
0 Inferior Vena Cava **1** Splenic Vein **2** Gastric Vein **3** Esophageal Vein **4** Hepatic Vein **5** Superior Mesenteric Vein **6** Inferior Mesenteric Vein **7** Colic Vein **8** Portal Vein **9** Renal Vein, Right **B** Renal Vein, Left **C** Common Iliac Vein, Right **D** Common Iliac Vein, Left **F** External Iliac Vein, Right **G** External Iliac Vein, Left **H** Hypogastric Vein, Right **J** Hypogastric Vein, Left **M** Femoral Vein, Right **N** Femoral Vein, Left **P** Saphenous Vein, Right **Q** Saphenous Vein, Left **T** Foot Vein, Right **V** Foot Vein, Left **Y** Lower Vein	**0** Open **3** Percutaneous **4** Percutaneous Endoscopic	**C** Extraluminal Device **D** Intraluminal Device **Z** No Device	**Z** No Qualifier

0   **Medical and Surgical**
6   **Lower Veins**
W   **Revision:** Correcting, to the extent possible, a portion of a malfunctioning device or the position of a displaced device

Body Part	Approach	Device	Qualifier
Character 4	Character 5	Character 6	Character 7
Y Lower Vein	**0** Open **3** Percutaneous **4** Percutaneous Endoscopic	**0** Drainage Device **2** Monitoring Device **3** Infusion Device **7** Autologous Tissue Substitute **C** Extraluminal Device **D** Intraluminal Device **J** Synthetic Substitute **K** Nonautologous Tissue Substitute **Y** Other Device	**Z** No Qualifier
Y Lower Vein	**X** External	**0** Drainage Device **2** Monitoring Device **3** Infusion Device **7** Autologous Tissue Substitute **C** Extraluminal Device **D** Intraluminal Device **J** Synthetic Substitute **K** Nonautologous Tissue Substitute	**Z** No Qualifier

LC Limited Coverage   NC Noncovered   HAC HAC-associated Procedure   CC Combination Cluster - See Appendix G for code lists
DRG Non-OR-Affecting MS-DRG Assignment   New/Revised Text in Orange   ♂ Male   ♀ Female

2021 ICD-10-PCS

267

NOTES

Lymphatic and Hemic Systems 072-07Y

0 Medical and Surgical
7 Lymphatic and Hemic Systems
2 **Change:** Taking out or off a device from a body part and putting back an identical or similar device in or on the same body part without cutting or puncturing the skin or a mucous membrane

Body Part	Approach	Device	Qualifier
Character 4	Character 5	Character 6	Character 7
K Thoracic Duct **L** Cisterna Chyli **M** Thymus **N** Lymphatic **P** Spleen **T** Bone Marrow	**X** External	**0** Drainage Device **Y** Other Device	**Z** No Qualifier

0 Medical and Surgical
7 Lymphatic and Hemic Systems
5 **Destruction:** Physical eradication of all or a portion of a body part by the direct use of energy, force, or a destructive agent

Body Part	Approach	Device	Qualifier
Character 4	Character 5	Character 6	Character 7
0 Lymphatic, Head **1** Lymphatic, Right Neck **2** Lymphatic, Left Neck **3** Lymphatic, Right Upper Extremity **4** Lymphatic, Left Upper Extremity **5** Lymphatic, Right Axillary **6** Lymphatic, Left Axillary **7** Lymphatic, Thorax **8** Lymphatic, Internal Mammary, Right **9** Lymphatic, Internal Mammary, Left **B** Lymphatic, Mesenteric **C** Lymphatic, Pelvis **D** Lymphatic, Aortic **F** Lymphatic, Right Lower Extremity **G** Lymphatic, Left Lower Extremity **H** Lymphatic, Right Inguinal **J** Lymphatic, Left Inguinal **K** Thoracic Duct **L** Cisterna Chyli **M** Thymus **P** Spleen	**0** Open **3** Percutaneous **4** Percutaneous Endoscopic	**Z** No Device	**Z** No Qualifier

0 **Medical and Surgical**
7 **Lymphatic and Hemic Systems**
9 **Drainage:** Taking or letting out fluids and/or gases from a body part

Body Part	Approach	Device	Qualifier
Character 4	Character 5	Character 6	Character 7
0 Lymphatic, Head 1 Lymphatic, Right Neck 2 Lymphatic, Left Neck 3 Lymphatic, Right Upper Extremity 4 Lymphatic, Left Upper Extremity 5 Lymphatic, Right Axillary 6 Lymphatic, Left Axillary 7 Lymphatic, Thorax 8 Lymphatic, Internal Mammary, Right 9 Lymphatic, Internal Mammary, Left B Lymphatic, Mesenteric C Lymphatic, Pelvis D Lymphatic, Aortic F Lymphatic, Right Lower Extremity G Lymphatic, Left Lower Extremity H Lymphatic, Right Inguinal J Lymphatic, Left Inguinal K Thoracic Duct L Cisterna Chyli	0 Open 3 Percutaneous 4 Percutaneous Endoscopic 8 Via Natural or Artificial Opening Endoscopic	0 Drainage Device	Z No Qualifier
0 Lymphatic, Head 1 Lymphatic, Right Neck 2 Lymphatic, Left Neck 3 Lymphatic, Right Upper Extremity 4 Lymphatic, Left Upper Extremity 5 Lymphatic, Right Axillary 6 Lymphatic, Left Axillary 7 Lymphatic, Thorax 8 Lymphatic, Internal Mammary, Right 9 Lymphatic, Internal Mammary, Left B Lymphatic, Mesenteric C Lymphatic, Pelvis D Lymphatic, Aortic F Lymphatic, Right Lower Extremity G Lymphatic, Left Lower Extremity H Lymphatic, Right Inguinal J Lymphatic, Left Inguinal K Thoracic Duct L Cisterna Chyli	0 Open 3 Percutaneous 4 Percutaneous Endoscopic 8 Via Natural or Artificial Opening Endoscopic	Z No Device	X Diagnostic Z No Qualifier
M Thymus P Spleen T Bone Marrow	0 Open 3 Percutaneous 4 Percutaneous Endoscopic	0 Drainage Device	Z No Qualifier
M Thymus P Spleen T Bone Marrow	0 Open 3 Percutaneous 4 Percutaneous Endoscopic	Z No Device	X Diagnostic Z No Qualifier

0 **Medical and Surgical**

7 **Lymphatic and Hemic Systems**

B **Excision:** Cutting out or off, without replacement, a portion of a body part

Body Part	Approach	Device	Qualifier
Character 4	Character 5	Character 6	Character 7
0 Lymphatic, Head **1** Lymphatic, Right Neck **2** Lymphatic, Left Neck **3** Lymphatic, Right Upper Extremity **4** Lymphatic, Left Upper Extremity **5** Lymphatic, Right Axillary **6** Lymphatic, Left Axillary **7** Lymphatic, Thorax **8** Lymphatic, Internal Mammary, Right **9** Lymphatic, Internal Mammary, Left **B** Lymphatic, Mesenteric **C** Lymphatic, Pelvis **D** Lymphatic, Aortic **F** Lymphatic, Right Lower Extremity **G** Lymphatic, Left Lower Extremity **H** Lymphatic, Right Inguinal ᴄᴄ **J** Lymphatic, Left Inguinal ᴄᴄ **K** Thoracic Duct **L** Cisterna Chyli **M** Thymus **P** Spleen	**0** Open **3** Percutaneous **4** Percutaneous Endoscopic	**Z** No Device	**X** Diagnostic **Z** No Qualifier

ᴄᴄ 07BH0ZZ   07BH4ZZ   07BJ0ZZ   07BJ4ZZ

0 **Medical and Surgical**

7 **Lymphatic and Hemic Systems**

C **Extirpation:** Taking or cutting out solid matter from a body part

Body Part	Approach	Device	Qualifier
Character 4	Character 5	Character 6	Character 7
0 Lymphatic, Head **1** Lymphatic, Right Neck **2** Lymphatic, Left Neck **3** Lymphatic, Right Upper Extremity **4** Lymphatic, Left Upper Extremity **5** Lymphatic, Right Axillary **6** Lymphatic, Left Axillary **7** Lymphatic, Thorax **8** Lymphatic, Internal Mammary, Right **9** Lymphatic, Internal Mammary, Left **B** Lymphatic, Mesenteric **C** Lymphatic, Pelvis **D** Lymphatic, Aortic **F** Lymphatic, Right Lower Extremity **G** Lymphatic, Left Lower Extremity **H** Lymphatic, Right Inguinal **J** Lymphatic, Left Inguinal **K** Thoracic Duct **L** Cisterna Chyli **M** Thymus **P** Spleen	**0** Open **3** Percutaneous **4** Percutaneous Endoscopic	**Z** No Device	**Z** No Qualifier

ᴸᴄ Limited Coverage   ᴺᶜ Noncovered   ᴴᴬᶜ HAC-associated Procedure   ᴄᴄ Combination Cluster - See Appendix G for code lists
ᴰᴿᴳ Non-OR-Affecting MS-DRG Assignment   New/Revised Text in **Orange**   ♂ Male   ♀ Female

0 **Medical and Surgical**
7 **Lymphatic and Hemic Systems**
D **Extraction:** Pulling or stripping out or off all or a portion of a body part by the use of force

Body Part	Approach	Device	Qualifier
Character 4	Character 5	Character 6	Character 7
0 Lymphatic, Head 1 Lymphatic, Right Neck 2 Lymphatic, Left Neck 3 Lymphatic, Right Upper Extremity 4 Lymphatic, Left Upper Extremity 5 Lymphatic, Right Axillary 6 Lymphatic, Left Axillary 7 Lymphatic, Thorax 8 Lymphatic, Internal Mammary, Right 9 Lymphatic, Internal Mammary, Left B Lymphatic, Mesenteric C Lymphatic, Pelvis D Lymphatic, Aortic F Lymphatic, Right Lower Extremity G Lymphatic, Left Lower Extremity H Lymphatic, Right Inguinal J Lymphatic, Left Inguinal K Thoracic Duct L Cisterna Chyli	3 Percutaneous 4 Percutaneous Endoscopic 8 Via Natural or Artificial Opening Endoscopic	Z No Device	X Diagnostic
M Thymus P Spleen	3 Percutaneous 4 Percutaneous Endoscopic	Z No Device	X Diagnostic
Q Bone Marrow, Sternum R Bone Marrow, Iliac S Bone Marrow, Vertebral	0 Open 3 Percutaneous	Z No Device	X Diagnostic Z No Qualifier

0 **Medical and Surgical**
7 **Lymphatic and Hemic Systems**
H **Insertion:** Putting in a nonbiological appliance that monitors, assists, performs, or prevents a physiological function but does not physically take the place of a body part

Body Part	Approach	Device	Qualifier
Character 4	Character 5	Character 6	Character 7
K Thoracic Duct L Cisterna Chyli M Thymus N Lymphatic P Spleen T Bone Marrow	0 Open 3 Percutaneous 4 Percutaneous Endoscopic	1 Radioactive Element 3 Infusion Device Y Other Device	Z No Qualifier

LC Limited Coverage   NC Noncovered   HAC HAC-associated Procedure   CC Combination Cluster - See Appendix G for code lists
Non-OR-Affecting MS-DRG Assignment   New/Revised Text in **Orange**   ♂ Male   ♀ Female

272

2021 ICD-10-PCS

0   Medical and Surgical
7   Lymphatic and Hemic Systems
J   Inspection: Visually and/or manually exploring a body part

Body Part	Approach	Device	Qualifier
Character 4	**Character 5**	**Character 6**	**Character 7**
K Thoracic Duct **L** Cisterna Chyli **M** Thymus **T** Bone Marrow	**0** Open **3** Percutaneous **4** Percutaneous Endoscopic	**Z** No Device	**Z** No Qualifier
N Lymphatic	**0** Open **3** Percutaneous **4** Percutaneous Endoscopic **8** Via Natural or Artificial Opening Endoscopic **X** External	**Z** No Device	**Z** No Qualifier
P Spleen	**0** Open **3** Percutaneous **4** Percutaneous Endoscopic **X** External	**Z** No Device	**Z** No Qualifier

0   Medical and Surgical
7   Lymphatic and Hemic Systems
L   Occlusion: Completely closing an orifice or the lumen of a tubular body part

Body Part	Approach	Device	Qualifier
Character 4	**Character 5**	**Character 6**	**Character 7**
0 Lymphatic, Head **1** Lymphatic, Right Neck **2** Lymphatic, Left Neck **3** Lymphatic, Right Upper Extremity **4** Lymphatic, Left Upper Extremity **5** Lymphatic, Right Axillary **6** Lymphatic, Left Axillary **7** Lymphatic, Thorax **8** Lymphatic, Internal Mammary, Right **9** Lymphatic, Internal Mammary, Left **B** Lymphatic, Mesenteric **C** Lymphatic, Pelvis **D** Lymphatic, Aortic **F** Lymphatic, Right Lower Extremity **G** Lymphatic, Left Lower Extremity **H** Lymphatic, Right Inguinal **J** Lymphatic, Left Inguinal **K** Thoracic Duct **L** Cisterna Chyli	**0** Open **3** Percutaneous **4** Percutaneous Endoscopic	**C** Extraluminal Device **D** Intraluminal Device **Z** No Device	**Z** No Qualifier

0 Medical and Surgical
7 Lymphatic and Hemic Systems
N Release: Freeing a body part from an abnormal physical constraint by cutting or by the use of force

Body Part	Approach	Device	Qualifier
Character 4	**Character 5**	**Character 6**	**Character 7**
0 Lymphatic, Head 1 Lymphatic, Right Neck 2 Lymphatic, Left Neck 3 Lymphatic, Right Upper Extremity 4 Lymphatic, Left Upper Extremity 5 Lymphatic, Right Axillary 6 Lymphatic, Left Axillary 7 Lymphatic, Thorax 8 Lymphatic, Internal Mammary, Right 9 Lymphatic, Internal Mammary, Left B Lymphatic, Mesenteric C Lymphatic, Pelvis D Lymphatic, Aortic F Lymphatic, Right Lower Extremity G Lymphatic, Left Lower Extremity H Lymphatic, Right Inguinal J Lymphatic, Left Inguinal K Thoracic Duct L Cisterna Chyli M Thymus P Spleen	0 Open 3 Percutaneous 4 Percutaneous Endoscopic	Z No Device	Z No Qualifier

0 Medical and Surgical
7 Lymphatic and Hemic Systems
P Removal: Taking out or off a device from a body part

Body Part	Approach	Device	Qualifier
Character 4	**Character 5**	**Character 6**	**Character 7**
K Thoracic Duct L Cisterna Chyli N Lymphatic	0 Open 3 Percutaneous 4 Percutaneous Endoscopic	0 Drainage Device 3 Infusion Device 7 Autologous Tissue Substitute C Extraluminal Device D Intraluminal Device J Synthetic Substitute K Nonautologous Tissue Substitute Y Other Device	Z No Qualifier
K Thoracic Duct L Cisterna Chyli N Lymphatic	X External	0 Drainage Device 3 Infusion Device D Intraluminal Device	Z No Qualifier
M Thymus P Spleen	0 Open 3 Percutaneous 4 Percutaneous Endoscopic	0 Drainage Device 3 Infusion Device Y Other Device	Z No Qualifier
M Thymus P Spleen	X External	0 Drainage Device 3 Infusion Device	Z No Qualifier
T Bone Marrow	0 Open 3 Percutaneous 4 Percutaneous Endoscopic X External	0 Drainage Device	Z No Qualifier

0 Medical and Surgical
7 Lymphatic and Hemic Systems
Q Repair: Restoring, to the extent possible, a body part to its normal anatomic structure and function

Body Part	Approach	Device	Qualifier
Character 4	Character 5	Character 6	Character 7
0 Lymphatic, Head **1** Lymphatic, Right Neck **2** Lymphatic, Left Neck **3** Lymphatic, Right Upper Extremity **4** Lymphatic, Left Upper Extremity **5** Lymphatic, Right Axillary **6** Lymphatic, Left Axillary **7** Lymphatic, Thorax **8** Lymphatic, Internal Mammary, Right **9** Lymphatic, Internal Mammary, Left **B** Lymphatic, Mesenteric **C** Lymphatic, Pelvis **D** Lymphatic, Aortic **F** Lymphatic, Right Lower Extremity **G** Lymphatic, Left Lower Extremity **H** Lymphatic, Right Inguinal **J** Lymphatic, Left Inguinal **K** Thoracic Duct **L** Cisterna Chyli	**0** Open **3** Percutaneous **4** Percutaneous Endoscopic **8** Via Natural or Artificial Opening Endoscopic	**Z** No Device	**Z** No Qualifier
M Thymus **P** Spleen	**0** Open **3** Percutaneous **4** Percutaneous Endoscopic	**Z** No Device	**Z** No Qualifier

0 Medical and Surgical
7 Lymphatic and Hemic Systems
S Reposition: Moving to its normal location, or other suitable location, all or a portion of a body part

Body Part	Approach	Device	Qualifier
Character 4	Character 5	Character 6	Character 7
M Thymus **P** Spleen	**0** Open	**Z** No Device	**Z** No Qualifier

LC Limited Coverage   **NC** Noncovered   **HAC** HAC-associated Procedure   **CC** Combination Cluster - See Appendix G for code lists
DRG Non-OR-Affecting MS-DRG Assignment   New/Revised Text in **Orange**   ♂ Male   ♀ Female

2021 ICD-10-PCS

275

LYMPHATIC AND HEMIC SYSTEMS 072-07Y

0   **Medical and Surgical**
7   **Lymphatic and Hemic Systems**
T   **Resection:** Cutting out or off, without replacement, all of a body part

Body Part	Approach	Device	Qualifier
Character 4	Character 5	Character 6	Character 7
0 Lymphatic, Head **1** Lymphatic, Right Neck **2** Lymphatic, Left Neck **3** Lymphatic, Right Upper Extremity **4** Lymphatic, Left Upper Extremity **5** Lymphatic, Right Axillary ◪ **6** Lymphatic, Left Axillary ◪ **7** Lymphatic, Thorax ◪ **8** Lymphatic, Internal Mammary, Right ◪ **9** Lymphatic, Internal Mammary, Left ◪ **B** Lymphatic, Mesenteric **C** Lymphatic, Pelvis **D** Lymphatic, Aortic **F** Lymphatic, Right Lower Extremity **G** Lymphatic, Left Lower Extremity **H** Lymphatic, Right Inguinal **J** Lymphatic, Left Inguinal **K** Thoracic Duct **L** Cisterna Chyli **M** Thymus **P** Spleen	**0** Open **4** Percutaneous Endoscopic	**Z** No Device	**Z** No Qualifier

◪   07T50ZZ   07T60ZZ   07T70ZZ   07T80ZZ   07T90ZZ

0   **Medical and Surgical**
7   **Lymphatic and Hemic Systems**
U   **Supplement:** Putting in or on biological or synthetic material that physically reinforces and/or augments the function of a portion of a body part

Body Part	Approach	Device	Qualifier
Character 4	Character 5	Character 6	Character 7
0 Lymphatic, Head **1** Lymphatic, Right Neck **2** Lymphatic, Left Neck **3** Lymphatic, Right Upper Extremity **4** Lymphatic, Left Upper Extremity **5** Lymphatic, Right Axillary **6** Lymphatic, Left Axillary **7** Lymphatic, Thorax **8** Lymphatic, Internal Mammary, Right **9** Lymphatic, Internal Mammary, Left **B** Lymphatic, Mesenteric **C** Lymphatic, Pelvis **D** Lymphatic, Aortic **F** Lymphatic, Right Lower Extremity **G** Lymphatic, Left Lower Extremity **H** Lymphatic, Right Inguinal **J** Lymphatic, Left Inguinal **K** Thoracic Duct **L** Cisterna Chyli	**0** Open **4** Percutaneous Endoscopic	**7** Autologous Tissue Substitute **J** Synthetic Substitute **K** Nonautologous Tissue Substitute	**Z** No Qualifier

0   **Medical and Surgical**

7   **Lymphatic and Hemic Systems**

V   **Restriction:** Partially closing an orifice or the lumen of a tubular body part

Body Part	Approach	Device	Qualifier
Character 4	Character 5	Character 6	Character 7
0 Lymphatic, Head **1** Lymphatic, Right Neck **2** Lymphatic, Left Neck **3** Lymphatic, Right Upper Extremity **4** Lymphatic, Left Upper Extremity **5** Lymphatic, Right Axillary **6** Lymphatic, Left Axillary **7** Lymphatic, Thorax **8** Lymphatic, Internal Mammary, Right **9** Lymphatic, Internal Mammary, Left **B** Lymphatic, Mesenteric **C** Lymphatic, Pelvis **D** Lymphatic, Aortic **F** Lymphatic, Right Lower Extremity **G** Lymphatic, Left Lower Extremity **H** Lymphatic, Right Inguinal **J** Lymphatic, Left Inguinal **K** Thoracic Duct **L** Cisterna Chyli	**0** Open **3** Percutaneous **4** Percutaneous Endoscopic	**C** Extraluminal Device **D** Intraluminal Device **Z** No Device	**Z** No Qualifier

0   **Medical and Surgical**

7   **Lymphatic and Hemic Systems**

W   **Revision:** Correcting, to the extent possible, a portion of a malfunctioning device or the position of a displaced device

Body Part	Approach	Device	Qualifier
Character 4	Character 5	Character 6	Character 7
K Thoracic Duct **L** Cisterna Chyli **N** Lymphatic	**0** Open **3** Percutaneous **4** Percutaneous Endoscopic	**0** Drainage Device **3** Infusion Device **7** Autologous Tissue Substitute **C** Extraluminal Device **D** Intraluminal Device **J** Synthetic Substitute **K** Nonautologous Tissue Substitute **Y** Other Device	**Z** No Qualifier
K Thoracic Duct **L** Cisterna Chyli **N** Lymphatic	**X** External	**0** Drainage Device **3** Infusion Device **7** Autologous Tissue Substitute **C** Extraluminal Device **D** Intraluminal Device **J** Synthetic Substitute **K** Nonautologous Tissue Substitute	**Z** No Qualifier
M Thymus **P** Spleen	**0** Open **3** Percutaneous **4** Percutaneous Endoscopic	**0** Drainage Device **3** Infusion Device **Y** Other Device	**Z** No Qualifier
M Thymus **P** Spleen	**X** External	**0** Drainage Device **3** Infusion Device	**Z** No Qualifier
T Bone Marrow	**0** Open **3** Percutaneous **4** Percutaneous Endoscopic **X** External	**0** Drainage Device	**Z** No Qualifier

0   **Medical and Surgical**
7   **Lymphatic and Hemic Systems**
Y   **Transplantation:** Putting in or on all or a portion of a living body part taken from another individual or animal to physically take the place and/or function of all or a portion of a similar body part

Body Part	Approach	Device	Qualifier
Character 4	Character 5	Character 6	Character 7
M Thymus **P** Spleen	**0** Open	**Z** No Device	**0** Allogeneic **1** Syngeneic **2** Zooplastic

NOTES

NOTES

Eye 080-08X

0 **Medical and Surgical**
8 **Eye**
0 **Alteration:** Modifying the anatomic structure of a body part without affecting the function of the body part

Body Part	Approach	Device	Qualifier
Character 4	Character 5	Character 6	Character 7
N Upper Eyelid, Right **P** Upper Eyelid, Left **Q** Lower Eyelid, Right **R** Lower Eyelid, Left	**0** Open **3** Percutaneous **X** External	**7** Autologous Tissue Substitute **J** Synthetic Substitute **K** Nonautologous Tissue Substitute **Z** No Device	**Z** No Qualifier

0 **Medical and Surgical**
8 **Eye**
1 **Bypass:** Altering the route of passage of the contents of a tubular body part

Body Part	Approach	Device	Qualifier
Character 4	Character 5	Character 6	Character 7
2 Anterior Chamber, Right **3** Anterior Chamber, Left	**3** Percutaneous	**J** Synthetic Substitute **K** Nonautologous Tissue Substitute **Z** No Device	**4** Sclera
X Lacrimal Duct, Right **Y** Lacrimal Duct, Left	**0** Open **3** Percutaneous	**J** Synthetic Substitute **K** Nonautologous Tissue Substitute **Z** No Device	**3** Nasal Cavity

0 **Medical and Surgical**
8 **Eye**
2 **Change:** Taking out or off a device from a body part and putting back an identical or similar device in or on the same body part without cutting or puncturing the skin or a mucous membrane

Body Part	Approach	Device	Qualifier
Character 4	Character 5	Character 6	Character 7
0 Eye, Right **1** Eye, Left	**X** External	**0** Drainage Device **Y** Other Device	**Z** No Qualifier

LC Limited Coverage   **NC** Noncovered   **HAC** HAC-associated Procedure   **CC** Combination Cluster - See Appendix G for code lists
DRG Non-OR-Affecting MS-DRG Assignment   New/Revised Text in Orange   ♂ Male   ♀ Female

2021 ICD-10-PCS   **281**

EYE 080-08X

0 Medical and Surgical

8 Eye

5 Destruction: Physical eradication of all or a portion of a body part by the direct use of energy, force, or a destructive agent

Body Part	Approach	Device	Qualifier
Character 4	Character 5	Character 6	Character 7
0 Eye, Right 1 Eye, Left 6 Sclera, Right 7 Sclera, Left 8 Cornea, Right 9 Cornea, Left S Conjunctiva, Right T Conjunctiva, Left	X External	Z No Device	Z No Qualifier
2 Anterior Chamber, Right 3 Anterior Chamber, Left 4 Vitreous, Right 5 Vitreous, Left C Iris, Right D Iris, Left E Retina, Right F Retina, Left G Retinal Vessel, Right H Retinal Vessel, Left J Lens, Right K Lens, Left	3 Percutaneous	Z No Device	Z No Qualifier
A Choroid, Right B Choroid, Left L Extraocular Muscle, Right M Extraocular Muscle, Left V Lacrimal Gland, Right W Lacrimal Gland, Left	0 Open 3 Percutaneous	Z No Device	Z No Qualifier
N Upper Eyelid, Right P Upper Eyelid, Left Q Lower Eyelid, Right R Lower Eyelid, Left	0 Open 3 Percutaneous X External	Z No Device	Z No Qualifier
X Lacrimal Duct, Right Y Lacrimal Duct, Left	0 Open 3 Percutaneous 7 Via Natural or Artificial Opening 8 Via Natural or Artificial Opening Endoscopic	Z No Device	Z No Qualifier

0 Medical and Surgical

8 Eye

7 Dilation: Expanding an orifice or the lumen of a tubular body part

Body Part	Approach	Device	Qualifier
Character 4	Character 5	Character 6	Character 7
X Lacrimal Duct, Right Y Lacrimal Duct, Left	0 Open 3 Percutaneous 7 Via Natural or Artificial Opening 8 Via Natural or Artificial Opening Endoscopic	D Intraluminal Device Z No Device	Z No Qualifier

0 Medical and Surgical
8 Eye
9 Drainage: Taking or letting out fluids and/or gases from a body part

Body Part	Approach	Device	Qualifier
Character 4	Character 5	Character 6	Character 7
0 Eye, Right **1** Eye, Left **6** Sclera, Right **7** Sclera, Left **8** Cornea, Right **9** Cornea, Left **S** Conjunctiva, Right **T** Conjunctiva, Left	**X** External	**0** Drainage Device	**Z** No Qualifier
0 Eye, Right **1** Eye, Left **6** Sclera, Right **7** Sclera, Left **8** Cornea, Right **9** Cornea, Left **S** Conjunctiva, Right **T** Conjunctiva, Left	**X** External	**Z** No Device	**X** Diagnostic **Z** No Qualifier
2 Anterior Chamber, Right **3** Anterior Chamber, Left **4** Vitreous, Right **5** Vitreous, Left **C** Iris, Right **D** Iris, Left **E** Retina, Right **F** Retina, Left **G** Retinal Vessel, Right **H** Retinal Vessel, Left **J** Lens, Right **K** Lens, Left	**3** Percutaneous	**0** Drainage Device	**Z** No Qualifier
2 Anterior Chamber, Right **3** Anterior Chamber, Left **4** Vitreous, Right **5** Vitreous, Left **C** Iris, Right **D** Iris, Left **E** Retina, Right **F** Retina, Left **G** Retinal Vessel, Right **H** Retinal Vessel, Left **J** Lens, Right **K** Lens, Left	**3** Percutaneous	**Z** No Device	**X** Diagnostic **Z** No Qualifier
A Choroid, Right **B** Choroid, Left **L** Extraocular Muscle, Right **M** Extraocular Muscle, Left **V** Lacrimal Gland, Right **W** Lacrimal Gland, Left	**0** Open **3** Percutaneous	**0** Drainage Device	**Z** No Qualifier
A Choroid, Right **B** Choroid, Left **L** Extraocular Muscle, Right **M** Extraocular Muscle, Left **V** Lacrimal Gland, Right **W** Lacrimal Gland, Left	**0** Open **3** Percutaneous	**Z** No Device	**X** Diagnostic **Z** No Qualifier
N Upper Eyelid, Right **P** Upper Eyelid, Left **Q** Lower Eyelid, Right **R** Lower Eyelid, Left	**0** Open **3** Percutaneous **X** External	**0** Drainage Device	**Z** No Qualifier

089 continued on next page

LC Limited Coverage   NC Noncovered   HAC HAC-associated Procedure   CC Combination Cluster - See Appendix G for code lists
DRG Non-OR-Affecting MS-DRG Assignment   New/Revised Text in **Orange**   ♂ Male   ♀ Female

0 **Medical and Surgical**

8 **Eye**

9 **Drainage:** Taking or letting out fluids and/or gases from a body part

089 continued from previous page

Body Part	Approach	Device	Qualifier
Character 4	Character 5	Character 6	Character 7
N Upper Eyelid, Right P Upper Eyelid, Left Q Lower Eyelid, Right R Lower Eyelid, Left	0 Open 3 Percutaneous X External	Z No Device	X Diagnostic Z No Qualifier
X Lacrimal Duct, Right Y Lacrimal Duct, Left	0 Open 3 Percutaneous 7 Via Natural or Artificial Opening 8 Via Natural or Artificial Opening Endoscopic	0 Drainage Device	Z No Qualifier
X Lacrimal Duct, Right Y Lacrimal Duct, Left	0 Open 3 Percutaneous 7 Via Natural or Artificial Opening 8 Via Natural or Artificial Opening Endoscopic	Z No Device	X Diagnostic Z No Qualifier

0 **Medical and Surgical**

8 **Eye**

B **Excision:** Cutting out or off, without replacement, a portion of a body part

Body Part	Approach	Device	Qualifier
Character 4	Character 5	Character 6	Character 7
0 Eye, Right 1 Eye, Left N Upper Eyelid, Right P Upper Eyelid, Left Q Lower Eyelid, Right R Lower Eyelid, Left	0 Open 3 Percutaneous X External	Z No Device	X Diagnostic Z No Qualifier
4 Vitreous, Right 5 Vitreous, Left C Iris, Right D Iris, Left E Retina, Right F Retina, Left J Lens, Right K Lens, Left	3 Percutaneous	Z No Device	X Diagnostic Z No Qualifier
6 Sclera, Right 7 Sclera, Left 8 Cornea, Right 9 Cornea, Left S Conjunctiva, Right T Conjunctiva, Left	X External	Z No Device	X Diagnostic Z No Qualifier
A Choroid, Right B Choroid, Left L Extraocular Muscle, Right M Extraocular Muscle, Left V Lacrimal Gland, Right W Lacrimal Gland, Left	0 Open 3 Percutaneous	Z No Device	X Diagnostic Z No Qualifier
X Lacrimal Duct, Right Y Lacrimal Duct, Left	0 Open 3 Percutaneous 7 Via Natural or Artificial Opening 8 Via Natural or Artificial Opening Endoscopic	Z No Device	X Diagnostic Z No Qualifier

2021 ICD-10-PCS

0 **Medical and Surgical**
8 **Eye**
C **Extirpation:** Taking or cutting out solid matter from a body part

Body Part	Approach	Device	Qualifier
Character 4	Character 5	Character 6	Character 7
0 Eye, Right 1 Eye, Left 6 Sclera, Right 7 Sclera, Left 8 Cornea, Right 9 Cornea, Left S Conjunctiva, Right T Conjunctiva, Left	X External	Z No Device	Z No Qualifier
2 Anterior Chamber, Right 3 Anterior Chamber, Left 4 Vitreous, Right 5 Vitreous, Left C Iris, Right D Iris, Left E Retina, Right F Retina, Left G Retinal Vessel, Right H Retinal Vessel, Left J Lens, Right K Lens, Left	3 Percutaneous X External	Z No Device	Z No Qualifier
A Choroid, Right B Choroid, Left L Extraocular Muscle, Right M Extraocular Muscle, Left N Upper Eyelid, Right P Upper Eyelid, Left Q Lower Eyelid, Right R Lower Eyelid, Left V Lacrimal Gland, Right W Lacrimal Gland, Left	0 Open 3 Percutaneous X External	Z No Device	Z No Qualifier
X Lacrimal Duct, Right Y Lacrimal Duct, Left	0 Open 3 Percutaneous 7 Via Natural or Artificial Opening 8 Via Natural or Artificial Opening Endoscopic	Z No Device	Z No Qualifier

0 **Medical and Surgical**
8 **Eye**
D **Extraction:** Pulling or stripping out or off all or a portion of a body part by the use of force

Body Part	Approach	Device	Qualifier
Character 4	Character 5	Character 6	Character 7
8 Cornea, Right 9 Cornea, Left	X External	Z No Device	X Diagnostic Z No Qualifier
J Lens, Right K Lens, Left	3 Percutaneous	Z No Device	Z No Qualifier

0 **Medical and Surgical**
8 **Eye**
F **Fragmentation:** Breaking solid matter in a body part into pieces

Body Part	Approach	Device	Qualifier
Character 4	Character 5	Character 6	Character 7
4 Vitreous, Right ℕℂ 5 Vitreous, Left ℕℂ	3 Percutaneous X External	Z No Device	Z No Qualifier

ℕℂ   08F4XZZ   08F5XZZ

ℂ Limited Coverage   ℕℂ Noncovered   ℍᴬℂ HAC-associated Procedure   ℂℂ Combination Cluster - See Appendix G for code lists
🔄 Non-OR-Affecting MS-DRG Assignment   New/Revised Text in **Orange**   ♂ Male   ♀ Female

0 Medical and Surgical

8 Eye

H Insertion: Putting in a nonbiological appliance that monitors, assists, performs, or prevents a physiological function but does not physically take the place of a body part

Body Part	Approach	Device	Qualifier
Character 4	Character 5	Character 6	Character 7
0 Eye, Right 1 Eye, Left	0 Open	5 Epiretinal Visual Prosthesis Y Other Device	Z No Qualifier
0 Eye, Right 1 Eye, Left	3 Percutaneous	1 Radioactive Element 3 Infusion Device Y Other Device	Z No Qualifier
0 Eye, Right 1 Eye, Left	7 Via Natural or Artificial Opening 8 Via Natural or Artificial Opening Endoscopic	Y Other Device	Z No Qualifier
0 Eye, Right 1 Eye, Left	X External	1 Radioactive Element 3 Infusion Device	Z No Qualifier

0 Medical and Surgical

8 Eye

J Inspection: Visually and/or manually exploring a body part

Body Part	Approach	Device	Qualifier
Character 4	Character 5	Character 6	Character 7
0 Eye, Right 1 Eye, Left J Lens, Right K Lens, Left	X External	Z No Device	Z No Qualifier
L Extraocular Muscle, Right M Extraocular Muscle, Left	0 Open X External	Z No Device	Z No Qualifier

0 Medical and Surgical

8 Eye

L Occlusion: Completely closing an orifice or the lumen of a tubular body part

Body Part	Approach	Device	Qualifier
Character 4	Character 5	Character 6	Character 7
X Lacrimal Duct, Right Y Lacrimal Duct, Left	0 Open 3 Percutaneous	C Extraluminal Device D Intraluminal Device Z No Device	Z No Qualifier
X Lacrimal Duct, Right Y Lacrimal Duct, Left	7 Via Natural or Artificial Opening 8 Via Natural or Artificial Opening Endoscopic	D Intraluminal Device Z No Device	Z No Qualifier

0 Medical and Surgical

8 Eye

M Reattachment: Putting back in or on all or a portion of a separated body part to its normal location or other suitable location

Body Part	Approach	Device	Qualifier
Character 4	Character 5	Character 6	Character 7
N Upper Eyelid, Right P Upper Eyelid, Left Q Lower Eyelid, Right R Lower Eyelid, Left	X External	Z No Device	Z No Qualifier

LC Limited Coverage   NC Noncovered   HAC HAC-associated Procedure   CC Combination Cluster - See Appendix G for code lists
DRG Non-OR-Affecting MS-DRG Assignment   New/Revised Text in Orange   ♂ Male   ♀ Female

286

2021 ICD-10-PCS

0   **Medical and Surgical**
8   **Eye**
N   **Release:** Freeing a body part from an abnormal physical constraint by cutting or by the use of force

Body Part	Approach	Device	Qualifier
Character 4	**Character 5**	**Character 6**	**Character 7**
0 Eye, Right 1 Eye, Left 6 Sclera, Right 7 Sclera, Left 8 Cornea, Right 9 Cornea, Left S Conjunctiva, Right T Conjunctiva, Left	**X** External	**Z** No Device	**Z** No Qualifier
2 Anterior Chamber, Right 3 Anterior Chamber, Left 4 Vitreous, Right 5 Vitreous, Left C Iris, Right D Iris, Left E Retina, Right F Retina, Left G Retinal Vessel, Right H Retinal Vessel, Left J Lens, Right K Lens, Left	**3** Percutaneous	**Z** No Device	**Z** No Qualifier
A Choroid, Right B Choroid, Left L Extraocular Muscle, Right M Extraocular Muscle, Left V Lacrimal Gland, Right W Lacrimal Gland, Left	**0** Open **3** Percutaneous	**Z** No Device	**Z** No Qualifier
N Upper Eyelid, Right P Upper Eyelid, Left Q Lower Eyelid, Right R Lower Eyelid, Left	**0** Open **3** Percutaneous **X** External	**Z** No Device	**Z** No Qualifier
X Lacrimal Duct, Right Y Lacrimal Duct, Left	**0** Open **3** Percutaneous **7** Via Natural or Artificial Opening **8** Via Natural or Artificial Opening Endoscopic	**Z** No Device	**Z** No Qualifier

LC Limited Coverage   **NC** Noncovered   **HAC** HAC-associated Procedure   **CC** Combination Cluster - See Appendix G for code lists
DRG Non-OR-Affecting MS-DRG Assignment   New/Revised Text in **Orange**   ♂ Male   ♀ Female

2021 ICD-10-PCS   287

EYE 080-08X

0   **Medical and Surgical**
8   **Eye**
P   **Removal:** Taking out or off a device from a body part

Body Part	Approach	Device	Qualifier
Character 4	**Character 5**	**Character 6**	**Character 7**
0 Eye, Right **1** Eye, Left	**0** Open **3** Percutaneous **7** Via Natural or Artificial Opening **8** Via Natural or Artificial Opening Endoscopic	**0** Drainage Device **1** Radioactive Element **3** Infusion Device **7** Autologous Tissue Substitute **C** Extraluminal Device **D** Intraluminal Device **J** Synthetic Substitute **K** Nonautologous Tissue Substitute **Y** Other Device	**Z** No Qualifier
0 Eye, Right **1** Eye, Left	**X** External	**0** Drainage Device **1** Radioactive Element **3** Infusion Device **7** Autologous Tissue Substitute **C** Extraluminal Device **D** Intraluminal Device **J** Synthetic Substitute **K** Nonautologous Tissue Substitute	**Z** No Qualifier
J Lens, Right **K** Lens, Left	**3** Percutaneous	**J** Synthetic Substitute **Y** Other Device	**Z** No Qualifier
L Extraocular Muscle, Right **M** Extraocular Muscle, Left	**0** Open **3** Percutaneous	**0** Drainage Device **7** Autologous Tissue Substitute **J** Synthetic Substitute **K** Nonautologous Tissue Substitute **Y** Other Device	**Z** No Qualifier

LC Limited Coverage   **NC** Noncovered   **HAC** HAC-associated Procedure   **CC** Combination Cluster - See Appendix G for code lists
DRG Non-OR-Affecting MS-DRG Assignment   New/Revised Text in **Orange**   ♂ Male   ♀ Female

288   **2021 ICD-10-PCS**

0 **Medical and Surgical**
8 **Eye**
Q **Repair:** Restoring, to the extent possible, a body part to its normal anatomic structure and function

Body Part		Approach		Device		Qualifier	
Character 4		**Character 5**		**Character 6**		**Character 7**	
0	Eye, Right	X	External	Z	No Device	Z	No Qualifier
1	Eye, Left						
6	Sclera, Right						
7	Sclera, Left						
8	Cornea, Right NC						
9	Cornea, Left NC						
S	Conjunctiva, Right						
T	Conjunctiva, Left						
2	Anterior Chamber, Right	3	Percutaneous	Z	No Device	Z	No Qualifier
3	Anterior Chamber, Left						
4	Vitreous, Right						
5	Vitreous, Left						
C	Iris, Right						
D	Iris, Left						
E	Retina, Right						
F	Retina, Left						
G	Retinal Vessel, Right						
H	Retinal Vessel, Left						
J	Lens, Right						
K	Lens, Left						
A	Choroid, Right	0	Open	Z	No Device	Z	No Qualifier
B	Choroid, Left	3	Percutaneous				
L	Extraocular Muscle, Right						
M	Extraocular Muscle, Left						
V	Lacrimal Gland, Right						
W	Lacrimal Gland, Left						
N	Upper Eyelid, Right	0	Open	Z	No Device	Z	No Qualifier
P	Upper Eyelid, Left	3	Percutaneous				
Q	Lower Eyelid, Right	X	External				
R	Lower Eyelid, Left						
X	Lacrimal Duct, Right	0	Open	Z	No Device	Z	No Qualifier
Y	Lacrimal Duct, Left	3	Percutaneous				
		7	Via Natural or Artificial Opening				
		8	Via Natural or Artificial Opening Endoscopic				

NC 08Q8XZZ   08Q9XZZ

0 Medical and Surgical
8 Eye
R Replacement: Putting in or on biological or synthetic material that physically takes the place and/or function of all or a portion of a body part

Body Part	Approach	Device	Qualifier
Character 4	**Character 5**	**Character 6**	**Character 7**
0 Eye, Right **1** Eye, Left **A** Choroid, Right **B** Choroid, Left	**0** Open **3** Percutaneous	**7** Autologous Tissue Substitute **J** Synthetic Substitute **K** Nonautologous Tissue Substitute	**Z** No Qualifier
4 Vitreous, Right **5** Vitreous, Left **C** Iris, Right **D** Iris, Left **G** Retinal Vessel, Right **H** Retinal Vessel, Left	**3** Percutaneous	**7** Autologous Tissue Substitute **J** Synthetic Substitute **K** Nonautologous Tissue Substitute	**Z** No Qualifier
6 Sclera, Right **7** Sclera, Left **S** Conjunctiva, Right **T** Conjunctiva, Left	**X** External	**7** Autologous Tissue Substitute **J** Synthetic Substitute **K** Nonautologous Tissue Substitute	**Z** No Qualifier
8 Cornea, Right **9** Cornea, Left	**3** Percutaneous **X** External	**7** Autologous Tissue Substitute **J** Synthetic Substitute **K** Nonautologous Tissue Substitute	**Z** No Qualifier
J Lens, Right **K** Lens, Left	**3** Percutaneous	**0** Synthetic Substitute, Intraocular Telescope **7** Autologous Tissue Substitute **J** Synthetic Substitute **K** Nonautologous Tissue Substitute	**Z** No Qualifier
N Upper Eyelid, Right **P** Upper Eyelid, Left **Q** Lower Eyelid, Right **R** Lower Eyelid, Left	**0** Open **3** Percutaneous **X** External	**7** Autologous Tissue Substitute **J** Synthetic Substitute **K** Nonautologous Tissue Substitute	**Z** No Qualifier
X Lacrimal Duct, Right **Y** Lacrimal Duct, Left	**0** Open **3** Percutaneous **7** Via Natural or Artificial Opening **8** Via Natural or Artificial Opening Endoscopic	**7** Autologous Tissue Substitute **J** Synthetic Substitute **K** Nonautologous Tissue Substitute	**Z** No Qualifier

LC Limited Coverage   NC Noncovered   HAC HAC-associated Procedure   CC Combination Cluster - See Appendix G for code lists
DRG Non-OR-Affecting MS-DRG Assignment   New/Revised Text in Orange   ♂ Male   ♀ Female

290

2021 ICD-10-PCS

0 **Medical and Surgical**

8 **Eye**

S **Reposition:** Moving to its normal location, or other suitable location, all or a portion of a body part

Body Part	Approach	Device	Qualifier
Character 4	Character 5	Character 6	Character 7
C Iris, Right **D** Iris, Left **G** Retinal Vessel, Right **H** Retinal Vessel, Left **J** Lens, Right **K** Lens, Left	**3** Percutaneous	**Z** No Device	**Z** No Qualifier
L Extraocular Muscle, Right **M** Extraocular Muscle, Left **V** Lacrimal Gland, Right **W** Lacrimal Gland, Left	**0** Open **3** Percutaneous	**Z** No Device	**Z** No Qualifier
N Upper Eyelid, Right **P** Upper Eyelid, Left **Q** Lower Eyelid, Right **R** Lower Eyelid, Left	**0** Open **3** Percutaneous **X** External	**Z** No Device	**Z** No Qualifier
X Lacrimal Duct, Right **Y** Lacrimal Duct, Left	**0** Open **3** Percutaneous **7** Via Natural or Artificial Opening **8** Via Natural or Artificial Opening Endoscopic	**Z** No Device	**Z** No Qualifier

0 **Medical and Surgical**

8 **Eye**

T **Resection:** Cutting out or off, without replacement, all of a body part

Body Part	Approach	Device	Qualifier
Character 4	Character 5	Character 6	Character 7
0 Eye, Right **1** Eye, Left **8** Cornea, Right **9** Cornea, Left	**X** External	**Z** No Device	**Z** No Qualifier
4 Vitreous, Right **5** Vitreous, Left **C** Iris, Right **D** Iris, Left **J** Lens, Right **K** Lens, Left	**3** Percutaneous	**Z** No Device	**Z** No Qualifier
L Extraocular Muscle, Right **M** Extraocular Muscle, Left **V** Lacrimal Gland, Right **W** Lacrimal Gland, Left	**0** Open **3** Percutaneous	**Z** No Device	**Z** No Qualifier
N Upper Eyelid, Right **P** Upper Eyelid, Left **Q** Lower Eyelid, Right **R** Lower Eyelid, Left	**0** Open **X** External	**Z** No Device	**Z** No Qualifier
X Lacrimal Duct, Right **Y** Lacrimal Duct, Left	**0** Open **3** Percutaneous **7** Via Natural or Artificial Opening **8** Via Natural or Artificial Opening Endoscopic	**Z** No Device	**Z** No Qualifier

LC Limited Coverage   NC Noncovered   HAC HAC-associated Procedure   CC Combination Cluster - See Appendix G for code lists
DRG Non-OR-Affecting MS-DRG Assignment   New/Revised Text in Orange   ♂ Male   ♀ Female

2021 ICD-10-PCS

291

EYE 080-08X

0 Medical and Surgical
8 Eye
U Supplement: Putting in or on biological or synthetic material that physically reinforces and/or augments the function of a portion of a body part

Body Part	Approach	Device	Qualifier
Character 4	Character 5	Character 6	Character 7
0 Eye, Right 1 Eye, Left C Iris, Right D Iris, Left E Retina, Right F Retina, Left G Retinal Vessel, Right H Retinal Vessel, Left L Extraocular Muscle, Right M Extraocular Muscle, Left	0 Open 3 Percutaneous	7 Autologous Tissue Substitute J Synthetic Substitute K Nonautologous Tissue Substitute	Z No Qualifier
8 Cornea, Right NC 9 Cornea, Left NC N Upper Eyelid, Right P Upper Eyelid, Left Q Lower Eyelid, Right R Lower Eyelid, Left	0 Open 3 Percutaneous X External	7 Autologous Tissue Substitute J Synthetic Substitute K Nonautologous Tissue Substitute	Z No Qualifier
X Lacrimal Duct, Right Y Lacrimal Duct, Left	0 Open 3 Percutaneous 7 Via Natural or Artificial Opening 8 Via Natural or Artificial Opening Endoscopic	7 Autologous Tissue Substitute J Synthetic Substitute K Nonautologous Tissue Substitute	Z No Qualifier

NC 08U80KZ   08U83KZ   08U8XKZ   08U90KZ   08U93KZ   08U9XKZ

0 Medical and Surgical
8 Eye
V Restriction: Partially closing an orifice or the lumen of a tubular body part

Body Part	Approach	Device	Qualifier
Character 4	Character 5	Character 6	Character 7
X Lacrimal Duct, Right Y Lacrimal Duct, Left	0 Open 3 Percutaneous	C Extraluminal Device D Intraluminal Device Z No Device	Z No Qualifier
X Lacrimal Duct, Right Y Lacrimal Duct, Left	7 Via Natural or Artificial Opening 8 Via Natural or Artificial Opening Endoscopic	D Intraluminal Device Z No Device	Z No Qualifier

LC Limited Coverage   NC Noncovered   HAC HAC-associated Procedure   CC Combination Cluster - See Appendix G for code lists
DRG Non-OR-Affecting MS-DRG Assignment   New/Revised Text in Orange   ♂ Male   ♀ Female

292

2021 ICD-10-PCS

0 Medical and Surgical
8 Eye
W Revision: Correcting, to the extent possible, a portion of a malfunctioning device or the position of a displaced device

Body Part	Approach	Device	Qualifier
Character 4	Character 5	Character 6	Character 7
0 Eye, Right **1** Eye, Left	**0** Open **3** Percutaneous **7** Via Natural or Artificial Opening **8** Via Natural or Artificial Opening Endoscopic	**0** Drainage Device **3** Infusion Device **7** Autologous Tissue Substitute **C** Extraluminal Device **D** Intraluminal Device **J** Synthetic Substitute **K** Nonautologous Tissue Substitute **Y** Other Device	**Z** No Qualifier
0 Eye, Right **1** Eye, Left	**X** External	**0** Drainage Device **3** Infusion Device **7** Autologous Tissue Substitute **C** Extraluminal Device **D** Intraluminal Device **J** Synthetic Substitute **K** Nonautologous Tissue Substitute	**Z** No Qualifier
J Lens, Right **K** Lens, Left	**3** Percutaneous	**J** Synthetic Substitute **Y** Other Device	**Z** No Qualifier
J Lens, Right **K** Lens, Left	**X** External	**J** Synthetic Substitute	**Z** No Qualifier
L Extraocular Muscle, Right **M** Extraocular Muscle, Left	**0** Open **3** Percutaneous	**0** Drainage Device **7** Autologous Tissue Substitute **J** Synthetic Substitute **K** Nonautologous Tissue Substitute **Y** Other Device	**Z** No Qualifier

0 Medical and Surgical
8 Eye
X Transfer: Moving, without taking out, all or a portion of a body part to another location to take over the function of all or a portion of a body part

Body Part	Approach	Device	Qualifier
Character 4	Character 5	Character 6	Character 7
L Extraocular Muscle, Right **M** Extraocular Muscle, Left	**0** Open **3** Percutaneous	**Z** No Device	**Z** No Qualifier

NOTES

Ear, Nose, Sinus 090-09W

0 Medical and Surgical
9 Ear, Nose, Sinus
0 Alteration: Modifying the anatomic structure of a body part without affecting the function of the body part

Body Part	Approach	Device	Qualifier
Character 4	Character 5	Character 6	Character 7
0 External Ear, Right 1 External Ear, Left 2 External Ear, Bilateral K Nasal Mucosa and Soft Tissue	0 Open 3 Percutaneous 4 Percutaneous Endoscopic X External	7 Autologous Tissue Substitute J Synthetic Substitute K Nonautologous Tissue Substitute Z No Device	Z No Qualifier

0 Medical and Surgical
9 Ear, Nose, Sinus
1 Bypass: Altering the route of passage of the contents of a tubular body part

Body Part	Approach	Device	Qualifier
Character 4	Character 5	Character 6	Character 7
D Inner Ear, Right E Inner Ear, Left	0 Open	7 Autologous Tissue Substitute J Synthetic Substitute K Nonautologous Tissue Substitute Z No Device	0 Endolymphatic

0 Medical and Surgical
9 Ear, Nose, Sinus
2 Change: Taking out or off a device from a body part and putting back an identical or similar device in or on the same body part without cutting or puncturing the skin or a mucous membrane

Body Part	Approach	Device	Qualifier
Character 4	Character 5	Character 6	Character 7
H Ear, Right J Ear, Left K Nasal Mucosa and Soft Tissue Y Sinus	X External	0 Drainage Device Y Other Device	Z No Qualifier

0 Medical and Surgical
9 Ear, Nose, Sinus
3 Control: Stopping, or attempting to stop, postprocedural or other acute bleeding

Body Part	Approach	Device	Qualifier
Character 4	Character 5	Character 6	Character 7
K Nasal Mucosa and Soft Tissue	7 Via Natural or Artificial Opening 8 Via Natural or Artificial Opening Endoscopic	Z No Device	Z No Qualifier

---

LC Limited Coverage   NC Noncovered   HAC HAC-associated Procedure   CC Combination Cluster - See Appendix G for code lists
DRG Non-OR-Affecting MS-DRG Assignment   New/Revised Text in **Orange**   ♂ Male   ♀ Female

095-097

EAR, NOSE, SINUS 090-09W

0   **Medical and Surgical**
9   **Ear, Nose, Sinus**
5   **Destruction:** Physical eradication of all or a portion of a body part by the direct use of energy, force, or a destructive agent

Body Part	Approach	Device	Qualifier
Character 4	Character 5	Character 6	Character 7
0 External Ear, Right **1** External Ear, Left	**0** Open **3** Percutaneous **4** Percutaneous Endoscopic **X** External	**Z** No Device	**Z** No Qualifier
3 External Auditory Canal, Right **4** External Auditory Canal, Left	**0** Open **3** Percutaneous **4** Percutaneous Endoscopic **7** Via Natural or Artificial Opening **8** Via Natural or Artificial Opening Endoscopic **X** External	**Z** No Device	**Z** No Qualifier
5 Middle Ear, Right **6** Middle Ear, Left **9** Auditory Ossicle, Right **A** Auditory Ossicle, Left **D** Inner Ear, Right **E** Inner Ear, Left	**0** Open **8** Via Natural or Artificial Opening Endoscopic	**Z** No Device	**Z** No Qualifier
7 Tympanic Membrane, Right **8** Tympanic Membrane, Left **F** Eustachian Tube, Right **G** Eustachian Tube, Left **L** Nasal Turbinate **N** Nasopharynx	**0** Open **3** Percutaneous **4** Percutaneous Endoscopic **7** Via Natural or Artificial Opening **8** Via Natural or Artificial Opening Endoscopic	**Z** No Device	**Z** No Qualifier
B Mastoid Sinus, Right **C** Mastoid Sinus, Left **M** Nasal Septum **P** Accessory Sinus **Q** Maxillary Sinus, Right **R** Maxillary Sinus, Left **S** Frontal Sinus, Right **T** Frontal Sinus, Left **U** Ethmoid Sinus, Right **V** Ethmoid Sinus, Left **W** Sphenoid Sinus, Right **X** Sphenoid Sinus, Left	**0** Open **3** Percutaneous **4** Percutaneous Endoscopic **8** Via Natural or Artificial Opening Endoscopic	**Z** No Device	**Z** No Qualifier
K Nasal Mucosa and Soft Tissue	**0** Open **3** Percutaneous **4** Percutaneous Endoscopic **8** Via Natural or Artificial Opening Endoscopic **X** External	**Z** No Device	**Z** No Qualifier

0   **Medical and Surgical**
9   **Ear, Nose, Sinus**
7   **Dilation:** Expanding an orifice or the lumen of a tubular body part

Body Part	Approach	Device	Qualifier
Character 4	Character 5	Character 6	Character 7
F Eustachian Tube, Right **G** Eustachian Tube, Left	**0** Open **7** Via Natural or Artificial Opening **8** Via Natural or Artificial Opening Endoscopic	**D** Intraluminal Device **Z** No Device	**Z** No Qualifier
F Eustachian Tube, Right **G** Eustachian Tube, Left	**3** Percutaneous **4** Percutaneous Endoscopic	**Z** No Device	**Z** No Qualifier

0 Medical and Surgical
9 Ear, Nose, Sinus
8 Division: Cutting into a body part, without draining fluids and/or gases from the body part, in order to separate or transect a body part

Body Part	Approach	Device	Qualifier
Character 4	Character 5	Character 6	Character 7
L Nasal Turbinate	**0** Open **3** Percutaneous **4** Percutaneous Endoscopic **7** Via Natural or Artificial Opening **8** Via Natural or Artificial Opening Endoscopic	**Z** No Device	**Z** No Qualifier

0 Medical and Surgical
9 Ear, Nose, Sinus
9 Drainage: Taking or letting out fluids and/or gases from a body part

Body Part	Approach	Device	Qualifier
Character 4	Character 5	Character 6	Character 7
0 External Ear, Right **1** External Ear, Left	**0** Open **3** Percutaneous **4** Percutaneous Endoscopic **X** External	**0** Drainage Device	**Z** No Qualifier
0 External Ear, Right **1** External Ear, Left	**0** Open **3** Percutaneous **4** Percutaneous Endoscopic **X** External	**Z** No Device	**X** Diagnostic **Z** No Qualifier
3 External Auditory Canal, Right **4** External Auditory Canal, Left **K** Nasal Mucosa and Soft Tissue	**0** Open **3** Percutaneous **4** Percutaneous Endoscopic **7** Via Natural or Artificial Opening **8** Via Natural or Artificial Opening Endoscopic **X** External	**0** Drainage Device	**Z** No Qualifier
3 External Auditory Canal, Right **4** External Auditory Canal, Left **K** Nasal Mucosa and Soft Tissue	**0** Open **3** Percutaneous **4** Percutaneous Endoscopic **7** Via Natural or Artificial Opening **8** Via Natural or Artificial Opening Endoscopic **X** External	**Z** No Device	**X** Diagnostic **Z** No Qualifier
5 Middle Ear, Right **6** Middle Ear, Left **9** Auditory Ossicle, Right **A** Auditory Ossicle, Left **D** Inner Ear, Right **E** Inner Ear, Left	**0** Open **7** Via Natural or Artificial Opening **8** Via Natural or Artificial Opening Endoscopic	**0** Drainage Device	**Z** No Qualifier
5 Middle Ear, Right **6** Middle Ear, Left **9** Auditory Ossicle, Right **A** Auditory Ossicle, Left **D** Inner Ear, Right **E** Inner Ear, Left	**0** Open **7** Via Natural or Artificial Opening **8** Via Natural or Artificial Opening Endoscopic	**Z** No Device	**X** Diagnostic **Z** No Qualifier

099 continued on next page

LC Limited Coverage   NC Noncovered   HAC HAC-associated Procedure   CC Combination Cluster - See Appendix G for code lists
DRG Non-OR-Affecting MS-DRG Assignment   New/Revised Text in **Orange**   ♂ Male   ♀ Female

0 **Medical and Surgical**
9 **Ear, Nose, Sinus**
9 **Drainage:** Taking or letting out fluids and/or gases from a body part

099 continued from previous page

Body Part	Approach	Device	Qualifier
Character 4	Character 5	Character 6	Character 7
7 Tympanic Membrane, Right 8 Tympanic Membrane, Left B Mastoid Sinus, Right C Mastoid Sinus, Left F Eustachian Tube, Right G Eustachian Tube, Left L Nasal Turbinate M Nasal Septum N Nasopharynx P Accessory Sinus Q Maxillary Sinus, Right R Maxillary Sinus, Left S Frontal Sinus, Right T Frontal Sinus, Left U Ethmoid Sinus, Right V Ethmoid Sinus, Left W Sphenoid Sinus, Right X Sphenoid Sinus, Left	0 Open 3 Percutaneous 4 Percutaneous Endoscopic 7 Via Natural or Artificial Opening 8 Via Natural or Artificial Opening Endoscopic	0 Drainage Device	Z No Qualifier
7 Tympanic Membrane, Right 8 Tympanic Membrane, Left B Mastoid Sinus, Right C Mastoid Sinus, Left F Eustachian Tube, Right G Eustachian Tube, Left L Nasal Turbinate M Nasal Septum N Nasopharynx P Accessory Sinus Q Maxillary Sinus, Right R Maxillary Sinus, Left S Frontal Sinus, Right T Frontal Sinus, Left U Ethmoid Sinus, Right V Ethmoid Sinus, Left W Sphenoid Sinus, Right X Sphenoid Sinus, Left	0 Open 3 Percutaneous 4 Percutaneous Endoscopic 7 Via Natural or Artificial Opening 8 Via Natural or Artificial Opening Endoscopic	Z No Device	X Diagnostic Z No Qualifier

LC Limited Coverage   NC Noncovered   HAC HAC-associated Procedure   CC Combination Cluster - See Appendix G for code lists
DRG Non-OR-Affecting MS-DRG Assignment   New/Revised Text in Orange   ♂ Male   ♀ Female

298   2021 ICD-10-PCS

0   **Medical and Surgical**
9   **Ear, Nose, Sinus**
B   **Excision:** Cutting out or off, without replacement, a portion of a body part

Body Part	Approach	Device	Qualifier
Character 4	Character 5	Character 6	Character 7
0 External Ear, Right **1** External Ear, Left	**0** Open **3** Percutaneous **4** Percutaneous Endoscopic **X** External	**Z** No Device	**X** Diagnostic **Z** No Qualifier
3 External Auditory Canal, Right **4** External Auditory Canal, Left	**0** Open **3** Percutaneous **4** Percutaneous Endoscopic **7** Via Natural or Artificial Opening **8** Via Natural or Artificial Opening Endoscopic **X** External	**Z** No Device	**X** Diagnostic **Z** No Qualifier
5 Middle Ear, Right **6** Middle Ear, Left **9** Auditory Ossicle, Right **A** Auditory Ossicle, Left **D** Inner Ear, Right **E** Inner Ear, Left	**0** Open **8** Via Natural or Artificial Opening Endoscopic	**Z** No Device	**X** Diagnostic **Z** No Qualifier
7 Tympanic Membrane, Right **8** Tympanic Membrane, Left **F** Eustachian Tube, Right **G** Eustachian Tube, Left **L** Nasal Turbinate **N** Nasopharynx	**0** Open **3** Percutaneous **4** Percutaneous Endoscopic **7** Via Natural or Artificial Opening **8** Via Natural or Artificial Opening Endoscopic	**Z** No Device	**X** Diagnostic **Z** No Qualifier
B Mastoid Sinus, Right **C** Mastoid Sinus, Left **M** Nasal Septum **P** Accessory Sinus **Q** Maxillary Sinus, Right **R** Maxillary Sinus, Left **S** Frontal Sinus, Right **T** Frontal Sinus, Left **U** Ethmoid Sinus, Right **V** Ethmoid Sinus, Left **W** Sphenoid Sinus, Right **X** Sphenoid Sinus, Left	**0** Open **3** Percutaneous **4** Percutaneous Endoscopic **8** Via Natural or Artificial Opening Endoscopic	**Z** No Device	**X** Diagnostic **Z** No Qualifier
K Nasal Mucosa and Soft Tissue	**0** Open **3** Percutaneous **4** Percutaneous Endoscopic **8** Via Natural or Artificial Opening Endoscopic **X** External	**Z** No Device	**X** Diagnostic **Z** No Qualifier

0 **Medical and Surgical**
9 **Ear, Nose, Sinus**
C **Extirpation:** Taking or cutting out solid matter from a body part

Body Part	Approach	Device	Qualifier
Character 4	Character 5	Character 6	Character 7
0 External Ear, Right 1 External Ear, Left	0 Open 3 Percutaneous 4 Percutaneous Endoscopic X External	Z No Device	Z No Qualifier
3 External Auditory Canal, Right 4 External Auditory Canal, Left	0 Open 3 Percutaneous 4 Percutaneous Endoscopic 7 Via Natural or Artificial Opening 8 Via Natural or Artificial Opening Endoscopic X External	Z No Device	Z No Qualifier
5 Middle Ear, Right 6 Middle Ear, Left 9 Auditory Ossicle, Right A Auditory Ossicle, Left D Inner Ear, Right E Inner Ear, Left	0 Open 8 Via Natural or Artificial Opening Endoscopic	Z No Device	Z No Qualifier
7 Tympanic Membrane, Right 8 Tympanic Membrane, Left F Eustachian Tube, Right G Eustachian Tube, Left L Nasal Turbinate N Nasopharynx	0 Open 3 Percutaneous 4 Percutaneous Endoscopic 7 Via Natural or Artificial Opening 8 Via Natural or Artificial Opening Endoscopic	Z No Device	Z No Qualifier
B Mastoid Sinus, Right C Mastoid Sinus, Left M Nasal Septum P Accessory Sinus Q Maxillary Sinus, Right R Maxillary Sinus, Left S Frontal Sinus, Right T Frontal Sinus, Left U Ethmoid Sinus, Right V Ethmoid Sinus, Left W Sphenoid Sinus, Right X Sphenoid Sinus, Left	0 Open 3 Percutaneous 4 Percutaneous Endoscopic 8 Via Natural or Artificial Opening Endoscopic	Z No Device	Z No Qualifier
K Nasal Mucosa and Soft Tissue	0 Open 3 Percutaneous 4 Percutaneous Endoscopic 8 Via Natural or Artificial Opening Endoscopic X External	Z No Device	Z No Qualifier

LC Limited Coverage **NC** Noncovered **HAC** HAC-associated Procedure **CC** Combination Cluster - See Appendix G for code lists
DRG Non-OR-Affecting MS-DRG Assignment New/Revised Text in **Orange** ♂ Male ♀ Female

300

2021 ICD-10-PCS

0 **Medical and Surgical**

9 **Ear, Nose, Sinus**

D **Extraction:** Pulling or stripping out or off all or a portion of a body part by the use of force

Body Part	Approach	Device	Qualifier
Character 4	Character 5	Character 6	Character 7
7 Tympanic Membrane, Right 8 Tympanic Membrane, Left L Nasal Turbinate	0 Open 3 Percutaneous 4 Percutaneous Endoscopic 7 Via Natural or Artificial Opening 8 Via Natural or Artificial Opening Endoscopic	Z No Device	Z No Qualifier
9 Auditory Ossicle, Right A Auditory Ossicle, Left	0 Open	Z No Device	Z No Qualifier
B Mastoid Sinus, Right C Mastoid Sinus, Left M Nasal Septum P Accessory Sinus Q Maxillary Sinus, Right R Maxillary Sinus, Left S Frontal Sinus, Right T Frontal Sinus, Left U Ethmoid Sinus, Right V Ethmoid Sinus, Left W Sphenoid Sinus, Right X Sphenoid Sinus, Left	0 Open 3 Percutaneous 4 Percutaneous Endoscopic	Z No Device	Z No Qualifier

0 **Medical and Surgical**

9 **Ear, Nose, Sinus**

H **Insertion:** Putting in a nonbiological appliance that monitors, assists, performs, or prevents a physiological function but does not physically take the place of a body part

Body Part	Approach	Device	Qualifier
Character 4	Character 5	Character 6	Character 7
D Inner Ear, Right E Inner Ear, Left	0 Open 3 Percutaneous 4 Percutaneous Endoscopic	1 Radioactive Element 4 Hearing Device, Bone Conduction 5 Hearing Device, Single Channel Cochlear Prosthesis 6 Hearing Device, Multiple Channel Cochlear Prosthesis S Hearing Device	Z No Qualifier
H Ear, Right J Ear, Left K Nasal Mucosa and Soft Tissue Y Sinus	0 Open 3 Percutaneous 4 Percutaneous Endoscopic 7 Via Natural or Artificial Opening 8 Via Natural or Artificial Opening Endoscopic	1 Radioactive Element Y Other Device	Z No Qualifier
N Nasopharynx	7 Via Natural or Artificial Opening 8 Via Natural or Artificial Opening Endoscopic	1 Radioactive Element B Intraluminal Device, Airway	Z No Qualifier

0 Medical and Surgical
9 Ear, Nose, Sinus
J Inspection: Visually and/or manually exploring a body part

Body Part	Approach	Device	Qualifier
Character 4	Character 5	Character 6	Character 7
7 Tympanic Membrane, Right 8 Tympanic Membrane, Left H Ear, Right J Ear, Left	0 Open 3 Percutaneous 4 Percutaneous Endoscopic 7 Via Natural or Artificial Opening 8 Via Natural or Artificial Opening Endoscopic X External	Z No Device	Z No Qualifier
D Inner Ear, Right E Inner Ear, Left K Nasal Mucosa and Soft tissue Y Sinus	0 Open 3 Percutaneous 4 Percutaneous Endoscopic 8 Via Natural or Artificial Opening Endoscopic X External	Z No Device	Z No Qualifier

0 Medical and Surgical
9 Ear, Nose, Sinus
M Reattachment: Putting back in or on all or a portion of a separated body part to its normal location or other suitable location

Body Part	Approach	Device	Qualifier
Character 4	Character 5	Character 6	Character 7
0 External Ear, Right 1 External Ear, Left K Nasal Mucosa and Soft Tissue	X External	Z No Device	Z No Qualifier

0 **Medical and Surgical**
9 **Ear, Nose, Sinus**
N **Release:** Freeing a body part from an abnormal physical constraint by cutting or by the use of force

Body Part	Approach	Device	Qualifier
Character 4	Character 5	Character 6	Character 7
0 External Ear, Right **1** External Ear, Left	**0** Open **3** Percutaneous **4** Percutaneous Endoscopic **X** External	**Z** No Device	**Z** No Qualifier
3 External Auditory Canal, Right **4** External Auditory Canal, Left	**0** Open **3** Percutaneous **4** Percutaneous Endoscopic **7** Via Natural or Artificial Opening **8** Via Natural or Artificial Opening Endoscopic **X** External	**Z** No Device	**Z** No Qualifier
5 Middle Ear, Right **6** Middle Ear, Left **9** Auditory Ossicle, Right **A** Auditory Ossicle, Left **D** Inner Ear, Right **E** Inner Ear, Left	**0** Open **8** Via Natural or Artificial Opening Endoscopic	**Z** No Device	**Z** No Qualifier
7 Tympanic Membrane, Right **8** Tympanic Membrane, Left **F** Eustachian Tube, Right **G** Eustachian Tube, Left **L** Nasal Turbinate **N** Nasopharynx	**0** Open **3** Percutaneous **4** Percutaneous Endoscopic **7** Via Natural or Artificial Opening **8** Via Natural or Artificial Opening Endoscopic	**Z** No Device	**Z** No Qualifier
B Mastoid Sinus, Right **C** Mastoid Sinus, Left **M** Nasal Septum **P** Accessory Sinus **Q** Maxillary Sinus, Right **R** Maxillary Sinus, Left **S** Frontal Sinus, Right **T** Frontal Sinus, Left **U** Ethmoid Sinus, Right **V** Ethmoid Sinus, Left **W** Sphenoid Sinus, Right **X** Sphenoid Sinus, Left	**0** Open **3** Percutaneous **4** Percutaneous Endoscopic **8** Via Natural or Artificial Opening Endoscopic	**Z** No Device	**Z** No Qualifier
K Nasal Mucosa and Soft Tissue	**0** Open **3** Percutaneous **4** Percutaneous Endoscopic **8** Via Natural or Artificial Opening Endoscopic **X** External	**Z** No Device	**Z** No Qualifier

0 **Medical and Surgical**
9 **Ear, Nose, Sinus**
P **Removal:** Taking out or off a device from a body part

Body Part	Approach	Device	Qualifier
Character 4	**Character 5**	**Character 6**	**Character 7**
7 Tympanic Membrane, Right 8 Tympanic Membrane, Left	0 Open 7 Via Natural or Artificial Opening 8 Via Natural or Artificial Opening Endoscopic X External	0 Drainage Device	Z No Qualifier
D Inner Ear, Right E Inner Ear, Left	0 Open 7 Via Natural or Artificial Opening 8 Via Natural or Artificial Opening Endoscopic	S Hearing Device	Z No Qualifier
H Ear, Right J Ear, Left K Nasal Mucosa and Soft Tissue	0 Open 3 Percutaneous 4 Percutaneous Endoscopic 7 Via Natural or Artificial Opening 8 Via Natural or Artificial Opening Endoscopic	0 Drainage Device 7 Autologous Tissue Substitute D Intraluminal Device J Synthetic Substitute K Nonautologous Tissue Substitute Y Other Device	Z No Qualifier
H Ear, Right J Ear, Left K Nasal Mucosa and Soft Tissue	X External	0 Drainage Device 7 Autologous Tissue Substitute D Intraluminal Device J Synthetic Substitute K Nonautologous Tissue Substitute	Z No Qualifier
Y Sinus	0 Open 3 Percutaneous 4 Percutaneous Endoscopic	0 Drainage Device Y Other Device	Z No Qualifier
Y Sinus	7 Via Natural or Artificial Opening 8 Via Natural or Artificial Opening Endoscopic	Y Other Device	Z No Qualifier
Y Sinus	X External	0 Drainage Device	Z No Qualifier

LC Limited Coverage   **NC** Noncovered   **HAC** HAC-associated Procedure   **CC** Combination Cluster - See Appendix G for code lists

Non-OR-Affecting MS-DRG Assignment   New/Revised Text in **Orange**   ♂ Male   ♀ Female

304   **2021 ICD-10-PCS**

0 Medical and Surgical
9 Ear, Nose, Sinus
Q Repair: Restoring, to the extent possible, a body part to its normal anatomic structure and function

Body Part	Approach	Device	Qualifier
Character 4	Character 5	Character 6	Character 7
0 External Ear, Right 1 External Ear, Left 2 External Ear, Bilateral	0 Open 3 Percutaneous 4 Percutaneous Endoscopic X External	Z No Device	Z No Qualifier
3 External Auditory Canal, Right 4 External Auditory Canal, Left F Eustachian Tube, Right G Eustachian Tube, Left	0 Open 3 Percutaneous 4 Percutaneous Endoscopic 7 Via Natural or Artificial Opening 8 Via Natural or Artificial Opening Endoscopic X External	Z No Device	Z No Qualifier
5 Middle Ear, Right 6 Middle Ear, Left 9 Auditory Ossicle, Right A Auditory Ossicle, Left D Inner Ear, Right E Inner Ear, Left	0 Open 8 Via Natural or Artificial Opening Endoscopic	Z No Device	Z No Qualifier
7 Tympanic Membrane, Right 8 Tympanic Membrane, Left L Nasal Turbinate N Nasopharynx	0 Open 3 Percutaneous 4 Percutaneous Endoscopic 7 Via Natural or Artificial Opening 8 Via Natural or Artificial Opening Endoscopic	Z No Device	Z No Qualifier
B Mastoid Sinus, Right C Mastoid Sinus, Left M Nasal Septum P Accessory Sinus Q Maxillary Sinus, Right R Maxillary Sinus, Left S Frontal Sinus, Right T Frontal Sinus, Left U Ethmoid Sinus, Right V Ethmoid Sinus, Left W Sphenoid Sinus, Right X Sphenoid Sinus, Left	0 Open 3 Percutaneous 4 Percutaneous Endoscopic 8 Via Natural or Artificial Opening Endoscopic	Z No Device	Z No Qualifier
K Nasal Mucosa and Soft Tissue	0 Open 3 Percutaneous 4 Percutaneous Endoscopic 8 Via Natural or Artificial Opening Endoscopic X External	Z No Device	Z No Qualifier

LC Limited Coverage   **NC** Noncovered   **HAC** HAC-associated Procedure   **CC** Combination Cluster - See Appendix G for code lists
DRG Non-OR-Affecting MS-DRG Assignment   New/Revised Text in **Orange**   ♂ Male   ♀ Female

2021 ICD-10-PCS

305

0 Medical and Surgical
9 Ear, Nose, Sinus
R Replacement: Putting in or on biological or synthetic material that physically takes the place and/or function of all or a portion of a body part

Body Part	Approach	Device	Qualifier
Character 4	Character 5	Character 6	Character 7
0 External Ear, Right 1 External Ear, Left 2 External Ear, Bilateral K Nasal Mucosa and Soft Tissue	0 Open X External	7 Autologous Tissue Substitute J Synthetic Substitute K Nonautologous Tissue Substitute	Z No Qualifier
5 Middle Ear, Right 6 Middle Ear, Left 9 Auditory Ossicle, Right A Auditory Ossicle, Left D Inner Ear, Right E Inner Ear, Left	0 Open	7 Autologous Tissue Substitute J Synthetic Substitute K Nonautologous Tissue Substitute	Z No Qualifier
7 Tympanic Membrane, Right 8 Tympanic Membrane, Left N Nasopharynx	0 Open 7 Via Natural or Artificial Opening 8 Via Natural or Artificial Opening Endoscopic	7 Autologous Tissue Substitute J Synthetic Substitute K Nonautologous Tissue Substitute	Z No Qualifier
L Nasal Turbinate	0 Open 3 Percutaneous 4 Percutaneous Endoscopic 7 Via Natural or Artificial Opening 8 Via Natural or Artificial Opening Endoscopic	7 Autologous Tissue Substitute J Synthetic Substitute K Nonautologous Tissue Substitute	Z No Qualifier
M Nasal Septum	0 Open 3 Percutaneous 4 Percutaneous Endoscopic	7 Autologous Tissue Substitute J Synthetic Substitute K Nonautologous Tissue Substitute	Z No Qualifier

0 Medical and Surgical
9 Ear, Nose, Sinus
S Reposition: Moving to its normal location, or other suitable location, all or a portion of a body part

Body Part	Approach	Device	Qualifier
Character 4	Character 5	Character 6	Character 7
0 External Ear, Right 1 External Ear, Left 2 External Ear, Bilateral K Nasal Mucosa and Soft Tissue	0 Open 4 Percutaneous Endoscopic X External	Z No Device	Z No Qualifier
7 Tympanic Membrane, Right 8 Tympanic Membrane, Left F Eustachian Tube, Right G Eustachian Tube, Left L Nasal Turbinate	0 Open 4 Percutaneous Endoscopic 7 Via Natural or Artificial Opening 8 Via Natural or Artificial Opening Endoscopic	Z No Device	Z No Qualifier
9 Auditory Ossicle, Right A Auditory Ossicle, Left M Nasal Septum	0 Open 4 Percutaneous Endoscopic	Z No Device	Z No Qualifier

0 Medical and Surgical
9 Ear, Nose, Sinus
T Resection: Cutting out or off, without replacement, all of a body part

Body Part	Approach	Device	Qualifier
Character 4	Character 5	Character 6	Character 7
0 External Ear, Right 1 External Ear, Left	0 Open 4 Percutaneous Endoscopic X External	Z No Device	Z No Qualifier
5 Middle Ear, Right 6 Middle Ear, Left 9 Auditory Ossicle, Right A Auditory Ossicle, Left D Inner Ear, Right E Inner Ear, Left	0 Open 8 Via Natural or Artificial Opening Endoscopic	Z No Device	Z No Qualifier
7 Tympanic Membrane, Right 8 Tympanic Membrane, Left F Eustachian Tube, Right G Eustachian Tube, Left L Nasal Turbinate N Nasopharynx	0 Open 4 Percutaneous Endoscopic 7 Via Natural or Artificial Opening 8 Via Natural or Artificial Opening Endoscopic	Z No Device	Z No Qualifier
B Mastoid Sinus, Right C Mastoid Sinus, Left M Nasal Septum P Accessory Sinus Q Maxillary Sinus, Right R Maxillary Sinus, Left S Frontal Sinus, Right T Frontal Sinus, Left U Ethmoid Sinus, Right V Ethmoid Sinus, Left W Sphenoid Sinus, Right X Sphenoid Sinus, Left	0 Open 4 Percutaneous Endoscopic 8 Via Natural or Artificial Opening Endoscopic	Z No Device	Z No Qualifier
K Nasal Mucosa and Soft Tissue	0 Open 4 Percutaneous Endoscopic 8 Via Natural or Artificial Opening Endoscopic X External	Z No Device	Z No Qualifier

LC Limited Coverage   NC Noncovered   HAC HAC-associated Procedure   CC Combination Cluster - See Appendix G for code lists
DRG Non-OR-Affecting MS-DRG Assignment   New/Revised Text in **Orange**   ♂ Male   ♀ Female

0 Medical and Surgical
9 Ear, Nose, Sinus
U Supplement: Putting in or on biological or synthetic material that physically reinforces and/or augments the function of a portion of a body part

Body Part	Approach	Device	Qualifier
Character 4	Character 5	Character 6	Character 7
0 External Ear, Right 1 External Ear, Left 2 External Ear, Bilateral	0 Open X External	7 Autologous Tissue Substitute J Synthetic Substitute K Nonautologous Tissue Substitute	Z No Qualifier
5 Middle Ear, Right 6 Middle Ear, Left 9 Auditory Ossicle, Right A Auditory Ossicle, Left D Inner Ear, Right E Inner Ear, Left	0 Open 8 Via Natural or Artificial Opening Endoscopic	7 Autologous Tissue Substitute J Synthetic Substitute K Nonautologous Tissue Substitute	Z No Qualifier
7 Tympanic Membrane, Right 8 Tympanic Membrane, Left N Nasopharynx	0 Open 7 Via Natural or Artificial Opening 8 Via Natural or Artificial Opening Endoscopic	7 Autologous Tissue Substitute J Synthetic Substitute K Nonautologous Tissue Substitute	Z No Qualifier
B Mastoid Sinus, Right C Mastoid Sinus, Left L Nasal Turbinate P Accessory Sinus Q Maxillary Sinus, Right R Maxillary Sinus, Left S Frontal Sinus, Right T Frontal Sinus, Left U Ethmoid Sinus, Right V Ethmoid Sinus, Left W Sphenoid Sinus, Right X Sphenoid Sinus, Left	0 Open 3 Percutaneous 4 Percutaneous Endoscopic 7 Via Natural or Artificial Opening 8 Via Natural or Artificial Opening Endoscopic	7 Autologous Tissue Substitute J Synthetic Substitute K Nonautologous Tissue Substitute	Z No Qualifier
K Nasal Mucosa and Soft Tissue	0 Open 8 Via Natural or Artificial Opening Endoscopic X External	7 Autologous Tissue Substitute J Synthetic Substitute K Nonautologous Tissue Substitute	Z No Qualifier
M Nasal Septum	0 Open 3 Percutaneous 4 Percutaneous Endoscopic 8 Via Natural or Artificial Opening Endoscopic	7 Autologous Tissue Substitute J Synthetic Substitute K Nonautologous Tissue Substitute	Z No Qualifier

0 Medical and Surgical
9 Ear, Nose, Sinus
W Revision: Correcting, to the extent possible, a portion of a malfunctioning device or the position of a displaced device

Body Part	Approach	Device	Qualifier
Character 4	Character 5	Character 6	Character 7
7 Tympanic Membrane, Right 8 Tympanic Membrane, Left 9 Auditory Ossicle, Right A Auditory Ossicle, Left	0 Open 7 Via Natural or Artificial Opening 8 Via Natural or Artificial Opening Endoscopic	7 Autologous Tissue Substitute J Synthetic Substitute K Nonautologous Tissue Substitute	Z No Qualifier
D Inner Ear, Right E Inner Ear, Left	0 Open 7 Via Natural or Artificial Opening 8 Via Natural or Artificial Opening Endoscopic	S Hearing Device	Z No Qualifier
H Ear, Right J Ear, Left K Nasal Mucosa and Soft Tissue	0 Open 3 Percutaneous 4 Percutaneous Endoscopic 7 Via Natural or Artificial Opening 8 Via Natural or Artificial Opening Endoscopic	0 Drainage Device 7 Autologous Tissue Substitute D Intraluminal Device J Synthetic Substitute K Nonautologous Tissue Substitute Y Other Device	Z No Qualifier
H Ear, Right J Ear, Left K Nasal Mucosa and Soft Tissue	X External	0 Drainage Device 7 Autologous Tissue Substitute D Intraluminal Device J Synthetic Substitute K Nonautologous Tissue Substitute	Z No Qualifier
Y Sinus	0 Open 3 Percutaneous 4 Percutaneous Endoscopic	0 Drainage Device Y Other Device	Z No Qualifier
Y Sinus	7 Via Natural or Artificial Opening 8 Via Natural or Artificial Opening Endoscopic	Y Other Device	Z No Qualifier
Y Sinus	X External	0 Drainage Device	Z No Qualifier

LC Limited Coverage **NC** Noncovered **HAC** HAC-associated Procedure **CC** Combination Cluster - See Appendix G for code lists
DRG Non-OR-Affecting MS-DRG Assignment New/Revised Text in **Orange** ♂ Male ♀ Female

2021 ICD-10-PCS

309

EAR, NOSE, SINUS 090-09W

NOTES

Respiratory System 0B1-0BY

0 Medical and Surgical
B Respiratory System
1 Bypass: Altering the route of passage of the contents of a tubular body part

Body Part	Approach	Device	Qualifier
Character 4	Character 5	Character 6	Character 7
1 Trachea	**0** Open	**D** Intraluminal Device	**6** Esophagus
1 Trachea	**0** Open	**F** Tracheostomy Device **Z** No Device	**4** Cutaneous
1 Trachea ⓭	**3** Percutaneous **4** Percutaneous Endoscopic	**F** Tracheostomy Device **Z** No Device	**4** Cutaneous

⓭ 0B113F4   0B113Z4

0 Medical and Surgical
B Respiratory System
2 Change: Taking out or off a device from a body part and putting back an identical or similar device in or on the same body part without cutting or puncturing the skin or a mucous membrane

Body Part	Approach	Device	Qualifier
Character 4	Character 5	Character 6	Character 7
0 Tracheobronchial Tree **K** Lung, Right **L** Lung, Left **Q** Pleura **T** Diaphragm	**X** External	**0** Drainage Device **Y** Other Device	**Z** No Qualifier
1 Trachea	**X** External	**0** Drainage Device **E** Intraluminal Device, Endotracheal Airway **F** Tracheostomy Device **Y** Other Device	**Z** No Qualifier

0 Medical and Surgical
B Respiratory System
5 Destruction: Physical eradication of all or a portion of a body part by the direct use of energy, force, or a destructive agent

Body Part	Approach	Device	Qualifier
Character 4	Character 5	Character 6	Character 7
1 Trachea **2** Carina **3** Main Bronchus, Right **4** Upper Lobe Bronchus, Right **5** Middle Lobe Bronchus, Right **6** Lower Lobe Bronchus, Right **7** Main Bronchus, Left **8** Upper Lobe Bronchus, Left **9** Lingula Bronchus **B** Lower Lobe Bronchus, Left **C** Upper Lung Lobe, Right **D** Middle Lung Lobe, Right **F** Lower Lung Lobe, Right **G** Upper Lung Lobe, Left **H** Lung Lingula **J** Lower Lung Lobe, Left **K** Lung, Right **L** Lung, Left **M** Lungs, Bilateral	**0** Open **3** Percutaneous **4** Percutaneous Endoscopic **7** Via Natural or Artificial Opening **8** Via Natural or Artificial Opening Endoscopic	**Z** No Device	**Z** No Qualifier
N Pleura, Right **P** Pleura, Left **T** Diaphragm	**0** Open **3** Percutaneous **4** Percutaneous Endoscopic	**Z** No Device	**Z** No Qualifier

0   Medical and Surgical
B   Respiratory System
7   Dilation: Expanding an orifice or the lumen of a tubular body part

Body Part	Approach	Device	Qualifier
Character 4	Character 5	Character 6	Character 7
1 Trachea 2 Carina 3 Main Bronchus, Right 4 Upper Lobe Bronchus, Right 5 Middle Lobe Bronchus, Right 6 Lower Lobe Bronchus, Right 7 Main Bronchus, Left 8 Upper Lobe Bronchus, Left 9 Lingula Bronchus B Lower Lobe Bronchus, Left	0 Open 3 Percutaneous 4 Percutaneous Endoscopic 7 Via Natural or Artificial Opening 8 Via Natural or Artificial Opening Endoscopic	D Intraluminal Device Z No Device	Z No Qualifier

0   Medical and Surgical
B   Respiratory System
9   Drainage: Taking or letting out fluids and/or gases from a body part

Body Part	Approach	Device	Qualifier
Character 4	Character 5	Character 6	Character 7
1 Trachea 2 Carina 3 Main Bronchus, Right 4 Upper Lobe Bronchus, Right 5 Middle Lobe Bronchus, Right 6 Lower Lobe Bronchus, Right 7 Main Bronchus, Left 8 Upper Lobe Bronchus, Left 9 Lingula Bronchus B Lower Lobe Bronchus, Left C Upper Lung Lobe, Right D Middle Lung Lobe, Right F Lower Lung Lobe, Right G Upper Lung Lobe, Left H Lung Lingula J Lower Lung Lobe, Left K Lung, Right L Lung, Left M Lungs, Bilateral	0 Open 3 Percutaneous 4 Percutaneous Endoscopic 7 Via Natural or Artificial Opening 8 Via Natural or Artificial Opening Endoscopic	0 Drainage Device	Z No Qualifier
1 Trachea 2 Carina 3 Main Bronchus, Right 4 Upper Lobe Bronchus, Right 5 Middle Lobe Bronchus, Right 6 Lower Lobe Bronchus, Right 7 Main Bronchus, Left 8 Upper Lobe Bronchus, Left 9 Lingula Bronchus B Lower Lobe Bronchus, Left C Upper Lung Lobe, Right D Middle Lung Lobe, Right F Lower Lung Lobe, Right G Upper Lung Lobe, Left H Lung Lingula J Lower Lung Lobe, Left K Lung, Right L Lung, Left M Lungs, Bilateral	0 Open 3 Percutaneous 4 Percutaneous Endoscopic 7 Via Natural or Artificial Opening 8 Via Natural or Artificial Opening Endoscopic	Z No Device	X Diagnostic Z No Qualifier

0B9 continued on next page

LC Limited Coverage   **NC** Noncovered   **HAC** HAC-associated Procedure   **CC** Combination Cluster - See Appendix G for code lists
DRG Non-OR-Affecting MS-DRG Assignment   New/Revised Text in **Orange**   ♂ Male   ♀ Female

312   **2021 ICD-10-PCS**

0 **Medical and Surgical**   0B9 continued from previous page
B **Respiratory System**
9 **Drainage:** Taking or letting out fluids and/or gases from a body part

Body Part	Approach	Device	Qualifier
Character 4	**Character 5**	**Character 6**	**Character 7**
N Pleura, Right P Pleura, Left	0 Open 3 Percutaneous 4 Percutaneous Endoscopic 8 Via Natural or Artificial Opening Endoscopic	0 Drainage Device	Z No Qualifier
N Pleura, Right P Pleura, Left	0 Open 3 Percutaneous 4 Percutaneous Endoscopic 8 Via Natural or Artificial Opening Endoscopic	Z No Device	X Diagnostic Z No Qualifier
T Diaphragm	0 Open 3 Percutaneous 4 Percutaneous Endoscopic	0 Drainage Device	Z No Qualifier
T Diaphragm	0 Open 3 Percutaneous 4 Percutaneous Endoscopic	Z No Device	X Diagnostic Z No Qualifier

0 **Medical and Surgical**
B **Respiratory System**
B **Excision:** Cutting out or off, without replacement, a portion of a body part

Body Part	Approach	Device	Qualifier
Character 4	**Character 5**	**Character 6**	**Character 7**
1 Trachea 2 Carina 3 Main Bronchus, Right 4 Upper Lobe Bronchus, Right 5 Middle Lobe Bronchus, Right 6 Lower Lobe Bronchus, Right 7 Main Bronchus, Left 8 Upper Lobe Bronchus, Left 9 Lingula Bronchus B Lower Lobe Bronchus, Left C Upper Lung Lobe, Right D Middle Lung Lobe, Right F Lower Lung Lobe, Right G Upper Lung Lobe, Left H Lung Lingula J Lower Lung Lobe, Left K Lung, Right L Lung, Left M Lungs, Bilateral	0 Open 3 Percutaneous 4 Percutaneous Endoscopic 7 Via Natural or Artificial Opening 8 Via Natural or Artificial Opening Endoscopic	Z No Device	X Diagnostic Z No Qualifier
N Pleura, Right P Pleura, Left	0 Open 3 Percutaneous 4 Percutaneous Endoscopic 8 Via Natural or Artificial Opening Endoscopic	Z No Device	X Diagnostic Z No Qualifier
T Diaphragm	0 Open 3 Percutaneous 4 Percutaneous Endoscopic	Z No Device	X Diagnostic Z No Qualifier

0   Medical and Surgical
B   Respiratory System
C   Extirpation: Taking or cutting out solid matter from a body part

Body Part	Approach	Device	Qualifier
Character 4	**Character 5**	**Character 6**	**Character 7**
1 Trachea 2 Carina 3 Main Bronchus, Right 4 Upper Lobe Bronchus, Right 5 Middle Lobe Bronchus, Right 6 Lower Lobe Bronchus, Right 7 Main Bronchus, Left 8 Upper Lobe Bronchus, Left 9 Lingula Bronchus B Lower Lobe Bronchus, Left C Upper Lung Lobe, Right D Middle Lung Lobe, Right F Lower Lung Lobe, Right G Upper Lung Lobe, Left H Lung Lingula J Lower Lung Lobe, Left K Lung, Right L Lung, Left M Lungs, Bilateral	0 Open 3 Percutaneous 4 Percutaneous Endoscopic 7 Via Natural or Artificial Opening 8 Via Natural or Artificial Opening Endoscopic	Z No Device	Z No Qualifier
N Pleura, Right P Pleura, Left T Diaphragm	0 Open 3 Percutaneous 4 Percutaneous Endoscopic	Z No Device	Z No Qualifier

0   Medical and Surgical
B   Respiratory System
D   Extraction: Pulling or stripping out or off all or a portion of a body part by the use of force

Body Part	Approach	Device	Qualifier
Character 4	**Character 5**	**Character 6**	**Character 7**
1 Trachea 2 Carina 3 Main Bronchus, Right 4 Upper Lobe Bronchus, Right 5 Middle Lobe Bronchus, Right 6 Lower Lobe Bronchus, Right 7 Main Bronchus, Left 8 Upper Lobe Bronchus, Left 9 Lingula Bronchus B Lower Lobe Bronchus, Left C Upper Lung Lobe, Right D Middle Lung Lobe, Right F Lower Lung Lobe, Right G Upper Lung Lobe, Left H Lung Lingula J Lower Lung Lobe, Left K Lung, Right L Lung, Left M Lungs, Bilateral	4 Percutaneous Endoscopic 8 Via Natural or Artificial Opening Endoscopic	Z No Device	X Diagnostic
N Pleura, Right P Pleura, Left	0 Open 3 Percutaneous 4 Percutaneous Endoscopic	Z No Device	X Diagnostic Z No Qualifier

LC Limited Coverage   **NC** Noncovered   **HAC** HAC-associated Procedure   **CC** Combination Cluster - See Appendix G for code lists

DRG Non-OR-Affecting MS-DRG Assignment   New/Revised Text in **Orange**   ♂ Male ♀ Female

314   **2021 ICD-10-PCS**

0 **Medical and Surgical**
B **Respiratory System**
F **Fragmentation:** Breaking solid matter in a body part into pieces

Body Part	Approach	Device	Qualifier
Character 4	Character 5	Character 6	Character 7
1 Trachea NC 2 Carina NC 3 Main Bronchus, Right NC 4 Upper Lobe Bronchus, Right NC 5 Middle Lobe Bronchus, Right NC 6 Lower Lobe Bronchus, Right NC 7 Main Bronchus, Left NC 8 Upper Lobe Bronchus, Left NC 9 Lingula Bronchus NC B Lower Lobe Bronchus, Left NC	0 Open 3 Percutaneous 4 Percutaneous Endoscopic 7 Via Natural or Artificial Opening 8 Via Natural or Artificial Opening Endoscopic X External	Z No Device	Z No Qualifier

NC 0BF1XZZ 0BF2XZZ 0BF3XZZ 0BF4XZZ 0BF5XZZ 0BF6XZZ 0BF7XZZ 0BF8XZZ 0BF9XZZ 0BFBXZZ

0 **Medical and Surgical**
B **Respiratory System**
H **Insertion:** Putting in a nonbiological appliance that monitors, assists, performs, or prevents a physiological function but does not physically take the place of a body part

Body Part	Approach	Device	Qualifier
Character 4	Character 5	Character 6	Character 7
0 Tracheobronchial Tree	0 Open 3 Percutaneous 4 Percutaneous Endoscopic 7 Via Natural or Artificial Opening 8 Via Natural or Artificial Opening Endoscopic	1 Radioactive Element 2 Monitoring Device 3 Infusion Device D Intraluminal Device Y Other Device	Z No Qualifier
1 Trachea	0 Open	2 Monitoring Device D Intraluminal Device Y Other Device	Z No Qualifier
1 Trachea	3 Percutaneous	D Intraluminal Device E Intraluminal Device, Endotracheal Airway Y Other Device	Z No Qualifier
1 Trachea	4 Percutaneous Endoscopic	D Intraluminal Device Y Other Device	Z No Qualifier

1 Trachea	7 Via Natural or Artificial Opening
	8 Via Natural or Artificial Opening
	   Endoscopic
		2 Monitoring Device
		D Intraluminal Device
		E Intraluminal Device,
		   Endotracheal Airway
		Y Other Device
			Z No Qualifier

3 Main Bronchus, Right DRG
4 Upper Lobe Bronchus, Right DRG
5 Middle Lobe Bronchus, Right DRG
6 Lower Lobe Bronchus, Right DRG
7 Main Bronchus, Left DRG
8 Upper Lobe Bronchus, Left DRG
9 Lingula Bronchus DRG
B Lower Lobe Bronchus, Left DRG
	0 Open
	3 Percutaneous
	4 Percutaneous Endoscopic
	7 Via Natural or Artificial Opening
	8 Via Natural or Artificial Opening
	   Endoscopic
		G Intraluminal Device,
		   Endobronchial Valve
			Z No Qualifier

K Lung, Right L Lung, Left	0 Open 3 Percutaneous 4 Percutaneous Endoscopic 7 Via Natural or Artificial Opening 8 Via Natural or Artificial Opening Endoscopic	1 Radioactive Element 2 Monitoring Device 3 Infusion Device Y Other Device	Z No Qualifier

0BH continued on next page

LC Limited Coverage   NC Noncovered   HAC HAC-associated Procedure   CC Combination Cluster - See Appendix G for code lists
DRG Non-OR-Affecting MS-DRG Assignment   New/Revised Text in **Orange**   ♂ Male   ♀ Female

0 Medical and Surgical
B Respiratory System
H Insertion: Putting in a nonbiological appliance that monitors, assists, performs, or prevents a physiological function but does not physically take the place of a body part

0BH continued from previous page

Body Part	Approach	Device	Qualifier
Character 4	Character 5	Character 6	Character 7
Q Pleura	**0** Open **3** Percutaneous **4** Percutaneous Endoscopic **7** Via Natural or Artificial Opening **8** Via Natural or Artificial Opening Endoscopic	**Y** Other Device	**Z** No Qualifier
T Diaphragm	**0** Open **3** Percutaneous **4** Percutaneous Endoscopic	**2** Monitoring Device **M** Diaphragmatic Pacemaker Lead **Y** Other Device	**Z** No Qualifier
T Diaphragm	**7** Via Natural or Artificial Opening **8** Via Natural or Artificial Opening Endoscopic	**Y** Other Device	**Z** No Qualifier

ORG 0BH38GZ   0BH48GZ   0BH58GZ   0BH68GZ   0BH78GZ   0BH88GZ   0BH98GZ   0BHB8GZ

0 Medical and Surgical
B Respiratory System
J Inspection: Visually and/or manually exploring a body part

Body Part	Approach	Device	Qualifier
Character 4	Character 5	Character 6	Character 7
0 Tracheobronchial Tree **1** Trachea **K** Lung, Right **L** Lung, Left **Q** Pleura **T** Diaphragm	**0** Open **3** Percutaneous **4** Percutaneous Endoscopic **7** Via Natural or Artificial Opening **8** Via Natural or Artificial Opening Endoscopic **X** External	**Z** No Device	**Z** No Qualifier

0 Medical and Surgical
B Respiratory System
L Occlusion: Completely closing an orifice or the lumen of a tubular body part

Body Part	Approach	Device	Qualifier
Character 4	Character 5	Character 6	Character 7
1 Trachea **2** Carina **3** Main Bronchus, Right **4** Upper Lobe Bronchus, Right **5** Middle Lobe Bronchus, Right **6** Lower Lobe Bronchus, Right **7** Main Bronchus, Left **8** Upper Lobe Bronchus, Left **9** Lingula Bronchus **B** Lower Lobe Bronchus, Left	**0** Open **3** Percutaneous **4** Percutaneous Endoscopic	**C** Extraluminal Device **D** Intraluminal Device **Z** No Device	**Z** No Qualifier
1 Trachea **2** Carina **3** Main Bronchus, Right **4** Upper Lobe Bronchus, Right **5** Middle Lobe Bronchus, Right **6** Lower Lobe Bronchus, Right **7** Main Bronchus, Left **8** Upper Lobe Bronchus, Left **9** Lingula Bronchus **B** Lower Lobe Bronchus, Left	**7** Via Natural or Artificial Opening **8** Via Natural or Artificial Opening Endoscopic	**D** Intraluminal Device **Z** No Device	**Z** No Qualifier

LC Limited Coverage   NC Noncovered   HAC HAC-associated Procedure   CC Combination Cluster - See Appendix G for code lists
ORG Non-OR-Affecting MS-DRG Assignment   New/Revised Text in Orange   ♂ Male   ♀ Female

316

2021 ICD-10-PCS

0 Medical and Surgical
B Respiratory System
M Reattachment: Putting back in or on all or a portion of a separated body part to its normal location or other suitable location

Body Part	Approach	Device	Qualifier
Character 4	Character 5	Character 6	Character 7
1 Trachea	0 Open	Z No Device	Z No Qualifier
2 Carina			
3 Main Bronchus, Right			
4 Upper Lobe Bronchus, Right			
5 Middle Lobe Bronchus, Right			
6 Lower Lobe Bronchus, Right			
7 Main Bronchus, Left			
8 Upper Lobe Bronchus, Left			
9 Lingula Bronchus			
B Lower Lobe Bronchus, Left			
C Upper Lung Lobe, Right			
D Middle Lung Lobe, Right			
F Lower Lung Lobe, Right			
G Upper Lung Lobe, Left			
H Lung Lingula			
J Lower Lung Lobe, Left			
K Lung, Right			
L Lung, Left			
T Diaphragm			

0 Medical and Surgical
B Respiratory System
N Release: Freeing a body part from an abnormal physical constraint by cutting or by the use of force

Body Part	Approach	Device	Qualifier
Character 4	Character 5	Character 6	Character 7
1 Trachea	0 Open	Z No Device	Z No Qualifier
2 Carina	3 Percutaneous		
3 Main Bronchus, Right	4 Percutaneous Endoscopic		
4 Upper Lobe Bronchus, Right	7 Via Natural or Artificial Opening		
5 Middle Lobe Bronchus, Right	8 Via Natural or Artificial Opening Endoscopic		
6 Lower Lobe Bronchus, Right			
7 Main Bronchus, Left			
8 Upper Lobe Bronchus, Left			
9 Lingula Bronchus			
B Lower Lobe Bronchus, Left			
C Upper Lung Lobe, Right			
D Middle Lung Lobe, Right			
F Lower Lung Lobe, Right			
G Upper Lung Lobe, Left			
H Lung Lingula			
J Lower Lung Lobe, Left			
K Lung, Right			
L Lung, Left			
M Lungs, Bilateral			
N Pleura, Right	0 Open	Z No Device	Z No Qualifier
P Pleura, Left	3 Percutaneous		
T Diaphragm	4 Percutaneous Endoscopic		

0 **Medical and Surgical**
B **Respiratory System**
P **Removal:** Taking out or off a device from a body part

Body Part	Approach	Device	Qualifier
Character 4	Character 5	Character 6	Character 7
0 Tracheobronchial Tree	**0** Open **3** Percutaneous **4** Percutaneous Endoscopic **7** Via Natural or Artificial Opening **8** Via Natural or Artificial Opening Endoscopic	**0** Drainage Device **1** Radioactive Element **2** Monitoring Device **3** Infusion Device **7** Autologous Tissue Substitute **C** Extraluminal Device **D** Intraluminal Device **J** Synthetic Substitute **K** Nonautologous Tissue Substitute **Y** Other Device	**Z** No Qualifier
0 Tracheobronchial Tree	**X** External	**0** Drainage Device **1** Radioactive Element **2** Monitoring Device **3** Infusion Device **D** Intraluminal Device	**Z** No Qualifier
1 Trachea	**0** Open **3** Percutaneous **4** Percutaneous Endoscopic **7** Via Natural or Artificial Opening **8** Via Natural or Artificial Opening Endoscopic	**0** Drainage Device **2** Monitoring Device **7** Autologous Tissue Substitute **C** Extraluminal Device **D** Intraluminal Device **F** Tracheostomy Device **J** Synthetic Substitute **K** Nonautologous Tissue Substitute	**Z** No Qualifier
1 Trachea	**X** External	**0** Drainage Device **2** Monitoring Device **D** Intraluminal Device **F** Tracheostomy Device	**Z** No Qualifier
K Lung, Right **L** Lung, Left	**0** Open **3** Percutaneous **4** Percutaneous Endoscopic **7** Via Natural or Artificial Opening **8** Via Natural or Artificial Opening Endoscopic	**0** Drainage Device **1** Radioactive Element **2** Monitoring Device **3** Infusion Device **Y** Other Device	**Z** No Qualifier
K Lung, Right **L** Lung, Left	**X** External	**0** Drainage Device **1** Radioactive Element **2** Monitoring Device **3** Infusion Device	**Z** No Qualifier
Q Pleura	**0** Open **3** Percutaneous **4** Percutaneous Endoscopic **7** Via Natural or Artificial Opening **8** Via Natural or Artificial Opening Endoscopic	**0** Drainage Device **1** Radioactive Element **2** Monitoring Device **Y** Other Device	**Z** No Qualifier
Q Pleura	**X** External	**0** Drainage Device **1** Radioactive Element **2** Monitoring Device	**Z** No Qualifier
T Diaphragm	**0** Open **3** Percutaneous **4** Percutaneous Endoscopic **7** Via Natural or Artificial Opening **8** Via Natural or Artificial Opening Endoscopic	**0** Drainage Device **2** Monitoring Device **7** Autologous Tissue Substitute **J** Synthetic Substitute **K** Nonautologous Tissue Substitute **M** Diaphragmatic Pacemaker Lead **Y** Other Device	**Z** No Qualifier
T Diaphragm	**X** External	**0** Drainage Device **2** Monitoring Device **M** Diaphragmatic Pacemaker Lead	**Z** No Qualifier

LC Limited Coverage   **NC** Noncovered   **HAC** HAC-associated Procedure   **CC** Combination Cluster - See Appendix G for code lists
DRG Non-OR-Affecting MS-DRG Assignment   New/Revised Text in **Orange**   ♂ Male   ♀ Female

318

2021 ICD-10-PCS

0 **Medical and Surgical**
B **Respiratory System**
Q **Repair:** Restoring, to the extent possible, a body part to its normal anatomic structure and function

Body Part	Approach	Device	Qualifier
Character 4	Character 5	Character 6	Character 7
1 Trachea 2 Carina 3 Main Bronchus, Right 4 Upper Lobe Bronchus, Right 5 Middle Lobe Bronchus, Right 6 Lower Lobe Bronchus, Right 7 Main Bronchus, Left 8 Upper Lobe Bronchus, Left 9 Lingula Bronchus B Lower Lobe Bronchus, Left C Upper Lung Lobe, Right D Middle Lung Lobe, Right F Lower Lung Lobe, Right G Upper Lung Lobe, Left H Lung Lingula J Lower Lung Lobe, Left K Lung, Right L Lung, Left M Lungs, Bilateral	0 Open 3 Percutaneous 4 Percutaneous Endoscopic 7 Via Natural or Artificial Opening 8 Via Natural or Artificial Opening Endoscopic	Z No Device	Z No Qualifier
N Pleura, Right P Pleura, Left T Diaphragm	0 Open 3 Percutaneous 4 Percutaneous Endoscopic	Z No Device	Z No Qualifier

0 **Medical and Surgical**
B **Respiratory System**
R **Replacement:** Putting in or on biological or synthetic material that physically takes the place and/or function of all or a portion of a body part

Body Part	Approach	Device	Qualifier
Character 4	Character 5	Character 6	Character 7
1 Trachea 2 Carina 3 Main Bronchus, Right 4 Upper Lobe Bronchus, Right 5 Middle Lobe Bronchus, Right 6 Lower Lobe Bronchus, Right 7 Main Bronchus, Left 8 Upper Lobe Bronchus, Left 9 Lingula Bronchus B Lower Lobe Bronchus, Left T Diaphragm	0 Open 4 Percutaneous Endoscopic	7 Autologous Tissue Substitute J Synthetic Substitute K Nonautologous Tissue Substitute	Z No Qualifier

LC Limited Coverage　NC Noncovered　HAC HAC-associated Procedure　CC Combination Cluster - See Appendix G for code lists
DRG Non-OR-Affecting MS-DRG Assignment　New/Revised Text in Orange　♂ Male　♀ Female

2021 ICD-10-PCS

319

0 **Medical and Surgical**
B **Respiratory System**
S **Reposition:** Moving to its normal location, or other suitable location, all or a portion of a body part

Body Part	Approach	Device	Qualifier
Character 4	Character 5	Character 6	Character 7
1 Trachea **2** Carina **3** Main Bronchus, Right **4** Upper Lobe Bronchus, Right **5** Middle Lobe Bronchus, Right **6** Lower Lobe Bronchus, Right **7** Main Bronchus, Left **8** Upper Lobe Bronchus, Left **9** Lingula Bronchus **B** Lower Lobe Bronchus, Left **C** Upper Lung Lobe, Right **D** Middle Lung Lobe, Right **F** Lower Lung Lobe, Right **G** Upper Lung Lobe, Left **H** Lung Lingula **J** Lower Lung Lobe, Left **K** Lung, Right **L** Lung, Left **T** Diaphragm	**0** Open	**Z** No Device	**Z** No Qualifier

0 **Medical and Surgical**
B **Respiratory System**
T **Resection:** Cutting out or off, without replacement, all of a body part

Body Part	Approach	Device	Qualifier
Character 4	Character 5	Character 6	Character 7
1 Trachea **2** Carina **3** Main Bronchus, Right **4** Upper Lobe Bronchus, Right **5** Middle Lobe Bronchus, Right **6** Lower Lobe Bronchus, Right **7** Main Bronchus, Left **8** Upper Lobe Bronchus, Left **9** Lingula Bronchus **B** Lower Lobe Bronchus, Left **C** Upper Lung Lobe, Right **D** Middle Lung Lobe, Right **F** Lower Lung Lobe, Right **G** Upper Lung Lobe, Left **H** Lung Lingula **J** Lower Lung Lobe, Left **K** Lung, Right **L** Lung, Left **M** Lungs, Bilateral **T** Diaphragm	**0** Open **4** Percutaneous Endoscopic	**Z** No Device	**Z** No Qualifier

0 Medical and Surgical
B Respiratory System
U Supplement: Putting in or on biological or synthetic material that physically reinforces and/or augments the function of a portion of a body part

Body Part	Approach	Device	Qualifier
Character 4	**Character 5**	**Character 6**	**Character 7**
1 Trachea 2 Carina 3 Main Bronchus, Right 4 Upper Lobe Bronchus, Right 5 Middle Lobe Bronchus, Right 6 Lower Lobe Bronchus, Right 7 Main Bronchus, Left 8 Upper Lobe Bronchus, Left 9 Lingula Bronchus B Lower Lobe Bronchus, Left	0 Open 4 Percutaneous Endoscopic 8 Via Natural or Artificial Opening Endoscopic	7 Autologous Tissue Substitute J Synthetic Substitute K Nonautologous Tissue Substitute	Z No Qualifier
T Diaphragm	0 Open 4 Percutaneous Endoscopic	7 Autologous Tissue Substitute J Synthetic Substitute K Nonautologous Tissue Substitute	Z No Qualifier

0 Medical and Surgical
B Respiratory System
V Restriction: Partially closing an orifice or the lumen of a tubular body part

Body Part	Approach	Device	Qualifier
Character 4	**Character 5**	**Character 6**	**Character 7**
1 Trachea 2 Carina 3 Main Bronchus, Right 4 Upper Lobe Bronchus, Right 5 Middle Lobe Bronchus, Right 6 Lower Lobe Bronchus, Right 7 Main Bronchus, Left 8 Upper Lobe Bronchus, Left 9 Lingula Bronchus B Lower Lobe Bronchus, Left	0 Open 3 Percutaneous 4 Percutaneous Endoscopic	C Extraluminal Device D Intraluminal Device Z No Device	Z No Qualifier
1 Trachea 2 Carina 3 Main Bronchus, Right 4 Upper Lobe Bronchus, Right 5 Middle Lobe Bronchus, Right 6 Lower Lobe Bronchus, Right 7 Main Bronchus, Left 8 Upper Lobe Bronchus, Left 9 Lingula Bronchus B Lower Lobe Bronchus, Left	7 Via Natural or Artificial Opening 8 Via Natural or Artificial Opening Endoscopic	D Intraluminal Device Z No Device	Z No Qualifier

LC Limited Coverage   NC Noncovered   HAC HAC-associated Procedure   CC Combination Cluster - See Appendix G for code lists
Non-OR-Affecting MS-DRG Assignment   New/Revised Text in **Orange**   ♂ Male   ♀ Female

2021 ICD-10-PCS 321

0 **Medical and Surgical**
B **Respiratory System**
W **Revision:** Correcting, to the extent possible, a portion of a malfunctioning device or the position of a displaced device

Body Part	Approach	Device	Qualifier
Character 4	Character 5	Character 6	Character 7
0 Tracheobronchial Tree	**0** Open **3** Percutaneous **4** Percutaneous Endoscopic **7** Via Natural or Artificial Opening **8** Via Natural or Artificial Opening Endoscopic	**0** Drainage Device **2** Monitoring Device **3** Infusion Device **7** Autologous Tissue Substitute **C** Extraluminal Device **D** Intraluminal Device **J** Synthetic Substitute **K** Nonautologous Tissue Substitute **Y** Other Device	**Z** No Qualifier
0 Tracheobronchial Tree	**X** External	**0** Drainage Device **2** Monitoring Device **3** Infusion Device **7** Autologous Tissue Substitute **C** Extraluminal Device **D** Intraluminal Device **J** Synthetic Substitute **K** Nonautologous Tissue Substitute	**Z** No Qualifier
1 Trachea	**0** Open **3** Percutaneous **4** Percutaneous Endoscopic **7** Via Natural or Artificial Opening **8** Via Natural or Artificial Opening Endoscopic **X** External	**0** Drainage Device **2** Monitoring Device **7** Autologous Tissue Substitute **C** Extraluminal Device **D** Intraluminal Device **F** Tracheostomy Device **J** Synthetic Substitute **K** Nonautologous Tissue Substitute	**Z** No Qualifier
K Lung, Right **L** Lung, Left	**0** Open **3** Percutaneous **4** Percutaneous Endoscopic **7** Via Natural or Artificial Opening **8** Via Natural or Artificial Opening Endoscopic	**0** Drainage Device **2** Monitoring Device **3** Infusion Device **Y** Other Device	**Z** No Qualifier
K Lung, Right **L** Lung, Left	**X** External	**0** Drainage Device **2** Monitoring Device **3** Infusion Device	**Z** No Qualifier
Q Pleura	**0** Open **3** Percutaneous **4** Percutaneous Endoscopic **7** Via Natural or Artificial Opening **8** Via Natural or Artificial Opening Endoscopic	**0** Drainage Device **2** Monitoring Device **Y** Other Device	**Z** No Qualifier
Q Pleura	**X** External	**0** Drainage Device **2** Monitoring Device	**Z** No Qualifier
T Diaphragm	**0** Open **3** Percutaneous **4** Percutaneous Endoscopic **7** Via Natural or Artificial Opening **8** Via Natural or Artificial Opening Endoscopic	**0** Drainage Device **2** Monitoring Device **7** Autologous Tissue Substitute **J** Synthetic Substitute **K** Nonautologous Tissue Substitute **M** Diaphragmatic Pacemaker Lead **Y** Other Device	**Z** No Qualifier
T Diaphragm	**X** External	**0** Drainage Device **2** Monitoring Device **7** Autologous Tissue Substitute **J** Synthetic Substitute **K** Nonautologous Tissue Substitute **M** Diaphragmatic Pacemaker Lead	**Z** No Qualifier

LC Limited Coverage   **NC** Noncovered   **HAC** HAC-associated Procedure   **CC** Combination Cluster - See Appendix G for code lists
DW Non-OR-Affecting MS-DRG Assignment   New/Revised Text in **Orange**   ♂ Male   ♀ Female

322

2021 ICD-10-PCS

0 **Medical and Surgical**
B **Respiratory System**
Y **Transplantation:** Putting in or on all or a portion of a living body part taken from another individual or animal to physically take the place and/or function of all or a portion of a similar body part

Body Part	Approach	Device	Qualifier
Character 4	Character 5	Character 6	Character 7
C Upper Lung Lobe, Right 🅛🅒	**0** Open	**Z** No Device	**0** Allogeneic
D Middle Lung Lobe, Right 🅛🅒			**1** Syngeneic
F Lower Lung Lobe, Right 🅛🅒			**2** Zooplastic
G Upper Lung Lobe, Left 🅛🅒			
H Lung Lingula 🅛🅒			
J Lower Lung Lobe, Left 🅛🅒			
K Lung, Right 🅛🅒			
L Lung, Left 🅛🅒			
M Lungs, Bilateral 🅛🅒			

🅛🅒   0BYC0Z0   0BYC0Z1   0BYC0Z2   0BYD0Z0   0BYD0Z1   0BYD0Z2   0BYF0Z0   0BYF0Z1   0BYF0Z2   0BYG0Z0   0BYG0Z1   0BYG0Z2   0BYH0Z0
    0BYH0Z1   0BYH0Z2   0BYJ0Z0   0BYJ0Z1   0BYJ0Z2   0BYK0Z0   0BYK0Z1   0BYK0Z2   0BYL0Z0   0BYL0Z1   0BYL0Z2   0BYM0Z0   0BYM0Z1
    0BYM0Z2

🅛🅒 Limited Coverage   🅝🅒 Noncovered   🅗🅐🅒 HAC-associated Procedure   🅒🅒 Combination Cluster - See Appendix G for code lists
🅳🅡🅖 Non-OR-Affecting MS-DRG Assignment   New/Revised Text in **Orange**   ♂ Male   ♀ Female

2021 ICD-10-PCS

323

RESPIRATORY SYSTEM 0B1-0BY

NOTES

Mouth and Throat 0C0-0CX

0 Medical and Surgical
C Mouth and Throat
0 Alteration: Modifying the anatomic structure of a body part without affecting the function of the body part

Body Part	Approach	Device	Qualifier
Character 4	Character 5	Character 6	Character 7
0 Upper Lip **1** Lower Lip	**X** External	**7** Autologous Tissue Substitute **J** Synthetic Substitute **K** Nonautologous Tissue Substitute **Z** No Device	**Z** No Qualifier

0 Medical and Surgical
C Mouth and Throat
2 Change: Taking out or off a device from a body part and putting back an identical or similar device in or on the same body part without cutting or puncturing the skin or a mucous membrane

Body Part	Approach	Device	Qualifier
Character 4	Character 5	Character 6	Character 7
A Salivary Gland **S** Larynx **Y** Mouth and Throat	**X** External	**0** Drainage Device **Y** Other Device	**Z** No Qualifier

0 Medical and Surgical
C Mouth and Throat
5 Destruction: Physical eradication of all or a portion of a body part by the direct use of energy, force, or a destructive agent

Body Part	Approach	Device	Qualifier
Character 4	Character 5	Character 6	Character 7
0 Upper Lip **1** Lower Lip **2** Hard Palate **3** Soft Palate **4** Buccal Mucosa **5** Upper Gingiva **6** Lower Gingiva **7** Tongue **N** Uvula **P** Tonsils **Q** Adenoids	**0** Open **3** Percutaneous **X** External	**Z** No Device	**Z** No Qualifier
8 Parotid Gland, Right **9** Parotid Gland, Left **B** Parotid Duct, Right **C** Parotid Duct, Left **D** Sublingual Gland, Right **F** Sublingual Gland, Left **G** Submaxillary Gland, Right **H** Submaxillary Gland, Left **J** Minor Salivary Gland	**0** Open **3** Percutaneous	**Z** No Device	**Z** No Qualifier
M Pharynx **R** Epiglottis **S** Larynx **T** Vocal Cord, Right **V** Vocal Cord, Left	**0** Open **3** Percutaneous **4** Percutaneous Endoscopic **7** Via Natural or Artificial Opening **8** Via Natural or Artificial Opening Endoscopic	**Z** No Device	**Z** No Qualifier
W Upper Tooth **X** Lower Tooth	**0** Open **X** External	**Z** No Device	**0** Single **1** Multiple **2** All

0C7-0C9

0 Medical and Surgical
C Mouth and Throat
7 Dilation: Expanding an orifice or the lumen of a tubular body part

Body Part	Approach	Device	Qualifier
Character 4	Character 5	Character 6	Character 7
B Parotid Duct, Right C Parotid Duct, Left	0 Open 3 Percutaneous 7 Via Natural or Artificial Opening	D Intraluminal Device Z No Device	Z No Qualifier
M Pharynx	7 Via Natural or Artificial Opening 8 Via Natural or Artificial Opening Endoscopic	D Intraluminal Device Z No Device	Z No Qualifier
S Larynx	0 Open 3 Percutaneous 4 Percutaneous Endoscopic 7 Via Natural or Artificial Opening 8 Via Natural or Artificial Opening Endoscopic	D Intraluminal Device Z No Device	Z No Qualifier

0 Medical and Surgical
C Mouth and Throat
9 Drainage: Taking or letting out fluids and/or gases from a body part

Body Part	Approach	Device	Qualifier
Character 4	Character 5	Character 6	Character 7
0 Upper Lip 1 Lower Lip 2 Hard Palate 3 Soft Palate 4 Buccal Mucosa 5 Upper Gingiva 6 Lower Gingiva 7 Tongue N Uvula P Tonsils Q Adenoids	0 Open 3 Percutaneous X External	0 Drainage Device	Z No Qualifier
0 Upper Lip 1 Lower Lip 2 Hard Palate 3 Soft Palate 4 Buccal Mucosa 5 Upper Gingiva 6 Lower Gingiva 7 Tongue N Uvula P Tonsils Q Adenoids	0 Open 3 Percutaneous X External	Z No Device	X Diagnostic Z No Qualifier
8 Parotid Gland, Right 9 Parotid Gland, Left B Parotid Duct, Right C Parotid Duct, Left D Sublingual Gland, Right F Sublingual Gland, Left G Submaxillary Gland, Right H Submaxillary Gland, Left J Minor Salivary Gland	0 Open 3 Percutaneous	0 Drainage Device	Z No Qualifier

0C9 continued on next page

MOUTH AND THROAT 0C0-0CX

0 Medical and Surgical
C Mouth and Throat
9 **Drainage:** Taking or letting out fluids and/or gases from a body part

0C9 continued from previous page

Body Part	Approach	Device	Qualifier
Character 4	**Character 5**	**Character 6**	**Character 7**
8 Parotid Gland, Right **9** Parotid Gland, Left **B** Parotid Duct, Right **C** Parotid Duct, Left **D** Sublingual Gland, Right **F** Sublingual Gland, Left **G** Submaxillary Gland, Right **H** Submaxillary Gland, Left **J** Minor Salivary Gland	**0** Open **3** Percutaneous	**Z** No Device	**X** Diagnostic **Z** No Qualifier
M Pharynx **R** Epiglottis **S** Larynx **T** Vocal Cord, Right **V** Vocal Cord, Left	**0** Open **3** Percutaneous **4** Percutaneous Endoscopic **7** Via Natural or Artificial Opening **8** Via Natural or Artificial Opening Endoscopic	**0** Drainage Device	**Z** No Qualifier
M Pharynx **R** Epiglottis **S** Larynx **T** Vocal Cord, Right **V** Vocal Cord, Left	**0** Open **3** Percutaneous **4** Percutaneous Endoscopic **7** Via Natural or Artificial Opening **8** Via Natural or Artificial Opening Endoscopic	**Z** No Device	**X** Diagnostic **Z** No Qualifier
W Upper Tooth **X** Lower Tooth	**0** Open **X** External	**0** Drainage Device **Z** No Device	**0** Single **1** Multiple **2** All

0 Medical and Surgical
C Mouth and Throat
B **Excision:** Cutting out or off, without replacement, a portion of a body part

Body Part	Approach	Device	Qualifier
Character 4	**Character 5**	**Character 6**	**Character 7**
0 Upper Lip **1** Lower Lip **2** Hard Palate **3** Soft Palate **4** Buccal Mucosa **5** Upper Gingiva **6** Lower Gingiva **7** Tongue **N** Uvula **P** Tonsils **Q** Adenoids	**0** Open **3** Percutaneous **X** External	**Z** No Device	**X** Diagnostic **Z** No Qualifier
8 Parotid Gland, Right **9** Parotid Gland, Left **B** Parotid Duct, Right **C** Parotid Duct, Left **D** Sublingual Gland, Right **F** Sublingual Gland, Left **G** Submaxillary Gland, Right **H** Submaxillary Gland, Left **J** Minor Salivary Gland	**0** Open **3** Percutaneous	**Z** No Device	**X** Diagnostic **Z** No Qualifier
M Pharynx **R** Epiglottis **S** Larynx **T** Vocal Cord, Right **V** Vocal Cord, Left	**0** Open **3** Percutaneous **4** Percutaneous Endoscopic **7** Via Natural or Artificial Opening **8** Via Natural or Artificial Opening Endoscopic	**Z** No Device	**X** Diagnostic **Z** No Qualifier
W Upper Tooth **X** Lower Tooth	**0** Open **X** External	**Z** No Device	**0** Single **1** Multiple **2** All

LC Limited Coverage **NC** Noncovered **HAC** HAC-associated Procedure **CC** Combination Cluster - See Appendix G for code lists
DRG Non-OR-Affecting MS-DRG Assignment New/Revised Text in **Orange** ♂ Male ♀ Female

0 **Medical and Surgical**
C **Mouth and Throat**
C **Extirpation:** Taking or cutting out solid matter from a body part

Body Part	Approach	Device	Qualifier
Character 4	Character 5	Character 6	Character 7
0 Upper Lip 1 Lower Lip 2 Hard Palate 3 Soft Palate 4 Buccal Mucosa 5 Upper Gingiva 6 Lower Gingiva 7 Tongue N Uvula P Tonsils Q Adenoids	0 Open 3 Percutaneous X External	Z No Device	Z No Qualifier
8 Parotid Gland, Right 9 Parotid Gland, Left B Parotid Duct, Right C Parotid Duct, Left D Sublingual Gland, Right F Sublingual Gland, Left G Submaxillary Gland, Right H Submaxillary Gland, Left J Minor Salivary Gland	0 Open 3 Percutaneous	Z No Device	Z No Qualifier
M Pharynx R Epiglottis S Larynx T Vocal Cord, Right V Vocal Cord, Left	0 Open 3 Percutaneous 4 Percutaneous Endoscopic 7 Via Natural or Artificial Opening 8 Via Natural or Artificial Opening Endoscopic	Z No Device	Z No Qualifier
W Upper Tooth X Lower Tooth	0 Open X External	Z No Device	0 Single 1 Multiple 2 All

0 **Medical and Surgical**
C **Mouth and Throat**
D **Extraction:** Pulling or stripping out or off all or a portion of a body part by the use of force

Body Part	Approach	Device	Qualifier
Character 4	Character 5	Character 6	Character 7
T Vocal Cord, Right V Vocal Cord, Left	0 Open 3 Percutaneous 4 Percutaneous Endoscopic 7 Via Natural or Artificial Opening 8 Via Natural or Artificial Opening Endoscopic	Z No Device	Z No Qualifier
W Upper Tooth X Lower Tooth	X External	Z No Device	0 Single 1 Multiple 2 All

0 **Medical and Surgical**
C **Mouth and Throat**
F **Fragmentation:** Breaking solid matter in a body part into pieces

Body Part	Approach	Device	Qualifier
Character 4	Character 5	Character 6	Character 7
B Parotid Duct, Right NC C Parotid Duct, Left NC	0 Open 3 Percutaneous 7 Via Natural or Artificial Opening X External	Z No Device	Z No Qualifier

NC 0CFBXZZ   0CFCXZZ

LC Limited Coverage   NC Noncovered   HAC HAC-associated Procedure   CC Combination Cluster - See Appendix G for code lists
DRG Non-OR-Affecting MS-DRG Assignment   New/Revised Text in **Orange**   ♂ Male   ♀ Female

328

2021 ICD-10-PCS

0 **Medical and Surgical**
C **Mouth and Throat**
H **Insertion:** Putting in a nonbiological appliance that monitors, assists, performs, or prevents a physiological function but does not physically take the place of a body part

Body Part	Approach	Device	Qualifier
Character 4	Character 5	Character 6	Character 7
7 Tongue	**0** Open **3** Percutaneous **X** External	**1** Radioactive Element	**Z** No Qualifier
A Salivary Gland **S** Larynx	**0** Open **3** Percutaneous **7** Via Natural or Artificial Opening **8** Via Natural or Artificial Opening Endoscopic	**1** Radioactive Element **Y** Other Device	**Z** No Qualifier
Y Mouth and Throat	**0** Open **3** Percutaneous	**1** Radioactive Element **Y** Other Device	**Z** No Qualifier
Y Mouth and Throat	**7** Via Natural or Artificial Opening **8** Via Natural or Artificial Opening Endoscopic	**1** Radioactive Element **B** Intraluminal Device, Airway **Y** Other Device	**Z** No Qualifier

0 **Medical and Surgical**
C **Mouth and Throat**
J **Inspection:** Visually and/or manually exploring a body part

Body Part	Approach	Device	Qualifier
Character 4	Character 5	Character 6	Character 7
A Salivary Gland	**0** Open **3** Percutaneous **X** External	**Z** No Device	**Z** No Qualifier
S Larynx **Y** Mouth and Throat	**0** Open **3** Percutaneous **4** Percutaneous Endoscopic **7** Via Natural or Artificial Opening **8** Via Natural or Artificial Opening Endoscopic **X** External	**Z** No Device	**Z** No Qualifier

0 **Medical and Surgical**
C **Mouth and Throat**
L **Occlusion:** Completely closing an orifice or the lumen of a tubular body part

Body Part	Approach	Device	Qualifier
Character 4	Character 5	Character 6	Character 7
B Parotid Duct, Right **C** Parotid Duct, Left	**0** Open **3** Percutaneous **4** Percutaneous Endoscopic	**C** Extraluminal Device **D** Intraluminal Device **Z** No Device	**Z** No Qualifier
B Parotid Duct, Right **C** Parotid Duct, Left	**7** Via Natural or Artificial Opening **8** Via Natural or Artificial Opening Endoscopic	**D** Intraluminal Device **Z** No Device	**Z** No Qualifier

0 **Medical and Surgical**
C **Mouth and Throat**
M **Reattachment:** Putting back in or on all or a portion of a separated body part to its normal location or other suitable location

Body Part	Approach	Device	Qualifier
Character 4	Character 5	Character 6	Character 7
0 Upper Lip **1** Lower Lip **3** Soft Palate **7** Tongue **N** Uvula	**0** Open	**Z** No Device	**Z** No Qualifier
W Upper Tooth **X** Lower Tooth	**0** Open **X** External	**Z** No Device	**0** Single **1** Multiple **2** All

0 **Medical and Surgical**
C **Mouth and Throat**
N **Release:** Freeing a body part from an abnormal physical constraint by cutting or by the use of force

Body Part	Approach	Device	Qualifier
Character 4	Character 5	Character 6	Character 7
0 Upper Lip **1** Lower Lip **2** Hard Palate **3** Soft Palate **4** Buccal Mucosa **5** Upper Gingiva **6** Lower Gingiva **7** Tongue **N** Uvula **P** Tonsils **Q** Adenoids	**0** Open **3** Percutaneous **X** External	**Z** No Device	**Z** No Qualifier
8 Parotid Gland, Right **9** Parotid Gland, Left **B** Parotid Duct, Right **C** Parotid Duct, Left **D** Sublingual Gland, Right **F** Sublingual Gland, Left **G** Submaxillary Gland, Right **H** Submaxillary Gland, Left **J** Minor Salivary Gland	**0** Open **3** Percutaneous	**Z** No Device	**Z** No Qualifier
M Pharynx **R** Epiglottis **S** Larynx **T** Vocal Cord, Right **V** Vocal Cord, Left	**0** Open **3** Percutaneous **4** Percutaneous Endoscopic **7** Via Natural or Artificial Opening **8** Via Natural or Artificial Opening Endoscopic	**Z** No Device	**Z** No Qualifier
W Upper Tooth **X** Lower Tooth	**0** Open **X** External	**Z** No Device	**0** Single **1** Multiple **2** All

0 **Medical and Surgical**
C **Mouth and Throat**
P **Removal:** Taking out or off a device from a body part

Body Part	Approach	Device	Qualifier
Character 4	Character 5	Character 6	Character 7
A Salivary Gland	**0** Open **3** Percutaneous	**0** Drainage Device **C** Extraluminal Device **Y** Other Device	**Z** No Qualifier
A Salivary Gland	**7** Via Natural or Artificial Opening **8** Via Natural or Artificial Opening Endoscopic	**Y** Other Device	**Z** No Qualifier
S Larynx	**0** Open **3** Percutaneous **7** Via Natural or Artificial Opening **8** Via Natural or Artificial Opening Endoscopic	**0** Drainage Device **7** Autologous Tissue Substitute **D** Intraluminal Device **J** Synthetic Substitute **K** Nonautologous Tissue Substitute **Y** Other Device	**Z** No Qualifier
S Larynx	**X** External	**0** Drainage Device **7** Autologous Tissue Substitute **D** Intraluminal Device **J** Synthetic Substitute **K** Nonautologous Tissue Substitute	**Z** No Qualifier

0CP continued on next page

LC Limited Coverage NC Noncovered HAC HAC-associated Procedure CC Combination Cluster - See Appendix G for code lists
Non-OR-Affecting MS-DRG Assignment New/Revised Text in **Orange** ♂ Male ♀ Female

0 **Medical and Surgical**
C **Mouth and Throat**
P **Removal:** Taking out or off a device from a body part

0CP continued from previous page

Body Part	Approach	Device	Qualifier
Character 4	Character 5	Character 6	Character 7
Y Mouth and Throat	0 Open 3 Percutaneous 7 Via Natural or Artificial Opening 8 Via Natural or Artificial Opening Endoscopic	0 Drainage Device 1 Radioactive Element 7 Autologous Tissue Substitute D Intraluminal Device J Synthetic Substitute K Nonautologous Tissue Substitute Y Other Device	Z No Qualifier
Y Mouth and Throat	X External	0 Drainage Device 1 Radioactive Element 7 Autologous Tissue Substitute D Intraluminal Device J Synthetic Substitute K Nonautologous Tissue Substitute	Z No Qualifier

0 **Medical and Surgical**
C **Mouth and Throat**
Q **Repair:** Restoring, to the extent possible, a body part to its normal anatomic structure and function

Body Part	Approach	Device	Qualifier
Character 4	Character 5	Character 6	Character 7
0 Upper Lip 1 Lower Lip 2 Hard Palate 3 Soft Palate 4 Buccal Mucosa 5 Upper Gingiva 6 Lower Gingiva 7 Tongue N Uvula P Tonsils Q Adenoids	0 Open 3 Percutaneous X External	Z No Device	Z No Qualifier
8 Parotid Gland, Right 9 Parotid Gland, Left B Parotid Duct, Right C Parotid Duct, Left D Sublingual Gland, Right F Sublingual Gland, Left G Submaxillary Gland, Right H Submaxillary Gland, Left J Minor Salivary Gland	0 Open 3 Percutaneous	Z No Device	Z No Qualifier
M Pharynx R Epiglottis S Larynx T Vocal Cord, Right V Vocal Cord, Left	0 Open 3 Percutaneous 4 Percutaneous Endoscopic 7 Via Natural or Artificial Opening 8 Via Natural or Artificial Opening Endoscopic	Z No Device	Z No Qualifier
W Upper Tooth X Lower Tooth	0 Open X External	Z No Device	0 Single 1 Multiple 2 All

LC Limited Coverage **NC** Noncovered **HAC** HAC-associated Procedure **CC** Combination Cluster - See Appendix G for code lists
DRG Non-OR-Affecting MS-DRG Assignment New/Revised Text in **Orange** ♂ Male ♀ Female

2021 ICD-10-PCS

331

MOUTH AND THROAT 0C0-0CX

0 Medical and Surgical
C Mouth and Throat
R Replacement: Putting in or on biological or synthetic material that physically takes the place and/or function of all or a portion of a body part

Body Part	Approach	Device	Qualifier
Character 4	Character 5	Character 6	Character 7
0 Upper Lip 1 Lower Lip 2 Hard Palate 3 Soft Palate 4 Buccal Mucosa 5 Upper Gingiva 6 Lower Gingiva 7 Tongue N Uvula	0 Open 3 Percutaneous X External	7 Autologous Tissue Substitute J Synthetic Substitute K Nonautologous Tissue Substitute	Z No Qualifier
B Parotid Duct, Right C Parotid Duct, Left	0 Open 3 Percutaneous	7 Autologous Tissue Substitute J Synthetic Substitute K Nonautologous Tissue Substitute	Z No Qualifier
M Pharynx R Epiglottis S Larynx T Vocal Cord, Right V Vocal Cord, Left	0 Open 7 Via Natural or Artificial Opening 8 Via Natural or Artificial Opening Endoscopic	7 Autologous Tissue Substitute J Synthetic Substitute K Nonautologous Tissue Substitute	Z No Qualifier
W Upper Tooth X Lower Tooth	0 Open X External	7 Autologous Tissue Substitute J Synthetic Substitute K Nonautologous Tissue Substitute	0 Single 1 Multiple 2 All

0 Medical and Surgical
C Mouth and Throat
S Reposition: Moving to its normal location, or other suitable location, all or a portion of a body part

Body Part	Approach	Device	Qualifier
Character 4	Character 5	Character 6	Character 7
0 Upper Lip 1 Lower Lip 2 Hard Palate 3 Soft Palate 7 Tongue N Uvula	0 Open X External	Z No Device	Z No Qualifier
B Parotid Duct, Right C Parotid Duct, Left	0 Open 3 Percutaneous	Z No Device	Z No Qualifier
R Epiglottis T Vocal Cord, Right V Vocal Cord, Left	0 Open 7 Via Natural or Artificial Opening 8 Via Natural or Artificial Opening Endoscopic	Z No Device	Z No Qualifier
W Upper Tooth X Lower Tooth	0 Open X External	5 External Fixation Device Z No Device	0 Single 1 Multiple 2 All

0   **Medical and Surgical**
C   **Mouth and Throat**
T   **Resection:** Cutting out or off, without replacement, all of a body part

Body Part	Approach	Device	Qualifier
Character 4	**Character 5**	**Character 6**	**Character 7**
0 Upper Lip **1** Lower Lip **2** Hard Palate **3** Soft Palate **7** Tongue **N** Uvula **P** Tonsils **Q** Adenoids	**0** Open **X** External	**Z** No Device	**Z** No Qualifier
8 Parotid Gland, Right **9** Parotid Gland, Left **B** Parotid Duct, Right **C** Parotid Duct, Left **D** Sublingual Gland, Right **F** Sublingual Gland, Left **G** Submaxillary Gland, Right **H** Submaxillary Gland, Left **J** Minor Salivary Gland	**0** Open	**Z** No Device	**Z** No Qualifier
M Pharynx **R** Epiglottis **S** Larynx **T** Vocal Cord, Right **V** Vocal Cord, Left	**0** Open **4** Percutaneous Endoscopic **7** Via Natural or Artificial Opening **8** Via Natural or Artificial Opening Endoscopic	**Z** No Device	**Z** No Qualifier
W Upper Tooth **X** Lower Tooth	**0** Open	**Z** No Device	**0** Single **1** Multiple **2** All

0   **Medical and Surgical**
C   **Mouth and Throat**
U   **Supplement:** Putting in or on biological or synthetic material that physically reinforces and/or augments the function of a portion of a body part

Body Part	Approach	Device	Qualifier
Character 4	**Character 5**	**Character 6**	**Character 7**
0 Upper Lip **1** Lower Lip **2** Hard Palate **3** Soft Palate **4** Buccal Mucosa **5** Upper Gingiva **6** Lower Gingiva **7** Tongue **N** Uvula	**0** Open **3** Percutaneous **X** External	**7** Autologous Tissue Substitute **J** Synthetic Substitute **K** Nonautologous Tissue Substitute	**Z** No Qualifier
M Pharynx **R** Epiglottis **S** Larynx **T** Vocal Cord, Right **V** Vocal Cord, Left	**0** Open **7** Via Natural or Artificial Opening **8** Via Natural or Artificial Opening Endoscopic	**7** Autologous Tissue Substitute **J** Synthetic Substitute **K** Nonautologous Tissue Substitute	**Z** No Qualifier

LC Limited Coverage   **NC** Noncovered   **HAC** HAC-associated Procedure   **CC** Combination Cluster - See Appendix G for code lists
DRG Non-OR-Affecting MS-DRG Assignment   New/Revised Text in **Orange**   ♂ Male   ♀ Female

2021 ICD-10-PCS

333

0CV-0CX

MOUTH AND THROAT 0C0-0CX

0   Medical and Surgical
C   Mouth and Throat
V   Restriction: Partially closing an orifice or the lumen of a tubular body part

Body Part	Approach	Device	Qualifier
Character 4	Character 5	Character 6	Character 7
B Parotid Duct, Right C Parotid Duct, Left	0 Open 3 Percutaneous	C Extraluminal Device D Intraluminal Device Z No Device	Z No Qualifier
B Parotid Duct, Right C Parotid Duct, Left	7 Via Natural or Artificial Opening 8 Via Natural or Artificial Opening Endoscopic	D Intraluminal Device Z No Device	Z No Qualifier

0   Medical and Surgical
C   Mouth and Throat
W   Revision: Correcting, to the extent possible, a portion of a malfunctioning device or the position of a displaced device

Body Part	Approach	Device	Qualifier
Character 4	Character 5	Character 6	Character 7
A Salivary Gland	0 Open 3 Percutaneous	0 Drainage Device C Extraluminal Device Y Other Device	Z No Qualifier
A Salivary Gland	7 Via Natural or Artificial Opening 8 Via Natural or Artificial Opening Endoscopic	Y Other Device	Z No Qualifier
A Salivary Gland	X External	0 Drainage Device C Extraluminal Device	Z No Qualifier
S Larynx	0 Open 3 Percutaneous 7 Via Natural or Artificial Opening 8 Via Natural or Artificial Opening Endoscopic	0 Drainage Device 7 Autologous Tissue Substitute D Intraluminal Device J Synthetic Substitute K Nonautologous Tissue Substitute Y Other Device	Z No Qualifier
S Larynx	X External	0 Drainage Device 7 Autologous Tissue Substitute D Intraluminal Device J Synthetic Substitute K Nonautologous Tissue Substitute	Z No Qualifier
Y Mouth and Throat	0 Open 3 Percutaneous 7 Via Natural or Artificial Opening 8 Via Natural or Artificial Opening Endoscopic	0 Drainage Device 1 Radioactive Element 7 Autologous Tissue Substitute D Intraluminal Device J Synthetic Substitute K Nonautologous Tissue Substitute Y Other Device	Z No Qualifier
Y Mouth and Throat	X External	0 Drainage Device 1 Radioactive Element 7 Autologous Tissue Substitute D Intraluminal Device J Synthetic Substitute K Nonautologous Tissue Substitute	Z No Qualifier

0   Medical and Surgical
C   Mouth and Throat
X   Transfer: Moving, without taking out, all or a portion of a body part to another location to take over the function of all or a portion of a body part

Body Part	Approach	Device	Qualifier
Character 4	Character 5	Character 6	Character 7
0 Upper Lip 1 Lower Lip 3 Soft Palate 4 Buccal Mucosa 5 Upper Gingiva 6 Lower Gingiva 7 Tongue	0 Open X External	Z No Device	Z No Qualifier

NOTES

NOTES

Gastrointestinal System 0D1-0DY

0 Medical and Surgical
D Gastrointestinal System
1 Bypass: Altering the route of passage of the contents of a tubular body part

Body Part	Approach	Device	Qualifier
Character 4	Character 5	Character 6	Character 7
1 Esophagus, Upper 2 Esophagus, Middle 3 Esophagus, Lower 5 Esophagus	0 Open 4 Percutaneous Endoscopic 8 Via Natural or Artificial Opening Endoscopic	7 Autologous Tissue Substitute J Synthetic Substitute K Nonautologous Tissue Substitute Z No Device	4 Cutaneous 6 Stomach 9 Duodenum A Jejunum B Ileum
1 Esophagus, Upper 2 Esophagus, Middle 3 Esophagus, Lower 5 Esophagus	3 Percutaneous	J Synthetic Substitute	4 Cutaneous
6 Stomach ⬛HAC 9 Duodenum	0 Open 4 Percutaneous Endoscopic 8 Via Natural or Artificial Opening Endoscopic	7 Autologous Tissue Substitute J Synthetic Substitute K Nonautologous Tissue Substitute Z No Device	4 Cutaneous 9 Duodenum A Jejunum B Ileum L Transverse Colon
6 Stomach 9 Duodenum	3 Percutaneous	J Synthetic Substitute	4 Cutaneous
8 Small Intestine	0 Open 4 Percutaneous Endoscopic 8 Via Natural or Artificial Opening Endoscopic	7 Autologous Tissue Substitute J Synthetic Substitute K Nonautologous Tissue Substitute Z No Device	4 Cutaneous 8 Small Intestine H Cecum K Ascending Colon L Transverse Colon M Descending Colon N Sigmoid Colon P Rectum Q Anus
A Jejunum	0 Open 4 Percutaneous Endoscopic 8 Via Natural or Artificial Opening Endoscopic	7 Autologous Tissue Substitute J Synthetic Substitute K Nonautologous Tissue Substitute Z No Device	4 Cutaneous A Jejunum B Ileum H Cecum K Ascending Colon L Transverse Colon M Descending Colon N Sigmoid Colon P Rectum Q Anus
A Jejunum	3 Percutaneous	J Synthetic Substitute	4 Cutaneous
B Ileum	0 Open 4 Percutaneous Endoscopic 8 Via Natural or Artificial Opening Endoscopic	7 Autologous Tissue Substitute J Synthetic Substitute K Nonautologous Tissue Substitute Z No Device	4 Cutaneous B Ileum H Cecum K Ascending Colon L Transverse Colon M Descending Colon N Sigmoid Colon P Rectum Q Anus
B Ileum	3 Percutaneous	J Synthetic Substitute	4 Cutaneous
E Large Intestine	0 Open 4 Percutaneous Endoscopic 8 Via Natural or Artificial Opening Endoscopic	7 Autologous Tissue Substitute J Synthetic Substitute K Nonautologous Tissue Substitute Z No Device	4 Cutaneous E Large Intestine P Rectum

0D1 continued on next page

⬛ Limited Coverage ⬛ Noncovered ⬛ HAC-associated Procedure ⬛ Combination Cluster - See Appendix G for code lists
⬛ Non-OR-Affecting MS-DRG Assignment   New/Revised Text in **Orange**   ♂ Male   ♀ Female

0 **Medical and Surgical**
D **Gastrointestinal System**
1 **Bypass:** Altering the route of passage of the contents of a tubular body part

0D1 continued from previous page

Body Part	Approach	Device	Qualifier
Character 4	Character 5	Character 6	Character 7
H Cecum	0 Open 4 Percutaneous Endoscopic 8 Via Natural or Artificial Opening Endoscopic	7 Autologous Tissue Substitute J Synthetic Substitute K Nonautologous Tissue Substitute Z No Device	4 Cutaneous H Cecum K Ascending Colon L Transverse Colon M Descending Colon N Sigmoid Colon P Rectum
H Cecum	3 Percutaneous	J Synthetic Substitute	4 Cutaneous
K Ascending Colon	0 Open 4 Percutaneous Endoscopic 8 Via Natural or Artificial Opening Endoscopic	7 Autologous Tissue Substitute J Synthetic Substitute K Nonautologous Tissue Substitute Z No Device	4 Cutaneous K Ascending Colon L Transverse Colon M Descending Colon N Sigmoid Colon P Rectum
K Ascending Colon	3 Percutaneous	J Synthetic Substitute	4 Cutaneous
L Transverse Colon	0 Open 4 Percutaneous Endoscopic 8 Via Natural or Artificial Opening Endoscopic	7 Autologous Tissue Substitute J Synthetic Substitute K Nonautologous Tissue Substitute Z No Device	4 Cutaneous L Transverse Colon M Descending Colon N Sigmoid Colon P Rectum
L Transverse Colon	3 Percutaneous	J Synthetic Substitute	4 Cutaneous
M Descending Colon	0 Open 4 Percutaneous Endoscopic 8 Via Natural or Artificial Opening Endoscopic	7 Autologous Tissue Substitute J Synthetic Substitute K Nonautologous Tissue Substitute Z No Device	4 Cutaneous M Descending Colon N Sigmoid Colon P Rectum
M Descending Colon	3 Percutaneous	J Synthetic Substitute	4 Cutaneous
N Sigmoid Colon	0 Open 4 Percutaneous Endoscopic 8 Via Natural or Artificial Opening Endoscopic	7 Autologous Tissue Substitute J Synthetic Substitute K Nonautologous Tissue Substitute Z No Device	4 Cutaneous N Sigmoid Colon P Rectum
N Sigmoid Colon	3 Percutaneous	J Synthetic Substitute	4 Cutaneous

HAC 0D16079   0D1607A   0D1607B   0D1607L   0D160J9   0D160JA   0D160JB   0D160JL   0D160K9   0D160KA   0D160KB   0D160KL   0D160Z9
0D160ZA   0D160ZB   0D160ZL   0D16479   0D1647A   0D1647B   0D1647L   0D164J9   0D164JA   0D164JB   0D164JL   0D164K9   0D164KA
0D164KB   0D164KL   0D164Z9   0D164ZA   0D164ZB   0D164ZL   0D16879   0D1687A   0D1687B   0D1687L   0D168J9   0D168JA   0D168JB
0D168JL   0D168K9   0D168KA   0D168KB   0D168KL   0D168Z9   0D168ZA   0D168ZB   0D168ZL

Surgical site infection following bariatric surgery procedures and principal diagnoses E66.01 and secondary diagnoses K68.11, K95.01, K95.81, T81.40XA, T81.41XA, T81.42XA,T81.43XA, T81.44XA,T81.49XA.

0 **Medical and Surgical**
D **Gastrointestinal System**
2 **Change:** Taking out or off a device from a body part and putting back an identical or similar device in or on the same body part without cutting or puncturing the skin or a mucous membrane

Body Part	Approach	Device	Qualifier
Character 4	Character 5	Character 6	Character 7
0 Upper Intestinal Tract D Lower Intestinal Tract	X External	0 Drainage Device U Feeding Device Y Other Device	Z No Qualifier
U Omentum V Mesentery W Peritoneum	X External	0 Drainage Device Y Other Device	Z No Qualifier

0 **Medical and Surgical**
D **Gastrointestinal System**
5 **Destruction:** Physical eradication of all or a portion of a body part by the direct use of energy, force, or a destructive agent

Body Part	Approach	Device	Qualifier
Character 4	Character 5	Character 6	Character 7
1 Esophagus, Upper **2** Esophagus, Middle **3** Esophagus, Lower **4** Esophagogastric Junction **5** Esophagus **6** Stomach **7** Stomach, Pylorus **8** Small Intestine **9** Duodenum **A** Jejunum **B** Ileum **C** Ileocecal Valve **E** Large Intestine **F** Large Intestine, Right **G** Large Intestine, Left **H** Cecum **J** Appendix **K** Ascending Colon **L** Transverse Colon **M** Descending Colon **N** Sigmoid Colon **P** Rectum	**0** Open **3** Percutaneous **4** Percutaneous Endoscopic **7** Via Natural or Artificial Opening **8** Via Natural or Artificial Opening Endoscopic	**Z** No Device	**Z** No Qualifier
Q Anus	**0** Open **3** Percutaneous **4** Percutaneous Endoscopic **7** Via Natural or Artificial Opening **8** Via Natural or Artificial Opening Endoscopic **X** External	**Z** No Device	**Z** No Qualifier
R Anal Sphincter **U** Omentum **V** Mesentery **W** Peritoneum	**0** Open **3** Percutaneous **4** Percutaneous Endoscopic	**Z** No Device	**Z** No Qualifier

0 Medical and Surgical
D Gastrointestinal System
7 Dilation: Expanding an orifice or the lumen of a tubular body part

Body Part	Approach	Device	Qualifier
Character 4	Character 5	Character 6	Character 7
1 Esophagus, Upper **2** Esophagus, Middle **3** Esophagus, Lower **4** Esophagogastric Junction **5** Esophagus **6** Stomach **7** Stomach, Pylorus **8** Small Intestine **9** Duodenum **A** Jejunum **B** Ileum **C** Ileocecal Valve **E** Large Intestine **F** Large Intestine, Right **G** Large Intestine, Left **H** Cecum **K** Ascending Colon **L** Transverse Colon **M** Descending Colon **N** Sigmoid Colon **P** Rectum **Q** Anus	**0** Open **3** Percutaneous **4** Percutaneous Endoscopic **7** Via Natural or Artificial Opening **8** Via Natural or Artificial Opening Endoscopic	**D** Intraluminal Device **Z** No Device	**Z** No Qualifier

0 Medical and Surgical
D Gastrointestinal System
8 Division: Cutting into a body part, without draining fluids and/or gases from the body part, in order to separate or transect a body part

Body Part	Approach	Device	Qualifier
Character 4	Character 5	Character 6	Character 7
4 Esophagogastric Junction **7** Stomach, Pylorus	**0** Open **3** Percutaneous **4** Percutaneous Endoscopic **7** Via Natural or Artificial Opening **8** Via Natural or Artificial Opening Endoscopic	**Z** No Device	**Z** No Qualifier
R Anal Sphincter	**0** Open **3** Percutaneous	**Z** No Device	**Z** No Qualifier

0 **Medical and Surgical**
D **Gastrointestinal System**
9 **Drainage:** Taking or letting out fluids and/or gases from a body part

Body Part	Approach	Device	Qualifier
Character 4	Character 5	Character 6	Character 7
1 Esophagus, Upper 2 Esophagus, Middle 3 Esophagus, Lower 4 Esophagogastric Junction 5 Esophagus 6 Stomach 7 Stomach, Pylorus 8 Small Intestine 9 Duodenum A Jejunum B Ileum C Ileocecal Valve E Large Intestine F Large Intestine, Right G Large Intestine, Left H Cecum J Appendix K Ascending Colon L Transverse Colon M Descending Colon N Sigmoid Colon P Rectum	0 Open 3 Percutaneous 4 Percutaneous Endoscopic 7 Via Natural or Artificial Opening 8 Via Natural or Artificial Opening Endoscopic	0 Drainage Device	Z No Qualifier
1 Esophagus, Upper 2 Esophagus, Middle 3 Esophagus, Lower 4 Esophagogastric Junction 5 Esophagus 6 Stomach 7 Stomach, Pylorus 8 Small Intestine 9 Duodenum A Jejunum B Ileum C Ileocecal Valve E Large Intestine F Large Intestine, Right G Large Intestine, Left H Cecum J Appendix K Ascending Colon L Transverse Colon M Descending Colon N Sigmoid Colon P Rectum	0 Open 3 Percutaneous 4 Percutaneous Endoscopic 7 Via Natural or Artificial Opening 8 Via Natural or Artificial Opening Endoscopic	Z No Device	X Diagnostic Z No Qualifier
Q Anus	0 Open 3 Percutaneous 4 Percutaneous Endoscopic 7 Via Natural or Artificial Opening 8 Via Natural or Artificial Opening Endoscopic X External	0 Drainage Device	Z No Qualifier
Q Anus	0 Open 3 Percutaneous 4 Percutaneous Endoscopic 7 Via Natural or Artificial Opening 8 Via Natural or Artificial Opening Endoscopic X External	Z No Device	X Diagnostic Z No Qualifier

0D9 continued on next page

LC Limited Coverage   NC Noncovered   HAC HAC-associated Procedure   CC Combination Cluster - See Appendix G for code lists
DRG Non-OR-Affecting MS-DRG Assignment   New/Revised Text in **Orange**   ♂ Male   ♀ Female

0 Medical and Surgical
D Gastrointestinal System
9 Drainage: Taking or letting out fluids and/or gases from a body part

0D9 continued from previous page

Body Part	Approach	Device	Qualifier
Character 4	Character 5	Character 6	Character 7
R Anal Sphincter **U** Omentum **V** Mesentery **W** Peritoneum	**0** Open **3** Percutaneous **4** Percutaneous Endoscopic	**0** Drainage Device	**Z** No Qualifier
R Anal Sphincter **U** Omentum **V** Mesentery **W** Peritoneum	**0** Open **3** Percutaneous **4** Percutaneous Endoscopic	**Z** No Device	**X** Diagnostic **Z** No Qualifier

0 Medical and Surgical
D Gastrointestinal System
B Excision: Cutting out or off, without replacement, a portion of a body part

Body Part	Approach	Device	Qualifier
Character 4	Character 5	Character 6	Character 7
1 Esophagus, Upper **2** Esophagus, Middle **3** Esophagus, Lower **4** Esophagogastric Junction **5** Esophagus **7** Stomach, Pylorus **8** Small Intestine **9** Duodenum **A** Jejunum **B** Ileum **C** Ileocecal Valve **E** Large Intestine **F** Large Intestine, Right **H** Cecum **J** Appendix **K** Ascending Colon **P** Rectum	**0** Open **3** Percutaneous **4** Percutaneous Endoscopic **7** Via Natural or Artificial Opening **8** Via Natural or Artificial Opening Endoscopic	**Z** No Device	**X** Diagnostic **Z** No Qualifier
6 Stomach	**0** Open **3** Percutaneous **4** Percutaneous Endoscopic **7** Via Natural or Artificial Opening **8** Via Natural or Artificial Opening Endoscopic	**Z** No Device	**3** Vertical **X** Diagnostic **Z** No Qualifier
G Large Intestine, Left **L** Transverse Colon **M** Descending Colon **N** Sigmoid Colon	**0** Open **3** Percutaneous **4** Percutaneous Endoscopic **7** Via Natural or Artificial Opening **8** Via Natural or Artificial Opening Endoscopic	**Z** No Device	**X** Diagnostic **Z** No Qualifier
G Large Intestine, Left **L** Transverse Colon **M** Descending Colon **N** Sigmoid Colon	**F** Via Natural or Artificial Opening With Percutaneous Endoscopic Assistance	**Z** No Device	**Z** No Qualifier
Q Anus	**0** Open **3** Percutaneous **4** Percutaneous Endoscopic **7** Via Natural or Artificial Opening **8** Via Natural or Artificial Opening Endoscopic **X** External	**Z** No Device	**X** Diagnostic **Z** No Qualifier

0DB continued on next page

0 Medical and Surgical
D Gastrointestinal System
B **Excision:** Cutting out or off, without replacement, a portion of a body part

0DB continued from previous page

Body Part	Approach	Device	Qualifier
Character 4	Character 5	Character 6	Character 7
R Anal Sphincter **U** Omentum **V** Mesentery **W** Peritoneum	**0** Open **3** Percutaneous **4** Percutaneous Endoscopic	**Z** No Device	**X** Diagnostic **Z** No Qualifier

0 Medical and Surgical
D Gastrointestinal System
C **Extirpation:** Taking or cutting out solid matter from a body part

Body Part	Approach	Device	Qualifier
Character 4	Character 5	Character 6	Character 7
1 Esophagus, Upper **2** Esophagus, Middle **3** Esophagus, Lower **4** Esophagogastric Junction **5** Esophagus **6** Stomach **7** Stomach, Pylorus **8** Small Intestine **9** Duodenum **A** Jejunum **B** Ileum **C** Ileocecal Valve **E** Large Intestine **F** Large Intestine, Right **G** Large Intestine, Left **H** Cecum **J** Appendix **K** Ascending Colon **L** Transverse Colon **M** Descending Colon **N** Sigmoid Colon **P** Rectum	**0** Open **3** Percutaneous **4** Percutaneous Endoscopic **7** Via Natural or Artificial Opening **8** Via Natural or Artificial Opening Endoscopic	**Z** No Device	**Z** No Qualifier
Q Anus	**0** Open **3** Percutaneous **4** Percutaneous Endoscopic **7** Via Natural or Artificial Opening **8** Via Natural or Artificial Opening Endoscopic **X** External	**Z** No Device	**Z** No Qualifier
R Anal Sphincter **U** Omentum **V** Mesentery **W** Peritoneum	**0** Open **3** Percutaneous **4** Percutaneous Endoscopic	**Z** No Device	**Z** No Qualifier

0 Medical and Surgical
D Gastrointestinal System
D Extraction: Pulling or stripping out or off all or a portion of a body part by the use of force

Body Part	Approach	Device	Qualifier
Character 4	Character 5	Character 6	Character 7
1 Esophagus, Upper 2 Esophagus, Middle 3 Esophagus, Lower 4 Esophagogastric Junction 5 Esophagus 6 Stomach 7 Stomach, Pylorus 8 Small Intestine 9 Duodenum A Jejunum B Ileum C Ileocecal Valve E Large Intestine F Large Intestine, Right G Large Intestine, Left H Cecum J Appendix K Ascending Colon L Transverse Colon M Descending Colon N Sigmoid Colon P Rectum	3 Percutaneous 4 Percutaneous Endoscopic 8 Via Natural or Artificial Opening Endoscopic	Z No Device	X Diagnostic
Q Anus	3 Percutaneous 4 Percutaneous Endoscopic 8 Via Natural or Artificial Opening Endoscopic X External	Z No Device	X Diagnostic

0 Medical and Surgical
D Gastrointestinal System
F Fragmentation: Breaking solid matter in a body part into pieces

Body Part	Approach	Device	Qualifier
Character 4	Character 5	Character 6	Character 7
5 Esophagus 🅝🅒 6 Stomach 🅝🅒 8 Small Intestine 🅝🅒 9 Duodenum 🅝🅒 A Jejunum 🅝🅒 B Ileum 🅝🅒 E Large Intestine 🅝🅒 F Large Intestine, Right 🅝🅒 G Large Intestine, Left 🅝🅒 H Cecum 🅝🅒 J Appendix 🅝🅒 K Ascending Colon 🅝🅒 L Transverse Colon 🅝🅒 M Descending Colon 🅝🅒 N Sigmoid Colon 🅝🅒 P Rectum 🅝🅒 Q Anus 🅝🅒	0 Open 3 Percutaneous 4 Percutaneous Endoscopic 7 Via Natural or Artificial Opening 8 Via Natural or Artificial Opening Endoscopic X External	Z No Device	Z No Qualifier

🅝🅒 0DF5XZZ　0DF6XZZ　0DF8XZZ　0DF9XZZ　0DFAXZZ　0DFBXZZ　0DFEXZZ　0DFFXZZ　0DFGXZZ　0DFHXZZ　0DFJXZZ　0DFKXZZ　0DFLXZZ
　　 0DFMXZZ　0DFNXZZ　0DFPXZZ　0DFQXZZ

0 **Medical and Surgical**
D **Gastrointestinal System**
H **Insertion:** Putting in a nonbiological appliance that monitors, assists, performs, or prevents a physiological function but does not physically take the place of a body part

Body Part	Approach	Device	Qualifier
Character 4	**Character 5**	**Character 6**	**Character 7**
0 Upper Intestinal Tract **D** Lower Intestinal Tract	**0** Open **3** Percutaneous **4** Percutaneous Endoscopic **7** Via Natural or Artificial Opening **8** Via Natural or Artificial Opening Endoscopic	**Y** Other Device	**Z** No Qualifier
5 Esophagus	**0** Open **3** Percutaneous **4** Percutaneous Endoscopic	**1** Radioactive Element **2** Monitoring Device **3** Infusion Device **D** Intraluminal Device **U** Feeding Device **Y** Other Device	**Z** No Qualifier
5 Esophagus	**7** Via Natural or Artificial Opening **8** Via Natural or Artificial Opening Endoscopic	**1** Radioactive Element **2** Monitoring Device **3** Infusion Device **B** Intraluminal Device, Airway **D** Intraluminal Device **U** Feeding Device **Y** Other Device	**Z** No Qualifier
6 Stomach ⊂⊂	**0** Open **3** Percutaneous **4** Percutaneous Endoscopic	**1** Radioactive Element **2** Monitoring Device **3** Infusion Device **D** Intraluminal Device **M** Stimulator Lead **U** Feeding Device **Y** Other Device	**Z** No Qualifier
6 Stomach	**7** Via Natural or Artificial Opening **8** Via Natural or Artificial Opening Endoscopic	**1** Radioactive Element **2** Monitoring Device **3** Infusion Device **D** Intraluminal Device **U** Feeding Device **Y** Other Device	**Z** No Qualifier
8 Small Intestine **9** Duodenum **A** Jejunum **B** Ileum	**0** Open **3** Percutaneous **4** Percutaneous Endoscopic **7** Via Natural or Artificial Opening **8** Via Natural or Artificial Opening Endoscopic	**1** Radioactive Element **2** Monitoring Device **3** Infusion Device **D** Intraluminal Device **U** Feeding Device	**Z** No Qualifier
E Large Intestine **P** Rectum	**0** Open **3** Percutaneous **4** Percutaneous Endoscopic **7** Via Natural or Artificial Opening **8** Via Natural or Artificial Opening Endoscopic	**1** Radioactive Element **D** Intraluminal Device	**Z** No Qualifier
Q Anus	**0** Open **3** Percutaneous **4** Percutaneous Endoscopic	**D** Intraluminal Device **L** Artificial Sphincter	**Z** No Qualifier
Q Anus	**7** Via Natural or Artificial Opening **8** Via Natural or Artificial Opening Endoscopic	**D** Intraluminal Device	**Z** No Qualifier
R Anal Sphincter	**0** Open **3** Percutaneous **4** Percutaneous Endoscopic	**M** Stimulator Lead	**Z** No Qualifier

⊂⊂ 0DH60MZ 0DH63MZ 0DH64MZ

0 **Medical and Surgical**
D **Gastrointestinal System**
J **Inspection:** Visually and/or manually exploring a body part

Body Part	Approach	Device	Qualifier
Character 4	Character 5	Character 6	Character 7
0 Upper Intestinal Tract 6 Stomach D Lower Intestinal Tract	0 Open 3 Percutaneous 4 Percutaneous Endoscopic 7 Via Natural or Artificial Opening 8 Via Natural or Artificial Opening Endoscopic X External	Z No Device	Z No Qualifier
U Omentum V Mesentery W Peritoneum	0 Open 3 Percutaneous 4 Percutaneous Endoscopic X External	Z No Device	Z No Qualifier

0 **Medical and Surgical**
D **Gastrointestinal System**
L **Occlusion:** Completely closing an orifice or the lumen of a tubular body part

Body Part	Approach	Device	Qualifier
Character 4	Character 5	Character 6	Character 7
1 Esophagus, Upper 2 Esophagus, Middle 3 Esophagus, Lower 4 Esophagogastric Junction 5 Esophagus 6 Stomach 7 Stomach, Pylorus 8 Small Intestine 9 Duodenum A Jejunum B Ileum C Ileocecal Valve E Large Intestine F Large Intestine, Right G Large Intestine, Left H Cecum K Ascending Colon L Transverse Colon M Descending Colon N Sigmoid Colon P Rectum	0 Open 3 Percutaneous 4 Percutaneous Endoscopic	C Extraluminal Device D Intraluminal Device Z No Device	Z No Qualifier
1 Esophagus, Upper 2 Esophagus, Middle 3 Esophagus, Lower 4 Esophagogastric Junction 5 Esophagus 6 Stomach 7 Stomach, Pylorus 8 Small Intestine 9 Duodenum A Jejunum B Ileum C Ileocecal Valve E Large Intestine F Large Intestine, Right G Large Intestine, Left H Cecum K Ascending Colon L Transverse Colon M Descending Colon N Sigmoid Colon P Rectum	7 Via Natural or Artificial Opening 8 Via Natural or Artificial Opening Endoscopic	D Intraluminal Device Z No Device	Z No Qualifier

0DL continued on next page

0 Medical and Surgical
D Gastrointestinal System
L Occlusion: Completely closing an orifice or the lumen of a tubular body part

0DL continued from previous page

Body Part	Approach	Device	Qualifier
Character 4	Character 5	Character 6	Character 7
Q Anus	**0** Open **3** Percutaneous **4** Percutaneous Endoscopic **X** External	**C** Extraluminal Device **D** Intraluminal Device **Z** No Device	**Z** No Qualifier
Q Anus	**7** Via Natural or Artificial Opening **8** Via Natural or Artificial Opening Endoscopic	**D** Intraluminal Device **Z** No Device	**Z** No Qualifier

0 Medical and Surgical
D Gastrointestinal System
M Reattachment: Putting back in or on all or a portion of a separated body part to its normal location or other suitable location

Body Part	Approach	Device	Qualifier
Character 4	Character 5	Character 6	Character 7
5 Esophagus **6** Stomach **8** Small Intestine **9** Duodenum **A** Jejunum **B** Ileum **E** Large Intestine **F** Large Intestine, Right **G** Large Intestine, Left **H** Cecum **K** Ascending Colon **L** Transverse Colon **M** Descending Colon **N** Sigmoid Colon **P** Rectum	**0** Open **4** Percutaneous Endoscopic	**Z** No Device	**Z** No Qualifier

0 Medical and Surgical
D Gastrointestinal System
N Release: Freeing a body part from an abnormal physical constraint by cutting or by the use of force

Body Part	Approach	Device	Qualifier
Character 4	Character 5	Character 6	Character 7
1 Esophagus, Upper **2** Esophagus, Middle **3** Esophagus, Lower **4** Esophagogastric Junction **5** Esophagus **6** Stomach **7** Stomach, Pylorus **8** Small Intestine **9** Duodenum **A** Jejunum **B** Ileum **C** Ileocecal Valve **E** Large Intestine **F** Large Intestine, Right **G** Large Intestine, Left **H** Cecum **J** Appendix **K** Ascending Colon **L** Transverse Colon **M** Descending Colon **N** Sigmoid Colon **P** Rectum	**0** Open **3** Percutaneous **4** Percutaneous Endoscopic **7** Via Natural or Artificial Opening **8** Via Natural or Artificial Opening Endoscopic	**Z** No Device	**Z** No Qualifier

0DN continued on next page

LC Limited Coverage   NC Noncovered   HAC HAC-associated Procedure   CC Combination Cluster - See Appendix G for code lists
Non-OR-Affecting MS-DRG Assignment   New/Revised Text in Orange   ♂ Male   ♀ Female

0 **Medical and Surgical**
D **Gastrointestinal System**
N **Release:** Freeing a body part from an abnormal physical constraint by cutting or by the use of force

0DN continued from previous page

Body Part	Approach	Device	Qualifier
Character 4	Character 5	Character 6	Character 7
Q Anus	**0** Open **3** Percutaneous **4** Percutaneous Endoscopic **7** Via Natural or Artificial Opening **8** Via Natural or Artificial Opening Endoscopic **X** External	**Z** No Device	**Z** No Qualifier
R Anal Sphincter **U** Omentum **V** Mesentery **W** Peritoneum	**0** Open **3** Percutaneous **4** Percutaneous Endoscopic	**Z** No Device	**Z** No Qualifier

0 **Medical and Surgical**
D **Gastrointestinal System**
P **Removal:** Taking out or off a device from a body part

Body Part	Approach	Device	Qualifier
Character 4	Character 5	Character 6	Character 7
0 Upper Intestinal Tract **D** Lower Intestinal Tract	**0** Open **3** Percutaneous **4** Percutaneous Endoscopic **7** Via Natural or Artificial Opening **8** Via Natural or Artificial Opening Endoscopic	**0** Drainage Device **2** Monitoring Device **3** Infusion Device **7** Autologous Tissue Substitute **C** Extraluminal Device **D** Intraluminal Device **J** Synthetic Substitute **K** Nonautologous Tissue Substitute **U** Feeding Device **Y** Other Device	**Z** No Qualifier
0 Upper Intestinal Tract **D** Lower Intestinal Tract	**X** External	**0** Drainage Device **2** Monitoring Device **3** Infusion Device **D** Intraluminal Device **U** Feeding Device	**Z** No Qualifier
5 Esophagus	**0** Open **3** Percutaneous **4** Percutaneous Endoscopic	**1** Radioactive Element **2** Monitoring Device **3** Infusion Device **U** Feeding Device **Y** Other Device	**Z** No Qualifier
5 Esophagus	**7** Via Natural or Artificial Opening **8** Via Natural or Artificial Opening Endoscopic	**1** Radioactive Element **D** Intraluminal Device **Y** Other Device	**Z** No Qualifier
5 Esophagus	**X** External	**1** Radioactive Element **2** Monitoring Device **3** Infusion Device **D** Intraluminal Device **U** Feeding Device	**Z** No Qualifier
6 Stomach	**0** Open **3** Percutaneous **4** Percutaneous Endoscopic	**0** Drainage Device **2** Monitoring Device **3** Infusion Device **7** Autologous Tissue Substitute **C** Extraluminal Device **D** Intraluminal Device **J** Synthetic Substitute **K** Nonautologous Tissue Substitute **M** Stimulator Lead **U** Feeding Device **Y** Other Device	**Z** No Qualifier

0DP continued on next page

0DP continued from previous page

0 **Medical and Surgical**
D **Gastrointestinal System**
P **Removal:** Taking out or off a device from a body part

Body Part	Approach	Device	Qualifier
Character 4	**Character 5**	**Character 6**	**Character 7**
6 Stomach	**7** Via Natural or Artificial Opening **8** Via Natural or Artificial Opening Endoscopic	**0** Drainage Device **2** Monitoring Device **3** Infusion Device **7** Autologous Tissue Substitute **C** Extraluminal Device **D** Intraluminal Device **J** Synthetic Substitute **K** Nonautologous Tissue Substitute **U** Feeding Device **Y** Other Device	**Z** No Qualifier
6 Stomach	**X** External	**0** Drainage Device **2** Monitoring Device **3** Infusion Device **D** Intraluminal Device **U** Feeding Device	**Z** No Qualifier
P Rectum	**0** Open **3** Percutaneous **4** Percutaneous Endoscopic **7** Via Natural or Artificial Opening **8** Via Natural or Artificial Opening Endoscopic **X** External	**1** Radioactive Element	**Z** No Qualifier
Q Anus	**0** Open **3** Percutaneous **4** Percutaneous Endoscopic **7** Via Natural or Artificial Opening **8** Via Natural or Artificial Opening Endoscopic	**L** Artificial Sphincter	**Z** No Qualifier
R Anal Sphincter	**0** Open **3** Percutaneous **4** Percutaneous Endoscopic	**M** Stimulator Lead	**Z** No Qualifier
U Omentum **V** Mesentery **W** Peritoneum	**0** Open **3** Percutaneous **4** Percutaneous Endoscopic	**0** Drainage Device **1** Radioactive Element **7** Autologous Tissue Substitute **J** Synthetic Substitute **K** Nonautologous Tissue Substitute	**Z** No Qualifier

LC Limited Coverage   **NC** Noncovered   **HAC** HAC-associated Procedure   **CC** Combination Cluster - See Appendix G for code lists
DRG Non-OR-Affecting MS-DRG Assignment   New/Revised Text in **Orange**   ♂ Male   ♀ Female

2021 ICD-10-PCS

349

0 Medical and Surgical

D Gastrointestinal System

Q **Repair:** Restoring, to the extent possible, a body part to its normal anatomic structure and function

Body Part	Approach	Device	Qualifier
Character 4	Character 5	Character 6	Character 7
1 Esophagus, Upper **2** Esophagus, Middle **3** Esophagus, Lower **4** Esophagogastric Junction **5** Esophagus **6** Stomach **7** Stomach, Pylorus **8** Small Intestine ㏄ **9** Duodenum ㏄ **A** Jejunum ㏄ **B** Ileum ㏄ **C** Ileocecal Valve **E** Large Intestine ㏄ **F** Large Intestine, Right ㏄ **G** Large Intestine, Left ㏄ **H** Cecum ㏄ **J** Appendix **K** Ascending Colon ㏄ **L** Transverse Colon ㏄ **M** Descending Colon ㏄ **N** Sigmoid Colon ㏄ **P** Rectum	**0** Open **3** Percutaneous **4** Percutaneous Endoscopic **7** Via Natural or Artificial Opening **8** Via Natural or Artificial Opening Endoscopic	**Z** No Device	**Z** No Qualifier
Q Anus	**0** Open **3** Percutaneous **4** Percutaneous Endoscopic **7** Via Natural or Artificial Opening **8** Via Natural or Artificial Opening Endoscopic **X** External	**Z** No Device	**Z** No Qualifier
R Anal Sphincter **U** Omentum **V** Mesentery **W** Peritoneum	**0** Open **3** Percutaneous **4** Percutaneous Endoscopic	**Z** No Device	**Z** No Qualifier

㏄ 0DQ80ZZ 0DQ90ZZ 0DQA0ZZ 0DQB0ZZ 0DQE0ZZ 0DQF0ZZ 0DQG0ZZ 0DQH0ZZ 0DQK0ZZ 0DQL0ZZ 0DQM0ZZ 0DQN0ZZ

0 Medical and Surgical

D Gastrointestinal System

R **Replacement:** Putting in or on biological or synthetic material that physically takes the place and/or function of all or a portion of a body part

Body Part	Approach	Device	Qualifier
Character 4	Character 5	Character 6	Character 7
5 Esophagus	**0** Open **4** Percutaneous Endoscopic **7** Via Natural or Artificial Opening **8** Via Natural or Artificial Opening Endoscopic	**7** Autologous Tissue Substitute **J** Synthetic Substitute **K** Nonautologous Tissue Substitute	**Z** No Qualifier
R Anal Sphincter **U** Omentum **V** Mesentery **W** Peritoneum	**0** Open **4** Percutaneous Endoscopic	**7** Autologous Tissue Substitute **J** Synthetic Substitute **K** Nonautologous Tissue Substitute	**Z** No Qualifier

0   **Medical and Surgical**
D   **Gastrointestinal System**
S   **Reposition:** Moving to its normal location, or other suitable location, all or a portion of a body part

Body Part	Approach	Device	Qualifier
Character 4	**Character 5**	**Character 6**	**Character 7**
5 Esophagus 6 Stomach 9 Duodenum A Jejunum B Ileum H Cecum K Ascending Colon L Transverse Colon M Descending Colon N Sigmoid Colon P Rectum Q Anus	0 Open 4 Percutaneous Endoscopic 7 Via Natural or Artificial Opening 8 Via Natural or Artificial Opening Endoscopic X External	Z No Device	Z No Qualifier
8 Small Intestine E Large Intestine	0 Open 4 Percutaneous Endoscopic 7 Via Natural or Artificial Opening 8 Via Natural or Artificial Opening Endoscopic	Z No Device	Z No Qualifier

0   **Medical and Surgical**
D   **Gastrointestinal System**
T   **Resection:** Cutting out or off, without replacement, all of a body part

Body Part	Approach	Device	Qualifier
Character 4	**Character 5**	**Character 6**	**Character 7**
1 Esophagus, Upper 2 Esophagus, Middle 3 Esophagus, Lower 4 Esophagogastric Junction 5 Esophagus 6 Stomach 7 Stomach, Pylorus 8 Small Intestine 9 Duodenum 🅒🅒 A Jejunum B Ileum C Ileocecal Valve E Large Intestine F Large Intestine, Right H Cecum J Appendix K Ascending Colon P Rectum Q Anus	0 Open 4 Percutaneous Endoscopic 7 Via Natural or Artificial Opening 8 Via Natural or Artificial Opening Endoscopic	Z No Device	Z No Qualifier
G Large Intestine, Left L Transverse Colon M Descending Colon N Sigmoid Colon	0 Open 4 Percutaneous Endoscopic 7 Via Natural or Artificial Opening 8 Via Natural or Artificial Opening Endoscopic F Via Natural or Artificial Opening With Percutaneous Endoscopic Assistance	Z No Device	Z No Qualifier
R Anal Sphincter U Omentum	0 Open 4 Percutaneous Endoscopic	Z No Device	Z No Qualifier

🅒🅒 0DT90ZZ

0 **Medical and Surgical**
D **Gastrointestinal System**
U **Supplement:** Putting in or on biological or synthetic material that physically reinforces and/or augments the function of a portion of a body part

Body Part	Approach	Device	Qualifier
Character 4	**Character 5**	**Character 6**	**Character 7**
1 Esophagus, Upper 2 Esophagus, Middle 3 Esophagus, Lower 4 Esophagogastric Junction 5 Esophagus 6 Stomach 7 Stomach, Pylorus 8 Small Intestine 9 Duodenum A Jejunum B Ileum C Ileocecal Valve E Large Intestine F Large Intestine, Right G Large Intestine, Left H Cecum K Ascending Colon L Transverse Colon M Descending Colon N Sigmoid Colon P Rectum	0 Open 4 Percutaneous Endoscopic 7 Via Natural or Artificial Opening 8 Via Natural or Artificial Opening Endoscopic	7 Autologous Tissue Substitute J Synthetic Substitute K Nonautologous Tissue Substitute	Z No Qualifier
Q Anus	0 Open 4 Percutaneous Endoscopic 7 Via Natural or Artificial Opening 8 Via Natural or Artificial Opening Endoscopic X External	7 Autologous Tissue Substitute J Synthetic Substitute K Nonautologous Tissue Substitute	Z No Qualifier
R Anal Sphincter U Omentum V Mesentery W Peritoneum	0 Open 4 Percutaneous Endoscopic	7 Autologous Tissue Substitute J Synthetic Substitute K Nonautologous Tissue Substitute	Z No Qualifier

0 **Medical and Surgical**
D **Gastrointestinal System**
V **Restriction:** Partially closing an orifice or the lumen of a tubular body part

Body Part	Approach	Device	Qualifier
Character 4	**Character 5**	**Character 6**	**Character 7**
1 Esophagus, Upper 2 Esophagus, Middle 3 Esophagus, Lower 4 Esophagogastric Junction 5 Esophagus 6 Stomach HAC 7 Stomach, Pylorus 8 Small Intestine 9 Duodenum A Jejunum B Ileum C Ileocecal Valve E Large Intestine F Large Intestine, Right G Large Intestine, Left H Cecum K Ascending Colon L Transverse Colon M Descending Colon N Sigmoid Colon P Rectum	0 Open 3 Percutaneous 4 Percutaneous Endoscopic	C Extraluminal Device D Intraluminal Device Z No Device	Z No Qualifier

0DV continued on next page

0 **Medical and Surgical**
D **Gastrointestinal System**
V **Restriction:** Partially closing an orifice or the lumen of a tubular body part

0DV continued from previous page

Body Part	Approach	Device	Qualifier
Character 4	**Character 5**	**Character 6**	**Character 7**
1 Esophagus, Upper 2 Esophagus, Middle 3 Esophagus, Lower 4 Esophagogastric Junction 5 Esophagus 6 Stomach 🔲 7 Stomach, Pylorus 8 Small Intestine 9 Duodenum A Jejunum B Ileum C Ileocecal Valve E Large Intestine F Large Intestine, Right G Large Intestine, Left H Cecum K Ascending Colon L Transverse Colon M Descending Colon N Sigmoid Colon P Rectum	7 Via Natural or Artificial Opening 8 Via Natural or Artificial Opening Endoscopic	D Intraluminal Device Z No Device	Z No Qualifier
Q Anus	0 Open 3 Percutaneous 4 Percutaneous Endoscopic X External	C Extraluminal Device D Intraluminal Device Z No Device	Z No Qualifier
Q Anus	7 Via Natural or Artificial Opening 8 Via Natural or Artificial Opening Endoscopic	D Intraluminal Device Z No Device	Z No Qualifier

🔲 0DV64CZ
Surgical site infection following bariatric surgery procedures and principal diagnoses E66.01 and secondary diagnoses K68.11, K95.01, K95.81, T81.40XA, T81.41XA, T81.42XA,T81.43XA, T81.44XA,T81.49XA.

🔲 0DV67DZ   0DV68DZ

0 **Medical and Surgical**
D **Gastrointestinal System**
W **Revision:** Correcting, to the extent possible, a portion of a malfunctioning device or the position of a displaced device

Body Part	Approach	Device	Qualifier
Character 4	**Character 5**	**Character 6**	**Character 7**
0 Upper Intestinal Tract D Lower Intestinal Tract	0 Open 3 Percutaneous 4 Percutaneous Endoscopic 7 Via Natural or Artificial Opening 8 Via Natural or Artificial Opening Endoscopic	0 Drainage Device 2 Monitoring Device 3 Infusion Device 7 Autologous Tissue Substitute C Extraluminal Device D Intraluminal Device J Synthetic Substitute K Nonautologous Tissue Substitute U Feeding Device Y Other Device	Z No Qualifier
0 Upper Intestinal Tract D Lower Intestinal Tract	X External	0 Drainage Device 2 Monitoring Device 3 Infusion Device 7 Autologous Tissue Substitute C Extraluminal Device D Intraluminal Device J Synthetic Substitute K Nonautologous Tissue Substitute U Feeding Device	Z No Qualifier

0DW continued on next page

🔲 Limited Coverage   🔲 Noncovered   🔲 HAC-associated Procedure   🔲 Combination Cluster - See Appendix G for code lists
🔲 Non-OR-Affecting MS-DRG Assignment   New/Revised Text in **Orange**   ♂ Male   ♀ Female

0   **Medical and Surgical**
D   **Gastrointestinal System**

0DW continued from previous page

W   **Revision:** Correcting, to the extent possible, a portion of a malfunctioning device or the position of a displaced device

Body Part	Approach	Device	Qualifier
Character 4	Character 5	Character 6	Character 7
5 Esophagus	0 Open 3 Percutaneous 4 Percutaneous Endoscopic	Y Other Device	Z No Qualifier
5 Esophagus	7 Via Natural or Artificial Opening 8 Via Natural or Artificial Opening Endoscopic	D Intraluminal Device Y Other Device	Z No Qualifier
5 Esophagus	X External	D Intraluminal Device	Z No Qualifier
6 Stomach	0 Open 3 Percutaneous 4 Percutaneous Endoscopic	0 Drainage Device 2 Monitoring Device 3 Infusion Device 7 Autologous Tissue Substitute C Extraluminal Device D Intraluminal Device J Synthetic Substitute K Nonautologous Tissue Substitute M Stimulator Lead U Feeding Device Y Other Device	Z No Qualifier
6 Stomach	7 Via Natural or Artificial Opening 8 Via Natural or Artificial Opening Endoscopic	0 Drainage Device 2 Monitoring Device 3 Infusion Device 7 Autologous Tissue Substitute C Extraluminal Device D Intraluminal Device J Synthetic Substitute K Nonautologous Tissue Substitute U Feeding Device Y Other Device	Z No Qualifier
6 Stomach	X External	0 Drainage Device 2 Monitoring Device 3 Infusion Device 7 Autologous Tissue Substitute C Extraluminal Device D Intraluminal Device J Synthetic Substitute K Nonautologous Tissue Substitute U Feeding Device	Z No Qualifier
8 Small Intestine E Large Intestine	0 Open 4 Percutaneous Endoscopic 7 Via Natural or Artificial Opening 8 Via Natural or Artificial Opening Endoscopic	7 Autologous Tissue Substitute J Synthetic Substitute K Nonautologous Tissue Substitute	Z No Qualifier
Q Anus	0 Open 3 Percutaneous 4 Percutaneous Endoscopic 7 Via Natural or Artificial Opening 8 Via Natural or Artificial Opening Endoscopic	L Artificial Sphincter	Z No Qualifier
R Anal Sphincter	0 Open 3 Percutaneous 4 Percutaneous Endoscopic	M Stimulator Lead	Z No Qualifier
U Omentum V Mesentery W Peritoneum	0 Open 3 Percutaneous 4 Percutaneous Endoscopic	0 Drainage Device 7 Autologous Tissue Substitute J Synthetic Substitute K Nonautologous Tissue Substitute	Z No Qualifier

LC Limited Coverage   **NC** Noncovered   **HAC** HAC-associated Procedure   **CC** Combination Cluster - See Appendix G for code lists
DRG Non-OR-Affecting MS-DRG Assignment   New/Revised Text in **Orange**   ♂ Male   ♀ Female

354

2021 ICD-10-PCS

0   **Medical and Surgical**

D   **Gastrointestinal System**

X   **Transfer:** Moving, without taking out, all or a portion of a body part to another location to take over the function of all or a portion of a body part

Body Part	Approach	Device	Qualifier
Character 4	Character 5	Character 6	Character 7
6 Stomach **8** Small Intestine	**0** Open **4** Percutaneous Endoscopic	**Z** No Device	**5** Esophagus
E Large Intestine ♀	**0** Open **4** Percutaneous Endoscopic	**Z** No Device	**5** Esophagus **7** Vagina

♀   0DXE0Z7   0DXE4Z7

0   **Medical and Surgical**

D   **Gastrointestinal System**

Y   **Transplantation:** Putting in or on all or a portion of a living body part taken from another individual or animal to physically take the place and/or function of all or a portion of a similar body part

Body Part	Approach	Device	Qualifier
Character 4	Character 5	Character 6	Character 7
5 Esophagus **6** Stomach **8** Small Intestine **LC** **E** Large Intestine **LC**	**0** Open	**Z** No Device	**0** Allogeneic **1** Syngeneic **2** Zooplastic

LC   0DY80Z0   0DY80Z1   0DY80Z2   0DYE0Z0   0DYE0Z1   0DYE0Z2

LC Limited Coverage   **NC** Noncovered   **HAC** HAC-associated Procedure   **CC** Combination Cluster - See Appendix G for code lists

DRG Non-OR-Affecting MS-DRG Assignment   New/Revised Text in **Orange**   ♂ Male   ♀ Female

2021 ICD-10-PCS

355

NOTES

Hepatobiliary System and Pancreas 0F1-0FY

0 Medical and Surgical
F Hepatobiliary System and Pancreas
1 Bypass: Altering the route of passage of the contents of a tubular body part

Body Part	Approach	Device	Qualifier
Character 4	Character 5	Character 6	Character 7
4 Gallbladder **5** Hepatic Duct, Right **6** Hepatic Duct, Left **7** Hepatic Duct, Common **8** Cystic Duct **9** Common Bile Duct	**0** Open **4** Percutaneous Endoscopic	**D** Intraluminal Device **Z** No Device	**3** Duodenum **4** Stomach **5** Hepatic Duct, Right **6** Hepatic Duct, Left **7** Hepatic Duct, Caudate **8** Cystic Duct **9** Common Bile Duct **B** Small Intestine
D Pancreatic Duct	**0** Open **4** Percutaneous Endoscopic	**D** Intraluminal Device **Z** No Device	**3** Duodenum **4** Stomach **B** Small Intestine **C** Large Intestine
F Pancreatic Duct, Accessory **G** Pancreas	**0** Open **4** Percutaneous Endoscopic	**D** Intraluminal Device **Z** No Device	**3** Duodenum **B** Small Intestine **C** Large Intestine

0 Medical and Surgical
F Hepatobiliary System and Pancreas
2 Change: Taking out or off a device from a body part and putting back an identical or similar device in or on the same body part without cutting or puncturing the skin or a mucous membrane

Body Part	Approach	Device	Qualifier
Character 4	Character 5	Character 6	Character 7
0 Liver **4** Gallbladder **B** Hepatobiliary Duct **D** Pancreatic Duct **G** Pancreas	**X** External	**0** Drainage Device **Y** Other Device	**Z** No Qualifier

0 Medical and Surgical
F Hepatobiliary System and Pancreas
5 Destruction: Physical eradication of all or a portion of a body part by the direct use of energy, force, or a destructive agent

Body Part	Approach	Device	Qualifier
Character 4	Character 5	Character 6	Character 7
0 Liver **1** Liver, Right Lobe **2** Liver, Left Lobe	**0** Open **3** Percutaneous **4** Percutaneous Endoscopic	**Z** No Device	**F** Irreversible Electroporation **Z** No Qualifier
4 Gallbladder	**0** Open **3** Percutaneous **4** Percutaneous Endoscopic **8** Via Natural or Artificial Opening Endoscopic	**Z** No Device	**Z** No Qualifier
5 Hepatic Duct, Right **6** Hepatic Duct, Left **7** Hepatic Duct, Common **8** Cystic Duct **9** Common Bile Duct **C** Ampulla of Vater **D** Pancreatic Duct **F** Pancreatic Duct, Accessory	**0** Open **3** Percutaneous **4** Percutaneous Endoscopic **7** Via Natural or Artificial Opening **8** Via Natural or Artificial Opening Endoscopic	**Z** No Device	**Z** No Qualifier
G Pancreas	**0** Open **3** Percutaneous **4** Percutaneous Endoscopic	**Z** No Device	**F** Irreversible Electroporation **Z** No Qualifier
G Pancreas	**8** Via Natural or Artificial Opening Endoscopic	**Z** No Device	**Z** No Qualifier

LC Limited Coverage   **NC** Noncovered   **HAC** HAC-associated Procedure   **CC** Combination Cluster - See Appendix G for code lists
DRG Non-OR-Affecting MS-DRG Assignment   New/Revised Text in **Orange**   ♂ Male   ♀ Female

0 Medical and Surgical
F Hepatobiliary System and Pancreas
7 **Dilation:** Expanding an orifice or the lumen of a tubular body part

Body Part	Approach	Device	Qualifier
Character 4	Character 5	Character 6	Character 7
5 Hepatic Duct, Right **6** Hepatic Duct, Left **7** Hepatic Duct, Common **8** Cystic Duct **9** Common Bile Duct **C** Ampulla of Vater **D** Pancreatic Duct **F** Pancreatic Duct, Accessory	**0** Open **3** Percutaneous **4** Percutaneous Endoscopic **7** Via Natural or Artificial Opening **8** Via Natural or Artificial Opening Endoscopic	**D** Intraluminal Device **Z** No Device	**Z** No Qualifier

0 Medical and Surgical
F Hepatobiliary System and Pancreas
8 **Division:** Cutting into a body part, without draining fluids and/or gases from the body part, in order to separate or transect a body part

Body Part	Approach	Device	Qualifier
Character 4	Character 5	Character 6	Character 7
G Pancreas	**0** Open **3** Percutaneous **4** Percutaneous Endoscopic	**Z** No Device	**Z** No Qualifier

0 Medical and Surgical
F Hepatobiliary System and Pancreas
9 **Drainage:** Taking or letting out fluids and/or gases from a body part

Body Part	Approach	Device	Qualifier
Character 4	Character 5	Character 6	Character 7
0 Liver **1** Liver, Right Lobe **2** Liver, Left Lobe	**0** Open **3** Percutaneous **4** Percutaneous Endoscopic	**0** Drainage Device	**Z** No Qualifier
0 Liver **1** Liver, Right Lobe **2** Liver, Left Lobe	**0** Open **3** Percutaneous **4** Percutaneous Endoscopic	**Z** No Device	**X** Diagnostic **Z** No Qualifier
4 Gallbladder **G** Pancreas	**0** Open **3** Percutaneous **4** Percutaneous Endoscopic **8** Via Natural or Artificial Opening Endoscopic	**0** Drainage Device	**Z** No Qualifier
4 Gallbladder **G** Pancreas	**0** Open **3** Percutaneous **4** Percutaneous Endoscopic **8** Via Natural or Artificial Opening Endoscopic	**Z** No Device	**X** Diagnostic **Z** No Qualifier
5 Hepatic Duct, Right **6** Hepatic Duct, Left **7** Hepatic Duct, Common **8** Cystic Duct **9** Common Bile Duct **C** Ampulla of Vater **D** Pancreatic Duct **F** Pancreatic Duct, Accessory	**0** Open **3** Percutaneous **4** Percutaneous Endoscopic **7** Via Natural or Artificial Opening **8** Via Natural or Artificial Opening Endoscopic	**0** Drainage Device	**Z** No Qualifier
5 Hepatic Duct, Right **6** Hepatic Duct, Left **7** Hepatic Duct, Common **8** Cystic Duct **9** Common Bile Duct **C** Ampulla of Vater **D** Pancreatic Duct **F** Pancreatic Duct, Accessory	**0** Open **3** Percutaneous **4** Percutaneous Endoscopic **7** Via Natural or Artificial Opening **8** Via Natural or Artificial Opening Endoscopic	**Z** No Device	**X** Diagnostic **Z** No Qualifier

LC Limited Coverage **NC** Noncovered **HAC** HAC-associated Procedure **CC** Combination Cluster - See Appendix G for code lists
DRG Non-OR-Affecting MS-DRG Assignment New/Revised Text in **Orange** ♂ Male ♀ Female

358

2021 ICD-10-PCS

0 Medical and Surgical
F Hepatobiliary System and Pancreas
B Excision: Cutting out or off, without replacement, a portion of a body part

Body Part	Approach	Device	Qualifier
Character 4	Character 5	Character 6	Character 7
0 Liver 1 Liver, Right Lobe 2 Liver, Left Lobe	0 Open 3 Percutaneous 4 Percutaneous Endoscopic	Z No Device	X Diagnostic Z No Qualifier
4 Gallbladder G Pancreas	0 Open 3 Percutaneous 4 Percutaneous Endoscopic 8 Via Natural or Artificial Opening Endoscopic	Z No Device	X Diagnostic Z No Qualifier
5 Hepatic Duct, Right 6 Hepatic Duct, Left 7 Hepatic Duct, Common 8 Cystic Duct 9 Common Bile Duct C Ampulla of Vater D Pancreatic Duct F Pancreatic Duct, Accessory	0 Open 3 Percutaneous 4 Percutaneous Endoscopic 7 Via Natural or Artificial Opening 8 Via Natural or Artificial Opening Endoscopic	Z No Device	X Diagnostic Z No Qualifier

0 Medical and Surgical
F Hepatobiliary System and Pancreas
C Extirpation: Taking or cutting out solid matter from a body part

Body Part	Approach	Device	Qualifier
Character 4	Character 5	Character 6	Character 7
0 Liver 1 Liver, Right Lobe 2 Liver, Left Lobe	0 Open 3 Percutaneous 4 Percutaneous Endoscopic	Z No Device	Z No Qualifier
4 Gallbladder G Pancreas	0 Open 3 Percutaneous 4 Percutaneous Endoscopic 8 Via Natural or Artificial Opening Endoscopic	Z No Device	Z No Qualifier
5 Hepatic Duct, Right 6 Hepatic Duct, Left 7 Hepatic Duct, Common 8 Cystic Duct 9 Common Bile Duct C Ampulla of Vater D Pancreatic Duct F Pancreatic Duct, Accessory	0 Open 3 Percutaneous 4 Percutaneous Endoscopic 7 Via Natural or Artificial Opening 8 Via Natural or Artificial Opening Endoscopic	Z No Device	Z No Qualifier

0 Medical and Surgical
F Hepatobiliary System and Pancreas
D Extraction: Pulling or stripping out or off all or a portion of a body part by the use of force

Body Part	Approach	Device	Qualifier
Character 4	Character 5	Character 6	Character 7
0 Liver 1 Liver, Right Lobe 2 Liver, Left Lobe	3 Percutaneous 4 Percutaneous Endoscopic	Z No Device	X Diagnostic
4 Gallbladder 5 Hepatic Duct, Right 6 Hepatic Duct, Left 7 Hepatic Duct, Common 8 Cystic Duct 9 Common Bile Duct C Ampulla of Vater D Pancreatic Duct F Pancreatic Duct, Accessory G Pancreas	3 Percutaneous 4 Percutaneous Endoscopic 8 Via Natural or Artificial Opening Endoscopic	Z No Device	X Diagnostic

LC Limited Coverage   NC Noncovered   HAC HAC-associated Procedure   CC Combination Cluster - See Appendix G for code lists
DRG Non-OR-Affecting MS-DRG Assignment   New/Revised Text in **Orange**   ♂ Male   ♀ Female

0 **Medical and Surgical**
F **Hepatobiliary System and Pancreas**
F **Fragmentation:** Breaking solid matter in a body part into pieces

Body Part	Approach	Device	Qualifier
Character 4	Character 5	Character 6	Character 7
4 Gallbladder NC **5** Hepatic Duct, Right NC **6** Hepatic Duct, Left NC **7** Hepatic Duct, Common **8** Cystic Duct NC **9** Common Bile Duct NC **C** Ampulla of Vater NC **D** Pancreatic Duct NC **F** Pancreatic Duct, Accessory NC	**0** Open **3** Percutaneous **4** Percutaneous Endoscopic **7** Via Natural or Artificial Opening **8** Via Natural or Artificial Opening Endoscopic **X** External	**Z** No Device	**Z** No Qualifier

NC 0FF4XZZ   0FF5XZZ   0FF6XZZ   0FF8XZZ   0FF9XZZ   0FFCXZZ   0FFDXZZ   0FFFXZZ

0 **Medical and Surgical**
F **Hepatobiliary System and Pancreas**
H **Insertion:** Putting in a nonbiological appliance that monitors, assists, performs, or prevents a physiological function but does not physically take the place of a body part

Body Part	Approach	Device	Qualifier
Character 4	Character 5	Character 6	Character 7
0 Liver **4** Gallbladder **G** Pancreas	**0** Open **3** Percutaneous **4** Percutaneous Endoscopic	**1** Radioactive Element **2** Monitoring Device **3** Infusion Device **Y** Other Device	**Z** No Qualifier
1 Liver, Right Lobe **2** Liver, Left Lobe	**0** Open **3** Percutaneous **4** Percutaneous Endoscopic	**2** Monitoring Device **3** Infusion Device	**Z** No Qualifier
B Hepatobiliary Duct **D** Pancreatic Duct	**0** Open **3** Percutaneous **4** Percutaneous Endoscopic **7** Via Natural or Artificial Opening **8** Via Natural or Artificial Opening Endoscopic	**1** Radioactive Element **2** Monitoring Device **3** Infusion Device **D** Intraluminal Device **Y** Other Device	**Z** No Qualifier

0 **Medical and Surgical**
F **Hepatobiliary System and Pancreas**
J **Inspection:** Visually and/or manually exploring a body part

Body Part	Approach	Device	Qualifier
Character 4	Character 5	Character 6	Character 7
0 Liver	**0** Open **3** Percutaneous **4** Percutaneous Endoscopic **X** External	**Z** No Device	**Z** No Qualifier
4 Gallbladder **G** Pancreas	**0** Open **3** Percutaneous **4** Percutaneous Endoscopic **8** Via Natural or Artificial Opening Endoscopic **X** External	**Z** No Device	**Z** No Qualifier
B Hepatobiliary Duct **D** Pancreatic Duct	**0** Open **3** Percutaneous **4** Percutaneous Endoscopic **7** Via Natural or Artificial Opening **8** Via Natural or Artificial Opening Endoscopic	**Z** No Device	**Z** No Qualifier

LC Limited Coverage   NC Noncovered   HAC HAC-associated Procedure   CC Combination Cluster - See Appendix G for code lists
DRG Non-OR-Affecting MS-DRG Assignment   New/Revised Text in **Orange**   ♂ Male   ♀ Female

360

2021 ICD-10-PCS

0 **Medical and Surgical**
F **Hepatobiliary System and Pancreas**
L **Occlusion:** Completely closing an orifice or the lumen of a tubular body part

Body Part	Approach	Device	Qualifier
Character 4	**Character 5**	**Character 6**	**Character 7**
5 Hepatic Duct, Right 6 Hepatic Duct, Left 7 Hepatic Duct, Common 8 Cystic Duct 9 Common Bile Duct C Ampulla of Vater D Pancreatic Duct F Pancreatic Duct, Accessory	0 Open 3 Percutaneous 4 Percutaneous Endoscopic	C Extraluminal Device D Intraluminal Device Z No Device	Z No Qualifier
5 Hepatic Duct, Right 6 Hepatic Duct, Left 7 Hepatic Duct, Common 8 Cystic Duct 9 Common Bile Duct C Ampulla of Vater D Pancreatic Duct F Pancreatic Duct, Accessory	7 Via Natural or Artificial Opening 8 Via Natural or Artificial Opening Endoscopic	D Intraluminal Device Z No Device	Z No Qualifier

0 **Medical and Surgical**
F **Hepatobiliary System and Pancreas**
M **Reattachment:** Putting back in or on all or a portion of a separated body part to its normal location or other suitable location

Body Part	Approach	Device	Qualifier
Character 4	**Character 5**	**Character 6**	**Character 7**
0 Liver 1 Liver, Right Lobe 2 Liver, Left Lobe 4 Gallbladder 5 Hepatic Duct, Right 6 Hepatic Duct, Left 7 Hepatic Duct, Common 8 Cystic Duct 9 Common Bile Duct C Ampulla of Vater D Pancreatic Duct F Pancreatic Duct, Accessory G Pancreas	0 Open 4 Percutaneous Endoscopic	Z No Device	Z No Qualifier

0 **Medical and Surgical**
F **Hepatobiliary System and Pancreas**
N **Release:** Freeing a body part from an abnormal physical constraint by cutting or by the use of force

Body Part	Approach	Device	Qualifier
Character 4	**Character 5**	**Character 6**	**Character 7**
0 Liver 1 Liver, Right Lobe 2 Liver, Left Lobe	0 Open 3 Percutaneous 4 Percutaneous Endoscopic	Z No Device	Z No Qualifier
4 Gallbladder G Pancreas	0 Open 3 Percutaneous 4 Percutaneous Endoscopic 8 Via Natural or Artificial Opening Endoscopic	Z No Device	Z No Qualifier
5 Hepatic Duct, Right 6 Hepatic Duct, Left 7 Hepatic Duct, Common 8 Cystic Duct 9 Common Bile Duct C Ampulla of Vater D Pancreatic Duct F Pancreatic Duct, Accessory	0 Open 3 Percutaneous 4 Percutaneous Endoscopic 7 Via Natural or Artificial Opening 8 Via Natural or Artificial Opening Endoscopic	Z No Device	Z No Qualifier

LC Limited Coverage   NC Noncovered   HAC HAC-associated Procedure   CC Combination Cluster - See Appendix G for code lists
NC Non-OR-Affecting MS-DRG Assignment   New/Revised Text in **Orange**   ♂ Male   ♀ Female

0 **Medical and Surgical**
F **Hepatobiliary System and Pancreas**
P **Removal:** Taking out or off a device from a body part

Body Part	Approach	Device	Qualifier
Character 4	Character 5	Character 6	Character 7
0 Liver	**0** Open **3** Percutaneous **4** Percutaneous Endoscopic	**0** Drainage Device **2** Monitoring Device **3** Infusion Device **Y** Other Device	**Z** No Qualifier
0 Liver	**X** External	**0** Drainage Device **2** Monitoring Device **3** Infusion Device	**Z** No Qualifier
4 Gallbladder **G** Pancreas	**0** Open **3** Percutaneous **4** Percutaneous Endoscopic	**0** Drainage Device **2** Monitoring Device **3** Infusion Device **D** Intraluminal Device **Y** Other Device	**Z** No Qualifier
4 Gallbladder **G** Pancreas	**X** External	**0** Drainage Device **2** Monitoring Device **3** Infusion Device **D** Intraluminal Device	**Z** No Qualifier
B Hepatobiliary Duct **D** Pancreatic Duct	**0** Open **3** Percutaneous **4** Percutaneous Endoscopic **7** Via Natural or Artificial Opening **8** Via Natural or Artificial Opening Endoscopic	**0** Drainage Device **1** Radioactive Element **2** Monitoring Device **3** Infusion Device **7** Autologous Tissue Substitute **C** Extraluminal Device **D** Intraluminal Device **J** Synthetic Substitute **K** Nonautologous Tissue Substitute **Y** Other Device	**Z** No Qualifier
B Hepatobiliary Duct **D** Pancreatic Duct	**X** External	**0** Drainage Device **1** Radioactive Element **2** Monitoring Device **3** Infusion Device **D** Intraluminal Device	**Z** No Qualifier

0 **Medical and Surgical**
F **Hepatobiliary System and Pancreas**
Q **Repair:** Restoring, to the extent possible, a body part to its normal anatomic structure and function

Body Part	Approach	Device	Qualifier
Character 4	Character 5	Character 6	Character 7
0 Liver **1** Liver, Right Lobe **2** Liver, Left Lobe	**0** Open **3** Percutaneous **4** Percutaneous Endoscopic	**Z** No Device	**Z** No Qualifier
4 Gallbladder **G** Pancreas	**0** Open **3** Percutaneous **4** Percutaneous Endoscopic **8** Via Natural or Artificial Opening Endoscopic	**Z** No Device	**Z** No Qualifier
5 Hepatic Duct, Right **6** Hepatic Duct, Left **7** Hepatic Duct, Common **8** Cystic Duct **9** Common Bile Duct **C** Ampulla of Vater **D** Pancreatic Duct **F** Pancreatic Duct, Accessory	**0** Open **3** Percutaneous **4** Percutaneous Endoscopic **7** Via Natural or Artificial Opening **8** Via Natural or Artificial Opening Endoscopic	**Z** No Device	**Z** No Qualifier

LC Limited Coverage   **NC** Noncovered   **HAC** HAC-associated Procedure   **CC** Combination Cluster - See Appendix G for code lists

⊕ Non-OR-Affecting MS-DRG Assignment   New/Revised Text in Orange   ♂ Male   ♀ Female

362

2021 ICD-10-PCS

0 Medical and Surgical
F Hepatobiliary System and Pancreas
R Replacement: Putting in or on biological or synthetic material that physically takes the place and/or function of all or a portion of a body part

Body Part	Approach	Device	Qualifier
Character 4	Character 5	Character 6	Character 7
5 Hepatic Duct, Right 6 Hepatic Duct, Left 7 Hepatic Duct, Common 8 Cystic Duct 9 Common Bile Duct C Ampulla of Vater D Pancreatic Duct F Pancreatic Duct, Accessory	0 Open 4 Percutaneous Endoscopic 8 Via Natural or Artificial Opening Endoscopic	7 Autologous Tissue Substitute J Synthetic Substitute K Nonautologous Tissue Substitute	Z No Qualifier

0 Medical and Surgical
F Hepatobiliary System and Pancreas
S Reposition: Moving to its normal location, or other suitable location, all or a portion of a body part

Body Part	Approach	Device	Qualifier
Character 4	Character 5	Character 6	Character 7
0 Liver 4 Gallbladder 5 Hepatic Duct, Right 6 Hepatic Duct, Left 7 Hepatic Duct, Common 8 Cystic Duct 9 Common Bile Duct C Ampulla of Vater D Pancreatic Duct F Pancreatic Duct, Accessory G Pancreas	0 Open 4 Percutaneous Endoscopic	Z No Device	Z No Qualifier

0 Medical and Surgical
F Hepatobiliary System and Pancreas
T Resection: Cutting out or off, without replacement, all of a body part

Body Part	Approach	Device	Qualifier
Character 4	Character 5	Character 6	Character 7
0 Liver 1 Liver, Right Lobe 2 Liver, Left Lobe 4 Gallbladder G Pancreas ⊠	0 Open 4 Percutaneous Endoscopic	Z No Device	Z No Qualifier
5 Hepatic Duct, Right 6 Hepatic Duct, Left 7 Hepatic Duct, Common 8 Cystic Duct 9 Common Bile Duct C Ampulla of Vater D Pancreatic Duct F Pancreatic Duct, Accessory	0 Open 4 Percutaneous Endoscopic 7 Via Natural or Artificial Opening 8 Via Natural or Artificial Opening Endoscopic	Z No Device	Z No Qualifier

⊠ 0FTG0ZZ

0 **Medical and Surgical**
F **Hepatobiliary System and Pancreas**
U **Supplement:** Putting in or on biological or synthetic material that physically reinforces and/or augments the function of a portion of a body part

Body Part	Approach	Device	Qualifier
Character 4	Character 5	Character 6	Character 7
5 Hepatic Duct, Right 6 Hepatic Duct, Left 7 Hepatic Duct, Common 8 Cystic Duct 9 Common Bile Duct C Ampulla of Vater D Pancreatic Duct F Pancreatic Duct, Accessory	0 Open 3 Percutaneous 4 Percutaneous Endoscopic 8 Via Natural or Artificial Opening Endoscopic	7 Autologous Tissue Substitute J Synthetic Substitute K Nonautologous Tissue Substitute	Z No Qualifier

0 **Medical and Surgical**
F **Hepatobiliary System and Pancreas**
V **Restriction:** Partially closing an orifice or the lumen of a tubular body part

Body Part	Approach	Device	Qualifier
Character 4	Character 5	Character 6	Character 7
5 Hepatic Duct, Right 6 Hepatic Duct, Left 7 Hepatic Duct, Common 8 Cystic Duct 9 Common Bile Duct C Ampulla of Vater D Pancreatic Duct F Pancreatic Duct, Accessory	0 Open 3 Percutaneous 4 Percutaneous Endoscopic	C Extraluminal Device D Intraluminal Device Z No Device	Z No Qualifier
5 Hepatic Duct, Right 6 Hepatic Duct, Left 7 Hepatic Duct, Common 8 Cystic Duct 9 Common Bile Duct C Ampulla of Vater D Pancreatic Duct F Pancreatic Duct, Accessory	7 Via Natural or Artificial Opening 8 Via Natural or Artificial Opening Endoscopic	D Intraluminal Device Z No Device	Z No Qualifier

0 **Medical and Surgical**
F **Hepatobiliary System and Pancreas**
W **Revision:** Correcting, to the extent possible, a portion of a malfunctioning device or the position of a displaced device

Body Part	Approach	Device	Qualifier
Character 4	Character 5	Character 6	Character 7
0 Liver	0 Open 3 Percutaneous 4 Percutaneous Endoscopic	0 Drainage Device 2 Monitoring Device 3 Infusion Device Y Other Device	Z No Qualifier
0 Liver	X External	0 Drainage Device 2 Monitoring Device 3 Infusion Device	Z No Qualifier
4 Gallbladder G Pancreas	0 Open 3 Percutaneous 4 Percutaneous Endoscopic	0 Drainage Device 2 Monitoring Device 3 Infusion Device D Intraluminal Device Y Other Device	Z No Qualifier
4 Gallbladder G Pancreas	X External	0 Drainage Device 2 Monitoring Device 3 Infusion Device D Intraluminal Device	Z No Qualifier

0FW continued on next page

0 **Medical and Surgical**
F **Hepatobiliary System and Pancreas**
W **Revision:** Correcting, to the extent possible, a portion of a malfunctioning device or the position of a displaced device

0FW continued from previous page

Body Part	Approach	Device	Qualifier
Character 4	Character 5	Character 6	Character 7
B Hepatobiliary Duct D Pancreatic Duct	0 Open 3 Percutaneous 4 Percutaneous Endoscopic 7 Via Natural or Artificial Opening 8 Via Natural or Artificial Opening Endoscopic	0 Drainage Device 2 Monitoring Device 3 Infusion Device 7 Autologous Tissue Substitute C Extraluminal Device D Intraluminal Device J Synthetic Substitute K Nonautologous Tissue Substitute Y Other Device	Z No Qualifier
B Hepatobiliary Duct D Pancreatic Duct	X External	0 Drainage Device 2 Monitoring Device 3 Infusion Device 7 Autologous Tissue Substitute C Extraluminal Device D Intraluminal Device J Synthetic Substitute K Nonautologous Tissue Substitute	Z No Qualifier

0 **Medical and Surgical**
F **Hepatobiliary System and Pancreas**
Y **Transplantation:** Putting in or on all or a portion of a living body part taken from another individual or animal to physically take the place and/or function of all or a portion of a similar body part

Body Part	Approach	Device	Qualifier
Character 4	Character 5	Character 6	Character 7
0 Liver 🄻🄲 G Pancreas 🄻🄲 🄽🄲 🄲🄲	0 Open	Z No Device	0 Allogeneic 1 Syngeneic 2 Zooplastic

🄻🄲 0FY00Z0   0FY00Z1   0FY00Z2   0FYG0Z0   0FYG0Z1

🄽🄲 0FYG0Z2

🄽🄲 0FYG0Z0   0FYG0Z1

Codes in this list are identified as noncovered procedure except when combined with procedures codes 0TY00Z0, 0TY00Z1, 0TY00Z2, 0TY10Z0, 0TY10Z1, 0TY10Z2 and with diagnosis codes: E10.10, E10.11, E10.21, E10.22, E10.29, E10.311, E10.319, E10.3211, E10.3212, E10.3213, E10.3219, E10.3291, E10.3292, E10.3293, E10.3299, E10.3311, E10.3312, E10.3313, E10.3319, E10.3391, E10.3392, E10.3393, E10.3399, E10.3411, E10.3412, E10.3413, E10.3419, E10.3491, E10.3492, E10.3493, E10.3499, E10.3511, E10.3512, E10.3513, E10.3519, E10.3521, E10.3522, E10.3523, E10.3529, E10.3531, E10.3532, E10.3533, E10.3539, E10.3541, E10.3542, E10.3543, E10.3549, E10.3551, E10.3552, E10.3553, E10.3559, E10.3591, E10.3592, E10.3593, E10.3599, E10.36, E10.37X1, E10.37X2, E10.37X3, E10.37X9, E10.39, E10.40, E10.41, E10.42, E10.43, E10.44, E10.49, E10.51, E10.52, E10.59, E10.610, E10.618, E10.620, E10.621, E10.622, E10.628, E10.630, E10.638, E10.641, E10.649, E10.65, E10.69, E10.8, E10.9, E89.1.

🄲🄲 0FYG0Z0   0FYG0Z1   0FYG0Z2

🄻🄲 Limited Coverage   🄽🄲 Noncovered   🄷🄰🄲 HAC-associated Procedure   🄲🄲 Combination Cluster - See Appendix G for code lists
🅳🆁🅶 Non-OR-Affecting MS-DRG Assignment   New/Revised Text in Orange   ♂ Male   ♀ Female

2021 ICD-10-PCS

365

NOTES

Endocrine System 0G2-0GW

0 Medical and Surgical
G Endocrine System
2 Change: Taking out or off a device from a body part and putting back an identical or similar device in or on the same body part without cutting or puncturing the skin or a mucous membrane

Body Part	Approach	Device	Qualifier
Character 4	**Character 5**	**Character 6**	**Character 7**
0 Pituitary Gland **1** Pineal Body **5** Adrenal Gland **K** Thyroid Gland **R** Parathyroid Gland **S** Endocrine Gland	**X** External	**0** Drainage Device **Y** Other Device	**Z** No Qualifier

0 Medical and Surgical
G Endocrine System
5 Destruction: Physical eradication of all or a portion of a body part by the direct use of energy, force, or a destructive agent

Body Part	Approach	Device	Qualifier
Character 4	**Character 5**	**Character 6**	**Character 7**
0 Pituitary Gland **1** Pineal Body **2** Adrenal Gland, Left **3** Adrenal Gland, Right **4** Adrenal Glands, Bilateral **6** Carotid Body, Left **7** Carotid Body, Right **8** Carotid Bodies, Bilateral **9** Para-aortic Body **B** Coccygeal Glomus **C** Glomus Jugulare **D** Aortic Body **F** Paraganglion Extremity **G** Thyroid Gland Lobe, Left **H** Thyroid Gland Lobe, Right **K** Thyroid Gland **L** Superior Parathyroid Gland, Right **M** Superior Parathyroid Gland, Left **N** Inferior Parathyroid Gland, Right **P** Inferior Parathyroid Gland, Left **Q** Parathyroid Glands, Multiple **R** Parathyroid Gland	**0** Open **3** Percutaneous **4** Percutaneous Endoscopic	**Z** No Device	**Z** No Qualifier

0 Medical and Surgical
G Endocrine System
8 Division: Cutting into a body part, without draining fluids and/or gases from the body part, in order to separate or transect a body part

Body Part	Approach	Device	Qualifier
Character 4	**Character 5**	**Character 6**	**Character 7**
0 Pituitary Gland **J** Thyroid Gland Isthmus	**0** Open **3** Percutaneous **4** Percutaneous Endoscopic	**Z** No Device	**Z** No Qualifier

LC Limited Coverage **NC** Noncovered **HAC** HAC-associated Procedure **CC** Combination Cluster - See Appendix G for code lists
DRG Non-OR-Affecting MS-DRG Assignment New/Revised Text in **Orange** ♂ Male ♀ Female

2021 ICD-10-PCS 367

0 Medical and Surgical
G Endocrine System
9 Drainage: Taking or letting out fluids and/or gases from a body part

Body Part	Approach	Device	Qualifier
Character 4	**Character 5**	**Character 6**	**Character 7**
0 Pituitary Gland **1** Pineal Body **2** Adrenal Gland, Left **3** Adrenal Gland, Right **4** Adrenal Glands, Bilateral **6** Carotid Body, Left **7** Carotid Body, Right **8** Carotid Bodies, Bilateral **9** Para-aortic Body **B** Coccygeal Glomus **C** Glomus Jugulare **D** Aortic Body **F** Paraganglion Extremity **G** Thyroid Gland Lobe, Left **H** Thyroid Gland Lobe, Right **K** Thyroid Gland **L** Superior Parathyroid Gland, Right **M** Superior Parathyroid Gland, Left **N** Inferior Parathyroid Gland, Right **P** Inferior Parathyroid Gland, Left **Q** Parathyroid Glands, Multiple **R** Parathyroid Gland	**0** Open **3** Percutaneous **4** Percutaneous Endoscopic	**0** Drainage Device	**Z** No Qualifier
0 Pituitary Gland **1** Pineal Body **2** Adrenal Gland, Left **3** Adrenal Gland, Right **4** Adrenal Glands, Bilateral **6** Carotid Body, Left **7** Carotid Body, Right **8** Carotid Bodies, Bilateral **9** Para-aortic Body **B** Coccygeal Glomus **C** Glomus Jugulare **D** Aortic Body **F** Paraganglion Extremity **G** Thyroid Gland Lobe, Left **H** Thyroid Gland Lobe, Right **K** Thyroid Gland **L** Superior Parathyroid Gland, Right **M** Superior Parathyroid Gland, Left **N** Inferior Parathyroid Gland, Right **P** Inferior Parathyroid Gland, Left **Q** Parathyroid Glands, Multiple **R** Parathyroid Gland	**0** Open **3** Percutaneous **4** Percutaneous Endoscopic	**Z** No Device	**X** Diagnostic **Z** No Qualifier

LC Limited Coverage **NC** Noncovered **HAC** HAC-associated Procedure **CC** Combination Cluster - See Appendix G for code lists
♦ Non-OR-Affecting MS-DRG Assignment New/Revised Text in **Orange** ♂ Male ♀ Female

368

2021 ICD-10-PCS

0   **Medical and Surgical**
G   **Endocrine System**
B   **Excision:** Cutting out or off, without replacement, a portion of a body part

Body Part	Approach	Device	Qualifier
Character 4	Character 5	Character 6	Character 7
0 Pituitary Gland **1** Pineal Body **2** Adrenal Gland, Left **3** Adrenal Gland, Right **4** Adrenal Glands, Bilateral **6** Carotid Body, Left **7** Carotid Body, Right **8** Carotid Bodies, Bilateral **9** Para-aortic Body **B** Coccygeal Glomus **C** Glomus Jugulare **D** Aortic Body **F** Paraganglion Extremity **G** Thyroid Gland Lobe, Left **H** Thyroid Gland Lobe, Right **J** Thyroid Gland Isthmus **L** Superior Parathyroid Gland, Right **M** Superior Parathyroid Gland, Left **N** Inferior Parathyroid Gland, Right **P** Inferior Parathyroid Gland, Left **Q** Parathyroid Glands, Multiple **R** Parathyroid Gland	**0** Open **3** Percutaneous **4** Percutaneous Endoscopic	**Z** No Device	**X** Diagnostic **Z** No Qualifier

0   **Medical and Surgical**
G   **Endocrine System**
C   **Extirpation:** Taking or cutting out solid matter from a body part

Body Part	Approach	Device	Qualifier
Character 4	Character 5	Character 6	Character 7
0 Pituitary Gland **1** Pineal Body **2** Adrenal Gland, Left **3** Adrenal Gland, Right **4** Adrenal Glands, Bilateral **6** Carotid Body, Left **7** Carotid Body, Right **8** Carotid Bodies, Bilateral **9** Para-aortic Body **B** Coccygeal Glomus **C** Glomus Jugulare **D** Aortic Body **F** Paraganglion Extremity **G** Thyroid Gland Lobe, Left **H** Thyroid Gland Lobe, Right **K** Thyroid Gland **L** Superior Parathyroid Gland, Right **M** Superior Parathyroid Gland, Left **N** Inferior Parathyroid Gland, Right **P** Inferior Parathyroid Gland, Left **Q** Parathyroid Glands, Multiple **R** Parathyroid Gland	**0** Open **3** Percutaneous **4** Percutaneous Endoscopic	**Z** No Device	**Z** No Qualifier

LC Limited Coverage   **NC** Noncovered   **HAC** HAC-associated Procedure   **CC** Combination Cluster - See Appendix G for code lists
DRG Non-OR-Affecting MS-DRG Assignment   New/Revised Text in Orange   ♂ Male   ♀ Female

2021 ICD-10-PCS   **369**

0 Medical and Surgical
G Endocrine System
H Insertion: Putting in a nonbiological appliance that monitors, assists, performs, or prevents a physiological function but does not physically take the place of a body part

Body Part	Approach	Device	Qualifier
Character 4	Character 5	Character 6	Character 7
S Endocrine Gland	0 Open 3 Percutaneous 4 Percutaneous Endoscopic	1 Radioactive Element 2 Monitoring Device 3 Infusion Device Y Other Device	Z No Qualifier

0 Medical and Surgical
G Endocrine System
J Inspection: Visually and/or manually exploring a body part

Body Part	Approach	Device	Qualifier
Character 4	Character 5	Character 6	Character 7
0 Pituitary Gland 1 Pineal Body 5 Adrenal Gland K Thyroid Gland R Parathyroid Gland S Endocrine Gland	0 Open 3 Percutaneous 4 Percutaneous Endoscopic	Z No Device	Z No Qualifier

0 Medical and Surgical
G Endocrine System
M Reattachment: Putting back in or on all or a portion of a separated body part to its normal location or other suitable location

Body Part	Approach	Device	Qualifier
Character 4	Character 5	Character 6	Character 7
2 Adrenal Gland, Left 3 Adrenal Gland, Right G Thyroid Gland Lobe, Left H Thyroid Gland Lobe, Right L Superior Parathyroid Gland, Right M Superior Parathyroid Gland, Left N Inferior Parathyroid Gland, Right P Inferior Parathyroid Gland, Left Q Parathyroid Glands, Multiple R Parathyroid Gland	0 Open 4 Percutaneous Endoscopic	Z No Device	Z No Qualifier

0 **Medical and Surgical**
G **Endocrine System**
N **Release:** Freeing a body part from an abnormal physical constraint by cutting or by the use of force

Body Part	Approach	Device	Qualifier
Character 4	Character 5	Character 6	Character 7
0 Pituitary Gland 1 Pineal Body 2 Adrenal Gland, Left 3 Adrenal Gland, Right 4 Adrenal Glands, Bilateral 6 Carotid Body, Left 7 Carotid Body, Right 8 Carotid Bodies, Bilateral 9 Para-aortic Body B Coccygeal Glomus C Glomus Jugulare D Aortic Body F Paraganglion Extremity G Thyroid Gland Lobe, Left H Thyroid Gland Lobe, Right K Thyroid Gland L Superior Parathyroid Gland, Right M Superior Parathyroid Gland, Left N Inferior Parathyroid Gland, Right P Inferior Parathyroid Gland, Left Q Parathyroid Glands, Multiple R Parathyroid Gland	0 Open 3 Percutaneous 4 Percutaneous Endoscopic	Z No Device	Z No Qualifier

0 **Medical and Surgical**
G **Endocrine System**
P **Removal:** Taking out or off a device from a body part

Body Part	Approach	Device	Qualifier
Character 4	Character 5	Character 6	Character 7
0 Pituitary Gland 1 Pineal Body 5 Adrenal Gland K Thyroid Gland R Parathyroid Gland	0 Open 3 Percutaneous 4 Percutaneous Endoscopic X External	0 Drainage Device	Z No Qualifier
S Endocrine Gland	0 Open 3 Percutaneous 4 Percutaneous Endoscopic	0 Drainage Device 2 Monitoring Device 3 Infusion Device Y Other Device	Z No Qualifier
S Endocrine Gland	X External	0 Drainage Device 2 Monitoring Device 3 Infusion Device	Z No Qualifier

IC Limited Coverage   **NC** Noncovered   **HAC** HAC-associated Procedure   **CC** Combination Cluster - See Appendix G for code lists
DRG Non-OR-Affecting MS-DRG Assignment   New/Revised Text in **Orange**   ♂ Male   ♀ Female

2021 ICD-10-PCS 371

0 Medical and Surgical
G Endocrine System
Q Repair: Restoring, to the extent possible, a body part to its normal anatomic structure and function

Body Part	Approach	Device	Qualifier
Character 4	**Character 5**	**Character 6**	**Character 7**
0 Pituitary Gland	0 Open	Z No Device	Z No Qualifier
1 Pineal Body	3 Percutaneous		
2 Adrenal Gland, Left	4 Percutaneous Endoscopic		
3 Adrenal Gland, Right			
4 Adrenal Glands, Bilateral			
6 Carotid Body, Left			
7 Carotid Body, Right			
8 Carotid Bodies, Bilateral			
9 Para-aortic Body			
B Coccygeal Glomus			
C Glomus Jugulare			
D Aortic Body			
F Paraganglion Extremity			
G Thyroid Gland Lobe, Left			
H Thyroid Gland Lobe, Right			
J Thyroid Gland Isthmus			
K Thyroid Gland			
L Superior Parathyroid Gland, Right			
M Superior Parathyroid Gland, Left			
N Inferior Parathyroid Gland, Right			
P Inferior Parathyroid Gland, Left			
Q Parathyroid Glands, Multiple			
R Parathyroid Gland			

0 Medical and Surgical
G Endocrine System
S Reposition: Moving to its normal location, or other suitable location, all or a portion of a body part

Body Part	Approach	Device	Qualifier
Character 4	**Character 5**	**Character 6**	**Character 7**
2 Adrenal Gland, Left	0 Open	Z No Device	Z No Qualifier
3 Adrenal Gland, Right	4 Percutaneous Endoscopic		
G Thyroid Gland Lobe, Left			
H Thyroid Gland Lobe, Right			
L Superior Parathyroid Gland, Right			
M Superior Parathyroid Gland, Left			
N Inferior Parathyroid Gland, Right			
P Inferior Parathyroid Gland, Left			
Q Parathyroid Glands, Multiple			
R Parathyroid Gland			

LC Limited Coverage   **NC** Noncovered   **HAC** HAC-associated Procedure   **CC** Combination Cluster - See Appendix G for code lists
DRG Non-OR-Affecting MS-DRG Assignment   New/Revised Text in **Orange**   ♂ Male   ♀ Female

372

2021 ICD-10-PCS

0 **Medical and Surgical**
G **Endocrine System**
T **Resection:** Cutting out or off, without replacement, all of a body part

Body Part	Approach	Device	Qualifier
Character 4	Character 5	Character 6	Character 7
0 Pituitary Gland **1** Pineal Body **2** Adrenal Gland, Left **3** Adrenal Gland, Right **4** Adrenal Glands, Bilateral **6** Carotid Body, Left **7** Carotid Body, Right **8** Carotid Bodies, Bilateral **9** Para-aortic Body **B** Coccygeal Glomus **C** Glomus Jugulare **D** Aortic Body **F** Paraganglion Extremity **G** Thyroid Gland Lobe, Left **H** Thyroid Gland Lobe, Right **J** Thyroid Gland Isthmus **K** Thyroid Gland **L** Superior Parathyroid Gland, Right **M** Superior Parathyroid Gland, Left **N** Inferior Parathyroid Gland, Right **P** Inferior Parathyroid Gland, Left **Q** Parathyroid Glands, Multiple **R** Parathyroid Gland	**0** Open **4** Percutaneous Endoscopic	**Z** No Device	**Z** No Qualifier

0 **Medical and Surgical**
G **Endocrine System**
W **Revision:** Correcting, to the extent possible, a portion of a malfunctioning device or the position of a displaced device

Body Part	Approach	Device	Qualifier
Character 4	Character 5	Character 6	Character 7
0 Pituitary Gland **1** Pineal Body **5** Adrenal Gland **K** Thyroid Gland **R** Parathyroid Gland	**0** Open **3** Percutaneous **4** Percutaneous Endoscopic **X** External	**0** Drainage Device	**Z** No Qualifier
S Endocrine Gland	**0** Open **3** Percutaneous **4** Percutaneous Endoscopic	**0** Drainage Device **2** Monitoring Device **3** Infusion Device **Y** Other Device	**Z** No Qualifier
S Endocrine Gland	**X** External	**0** Drainage Device **2** Monitoring Device **3** Infusion Device	**Z** No Qualifier

NOTES

0 Medical and Surgical

H Skin and Breast

0 Alteration: Modifying the anatomic structure of a body part without affecting the function of the body part

Body Part	Approach	Device	Qualifier
Character 4	Character 5	Character 6	Character 7
T Breast, Right U Breast, Left V Breast, Bilateral	0 Open 3 Percutaneous	7 Autologous Tissue Substitute J Synthetic Substitute K Nonautologous Tissue Substitute Z No Device	Z No Qualifier

0 Medical and Surgical

H Skin and Breast

2 Change: Taking out or off a device from a body part and putting back an identical or similar device in or on the same body part without cutting or puncturing the skin or a mucous membrane

Body Part	Approach	Device	Qualifier
Character 4	Character 5	Character 6	Character 7
P Skin T Breast, Right U Breast, Left	X External	0 Drainage Device Y Other Device	Z No Qualifier

0 Medical and Surgical

H Skin and Breast

5 Destruction: Physical eradication of all or a portion of a body part by the direct use of energy, force, or a destructive agent

Body Part	Approach	Device	Qualifier
Character 4	Character 5	Character 6	Character 7
0 Skin, Scalp ᴰᴿᴳ 1 Skin, Face ᴰᴿᴳ 2 Skin, Right Ear 3 Skin, Left Ear 4 Skin, Neck ᴰᴿᴳ 5 Skin, Chest ᴰᴿᴳ 6 Skin, Back ᴰᴿᴳ 7 Skin, Abdomen ᴰᴿᴳ 8 Skin, Buttock ᴰᴿᴳ 9 Skin, Perineum ᴰᴿᴳ A Skin, Inguinal ᴰᴿᴳ B Skin, Right Upper Arm ᴰᴿᴳ C Skin, Left Upper Arm ᴰᴿᴳ D Skin, Right Lower Arm ᴰᴿᴳ E Skin, Left Lower Arm ᴰᴿᴳ F Skin, Right Hand ᴰᴿᴳ G Skin, Left Hand ᴰᴿᴳ H Skin, Right Upper Leg ᴰᴿᴳ J Skin, Left Upper Leg ᴰᴿᴳ K Skin, Right Lower Leg ᴰᴿᴳ L Skin, Left Lower Leg ᴰᴿᴳ M Skin, Right Foot ᴰᴿᴳ N Skin, Left Foot ᴰᴿᴳ	X External	Z No Device	D Multiple Z No Qualifier
Q Finger Nail ᴰᴿᴳ R Toe Nail ᴰᴿᴳ	X External	Z No Device	Z No Qualifier
T Breast, Right U Breast, Left V Breast, Bilateral	0 Open 3 Percutaneous 7 Via Natural or Artificial Opening 8 Via Natural or Artificial Opening Endoscopic	Z No Device	Z No Qualifier

0H5 continued on next page

---

0 **Medical and Surgical**

H **Skin and Breast**

5 **Destruction:** Physical eradication of all or a portion of a body part by the direct use of energy, force, or a destructive agent

0H5 continued from previous page

Body Part	Approach	Device	Qualifier
Character 4	Character 5	Character 6	Character 7
W Nipple, Right **X** Nipple, Left	**0** Open **3** Percutaneous **7** Via Natural or Artificial Opening **8** Via Natural or Artificial Opening Endoscopic **X** External	**Z** No Device	**Z** No Qualifier

ᴏʀɢ 0H50XZD 0H50XZZ 0H51XZD 0H51XZZ 0H54XZD 0H54XZZ 0H55XZD 0H55XZZ 0H56XZD 0H56XZZ 0H57XZD 0H57XZZ 0H58XZD
0H58XZZ 0H59XZD 0H59XZZ 0H5AXZD 0H5AXZZ 0H5BXZD 0H5BXZZ 0H5CXZD 0H5CXZZ 0H5DXZD 0H5DXZZ 0H5EXZD 0H5EXZZ
0H5FXZD 0H5FXZZ 0H5GXZD 0H5GXZZ 0H5HXZD 0H5HXZZ 0H5JXZD 0H5JXZZ 0H5KXZD 0H5KXZZ 0H5LXZD 0H5LXZZ 0H5MXZD
0H5MXZZ 0H5NXZD 0H5NXZZ 0H5QXZZ 0H5RXZZ

0 **Medical and Surgical**

H **Skin and Breast**

8 **Division:** Cutting into a body part, without draining fluids and/or gases from the body part, in order to separate or transect a body part

Body Part	Approach	Device	Qualifier
Character 4	Character 5	Character 6	Character 7
0 Skin, Scalp **1** Skin, Face **2** Skin, Right Ear **3** Skin, Left Ear **4** Skin, Neck **5** Skin, Chest **6** Skin, Back **7** Skin, Abdomen **8** Skin, Buttock **9** Skin, Perineum **A** Skin, Inguinal **B** Skin, Right Upper Arm **C** Skin, Left Upper Arm **D** Skin, Right Lower Arm **E** Skin, Left Lower Arm **F** Skin, Right Hand **G** Skin, Left Hand **H** Skin, Right Upper Leg **J** Skin, Left Upper Leg **K** Skin, Right Lower Leg **L** Skin, Left Lower Leg **M** Skin, Right Foot **N** Skin, Left Foot	**X** External	**Z** No Device	**Z** No Qualifier

ʟᴄ Limited Coverage   ɴᴄ Noncovered   ʜᴀᴄ HAC-associated Procedure   ᴄᴄ Combination Cluster - See Appendix G for code lists
ᴏʀɢ Non-OR-Affecting MS-DRG Assignment   New/Revised Text in **Orange**   ♂ Male   ♀ Female

376

2021 ICD-10-PCS

0 **Medical and Surgical**
H **Skin and Breast**
9 **Drainage:** Taking or letting out fluids and/or gases from a body part

Body Part	Approach	Device	Qualifier
Character 4	Character 5	Character 6	Character 7
0 Skin, Scalp 1 Skin, Face 2 Skin, Right Ear 3 Skin, Left Ear 4 Skin, Neck 5 Skin, Chest 6 Skin, Back 7 Skin, Abdomen 8 Skin, Buttock 9 Skin, Perineum A Skin, Inguinal B Skin, Right Upper Arm C Skin, Left Upper Arm D Skin, Right Lower Arm E Skin, Left Lower Arm F Skin, Right Hand G Skin, Left Hand H Skin, Right Upper Leg J Skin, Left Upper Leg K Skin, Right Lower Leg L Skin, Left Lower Leg M Skin, Right Foot N Skin, Left Foot Q Finger Nail R Toe Nail	X External	0 Drainage Device	Z No Qualifier
0 Skin, Scalp 1 Skin, Face 2 Skin, Right Ear 3 Skin, Left Ear 4 Skin, Neck 5 Skin, Chest 6 Skin, Back 7 Skin, Abdomen 8 Skin, Buttock 9 Skin, Perineum A Skin, Inguinal B Skin, Right Upper Arm C Skin, Left Upper Arm D Skin, Right Lower Arm E Skin, Left Lower Arm F Skin, Right Hand G Skin, Left Hand H Skin, Right Upper Leg J Skin, Left Upper Leg K Skin, Right Lower Leg L Skin, Left Lower Leg M Skin, Right Foot N Skin, Left Foot Q Finger Nail R Toe Nail	X External	Z No Device	X Diagnostic Z No Qualifier
T Breast, Right U Breast, Left V Breast, Bilateral	0 Open 3 Percutaneous 7 Via Natural or Artificial Opening 8 Via Natural or Artificial Opening Endoscopic	0 Drainage Device	Z No Qualifier

0H9 continued on next page

LC Limited Coverage   NC Noncovered   HAC HAC-associated Procedure   CC Combination Cluster - See Appendix G for code lists
DRG Non-OR-Affecting MS-DRG Assignment   New/Revised Text in **Orange**   ♂ Male   ♀ Female

0 **Medical and Surgical**
H **Skin and Breast**
9 **Drainage:** Taking or letting out fluids and/or gases from a body part

0H9 continued from previous page

Body Part	Approach	Device	Qualifier
Character 4	Character 5	Character 6	Character 7
T Breast, Right **U** Breast, Left **V** Breast, Bilateral	**0** Open **3** Percutaneous **7** Via Natural or Artificial Opening **8** Via Natural or Artificial Opening Endoscopic	**Z** No Device	**X** Diagnostic **Z** No Qualifier
W Nipple, Right **X** Nipple, Left	**0** Open **3** Percutaneous **7** Via Natural or Artificial Opening **8** Via Natural or Artificial Opening Endoscopic **X** External	**0** Drainage Device	**Z** No Qualifier
W Nipple, Right **X** Nipple, Left	**0** Open **3** Percutaneous **7** Via Natural or Artificial Opening **8** Via Natural or Artificial Opening Endoscopic **X** External	**Z** No Device	**X** Diagnostic **Z** No Qualifier

0 **Medical and Surgical**
H **Skin and Breast**
B **Excision:** Cutting out or off, without replacement, a portion of a body part

Body Part	Approach	Device	Qualifier
Character 4	Character 5	Character 6	Character 7
0 Skin, Scalp **1** Skin, Face **2** Skin, Right Ear **3** Skin, Left Ear **4** Skin, Neck **5** Skin, Chest **6** Skin, Back **7** Skin, Abdomen **8** Skin, Buttock **9** Skin, Perineum 🆖 **A** Skin, Inguinal **B** Skin, Right Upper Arm **C** Skin, Left Upper Arm **D** Skin, Right Lower Arm **E** Skin, Left Lower Arm **F** Skin, Right Hand **G** Skin, Left Hand **H** Skin, Right Upper Leg **J** Skin, Left Upper Leg **K** Skin, Right Lower Leg **L** Skin, Left Lower Leg **M** Skin, Right Foot **N** Skin, Left Foot **Q** Finger Nail **R** Toe Nail	**X** External	**Z** No Device	**X** Diagnostic **Z** No Qualifier
T Breast, Right **U** Breast, Left **V** Breast, Bilateral **Y** Supernumerary Breast	**0** Open **3** Percutaneous **7** Via Natural or Artificial Opening **8** Via Natural or Artificial Opening Endoscopic	**Z** No Device	**X** Diagnostic **Z** No Qualifier
W Nipple, Right **X** Nipple, Left	**0** Open **3** Percutaneous **7** Via Natural or Artificial Opening **8** Via Natural or Artificial Opening Endoscopic **X** External	**Z** No Device	**X** Diagnostic **Z** No Qualifier

🆖 0HB9XZZ

🆖 Limited Coverage   🆖 Noncovered   🆖 HAC-associated Procedure   🆖 Combination Cluster - See Appendix G for code lists
🆖 Non-OR-Affecting MS-DRG Assignment   New/Revised Text in **Orange**   ♂ Male   ♀ Female

378

2021 ICD-10-PCS

0 **Medical and Surgical**
H **Skin and Breast**
C **Extirpation:** Taking or cutting out solid matter from a body part

Body Part	Approach	Device	Qualifier
Character 4	**Character 5**	**Character 6**	**Character 7**
0 Skin, Scalp **1** Skin, Face **2** Skin, Right Ear **3** Skin, Left Ear **4** Skin, Neck **5** Skin, Chest **6** Skin, Back **7** Skin, Abdomen **8** Skin, Buttock **9** Skin, Perineum **A** Skin, Inguinal **B** Skin, Right Upper Arm **C** Skin, Left Upper Arm **D** Skin, Right Lower Arm **E** Skin, Left Lower Arm **F** Skin, Right Hand **G** Skin, Left Hand **H** Skin, Right Upper Leg **J** Skin, Left Upper Leg **K** Skin, Right Lower Leg **L** Skin, Left Lower Leg **M** Skin, Right Foot **N** Skin, Left Foot **Q** Finger Nail **R** Toe Nail	**X** External	**Z** No Device	**Z** No Qualifier
T Breast, Right **U** Breast, Left **V** Breast, Bilateral	**0** Open **3** Percutaneous **7** Via Natural or Artificial Opening **8** Via Natural or Artificial Opening Endoscopic	**Z** No Device	**Z** No Qualifier
W Nipple, Right **X** Nipple, Left	**0** Open **3** Percutaneous **7** Via Natural or Artificial Opening **8** Via Natural or Artificial Opening Endoscopic **X** External	**Z** No Device	**Z** No Qualifier

IC Limited Coverage   **NC** Noncovered   **HAC** HAC-associated Procedure   **CC** Combination Cluster - See Appendix G for code lists
⬛ Non-OR-Affecting MS-DRG Assignment   New/Revised Text in **Orange**   ♂ Male   ♀ Female

2021 ICD-10-PCS

379

0   Medical and Surgical
H   Skin and Breast
D   Extraction: Pulling or stripping out or off all or a portion of a body part by the use of force

Body Part	Approach	Device	Qualifier
Character 4	**Character 5**	**Character 6**	**Character 7**
0 Skin, Scalp **1** Skin, Face **2** Skin, Right Ear **3** Skin, Left Ear **4** Skin, Neck **5** Skin, Chest **6** Skin, Back **7** Skin, Abdomen **8** Skin, Buttock **9** Skin, Perineum **A** Skin, Inguinal **B** Skin, Right Upper Arm **C** Skin, Left Upper Arm **D** Skin, Right Lower Arm **E** Skin, Left Lower Arm **F** Skin, Right Hand **G** Skin, Left Hand **H** Skin, Right Upper Leg **J** Skin, Left Upper Leg **K** Skin, Right Lower Leg **L** Skin, Left Lower Leg **M** Skin, Right Foot **N** Skin, Left Foot **Q** Finger Nail **R** Toe Nail **S** Hair	**X** External	**Z** No Device	**Z** No Qualifier
T Breast, Right **U** Breast, Left **V** Breast, Bilateral **Y** Supernumerary Breast	**0** Open	**Z** No Device	**Z** No Qualifier

0   Medical and Surgical
H   Skin and Breast
H   Insertion: Putting in a nonbiological appliance that monitors, assists, performs, or prevents a physiological function but does not physically take the place of a body part

Body Part	Approach	Device	Qualifier
Character 4	**Character 5**	**Character 6**	**Character 7**
P Skin	**X** External	**Y** Other Device	**Z** No Qualifier
T Breast, Right **U** Breast, Left	**0** Open **3** Percutaneous **7** Via Natural or Artificial Opening **8** Via Natural or Artificial Opening Endoscopic	**1** Radioactive Element **N** Tissue Expander **Y** Other Device	**Z** No Qualifier
V Breast, Bilateral	**0** Open **3** Percutaneous **7** Via Natural or Artificial Opening **8** Via Natural or Artificial Opening Endoscopic	**1** Radioactive Element **N** Tissue	**Z** No Qualifier
W Nipple, Right **X** Nipple, Left	**0** Open **3** Percutaneous **7** Via Natural or Artificial Opening **8** Via Natural or Artificial Opening Endoscopic	**1** Radioactive Element **N** Tissue Expander	**Z** No Qualifier
W Nipple, Right **X** Nipple, Left	**X** External	**1** Radioactive Element	**Z** No Qualifier

LC Limited Coverage   **NC** Noncovered   **HAC** HAC-associated Procedure   **CC** Combination Cluster - See Appendix G for code lists
DRG Non-OR-Affecting MS-DRG Assignment   New/Revised Text in **Orange**   ♂ Male   ♀ Female

380   **2021 ICD-10-PCS**

0 Medical and Surgical

H Skin and Breast

J Inspection: Visually and/or manually exploring a body part

Body Part	Approach	Device	Qualifier
Character 4	Character 5	Character 6	Character 7
P Skin **Q** Finger Nail **R** Toe Nail	**X** External	**Z** No Device	**Z** No Qualifier
T Breast, Right **U** Breast, Left	**0** Open **3** Percutaneous **7** Via Natural or Artificial Opening **8** Via Natural or Artificial Opening Endoscopic	**Z** No Device	**Z** No Qualifier

0 Medical and Surgical

H Skin and Breast

M Reattachment: Putting back in or on all or a portion of a separated body part to its normal location or other suitable location

Body Part	Approach	Device	Qualifier
Character 4	Character 5	Character 6	Character 7
0 Skin, Scalp **1** Skin, Face **2** Skin, Right Ear **3** Skin, Left Ear **4** Skin, Neck **5** Skin, Chest **6** Skin, Back **7** Skin, Abdomen **8** Skin, Buttock **9** Skin, Perineum **A** Skin, Inguinal **B** Skin, Right Upper Arm **C** Skin, Left Upper Arm **D** Skin, Right Lower Arm **E** Skin, Left Lower Arm **F** Skin, Right Hand **G** Skin, Left Hand **H** Skin, Right Upper Leg **J** Skin, Left Upper Leg **K** Skin, Right Lower Leg **L** Skin, Left Lower Leg **M** Skin, Right Foot **N** Skin, Left Foot **T** Breast, Right **U** Breast, Left **V** Breast, Bilateral **W** Nipple, Right **X** Nipple, Left	**X** External	**Z** No Device	**Z** No Qualifier

0   Medical and Surgical
H   Skin and Breast
N   Release: Freeing a body part from an abnormal physical constraint by cutting or by the use of force

Body Part	Approach	Device	Qualifier
Character 4	**Character 5**	**Character 6**	**Character 7**
0 Skin, Scalp **1** Skin, Face **2** Skin, Right Ear **3** Skin, Left Ear **4** Skin, Neck **5** Skin, Chest **6** Skin, Back **7** Skin, Abdomen **8** Skin, Buttock **9** Skin, Perineum **A** Skin, Inguinal **B** Skin, Right Upper Arm **C** Skin, Left Upper Arm **D** Skin, Right Lower Arm **E** Skin, Left Lower Arm **F** Skin, Right Hand **G** Skin, Left Hand **H** Skin, Right Upper Leg **J** Skin, Left Upper Leg **K** Skin, Right Lower Leg **L** Skin, Left Lower Leg **M** Skin, Right Foot **N** Skin, Left Foot **Q** Finger Nail **R** Toe Nail	**X** External	**Z** No Device	**Z** No Qualifier
T Breast, Right **U** Breast, Left **V** Breast, Bilateral	**0** Open **3** Percutaneous **7** Via Natural or Artificial Opening **8** Via Natural or Artificial Opening Endoscopic	**Z** No Device	**Z** No Qualifier
W Nipple, Right **X** Nipple, Left	**0** Open **3** Percutaneous **7** Via Natural or Artificial Opening **8** Via Natural or Artificial Opening Endoscopic **X** External	**Z** No Device	**Z** No Qualifier

LC Limited Coverage   NC Noncovered   HAC HAC-associated Procedure   CC Combination Cluster - See Appendix G for code lists
Non-OR-Affecting MS-DRG Assignment   New/Revised Text in **Orange**   ♂ Male   ♀ Female

382

2021 ICD-10-PCS

0   **Medical and Surgical**
H   **Skin and Breast**
P   **Removal:** Taking out or off a device from a body part

Body Part	Approach	Device	Qualifier
Character 4	**Character 5**	**Character 6**	**Character 7**
P Skin	**X** External	**0** Drainage Device **7** Autologous Tissue Substitute **J** Synthetic Substitute **K** Nonautologous Tissue Substitute **Y** Other Device	**Z** No Qualifier
Q Finger Nail **R** Toe Nail	**X** External	**0** Drainage Device **7** Autologous Tissue Substitute **J** Synthetic Substitute **K** Nonautologous Tissue Substitute	**Z** No Qualifier
S Hair	**X** External	**7** Autologous Tissue Substitute **J** Synthetic Substitute **K** Nonautologous Tissue Substitute	**Z** No Qualifier
T Breast, Right **U** Breast, Left	**0** Open **3** Percutaneous **7** Via Natural or Artificial Opening **8** Via Natural or Artificial Opening Endoscopic	**0** Drainage Device **1** Radioactive Element **7** Autologous Tissue Substitute **J** Synthetic Substitute **K** Nonautologous Tissue Substitute **N** Tissue Expander **Y** Other Device	**Z** No Qualifier

LC Limited Coverage   **NC** Noncovered   **HAC** HAC-associated Procedure   **CC** Combination Cluster - See Appendix G for code lists
DRG Non-OR-Affecting MS-DRG Assignment   New/Revised Text in **Orange**   ♂ Male   ♀ Female

2021 ICD-10-PCS

383

0 Medical and Surgical
H Skin and Breast
Q Repair: Restoring, to the extent possible, a body part to its normal anatomic structure and function

Body Part	Approach	Device	Qualifier
Character 4	Character 5	Character 6	Character 7
0 Skin, Scalp	**X** External	**Z** No Device	**Z** No Qualifier
1 Skin, Face			
2 Skin, Right Ear			
3 Skin, Left Ear			
4 Skin, Neck			
5 Skin, Chest			
6 Skin, Back			
7 Skin, Abdomen			
8 Skin, Buttock			
9 Skin, Perineum ᴰᴿᴳ			
A Skin, Inguinal			
B Skin, Right Upper Arm			
C Skin, Left Upper Arm			
D Skin, Right Lower Arm			
E Skin, Left Lower Arm			
F Skin, Right Hand			
G Skin, Left Hand			
H Skin, Right Upper Leg			
J Skin, Left Upper Leg			
K Skin, Right Lower Leg			
L Skin, Left Lower Leg			
M Skin, Right Foot			
N Skin, Left Foot			
Q Finger Nail			
R Toe Nail			
T Breast, Right	**0** Open	**Z** No Device	**Z** No Qualifier
U Breast, Left	**3** Percutaneous		
V Breast, Bilateral	**7** Via Natural or Artificial Opening		
Y Supernumerary Breast	**8** Via Natural or Artificial Opening Endoscopic		
W Nipple, Right	**0** Open	**Z** No Device	**Z** No Qualifier
X Nipple, Left	**3** Percutaneous		
	7 Via Natural or Artificial Opening		
	8 Via Natural or Artificial Opening Endoscopic		
	X External		

ᴰᴿᴳ 0HQ9XZZ

ᴸᶜ Limited Coverage   ᴺᶜ Noncovered   ᴴᴬᶜ HAC-associated Procedure   ᶜᶜ Combination Cluster - See Appendix G for code lists
ᴰᴿᴳ Non-OR-Affecting MS-DRG Assignment   New/Revised Text in Orange   ♂ Male   ♀ Female

0   Medical and Surgical
H   Skin and Breast
R   Replacement: Putting in or on biological or synthetic material that physically takes the place and/or function of all or a portion of a body part

Body Part	Approach	Device	Qualifier
Character 4	Character 5	Character 6	Character 7
0 Skin, Scalp 1 Skin, Face 2 Skin, Right Ear 3 Skin, Left Ear 4 Skin, Neck 5 Skin, Chest 6 Skin, Back 7 Skin, Abdomen 8 Skin, Buttock 9 Skin, Perineum A Skin, Inguinal B Skin, Right Upper Arm C Skin, Left Upper Arm D Skin, Right Lower Arm E Skin, Left Lower Arm F Skin, Right Hand G Skin, Left Hand H Skin, Right Upper Leg J Skin, Left Upper Leg K Skin, Right Lower Leg L Skin, Left Lower Leg M Skin, Right Foot N Skin, Left Foot	X External	7 Autologous Tissue Substitute	2 Cell Suspension Technique 3 Full Thickness 4 Partial Thickness
0 Skin, Scalp 1 Skin, Face 2 Skin, Right Ear 3 Skin, Left Ear 4 Skin, Neck 5 Skin, Chest 6 Skin, Back 7 Skin, Abdomen 8 Skin, Buttock 9 Skin, Perineum A Skin, Inguinal B Skin, Right Upper Arm C Skin, Left Upper Arm D Skin, Right Lower Arm E Skin, Left Lower Arm F Skin, Right Hand G Skin, Left Hand H Skin, Right Upper Leg J Skin, Left Upper Leg K Skin, Right Lower Leg L Skin, Left Lower Leg M Skin, Right Foot N Skin, Left Foot	X External	J Synthetic Substitute	3 Full Thickness 4 Partial Thickness Z No Qualifier

0HR continued on next page

LC Limited Coverage   NC Noncovered   HAC HAC-associated Procedure   CC Combination Cluster - See Appendix G for code lists
DRG Non-OR-Affecting MS-DRG Assignment   New/Revised Text in **Orange**   ♂ Male   ♀ Female

2021 ICD-10-PCS   **385**

0   **Medical and Surgical**   0HR continued from previous page
H   **Skin and Breast**
R   **Replacement:** Putting in or on biological or synthetic material that physically takes the place and/or function of all or a portion of a body part

Body Part	Approach	Device	Qualifier
Character 4	**Character 5**	**Character 6**	**Character 7**
0 Skin, Scalp 1 Skin, Face 2 Skin, Right Ear 3 Skin, Left Ear 4 Skin, Neck 5 Skin, Chest 6 Skin, Back 7 Skin, Abdomen 8 Skin, Buttock 9 Skin, Perineum A Skin, Inguinal B Skin, Right Upper Arm C Skin, Left Upper Arm D Skin, Right Lower Arm E Skin, Left Lower Arm F Skin, Right Hand G Skin, Left Hand H Skin, Right Upper Leg J Skin, Left Upper Leg K Skin, Right Lower Leg L Skin, Left Lower Leg M Skin, Right Foot N Skin, Left Foot	X External	K Nonautologous Tissue Substitute	3 Full Thickness 4 Partial Thickness
Q Finger Nail R Toe Nail S Hair	X External	7 Autologous Tissue Substitute J Synthetic Substitute K Nonautologous Tissue Substitute	Z No Qualifier
T Breast, Right U Breast, Left V Breast, Bilateral	0 Open	7 Autologous Tissue Substitute	5 Latissimus Dorsi Myocutaneous Flap 6 Transverse Rectus Abdominis Myocutaneous Flap 7 Deep Inferior Epigastric Artery Perforator Flap 8 Superficial Inferior Epigastric Artery Flap 9 Gluteal Artery Perforator Flap Z No Qualifier
T Breast, Right U Breast, Left V Breast, Bilateral	0 Open	J Synthetic Substitute K Nonautologous Tissue Substitute	Z No Qualifier
T Breast, Right ᴄᴄ U Breast, Left ᴄᴄ V Breast, Bilateral ᴄᴄ	3 Percutaneous	7 Autologous Tissue Substitute J Synthetic Substitute K Nonautologous Tissue Substitute	Z No Qualifier
W Nipple, Right X Nipple, Left	0 Open 3 Percutaneous X External	7 Autologous Tissue Substitute J Synthetic Substitute K Nonautologous Tissue Substitute	Z No Qualifier

ᴄᴄ   0HRT37Z   0HRU37Z   0HRV37Z

---

0 Medical and Surgical
H Skin and Breast
S Reposition: Moving to its normal location, or other suitable location, all or a portion of a body part

Body Part	Approach	Device	Qualifier
Character 4	Character 5	Character 6	Character 7
S Hair W Nipple, Right X Nipple, Left	X External	Z No Device	Z No Qualifier
T Breast, Right U Breast, Left V Breast, Bilateral	0 Open	Z No Device	Z No Qualifier

0 Medical and Surgical
H Skin and Breast
T Resection: Cutting out or off, without replacement, all of a body part

Body Part	Approach	Device	Qualifier
Character 4	Character 5	Character 6	Character 7
Q Finger Nail R Toe Nail W Nipple, Right X Nipple, Left	X External	Z No Device	Z No Qualifier
T Breast, Right ◰ U Breast, Left ◰ V Breast, Bilateral ◰ Y Supernumerary Breast	0 Open	Z No Device	Z No Qualifier

◰ 0HTT0ZZ   0HTU0ZZ   0HTV0ZZ

0 Medical and Surgical
H Skin and Breast
U Supplement: Putting in or on biological or synthetic material that physically reinforces and/or augments the function of a portion of a body part

Body Part	Approach	Device	Qualifier
Character 4	Character 5	Character 6	Character 7
T Breast, Right U Breast, Left V Breast, Bilateral	0 Open 3 Percutaneous 7 Via Natural or Artificial Opening 8 Via Natural or Artificial Opening Endoscopic	7 Autologous Tissue Substitute J Synthetic Substitute K Nonautologous Tissue Substitute	Z No Qualifier
W Nipple, Right X Nipple, Left	0 Open 3 Percutaneous 7 Via Natural or Artificial Opening 8 Via Natural or Artificial Opening Endoscopic X External	7 Autologous Tissue Substitute J Synthetic Substitute K Nonautologous Tissue Substitute	Z No Qualifier

LC Limited Coverage   NC Noncovered   HAC HAC-associated Procedure   CC Combination Cluster - See Appendix G for code lists
DRG Non-OR-Affecting MS-DRG Assignment   New/Revised Text in **Orange**   ♂ Male   ♀ Female

2021 ICD-10-PCS

387

0 Medical and Surgical
H Skin and Breast
W Revision: Correcting, to the extent possible, a portion of a malfunctioning device or the position of a displaced device

Body Part	Approach	Device	Qualifier
Character 4	Character 5	Character 6	Character 7
P Skin	**X** External	**0** Drainage Device **7** Autologous Tissue Substitute **J** Synthetic Substitute **K** Nonautologous Tissue Substitute **Y** Other Device	**Z** No Qualifier
Q Finger Nail **R** Toe Nail	**X** External	**0** Drainage Device **7** Autologous Tissue Substitute **J** Synthetic Substitute **K** Nonautologous Tissue Substitute	**Z** No Qualifier
S Hair	**X** External	**7** Autologous Tissue Substitute **J** Synthetic Substitute **K** Nonautologous Tissue Substitute	**Z** No Qualifier
T Breast, Right **U** Breast, Left	**0** Open **3** Percutaneous **7** Via Natural or Artificial Opening **8** Via Natural or Artificial Opening Endoscopic	**0** Drainage Device **7** Autologous Tissue Substitute **J** Synthetic Substitute **K** Nonautologous Tissue Substitute **N** Tissue Expander **Y** Other Device	**Z** No Qualifier

0 Medical and Surgical
H Skin and Breast
X Transfer: Moving, without taking out, all or a portion of a body part to another location to take over the function of all or a portion of a body part

Body Part	Approach	Device	Qualifier
Character 4	Character 5	Character 6	Character 7
0 Skin, Scalp **1** Skin, Face **2** Skin, Right Ear **3** Skin, Left Ear **4** Skin, Neck **5** Skin, Chest **6** Skin, Back **7** Skin, Abdomen **8** Skin, Buttock **9** Skin, Perineum **A** Skin, Inguinal **B** Skin, Right Upper Arm **C** Skin, Left Upper Arm **D** Skin, Right Lower Arm **E** Skin, Left Lower Arm **F** Skin, Right Hand **G** Skin, Left Hand **H** Skin, Right Upper Leg **J** Skin, Left Upper Leg **K** Skin, Right Lower Leg **L** Skin, Left Lower Leg **M** Skin, Right Foot **N** Skin, Left Foot	**X** External	**Z** No Device	**Z** No Qualifier

LC Limited Coverage   NC Noncovered   HAC HAC-associated Procedure   CC Combination Cluster - See Appendix G for code lists
Non-OR-Affecting MS-DRG Assignment   New/Revised Text in Orange   ♂ Male   ♀ Female

388

2021 ICD-10-PCS

NOTES

NOTES

Subcutaneous Tissue and Fascia 0J0-0JX

0 **Medical and Surgical**
J **Subcutaneous Tissue and Fascia**
0 **Alteration:** Modifying the anatomic structure of a body part without affecting the function of the body part

Body Part	Approach	Device	Qualifier
Character 4	**Character 5**	**Character 6**	**Character 7**
1 Subcutaneous Tissue and Fascia, Face	**0** Open	**Z** No Device	**Z** No Qualifier
4 Subcutaneous Tissue and Fascia, Right Neck	**3** Percutaneous		
5 Subcutaneous Tissue and Fascia, Left Neck			
6 Subcutaneous Tissue and Fascia, Chest			
7 Subcutaneous Tissue and Fascia, Back			
8 Subcutaneous Tissue and Fascia, Abdomen			
9 Subcutaneous Tissue and Fascia, Buttock			
D Subcutaneous Tissue and Fascia, Right Upper Arm			
F Subcutaneous Tissue and Fascia, Left Upper Arm			
G Subcutaneous Tissue and Fascia, Right Lower Arm			
H Subcutaneous Tissue and Fascia, Left Lower Arm			
L Subcutaneous Tissue and Fascia, Right Upper Leg			
M Subcutaneous Tissue and Fascia, Left Upper Leg			
N Subcutaneous Tissue and Fascia, Right Lower Leg			
P Subcutaneous Tissue and Fascia, Left Lower Leg			

0 **Medical and Surgical**
J **Subcutaneous Tissue and Fascia**
2 **Change:** Taking out or off a device from a body part and putting back an identical or similar device in or on the same body part without cutting or puncturing the skin or a mucous membrane

Body Part	Approach	Device	Qualifier
Character 4	**Character 5**	**Character 6**	**Character 7**
S Subcutaneous Tissue and Fascia, Head and Neck	**X** External	**0** Drainage Device	**Z** No Qualifier
T Subcutaneous Tissue and Fascia, Trunk		**Y** Other Device	
V Subcutaneous Tissue and Fascia, Upper Extremity			
W Subcutaneous Tissue and Fascia, Lower Extremity			

LC Limited Coverage NC Noncovered HAC HAC-associated Procedure CC Combination Cluster - See Appendix G for code lists
DRG Non-OR-Affecting MS-DRG Assignment New/Revised Text in Orange ♂ Male ♀ Female

0 **Medical and Surgical**
J **Subcutaneous Tissue and Fascia**
5 **Destruction:** Physical eradication of all or a portion of a body part by the direct use of energy, force, or a destructive agent

Body Part	Approach	Device	Qualifier
Character 4	Character 5	Character 6	Character 7
0 Subcutaneous Tissue and Fascia, Scalp ᴼᴿᴳ 1 Subcutaneous Tissue and Fascia, Face ᴼᴿᴳ 4 Subcutaneous Tissue and Fascia, Right Neck ᴼᴿᴳ 5 Subcutaneous Tissue and Fascia, Left Neck ᴼᴿᴳ 6 Subcutaneous Tissue and Fascia, Chest ᴼᴿᴳ 7 Subcutaneous Tissue and Fascia, Back ᴼᴿᴳ 8 Subcutaneous Tissue and Fascia, Abdomen ᴼᴿᴳ 9 Subcutaneous Tissue and Fascia, Buttock ᴼᴿᴳ B Subcutaneous Tissue and Fascia, Perineum ᴼᴿᴳ C Subcutaneous Tissue and Fascia, Pelvic Region ᴼᴿᴳ D Subcutaneous Tissue and Fascia, Right Upper Arm ᴼᴿᴳ F Subcutaneous Tissue and Fascia, Left Upper Arm ᴼᴿᴳ G Subcutaneous Tissue and Fascia, Right Lower Arm ᴼᴿᴳ H Subcutaneous Tissue and Fascia, Left Lower Arm ᴼᴿᴳ J Subcutaneous Tissue and Fascia, Right Hand ᴼᴿᴳ K Subcutaneous Tissue and Fascia, Left Hand ᴼᴿᴳ L Subcutaneous Tissue and Fascia, Right Upper Leg ᴼᴿᴳ M Subcutaneous Tissue and Fascia, Left Upper Leg ᴼᴿᴳ N Subcutaneous Tissue and Fascia, Right Lower Leg ᴼᴿᴳ P Subcutaneous Tissue and Fascia, Left Lower Leg ᴼᴿᴳ Q Subcutaneous Tissue and Fascia, Right Foot ᴼᴿᴳ R Subcutaneous Tissue and Fascia, Left Foot ᴼᴿᴳ	0 Open 3 Percutaneous	Z No Device	Z No Qualifier

ᴼᴿᴳ

0J500ZZ	0J503ZZ	0J510ZZ	0J513ZZ	0J540ZZ	0J543ZZ	0J550ZZ	0J553ZZ	0J560ZZ	0J563ZZ	0J570ZZ	0J573ZZ	0J580ZZ
0J583ZZ	0J590ZZ	0J593ZZ	0J5B0ZZ	0J5B3ZZ	0J5C0ZZ	0J5C3ZZ	0J5D0ZZ	0J5D3ZZ	0J5F0ZZ	0J5F3ZZ	0J5G0ZZ	0J5G3ZZ
0J5H0ZZ	0J5H3ZZ	0J5J0ZZ	0J5J3ZZ	0J5K0ZZ	0J5K3ZZ	0J5L0ZZ	0J5L3ZZ	0J5M0ZZ	0J5M3ZZ	0J5N0ZZ	0J5N3ZZ	0J5P0ZZ
0J5P3ZZ	0J5Q0ZZ	0J5Q3ZZ	0J5R0ZZ	0J5R3ZZ								

LC Limited Coverage **NC** Noncovered **HAC** HAC-associated Procedure **CC** Combination Cluster - See Appendix G for code lists
ᴼᴿᴳ Non-OR-Affecting MS-DRG Assignment New/Revised Text in **Orange** ♂ Male ♀ Female

392

2021 ICD-10-PCS

0 **Medical and Surgical**
J **Subcutaneous Tissue and Fascia**
8 **Division:** Cutting into a body part, without draining fluids and/or gases from the body part, in order to separate or transect a body part

Body Part	Approach	Device	Qualifier
Character 4	Character 5	Character 6	Character 7
0 Subcutaneous Tissue and Fascia, Scalp	**0** Open	**Z** No Device	**Z** No Qualifier
1 Subcutaneous Tissue and Fascia, Face	**3** Percutaneous		
4 Subcutaneous Tissue and Fascia, Right Neck			
5 Subcutaneous Tissue and Fascia, Left Neck			
6 Subcutaneous Tissue and Fascia, Chest			
7 Subcutaneous Tissue and Fascia, Back			
8 Subcutaneous Tissue and Fascia, Abdomen			
9 Subcutaneous Tissue and Fascia, Buttock			
B Subcutaneous Tissue and Fascia, Perineum			
C Subcutaneous Tissue and Fascia, Pelvic Region			
D Subcutaneous Tissue and Fascia, Right Upper Arm			
F Subcutaneous Tissue and Fascia, Left Upper Arm			
G Subcutaneous Tissue and Fascia, Right Lower Arm			
H Subcutaneous Tissue and Fascia, Left Lower Arm			
J Subcutaneous Tissue and Fascia, Right Hand			
K Subcutaneous Tissue and Fascia, Left Hand			
L Subcutaneous Tissue and Fascia, Right Upper Leg			
M Subcutaneous Tissue and Fascia, Left Upper Leg			
N Subcutaneous Tissue and Fascia, Right Lower Leg			
P Subcutaneous Tissue and Fascia, Left Lower Leg			
Q Subcutaneous Tissue and Fascia, Right Foot			
R Subcutaneous Tissue and Fascia, Left Foot			
S Subcutaneous Tissue and Fascia, Head and Neck			
T Subcutaneous Tissue and Fascia, Trunk			
V Subcutaneous Tissue and Fascia, Upper Extremity			
W Subcutaneous Tissue and Fascia, Lower Extremity			

0   **Medical and Surgical**
J   **Subcutaneous Tissue and Fascia**
9   **Drainage:** Taking or letting out fluids and/or gases from a body part

Body Part	Approach	Device	Qualifier
Character 4	**Character 5**	**Character 6**	**Character 7**
0 Subcutaneous Tissue and Fascia, Scalp	**0** Open	**0** Drainage Device	**Z** No Qualifier
1 Subcutaneous Tissue and Fascia, Face	**3** Percutaneous		
4 Subcutaneous Tissue and Fascia, Right Neck			
5 Subcutaneous Tissue and Fascia, Left Neck			
6 Subcutaneous Tissue and Fascia, Chest			
7 Subcutaneous Tissue and Fascia, Back			
8 Subcutaneous Tissue and Fascia, Abdomen			
9 Subcutaneous Tissue and Fascia, Buttock			
B Subcutaneous Tissue and Fascia, Perineum			
C Subcutaneous Tissue and Fascia, Pelvic Region			
D Subcutaneous Tissue and Fascia, Right Upper Arm			
F Subcutaneous Tissue and Fascia, Left Upper Arm			
G Subcutaneous Tissue and Fascia, Right Lower Arm			
H Subcutaneous Tissue and Fascia, Left Lower Arm			
J Subcutaneous Tissue and Fascia, Right Hand			
K Subcutaneous Tissue and Fascia, Left Hand			
L Subcutaneous Tissue and Fascia, Right Upper Leg			
M Subcutaneous Tissue and Fascia, Left Upper Leg			
N Subcutaneous Tissue and Fascia, Right Lower Leg			
P Subcutaneous Tissue and Fascia, Left Lower Leg			
Q Subcutaneous Tissue and Fascia, Right Foot			
R Subcutaneous Tissue and Fascia, Left Foot			

0J9 continued on next page

0 **Medical and Surgical**
J **Subcutaneous Tissue and Fascia**
9 **Drainage:** Taking or letting out fluids and/or gases from a body part

0J9 continued from previous page

Body Part	Approach	Device	Qualifier
Character 4	**Character 5**	**Character 6**	**Character 7**
0 Subcutaneous Tissue and Fascia, Scalp 1 Subcutaneous Tissue and Fascia, Face 4 Subcutaneous Tissue and Fascia, Right Neck 5 Subcutaneous Tissue and Fascia, Left Neck 6 Subcutaneous Tissue and Fascia, Chest 7 Subcutaneous Tissue and Fascia, Back 8 Subcutaneous Tissue and Fascia, Abdomen 9 Subcutaneous Tissue and Fascia, Buttock B Subcutaneous Tissue and Fascia, Perineum C Subcutaneous Tissue and Fascia, Pelvic Region D Subcutaneous Tissue and Fascia, Right Upper Arm F Subcutaneous Tissue and Fascia, Left Upper Arm G Subcutaneous Tissue and Fascia, Right Lower Arm H Subcutaneous Tissue and Fascia, Left Lower Arm J Subcutaneous Tissue and Fascia, Right Hand K Subcutaneous Tissue and Fascia, Left Hand L Subcutaneous Tissue and Fascia, Right Upper Leg M Subcutaneous Tissue and Fascia, Left Upper Leg N Subcutaneous Tissue and Fascia, Right Lower Leg P Subcutaneous Tissue and Fascia, Left Lower Leg Q Subcutaneous Tissue and Fascia, Right Foot R Subcutaneous Tissue and Fascia, Left Foot	0 Open 3 Percutaneous	Z No Device	X Diagnostic Z No Qualifier

IC Limited Coverage   NC Noncovered   HAC HAC-associated Procedure   CC Combination Cluster - See Appendix G for code lists
DRG Non-OR-Affecting MS-DRG Assignment   New/Revised Text in **Orange**   ♂ Male   ♀ Female

0 **Medical and Surgical**
J **Subcutaneous Tissue and Fascia**
B **Excision:** Cutting out or off, without replacement, a portion of a body part

Body Part	Approach	Device	Qualifier
Character 4	Character 5	Character 6	Character 7
0 Subcutaneous Tissue and Fascia, Scalp ᴼᴿᴳ	**0** Open	**Z** No Device	**X** Diagnostic
1 Subcutaneous Tissue and Fascia, Face	**3** Percutaneous		**Z** No Qualifier
4 Subcutaneous Tissue and Fascia, Right Neck ᴼᴿᴳ			
5 Subcutaneous Tissue and Fascia, Left Neck ᴼᴿᴳ			
6 Subcutaneous Tissue and Fascia, Chest ᴼᴿᴳ			
7 Subcutaneous Tissue and Fascia, Back ᴼᴿᴳ			
8 Subcutaneous Tissue and Fascia, Abdomen ᴼᴿᴳ			
9 Subcutaneous Tissue and Fascia, Buttock ᴼᴿᴳ			
B Subcutaneous Tissue and Fascia, Perineum ᴼᴿᴳ			
C Subcutaneous Tissue and Fascia, Pelvic Region ᴼᴿᴳ			
D Subcutaneous Tissue and Fascia, Right Upper Arm ᴼᴿᴳ			
F Subcutaneous Tissue and Fascia, Left Upper Arm ᴼᴿᴳ			
G Subcutaneous Tissue and Fascia, Right Lower Arm ᴼᴿᴳ			
H Subcutaneous Tissue and Fascia, Left Lower Arm ᴼᴿᴳ			
J Subcutaneous Tissue and Fascia, Right Hand			
K Subcutaneous Tissue and Fascia, Left Hand			
L Subcutaneous Tissue and Fascia, Right Upper Leg ᴼᴿᴳ			
M Subcutaneous Tissue and Fascia, Left Upper Leg ᴼᴿᴳ			
N Subcutaneous Tissue and Fascia, Right Lower Leg ᴼᴿᴳ			
P Subcutaneous Tissue and Fascia, Left Lower Leg ᴼᴿᴳ			
Q Subcutaneous Tissue and Fascia, Right Foot ᴼᴿᴳ			
R Subcutaneous Tissue and Fascia, Left Foot ᴼᴿᴳ			

ᴼᴿᴳ 0JB03ZZ   0JB43ZZ   0JB53ZZ   0JB63ZZ   0JB73ZZ   0JB83ZZ   0JB93ZZ   0JBB3ZZ   0JBC3ZZ   0JBD3ZZ   0JBF3ZZ   0JBG3ZZ   0JBH3ZZ
0JBL3ZZ   0JBM3ZZ   0JBN3ZZ   0JBP3ZZ   0JBQ3ZZ   0JBR3ZZ

0 **Medical and Surgical**
J **Subcutaneous Tissue and Fascia**
C **Extirpation:** Taking or cutting out solid matter from a body part

Body Part	Approach	Device	Qualifier
Character 4	Character 5	Character 6	Character 7
0 Subcutaneous Tissue and Fascia, Scalp	0 Open	Z No Device	Z No Qualifier
1 Subcutaneous Tissue and Fascia, Face	3 Percutaneous		
4 Subcutaneous Tissue and Fascia, Right Neck			
5 Subcutaneous Tissue and Fascia, Left Neck			
6 Subcutaneous Tissue and Fascia, Chest			
7 Subcutaneous Tissue and Fascia, Back			
8 Subcutaneous Tissue and Fascia, Abdomen			
9 Subcutaneous Tissue and Fascia, Buttock			
B Subcutaneous Tissue and Fascia, Perineum			
C Subcutaneous Tissue and Fascia, Pelvic Region			
D Subcutaneous Tissue and Fascia, Right Upper Arm			
F Subcutaneous Tissue and Fascia, Left Upper Arm			
G Subcutaneous Tissue and Fascia, Right Lower Arm			
H Subcutaneous Tissue and Fascia, Left Lower Arm			
J Subcutaneous Tissue and Fascia, Right Hand			
K Subcutaneous Tissue and Fascia, Left Hand			
L Subcutaneous Tissue and Fascia, Right Upper Leg			
M Subcutaneous Tissue and Fascia, Left Upper Leg			
N Subcutaneous Tissue and Fascia, Right Lower Leg			
P Subcutaneous Tissue and Fascia, Left Lower Leg			
Q Subcutaneous Tissue and Fascia, Right Foot			
R Subcutaneous Tissue and Fascia, Left Foot			

0 Medical and Surgical
J Subcutaneous Tissue and Fascia
D Extraction: Pulling or stripping out or off all or a portion of a body part by the use of force

Body Part	Approach	Device	Qualifier
Character 4	Character 5	Character 6	Character 7
0 Subcutaneous Tissue and Fascia, Scalp	**0** Open	**Z** No Device	**Z** No Qualifier
1 Subcutaneous Tissue and Fascia, Face	**3** Percutaneous		
4 Subcutaneous Tissue and Fascia, Right Neck			
5 Subcutaneous Tissue and Fascia, Left Neck			
6 Subcutaneous Tissue and Fascia, Chest ⬛ ⬛			
7 Subcutaneous Tissue and Fascia, Back ⬛ ⬛			
8 Subcutaneous Tissue and Fascia, Abdomen ⬛ ⬛			
9 Subcutaneous Tissue and Fascia, Buttock ⬛ ⬛			
B Subcutaneous Tissue and Fascia, Perineum			
C Subcutaneous Tissue and Fascia, Pelvic Region			
D Subcutaneous Tissue and Fascia, Right Upper Arm			
F Subcutaneous Tissue and Fascia, Left Upper Arm			
G Subcutaneous Tissue and Fascia, Right Lower Arm			
H Subcutaneous Tissue and Fascia, Left Lower Arm			
J Subcutaneous Tissue and Fascia, Right Hand			
K Subcutaneous Tissue and Fascia, Left Hand			
L Subcutaneous Tissue and Fascia, Right Upper Leg ⬛ ⬛			
M Subcutaneous Tissue and Fascia, Left Upper Leg ⬛ ⬛			
N Subcutaneous Tissue and Fascia, Right Lower Leg			
P Subcutaneous Tissue and Fascia, Left Lower Leg			
Q Subcutaneous Tissue and Fascia, Right Foot			
R Subcutaneous Tissue and Fascia, Left Foot			

⬛ 0JD63ZZ   0JD73ZZ   0JD83ZZ   0JD93ZZ   0JDL3ZZ   0JDM3ZZ
⬛ 0JD63ZZ   0JD73ZZ   0JD83ZZ   0JD93ZZ   0JDL3ZZ   0JDM3ZZ

⬛ Limited Coverage   ⬛ Noncovered   ⬛ HAC-associated Procedure   ⬛ Combination Cluster - See Appendix G for code lists
⬛ Non-OR-Affecting MS-DRG Assignment   New/Revised Text in **Orange**   ♂ Male   ♀ Female

398

2021 ICD-10-PCS

0 **Medical and Surgical**
J **Subcutaneous Tissue and Fascia**
H **Insertion:** Putting in a nonbiological appliance that monitors, assists, performs, or prevents a physiological function but does not physically take the place of a body part

Body Part	Approach	Device	Qualifier
Character 4	**Character 5**	**Character 6**	**Character 7**
0 Subcutaneous Tissue and Fascia, Scalp 1 Subcutaneous Tissue and Fascia, Face 4 Subcutaneous Tissue and Fascia, Right Neck 5 Subcutaneous Tissue and Fascia, Left Neck 9 Subcutaneous Tissue and Fascia, Buttock B Subcutaneous Tissue and Fascia, Perineum C Subcutaneous Tissue and Fascia, Pelvic Region J Subcutaneous Tissue and Fascia, Right Hand K Subcutaneous Tissue and Fascia, Left Hand Q Subcutaneous Tissue and Fascia, Right Foot R Subcutaneous Tissue and Fascia, Left Foot	0 Open 3 Percutaneous	N Tissue Expander	Z No Qualifier
6 Subcutaneous Tissue and Fascia, Chest **HAC CC DRG**	0 Open 3 Percutaneous	0 Monitoring Device, Hemodynamic 2 Monitoring Device 4 Pacemaker, Single Chamber 5 Pacemaker, Single Chamber Rate Responsive 6 Pacemaker, Dual Chamber 7 Cardiac Resynchronization Pacemaker Pulse Generator 8 Defibrillator Generator 9 Cardiac Resynchronization Defibrillator Pulse Generator A Contractility Modulation Device B Stimulator Generator, Single Array C Stimulator Generator, Single Array Rechargeable D Stimulator Generator, Multiple Array E Stimulator Generator, Multiple Array Rechargeable F Subcutaneous Defibrillator Lead H Contraceptive Device M Stimulator Generator N Tissue Expander P Cardiac Rhythm Related Device V Infusion Device, Pump W Vascular Access Device, Totally Implantable X Vascular Access Device, Tunneled Y Other Device	Z No Qualifier

0JH continued on next page

LC Limited Coverage   **NC** Noncovered   **HAC** HAC-associated Procedure   **CC** Combination Cluster - See Appendix G for code lists
 DRG Non-OR-Affecting MS-DRG Assignment   New/Revised Text in **Orange**   ♂ Male   ♀ Female

2021 ICD-10-PCS

399

SUBCUTANEOUS TISSUE AND FASCIA 0J0-0JX

0   **Medical and Surgical**
J   **Subcutaneous Tissue and Fascia**
H   **Insertion:** Putting in a nonbiological appliance that monitors, assists, performs, or prevents a physiological function but does not physically take the place of a body part

0JH continued from previous page

Body Part		Approach		Device		Qualifier	
Character 4		**Character 5**		**Character 6**		**Character 7**	
7	Subcutaneous Tissue and Fascia, Back **CC NC**	0	Open	B	Stimulator Generator, Single Array	Z	No Qualifier
		3	Percutaneous	C	Stimulator Generator, Single Array Rechargeable		
				D	Stimulator Generator, Multiple Array		
				E	Stimulator Generator, Multiple Array Rechargeable		
				M	Stimulator Generator		
				N	Tissue Expander		
				V	Infusion Device, Pump		
				Y	Other Device		
8	Subcutaneous Tissue and Fascia, Abdomen **NC HAC CC DRG**	0	Open	0	Monitoring Device, Hemodynamic	Z	No Qualifier
		3	Percutaneous	2	Monitoring Device		
				4	Pacemaker, Single Chamber		
				5	Pacemaker, Single Chamber Rate Responsive		
				6	Pacemaker, Dual Chamber		
				7	Cardiac Resynchronization Pacemaker Pulse Generator		
				8	Defibrillator Generator		
				9	Cardiac Resynchronization Defibrillator Pulse Generator		
				A	Contractility Modulation Device		
				B	Stimulator Generator, Single Array		
				C	Stimulator Generator, Single Array Rechargeable		
				D	Stimulator Generator, Multiple Array		
				E	Stimulator Generator, Multiple Array Rechargeable		
				H	Contraceptive Device		
				M	Stimulator Generator		
				N	Tissue Expander		
				P	Cardiac Rhythm Related Device		
				V	Infusion Device, Pump		
				W	Vascular Access Device, Totally Implantable		
				X	Vascular Access Device, Tunneled		
				Y	Other Device		
D	Subcutaneous Tissue and Fascia, Right Upper Arm **DRG**	0	Open	H	Contraceptive Device	Z	No Qualifier
F	Subcutaneous Tissue and Fascia, Left Upper Arm **DRG**	3	Percutaneous	N	Tissue Expander		
G	Subcutaneous Tissue and Fascia, Right Lower Arm **DRG**			V	Infusion Device, Pump		
H	Subcutaneous Tissue and Fascia, Left Lower Arm **DRG**			W	Vascular Access Device, Totally Implantable		
L	Subcutaneous Tissue and Fascia, Right Upper Leg **DRG**			X	Vascular Access Device, Tunneled		
M	Subcutaneous Tissue and Fascia, Left Upper Leg **DRG**						
N	Subcutaneous Tissue and Fascia, Right Lower Leg **DRG**						
P	Subcutaneous Tissue and Fascia, Left Lower Leg **DRG**						

0JH continued on next page

LC Limited Coverage   **NC** Noncovered   **HAC** HAC-associated Procedure   **CC** Combination Cluster - See Appendix G for code lists
DRG Non-OR-Affecting MS-DRG Assignment   New/Revised Text in Orange   ♂ Male   ♀ Female

0   **Medical and Surgical**
J   **Subcutaneous Tissue and Fascia**
H   **Insertion:** Putting in a nonbiological appliance that monitors, assists, performs, or prevents a physiological function but does not physically take the place of a body part

0JH continued from previous page

Body Part	Approach	Device	Qualifier
Character 4	Character 5	Character 6	Character 7
S Subcutaneous Tissue and Fascia, Head and Neck **V** Subcutaneous Tissue and Fascia, Upper Extremity **W** Subcutaneous Tissue and Fascia, Lower Extremity	**0** Open **3** Percutaneous	**1** Radioactive Element **3** Infusion Device **Y** Other Device	**Z** No Qualifier
T Subcutaneous Tissue and Fascia, Trunk	**0** Open **3** Percutaneous	**1** Radioactive Element **3** Infusion Device **V** Infusion Device, Pump **Y** Other Device	**Z** No Qualifier

NC 0JH70MZ   0JH73MZ   0JH80MZ   0JH83MZ

HAC 0JH604Z   0JH605Z   0JH606Z   0JH607Z   0JH608Z   0JH609Z   0JH60PZ   0JH634Z   0JH635Z   0JH636Z   0JH637Z   0JH638Z   0JH639Z
0JH63PZ

Surgical site infection (SSI) following cardiac implantable electronic device (CIED) procedures and secondary diagnosis K68.11, T81.40XA, T81.41XA, T81.42XA, T81.43XA, T81.44XA, T81.49XA, T82.6XXA, T82.7XXA.

HAC 0JH63XZ

Iatrogenic pneumothorax w/ venous catheterization procedures and secondary diagnosis J95.811.

HAC 0JH804Z   0JH805Z   0JH806Z   0JH807Z   0JH808Z   0JH809Z   0JH80PZ   0JH834Z   0JH835Z   0JH836Z   0JH837Z   0JH838Z   0JH839Z
0JH83PZ

Surgical site infection (SSI) following cardiac implantable electronic device (CIED) procedures and secondary diagnosis K68.11, T81.40XA, T81.41XA, T81.42XA, T81.43XA, T81.44XA, T81.49XA, T82.6XXA, T82.7XXA.

CC
0JH604Z	0JH605Z	0JH606Z	0JH607Z	0JH608Z	0JH609Z	0JH60AZ	0JH60BZ	0JH60CZ	0JH60DZ	0JH60EZ	0JH60FZ	0JH60PZ
0JH634Z	0JH635Z	0JH636Z	0JH637Z	0JH638Z	0JH639Z	0JH63AZ	0JH63BZ	0JH63CZ	0JH63DZ	0JH63EZ	0JH63FZ	0JH63PZ
0JH70BZ	0JH70CZ	0JH70DZ	0JH70EZ	0JH73BZ	0JH73CZ	0JH73DZ	0JH73EZ	0JH804Z	0JH805Z	0JH806Z	0JH807Z	0JH808Z
0JH809Z	0JH80AZ	0JH80BZ	0JH80CZ	0JH80DZ	0JH80EZ	0JH80PZ	0JH834Z	0JH835Z	0JH836Z	0JH837Z	0JH838Z	0JH839Z
0JH83AZ	0JH83BZ	0JH83CZ	0JH83DZ	0JH83EZ	0JH83PZ							

DRG
0JH604Z	0JH605Z	0JH606Z	0JH607Z	0JH60HZ	0JH60PZ	0JH60XZ	0JH634Z	0JH635Z	0JH636Z	0JH637Z	0JH63HZ	0JH63PZ
0JH63WZ	0JH63XZ	0JH802Z	0JH804Z	0JH805Z	0JH806Z	0JH807Z	0JH80HZ	0JH80PZ	0JH80XZ	0JH832Z	0JH834Z	0JH835Z
0JH836Z	0JH837Z	0JH83HZ	0JH83PZ	0JH83WZ	0JH83XZ	0JHD0XZ	0JHD3WZ	0JHD3XZ	0JHF0XZ	0JHF3WZ	0JHF3XZ	0JHG0XZ
0JHG3WZ	0JHG3XZ	0JHH0XZ	0JHH3WZ	0JHH3XZ	0JHL0XZ	0JHL3WZ	0JHL3XZ	0JHM0XZ	0JHM3WZ	0JHM3XZ	0JHN0XZ	0JHN3HZ
0JHN3WZ	0JHN3XZ	0JHP0HZ	0JHP0XZ	0JHP3HZ	0JHP3WZ	0JHP3XZ						

0   **Medical and Surgical**
J   **Subcutaneous Tissue and Fascia**
J   **Inspection:** Visually and/or manually exploring a body part

Body Part	Approach	Device	Qualifier
Character 4	Character 5	Character 6	Character 7
S Subcutaneous Tissue and Fascia, Head and Neck **T** Subcutaneous Tissue and Fascia, Trunk **V** Subcutaneous Tissue and Fascia, Upper Extremity **W** Subcutaneous Tissue and Fascia, Lower Extremity	**0** Open **3** Percutaneous **X** External	**Z** No Device	**Z** No Qualifier

---

LC Limited Coverage   **NC** Noncovered   **HAC** HAC-associated Procedure   **CC** Combination Cluster - See Appendix G for code lists
DRG Non-OR-Affecting MS-DRG Assignment   New/Revised Text in **Orange**   ♂ Male   ♀ Female

0 Medical and Surgical
J Subcutaneous Tissue and Fascia
N Release: Freeing a body part from an abnormal physical constraint by cutting or by the use of force

Body Part	Approach	Device	Qualifier
Character 4	Character 5	Character 6	Character 7
0 Subcutaneous Tissue and Fascia, Scalp	0 Open	Z No Device	Z No Qualifier
1 Subcutaneous Tissue and Fascia, Face	3 Percutaneous		
4 Subcutaneous Tissue and Fascia, Right Neck	X External		
5 Subcutaneous Tissue and Fascia, Left Neck			
6 Subcutaneous Tissue and Fascia, Chest			
7 Subcutaneous Tissue and Fascia, Back			
8 Subcutaneous Tissue and Fascia, Abdomen			
9 Subcutaneous Tissue and Fascia, Buttock			
B Subcutaneous Tissue and Fascia, Perineum			
C Subcutaneous Tissue and Fascia, Pelvic Region			
D Subcutaneous Tissue and Fascia, Right Upper Arm			
F Subcutaneous Tissue and Fascia, Left Upper Arm			
G Subcutaneous Tissue and Fascia, Right Lower Arm			
H Subcutaneous Tissue and Fascia, Left Lower Arm			
J Subcutaneous Tissue and Fascia, Right Hand			
K Subcutaneous Tissue and Fascia, Left Hand			
L Subcutaneous Tissue and Fascia, Right Upper Leg			
M Subcutaneous Tissue and Fascia, Left Upper Leg			
N Subcutaneous Tissue and Fascia, Right Lower Leg			
P Subcutaneous Tissue and Fascia, Left Lower Leg			
Q Subcutaneous Tissue and Fascia, Right Foot			
R Subcutaneous Tissue and Fascia, Left Foot			

0 **Medical and Surgical**
J **Subcutaneous Tissue and Fascia**
P **Removal:** Taking out or off a device from a body part

Body Part	Approach	Device	Qualifier
Character 4	Character 5	Character 6	Character 7
S Subcutaneous Tissue and Fascia, Head and Neck	**0** Open **3** Percutaneous	**0** Drainage Device **1** Radioactive Element **3** Infusion Device **7** Autologous Tissue Substitute **J** Synthetic Substitute **K** Nonautologous Tissue Substitute **N** Tissue Expander **Y** Other Device	**Z** No Qualifier
S Subcutaneous Tissue and Fascia, Head and Neck	**X** External	**0** Drainage Device **1** Radioactive Element **3** Infusion Device	**Z** No Qualifier
T Subcutaneous Tissue and Fascia, Trunk **HAC**	**0** Open **3** Percutaneous	**0** Drainage Device **1** Radioactive Element **2** Monitoring Device **3** Infusion Device **7** Autologous Tissue Substitute **F** Subcutaneous Defibrillator Lead **H** Contraceptive Device **J** Synthetic Substitute **K** Nonautologous Tissue Substitute **M** Stimulator Generator **N** Tissue Expander **P** Cardiac Rhythm Related Device **V** Infusion Device, Pump **W** Vascular Access Device, Totally Implantable **X** Vascular Access Device, Tunneled **Y** Other Device	**Z** No Qualifier
T Subcutaneous Tissue and Fascia, Trunk	**X** External	**0** Drainage Device **1** Radioactive Element **2** Monitoring Device **3** Infusion Device **H** Contraceptive Device **V** Infusion Device, Pump **X** Vascular Access Device, Tunneled	**Z** No Qualifier
V Subcutaneous Tissue and Fascia, Upper Extremity **W** Subcutaneous Tissue and Fascia, Lower Extremity	**0** Open **3** Percutaneous	**0** Drainage Device **1** Radioactive Element **3** Infusion Device **7** Autologous Tissue Substitute **H** Contraceptive Device **J** Synthetic Substitute **K** Nonautologous Tissue Substitute **N** Tissue Expander **V** Infusion Device, Pump **W** Vascular Access Device, Totally Implantable **X** Vascular Access Device, Tunneled **Y** Other Device	**Z** No Qualifier
V Subcutaneous Tissue and Fascia, Upper Extremity **W** Subcutaneous Tissue and Fascia, Lower Extremity	**X** External	**0** Drainage Device **1** Radioactive Element **3** Infusion Device **H** Contraceptive Device **V** Infusion Device, Pump **X** Vascular Access Device, Tunneled	**Z** No Qualifier

HAC 0JPT0FZ   0JPT0PZ   0JPT3FZ   0JPT3PZ
Surgical site infection (SSI) following cardiac implantable electronic device (CIED) procedures and secondary diagnosis K68.11, T81.40XA, T81.41XA, T81.42XA, T81.43XA, T81.44XA, T81.49XA, T82.6XXA, T82.7XXA.

LC Limited Coverage   **NC** Noncovered   **HAC** HAC-associated Procedure   **CC** Combination Cluster - See Appendix G for code lists
DRG Non-OR-Affecting MS-DRG Assignment   New/Revised Text in **Orange**   ♂ Male   ♀ Female

0   **Medical and Surgical**
J   **Subcutaneous Tissue and Fascia**
Q   **Repair:** Restoring, to the extent possible, a body part to its normal anatomic structure and function

Body Part	Approach	Device	Qualifier
Character 4	**Character 5**	**Character 6**	**Character 7**
0 Subcutaneous Tissue and Fascia, Scalp	**0** Open	**Z** No Device	**Z** No Qualifier
1 Subcutaneous Tissue and Fascia, Face	**3** Percutaneous		
4 Subcutaneous Tissue and Fascia, Right Neck			
5 Subcutaneous Tissue and Fascia, Left Neck			
6 Subcutaneous Tissue and Fascia, Chest			
7 Subcutaneous Tissue and Fascia, Back			
8 Subcutaneous Tissue and Fascia, Abdomen			
9 Subcutaneous Tissue and Fascia, Buttock			
B Subcutaneous Tissue and Fascia, Perineum			
C Subcutaneous Tissue and Fascia, Pelvic Region			
D Subcutaneous Tissue and Fascia, Right Upper Arm			
F Subcutaneous Tissue and Fascia, Left Upper Arm			
G Subcutaneous Tissue and Fascia, Right Lower Arm			
H Subcutaneous Tissue and Fascia, Left Lower Arm			
J Subcutaneous Tissue and Fascia, Right Hand			
K Subcutaneous Tissue and Fascia, Left Hand			
L Subcutaneous Tissue and Fascia, Right Upper Leg			
M Subcutaneous Tissue and Fascia, Left Upper Leg			
N Subcutaneous Tissue and Fascia, Right Lower Leg			
P Subcutaneous Tissue and Fascia, Left Lower Leg			
Q Subcutaneous Tissue and Fascia, Right Foot			
R Subcutaneous Tissue and Fascia, Left Foot			

LC Limited Coverage   **NC** Noncovered   **HAC** HAC-associated Procedure   **CC** Combination Cluster - See Appendix G for code lists
DRG Non-OR-Affecting MS-DRG Assignment   New/Revised Text in **Orange**   ♂ Male   ♀ Female

404   **2021 ICD-10-PCS**

0 **Medical and Surgical**
J **Subcutaneous Tissue and Fascia**
R **Replacement:** Putting in or on biological or synthetic material that physically takes the place and/or function of all or a portion of a body part

Body Part	Approach	Device	Qualifier
Character 4	Character 5	Character 6	Character 7
0 Subcutaneous Tissue and Fascia, Scalp **1** Subcutaneous Tissue and Fascia, Face **4** Subcutaneous Tissue and Fascia, Right Neck **5** Subcutaneous Tissue and Fascia, Left Neck **6** Subcutaneous Tissue and Fascia, Chest **7** Subcutaneous Tissue and Fascia, Back **8** Subcutaneous Tissue and Fascia, Abdomen **9** Subcutaneous Tissue and Fascia, Buttock **B** Subcutaneous Tissue and Fascia, Perineum **C** Subcutaneous Tissue and Fascia, Pelvic Region **D** Subcutaneous Tissue and Fascia, Right Upper Arm **F** Subcutaneous Tissue and Fascia, Left Upper Arm **G** Subcutaneous Tissue and Fascia, Right Lower Arm **H** Subcutaneous Tissue and Fascia, Left Lower Arm **J** Subcutaneous Tissue and Fascia, Right Hand **K** Subcutaneous Tissue and Fascia, Left Hand **L** Subcutaneous Tissue and Fascia, Right Upper Leg **M** Subcutaneous Tissue and Fascia, Left Upper Leg **N** Subcutaneous Tissue and Fascia, Right Lower Leg **P** Subcutaneous Tissue and Fascia, Left Lower Leg **Q** Subcutaneous Tissue and Fascia, Right Foot **R** Subcutaneous Tissue and Fascia, Left Foot	**0** Open **3** Percutaneous	**7** Autologous Tissue Substitute **J** Synthetic Substitute **K** Nonautologous Tissue Substitute	**Z** No Qualifier

EC Limited Coverage   **NC** Noncovered   **HAC** HAC-associated Procedure   **CC** Combination Cluster - See Appendix G for code lists
DRG Non-OR-Affecting MS-DRG Assignment   New/Revised Text in **Orange**   ♂ Male   ♀ Female

2021 ICD-10-PCS

405

0 **Medical and Surgical**
J **Subcutaneous Tissue and Fascia**
U **Supplement:** Putting in or on biological or synthetic material that physically reinforces and/or augments the function of a portion of a body part

Body Part	Approach	Device	Qualifier
Character 4	Character 5	Character 6	Character 7
0 Subcutaneous Tissue and Fascia, Scalp	0 Open	7 Autologous Tissue Substitute	Z No Qualifier
1 Subcutaneous Tissue and Fascia, Face	3 Percutaneous	J Synthetic Substitute	
4 Subcutaneous Tissue and Fascia, Right Neck		K Nonautologous Tissue Substitute	
5 Subcutaneous Tissue and Fascia, Left Neck			
6 Subcutaneous Tissue and Fascia, Chest			
7 Subcutaneous Tissue and Fascia, Back			
8 Subcutaneous Tissue and Fascia, Abdomen			
9 Subcutaneous Tissue and Fascia, Buttock			
B Subcutaneous Tissue and Fascia, Perineum			
C Subcutaneous Tissue and Fascia, Pelvic Region			
D Subcutaneous Tissue and Fascia, Right Upper Arm			
F Subcutaneous Tissue and Fascia, Left Upper Arm			
G Subcutaneous Tissue and Fascia, Right Lower Arm			
H Subcutaneous Tissue and Fascia, Left Lower Arm			
J Subcutaneous Tissue and Fascia, Right Hand			
K Subcutaneous Tissue and Fascia, Left Hand			
L Subcutaneous Tissue and Fascia, Right Upper Leg			
M Subcutaneous Tissue and Fascia, Left Upper Leg			
N Subcutaneous Tissue and Fascia, Right Lower Leg			
P Subcutaneous Tissue and Fascia, Left Lower Leg			
Q Subcutaneous Tissue and Fascia, Right Foot			
R Subcutaneous Tissue and Fascia, Left Foot			

LC Limited Coverage   **NC** Noncovered   **HAC** HAC-associated Procedure   **CC** Combination Cluster - See Appendix G for code lists
DRG Non-OR-Affecting MS-DRG Assignment   New/Revised Text in **Orange**   ♂ Male   ♀ Female

406

2021 ICD-10-PCS

0 **Medical and Surgical**
J **Subcutaneous Tissue and Fascia**
W **Revision:** Correcting, to the extent possible, a portion of a malfunctioning device or the position of a displaced device

Body Part	Approach	Device	Qualifier
Character 4	Character 5	Character 6	Character 7
S Subcutaneous Tissue and Fascia, Head and Neck ⓓⓡⓖ	0 Open 3 Percutaneous	0 Drainage Device 3 Infusion Device 7 Autologous Tissue Substitute J Synthetic Substitute K Nonautologous Tissue Substitute N Tissue Expander Y Other Device	Z No Qualifier
S Subcutaneous Tissue and Fascia, Head and Neck	X External	0 Drainage Device 3 Infusion Device 7 Autologous Tissue Substitute J Synthetic Substitute K Nonautologous Tissue Substitute N Tissue Expander	Z No Qualifier
T Subcutaneous Tissue and Fascia, Trunk ⒽⒶⒸ ⓓⓡⓖ	0 Open 3 Percutaneous	0 Drainage Device 2 Monitoring Device 3 Infusion Device 7 Autologous Tissue Substitute F Subcutaneous Defibrillator Lead H Contraceptive Device J Synthetic Substitute K Nonautologous Tissue Substitute M Stimulator Generator N Tissue Expander P Cardiac Rhythm Related Device V Infusion Device, Pump W Vascular Access Device, Totally Implantable X Vascular Access Device, Tunneled Y Other Device	Z No Qualifier
T Subcutaneous Tissue and Fascia, Trunk ⓓⓡⓖ	X External	0 Drainage Device 2 Monitoring Device 3 Infusion Device 7 Autologous Tissue Substitute F Subcutaneous Defibrillator Lead H Contraceptive Device J Synthetic Substitute K Nonautologous Tissue Substitute M Stimulator Generator N Tissue Expander P Cardiac Rhythm Related Device V Infusion Device, Pump W Vascular Access Device, Totally Implantable X Vascular Access Device, Tunneled	Z No Qualifier

0JW continued on next page

LC Limited Coverage   NC Noncovered   HAC HAC-associated Procedure   CC Combination Cluster - See Appendix G for code lists
ⓓⓡⓖ Non-OR-Affecting MS-DRG Assignment   New/Revised Text in **Orange**   ♂ Male   ♀ Female

0 Medical and Surgical
J Subcutaneous Tissue and Fascia

0JW continued from previous page

W Revision: Correcting, to the extent possible, a portion of a malfunctioning device or the position of a displaced device

Body Part	Approach	Device	Qualifier
Character 4	Character 5	Character 6	Character 7
V Subcutaneous Tissue and Fascia, Upper Extremity ᴰᴿᴳ **W** Subcutaneous Tissue and Fascia, Lower Extremity ᴰᴿᴳ	**0** Open **3** Percutaneous	**0** Drainage Device **3** Infusion Device **7** Autologous Tissue Substitute **H** Contraceptive Device **J** Synthetic Substitute **K** Nonautologous Tissue Substitute **N** Tissue Expander **V** Infusion Device, Pump **W** Vascular Access Device, Totally Implantable **X** Vascular Access Device, Tunneled **Y** Other Device	**Z** No Qualifier
V Subcutaneous Tissue and Fascia, Upper Extremity **W** Subcutaneous Tissue and Fascia, Lower Extremity	**X** External	**0** Drainage Device **3** Infusion Device **7** Autologous Tissue Substitute **H** Contraceptive Device **J** Synthetic Substitute **K** Nonautologous Tissue Substitute **N** Tissue Expander **V** Infusion Device, Pump **W** Vascular Access Device, Totally Implantable **X** Vascular Access Device, Tunneled	**Z** No Qualifier

ᴴᴬᶜ OJWT0FZ   OJWT0PZ   OJWT3FZ   OJWT3PZ

Surgical site infection (SSI) following cardiac implantable electronic device (CIED) procedures and secondary diagnosis K68.11, T81.40XA, T81.41XA, T81.42XA, T81.43XA, T81.44XA, T81.49XA, T82.6XXA, T82.7XXA.

ᴰᴿᴳ
OJWS00Z	OJWS03Z	OJWS07Z	OJWS0JZ	OJWS0KZ	OJWS0NZ	OJWS0YZ	OJWS30Z	OJWS33Z	OJWS37Z	OJWS3JZ	OJWS3KZ	OJWS3NZ
OJWS3YZ	OJWT00Z	OJWT03Z	OJWT07Z	OJWT0HZ	OJWT0JZ	OJWT0KZ	OJWT0MZ	OJWT0NZ	OJWT0VZ	OJWT0WZ	OJWT0XZ	OJWT30Z
OJWT33Z	OJWT37Z	OJWT3HZ	OJWT3JZ	OJWT3KZ	OJWT3MZ	OJWT3NZ	OJWT3VZ	OJWT3WZ	OJWT3XZ	OJWTXMZ	OJWV00Z	OJWV03Z
OJWV07Z	OJWV0HZ	OJWV0JZ	OJWV0KZ	OJWV0NZ	OJWV0VZ	OJWV0WZ	OJWV0XZ	OJWV0YZ	OJWV30Z	OJWV33Z	OJWV37Z	OJWV3HZ
OJWV3JZ	OJWV3KZ	OJWV3NZ	OJWV3VZ	OJWV3WZ	OJWV3XZ	OJWV3YZ	OJWW00Z	OJWW03Z	OJWW07Z	OJWW0HZ	OJWW0JZ	OJWW0KZ
OJWW0NZ	OJWW0VZ	OJWW0WZ	OJWW0XZ	OJWW0YZ	OJWW30Z	OJWW33Z	OJWW37Z	OJWW3HZ	OJWW3JZ	OJWW3KZ	OJWW3NZ	OJWW3VZ
OJWW3WZ	OJWW3XZ	OJWW3YZ										

ᴸᶜ Limited Coverage   ᴺᶜ Noncovered   ᴴᴬᶜ HAC-associated Procedure   ᶜᶜ Combination Cluster - See Appendix G for code lists
ᴰᴿᴳ Non-OR-Affecting MS-DRG Assignment   New/Revised Text in **Orange**   ♂ Male   ♀ Female

0 Medical and Surgical
J Subcutaneous Tissue and Fascia
X Transfer: Moving, without taking out, all or a portion of a body part to another location to take over the function of all or a portion of a body part

Body Part	Approach	Device	Qualifier
Character 4	Character 5	Character 6	Character 7
0 Subcutaneous Tissue and Fascia, Scalp	**0** Open	**Z** No Device	**B** Skin and Subcutaneous Tissue
1 Subcutaneous Tissue and Fascia, Face	**3** Percutaneous		**C** Skin, Subcutaneous Tissue and Fascia
4 Subcutaneous Tissue and Fascia, Right Neck			**Z** No Qualifier
5 Subcutaneous Tissue and Fascia, Left Neck			
6 Subcutaneous Tissue and Fascia, Chest			
7 Subcutaneous Tissue and Fascia, Back			
8 Subcutaneous Tissue and Fascia, Abdomen			
9 Subcutaneous Tissue and Fascia, Buttock			
B Subcutaneous Tissue and Fascia, Perineum			
C Subcutaneous Tissue and Fascia, Pelvic Region			
D Subcutaneous Tissue and Fascia, Right Upper Arm			
F Subcutaneous Tissue and Fascia, Left Upper Arm			
G Subcutaneous Tissue and Fascia, Right Lower Arm			
H Subcutaneous Tissue and Fascia, Left Lower Arm			
J Subcutaneous Tissue and Fascia, Right Hand			
K Subcutaneous Tissue and Fascia, Left Hand			
L Subcutaneous Tissue and Fascia, Right Upper Leg			
M Subcutaneous Tissue and Fascia, Left Upper Leg			
N Subcutaneous Tissue and Fascia, Right Lower Leg			
P Subcutaneous Tissue and Fascia, Left Lower Leg			
Q Subcutaneous Tissue and Fascia, Right Foot			
R Subcutaneous Tissue and Fascia, Left Foot			

NOTES

Muscles 0K2-0KX

0 **Medical and Surgical**
K **Muscles**
2 **Change:** Taking out or off a device from a body part and putting back an identical or similar device in or on the same body part without cutting or puncturing the skin or a mucous membrane

Body Part	Approach	Device	Qualifier
Character 4	Character 5	Character 6	Character 7
X Upper Muscle **Y** Lower Muscle	**X** External	**0** Drainage Device **Y** Other Device	**Z** No Qualifier

0 **Medical and Surgical**
K **Muscles**
5 **Destruction:** Physical eradication of all or a portion of a body part by the direct use of energy, force, or a destructive agent

Body Part	Approach	Device	Qualifier
Character 4	Character 5	Character 6	Character 7
0 Head Muscle **1** Facial Muscle **2** Neck Muscle, Right **3** Neck Muscle, Left **4** Tongue, Palate, Pharynx Muscle **5** Shoulder Muscle, Right **6** Shoulder Muscle, Left **7** Upper Arm Muscle, Right **8** Upper Arm Muscle, Left **9** Lower Arm and Wrist Muscle, Right **B** Lower Arm and Wrist Muscle, Left **C** Hand Muscle, Right **D** Hand Muscle, Left **F** Trunk Muscle, Right **G** Trunk Muscle, Left **H** Thorax Muscle, Right **J** Thorax Muscle, Left **K** Abdomen Muscle, Right **L** Abdomen Muscle, Left **M** Perineum Muscle **N** Hip Muscle, Right **P** Hip Muscle, Left **Q** Upper Leg Muscle, Right **R** Upper Leg Muscle, Left **S** Lower Leg Muscle, Right **T** Lower Leg Muscle, Left **V** Foot Muscle, Right **W** Foot Muscle, Left	**0** Open **3** Percutaneous **4** Percutaneous Endoscopic	**Z** No Device	**Z** No Qualifier

Non-OR-Affecting MS-DRG Assignment   New/Revised Text in **Orange**   ♂ Male   ♀ Female

0 **Medical and Surgical**
K **Muscles**
8 **Division:** Cutting into a body part, without draining fluids and/or gases from the body part, in order to separate or transect a body part

Body Part	Approach	Device	Qualifier
Character 4	Character 5	Character 6	Character 7
0 Head Muscle 1 Facial Muscle 2 Neck Muscle, Right 3 Neck Muscle, Left 4 Tongue, Palate, Pharynx Muscle 5 Shoulder Muscle, Right 6 Shoulder Muscle, Left 7 Upper Arm Muscle, Right 8 Upper Arm Muscle, Left 9 Lower Arm and Wrist Muscle, Right B Lower Arm and Wrist Muscle, Left C Hand Muscle, Right D Hand Muscle, Left F Trunk Muscle, Right G Trunk Muscle, Left H Thorax Muscle, Right J Thorax Muscle, Left K Abdomen Muscle, Right L Abdomen Muscle, Left M Perineum Muscle N Hip Muscle, Right P Hip Muscle, Left Q Upper Leg Muscle, Right R Upper Leg Muscle, Left S Lower Leg Muscle, Right T Lower Leg Muscle, Left V Foot Muscle, Right W Foot Muscle, Left	0 Open 3 Percutaneous 4 Percutaneous Endoscopic	Z No Device	Z No Qualifier

LC Limited Coverage   NC Noncovered   HAC HAC-associated Procedure   CC Combination Cluster - See Appendix G for code lists
DRG Non-OR-Affecting MS-DRG Assignment   New/Revised Text in Orange   ♂ Male   ♀ Female

412

2021 ICD-10-PCS

0   **Medical and Surgical**
K   **Muscles**
9   **Drainage:** Taking or letting out fluids and/or gases from a body part

Body Part		Approach		Device		Qualifier	
Character 4		**Character 5**		**Character 6**		**Character 7**	
0	Head Muscle	**0**	Open	**0**	Drainage Device	**Z**	No Qualifier
1	Facial Muscle	**3**	Percutaneous				
2	Neck Muscle, Right	**4**	Percutaneous Endoscopic				
3	Neck Muscle, Left						
4	Tongue, Palate, Pharynx Muscle						
5	Shoulder Muscle, Right						
6	Shoulder Muscle, Left						
7	Upper Arm Muscle, Right						
8	Upper Arm Muscle, Left						
9	Lower Arm and Wrist Muscle, Right						
B	Lower Arm and Wrist Muscle, Left						
C	Hand Muscle, Right						
D	Hand Muscle, Left						
F	Trunk Muscle, Right						
G	Trunk Muscle, Left						
H	Thorax Muscle, Right						
J	Thorax Muscle, Left						
K	Abdomen Muscle, Right						
L	Abdomen Muscle, Left						
M	Perineum Muscle						
N	Hip Muscle, Right						
P	Hip Muscle, Left						
Q	Upper Leg Muscle, Right						
R	Upper Leg Muscle, Left						
S	Lower Leg Muscle, Right						
T	Lower Leg Muscle, Left						
V	Foot Muscle, Right						
W	Foot Muscle, Left						
0	Head Muscle	**0**	Open	**Z**	No Device	**X**	Diagnostic
1	Facial Muscle	**3**	Percutaneous			**Z**	No Qualifier
2	Neck Muscle, Right	**4**	Percutaneous Endoscopic				
3	Neck Muscle, Left						
4	Tongue, Palate, Pharynx Muscle						
5	Shoulder Muscle, Right						
6	Shoulder Muscle, Left						
7	Upper Arm Muscle, Right						
8	Upper Arm Muscle, Left						
9	Lower Arm and Wrist Muscle, Right						
B	Lower Arm and Wrist Muscle, Left						
C	Hand Muscle, Right						
D	Hand Muscle, Left						
F	Trunk Muscle, Right						
G	Trunk Muscle, Left						
H	Thorax Muscle, Right						
J	Thorax Muscle, Left						
K	Abdomen Muscle, Right						
L	Abdomen Muscle, Left						
M	Perineum Muscle						
N	Hip Muscle, Right						
P	Hip Muscle, Left						
Q	Upper Leg Muscle, Right						
R	Upper Leg Muscle, Left						
S	Lower Leg Muscle, Right						
T	Lower Leg Muscle, Left						
V	Foot Muscle, Right						
W	Foot Muscle, Left						

0 Medical and Surgical
K Muscles
B **Excision:** Cutting out or off, without replacement, a portion of a body part

Body Part	Approach	Device	Qualifier
Character 4	**Character 5**	**Character 6**	**Character 7**
0 Head Muscle	0 Open	Z No Device	X Diagnostic
1 Facial Muscle	3 Percutaneous		Z No Qualifier
2 Neck Muscle, Right	4 Percutaneous Endoscopic		
3 Neck Muscle, Left			
4 Tongue, Palate, Pharynx Muscle			
5 Shoulder Muscle, Right			
6 Shoulder Muscle, Left			
7 Upper Arm Muscle, Right			
8 Upper Arm Muscle, Left			
9 Lower Arm and Wrist Muscle, Right			
B Lower Arm and Wrist Muscle, Left			
C Hand Muscle, Right			
D Hand Muscle, Left			
F Trunk Muscle, Right			
G Trunk Muscle, Left			
H Thorax Muscle, Right			
J Thorax Muscle, Left			
K Abdomen Muscle, Right			
L Abdomen Muscle, Left			
M Perineum Muscle			
N Hip Muscle, Right			
P Hip Muscle, Left			
Q Upper Leg Muscle, Right			
R Upper Leg Muscle, Left			
S Lower Leg Muscle, Right			
T Lower Leg Muscle, Left			
V Foot Muscle, Right			
W Foot Muscle, Left			

0 Medical and Surgical
K Muscles
C **Extirpation:** Taking or cutting out solid matter from a body part

Body Part	Approach	Device	Qualifier
Character 4	**Character 5**	**Character 6**	**Character 7**
0 Head Muscle	0 Open	Z No Device	Z No Qualifier
1 Facial Muscle	3 Percutaneous		
2 Neck Muscle, Right	4 Percutaneous Endoscopic		
3 Neck Muscle, Left			
4 Tongue, Palate, Pharynx Muscle			
5 Shoulder Muscle, Right			
6 Shoulder Muscle, Left			
7 Upper Arm Muscle, Right			
8 Upper Arm Muscle, Left			
9 Lower Arm and Wrist Muscle, Right			
B Lower Arm and Wrist Muscle, Left			
C Hand Muscle, Right			
D Hand Muscle, Left			
F Trunk Muscle, Right			
G Trunk Muscle, Left			
H Thorax Muscle, Right			
J Thorax Muscle, Left			
K Abdomen Muscle, Right			
L Abdomen Muscle, Left			
M Perineum Muscle			
N Hip Muscle, Right			
P Hip Muscle, Left			
Q Upper Leg Muscle, Right			
R Upper Leg Muscle, Left			
S Lower Leg Muscle, Right			
T Lower Leg Muscle, Left			
V Foot Muscle, Right			
W Foot Muscle, Left			

LC Limited Coverage   **NC** Noncovered   **HAC** HAC-associated Procedure   **CC** Combination Cluster - See Appendix G for code lists
DRG Non-OR-Affecting MS-DRG Assignment   New/Revised Text in **Orange**   ♂ Male   ♀ Female

414

2021 ICD-10-PCS

0 **Medical and Surgical**
K **Muscles**
D **Extraction:** Pulling or stripping out or off all or a portion of a body part by the use of force

Body Part	Approach	Device	Qualifier
Character 4	Character 5	Character 6	Character 7
0 Head Muscle	0 Open	Z No Device	Z No Qualifier
1 Facial Muscle			
2 Neck Muscle, Right			
3 Neck Muscle, Left			
4 Tongue, Palate, Pharynx Muscle			
5 Shoulder Muscle, Right			
6 Shoulder Muscle, Left			
7 Upper Arm Muscle, Right			
8 Upper Arm Muscle, Left			
9 Lower Arm and Wrist Muscle, Right			
B Lower Arm and Wrist Muscle, Left			
C Hand Muscle, Right			
D Hand Muscle, Left			
F Trunk Muscle, Right			
G Trunk Muscle, Left			
H Thorax Muscle, Right			
J Thorax Muscle, Left			
K Abdomen Muscle, Right			
L Abdomen Muscle, Left			
M Perineum Muscle			
N Hip Muscle, Right			
P Hip Muscle, Left			
Q Upper Leg Muscle, Right			
R Upper Leg Muscle, Left			
S Lower Leg Muscle, Right			
T Lower Leg Muscle, Left			
V Foot Muscle, Right			
W Foot Muscle, Left			

0 **Medical and Surgical**
K **Muscles**
H **Insertion:** Putting in a nonbiological appliance that monitors, assists, performs, or prevents a physiological function but does not physically take the place of a body part

Body Part	Approach	Device	Qualifier
Character 4	Character 5	Character 6	Character 7
X Upper Muscle	0 Open	M Stimulator Lead	Z No Qualifier
Y Lower Muscle	3 Percutaneous	Y Other Device	
	4 Percutaneous Endoscopic		

0 **Medical and Surgical**
K **Muscles**
J **Inspection:** Visually and/or manually exploring a body part

Body Part	Approach	Device	Qualifier
Character 4	Character 5	Character 6	Character 7
X Upper Muscle	0 Open	Z No Device	Z No Qualifier
Y Lower Muscle	3 Percutaneous		
	4 Percutaneous Endoscopic		
	X External		

0 **Medical and Surgical**
K **Muscles**
M **Reattachment:** Putting back in or on all or a portion of a separated body part to its normal location or other suitable location

Body Part	Approach	Device	Qualifier
Character 4	Character 5	Character 6	Character 7
0 Head Muscle	0 Open	Z No Device	Z No Qualifier
1 Facial Muscle	4 Percutaneous Endoscopic		
2 Neck Muscle, Right			
3 Neck Muscle, Left			
4 Tongue, Palate, Pharynx Muscle			
5 Shoulder Muscle, Right			
6 Shoulder Muscle, Left			
7 Upper Arm Muscle, Right			
8 Upper Arm Muscle, Left			
9 Lower Arm and Wrist Muscle, Right			
B Lower Arm and Wrist Muscle, Left			
C Hand Muscle, Right			
D Hand Muscle, Left			
F Trunk Muscle, Right			
G Trunk Muscle, Left			
H Thorax Muscle, Right			
J Thorax Muscle, Left			
K Abdomen Muscle, Right			
L Abdomen Muscle, Left			
M Perineum Muscle			
N Hip Muscle, Right			
P Hip Muscle, Left			
Q Upper Leg Muscle, Right			
R Upper Leg Muscle, Left			
S Lower Leg Muscle, Right			
T Lower Leg Muscle, Left			
V Foot Muscle, Right			
W Foot Muscle, Left			

LC Limited Coverage   **NC** Noncovered   **HAC** HAC-associated Procedure   **CC** Combination Cluster - See Appendix G for code lists

DRG Non-OR-Affecting MS-DRG Assignment   New/Revised Text in **Orange**   ♂ Male   ♀ Female

416

2021 ICD-10-PCS

0 Medical and Surgical
K Muscles
N Release: Freeing a body part from an abnormal physical constraint by cutting or by the use of force

Body Part	Approach	Device	Qualifier
Character 4	Character 5	Character 6	Character 7
0 Head Muscle 1 Facial Muscle 2 Neck Muscle, Right 3 Neck Muscle, Left 4 Tongue, Palate, Pharynx Muscle 5 Shoulder Muscle, Right 6 Shoulder Muscle, Left 7 Upper Arm Muscle, Right 8 Upper Arm Muscle, Left 9 Lower Arm and Wrist Muscle, Right B Lower Arm and Wrist Muscle, Left C Hand Muscle, Right D Hand Muscle, Left F Trunk Muscle, Right G Trunk Muscle, Left H Thorax Muscle, Right J Thorax Muscle, Left K Abdomen Muscle, Right L Abdomen Muscle, Left M Perineum Muscle N Hip Muscle, Right P Hip Muscle, Left Q Upper Leg Muscle, Right R Upper Leg Muscle, Left S Lower Leg Muscle, Right T Lower Leg Muscle, Left V Foot Muscle, Right W Foot Muscle, Left	0 Open 3 Percutaneous 4 Percutaneous Endoscopic X External	Z No Device	Z No Qualifier

0 Medical and Surgical
K Muscles
P Removal: Taking out or off a device from a body part

Body Part	Approach	Device	Qualifier
Character 4	Character 5	Character 6	Character 7
X Upper Muscle Y Lower Muscle	0 Open 3 Percutaneous 4 Percutaneous Endoscopic	0 Drainage Device 7 Autologous Tissue Substitute J Synthetic Substitute K Nonautologous Tissue Substitute M Stimulator Lead Y Other Device	Z No Qualifier
X Upper Muscle Y Lower Muscle	X External	0 Drainage Device M Stimulator Lead	Z No Qualifier

0   Medical and Surgical
K   Muscles
Q   Repair: Restoring, to the extent possible, a body part to its normal anatomic structure and function

Body Part	Approach	Device	Qualifier
Character 4	Character 5	Character 6	Character 7
0 Head Muscle 1 Facial Muscle 2 Neck Muscle, Right 3 Neck Muscle, Left 4 Tongue, Palate, Pharynx Muscle 5 Shoulder Muscle, Right 6 Shoulder Muscle, Left 7 Upper Arm Muscle, Right 8 Upper Arm Muscle, Left 9 Lower Arm and Wrist Muscle, Right B Lower Arm and Wrist Muscle, Left C Hand Muscle, Right D Hand Muscle, Left F Trunk Muscle, Right G Trunk Muscle, Left H Thorax Muscle, Right J Thorax Muscle, Left K Abdomen Muscle, Right L Abdomen Muscle, Left M Perineum Muscle N Hip Muscle, Right P Hip Muscle, Left Q Upper Leg Muscle, Right R Upper Leg Muscle, Left S Lower Leg Muscle, Right T Lower Leg Muscle, Left V Foot Muscle, Right W Foot Muscle, Left	0 Open 3 Percutaneous 4 Percutaneous Endoscopic	Z No Device	Z No Qualifier

0   Medical and Surgical
K   Muscles
R   Replacement: Putting in or on biological or synthetic material that physically takes the place and/or function of all or a portion of a body part

Body Part	Approach	Device	Qualifier
Character 4	Character 5	Character 6	Character 7
0 Head Muscle 1 Facial Muscle 2 Neck Muscle, Right 3 Neck Muscle, Left 4 Tongue, Palate, Pharynx Muscle 5 Shoulder Muscle, Right 6 Shoulder Muscle, Left 7 Upper Arm Muscle, Right 8 Upper Arm Muscle, Left 9 Lower Arm and Wrist Muscle, Right B Lower Arm and Wrist Muscle, Left C Hand Muscle, Right D Hand Muscle, Left F Trunk Muscle, Right G Trunk Muscle, Left H Thorax Muscle, Right J Thorax Muscle, Left K Abdomen Muscle, Right L Abdomen Muscle, Left M Perineum Muscle N Hip Muscle, Right P Hip Muscle, Left Q Upper Leg Muscle, Right R Upper Leg Muscle, Left S Lower Leg Muscle, Right T Lower Leg Muscle, Left V Foot Muscle, Right W Foot Muscle, Left	0 Open 4 Percutaneous Endoscopic	7 Autologous Tissue Substitute J Synthetic Substitute K Nonautologous Tissue Substitute	Z No Qualifier

0 Medical and Surgical

K Muscles

S Reposition: Moving to its normal location, or other suitable location, all or a portion of a body part

Body Part	Approach	Device	Qualifier
Character 4	Character 5	Character 6	Character 7
0 Head Muscle 1 Facial Muscle 2 Neck Muscle, Right 3 Neck Muscle, Left 4 Tongue, Palate, Pharynx Muscle 5 Shoulder Muscle, Right 6 Shoulder Muscle, Left 7 Upper Arm Muscle, Right 8 Upper Arm Muscle, Left 9 Lower Arm and Wrist Muscle, Right B Lower Arm and Wrist Muscle, Left C Hand Muscle, Right D Hand Muscle, Left F Trunk Muscle, Right G Trunk Muscle, Left H Thorax Muscle, Right J Thorax Muscle, Left K Abdomen Muscle, Right L Abdomen Muscle, Left M Perineum Muscle N Hip Muscle, Right P Hip Muscle, Left Q Upper Leg Muscle, Right R Upper Leg Muscle, Left S Lower Leg Muscle, Right T Lower Leg Muscle, Left V Foot Muscle, Right W Foot Muscle, Left	0 Open 4 Percutaneous Endoscopic	Z No Device	Z No Qualifier

0 Medical and Surgical

K Muscles

T Resection: Cutting out or off, without replacement, all of a body part

Body Part	Approach	Device	Qualifier
Character 4	Character 5	Character 6	Character 7
0 Head Muscle 1 Facial Muscle 2 Neck Muscle, Right 3 Neck Muscle, Left 4 Tongue, Palate, Pharynx Muscle 5 Shoulder Muscle, Right 6 Shoulder Muscle, Left 7 Upper Arm Muscle, Right 8 Upper Arm Muscle, Left 9 Lower Arm and Wrist Muscle, Right B Lower Arm and Wrist Muscle, Left C Hand Muscle, Right D Hand Muscle, Left F Trunk Muscle, Right G Trunk Muscle, Left H Thorax Muscle, Right ᴄᴄ J Thorax Muscle, Left ᴄᴄ K Abdomen Muscle, Right L Abdomen Muscle, Left M Perineum Muscle N Hip Muscle, Right P Hip Muscle, Left Q Upper Leg Muscle, Right R Upper Leg Muscle, Left S Lower Leg Muscle, Right T Lower Leg Muscle, Left V Foot Muscle, Right W Foot Muscle, Left	0 Open 4 Percutaneous Endoscopic	Z No Device	Z No Qualifier

ᴄᴄ 0KTH0ZZ   0KTJ0ZZ

ᴸᴄ Limited Coverage   ᴺᶜ Noncovered   ᴴᴬᶜ HAC-associated Procedure   ᴄᴄ Combination Cluster - See Appendix G for code lists
ᴰᴿᴳ Non-OR-Affecting MS-DRG Assignment   New/Revised Text in **Orange**   ♂ Male   ♀ Female

0 Medical and Surgical
K Muscles
U Supplement: Putting in or on biological or synthetic material that physically reinforces and/or augments the function of a portion of a body part

Body Part	Approach	Device	Qualifier
Character 4	Character 5	Character 6	Character 7
0 Head Muscle **1** Facial Muscle **2** Neck Muscle, Right **3** Neck Muscle, Left **4** Tongue, Palate, Pharynx Muscle **5** Shoulder Muscle, Right **6** Shoulder Muscle, Left **7** Upper Arm Muscle, Right **8** Upper Arm Muscle, Left **9** Lower Arm and Wrist Muscle, Right **B** Lower Arm and Wrist Muscle, Left **C** Hand Muscle, Right **D** Hand Muscle, Left **F** Trunk Muscle, Right **G** Trunk Muscle, Left **H** Thorax Muscle, Right **J** Thorax Muscle, Left **K** Abdomen Muscle, Right **L** Abdomen Muscle, Left **M** Perineum Muscle **N** Hip Muscle, Right **P** Hip Muscle, Left **Q** Upper Leg Muscle, Right **R** Upper Leg Muscle, Left **S** Lower Leg Muscle, Right **T** Lower Leg Muscle, Left **V** Foot Muscle, Right **W** Foot Muscle, Left	**0** Open **4** Percutaneous Endoscopic	**7** Autologous Tissue Substitute **J** Synthetic Substitute **K** Nonautologous Tissue Substitute	**Z** No Qualifier

0 Medical and Surgical
K Muscles
W Revision: Correcting, to the extent possible, a portion of a malfunctioning device or the position of a displaced device

Body Part	Approach	Device	Qualifier
Character 4	Character 5	Character 6	Character 7
X Upper Muscle **Y** Lower Muscle	**0** Open **3** Percutaneous **4** Percutaneous Endoscopic	**0** Drainage Device **7** Autologous Tissue Substitute **J** Synthetic Substitute **K** Nonautologous Tissue Substitute **M** Stimulator Lead **Y** Other Device	**Z** No Qualifier
X Upper Muscle **Y** Lower Muscle	**X** External	**0** Drainage Device **7** Autologous Tissue Substitute **J** Synthetic Substitute **K** Nonautologous Tissue Substitute **M** Stimulator Lead	**Z** No Qualifier

0 **Medical and Surgical**
K **Muscles**
X **Transfer:** Moving, without taking out, all or a portion of a body part to another location to take over the function of all or a portion of a body part

Body Part	Approach	Device	Qualifier
Character 4	Character 5	Character 6	Character 7
0 Head Muscle 1 Facial Muscle 2 Neck Muscle, Right 3 Neck Muscle, Left 4 Tongue, Palate, Pharynx Muscle 5 Shoulder Muscle, Right 6 Shoulder Muscle, Left 7 Upper Arm Muscle, Right 8 Upper Arm Muscle, Left 9 Lower Arm and Wrist Muscle, Right B Lower Arm and Wrist Muscle, Left C Hand Muscle, Right D Hand Muscle, Left H Thorax Muscle, Right J Thorax Muscle, Left M Perineum Muscle N Hip Muscle, Right P Hip Muscle, Left Q Upper Leg Muscle, Right R Upper Leg Muscle, Left S Lower Leg Muscle, Right T Lower Leg Muscle, Left V Foot Muscle, Right W Foot Muscle, Left	0 Open 4 Percutaneous Endoscopic	Z No Device	0 Skin 1 Subcutaneous Tissue 2 Skin and Subcutaneous Tissue Z No Qualifier
F Trunk Muscle, Right G Trunk Muscle, Left	0 Open 4 Percutaneous Endoscopic	Z No Device	0 Skin 1 Subcutaneous Tissue 2 Skin and Subcutaneous Tissue 5 Latissimus Dorsi Myocutaneous Flap 7 Deep Inferior Epigastric Artery Perforator Flap 8 Superficial Inferior Epigastric Artery Flap 9 Gluteal Artery Perforator Flap Z No Qualifier
K Abdomen Muscle, Right L Abdomen Muscle, Left	0 Open 4 Percutaneous Endoscopic	Z No Device	0 Skin 1 Subcutaneous Tissue 2 Skin and Subcutaneous Tissue 6 Transverse Rectus Abdominis Myocutaneous Flap Z No Qualifier

LC Limited Coverage   **NC** Noncovered   **HAC** HAC-associated Procedure   **CC** Combination Cluster - See Appendix G for code lists
DRG Non-OR-Affecting MS-DRG Assignment   New/Revised Text in **Orange**   ♂ Male   ♀ Female

2021 ICD-10-PCS   **421**

MUSCLES 0K2-0KX

NOTES

0 **Medical and Surgical**
L **Tendons**
2 **Change:** Taking out or off a device from a body part and putting back an identical or similar device in or on the same body part without cutting or puncturing the skin or a mucous membrane

Body Part	Approach	Device	Qualifier
Character 4	Character 5	Character 6	Character 7
X Upper Tendon Y Lower Tendon	X External	0 Drainage Device Y Other Device	Z No Qualifier

0 **Medical and Surgical**
L **Tendons**
5 **Destruction:** Physical eradication of all or a portion of a body part by the direct use of energy, force, or a destructive agent

Body Part	Approach	Device	Qualifier
Character 4	Character 5	Character 6	Character 7
0 Head and Neck Tendon 1 Shoulder Tendon, Right 2 Shoulder Tendon, Left 3 Upper Arm Tendon, Right 4 Upper Arm Tendon, Left 5 Lower Arm and Wrist Tendon, Right 6 Lower Arm and Wrist Tendon, Left 7 Hand Tendon, Right 8 Hand Tendon, Left 9 Trunk Tendon, Right B Trunk Tendon, Left C Thorax Tendon, Right D Thorax Tendon, Left F Abdomen Tendon, Right G Abdomen Tendon, Left H Perineum Tendon J Hip Tendon, Right K Hip Tendon, Left L Upper Leg Tendon, Right M Upper Leg Tendon, Left N Lower Leg Tendon, Right P Lower Leg Tendon, Left Q Knee Tendon, Right R Knee Tendon, Left S Ankle Tendon, Right T Ankle Tendon, Left V Foot Tendon, Right W Foot Tendon, Left	0 Open 3 Percutaneous 4 Percutaneous Endoscopic	Z No Device	Z No Qualifier

LC Limited Coverage   **NC** Noncovered   **HAC** HAC-associated Procedure   **CC** Combination Cluster - See Appendix G for code lists
DRG Non-OR-Affecting MS-DRG Assignment   New/Revised Text in **Orange**   ♂ Male   ♀ Female

2021 ICD-10-PCS

423

0 **Medical and Surgical**
L **Tendons**
8 **Division:** Cutting into a body part, without draining fluids and/or gases from the body part, in order to separate or transect a body part

Body Part	Approach	Device	Qualifier
Character 4	Character 5	Character 6	Character 7
0 Head and Neck Tendon	0 Open	Z No Device	Z No Qualifier
1 Shoulder Tendon, Right	3 Percutaneous		
2 Shoulder Tendon, Left	4 Percutaneous Endoscopic		
3 Upper Arm Tendon, Right			
4 Upper Arm Tendon, Left			
5 Lower Arm and Wrist Tendon, Right			
6 Lower Arm and Wrist Tendon, Left			
7 Hand Tendon, Right			
8 Hand Tendon, Left			
9 Trunk Tendon, Right			
B Trunk Tendon, Left			
C Thorax Tendon, Right			
D Thorax Tendon, Left			
F Abdomen Tendon, Right			
G Abdomen Tendon, Left			
H Perineum Tendon			
J Hip Tendon, Right			
K Hip Tendon, Left			
L Upper Leg Tendon, Right			
M Upper Leg Tendon, Left			
N Lower Leg Tendon, Right			
P Lower Leg Tendon, Left			
Q Knee Tendon, Right			
R Knee Tendon, Left			
S Ankle Tendon, Right			
T Ankle Tendon, Left			
V Foot Tendon, Right			
W Foot Tendon, Left			

0 **Medical and Surgical**
L **Tendons**
9 **Drainage:** Taking or letting out fluids and/or gases from a body part

Body Part	Approach	Device	Qualifier
Character 4	Character 5	Character 6	Character 7
0 Head and Neck Tendon 1 Shoulder Tendon, Right 2 Shoulder Tendon, Left 3 Upper Arm Tendon, Right 4 Upper Arm Tendon, Left 5 Lower Arm and Wrist Tendon, Right 6 Lower Arm and Wrist Tendon, Left 7 Hand Tendon, Right 8 Hand Tendon, Left 9 Trunk Tendon, Right B Trunk Tendon, Left C Thorax Tendon, Right D Thorax Tendon, Left F Abdomen Tendon, Right G Abdomen Tendon, Left H Perineum Tendon J Hip Tendon, Right K Hip Tendon, Left L Upper Leg Tendon, Right M Upper Leg Tendon, Left N Lower Leg Tendon, Right P Lower Leg Tendon, Left Q Knee Tendon, Right R Knee Tendon, Left S Ankle Tendon, Right T Ankle Tendon, Left V Foot Tendon, Right W Foot Tendon, Left	0 Open 3 Percutaneous 4 Percutaneous Endoscopic	0 Drainage Device	Z No Qualifier
0 Head and Neck Tendon 1 Shoulder Tendon, Right 2 Shoulder Tendon, Left 3 Upper Arm Tendon, Right 4 Upper Arm Tendon, Left 5 Lower Arm and Wrist Tendon, Right 6 Lower Arm and Wrist Tendon, Left 7 Hand Tendon, Right 8 Hand Tendon, Left 9 Trunk Tendon, Right B Trunk Tendon, Left C Thorax Tendon, Right D Thorax Tendon, Left F Abdomen Tendon, Right G Abdomen Tendon, Left H Perineum Tendon J Hip Tendon, Right K Hip Tendon, Left L Upper Leg Tendon, Right M Upper Leg Tendon, Left N Lower Leg Tendon, Right P Lower Leg Tendon, Left Q Knee Tendon, Right R Knee Tendon, Left S Ankle Tendon, Right T Ankle Tendon, Left V Foot Tendon, Right W Foot Tendon, Left	0 Open 3 Percutaneous 4 Percutaneous Endoscopic	Z No Device	X Diagnostic Z No Qualifier

LC Limited Coverage **NC** Noncovered **HAC** HAC-associated Procedure **CC** Combination Cluster - See Appendix G for code lists
NR Non-OR-Affecting MS-DRG Assignment New/Revised Text in **Orange** ♂ Male ♀ Female

2021 ICD-10-PCS

425

TENDONS 0L2-0LX

0L9

0 **Medical and Surgical**
L **Tendons**
B **Excision:** Cutting out or off, without replacement, a portion of a body part

Body Part	Approach	Device	Qualifier
Character 4	Character 5	Character 6	Character 7
0 Head and Neck Tendon	**0** Open	**Z** No Device	**X** Diagnostic
1 Shoulder Tendon, Right	**3** Percutaneous		**Z** No Qualifier
2 Shoulder Tendon, Left	**4** Percutaneous Endoscopic		
3 Upper Arm Tendon, Right			
4 Upper Arm Tendon, Left			
5 Lower Arm and Wrist Tendon, Right			
6 Lower Arm and Wrist Tendon, Left			
7 Hand Tendon, Right			
8 Hand Tendon, Left			
9 Trunk Tendon, Right			
B Trunk Tendon, Left			
C Thorax Tendon, Right			
D Thorax Tendon, Left			
F Abdomen Tendon, Right			
G Abdomen Tendon, Left			
H Perineum Tendon			
J Hip Tendon, Right			
K Hip Tendon, Left			
L Upper Leg Tendon, Right			
M Upper Leg Tendon, Left			
N Lower Leg Tendon, Right			
P Lower Leg Tendon, Left			
Q Knee Tendon, Right			
R Knee Tendon, Left			
S Ankle Tendon, Right			
T Ankle Tendon, Left			
V Foot Tendon, Right			
W Foot Tendon, Left			

0 **Medical and Surgical**
L **Tendons**
C **Extirpation:** Taking or cutting out solid matter from a body part

Body Part	Approach	Device	Qualifier
Character 4	Character 5	Character 6	Character 7
0 Head and Neck Tendon	**0** Open	**Z** No Device	**Z** No Qualifier
1 Shoulder Tendon, Right	**3** Percutaneous		
2 Shoulder Tendon, Left	**4** Percutaneous Endoscopic		
3 Upper Arm Tendon, Right			
4 Upper Arm Tendon, Left			
5 Lower Arm and Wrist Tendon, Right			
6 Lower Arm and Wrist Tendon, Left			
7 Hand Tendon, Right			
8 Hand Tendon, Left			
9 Trunk Tendon, Right			
B Trunk Tendon, Left			
C Thorax Tendon, Right			
D Thorax Tendon, Left			
F Abdomen Tendon, Right			
G Abdomen Tendon, Left			
H Perineum Tendon			
J Hip Tendon, Right			
K Hip Tendon, Left			
L Upper Leg Tendon, Right			
M Upper Leg Tendon, Left			
N Lower Leg Tendon, Right			
P Lower Leg Tendon, Left			
Q Knee Tendon, Right			
R Knee Tendon, Left			
S Ankle Tendon, Right			
T Ankle Tendon, Left			
V Foot Tendon, Right			
W Foot Tendon, Left			

LC Limited Coverage   **NC** Noncovered   **HAC** HAC-associated Procedure   **CC** Combination Cluster - See Appendix G for code lists
DRG Non-OR-Affecting MS-DRG Assignment   New/Revised Text in **Orange**   ♂ Male   ♀ Female

426

2021 ICD-10-PCS

0   Medical and Surgical
L   Tendons
D   Extraction: Pulling or stripping out or off all or a portion of a body part by the use of force

Body Part	Approach	Device	Qualifier
Character 4	Character 5	Character 6	Character 7
0 Head and Neck Tendon **1** Shoulder Tendon, Right **2** Shoulder Tendon, Left **3** Upper Arm Tendon, Right **4** Upper Arm Tendon, Left **5** Lower Arm and Wrist Tendon, Right **6** Lower Arm and Wrist Tendon, Left **7** Hand Tendon, Right **8** Hand Tendon, Left **9** Trunk Tendon, Right **B** Trunk Tendon, Left **C** Thorax Tendon, Right **D** Thorax Tendon, Left **F** Abdomen Tendon, Right **G** Abdomen Tendon, Left **H** Perineum Tendon **J** Hip Tendon, Right **K** Hip Tendon, Left **L** Upper Leg Tendon, Right **M** Upper Leg Tendon, Left **N** Lower Leg Tendon, Right **P** Lower Leg Tendon, Left **Q** Knee Tendon, Right **R** Knee Tendon, Left **S** Ankle Tendon, Right **T** Ankle Tendon, Left **V** Foot Tendon, Right **W** Foot Tendon, Left	**0** Open	**Z** No Device	**Z** No Qualifier

0   Medical and Surgical
L   Tendons
H   Insertion: Putting in a nonbiological appliance that monitors, assists, performs, or prevents a physiological function but does not physically take the place of a body part

Body Part	Approach	Device	Qualifier
Character 4	Character 5	Character 6	Character 7
X Upper Tendon **Y** Lower Tendon	**0** Open **3** Percutaneous **4** Percutaneous Endoscopic	**Y** Other Device	**Z** No Qualifier

0   Medical and Surgical
L   Tendons
J   Inspection: Visually and/or manually exploring a body part

Body Part	Approach	Device	Qualifier
Character 4	Character 5	Character 6	Character 7
X Upper Tendon **Y** Lower Tendon	**0** Open **3** Percutaneous **4** Percutaneous Endoscopic **X** External	**Z** No Device	**Z** No Qualifier

LC Limited Coverage   **NC** Noncovered   **HAC** HAC-associated Procedure   **CC** Combination Cluster - See Appendix G for code lists
DRG Non-OR-Affecting MS-DRG Assignment   New/Revised Text in **Orange**   ♂ Male   ♀ Female

2021 ICD-10-PCS   **427**

0 **Medical and Surgical**
L **Tendons**
M **Reattachment:** Putting back in or on all or a portion of a separated body part to its normal location or other suitable location

Body Part	Approach	Device	Qualifier
Character 4	**Character 5**	**Character 6**	**Character 7**
0 Head and Neck Tendon	**0** Open	**Z** No Device	**Z** No Qualifier
1 Shoulder Tendon, Right	**4** Percutaneous Endoscopic		
2 Shoulder Tendon, Left			
3 Upper Arm Tendon, Right			
4 Upper Arm Tendon, Left			
5 Lower Arm and Wrist Tendon, Right			
6 Lower Arm and Wrist Tendon, Left			
7 Hand Tendon, Right			
8 Hand Tendon, Left			
9 Trunk Tendon, Right			
B Trunk Tendon, Left			
C Thorax Tendon, Right			
D Thorax Tendon, Left			
F Abdomen Tendon, Right			
G Abdomen Tendon, Left			
H Perineum Tendon			
J Hip Tendon, Right			
K Hip Tendon, Left			
L Upper Leg Tendon, Right			
M Upper Leg Tendon, Left			
N Lower Leg Tendon, Right			
P Lower Leg Tendon, Left			
Q Knee Tendon, Right			
R Knee Tendon, Left			
S Ankle Tendon, Right			
T Ankle Tendon, Left			
V Foot Tendon, Right			
W Foot Tendon, Left			

0   Medical and Surgical
L   Tendons
N   Release: Freeing a body part from an abnormal physical constraint by cutting or by the use of force

Body Part	Approach	Device	Qualifier
Character 4	Character 5	Character 6	Character 7
0 Head and Neck Tendon **1** Shoulder Tendon, Right **2** Shoulder Tendon, Left **3** Upper Arm Tendon, Right **4** Upper Arm Tendon, Left **5** Lower Arm and Wrist Tendon, Right **6** Lower Arm and Wrist Tendon, Left **7** Hand Tendon, Right **8** Hand Tendon, Left **9** Trunk Tendon, Right **B** Trunk Tendon, Left **C** Thorax Tendon, Right **D** Thorax Tendon, Left **F** Abdomen Tendon, Right **G** Abdomen Tendon, Left **H** Perineum Tendon **J** Hip Tendon, Right **K** Hip Tendon, Left **L** Upper Leg Tendon, Right **M** Upper Leg Tendon, Left **N** Lower Leg Tendon, Right **P** Lower Leg Tendon, Left **Q** Knee Tendon, Right **R** Knee Tendon, Left **S** Ankle Tendon, Right **T** Ankle Tendon, Left **V** Foot Tendon, Right **W** Foot Tendon, Left	**0** Open **3** Percutaneous **4** Percutaneous Endoscopic **X** External	**Z** No Device	**Z** No Qualifier

0   Medical and Surgical
L   Tendons
P   Removal: Taking out or off a device from a body part

Body Part	Approach	Device	Qualifier
Character 4	Character 5	Character 6	Character 7
X Upper Tendon **Y** Lower Tendon	**0** Open **3** Percutaneous **4** Percutaneous Endoscopic	**0** Drainage Device **7** Autologous Tissue Substitute **J** Synthetic Substitute **K** Nonautologous Tissue Substitute **Y** Other Device	**Z** No Qualifier
X Upper Tendon **Y** Lower Tendon	**X** External	**0** Drainage Device	**Z** No Qualifier

0 Medical and Surgical
L Tendons
Q Repair: Restoring, to the extent possible, a body part to its normal anatomic structure and function

Body Part	Approach	Device	Qualifier
Character 4	**Character 5**	**Character 6**	**Character 7**
0 Head and Neck Tendon	0 Open	Z No Device	Z No Qualifier
1 Shoulder Tendon, Right	3 Percutaneous		
2 Shoulder Tendon, Left	4 Percutaneous Endoscopic		
3 Upper Arm Tendon, Right			
4 Upper Arm Tendon, Left			
5 Lower Arm and Wrist Tendon, Right			
6 Lower Arm and Wrist Tendon, Left			
7 Hand Tendon, Right			
8 Hand Tendon, Left			
9 Trunk Tendon, Right			
B Trunk Tendon, Left			
C Thorax Tendon, Right			
D Thorax Tendon, Left			
F Abdomen Tendon, Right			
G Abdomen Tendon, Left			
H Perineum Tendon			
J Hip Tendon, Right			
K Hip Tendon, Left			
L Upper Leg Tendon, Right			
M Upper Leg Tendon, Left			
N Lower Leg Tendon, Right			
P Lower Leg Tendon, Left			
Q Knee Tendon, Right			
R Knee Tendon, Left			
S Ankle Tendon, Right			
T Ankle Tendon, Left			
V Foot Tendon, Right			
W Foot Tendon, Left			

0 Medical and Surgical
L Tendons
R Replacement: Putting in or on biological or synthetic material that physically takes the place and/or function of all or a portion of a body part

Body Part	Approach	Device	Qualifier
Character 4	**Character 5**	**Character 6**	**Character 7**
0 Head and Neck Tendon	0 Open	7 Autologous Tissue Substitute	Z No Qualifier
1 Shoulder Tendon, Right	4 Percutaneous Endoscopic	J Synthetic Substitute	
2 Shoulder Tendon, Left		K Nonautologous Tissue Substitute	
3 Upper Arm Tendon, Right			
4 Upper Arm Tendon, Left			
5 Lower Arm and Wrist Tendon, Right			
6 Lower Arm and Wrist Tendon, Left			
7 Hand Tendon, Right			
8 Hand Tendon, Left			
9 Trunk Tendon, Right			
B Trunk Tendon, Left			
C Thorax Tendon, Right			
D Thorax Tendon, Left			
F Abdomen Tendon, Right			
G Abdomen Tendon, Left			
H Perineum Tendon			
J Hip Tendon, Right			
K Hip Tendon, Left			
L Upper Leg Tendon, Right			
M Upper Leg Tendon, Left			
N Lower Leg Tendon, Right			
P Lower Leg Tendon, Left			
Q Knee Tendon, Right			
R Knee Tendon, Left			
S Ankle Tendon, Right			
T Ankle Tendon, Left			
V Foot Tendon, Right			
W Foot Tendon, Left			

LC Limited Coverage   NC Noncovered   HAC HAC-associated Procedure   CC Combination Cluster - See Appendix G for code lists
DRG Non-OR-Affecting MS-DRG Assignment   New/Revised Text in Orange   ♂ Male   ♀ Female

0 Medical and Surgical
L Tendons
S Reposition: Moving to its normal location, or other suitable location, all or a portion of a body part

Body Part	Approach	Device	Qualifier
Character 4	Character 5	Character 6	Character 7
0 Head and Neck Tendon	0 Open	Z No Device	Z No Qualifier
1 Shoulder Tendon, Right	4 Percutaneous Endoscopic		
2 Shoulder Tendon, Left			
3 Upper Arm Tendon, Right			
4 Upper Arm Tendon, Left			
5 Lower Arm and Wrist Tendon, Right			
6 Lower Arm and Wrist Tendon, Left			
7 Hand Tendon, Right			
8 Hand Tendon, Left			
9 Trunk Tendon, Right			
B Trunk Tendon, Left			
C Thorax Tendon, Right			
D Thorax Tendon, Left			
F Abdomen Tendon, Right			
G Abdomen Tendon, Left			
H Perineum Tendon			
J Hip Tendon, Right			
K Hip Tendon, Left			
L Upper Leg Tendon, Right			
M Upper Leg Tendon, Left			
N Lower Leg Tendon, Right			
P Lower Leg Tendon, Left			
Q Knee Tendon, Right			
R Knee Tendon, Left			
S Ankle Tendon, Right			
T Ankle Tendon, Left			
V Foot Tendon, Right			
W Foot Tendon, Left			

0 Medical and Surgical
L Tendons
T Resection: Cutting out or off, without replacement, all of a body part

Body Part	Approach	Device	Qualifier
Character 4	Character 5	Character 6	Character 7
0 Head and Neck Tendon	0 Open	Z No Device	Z No Qualifier
1 Shoulder Tendon, Right	4 Percutaneous Endoscopic		
2 Shoulder Tendon, Left			
3 Upper Arm Tendon, Right			
4 Upper Arm Tendon, Left			
5 Lower Arm and Wrist Tendon, Right			
6 Lower Arm and Wrist Tendon, Left			
7 Hand Tendon, Right			
8 Hand Tendon, Left			
9 Trunk Tendon, Right			
B Trunk Tendon, Left			
C Thorax Tendon, Right			
D Thorax Tendon, Left			
F Abdomen Tendon, Right			
G Abdomen Tendon, Left			
H Perineum Tendon			
J Hip Tendon, Right			
K Hip Tendon, Left			
L Upper Leg Tendon, Right			
M Upper Leg Tendon, Left			
N Lower Leg Tendon, Right			
P Lower Leg Tendon, Left			
Q Knee Tendon, Right			
R Knee Tendon, Left			
S Ankle Tendon, Right			
T Ankle Tendon, Left			
V Foot Tendon, Right			
W Foot Tendon, Left			

LC Limited Coverage   NC Noncovered   HAC HAC-associated Procedure   CC Combination Cluster - See Appendix G for code lists
Non-OR-Affecting MS-DRG Assignment   New/Revised Text in Orange   ♂ Male   ♀ Female

0 Medical and Surgical

L Tendons

U Supplement: Putting in or on biological or synthetic material that physically reinforces and/or augments the function of a portion of a body part

Body Part	Approach	Device	Qualifier
Character 4	Character 5	Character 6	Character 7
0 Head and Neck Tendon 1 Shoulder Tendon, Right 2 Shoulder Tendon, Left 3 Upper Arm Tendon, Right 4 Upper Arm Tendon, Left 5 Lower Arm and Wrist Tendon, Right 6 Lower Arm and Wrist Tendon, Left 7 Hand Tendon, Right 8 Hand Tendon, Left 9 Trunk Tendon, Right B Trunk Tendon, Left C Thorax Tendon, Right D Thorax Tendon, Left F Abdomen Tendon, Right G Abdomen Tendon, Left H Perineum Tendon J Hip Tendon, Right K Hip Tendon, Left L Upper Leg Tendon, Right M Upper Leg Tendon, Left N Lower Leg Tendon, Right P Lower Leg Tendon, Left Q Knee Tendon, Right R Knee Tendon, Left S Ankle Tendon, Right T Ankle Tendon, Left V Foot Tendon, Right W Foot Tendon, Left	0 Open 4 Percutaneous Endoscopic	7 Autologous Tissue Substitute J Synthetic Substitute K Nonautologous Tissue Substitute	Z No Qualifier

0 Medical and Surgical

L Tendons

W Revision: Correcting, to the extent possible, a portion of a malfunctioning device or the position of a displaced device

Body Part	Approach	Device	Qualifier
Character 4	Character 5	Character 6	Character 7
X Upper Tendon Y Lower Tendon	0 Open 3 Percutaneous 4 Percutaneous Endoscopic	0 Drainage Device 7 Autologous Tissue Substitute J Synthetic Substitute K Nonautologous Tissue Substitute Y Other Device	Z No Qualifier
X Upper Tendon Y Lower Tendon	X External	0 Drainage Device 7 Autologous Tissue Substitute J Synthetic Substitute K Nonautologous Tissue Substitute	Z No Qualifier

IC Limited Coverage   **NC** Noncovered   **HAC** HAC-associated Procedure   **CC** Combination Cluster - See Appendix G for code lists

Non-OR-Affecting MS-DRG Assignment   New/Revised Text in **Orange**   ♂ Male   ♀ Female

432

2021 ICD-10-PCS

0 Medical and Surgical
L Tendons
X **Transfer:** Moving, without taking out, all or a portion of a body part to another location to take over the function of all or a portion of a body part

Body Part	Approach	Device	Qualifier
Character 4	Character 5	Character 6	Character 7
0 Head and Neck Tendon	**0** Open	**Z** No Device	**Z** No Qualifier
1 Shoulder Tendon, Right	**4** Percutaneous Endoscopic		
2 Shoulder Tendon, Left			
3 Upper Arm Tendon, Right			
4 Upper Arm Tendon, Left			
5 Lower Arm and Wrist Tendon, Right			
6 Lower Arm and Wrist Tendon, Left			
7 Hand Tendon, Right			
8 Hand Tendon, Left			
9 Trunk Tendon, Right			
B Trunk Tendon, Left			
C Thorax Tendon, Right			
D Thorax Tendon, Left			
F Abdomen Tendon, Right			
G Abdomen Tendon, Left			
H Perineum Tendon			
J Hip Tendon, Right			
K Hip Tendon, Left			
L Upper Leg Tendon, Right			
M Upper Leg Tendon, Left			
N Lower Leg Tendon, Right			
P Lower Leg Tendon, Left			
Q Knee Tendon, Right			
R Knee Tendon, Left			
S Ankle Tendon, Right			
T Ankle Tendon, Left			
V Foot Tendon, Right			
W Foot Tendon, Left			

LC Limited Coverage   **NC** Noncovered   **HAC** HAC-associated Procedure   **CC** Combination Cluster - See Appendix G for code lists
DRG Non-OR-Affecting MS-DRG Assignment   New/Revised Text in **Orange**   ♂ Male   ♀ Female

2021 ICD-10-PCS

433

NOTES

Bursae and Ligaments 0M2-0MX

0 **Medical and Surgical**
M **Bursae and Ligaments**
2 **Change:** Taking out or off a device from a body part and putting back an identical or similar device in or on the same body part without cutting or puncturing the skin or a mucous membrane

Body Part	Approach	Device	Qualifier
Character 4	Character 5	Character 6	Character 7
X Upper Bursa and Ligament **Y** Lower Bursa and Ligament	**X** External	**0** Drainage Device **Y** Other Device	**Z** No Qualifier

0 **Medical and Surgical**
M **Bursae and Ligaments**
5 **Destruction:** Physical eradication of all or a portion of a body part by the direct use of energy, force, or a destructive agent

Body Part	Approach	Device	Qualifier
Character 4	Character 5	Character 6	Character 7
0 Head and Neck Bursa and Ligament **1** Shoulder Bursa and Ligament, Right **2** Shoulder Bursa and Ligament, Left **3** Elbow Bursa and Ligament, Right **4** Elbow Bursa and Ligament, Left **5** Wrist Bursa and Ligament, Right **6** Wrist Bursa and Ligament, Left **7** Hand Bursa and Ligament, Right **8** Hand Bursa and Ligament, Left **9** Upper Extremity Bursa and Ligament, Right **B** Upper Extremity Bursa and Ligament, Left **C** Upper Spine Bursa and Ligament **D** Lower Spine Bursa and Ligament **F** Sternum Bursa and Ligament **G** Rib(s) Bursa and Ligament **H** Abdomen Bursa and Ligament, Right **J** Abdomen Bursa and Ligament, Left **K** Perineum Bursa and Ligament **L** Hip Bursa and Ligament, Right **M** Hip Bursa and Ligament, Left **N** Knee Bursa and Ligament, Right **P** Knee Bursa and Ligament, Left **Q** Ankle Bursa and Ligament, Right **R** Ankle Bursa and Ligament, Left **S** Foot Bursa and Ligament, Right **T** Foot Bursa and Ligament, Left **V** Lower Extremity Bursa and Ligament, Right **W** Lower Extremity Bursa and Ligament, Left	**0** Open **3** Percutaneous **4** Percutaneous Endoscopic	**Z** No Device	**Z** No Qualifier

LC Limited Coverage **NC** Noncovered **HAC** HAC-associated Procedure **CC** Combination Cluster - See Appendix G for code lists
DRG Non-OR-Affecting MS-DRG Assignment New/Revised Text in Orange ♂ Male ♀ Female

2021 ICD-10-PCS 435

0 **Medical and Surgical**
M **Bursae and Ligaments**
8 **Division:** Cutting into a body part, without draining fluids and/or gases from the body part, in order to separate or transect a body part

Body Part	Approach	Device	Qualifier
Character 4	Character 5	Character 6	Character 7
0 Head and Neck Bursa and Ligament	0 Open	Z No Device	Z No Qualifier
1 Shoulder Bursa and Ligament, Right	3 Percutaneous		
2 Shoulder Bursa and Ligament, Left	4 Percutaneous Endoscopic		
3 Elbow Bursa and Ligament, Right			
4 Elbow Bursa and Ligament, Left			
5 Wrist Bursa and Ligament, Right			
6 Wrist Bursa and Ligament, Left			
7 Hand Bursa and Ligament, Right			
8 Hand Bursa and Ligament, Left			
9 Upper Extremity Bursa and Ligament, Right			
B Upper Extremity Bursa and Ligament, Left			
C Upper Spine Bursa and Ligament			
D Lower Spine Bursa and Ligament			
F Sternum Bursa and Ligament			
G Rib(s) Bursa and Ligament			
H Abdomen Bursa and Ligament, Right			
J Abdomen Bursa and Ligament, Left			
K Perineum Bursa and Ligament			
L Hip Bursa and Ligament, Right			
M Hip Bursa and Ligament, Left			
N Knee Bursa and Ligament, Right			
P Knee Bursa and Ligament, Left			
Q Ankle Bursa and Ligament, Right			
R Ankle Bursa and Ligament, Left			
S Foot Bursa and Ligament, Right			
T Foot Bursa and Ligament, Left			
V Lower Extremity Bursa and Ligament, Right			
W Lower Extremity Bursa and Ligament, Left			

LC Limited Coverage   NC Noncovered   HAC HAC-associated Procedure   CC Combination Cluster - See Appendix G for code lists
DRG Non-OR-Affecting MS-DRG Assignment   New/Revised Text in Orange   ♂ Male   ♀ Female

436

2021 ICD-10-PCS

0 **Medical and Surgical**
M **Bursae and Ligaments**
9 **Drainage:** Taking or letting out fluids and/or gases from a body part

Body Part	Approach	Device	Qualifier
Character 4	Character 5	Character 6	Character 7
0 Head and Neck Bursa and Ligament	0 Open	0 Drainage Device	Z No Qualifier
1 Shoulder Bursa and Ligament, Right	3 Percutaneous		
2 Shoulder Bursa and Ligament, Left	4 Percutaneous Endoscopic		
3 Elbow Bursa and Ligament, Right			
4 Elbow Bursa and Ligament, Left			
5 Wrist Bursa and Ligament, Right			
6 Wrist Bursa and Ligament, Left			
7 Hand Bursa and Ligament, Right			
8 Hand Bursa and Ligament, Left			
9 Upper Extremity Bursa and Ligament, Right			
B Upper Extremity Bursa and Ligament, Left			
C Upper Spine Bursa and Ligament			
D Lower Spine Bursa and Ligament			
F Sternum Bursa and Ligament			
G Rib(s) Bursa and Ligament			
H Abdomen Bursa and Ligament, Right			
J Abdomen Bursa and Ligament, Left			
K Perineum Bursa and Ligament			
L Hip Bursa and Ligament, Right			
M Hip Bursa and Ligament, Left			
N Knee Bursa and Ligament, Right			
P Knee Bursa and Ligament, Left			
Q Ankle Bursa and Ligament, Right			
R Ankle Bursa and Ligament, Left			
S Foot Bursa and Ligament, Right			
T Foot Bursa and Ligament, Left			
V Lower Extremity Bursa and Ligament, Right			
W Lower Extremity Bursa and Ligament, Left			

0M9 continued on next page

0 **Medical and Surgical**
M **Bursae and Ligaments**
9 **Drainage:** Taking or letting out fluids and/or gases from a body part

0M9 continued from previous page

Body Part	Approach	Device	Qualifier
Character 4	Character 5	Character 6	Character 7
0 Head and Neck Bursa and Ligament	0 Open	Z No Device	X Diagnostic
1 Shoulder Bursa and Ligament, Right	3 Percutaneous		Z No Qualifier
2 Shoulder Bursa and Ligament, Left	4 Percutaneous Endoscopic		
3 Elbow Bursa and Ligament, Right			
4 Elbow Bursa and Ligament, Left			
5 Wrist Bursa and Ligament, Right			
6 Wrist Bursa and Ligament, Left			
7 Hand Bursa and Ligament, Right			
8 Hand Bursa and Ligament, Left			
9 Upper Extremity Bursa and Ligament, Right			
B Upper Extremity Bursa and Ligament, Left			
C Upper Spine Bursa and Ligament			
D Lower Spine Bursa and Ligament			
F Sternum Bursa and Ligament			
G Rib(s) Bursa and Ligament			
H Abdomen Bursa and Ligament, Right			
J Abdomen Bursa and Ligament, Left			
K Perineum Bursa and Ligament			
L Hip Bursa and Ligament, Right			
M Hip Bursa and Ligament, Left			
N Knee Bursa and Ligament, Right			
P Knee Bursa and Ligament, Left			
Q Ankle Bursa and Ligament, Right			
R Ankle Bursa and Ligament, Left			
S Foot Bursa and Ligament, Right			
T Foot Bursa and Ligament, Left			
V Lower Extremity Bursa and Ligament, Right			
W Lower Extremity Bursa and Ligament, Left			

0   **Medical and Surgical**
M   **Bursae and Ligaments**
B   **Excision:** Cutting out or off, without replacement, a portion of a body part

Body Part	Approach	Device	Qualifier
Character 4	Character 5	Character 6	Character 7
0 Head and Neck Bursa and Ligament 1 Shoulder Bursa and Ligament, Right 2 Shoulder Bursa and Ligament, Left 3 Elbow Bursa and Ligament, Right 4 Elbow Bursa and Ligament, Left 5 Wrist Bursa and Ligament, Right 6 Wrist Bursa and Ligament, Left 7 Hand Bursa and Ligament, Right 8 Hand Bursa and Ligament, Left 9 Upper Extremity Bursa and Ligament, Right B Upper Extremity Bursa and Ligament, Left C Upper Spine Bursa and Ligament D Lower Spine Bursa and Ligament F Sternum Bursa and Ligament G Rib(s) Bursa and Ligament H Abdomen Bursa and Ligament, Right J Abdomen Bursa and Ligament, Left K Perineum Bursa and Ligament L Hip Bursa and Ligament, Right M Hip Bursa and Ligament, Left N Knee Bursa and Ligament, Right P Knee Bursa and Ligament, Left Q Ankle Bursa and Ligament, Right R Ankle Bursa and Ligament, Left S Foot Bursa and Ligament, Right T Foot Bursa and Ligament, Left V Lower Extremity Bursa and Ligament, Right W Lower Extremity Bursa and Ligament, Left	0 Open 3 Percutaneous 4 Percutaneous Endoscopic	Z No Device	X Diagnostic Z No Qualifier

0 Medical and Surgical
M Bursae and Ligaments
C **Extirpation:** Taking or cutting out solid matter from a body part

Body Part	Approach	Device	Qualifier
Character 4	Character 5	Character 6	Character 7
0 Head and Neck Bursa and Ligament	**0** Open	**Z** No Device	**Z** No Qualifier
1 Shoulder Bursa and Ligament, Right	**3** Percutaneous		
2 Shoulder Bursa and Ligament, Left	**4** Percutaneous Endoscopic		
3 Elbow Bursa and Ligament, Right			
4 Elbow Bursa and Ligament, Left			
5 Wrist Bursa and Ligament, Right			
6 Wrist Bursa and Ligament, Left			
7 Hand Bursa and Ligament, Right			
8 Hand Bursa and Ligament, Left			
9 Upper Extremity Bursa and Ligament, Right			
B Upper Extremity Bursa and Ligament, Left			
C Upper Spine Bursa and Ligament			
D Lower Spine Bursa and Ligament			
F Sternum Bursa and Ligament			
G Rib(s) Bursa and Ligament			
H Abdomen Bursa and Ligament, Right			
J Abdomen Bursa and Ligament, Left			
K Perineum Bursa and Ligament			
L Hip Bursa and Ligament, Right			
M Hip Bursa and Ligament, Left			
N Knee Bursa and Ligament, Right			
P Knee Bursa and Ligament, Left			
Q Ankle Bursa and Ligament, Right			
R Ankle Bursa and Ligament, Left			
S Foot Bursa and Ligament, Right			
T Foot Bursa and Ligament, Left			
V Lower Extremity Bursa and Ligament, Right			
W Lower Extremity Bursa and Ligament, Left			

0 **Medical and Surgical**
M **Bursae and Ligaments**
D **Extraction:** Pulling or stripping out or off all or a portion of a body part by the use of force

Body Part	Approach	Device	Qualifier
Character 4	Character 5	Character 6	Character 7
0 Head and Neck Bursa and Ligament	0 Open	Z No Device	Z No Qualifier
1 Shoulder Bursa and Ligament, Right	3 Percutaneous		
2 Shoulder Bursa and Ligament, Left	4 Percutaneous Endoscopic		
3 Elbow Bursa and Ligament, Right			
4 Elbow Bursa and Ligament, Left			
5 Wrist Bursa and Ligament, Right			
6 Wrist Bursa and Ligament, Left			
7 Hand Bursa and Ligament, Right			
8 Hand Bursa and Ligament, Left			
9 Upper Extremity Bursa and Ligament, Right			
B Upper Extremity Bursa and Ligament, Left			
C Upper Spine Bursa and Ligament			
D Lower Spine Bursa and Ligament			
F Sternum Bursa and Ligament			
G Rib(s) Bursa and Ligament			
H Abdomen Bursa and Ligament, Right			
J Abdomen Bursa and Ligament, Left			
K Perineum Bursa and Ligament			
L Hip Bursa and Ligament, Right			
M Hip Bursa and Ligament, Left			
N Knee Bursa and Ligament, Right			
P Knee Bursa and Ligament, Left			
Q Ankle Bursa and Ligament, Right			
R Ankle Bursa and Ligament, Left			
S Foot Bursa and Ligament, Right			
T Foot Bursa and Ligament, Left			
V Lower Extremity Bursa and Ligament, Right			
W Lower Extremity Bursa and Ligament, Left			

0 **Medical and Surgical**
M **Bursae and Ligaments**
H **Insertion:** Putting in a nonbiological appliance that monitors, assists, performs, or prevents a physiological function but does not physically take the place of a body part

Body Part	Approach	Device	Qualifier
Character 4	Character 5	Character 6	Character 7
X Upper Bursa and Ligament	0 Open	Y Other Device	Z No Qualifier
Y Lower Bursa and Ligament	3 Percutaneous		
	4 Percutaneous Endoscopic		

0 Medical and Surgical
M Bursae and Ligaments
J Inspection: Visually and/or manually exploring a body part

Body Part	Approach	Device	Qualifier
Character 4	Character 5	Character 6	Character 7
X Upper Bursa and Ligament Y Lower Bursa and Ligament	0 Open 3 Percutaneous 4 Percutaneous Endoscopic X External	Z No Device	Z No Qualifier

0 Medical and Surgical
M Bursae and Ligaments
M Reattachment: Putting back in or on all or a portion of a separated body part to its normal location or other suitable location

Body Part	Approach	Device	Qualifier
Character 4	Character 5	Character 6	Character 7
0 Head and Neck Bursa and Ligament 1 Shoulder Bursa and Ligament, Right 2 Shoulder Bursa and Ligament, Left 3 Elbow Bursa and Ligament, Right 4 Elbow Bursa and Ligament, Left 5 Wrist Bursa and Ligament, Right 6 Wrist Bursa and Ligament, Left 7 Hand Bursa and Ligament, Right 8 Hand Bursa and Ligament, Left 9 Upper Extremity Bursa and Ligament, Right B Upper Extremity Bursa and Ligament, Left C Upper Spine Bursa and Ligament D Lower Spine Bursa and Ligament F Sternum Bursa and Ligament G Rib(s) Bursa and Ligament H Abdomen Bursa and Ligament, Right J Abdomen Bursa and Ligament, Left K Perineum Bursa and Ligament L Hip Bursa and Ligament, Right M Hip Bursa and Ligament, Left N Knee Bursa and Ligament, Right P Knee Bursa and Ligament, Left Q Ankle Bursa and Ligament, Right R Ankle Bursa and Ligament, Left S Foot Bursa and Ligament, Right T Foot Bursa and Ligament, Left V Lower Extremity Bursa and Ligament, Right W Lower Extremity Bursa and Ligament, Left	0 Open 4 Percutaneous Endoscopic	Z No Device	Z No Qualifier

0 **Medical and Surgical**
M **Bursae and Ligaments**
N **Release:** Freeing a body part from an abnormal physical constraint by cutting or by the use of force

Body Part	Approach	Device	Qualifier
Character 4	Character 5	Character 6	Character 7
0 Head and Neck Bursa and Ligament **1** Shoulder Bursa and Ligament, Right **2** Shoulder Bursa and Ligament, Left **3** Elbow Bursa and Ligament, Right **4** Elbow Bursa and Ligament, Left **5** Wrist Bursa and Ligament, Right **6** Wrist Bursa and Ligament, Left **7** Hand Bursa and Ligament, Right **8** Hand Bursa and Ligament, Left **9** Upper Extremity Bursa and Ligament, Right **B** Upper Extremity Bursa and Ligament, Left **C** Upper Spine Bursa and Ligament **D** Lower Spine Bursa and Ligament **F** Sternum Bursa and Ligament **G** Rib(s) Bursa and Ligament **H** Abdomen Bursa and Ligament, Right **J** Abdomen Bursa and Ligament, Left **K** Perineum Bursa and Ligament **L** Hip Bursa and Ligament, Right **M** Hip Bursa and Ligament, Left **N** Knee Bursa and Ligament, Right **P** Knee Bursa and Ligament, Left **Q** Ankle Bursa and Ligament, Right **R** Ankle Bursa and Ligament, Left **S** Foot Bursa and Ligament, Right **T** Foot Bursa and Ligament, Left **V** Lower Extremity Bursa and Ligament, Right **W** Lower Extremity Bursa and Ligament, Left	**0** Open **3** Percutaneous **4** Percutaneous Endoscopic **X** External	**Z** No Device	**Z** No Qualifier

0 **Medical and Surgical**
M **Bursae and Ligaments**
P **Removal:** Taking out or off a device from a body part

Body Part	Approach	Device	Qualifier
Character 4	Character 5	Character 6	Character 7
X Upper Bursa and Ligament **Y** Lower Bursa and Ligament	**0** Open **3** Percutaneous **4** Percutaneous Endoscopic	**0** Drainage Device **7** Autologous Tissue Substitute **J** Synthetic Substitute **K** Nonautologous Tissue Substitute **Y** Other Device	**Z** No Qualifier
X Upper Bursa and Ligament **Y** Lower Bursa and Ligament	**X** External	**0** Drainage Device	**Z** No Qualifier

LC Limited Coverage NC Noncovered HAC HAC-associated Procedure CC Combination Cluster - See Appendix G for code lists
Non-OR-Affecting MS-DRG Assignment New/Revised Text in **Orange** ♂ Male ♀ Female

2021 ICD-10-PCS

443

BURSAE AND LIGAMENTS 0M2-0MX

0 **Medical and Surgical**
M **Bursae and Ligaments**
Q **Repair:** Restoring, to the extent possible, a body part to its normal anatomic structure and function

Body Part	Approach	Device	Qualifier
Character 4	Character 5	Character 6	Character 7
0 Head and Neck Bursa and Ligament	0 Open	Z No Device	Z No Qualifier
1 Shoulder Bursa and Ligament, Right	3 Percutaneous		
2 Shoulder Bursa and Ligament, Left	4 Percutaneous Endoscopic		
3 Elbow Bursa and Ligament, Right			
4 Elbow Bursa and Ligament, Left			
5 Wrist Bursa and Ligament, Right			
6 Wrist Bursa and Ligament, Left			
7 Hand Bursa and Ligament, Right			
8 Hand Bursa and Ligament, Left			
9 Upper Extremity Bursa and Ligament, Right			
B Upper Extremity Bursa and Ligament, Left			
C Upper Spine Bursa and Ligament			
D Lower Spine Bursa and Ligament			
F Sternum Bursa and Ligament			
G Rib(s) Bursa and Ligament			
H Abdomen Bursa and Ligament, Right			
J Abdomen Bursa and Ligament, Left			
K Perineum Bursa and Ligament			
L Hip Bursa and Ligament, Right			
M Hip Bursa and Ligament, Left			
N Knee Bursa and Ligament, Right			
P Knee Bursa and Ligament, Left			
Q Ankle Bursa and Ligament, Right			
R Ankle Bursa and Ligament, Left			
S Foot Bursa and Ligament, Right			
T Foot Bursa and Ligament, Left			
V Lower Extremity Bursa and Ligament, Right			
W Lower Extremity Bursa and Ligament, Left			

LC Limited Coverage   **NC** Noncovered   **HAC** HAC-associated Procedure   **CC** Combination Cluster - See Appendix G for code lists
DRG Non-OR-Affecting MS-DRG Assignment   New/Revised Text in **Orange**   ♂ Male   ♀ Female

444

2021 ICD-10-PCS

0 **Medical and Surgical**
M **Bursae and Ligaments**
R **Replacement:** Putting in or on biological or synthetic material that physically takes the place and/or function of all or a portion of a body part

Body Part	Approach	Device	Qualifier
Character 4	Character 5	Character 6	Character 7
0 Head and Neck Bursa and Ligament 1 Shoulder Bursa and Ligament, Right 2 Shoulder Bursa and Ligament, Left 3 Elbow Bursa and Ligament, Right 4 Elbow Bursa and Ligament, Left 5 Wrist Bursa and Ligament, Right 6 Wrist Bursa and Ligament, Left 7 Hand Bursa and Ligament, Right 8 Hand Bursa and Ligament, Left 9 Upper Extremity Bursa and Ligament, Right B Upper Extremity Bursa and Ligament, Left C Upper Spine Bursa and Ligament D Lower Spine Bursa and Ligament F Sternum Bursa and Ligament G Rib(s) Bursa and Ligament H Abdomen Bursa and Ligament, Right J Abdomen Bursa and Ligament, Left K Perineum Bursa and Ligament L Hip Bursa and Ligament, Right M Hip Bursa and Ligament, Left N Knee Bursa and Ligament, Right P Knee Bursa and Ligament, Left Q Ankle Bursa and Ligament, Right R Ankle Bursa and Ligament, Left S Foot Bursa and Ligament, Right T Foot Bursa and Ligament, Left V Lower Extremity Bursa and Ligament, Right W Lower Extremity Bursa and Ligament, Left	0 Open 4 Percutaneous Endoscopic	7 Autologous Tissue Substitute J Synthetic Substitute K Nonautologous Tissue Substitute	Z No Qualifier

LC Limited Coverage   **NC** Noncovered   **HAC** HAC-associated Procedure   **CC** Combination Cluster - See Appendix G for code lists

⊕ Non-OR-Affecting MS-DRG Assignment   New/Revised Text in Orange   ♂ Male   ♀ Female

2021 ICD-10-PCS

445

0 **Medical and Surgical**
M **Bursae and Ligaments**
S **Reposition:** Moving to its normal location, or other suitable location, all or a portion of a body part

Body Part	Approach	Device	Qualifier
Character 4	Character 5	Character 6	Character 7
0 Head and Neck Bursa and Ligament	**0** Open **4** Percutaneous Endoscopic	**Z** No Device	**Z** No Qualifier
1 Shoulder Bursa and Ligament, Right			
2 Shoulder Bursa and Ligament, Left			
3 Elbow Bursa and Ligament, Right			
4 Elbow Bursa and Ligament, Left			
5 Wrist Bursa and Ligament, Right			
6 Wrist Bursa and Ligament, Left			
7 Hand Bursa and Ligament, Right			
8 Hand Bursa and Ligament, Left			
9 Upper Extremity Bursa and Ligament, Right			
B Upper Extremity Bursa and Ligament, Left			
C Upper Spine Bursa and Ligament			
D Lower Spine Bursa and Ligament			
F Sternum Bursa and Ligament			
G Rib(s) Bursa and Ligament			
H Abdomen Bursa and Ligament, Right			
J Abdomen Bursa and Ligament, Left			
K Perineum Bursa and Ligament			
L Hip Bursa and Ligament, Right			
M Hip Bursa and Ligament, Left			
N Knee Bursa and Ligament, Right			
P Knee Bursa and Ligament, Left			
Q Ankle Bursa and Ligament, Right			
R Ankle Bursa and Ligament, Left			
S Foot Bursa and Ligament, Right			
T Foot Bursa and Ligament, Left			
V Lower Extremity Bursa and Ligament, Right			
W Lower Extremity Bursa and Ligament, Left			

LC Limited Coverage **NC** Noncovered **HAC** HAC-associated Procedure **CC** Combination Cluster - See Appendix G for code lists
DRG Non-OR-Affecting MS-DRG Assignment New/Revised Text in **Orange** ♂ Male ♀ Female

446

2021 ICD-10-PCS

0   Medical and Surgical
M   Bursae and Ligaments
T   Resection: Cutting out or off, without replacement, all of a body part

Body Part	Approach	Device	Qualifier
Character 4	**Character 5**	**Character 6**	**Character 7**
0 Head and Neck Bursa and Ligament	**0** Open	**Z** No Device	**Z** No Qualifier
1 Shoulder Bursa and Ligament, Right	**4** Percutaneous Endoscopic		
2 Shoulder Bursa and Ligament, Left			
3 Elbow Bursa and Ligament, Right			
4 Elbow Bursa and Ligament, Left			
5 Wrist Bursa and Ligament, Right			
6 Wrist Bursa and Ligament, Left			
7 Hand Bursa and Ligament, Right			
8 Hand Bursa and Ligament, Left			
9 Upper Extremity Bursa and Ligament, Right			
B Upper Extremity Bursa and Ligament, Left			
C Upper Spine Bursa and Ligament			
D Lower Spine Bursa and Ligament			
F Sternum Bursa and Ligament			
G Rib(s) Bursa and Ligament			
H Abdomen Bursa and Ligament, Right			
J Abdomen Bursa and Ligament, Left			
K Perineum Bursa and Ligament			
L Hip Bursa and Ligament, Right			
M Hip Bursa and Ligament, Left			
N Knee Bursa and Ligament, Right			
P Knee Bursa and Ligament, Left			
Q Ankle Bursa and Ligament, Right			
R Ankle Bursa and Ligament, Left			
S Foot Bursa and Ligament, Right			
T Foot Bursa and Ligament, Left			
V Lower Extremity Bursa and Ligament, Right			
W Lower Extremity Bursa and Ligament, Left			

0 **Medical and Surgical**
M **Bursae and Ligaments**
U **Supplement:** Putting in or on biological or synthetic material that physically reinforces and/or augments the function of a portion of a body part

Body Part	Approach	Device	Qualifier
Character 4	Character 5	Character 6	Character 7
0 Head and Neck Bursa and Ligament **1** Shoulder Bursa and Ligament, Right **2** Shoulder Bursa and Ligament, Left **3** Elbow Bursa and Ligament, Right **4** Elbow Bursa and Ligament, Left **5** Wrist Bursa and Ligament, Right **6** Wrist Bursa and Ligament, Left **7** Hand Bursa and Ligament, Right **8** Hand Bursa and Ligament, Left **9** Upper Extremity Bursa and Ligament, Right **B** Upper Extremity Bursa and Ligament, Left **C** Upper Spine Bursa and Ligament **D** Lower Spine Bursa and Ligament **F** Sternum Bursa and Ligament **G** Rib(s) Bursa and Ligament **H** Abdomen Bursa and Ligament, Right **J** Abdomen Bursa and Ligament, Left **K** Perineum Bursa and Ligament **L** Hip Bursa and Ligament, Right **M** Hip Bursa and Ligament, Left **N** Knee Bursa and Ligament, Right **P** Knee Bursa and Ligament, Left **Q** Ankle Bursa and Ligament, Right **R** Ankle Bursa and Ligament, Left **S** Foot Bursa and Ligament, Right **T** Foot Bursa and Ligament, Left **V** Lower Extremity Bursa and Ligament, Right **W** Lower Extremity Bursa and Ligament, Left	**0** Open **4** Percutaneous Endoscopic	**7** Autologous Tissue Substitute **J** Synthetic Substitute **K** Nonautologous Tissue Substitute	**Z** No Qualifier

0 **Medical and Surgical**
M **Bursae and Ligaments**
W **Revision:** Correcting, to the extent possible, a portion of a malfunctioning device or the position of a displaced device

Body Part	Approach	Device	Qualifier
Character 4	Character 5	Character 6	Character 7
X Upper Bursa and Ligament **Y** Lower Bursa and Ligament	**0** Open **3** Percutaneous **4** Percutaneous Endoscopic	**0** Drainage Device **7** Autologous Tissue Substitute **J** Synthetic Substitute **K** Nonautologous Tissue Substitute **Y** Other Device	**Z** No Qualifier
X Upper Bursa and Ligament **Y** Lower Bursa and Ligament	**X** External	**0** Drainage Device **7** Autologous Tissue Substitute **J** Synthetic Substitute **K** Nonautologous Tissue Substitute	**Z** No Qualifier

0 **Medical and Surgical**
M **Bursae and Ligaments**
X **Transfer:** Moving, without taking out, all or a portion of a body part to another location to take over the function of all or a portion of a body part

Body Part	Approach	Device	Qualifier
Character 4	Character 5	Character 6	Character 7
0 Head and Neck Bursa and Ligament	**0** Open	**Z** No Device	**Z** No Qualifier
1 Shoulder Bursa and Ligament, Right	**4** Percutaneous Endoscopic		
2 Shoulder Bursa and Ligament, Left			
3 Elbow Bursa and Ligament, Right			
4 Elbow Bursa and Ligament, Left			
5 Wrist Bursa and Ligament, Right			
6 Wrist Bursa and Ligament, Left			
7 Hand Bursa and Ligament, Right			
8 Hand Bursa and Ligament, Left			
9 Upper Extremity Bursa and Ligament, Right			
B Upper Extremity Bursa and Ligament, Left			
C Upper Spine Bursa and Ligament			
D Lower Spine Bursa and Ligament			
F Sternum Bursa and Ligament			
G Rib(s) Bursa and Ligament			
H Abdomen Bursa and Ligament, Right			
J Abdomen Bursa and Ligament, Left			
K Perineum Bursa and Ligament			
L Hip Bursa and Ligament, Right			
M Hip Bursa and Ligament, Left			
N Knee Bursa and Ligament, Right			
P Knee Bursa and Ligament, Left			
Q Ankle Bursa and Ligament, Right			
R Ankle Bursa and Ligament, Left			
S Foot Bursa and Ligament, Right			
T Foot Bursa and Ligament, Left			
V Lower Extremity Bursa and Ligament, Right			
W Lower Extremity Bursa and Ligament, Left			

LC Limited Coverage   **NC** Noncovered   **HAC** HAC-associated Procedure   **CC** Combination Cluster - See Appendix G for code lists
∞ Non-OR-Affecting MS-DRG Assignment   New/Revised Text in **Orange**   ♂ Male   ♀ Female

2021 ICD-10-PCS   **449**

NOTES

Head and Facial Bones 0N2-0NW

0 Medical and Surgical
N Head and Facial Bones
2 Change: Taking out or off a device from a body part and putting back an identical or similar device in or on the same body part without cutting or puncturing the skin or a mucous membrane

Body Part	Approach	Device	Qualifier
Character 4	Character 5	Character 6	Character 7
0 Skull B Nasal Bone W Facial Bone	X External	0 Drainage Device Y Other Device	Z No Qualifier

0 Medical and Surgical
N Head and Facial Bones
5 Destruction: Physical eradication of all or a portion of a body part by the direct use of energy, force, or a destructive agent

Body Part	Approach	Device	Qualifier
Character 4	Character 5	Character 6	Character 7
0 Skull 1 Frontal Bone 3 Parietal Bone, Right 4 Parietal Bone, Left 5 Temporal Bone, Right 6 Temporal Bone, Left 7 Occipital Bone B Nasal Bone C Sphenoid Bone F Ethmoid Bone, Right G Ethmoid Bone, Left H Lacrimal Bone, Right J Lacrimal Bone, Left K Palatine Bone, Right L Palatine Bone, Left M Zygomatic Bone, Right N Zygomatic Bone, Left P Orbit, Right Q Orbit, Left R Maxilla T Mandible, Right V Mandible, Left X Hyoid Bone	0 Open 3 Percutaneous 4 Percutaneous Endoscopic	Z No Device	Z No Qualifier

0 **Medical and Surgical**
N **Head and Facial Bones**
8 **Division:** Cutting into a body part, without draining fluids and/or gases from the body part, in order to separate or transect a body part

Body Part	Approach	Device	Qualifier
Character 4	**Character 5**	**Character 6**	**Character 7**
0 Skull	0 Open	Z No Device	Z No Qualifier
1 Frontal Bone	3 Percutaneous		
3 Parietal Bone, Right	4 Percutaneous Endoscopic		
4 Parietal Bone, Left			
5 Temporal Bone, Right			
6 Temporal Bone, Left			
7 Occipital Bone			
B Nasal Bone			
C Sphenoid Bone			
F Ethmoid Bone, Right			
G Ethmoid Bone, Left			
H Lacrimal Bone, Right			
J Lacrimal Bone, Left			
K Palatine Bone, Right			
L Palatine Bone, Left			
M Zygomatic Bone, Right			
N Zygomatic Bone, Left			
P Orbit, Right			
Q Orbit, Left			
R Maxilla			
T Mandible, Right			
V Mandible, Left			
X Hyoid Bone			

0   **Medical and Surgical**
N   **Head and Facial Bones**
9   **Drainage:** Taking or letting out fluids and/or gases from a body part

Body Part	Approach	Device	Qualifier
Character 4	**Character 5**	**Character 6**	**Character 7**
0 Skull **1** Frontal Bone **3** Parietal Bone, Right **4** Parietal Bone, Left **5** Temporal Bone, Right **6** Temporal Bone, Left **7** Occipital Bone **B** Nasal Bone **C** Sphenoid Bone **F** Ethmoid Bone, Right **G** Ethmoid Bone, Left **H** Lacrimal Bone, Right **J** Lacrimal Bone, Left **K** Palatine Bone, Right **L** Palatine Bone, Left **M** Zygomatic Bone, Right **N** Zygomatic Bone, Left **P** Orbit, Right **Q** Orbit, Left **R** Maxilla **T** Mandible, Right **V** Mandible, Left **X** Hyoid Bone	**0** Open **3** Percutaneous **4** Percutaneous Endoscopic	**0** Drainage Device	**Z** No Qualifier
0 Skull **1** Frontal Bone **3** Parietal Bone, Right **4** Parietal Bone, Left **5** Temporal Bone, Right **6** Temporal Bone, Left **7** Occipital Bone **B** Nasal Bone **C** Sphenoid Bone **F** Ethmoid Bone, Right **G** Ethmoid Bone, Left **H** Lacrimal Bone, Right **J** Lacrimal Bone, Left **K** Palatine Bone, Right **L** Palatine Bone, Left **M** Zygomatic Bone, Right **N** Zygomatic Bone, Left **P** Orbit, Right **Q** Orbit, Left **R** Maxilla **T** Mandible, Right **V** Mandible, Left **X** Hyoid Bone	**0** Open **3** Percutaneous **4** Percutaneous Endoscopic	**Z** No Device	**X** Diagnostic **Z** No Qualifier

0   Medical and Surgical
N   Head and Facial Bones
B   Excision: Cutting out or off, without replacement, a portion of a body part

Body Part	Approach	Device	Qualifier
Character 4	Character 5	Character 6	Character 7
0 Skull 1 Frontal Bone 3 Parietal Bone, Right 4 Parietal Bone, Left 5 Temporal Bone, Right 6 Temporal Bone, Left 7 Occipital Bone B Nasal Bone C Sphenoid Bone F Ethmoid Bone, Right G Ethmoid Bone, Left H Lacrimal Bone, Right J Lacrimal Bone, Left K Palatine Bone, Right L Palatine Bone, Left M Zygomatic Bone, Right N Zygomatic Bone, Left P Orbit, Right Q Orbit, Left R Maxilla T Mandible, Right V Mandible, Left X Hyoid Bone	0 Open 3 Percutaneous 4 Percutaneous Endoscopic	Z No Device	X Diagnostic Z No Qualifier

0   Medical and Surgical
N   Head and Facial Bones
C   Extirpation: Taking or cutting out solid matter from a body part

Body Part	Approach	Device	Qualifier
Character 4	Character 5	Character 6	Character 7
1 Frontal Bone 3 Parietal Bone, Right 4 Parietal Bone, Left 5 Temporal Bone, Right 6 Temporal Bone, Left 7 Occipital Bone B Nasal Bone C Sphenoid Bone F Ethmoid Bone, Right G Ethmoid Bone, Left H Lacrimal Bone, Right J Lacrimal Bone, Left K Palatine Bone, Right L Palatine Bone, Left M Zygomatic Bone, Right N Zygomatic Bone, Left P Orbit, Right Q Orbit, Left R Maxilla T Mandible, Right V Mandible, Left X Hyoid Bone	0 Open 3 Percutaneous 4 Percutaneous Endoscopic	Z No Device	Z No Qualifier

LC Limited Coverage   NC Noncovered   HAC HAC-associated Procedure   CC Combination Cluster - See Appendix G for code lists
DRG Non-OR-Affecting MS-DRG Assignment   New/Revised Text in **Orange**   ♂ Male   ♀ Female

454

2021 ICD-10-PCS

0 **Medical and Surgical**
N **Head and Facial Bones**
D **Extraction:** Pulling or stripping out or off all or a portion of a body part by the use of force

Body Part	Approach	Device	Qualifier
Character 4	**Character 5**	**Character 6**	**Character 7**
0 Skull	**0** Open	**Z** No Device	**Z** No Qualifier
1 Frontal Bone			
3 Parietal Bone, Right			
4 Parietal Bone, Left			
5 Temporal Bone, Right			
6 Temporal Bone, Left			
7 Occipital Bone			
B Nasal Bone			
C Sphenoid Bone			
F Ethmoid Bone, Right			
G Ethmoid Bone, Left			
H Lacrimal Bone, Right			
J Lacrimal Bone, Left			
K Palatine Bone, Right			
L Palatine Bone, Left			
M Zygomatic Bone, Right			
N Zygomatic Bone, Left			
P Orbit, Right			
Q Orbit, Left			
R Maxilla			
T Mandible, Right			
V Mandible, Left			
X Hyoid Bone			

LC Limited Coverage   **NC** Noncovered   **HAC** HAC-associated Procedure   **CC** Combination Cluster - See Appendix G for code lists
DRG Non-OR-Affecting MS-DRG Assignment   New/Revised Text in **Orange**   ♂ Male   ♀ Female

2021 ICD-10-PCS

455

0   **Medical and Surgical**
N   **Head and Facial Bones**
H   **Insertion:** Putting in a nonbiological appliance that monitors, assists, performs, or prevents a physiological function but does not physically take the place of a body part

Body Part	Approach	Device	Qualifier
Character 4	Character 5	Character 6	Character 7
0 Skull ◨	**0** Open	**4** Internal Fixation Device **5** External Fixation Device **M** Bone Growth Stimulator **N** Neurostimulator Generator	**Z** No Qualifier
0 Skull	**3** Percutaneous **4** Percutaneous Endoscopic	**4** Internal Fixation Device **5** External Fixation Device **M** Bone Growth Stimulator	**Z** No Qualifier
1 Frontal Bone **3** Parietal Bone, Right **4** Parietal Bone, Left **7** Occipital Bone **C** Sphenoid Bone **F** Ethmoid Bone, Right **G** Ethmoid Bone, Left **H** Lacrimal Bone, Right **J** Lacrimal Bone, Left **K** Palatine Bone, Right **L** Palatine Bone, Left **M** Zygomatic Bone, Right **N** Zygomatic Bone, Left **P** Orbit, Right **Q** Orbit, Left **X** Hyoid Bone	**0** Open **3** Percutaneous **4** Percutaneous Endoscopic	**4** Internal Fixation Device	**Z** No Qualifier
5 Temporal Bone, Right **6** Temporal Bone, Left	**0** Open **3** Percutaneous **4** Percutaneous Endoscopic	**4** Internal Fixation Device **S** Hearing Device	**Z** No Qualifier
B Nasal Bone	**0** Open **3** Percutaneous **4** Percutaneous Endoscopic	**4** Internal Fixation Device **M** Bone Growth Stimulator	**Z** No Qualifier
R Maxilla **T** Mandible, Right **V** Mandible, Left	**0** Open **3** Percutaneous **4** Percutaneous Endoscopic	**4** Internal Fixation Device **5** External Fixation Device	**Z** No Qualifier
W Facial Bone	**0** Open **3** Percutaneous **4** Percutaneous Endoscopic	**M** Bone Growth Stimulator	**Z** No Qualifier

◨   0NH00NZ

0   **Medical and Surgical**
N   **Head and Facial Bones**
J   **Inspection:** Visually and/or manually exploring a body part

Body Part	Approach	Device	Qualifier
Character 4	Character 5	Character 6	Character 7
0 Skull **B** Nasal Bone **W** Facial Bone	**0** Open **3** Percutaneous **4** Percutaneous Endoscopic **X** External	**Z** No Device	**Z** No Qualifier

0 **Medical and Surgical**
N **Head and Facial Bones**
N **Release:** Freeing a body part from an abnormal physical constraint by cutting or by the use of force

Body Part	Approach	Device	Qualifier
Character 4	Character 5	Character 6	Character 7
1 Frontal Bone **3** Parietal Bone, Right **4** Parietal Bone, Left **5** Temporal Bone, Right **6** Temporal Bone, Left **7** Occipital Bone **B** Nasal Bone **C** Sphenoid Bone **F** Ethmoid Bone, Right **G** Ethmoid Bone, Left **H** Lacrimal Bone, Right **J** Lacrimal Bone, Left **K** Palatine Bone, Right **L** Palatine Bone, Left **M** Zygomatic Bone, Right **N** Zygomatic Bone, Left **P** Orbit, Right **Q** Orbit, Left **R** Maxilla **T** Mandible, Right **V** Mandible, Left **X** Hyoid Bone	**0** Open **3** Percutaneous **4** Percutaneous Endoscopic	**Z** No Device	**Z** No Qualifier

0 **Medical and Surgical**
N **Head and Facial Bones**
P **Removal:** Taking out or off a device from a body part

Body Part	Approach	Device	Qualifier
Character 4	Character 5	Character 6	Character 7
0 Skull	**0** Open	**0** Drainage Device **4** Internal Fixation Device **5** External Fixation Device **7** Autologous Tissue Substitute **J** Synthetic Substitute **K** Nonautologous Tissue Substitute **M** Bone Growth Stimulator **N** Neurostimulator Generator **S** Hearing Device	**Z** No Qualifier
0 Skull	**3** Percutaneous **4** Percutaneous Endoscopic	**0** Drainage Device **4** Internal Fixation Device **5** External Fixation Device **7** Autologous Tissue Substitute **J** Synthetic Substitute **K** Nonautologous Tissue Substitute **M** Bone Growth Stimulator **S** Hearing Device	**Z** No Qualifier
0 Skull	**X** External	**0** Drainage Device **4** Internal Fixation Device **5** External Fixation Device **M** Bone Growth Stimulator **S** Hearing Device	**Z** No Qualifier
B Nasal Bone **W** Facial Bone	**0** Open **3** Percutaneous **4** Percutaneous Endoscopic	**0** Drainage Device **4** Internal Fixation Device **7** Autologous Tissue Substitute **J** Synthetic Substitute **K** Nonautologous Tissue Substitute **M** Bone Growth Stimulator	**Z** No Qualifier
B Nasal Bone **W** Facial Bone	**X** External	**0** Drainage Device **4** Internal Fixation Device **M** Bone Growth Stimulator	**Z** No Qualifier

0 Medical and Surgical

N Head and Facial Bones

Q Repair: Restoring, to the extent possible, a body part to its normal anatomic structure and function

Body Part	Approach	Device	Qualifier
Character 4	Character 5	Character 6	Character 7
0 Skull 1 Frontal Bone 3 Parietal Bone, Right 4 Parietal Bone, Left 5 Temporal Bone, Right 6 Temporal Bone, Left 7 Occipital Bone B Nasal Bone C Sphenoid Bone F Ethmoid Bone, Right G Ethmoid Bone, Left H Lacrimal Bone, Right J Lacrimal Bone, Left K Palatine Bone, Right L Palatine Bone, Left M Zygomatic Bone, Right N Zygomatic Bone, Left P Orbit, Right Q Orbit, Left R Maxilla T Mandible, Right V Mandible, Left X Hyoid Bone	0 Open 3 Percutaneous 4 Percutaneous Endoscopic X External	Z No Device	Z No Qualifier

0 Medical and Surgical

N Head and Facial Bones

R Replacement: Putting in or on biological or synthetic material that physically takes the place and/or function of all or a portion of a body part

Body Part	Approach	Device	Qualifier
Character 4	Character 5	Character 6	Character 7
0 Skull 1 Frontal Bone 3 Parietal Bone, Right 4 Parietal Bone, Left 5 Temporal Bone, Right 6 Temporal Bone, Left 7 Occipital Bone B Nasal Bone C Sphenoid Bone F Ethmoid Bone, Right G Ethmoid Bone, Left H Lacrimal Bone, Right J Lacrimal Bone, Left K Palatine Bone, Right L Palatine Bone, Left M Zygomatic Bone, Right N Zygomatic Bone, Left P Orbit, Right Q Orbit, Left R Maxilla T Mandible, Right V Mandible, Left X Hyoid Bone	0 Open 3 Percutaneous 4 Percutaneous Endoscopic	7 Autologous Tissue Substitute J Synthetic Substitute K Nonautologous Tissue Substitute	Z No Qualifier

0 Medical and Surgical
N Head and Facial Bones
S Reposition: Moving to its normal location, or other suitable location, all or a portion of a body part

Body Part		Approach		Device		Qualifier	
Character 4		**Character 5**		**Character 6**		**Character 7**	
0 Skull **R** Maxilla **T** Mandible, Right **V** Mandible, Left		**0** Open **3** Percutaneous **4** Percutaneous Endoscopic		**4** Internal Fixation Device **5** External Fixation Device **Z** No Device		**Z** No Qualifier	
0 Skull **R** Maxilla **T** Mandible, Right **V** Mandible, Left		**X** External		**Z** No Device		**Z** No Qualifier	
1 Frontal Bone **3** Parietal Bone, Right **4** Parietal Bone, Left **5** Temporal Bone, Right **6** Temporal Bone, Left **7** Occipital Bone **B** Nasal Bone **C** Sphenoid Bone **F** Ethmoid Bone, Right **G** Ethmoid Bone, Left **H** Lacrimal Bone, Right **J** Lacrimal Bone, Left **K** Palatine Bone, Right **L** Palatine Bone, Left **M** Zygomatic Bone, Right **N** Zygomatic Bone, Left **P** Orbit, Right **Q** Orbit, Left **X** Hyoid Bone		**0** Open **3** Percutaneous **4** Percutaneous Endoscopic		**4** Internal Fixation Device **Z** No Device		**Z** No Qualifier	
1 Frontal Bone **3** Parietal Bone, Right **4** Parietal Bone, Left **5** Temporal Bone, Right **6** Temporal Bone, Left **7** Occipital Bone **B** Nasal Bone **C** Sphenoid Bone **F** Ethmoid Bone, Right **G** Ethmoid Bone, Left **H** Lacrimal Bone, Right **J** Lacrimal Bone, Left **K** Palatine Bone, Right **L** Palatine Bone, Left **M** Zygomatic Bone, Right **N** Zygomatic Bone, Left **P** Orbit, Right **Q** Orbit, Left **X** Hyoid Bone		**X** External		**Z** No Device		**Z** No Qualifier	

0 Medical and Surgical
N Head and Facial Bones
T Resection: Cutting out or off, without replacement, all of a body part

Body Part	Approach	Device	Qualifier
Character 4	Character 5	Character 6	Character 7
1 Frontal Bone **3** Parietal Bone, Right **4** Parietal Bone, Left **5** Temporal Bone, Right **6** Temporal Bone, Left **7** Occipital Bone **B** Nasal Bone **C** Sphenoid Bone **F** Ethmoid Bone, Right **G** Ethmoid Bone, Left **H** Lacrimal Bone, Right **J** Lacrimal Bone, Left **K** Palatine Bone, Right **L** Palatine Bone, Left **M** Zygomatic Bone, Right **N** Zygomatic Bone, Left **P** Orbit, Right **Q** Orbit, Left **R** Maxilla **T** Mandible, Right **V** Mandible, Left **X** Hyoid Bone	**0** Open	**Z** No Device	**Z** No Qualifier

0 Medical and Surgical
N Head and Facial Bones
U Supplement: Putting in or on biological or synthetic material that physically reinforces and/or augments the function of a portion of a body part

Body Part	Approach	Device	Qualifier
Character 4	Character 5	Character 6	Character 7
0 Skull **1** Frontal Bone **3** Parietal Bone, Right **4** Parietal Bone, Left **5** Temporal Bone, Right **6** Temporal Bone, Left **7** Occipital Bone **B** Nasal Bone **C** Sphenoid Bone **F** Ethmoid Bone, Right **G** Ethmoid Bone, Left **H** Lacrimal Bone, Right **J** Lacrimal Bone, Left **K** Palatine Bone, Right **L** Palatine Bone, Left **M** Zygomatic Bone, Right **N** Zygomatic Bone, Left **P** Orbit, Right **Q** Orbit, Left **R** Maxilla **T** Mandible, Right **V** Mandible, Left **X** Hyoid Bone	**0** Open **3** Percutaneous **4** Percutaneous Endoscopic	**7** Autologous Tissue Substitute **J** Synthetic Substitute **K** Nonautologous Tissue Substitute	**Z** No Qualifier

LC Limited Coverage   NC Noncovered   HAC HAC-associated Procedure   CC Combination Cluster - See Appendix G for code lists
DRG Non-OR-Affecting MS-DRG Assignment   New/Revised Text in Orange   ♂ Male   ♀ Female

0 **Medical and Surgical**
N **Head and Facial Bones**
W **Revision:** Correcting, to the extent possible, a portion of a malfunctioning device or the position of a displaced device

Body Part	Approach	Device	Qualifier
Character 4	Character 5	Character 6	Character 7
0 Skull	**0** Open	**0** Drainage Device **4** Internal Fixation Device **5** External Fixation Device **7** Autologous Tissue Substitute **J** Synthetic Substitute **K** Nonautologous Tissue Substitute **M** Bone Growth Stimulator **N** Neurostimulator Generator **S** Hearing Device	**Z** No Qualifier
0 Skull	**3** Percutaneous **4** Percutaneous Endoscopic **X** External	**0** Drainage Device **4** Internal Fixation Device **5** External Fixation Device **7** Autologous Tissue Substitute **J** Synthetic Substitute **K** Nonautologous Tissue Substitute **M** Bone Growth Stimulator **S** Hearing Device	**Z** No Qualifier
B Nasal Bone **W** Facial Bone	**0** Open **3** Percutaneous **4** Percutaneous Endoscopic **X** External	**0** Drainage Device **4** Internal Fixation Device **7** Autologous Tissue Substitute **J** Synthetic Substitute **K** Nonautologous Tissue Substitute **M** Bone Growth Stimulator	**Z** No Qualifier

NOTES

Upper Bones 0P2-0PW

0 **Medical and Surgical**
P **Upper Bones**
2 **Change:** Taking out or off a device from a body part and putting back an identical or similar device in or on the same body part without cutting or puncturing the skin or a mucous membrane

Body Part	Approach	Device	Qualifier
Character 4	Character 5	Character 6	Character 7
Y Upper Bone	X External	0 Drainage Device Y Other Device	Z No Qualifier

0 **Medical and Surgical**
P **Upper Bones**
5 **Destruction:** Physical eradication of all or a portion of a body part by the direct use of energy, force, or a destructive agent

Body Part	Approach	Device	Qualifier
Character 4	Character 5	Character 6	Character 7
0 Sternum 1 Ribs, 1 to 2 2 Ribs, 3 or More 3 Cervical Vertebra 4 Thoracic Vertebra 5 Scapula, Right 6 Scapula, Left 7 Glenoid Cavity, Right 8 Glenoid Cavity, Left 9 Clavicle, Right B Clavicle, Left C Humeral Head, Right D Humeral Head, Left F Humeral Shaft, Right G Humeral Shaft, Left H Radius, Right J Radius, Left K Ulna, Right L Ulna, Left M Carpal, Right N Carpal, Left P Metacarpal, Right Q Metacarpal, Left R Thumb Phalanx, Right S Thumb Phalanx, Left T Finger Phalanx, Right V Finger Phalanx, Left	0 Open 3 Percutaneous 4 Percutaneous Endoscopic	Z No Device	Z No Qualifier

LC Limited Coverage **NC** Noncovered **HAC** HAC-associated Procedure **CC** Combination Cluster - See Appendix G for code lists
DRG Non-OR-Affecting MS-DRG Assignment   New/Revised Text in **Orange**   ♂ Male   ♀ Female

2021 ICD-10-PCS

463

UPPER BONES 0P2-0PW

0 **Medical and Surgical**
P **Upper Bones**
8 **Division:** Cutting into a body part, without draining fluids and/or gases from the body part, in order to separate or transect a body part

Body Part	Approach	Device	Qualifier
Character 4	Character 5	Character 6	Character 7
0 Sternum	**0** Open	**Z** No Device	**Z** No Qualifier
1 Ribs, 1 to 2	**3** Percutaneous		
2 Ribs, 3 or More	**4** Percutaneous Endoscopic		
3 Cervical Vertebra			
4 Thoracic Vertebra			
5 Scapula, Right			
6 Scapula, Left			
7 Glenoid Cavity, Right			
8 Glenoid Cavity, Left			
9 Clavicle, Right			
B Clavicle, Left			
C Humeral Head, Right			
D Humeral Head, Left			
F Humeral Shaft, Right			
G Humeral Shaft, Left			
H Radius, Right			
J Radius, Left			
K Ulna, Right			
L Ulna, Left			
M Carpal, Right			
N Carpal, Left			
P Metacarpal, Right			
Q Metacarpal, Left			
R Thumb Phalanx, Right			
S Thumb Phalanx, Left			
T Finger Phalanx, Right			
V Finger Phalanx, Left			

LC Limited Coverage   NC Noncovered   HAC HAC-associated Procedure   CC Combination Cluster - See Appendix G for code lists
Non-OR-Affecting MS-DRG Assignment   New/Revised Text in **Orange**   ♂ Male   ♀ Female

464   **2021 ICD-10-PCS**

0 **Medical and Surgical**
P **Upper Bones**
9 **Drainage:** Taking or letting out fluids and/or gases from a body part

Body Part	Approach	Device	Qualifier
Character 4	**Character 5**	**Character 6**	**Character 7**
0 Sternum 1 Ribs, 1 to 2 2 Ribs, 3 or More 3 Cervical Vertebra 4 Thoracic Vertebra 5 Scapula, Right 6 Scapula, Left 7 Glenoid Cavity, Right 8 Glenoid Cavity, Left 9 Clavicle, Right B Clavicle, Left C Humeral Head, Right D Humeral Head, Left F Humeral Shaft, Right G Humeral Shaft, Left H Radius, Right J Radius, Left K Ulna, Right L Ulna, Left M Carpal, Right N Carpal, Left P Metacarpal, Right Q Metacarpal, Left R Thumb Phalanx, Right S Thumb Phalanx, Left T Finger Phalanx, Right V Finger Phalanx, Left	0 Open 3 Percutaneous 4 Percutaneous Endoscopic	0 Drainage Device	Z No Qualifier
0 Sternum 1 Ribs, 1 to 2 2 Ribs, 3 or More 3 Cervical Vertebra 4 Thoracic Vertebra 5 Scapula, Right 6 Scapula, Left 7 Glenoid Cavity, Right 8 Glenoid Cavity, Left 9 Clavicle, Right B Clavicle, Left C Humeral Head, Right D Humeral Head, Left F Humeral Shaft, Right G Humeral Shaft, Left H Radius, Right J Radius, Left K Ulna, Right L Ulna, Left M Carpal, Right N Carpal, Left P Metacarpal, Right Q Metacarpal, Left R Thumb Phalanx, Right S Thumb Phalanx, Left T Finger Phalanx, Right V Finger Phalanx, Left	0 Open 3 Percutaneous 4 Percutaneous Endoscopic	Z No Device	X Diagnostic Z No Qualifier

0 Medical and Surgical

P Upper Bones

B Excision: Cutting out or off, without replacement, a portion of a body part

Body Part	Approach	Device	Qualifier
Character 4	Character 5	Character 6	Character 7
0 Sternum	0 Open	Z No Device	X Diagnostic
1 Ribs, 1 to 2	3 Percutaneous		Z No Qualifier
2 Ribs, 3 or More	4 Percutaneous Endoscopic		
3 Cervical Vertebra			
4 Thoracic Vertebra			
5 Scapula, Right			
6 Scapula, Left			
7 Glenoid Cavity, Right			
8 Glenoid Cavity, Left			
9 Clavicle, Right			
B Clavicle, Left			
C Humeral Head, Right			
D Humeral Head, Left			
F Humeral Shaft, Right			
G Humeral Shaft, Left			
H Radius, Right			
J Radius, Left			
K Ulna, Right			
L Ulna, Left			
M Carpal, Right			
N Carpal, Left			
P Metacarpal, Right			
Q Metacarpal, Left			
R Thumb Phalanx, Right			
S Thumb Phalanx, Left			
T Finger Phalanx, Right			
V Finger Phalanx, Left			

0 Medical and Surgical

P Upper Bones

C Extirpation: Taking or cutting out solid matter from a body part

Body Part	Approach	Device	Qualifier
Character 4	Character 5	Character 6	Character 7
0 Sternum	0 Open	Z No Device	Z No Qualifier
1 Ribs, 1 to 2	3 Percutaneous		
2 Ribs, 3 or More	4 Percutaneous Endoscopic		
3 Cervical Vertebra			
4 Thoracic Vertebra			
5 Scapula, Right			
6 Scapula, Left			
7 Glenoid Cavity, Right			
8 Glenoid Cavity, Left			
9 Clavicle, Right			
B Clavicle, Left			
C Humeral Head, Right			
D Humeral Head, Left			
F Humeral Shaft, Right			
G Humeral Shaft, Left			
H Radius, Right			
J Radius, Left			
K Ulna, Right			
L Ulna, Left			
M Carpal, Right			
N Carpal, Left			
P Metacarpal, Right			
Q Metacarpal, Left			
R Thumb Phalanx, Right			
S Thumb Phalanx, Left			
T Finger Phalanx, Right			
V Finger Phalanx, Left			

0 **Medical and Surgical**
P **Upper Bones**
D **Extraction:** Pulling or stripping out or off all or a portion of a body part by the use of force

Body Part	Approach	Device	Qualifier
Character 4	Character 5	Character 6	Character 7
0 Sternum	0 Open	Z No Device	Z No Qualifier
1 Ribs, 1 to 2			
2 Ribs, 3 or More			
3 Cervical Vertebra			
4 Thoracic Vertebra			
5 Scapula, Right			
6 Scapula, Left			
7 Glenoid Cavity, Right			
8 Glenoid Cavity, Left			
9 Clavicle, Right			
B Clavicle, Left			
C Humeral Head, Right			
D Humeral Head, Left			
F Humeral Shaft, Right			
G Humeral Shaft, Left			
H Radius, Right			
J Radius, Left			
K Ulna, Right			
L Ulna, Left			
M Carpal, Right			
N Carpal, Left			
P Metacarpal, Right			
Q Metacarpal, Left			
R Thumb Phalanx, Right			
S Thumb Phalanx, Left			
T Finger Phalanx, Right			
V Finger Phalanx, Left			

LC Limited Coverage   NC Noncovered   HAC HAC-associated Procedure   CC Combination Cluster - See Appendix G for code lists
DRG Non-OR-Affecting MS-DRG Assignment   New/Revised Text in **Orange**   ♂ Male   ♀ Female

2021 ICD-10-PCS

467

0 **Medical and Surgical**
P **Upper Bones**
H **Insertion:** Putting in a nonbiological appliance that monitors, assists, performs, or prevents a physiological function but does not physically take the place of a body part

Body Part	Approach	Device	Qualifier
Character 4	Character 5	Character 6	Character 7
0 Sternum	0 Open 3 Percutaneous 4 Percutaneous Endoscopic	0 Internal Fixation Device, Rigid Plate 4 Internal Fixation Device	Z No Qualifier
1 Ribs, 1 to 2 2 Ribs, 3 or More 3 Cervical Vertebra 4 Thoracic Vertebra 5 Scapula, Right 6 Scapula, Left 7 Glenoid Cavity, Right 8 Glenoid Cavity, Left 9 Clavicle, Right B Clavicle, Left	0 Open 3 Percutaneous 4 Percutaneous Endoscopic	4 Internal Fixation Device	Z No Qualifier
C Humeral Head, Right D Humeral Head, Left H Radius, Right J Radius, Left K Ulna, Right L Ulna, Left	0 Open 3 Percutaneous 4 Percutaneous Endoscopic	4 Internal Fixation Device 5 External Fixation Device 6 Internal Fixation Device, Intramedullary 8 External Fixation Device, Limb Lengthening B External Fixation Device, Monoplanar C External Fixation Device, Ring D External Fixation Device, Hybrid	Z No Qualifier
F Humeral Shaft, Right G Humeral Shaft, Left	0 Open 3 Percutaneous 4 Percutaneous Endoscopic	4 Internal Fixation Device 5 External Fixation Device 6 Internal Fixation Device, Intramedullary 7 Internal Fixation Device, Intramedullary Limb Lengthening 8 External Fixation Device, Limb Lengthening B External Fixation Device, Monoplanar C External Fixation Device, Ring D External Fixation Device, Hybrid	Z No Qualifier
M Carpal, Right N Carpal, Left P Metacarpal, Right Q Metacarpal, Left R Thumb Phalanx, Right S Thumb Phalanx, Left T Finger Phalanx, Right V Finger Phalanx, Left	0 Open 3 Percutaneous 4 Percutaneous Endoscopic	4 Internal Fixation Device 5 External Fixation Device	Z No Qualifier
Y Upper Bone	0 Open 3 Percutaneous 4 Percutaneous Endoscopic	M Bone Growth Stimulator	Z No Qualifier

0 **Medical and Surgical**
P **Upper Bones**
J **Inspection:** Visually and/or manually exploring a body part

Body Part	Approach	Device	Qualifier
Character 4	Character 5	Character 6	Character 7
Y Upper Bone	0 Open 3 Percutaneous 4 Percutaneous Endoscopic X External	Z No Device	Z No Qualifier

0 **Medical and Surgical**
P **Upper Bones**
N **Release:** Freeing a body part from an abnormal physical constraint by cutting or by the use of force

Body Part	Approach	Device	Qualifier
Character 4	Character 5	Character 6	Character 7
0 Sternum 1 Ribs, 1 to 2 2 Ribs, 3 or More 3 Cervical Vertebra 4 Thoracic Vertebra 5 Scapula, Right 6 Scapula, Left 7 Glenoid Cavity, Right 8 Glenoid Cavity, Left 9 Clavicle, Right B Clavicle, Left C Humeral Head, Right D Humeral Head, Left F Humeral Shaft, Right G Humeral Shaft, Left H Radius, Right J Radius, Left K Ulna, Right L Ulna, Left M Carpal, Right N Carpal, Left P Metacarpal, Right Q Metacarpal, Left R Thumb Phalanx, Right S Thumb Phalanx, Left T Finger Phalanx, Right V Finger Phalanx, Left	0 Open 3 Percutaneous 4 Percutaneous Endoscopic	Z No Device	Z No Qualifier

0 **Medical and Surgical**
P **Upper Bones**
P **Removal:** Taking out or off a device from a body part

Body Part	Approach	Device	Qualifier
Character 4	Character 5	Character 6	Character 7
0 Sternum 1 Ribs, 1 to 2 2 Ribs, 3 or More 3 Cervical Vertebra 4 Thoracic Vertebra 5 Scapula, Right 6 Scapula, Left 7 Glenoid Cavity, Right 8 Glenoid Cavity, Left 9 Clavicle, Right B Clavicle, Left	0 Open 3 Percutaneous 4 Percutaneous Endoscopic	4 Internal Fixation Device 7 Autologous Tissue Substitute J Synthetic Substitute K Nonautologous Tissue Substitute	Z No Qualifier
0 Sternum 1 Ribs, 1 to 2 2 Ribs, 3 or More 3 Cervical Vertebra 4 Thoracic Vertebra 5 Scapula, Right 6 Scapula, Left 7 Glenoid Cavity, Right 8 Glenoid Cavity, Left 9 Clavicle, Right B Clavicle, Left	X External	4 Internal Fixation Device	Z No Qualifier

0PP continued on next page

0 Medical and Surgical
P Upper Bones
P Removal: Taking out or off a device from a body part

0PP continued from previous page

Body Part	Approach	Device	Qualifier
Character 4	Character 5	Character 6	Character 7
C Humeral Head, Right D Humeral Head, Left F Humeral Shaft, Right G Humeral Shaft, Left H Radius, Right J Radius, Left K Ulna, Right L Ulna, Left M Carpal, Right N Carpal, Left P Metacarpal, Right Q Metacarpal, Left R Thumb Phalanx, Right S Thumb Phalanx, Left T Finger Phalanx, Right V Finger Phalanx, Left	0 Open 3 Percutaneous 4 Percutaneous Endoscopic	4 Internal Fixation Device 5 External Fixation Device 7 Autologous Tissue Substitute J Synthetic Substitute K Nonautologous Tissue Substitute	Z No Qualifier
C Humeral Head, Right D Humeral Head, Left F Humeral Shaft, Right G Humeral Shaft, Left H Radius, Right J Radius, Left K Ulna, Right L Ulna, Left M Carpal, Right N Carpal, Left P Metacarpal, Right Q Metacarpal, Left R Thumb Phalanx, Right S Thumb Phalanx, Left T Finger Phalanx, Right V Finger Phalanx, Left	X External	4 Internal Fixation Device 5 External Fixation Device	Z No Qualifier
Y Upper Bone	0 Open 3 Percutaneous 4 Percutaneous Endoscopic X External	0 Drainage Device M Bone Growth Stimulator	Z No Qualifier

LC Limited Coverage   NC Noncovered   HAC HAC-associated Procedure   CC Combination Cluster - See Appendix G for code lists
DRG Non-OR-Affecting MS-DRG Assignment   New/Revised Text in Orange   ♂ Male   ♀ Female

UPPER BONES 0P2-0PW

470

2021 ICD-10-PCS

0 **Medical and Surgical**
P **Upper Bones**
Q **Repair:** Restoring, to the extent possible, a body part to its normal anatomic structure and function

Body Part	Approach	Device	Qualifier
Character 4	Character 5	Character 6	Character 7
0 Sternum 1 Ribs, 1 to 2 2 Ribs, 3 or More 3 Cervical Vertebra 4 Thoracic Vertebra 5 Scapula, Right 6 Scapula, Left 7 Glenoid Cavity, Right 8 Glenoid Cavity, Left 9 Clavicle, Right B Clavicle, Left C Humeral Head, Right D Humeral Head, Left F Humeral Shaft, Right G Humeral Shaft, Left H Radius, Right J Radius, Left K Ulna, Right L Ulna, Left M Carpal, Right N Carpal, Left P Metacarpal, Right Q Metacarpal, Left R Thumb Phalanx, Right S Thumb Phalanx, Left T Finger Phalanx, Right V Finger Phalanx, Left	0 Open 3 Percutaneous 4 Percutaneous Endoscopic X External	Z No Device	Z No Qualifier

0 **Medical and Surgical**
P **Upper Bones**
R **Replacement:** Putting in or on biological or synthetic material that physically takes the place and/or function of all or a portion of a body part

Body Part	Approach	Device	Qualifier
Character 4	Character 5	Character 6	Character 7
0 Sternum 1 Ribs, 1 to 2 2 Ribs, 3 or More 3 Cervical Vertebra 4 Thoracic Vertebra 5 Scapula, Right 6 Scapula, Left 7 Glenoid Cavity, Right 8 Glenoid Cavity, Left 9 Clavicle, Right B Clavicle, Left C Humeral Head, Right D Humeral Head, Left F Humeral Shaft, Right G Humeral Shaft, Left H Radius, Right J Radius, Left K Ulna, Right L Ulna, Left M Carpal, Right N Carpal, Left P Metacarpal, Right Q Metacarpal, Left R Thumb Phalanx, Right S Thumb Phalanx, Left T Finger Phalanx, Right V Finger Phalanx, Left	0 Open 3 Percutaneous 4 Percutaneous Endoscopic	7 Autologous Tissue Substitute J Synthetic Substitute K Nonautologous Tissue Substitute	Z No Qualifier

0 Medical and Surgical
P Upper Bones
S Reposition: Moving to its normal location, or other suitable location, all or a portion of a body part

Body Part	Approach	Device	Qualifier
Character 4	Character 5	Character 6	Character 7
0 Sternum	**0** Open **3** Percutaneous **4** Percutaneous Endoscopic	**0** Internal Fixation Device, Rigid Plate **4** Internal Fixation Device **Z** No Device	**Z** No Qualifier
0 Sternum	**X** External	**Z** No Device	**Z** No Qualifier
1 Ribs, 1 to 2 **2** Ribs, 3 or More **3** Cervical Vertebra **4** Thoracic Vertebra **5** Scapula, Right **6** Scapula, Left **7** Glenoid Cavity, Right **8** Glenoid Cavity, Left **9** Clavicle, Right **B** Clavicle, Left	**0** Open **3** Percutaneous **4** Percutaneous Endoscopic	**4** Internal Fixation Device **Z** No Device	**Z** No Qualifier
1 Ribs, 1 to 2 **2** Ribs, 3 or More **3** Cervical Vertebra **4** Thoracic Vertebra **5** Scapula, Right **6** Scapula, Left **7** Glenoid Cavity, Right **8** Glenoid Cavity, Left **9** Clavicle, Right **B** Clavicle, Left	**X** External	**Z** No Device	**Z** No Qualifier
C Humeral Head, Right **D** Humeral Head, Left **F** Humeral Shaft, Right **G** Humeral Shaft, Left **H** Radius, Right **J** Radius, Left **K** Ulna, Right **L** Ulna, Left	**0** Open **3** Percutaneous **4** Percutaneous Endoscopic	**4** Internal Fixation Device **5** External Fixation Device **6** Internal Fixation Device, Intramedullary **B** External Fixation Device, Monoplanar **C** External Fixation Device, Ring **D** External Fixation Device, Hybrid **Z** No Device	**Z** No Qualifier
C Humeral Head, Right **D** Humeral Head, Left **F** Humeral Shaft, Right **G** Humeral Shaft, Left **H** Radius, Right **J** Radius, Left **K** Ulna, Right **L** Ulna, Left	**X** External	**Z** No Device	**Z** No Qualifier
M Carpal, Right **N** Carpal, Left **P** Metacarpal, Right **Q** Metacarpal, Left **R** Thumb Phalanx, Right **S** Thumb Phalanx, Left **T** Finger Phalanx, Right **V** Finger Phalanx, Left	**0** Open **3** Percutaneous **4** Percutaneous Endoscopic	**4** Internal Fixation Device **5** External Fixation Device **Z** No Device	**Z** No Qualifier
M Carpal, Right **N** Carpal, Left **P** Metacarpal, Right **Q** Metacarpal, Left **R** Thumb Phalanx, Right **S** Thumb Phalanx, Left **T** Finger Phalanx, Right **V** Finger Phalanx, Left	**X** External	**Z** No Device	**Z** No Qualifier

0 **Medical and Surgical**
P **Upper Bones**
T **Resection:** Cutting out or off, without replacement, all of a body part

Body Part	Approach	Device	Qualifier
Character 4	Character 5	Character 6	Character 7
0 Sternum	0 Open	Z No Device	Z No Qualifier
1 Ribs, 1 to 2			
2 Ribs, 3 or More			
5 Scapula, Right			
6 Scapula, Left			
7 Glenoid Cavity, Right			
8 Glenoid Cavity, Left			
9 Clavicle, Right			
B Clavicle, Left			
C Humeral Head, Right			
D Humeral Head, Left			
F Humeral Shaft, Right			
G Humeral Shaft, Left			
H Radius, Right			
J Radius, Left			
K Ulna, Right			
L Ulna, Left			
M Carpal, Right			
N Carpal, Left			
P Metacarpal, Right			
Q Metacarpal, Left			
R Thumb Phalanx, Right			
S Thumb Phalanx, Left			
T Finger Phalanx, Right			
V Finger Phalanx, Left			

0 **Medical and Surgical**
P **Upper Bones**
U **Supplement:** Putting in or on biological or synthetic material that physically reinforces and/or augments the function of a portion of a body part

Body Part	Approach	Device	Qualifier
Character 4	Character 5	Character 6	Character 7
0 Sternum	0 Open	7 Autologous Tissue Substitute	Z No Qualifier
1 Ribs, 1 to 2	3 Percutaneous	J Synthetic Substitute	
2 Ribs, 3 or More	4 Percutaneous Endoscopic	K Nonautologous Tissue Substitute	
3 Cervical Vertebra ᴄᴄ			
4 Thoracic Vertebra ᴄᴄ			
5 Scapula, Right			
6 Scapula, Left			
7 Glenoid Cavity, Right			
8 Glenoid Cavity, Left			
9 Clavicle, Right			
B Clavicle, Left			
C Humeral Head, Right			
D Humeral Head, Left			
F Humeral Shaft, Right			
G Humeral Shaft, Left			
H Radius, Right			
J Radius, Left			
K Ulna, Right			
L Ulna, Left			
M Carpal, Right			
N Carpal, Left			
P Metacarpal, Right			
Q Metacarpal, Left			
R Thumb Phalanx, Right			
S Thumb Phalanx, Left			
T Finger Phalanx, Right			
V Finger Phalanx, Left			

ᴄᴄ   0PU33JZ   0PU43JZ

0   **Medical and Surgical**
P   **Upper Bones**
W   **Revision:** Correcting, to the extent possible, a portion of a malfunctioning device or the position of a displaced device

Body Part		Approach		Device		Qualifier	
Character 4		**Character 5**		**Character 6**		**Character 7**	
0 Sternum 1 Ribs, 1 to 2 2 Ribs, 3 or More 3 Cervical Vertebra 4 Thoracic Vertebra 5 Scapula, Right 6 Scapula, Left 7 Glenoid Cavity, Right 8 Glenoid Cavity, Left 9 Clavicle, Right B Clavicle, Left		0 Open 3 Percutaneous 4 Percutaneous Endoscopic X External		4 Internal Fixation Device 7 Autologous Tissue Substitute J Synthetic Substitute K Nonautologous Tissue Substitute		Z No Qualifier	
C Humeral Head, Right D Humeral Head, Left F Humeral Shaft, Right G Humeral Shaft, Left H Radius, Right J Radius, Left K Ulna, Right L Ulna, Left M Carpal, Right N Carpal, Left P Metacarpal, Right Q Metacarpal, Left R Thumb Phalanx, Right S Thumb Phalanx, Left T Finger Phalanx, Right V Finger Phalanx, Left		0 Open 3 Percutaneous 4 Percutaneous Endoscopic X External		4 Internal Fixation Device 5 External Fixation Device 7 Autologous Tissue Substitute J Synthetic Substitute K Nonautologous Tissue Substitute		Z No Qualifier	
Y Upper Bone		0 Open 3 Percutaneous 4 Percutaneous Endoscopic X External		0 Drainage Device M Bone Growth Stimulator		Z No Qualifier	

LC Limited Coverage   NC Noncovered   HAC HAC-associated Procedure   CC Combination Cluster - See Appendix G for code lists
DRG Non-OR-Affecting MS-DRG Assignment   New/Revised Text in Orange   ♂ Male   ♀ Female

474

2021 ICD-10-PCS

NOTES

NOTES

Lower Bones 0Q2-0QW

0 Medical and Surgical
Q Lower Bones
2 Change: Taking out or off a device from a body part and putting back an identical or similar device in or on the same body part without cutting or puncturing the skin or a mucous membrane

Body Part	Approach	Device	Qualifier
Character 4	**Character 5**	**Character 6**	**Character 7**
Y Lower Bone	**X** External	**0** Drainage Device **Y** Other Device	**Z** No Qualifier

0 Medical and Surgical
Q Lower Bones
5 Destruction: Physical eradication of all or a portion of a body part by the direct use of energy, force, or a destructive agent

Body Part	Approach	Device	Qualifier
Character 4	**Character 5**	**Character 6**	**Character 7**
0 Lumbar Vertebra **1** Sacrum **2** Pelvic Bone, Right **3** Pelvic Bone, Left **4** Acetabulum, Right **5** Acetabulum, Left **6** Upper Femur, Right **7** Upper Femur, Left **8** Femoral Shaft, Right **9** Femoral Shaft, Left **B** Lower Femur, Right **C** Lower Femur, Left **D** Patella, Right **F** Patella, Left **G** Tibia, Right **H** Tibia, Left **J** Fibula, Right **K** Fibula, Left **L** Tarsal, Right **M** Tarsal, Left **N** Metatarsal, Right **P** Metatarsal, Left **Q** Toe Phalanx, Right **R** Toe Phalanx, Left **S** Coccyx	**0** Open **3** Percutaneous **4** Percutaneous Endoscopic	**Z** No Device	**Z** No Qualifier

0 **Medical and Surgical**
Q **Lower Bones**
8 **Division:** Cutting into a body part, without draining fluids and/or gases from the body part, in order to separate or transect a body part

Body Part	Approach	Device	Qualifier
Character 4	Character 5	Character 6	Character 7
0 Lumbar Vertebra	0 Open	Z No Device	Z No Qualifier
1 Sacrum	3 Percutaneous		
2 Pelvic Bone, Right	4 Percutaneous Endoscopic		
3 Pelvic Bone, Left			
4 Acetabulum, Right			
5 Acetabulum, Left			
6 Upper Femur, Right			
7 Upper Femur, Left			
8 Femoral Shaft, Right			
9 Femoral Shaft, Left			
B Lower Femur, Right			
C Lower Femur, Left			
D Patella, Right			
F Patella, Left			
G Tibia, Right			
H Tibia, Left			
J Fibula, Right			
K Fibula, Left			
L Tarsal, Right			
M Tarsal, Left			
N Metatarsal, Right			
P Metatarsal, Left			
Q Toe Phalanx, Right			
R Toe Phalanx, Left			
S Coccyx			

LC Limited Coverage   NC Noncovered   HAC HAC-associated Procedure   CC Combination Cluster - See Appendix G for code lists
DRG Non-OR-Affecting MS-DRG Assignment   New/Revised Text in **Orange**   ♂ Male   ♀ Female

478

2021 ICD-10-PCS

0 **Medical and Surgical**
Q **Lower Bones**
9 **Drainage:** Taking or letting out fluids and/or gases from a body part

Body Part	Approach	Device	Qualifier
Character 4	Character 5	Character 6	Character 7
0 Lumbar Vertebra 1 Sacrum 2 Pelvic Bone, Right 3 Pelvic Bone, Left 4 Acetabulum, Right 5 Acetabulum, Left 6 Upper Femur, Right 7 Upper Femur, Left 8 Femoral Shaft, Right 9 Femoral Shaft, Left B Lower Femur, Right C Lower Femur, Left D Patella, Right F Patella, Left G Tibia, Right H Tibia, Left J Fibula, Right K Fibula, Left L Tarsal, Right M Tarsal, Left N Metatarsal, Right P Metatarsal, Left Q Toe Phalanx, Right R Toe Phalanx, Left S Coccyx	0 Open 3 Percutaneous 4 Percutaneous Endoscopic	0 Drainage Device	Z No Qualifier
0 Lumbar Vertebra 1 Sacrum 2 Pelvic Bone, Right 3 Pelvic Bone, Left 4 Acetabulum, Right 5 Acetabulum, Left 6 Upper Femur, Right 7 Upper Femur, Left 8 Femoral Shaft, Right 9 Femoral Shaft, Left B Lower Femur, Right C Lower Femur, Left D Patella, Right F Patella, Left G Tibia, Right H Tibia, Left J Fibula, Right K Fibula, Left L Tarsal, Right M Tarsal, Left N Metatarsal, Right P Metatarsal, Left Q Toe Phalanx, Right R Toe Phalanx, Left S Coccyx	0 Open 3 Percutaneous 4 Percutaneous Endoscopic	Z No Device	X Diagnostic Z No Qualifier

LC Limited Coverage   NC Noncovered   HAC HAC-associated Procedure   CC Combination Cluster - See Appendix G for code lists
DRG Non-OR-Affecting MS-DRG Assignment   New/Revised Text in Orange   ♂ Male   ♀ Female

2021 ICD-10-PCS 479

0   Medical and Surgical
Q   Lower Bones
B   Excision: Cutting out or off, without replacement, a portion of a body part

Body Part	Approach	Device	Qualifier
Character 4	Character 5	Character 6	Character 7
0 Lumbar Vertebra 1 Sacrum 2 Pelvic Bone, Right 3 Pelvic Bone, Left 4 Acetabulum, Right 5 Acetabulum, Left 6 Upper Femur, Right 7 Upper Femur, Left 8 Femoral Shaft, Right 9 Femoral Shaft, Left B Lower Femur, Right C Lower Femur, Left D Patella, Right F Patella, Left G Tibia, Right H Tibia, Left J Fibula, Right K Fibula, Left L Tarsal, Right M Tarsal, Left N Metatarsal, Right P Metatarsal, Left Q Toe Phalanx, Right R Toe Phalanx, Left S Coccyx	0 Open 3 Percutaneous 4 Percutaneous Endoscopic	Z No Device	X Diagnostic Z No Qualifier

0   Medical and Surgical
Q   Lower Bones
C   Extirpation: Taking or cutting out solid matter from a body part

Body Part	Approach	Device	Qualifier
Character 4	Character 5	Character 6	Character 7
0 Lumbar Vertebra 1 Sacrum 2 Pelvic Bone, Right 3 Pelvic Bone, Left 4 Acetabulum, Right 5 Acetabulum, Left 6 Upper Femur, Right 7 Upper Femur, Left 8 Femoral Shaft, Right 9 Femoral Shaft, Left B Lower Femur, Right C Lower Femur, Left D Patella, Right F Patella, Left G Tibia, Right H Tibia, Left J Fibula, Right K Fibula, Left L Tarsal, Right M Tarsal, Left N Metatarsal, Right P Metatarsal, Left Q Toe Phalanx, Right R Toe Phalanx, Left S Coccyx	0 Open 3 Percutaneous 4 Percutaneous Endoscopic	Z No Device	Z No Qualifier

0 Medical and Surgical

Q Lower Bones

D Extraction: Pulling or stripping out or off all or a portion of a body part by the use of force

Body Part	Approach	Device	Qualifier
Character 4	Character 5	Character 6	Character 7
0 Lumbar Vertebra 1 Sacrum 2 Pelvic Bone, Right 3 Pelvic Bone, Left 4 Acetabulum, Right 5 Acetabulum, Left 6 Upper Femur, Right 7 Upper Femur, Left 8 Femoral Shaft, Right 9 Femoral Shaft, Left B Lower Femur, Right C Lower Femur, Left D Patella, Right F Patella, Left G Tibia, Right H Tibia, Left J Fibula, Right K Fibula, Left L Tarsal, Right M Tarsal, Left N Metatarsal, Right P Metatarsal, Left Q Toe Phalanx, Right R Toe Phalanx, Left S Coccyx	0 Open	Z No Device	Z No Qualifier

0 Medical and Surgical

Q Lower Bones

H Insertion: Putting in a nonbiological appliance that monitors, assists, performs, or prevents a physiological function but does not physically take the place of a body part

Body Part	Approach	Device	Qualifier
Character 4	Character 5	Character 6	Character 7
0 Lumbar Vertebra 1 Sacrum 2 Pelvic Bone, Right 3 Pelvic Bone, Left 4 Acetabulum, Right 5 Acetabulum, Left D Patella, Right F Patella, Left L Tarsal, Right M Tarsal, Left N Metatarsal, Right P Metatarsal, Left Q Toe Phalanx, Right R Toe Phalanx, Left S Coccyx	0 Open 3 Percutaneous 4 Percutaneous Endoscopic	4 Internal Fixation Device 5 External Fixation Device	Z No Qualifier
6 Upper Femur, Right 7 Upper Femur, Left B Lower Femur, Right C Lower Femur, Left J Fibula, Right K Fibula, Left	0 Open 3 Percutaneous 4 Percutaneous Endoscopic	4 Internal Fixation Device 5 External Fixation Device 6 Internal Fixation Device, Intramedullary 8 External Fixation Device, Limb Lengthening B External Fixation Device, Monoplanar C External Fixation Device, Ring D External Fixation Device, Hybrid	Z No Qualifier

0QH continued on next page

0 Medical and Surgical

0QH continued from previous page

Q Lower Bones

H Insertion: Putting in a nonbiological appliance that monitors, assists, performs, or prevents a physiological function but does not physically take the place of a body part

Body Part	Approach	Device	Qualifier
Character 4	Character 5	Character 6	Character 7
8 Femoral Shaft, Right 9 Femoral Shaft, Left G Tibia, Right H Tibia, Left	0 Open 3 Percutaneous 4 Percutaneous Endoscopic	4 Internal Fixation Device 5 External Fixation Device 6 Internal Fixation Device, Intramedullary 7 Internal Fixation Device, Intramedullary Limb Lengthening 8 External Fixation Device, Limb Lengthening B External Fixation Device, Monoplanar C External Fixation Device, Ring D External Fixation Device, Hybrid	Z No Qualifier
Y Lower Bone	0 Open 3 Percutaneous 4 Percutaneous Endoscopic	M Bone Growth Stimulator	Z No Qualifier

0 Medical and Surgical

Q Lower Bones

J Inspection: Visually and/or manually exploring a body part

Body Part	Approach	Device	Qualifier
Character 4	Character 5	Character 6	Character 7
Y Lower Bone	0 Open 3 Percutaneous 4 Percutaneous Endoscopic X External	Z No Device	Z No Qualifier

0 Medical and Surgical

Q Lower Bones

N Release: Freeing a body part from an abnormal physical constraint by cutting or by the use of force

Body Part	Approach	Device	Qualifier
Character 4	Character 5	Character 6	Character 7
0 Lumbar Vertebra 1 Sacrum 2 Pelvic Bone, Right 3 Pelvic Bone, Left 4 Acetabulum, Right 5 Acetabulum, Left 6 Upper Femur, Right 7 Upper Femur, Left 8 Femoral Shaft, Right 9 Femoral Shaft, Left B Lower Femur, Right C Lower Femur, Left D Patella, Right F Patella, Left G Tibia, Right H Tibia, Left J Fibula, Right K Fibula, Left L Tarsal, Right M Tarsal, Left N Metatarsal, Right P Metatarsal, Left Q Toe Phalanx, Right R Toe Phalanx, Left S Coccyx	0 Open 3 Percutaneous 4 Percutaneous Endoscopic	Z No Device	Z No Qualifier

0 **Medical and Surgical**
Q **Lower Bones**
P **Removal:** Taking out or off a device from a body part

Body Part	Approach	Device	Qualifier
Character 4	**Character 5**	**Character 6**	**Character 7**
0 Lumbar Vertebra 1 Sacrum 2 Pelvic Bone, Right 3 Pelvic Bone, Left 4 Acetabulum, Right 5 Acetabulum, Left 6 Upper Femur, Right 7 Upper Femur, Left 8 Femoral Shaft, Right 9 Femoral Shaft, Left B Lower Femur, Right C Lower Femur, Left D Patella, Right F Patella, Left G Tibia, Right H Tibia, Left J Fibula, Right K Fibula, Left L Tarsal, Right M Tarsal, Left N Metatarsal, Right P Metatarsal, Left Q Toe Phalanx, Right R Toe Phalanx, Left S Coccyx	0 Open 3 Percutaneous 4 Percutaneous Endoscopic	4 Internal Fixation Device 5 External Fixation Device 7 Autologous Tissue Substitute J Synthetic Substitute K Nonautologous Tissue Substitute	Z No Qualifier
0 Lumbar Vertebra 1 Sacrum 2 Pelvic Bone, Right 3 Pelvic Bone, Left 4 Acetabulum, Right 5 Acetabulum, Left 6 Upper Femur, Right 7 Upper Femur, Left 8 Femoral Shaft, Right 9 Femoral Shaft, Left B Lower Femur, Right C Lower Femur, Left D Patella, Right F Patella, Left G Tibia, Right H Tibia, Left J Fibula, Right K Fibula, Left L Tarsal, Right M Tarsal, Left N Metatarsal, Right P Metatarsal, Left Q Toe Phalanx, Right R Toe Phalanx, Left S Coccyx	X External	4 Internal Fixation Device 5 External Fixation Device	Z No Qualifier
Y Lower Bone	0 Open 3 Percutaneous 4 Percutaneous Endoscopic X External	0 Drainage Device M Bone Growth Stimulator	Z No Qualifier

0 Medical and Surgical
Q Lower Bones
Q **Repair:** Restoring, to the extent possible, a body part to its normal anatomic structure and function

Body Part	Approach	Device	Qualifier
Character 4	**Character 5**	**Character 6**	**Character 7**
0 Lumbar Vertebra **1** Sacrum **2** Pelvic Bone, Right **3** Pelvic Bone, Left **4** Acetabulum, Right **5** Acetabulum, Left **6** Upper Femur, Right **7** Upper Femur, Left **8** Femoral Shaft, Right **9** Femoral Shaft, Left **B** Lower Femur, Right **C** Lower Femur, Left **D** Patella, Right **F** Patella, Left **G** Tibia, Right **H** Tibia, Left **J** Fibula, Right **K** Fibula, Left **L** Tarsal, Right **M** Tarsal, Left **N** Metatarsal, Right **P** Metatarsal, Left **Q** Toe Phalanx, Right **R** Toe Phalanx, Left **S** Coccyx	**0** Open **3** Percutaneous **4** Percutaneous Endoscopic **X** External	**Z** No Device	**Z** No Qualifier

0 Medical and Surgical
Q Lower Bones
R **Replacement:** Putting in or on biological or synthetic material that physically takes the place and/or function of all or a portion of a body part

Body Part	Approach	Device	Qualifier
Character 4	**Character 5**	**Character 6**	**Character 7**
0 Lumbar Vertebra **1** Sacrum **2** Pelvic Bone, Right **3** Pelvic Bone, Left **4** Acetabulum, Right **5** Acetabulum, Left **6** Upper Femur, Right **7** Upper Femur, Left **8** Femoral Shaft, Right **9** Femoral Shaft, Left **B** Lower Femur, Right **C** Lower Femur, Left **D** Patella, Right **F** Patella, Left **G** Tibia, Right **H** Tibia, Left **J** Fibula, Right **K** Fibula, Left **L** Tarsal, Right **M** Tarsal, Left **N** Metatarsal, Right **P** Metatarsal, Left **Q** Toe Phalanx, Right **R** Toe Phalanx, Left **S** Coccyx	**0** Open **3** Percutaneous **4** Percutaneous Endoscopic	**7** Autologous Tissue Substitute **J** Synthetic Substitute **K** Nonautologous Tissue Substitute	**Z** No Qualifier

0 **Medical and Surgical**
Q **Lower Bones**
S **Reposition:** Moving to its normal location, or other suitable location, all or a portion of a body part

Body Part	Approach	Device	Qualifier
Character 4	Character 5	Character 6	Character 7
0 Lumbar Vertebra ⓒ 1 Sacrum ⓒ 4 Acetabulum, Right 5 Acetabulum, Left S Coccyx ⓒ	0 Open 3 Percutaneous 4 Percutaneous Endoscopic	4 Internal Fixation Device Z No Device	Z No Qualifier
0 Lumbar Vertebra 1 Sacrum 4 Acetabulum, Right 5 Acetabulum, Left S Coccyx	X External	Z No Device	Z No Qualifier
2 Pelvic Bone, Right 3 Pelvic Bone, Left D Patella, Right F Patella, Left L Tarsal, Right M Tarsal, Left Q Toe Phalanx, Right R Toe Phalanx, Left	0 Open 3 Percutaneous 4 Percutaneous Endoscopic	4 Internal Fixation Device 5 External Fixation Device Z No Device	Z No Qualifier
2 Pelvic Bone, Right 3 Pelvic Bone, Left D Patella, Right F Patella, Left L Tarsal, Right M Tarsal, Left Q Toe Phalanx, Right R Toe Phalanx, Left	X External	Z No Device	Z No Qualifier
6 Upper Femur, Right 7 Upper Femur, Left 8 Femoral Shaft, Right 9 Femoral Shaft, Left B Lower Femur, Right C Lower Femur, Left G Tibia, Right H Tibia, Left J Fibula, Right K Fibula, Left	0 Open 3 Percutaneous 4 Percutaneous Endoscopic	4 Internal Fixation Device 5 External Fixation Device 6 Internal Fixation Device, Intramedullary B External Fixation Device, Monoplanar C External Fixation Device, Ring D External Fixation Device, Hybrid Z No Device	Z No Qualifier
6 Upper Femur, Right 7 Upper Femur, Left 8 Femoral Shaft, Right 9 Femoral Shaft, Left B Lower Femur, Right C Lower Femur, Left G Tibia, Right H Tibia, Left J Fibula, Right K Fibula, Left	X External	Z No Device	Z No Qualifier
N Metatarsal, Right P Metatarsal, Left	0 Open 3 Percutaneous 4 Percutaneous Endoscopic	4 Internal Fixation Device 5 External Fixation Device Z No Device	2 Sesamoid Bone(s) 1st Toe Z No Qualifier
N Metatarsal, Right P Metatarsal, Left	X External	Z No Device	2 Sesamoid Bone(s) 1st Toe Z No Qualifier

ⓒ 0QS03ZZ   0QS13ZZ   0QSS3ZZ

ⓒ Limited Coverage ⓝ Noncovered ⓗ HAC-associated Procedure ⓒ Combination Cluster - See Appendix G for code lists
Non-OR-Affecting MS-DRG Assignment   New/Revised Text in **Orange**   ♂ Male   ♀ Female

2021 ICD-10-PCS

485

LOWER BONES 0Q2-0QW

0QT-0QU

0   Medical and Surgical
Q   Lower Bones
T   Resection: Cutting out or off, without replacement, all of a body part

Body Part	Approach	Device	Qualifier
Character 4	Character 5	Character 6	Character 7
2 Pelvic Bone, Right 3 Pelvic Bone, Left 4 Acetabulum, Right 5 Acetabulum, Left 6 Upper Femur, Right 7 Upper Femur, Left 8 Femoral Shaft, Right 9 Femoral Shaft, Left B Lower Femur, Right C Lower Femur, Left D Patella, Right F Patella, Left G Tibia, Right H Tibia, Left J Fibula, Right K Fibula, Left L Tarsal, Right M Tarsal, Left N Metatarsal, Right P Metatarsal, Left Q Toe Phalanx, Right R Toe Phalanx, Left S Coccyx	0 Open	Z No Device	Z No Qualifier

0   Medical and Surgical
Q   Lower Bones
U   Supplement: Putting in or on biological or synthetic material that physically reinforces and/or augments the function of a portion of a body part

Body Part	Approach	Device	Qualifier
Character 4	Character 5	Character 6	Character 7
0 Lumbar Vertebra ㏄ 1 Sacrum ㏄ 2 Pelvic Bone, Right 3 Pelvic Bone, Left 4 Acetabulum, Right 5 Acetabulum, Left 6 Upper Femur, Right 7 Upper Femur, Left 8 Femoral Shaft, Right 9 Femoral Shaft, Left B Lower Femur, Right C Lower Femur, Left D Patella, Right F Patella, Left G Tibia, Right H Tibia, Left J Fibula, Right K Fibula, Left L Tarsal, Right M Tarsal, Left N Metatarsal, Right P Metatarsal, Left Q Toe Phalanx, Right R Toe Phalanx, Left S Coccyx ㏄	0 Open 3 Percutaneous 4 Percutaneous Endoscopic	7 Autologous Tissue Substitute J Synthetic Substitute K Nonautologous Tissue Substitute	Z No Qualifier

㏄   0QU03JZ   0QU13JZ   0QUS3JZ

0 **Medical and Surgical**
Q **Lower Bones**
W **Revision:** Correcting, to the extent possible, a portion of a malfunctioning device or the position of a displaced device

Body Part	Approach	Device	Qualifier
Character 4	Character 5	Character 6	Character 7
0 Lumbar Vertebra **1** Sacrum **4** Acetabulum, Right **5** Acetabulum, Left **S** Coccyx	**0** Open **3** Percutaneous **4** Percutaneous Endoscopic **X** External	**4** Internal Fixation Device **7** Autologous Tissue Substitute **J** Synthetic Substitute **K** Nonautologous Tissue Substitute	**Z** No Qualifier
2 Pelvic Bone, Right **3** Pelvic Bone, Left **6** Upper Femur, Right **7** Upper Femur, Left **8** Femoral Shaft, Right **9** Femoral Shaft, Left **B** Lower Femur, Right **C** Lower Femur, Left **D** Patella, Right **F** Patella, Left **G** Tibia, Right **H** Tibia, Left **J** Fibula, Right **K** Fibula, Left **L** Tarsal, Right **M** Tarsal, Left **N** Metatarsal, Right **P** Metatarsal, Left **Q** Toe Phalanx, Right **R** Toe Phalanx, Left	**0** Open **3** Percutaneous **4** Percutaneous Endoscopic **X** External	**4** Internal Fixation Device **5** External Fixation Device **7** Autologous Tissue Substitute **J** Synthetic Substitute **K** Nonautologous Tissue Substitute	**Z** No Qualifier
Y Lower Bone	**0** Open **3** Percutaneous **4** Percutaneous Endoscopic **X** External	**0** Drainage Device **M** Bone Growth Stimulator	**Z** No Qualifier

NOTES

Upper Joints 0R2-0RW

0 Medical and Surgical
R Upper Joints
2 Change: Taking out or off a device from a body part and putting back an identical or similar device in or on the same body part without cutting or puncturing the skin or a mucous membrane

Body Part	Approach	Device	Qualifier
Character 4	Character 5	Character 6	Character 7
Y Upper Joint	X External	0 Drainage Device Y Other Device	Z No Qualifier

0 Medical and Surgical
R Upper Joints
5 Destruction: Physical eradication of all or a portion of a body part by the direct use of energy, force, or a destructive agent

Body Part	Approach	Device	Qualifier
Character 4	Character 5	Character 6	Character 7
0 Occipital-cervical Joint 1 Cervical Vertebral Joint 3 Cervical Vertebral Disc 4 Cervicothoracic Vertebral Joint 5 Cervicothoracic Vertebral Disc 6 Thoracic Vertebral Joint 9 Thoracic Vertebral Disc A Thoracolumbar Vertebral Joint B Thoracolumbar Vertebral Disc C Temporomandibular Joint, Right D Temporomandibular Joint, Left E Sternoclavicular Joint, Right F Sternoclavicular Joint, Left G Acromioclavicular Joint, Right H Acromioclavicular Joint, Left J Shoulder Joint, Right K Shoulder Joint, Left L Elbow Joint, Right M Elbow Joint, Left N Wrist Joint, Right P Wrist Joint, Left Q Carpal Joint, Right R Carpal Joint, Left S Carpometacarpal Joint, Right T Carpometacarpal Joint, Left U Metacarpophalangeal Joint, Right V Metacarpophalangeal Joint, Left W Finger Phalangeal Joint, Right X Finger Phalangeal Joint, Left	0 Open 3 Percutaneous 4 Percutaneous Endoscopic	Z No Device	Z No Qualifier

LC Limited Coverage   **NC** Noncovered   **HAC** HAC-associated Procedure   **CC** Combination Cluster - See Appendix G for code lists
DRG Non-OR-Affecting MS-DRG Assignment   New/Revised Text in Orange   ♂ Male   ♀ Female

2021 ICD-10-PCS

489

0 Medical and Surgical
R Upper Joints
9 Drainage: Taking or letting out fluids and/or gases from a body part

Body Part	Approach	Device	Qualifier
Character 4	Character 5	Character 6	Character 7
0 Occipital-cervical Joint 1 Cervical Vertebral Joint 3 Cervical Vertebral Disc 4 Cervicothoracic Vertebral Joint 5 Cervicothoracic Vertebral Disc 6 Thoracic Vertebral Joint 9 Thoracic Vertebral Disc A Thoracolumbar Vertebral Joint B Thoracolumbar Vertebral Disc C Temporomandibular Joint, Right D Temporomandibular Joint, Left E Sternoclavicular Joint, Right F Sternoclavicular Joint, Left G Acromioclavicular Joint, Right H Acromioclavicular Joint, Left J Shoulder Joint, Right K Shoulder Joint, Left L Elbow Joint, Right M Elbow Joint, Left N Wrist Joint, Right P Wrist Joint, Left Q Carpal Joint, Right R Carpal Joint, Left S Carpometacarpal Joint, Right T Carpometacarpal Joint, Left U Metacarpophalangeal Joint, Right V Metacarpophalangeal Joint, Left W Finger Phalangeal Joint, Right X Finger Phalangeal Joint, Left	0 Open 3 Percutaneous 4 Percutaneous Endoscopic	0 Drainage Device	Z No Qualifier
0 Occipital-cervical Joint 1 Cervical Vertebral Joint 3 Cervical Vertebral Disc 4 Cervicothoracic Vertebral Joint 5 Cervicothoracic Vertebral Disc 6 Thoracic Vertebral Joint 9 Thoracic Vertebral Disc A Thoracolumbar Vertebral Joint B Thoracolumbar Vertebral Disc C Temporomandibular Joint, Right D Temporomandibular Joint, Left E Sternoclavicular Joint, Right F Sternoclavicular Joint, Left G Acromioclavicular Joint, Right H Acromioclavicular Joint, Left J Shoulder Joint, Right K Shoulder Joint, Left L Elbow Joint, Right M Elbow Joint, Left N Wrist Joint, Right P Wrist Joint, Left Q Carpal Joint, Right R Carpal Joint, Left S Carpometacarpal Joint, Right T Carpometacarpal Joint, Left U Metacarpophalangeal Joint, Right V Metacarpophalangeal Joint, Left W Finger Phalangeal Joint, Right X Finger Phalangeal Joint, Left	0 Open 3 Percutaneous 4 Percutaneous Endoscopic	Z No Device	X Diagnostic Z No Qualifier

LC Limited Coverage **NC** Noncovered **HAC** HAC-associated Procedure **CC** Combination Cluster - See Appendix G for code lists

⊞ Non-OR-Affecting MS-DRG Assignment New/Revised Text in **Orange** ♂ Male ♀ Female

490

2021 ICD-10-PCS

0   **Medical and Surgical**
R   **Upper Joints**
B   **Excision:** Cutting out or off, without replacement, a portion of a body part

Body Part	Approach	Device	Qualifier
Character 4	Character 5	Character 6	Character 7
0 Occipital-cervical Joint	**0** Open	**Z** No Device	**X** Diagnostic
1 Cervical Vertebral Joint	**3** Percutaneous		**Z** No Qualifier
3 Cervical Vertebral Disc	**4** Percutaneous Endoscopic		
4 Cervicothoracic Vertebral Joint			
5 Cervicothoracic Vertebral Disc			
6 Thoracic Vertebral Joint			
9 Thoracic Vertebral Disc			
A Thoracolumbar Vertebral Joint			
B Thoracolumbar Vertebral Disc			
C Temporomandibular Joint, Right			
D Temporomandibular Joint, Left			
E Sternoclavicular Joint, Right			
F Sternoclavicular Joint, Left			
G Acromioclavicular Joint, Right			
H Acromioclavicular Joint, Left			
J Shoulder Joint, Right			
K Shoulder Joint, Left			
L Elbow Joint, Right			
M Elbow Joint, Left			
N Wrist Joint, Right			
P Wrist Joint, Left			
Q Carpal Joint, Right			
R Carpal Joint, Left			
S Carpometacarpal Joint, Right			
T Carpometacarpal Joint, Left			
U Metacarpophalangeal Joint, Right			
V Metacarpophalangeal Joint, Left			
W Finger Phalangeal Joint, Right			
X Finger Phalangeal Joint, Left			

0   **Medical and Surgical**
R   **Upper Joints**
C   **Extirpation:** Taking or cutting out solid matter from a body part

Body Part	Approach	Device	Qualifier
Character 4	Character 5	Character 6	Character 7
0 Occipital-cervical Joint	**0** Open	**Z** No Device	**Z** No Qualifier
1 Cervical Vertebral Joint	**3** Percutaneous		
3 Cervical Vertebral Disc	**4** Percutaneous Endoscopic		
4 Cervicothoracic Vertebral Joint			
5 Cervicothoracic Vertebral Disc			
6 Thoracic Vertebral Joint			
9 Thoracic Vertebral Disc			
A Thoracolumbar Vertebral Joint			
B Thoracolumbar Vertebral Disc			
C Temporomandibular Joint, Right			
D Temporomandibular Joint, Left			
E Sternoclavicular Joint, Right			
F Sternoclavicular Joint, Left			
G Acromioclavicular Joint, Right			
H Acromioclavicular Joint, Left			
J Shoulder Joint, Right			
K Shoulder Joint, Left			
L Elbow Joint, Right			
M Elbow Joint, Left			
N Wrist Joint, Right			
P Wrist Joint, Left			
Q Carpal Joint, Right			
R Carpal Joint, Left			
S Carpometacarpal Joint, Right			
T Carpometacarpal Joint, Left			
U Metacarpophalangeal Joint, Right			
V Metacarpophalangeal Joint, Left			
W Finger Phalangeal Joint, Right			
X Finger Phalangeal Joint, Left			

0   **Medical and Surgical**
R   **Upper Joints**
G   **Fusion:** Joining together portions of an articular body part rendering the articular body part immobile

Body Part	Approach	Device	Qualifier
Character 4	Character 5	Character 6	Character 7
0 Occipital-cervical Joint HAC	**0** Open	**7** Autologous Tissue Substitute	**0** Anterior Approach, Anterior Column
1 Cervical Vertebral Joint HAC	**3** Percutaneous	**J** Synthetic Substitute	**1** Posterior Approach, Posterior Column
2 Cervical Vertebral Joints, 2 or more HAC	**4** Percutaneous Endoscopic	**K** Nonautologous Tissue Substitute	**J** Posterior Approach, Anterior Column
4 Cervicothoracic Vertebral Joint HAC			
6 Thoracic Vertebral Joint HAC			
7 Thoracic Vertebral Joints, 2 to 7 HAC CC			
8 Thoracic Vertebral Joints, 8 or more HAC			
A Thoracolumbar Vertebral Joint HAC			
0 Occipital-cervical Joint HAC	**0** Open	**A** Interbody Fusion Device	**0** Anterior Approach, Anterior Column
1 Cervical Vertebral Joint HAC	**3** Percutaneous		**J** Posterior Approach, Anterior Column
2 Cervical Vertebral Joints, 2 or more HAC	**4** Percutaneous Endoscopic		
4 Cervicothoracic Vertebral Joint HAC			
6 Thoracic Vertebral Joint HAC			
7 Thoracic Vertebral Joints, 2 to 7 HAC CC			
8 Thoracic Vertebral Joints, 8 or more HAC			
A Thoracolumbar Vertebral Joint HAC			

0RG continued on next page

LC Limited Coverage   NC Noncovered   HAC HAC-associated Procedure   CC Combination Cluster - See Appendix G for code lists
ORG Non-OR-Affecting MS-DRG Assignment   New/Revised Text in **Orange**   ♂ Male   ♀ Female

0 Medical and Surgical

0RG continued from previous page

R Upper Joints

G **Fusion:** Joining together portions of an articular body part rendering the articular body part immobile

Body Part	Approach	Device	Qualifier
Character 4	**Character 5**	**Character 6**	**Character 7**
C Temporomandibular Joint, Right **D** Temporomandibular Joint, Left **E** Sternoclavicular Joint, Right HAC **F** Sternoclavicular Joint, Left HAC **G** Acromioclavicular Joint, Right HAC **H** Acromioclavicular Joint, Left HAC **J** Shoulder Joint, Right HAC **K** Shoulder Joint, Left HAC	**0** Open **3** Percutaneous **4** Percutaneous Endoscopic	**4** Internal Fixation Device **7** Autologous Tissue Substitute **J** Synthetic Substitute **K** Nonautologous Tissue Substitute	**Z** No Qualifier
L Elbow Joint, Right HAC **M** Elbow Joint, Left HAC **N** Wrist Joint, Right **P** Wrist Joint, Left **Q** Carpal Joint, Right **R** Carpal Joint, Left **S** Carpometacarpal Joint, Right **T** Carpometacarpal Joint, Left **U** Metacarpophalangeal Joint, Right **V** Metacarpophalangeal Joint, Left **W** Finger Phalangeal Joint, Right **X** Finger Phalangeal Joint, Left	**0** Open **3** Percutaneous **4** Percutaneous Endoscopic	**3** Internal Fixation Device, Sustained Compression **4** Internal Fixation Device **5** External Fixation Device **7** Autologous Tissue Substitute **J** Synthetic Substitute **K** Nonautologous Tissue Substitute	**Z** No Qualifier

HAC

0RG0070	0RG0071	0RG007J	0RG00A0	0RG00AJ	0RG00J0	0RG00J1	0RG00JJ	0RG00K0	0RG00K1	0RG00KJ	0RG0370	0RG0371
0RG037J	0RG03A0	0RG03AJ	0RG03J0	0RG03J1	0RG03JJ	0RG03K0	0RG03K1	0RG03KJ	0RG0470	0RG0471	0RG047J	0RG04A0
0RG04AJ	0RG04J0	0RG04J1	0RG04JJ	0RG04K0	0RG04K1	0RG04KJ	0RG1070	0RG1071	0RG107J	0RG10A0	0RG10AJ	0RG10J0
0RG10J1	0RG10JJ	0RG10K0	0RG10K1	0RG10KJ	0RG1370	0RG1371	0RG137J	0RG13A0	0RG13AJ	0RG13J0	0RG13J1	0RG13JJ
0RG13K0	0RG13K1	0RG13KJ	0RG1470	0RG1471	0RG147J	0RG14A0	0RG14AJ	0RG14J0	0RG14J1	0RG14JJ	0RG14K0	0RG14K1
0RG14KJ	0RG2070	0RG2071	0RG207J	0RG20A0	0RG20AJ	0RG20J0	0RG20J1	0RG20JJ	0RG20K0	0RG20K1	0RG20KJ	0RG2370
0RG2371	0RG237J	0RG23A0	0RG23AJ	0RG23J0	0RG23J1	0RG23JJ	0RG23K0	0RG23K1	0RG23KJ	0RG2470	0RG2471	0RG247J
0RG24A0	0RG24AJ	0RG24J0	0RG24J1	0RG24JJ	0RG24K0	0RG24K1	0RG24KJ	0RG4070	0RG4071	0RG407J	0RG40A0	0RG40AJ
0RG40J0	0RG40J1	0RG40JJ	0RG40K0	0RG40K1	0RG40KJ	0RG4370	0RG4371	0RG437J	0RG43A0	0RG43AJ	0RG43J0	0RG43J1
0RG43JJ	0RG43K0	0RG43K1	0RG43KJ	0RG4470	0RG4471	0RG447J	0RG44A0	0RG44AJ	0RG44J0	0RG44J1	0RG44JJ	0RG44K0
0RG44K1	0RG44KJ	0RG6070	0RG6071	0RG607J	0RG60A0	0RG60AJ	0RG60J0	0RG60J1	0RG60JJ	0RG60K0	0RG60K1	0RG60KJ
0RG6370	0RG6371	0RG637J	0RG63A0	0RG63AJ	0RG63J0	0RG63J1	0RG63JJ	0RG63K0	0RG63K1	0RG63KJ	0RG6470	0RG6471
0RG647J	0RG64A0	0RG64AJ	0RG64J0	0RG64J1	0RG64JJ	0RG64K0	0RG64K1	0RG64KJ	0RG7070	0RG7071	0RG707J	0RG70A0
0RG70AJ	0RG70J0	0RG70J1	0RG70JJ	0RG70K0	0RG70K1	0RG70KJ	0RG7370	0RG7371	0RG737J	0RG73A0	0RG73AJ	0RG73J0
0RG73J1	0RG73JJ	0RG73K0	0RG73K1	0RG73KJ	0RG7470	0RG7471	0RG747J	0RG74A0	0RG74AJ	0RG74J0	0RG74J1	0RG74JJ
0RG74K0	0RG74K1	0RG74KJ	0RG8070	0RG8071	0RG807J	0RG80A0	0RG80AJ	0RG80J0	0RG80J1	0RG80JJ	0RG80K0	0RG80K1
0RG80KJ	0RG8370	0RG8371	0RG837J	0RG83A0	0RG83AJ	0RG83J0	0RG83J1	0RG83JJ	0RG83K0	0RG83K1	0RG83KJ	0RG8470
0RG8471	0RG847J	0RG84A0	0RG84AJ	0RG84J0	0RG84J1	0RG84JJ	0RG84K0	0RG84K1	0RG84KJ	0RGA070	0RGA071	0RGA07J
0RGA0A0	0RGA0AJ	0RGA0J0	0RGA0J1	0RGA0JJ	0RGA0K0	0RGA0K1	0RGA0KJ	0RGA370	0RGA371	0RGA37J	0RGA3A0	0RGA3AJ
0RGA3J0	0RGA3J1	0RGA3JJ	0RGA3K0	0RGA3K1	0RGA3KJ	0RGA470	0RGA471	0RGA47J	0RGA4A0	0RGA4AJ	0RGA4J0	0RGA4J1
0RGA4JJ	0RGA4K0	0RGA4K1	0RGA4KJ	0RGE04Z	0RGE07Z	0RGE0JZ	0RGE0KZ	0RGE34Z	0RGE37Z	0RGE3JZ	0RGE3KZ	0RGE44Z
0RGE47Z	0RGE4JZ	0RGE4KZ	0RGF04Z	0RGF07Z	0RGF0JZ	0RGF0KZ	0RGF34Z	0RGF37Z	0RGF3JZ	0RGF3KZ	0RGF44Z	0RGF47Z
0RGF4JZ	0RGF4KZ	0RGG04Z	0RGG07Z	0RGG0JZ	0RGG0KZ	0RGG34Z	0RGG37Z	0RGG3JZ	0RGG3KZ	0RGG44Z	0RGG47Z	0RGG4JZ
0RGG4KZ	0RGH04Z	0RGH07Z	0RGH0JZ	0RGH0KZ	0RGH34Z	0RGH37Z	0RGH3JZ	0RGH3KZ	0RGH44Z	0RGH47Z	0RGH4JZ	0RGH4KZ
0RGJ04Z	0RGJ07Z	0RGJ0JZ	0RGJ0KZ	0RGJ34Z	0RGJ37Z	0RGJ3JZ	0RGJ3KZ	0RGJ44Z	0RGJ47Z	0RGJ4JZ	0RGJ4KZ	0RGK04Z
0RGK07Z	0RGK0JZ	0RGK0KZ	0RGK34Z	0RGK37Z	0RGK3JZ	0RGK3KZ	0RGK44Z	0RGK47Z	0RGK4JZ	0RGK4KZ	0RGL04Z	0RGL05Z
0RGL07Z	0RGL0JZ	0RGL0KZ	0RGL34Z	0RGL35Z	0RGL37Z	0RGL3JZ	0RGL3KZ	0RGL44Z	0RGL45Z	0RGL47Z	0RGL4JZ	0RGL4KZ
0RGM04Z	0RGM05Z	0RGM07Z	0RGM0JZ	0RGM0KZ	0RGM34Z	0RGM35Z	0RGM37Z	0RGM3JZ	0RGM3KZ	0RGM44Z	0RGM45Z	0RGM47Z
0RGM4JZ	0RGM4KZ											

Surgical site infection following certain orthopedic procedures of spine, shoulder and elbow procedures and secondary diagnosis K68.11, T81.40XA, T81.41XA, T81.42XA, T81.43XA, T81.44XA, T81.49XA, T84.60XA, T84.610A, T84.611A, T84.612A, T84.613A, T84.614A, T84.615A, T84.619A, T84.63XA, T84.69XA, T84.7XXA.

CC

0RG7070	0RG7071	0RG707J	0RG70A0	0RG70AJ	0RG70J0	0RG70J1	0RG70JJ	0RG70K0	0RG70K1	0RG70KJ	0RG7370	0RG7371
0RG737J	0RG73A0	0RG73AJ	0RG73J0	0RG73J1	0RG73JJ	0RG73K0	0RG73K1	0RG73KJ	0RG7470	0RG7471	0RG747J	0RG74A0
0RG74AJ	0RG74J0	0RG74J1	0RG74JJ	0RG74K0	0RG74K1	0RG74KJ						

0 Medical and Surgical

R Upper Joints

H Insertion: Putting in a nonbiological appliance that monitors, assists, performs, or prevents a physiological function but does not physically take the place of a body part

Body Part	Approach	Device	Qualifier
Character 4	Character 5	Character 6	Character 7
0 Occipital-cervical Joint **1** Cervical Vertebral Joint **4** Cervicothoracic Vertebral Joint **6** Thoracic Vertebral Joint **A** Thoracolumbar Vertebral Joint	**0** Open **3** Percutaneous **4** Percutaneous Endoscopic	**3** Infusion Device **4** Internal Fixation Device **8** Spacer **B** Spinal Stabilization Device, Interspinous Process **C** Spinal Stabilization Device, Pedicle-Based **D** Spinal Stabilization Device, Facet Replacement	**Z** No Qualifier
3 Cervical Vertebral Disc **5** Cervicothoracic Vertebral Disc **9** Thoracic Vertebral Disc **B** Thoracolumbar Vertebral Disc	**0** Open **3** Percutaneous **4** Percutaneous Endoscopic	**3** Infusion Device	**Z** No Qualifier
C Temporomandibular Joint, Right **D** Temporomandibular Joint, Left **E** Sternoclavicular Joint, Right **F** Sternoclavicular Joint, Left **G** Acromioclavicular Joint, Right **H** Acromioclavicular Joint, Left **J** Shoulder Joint, Right **K** Shoulder Joint, Left	**0** Open **3** Percutaneous **4** Percutaneous Endoscopic	**3** Infusion Device **4** Internal Fixation Device **8** Spacer	**Z** No Qualifier
L Elbow Joint, Right **M** Elbow Joint, Left **N** Wrist Joint, Right **P** Wrist Joint, Left **Q** Carpal Joint, Right **R** Carpal Joint, Left **S** Carpometacarpal Joint, Right **T** Carpometacarpal Joint, Left **U** Metacarpophalangeal Joint, Right **V** Metacarpophalangeal Joint, Left **W** Finger Phalangeal Joint, Right **X** Finger Phalangeal Joint, Left	**0** Open **3** Percutaneous **4** Percutaneous Endoscopic	**3** Infusion Device **4** Internal Fixation Device **5** External Fixation Device **8** Spacer	**Z** No Qualifier

LC Limited Coverage   **NC** Noncovered   **HAC** HAC-associated Procedure   **CC** Combination Cluster - See Appendix G for code lists

Non-OR Non-OR-Affecting MS-DRG Assignment   New/Revised Text in **Orange**   ♂ Male   ♀ Female

494   **2021 ICD-10-PCS**

0 Medical and Surgical
R Upper Joints
J Inspection: Visually and/or manually exploring a body part

Body Part	Approach	Device	Qualifier
Character 4	Character 5	Character 6	Character 7
0 Occipital-cervical Joint **1** Cervical Vertebral Joint **3** Cervical Vertebral Disc **4** Cervicothoracic Vertebral Joint **5** Cervicothoracic Vertebral Disc **6** Thoracic Vertebral Joint **9** Thoracic Vertebral Disc **A** Thoracolumbar Vertebral Joint **B** Thoracolumbar Vertebral Disc **C** Temporomandibular Joint, Right **D** Temporomandibular Joint, Left **E** Sternoclavicular Joint, Right **F** Sternoclavicular Joint, Left **G** Acromioclavicular Joint, Right **H** Acromioclavicular Joint, Left **J** Shoulder Joint, Right **K** Shoulder Joint, Left **L** Elbow Joint, Right **M** Elbow Joint, Left **N** Wrist Joint, Right **P** Wrist Joint, Left **Q** Carpal Joint, Right **R** Carpal Joint, Left **S** Carpometacarpal Joint, Right **T** Carpometacarpal Joint, Left **U** Metacarpophalangeal Joint, Right **V** Metacarpophalangeal Joint, Left **W** Finger Phalangeal Joint, Right **X** Finger Phalangeal Joint, Left	**0** Open **3** Percutaneous **4** Percutaneous Endoscopic **X** External	**Z** No Device	**Z** No Qualifier

0 **Medical and Surgical**
R **Upper Joints**
N **Release:** Freeing a body part from an abnormal physical constraint by cutting or by the use of force

Body Part	Approach	Device	Qualifier
Character 4	Character 5	Character 6	Character 7
0 Occipital-cervical Joint	**0** Open	**Z** No Device	**Z** No Qualifier
1 Cervical Vertebral Joint	**3** Percutaneous		
3 Cervical Vertebral Disc	**4** Percutaneous Endoscopic		
4 Cervicothoracic Vertebral Joint	**X** External		
5 Cervicothoracic Vertebral Disc			
6 Thoracic Vertebral Joint			
9 Thoracic Vertebral Disc			
A Thoracolumbar Vertebral Joint			
B Thoracolumbar Vertebral Disc			
C Temporomandibular Joint, Right			
D Temporomandibular Joint, Left			
E Sternoclavicular Joint, Right			
F Sternoclavicular Joint, Left			
G Acromioclavicular Joint, Right			
H Acromioclavicular Joint, Left			
J Shoulder Joint, Right			
K Shoulder Joint, Left			
L Elbow Joint, Right			
M Elbow Joint, Left			
N Wrist Joint, Right			
P Wrist Joint, Left			
Q Carpal Joint, Right			
R Carpal Joint, Left			
S Carpometacarpal Joint, Right			
T Carpometacarpal Joint, Left			
U Metacarpophalangeal Joint, Right			
V Metacarpophalangeal Joint, Left			
W Finger Phalangeal Joint, Right			
X Finger Phalangeal Joint, Left			

0 **Medical and Surgical**
R **Upper Joints**
P **Removal:** Taking out or off a device from a body part

Body Part	Approach	Device	Qualifier
Character 4	Character 5	Character 6	Character 7
0 Occipital-cervical Joint	**0** Open	**0** Drainage Device	**Z** No Qualifier
1 Cervical Vertebral Joint	**3** Percutaneous	**3** Infusion Device	
4 Cervicothoracic Vertebral Joint	**4** Percutaneous Endoscopic	**4** Internal Fixation Device	
6 Thoracic Vertebral Joint		**7** Autologous Tissue Substitute	
A Thoracolumbar Vertebral Joint		**8** Spacer	
		A Interbody Fusion Device	
		J Synthetic Substitute	
		K Nonautologous Tissue Substitute	
0 Occipital-cervical Joint	**X** External	**0** Drainage Device	**Z** No Qualifier
1 Cervical Vertebral Joint		**3** Infusion Device	
4 Cervicothoracic Vertebral Joint		**4** Internal Fixation Device	
6 Thoracic Vertebral Joint			
A Thoracolumbar Vertebral Joint			
3 Cervical Vertebral Disc	**0** Open	**0** Drainage Device	**Z** No Qualifier
5 Cervicothoracic Vertebral Disc	**3** Percutaneous	**3** Infusion Device	
9 Thoracic Vertebral Disc	**4** Percutaneous Endoscopic	**7** Autologous Tissue Substitute	
B Thoracolumbar Vertebral Disc		**J** Synthetic Substitute	
		K Nonautologous Tissue Substitute	

0RP continued on next page

LC Limited Coverage   **NC** Noncovered   **HAC** HAC-associated Procedure   **CC** Combination Cluster - See Appendix G for code lists
⬛ Non-OR-Affecting MS-DRG Assignment   New/Revised Text in **Orange**   ♂ Male   ♀ Female

496

2021 ICD-10-PCS

0 **Medical and Surgical**
R **Upper Joints**
P **Removal:** Taking out or off a device from a body part

0RP continued from previous page

Body Part	Approach	Device	Qualifier
Character 4	**Character 5**	**Character 6**	**Character 7**
3 Cervical Vertebral Disc 5 Cervicothoracic Vertebral Disc 9 Thoracic Vertebral Disc B Thoracolumbar Vertebral Disc	X External	0 Drainage Device 3 Infusion Device	Z No Qualifier
C Temporomandibular Joint, Right D Temporomandibular Joint, Left E Sternoclavicular Joint, Right F Sternoclavicular Joint, Left G Acromioclavicular Joint, Right H Acromioclavicular Joint, Left J Shoulder Joint, Right K Shoulder Joint, Left	0 Open 3 Percutaneous 4 Percutaneous Endoscopic	0 Drainage Device 3 Infusion Device 4 Internal Fixation Device 7 Autologous Tissue Substitute 8 Spacer J Synthetic Substitute K Nonautologous Tissue Substitute	Z No Qualifier
C Temporomandibular Joint, Right D Temporomandibular Joint, Left E Sternoclavicular Joint, Right F Sternoclavicular Joint, Left G Acromioclavicular Joint, Right H Acromioclavicular Joint, Left J Shoulder Joint, Right K Shoulder Joint, Left	X External	0 Drainage Device 3 Infusion Device 4 Internal Fixation Device	Z No Qualifier
L Elbow Joint, Right M Elbow Joint, Left N Wrist Joint, Right P Wrist Joint, Left Q Carpal Joint, Right R Carpal Joint, Left S Carpometacarpal Joint, Right T Carpometacarpal Joint, Left U Metacarpophalangeal Joint, Right V Metacarpophalangeal Joint, Left W Finger Phalangeal Joint, Right X Finger Phalangeal Joint, Left	0 Open 3 Percutaneous 4 Percutaneous Endoscopic	0 Drainage Device 3 Infusion Device 4 Internal Fixation Device 5 External Fixation Device 7 Autologous Tissue Substitute 8 Spacer J Synthetic Substitute K Nonautologous Tissue Substitute	Z No Qualifier
L Elbow Joint, Right M Elbow Joint, Left N Wrist Joint, Right P Wrist Joint, Left Q Carpal Joint, Right R Carpal Joint, Left S Carpometacarpal Joint, Right T Carpometacarpal Joint, Left U Metacarpophalangeal Joint, Right V Metacarpophalangeal Joint, Left W Finger Phalangeal Joint, Right X Finger Phalangeal Joint, Left	X External	0 Drainage Device 3 Infusion Device 4 Internal Fixation Device 5 External Fixation Device	Z No Qualifier

0 **Medical and Surgical**
R **Upper Joints**
Q **Repair:** Restoring, to the extent possible, a body part to its normal anatomic structure and function

Body Part	Approach	Device	Qualifier
Character 4	Character 5	Character 6	Character 7
0 Occipital-cervical Joint 1 Cervical Vertebral Joint 3 Cervical Vertebral Disc 4 Cervicothoracic Vertebral Joint 5 Cervicothoracic Vertebral Disc 6 Thoracic Vertebral Joint 9 Thoracic Vertebral Disc A Thoracolumbar Vertebral Joint B Thoracolumbar Vertebral Disc C Temporomandibular Joint, Right D Temporomandibular Joint, Left E Sternoclavicular Joint, Right HAC F Sternoclavicular Joint, Left HAC G Acromioclavicular Joint, Right HAC H Acromioclavicular Joint, Left HAC J Shoulder Joint, Right HAC K Shoulder Joint, Left HAC L Elbow Joint, Right HAC M Elbow Joint, Left HAC N Wrist Joint, Right P Wrist Joint, Left Q Carpal Joint, Right R Carpal Joint, Left S Carpometacarpal Joint, Right T Carpometacarpal Joint, Left U Metacarpophalangeal Joint, Right V Metacarpophalangeal Joint, Left W Finger Phalangeal Joint, Right X Finger Phalangeal Joint, Left	0 Open 3 Percutaneous 4 Percutaneous Endoscopic X External	Z No Device	Z No Qualifier

HAC 0RQE0ZZ 0RQE3ZZ 0RQE4ZZ 0RQEXZZ 0RQF0ZZ 0RQF3ZZ 0RQF4ZZ 0RQFXZZ 0RQG0ZZ 0RQG3ZZ 0RQG4ZZ 0RQGXZZ 0RQH0ZZ
0RQH3ZZ 0RQH4ZZ 0RQHXZZ 0RQJ0ZZ 0RQJ3ZZ 0RQJ4ZZ 0RQJXZZ 0RQK0ZZ 0RQK3ZZ 0RQK4ZZ 0RQKXZZ 0RQL0ZZ 0RQL3ZZ
0RQL4ZZ 0RQLXZZ 0RQM0ZZ 0RQM3ZZ 0RQM4ZZ 0RQMXZZ
Surgical site infection following certain orthopedic procedures of spine, shoulder and elbow procedures and secondary diagnosis K68.11, T81.40XA, T81.41XA, T81.42XA, T81.43XA, T81.44XA, T81.49XA, T84.60XA, T84.610A, T84.611A, T84.612A, T84.613A, T84.614A, T84.615A, T84.619A, T84.63XA, T84.69XA, T84.7XXA.

0   **Medical and Surgical**
R   **Upper Joints**
R   **Replacement:** Putting in or on biological or synthetic material that physically takes the place and/or function of all or a portion of a body part

Body Part	Approach	Device	Qualifier
Character 4	Character 5	Character 6	Character 7
0 Occipital-cervical Joint 1 Cervical Vertebral Joint 3 Cervical Vertebral Disc 4 Cervicothoracic Vertebral Joint 5 Cervicothoracic Vertebral Disc 6 Thoracic Vertebral Joint 9 Thoracic Vertebral Disc A Thoracolumbar Vertebral Joint B Thoracolumbar Vertebral Disc C Temporomandibular Joint, Right D Temporomandibular Joint, Left E Sternoclavicular Joint, Right F Sternoclavicular Joint, Left G Acromioclavicular Joint, Right H Acromioclavicular Joint, Left L Elbow Joint, Right M Elbow Joint, Left N Wrist Joint, Right P Wrist Joint, Left Q Carpal Joint, Right R Carpal Joint, Left S Carpometacarpal Joint, Right T Carpometacarpal Joint, Left U Metacarpophalangeal Joint, Right V Metacarpophalangeal Joint, Left W Finger Phalangeal Joint, Right X Finger Phalangeal Joint, Left	0 Open	7 Autologous Tissue Substitute J Synthetic Substitute K Nonautologous Tissue Substitute	Z No Qualifier
J Shoulder Joint, Right K Shoulder Joint, Left	0 Open	0 Synthetic Substitute, Reverse Ball and Socket 7 Autologous Tissue Substitute K Nonautologous Tissue Substitute	Z No Qualifier
J Shoulder Joint, Right K Shoulder Joint, Left	0 Open	J Synthetic Substitute	6 Humeral Surface 7 Glenoid Surface Z No Qualifier

LC Limited Coverage   **NC** Noncovered   **HAC** HAC-associated Procedure   **CC** Combination Cluster - See Appendix G for code lists

**Non-OR-Affecting MS-DRG Assignment   New/Revised Text in Orange   ♂ Male   ♀ Female

2021 ICD-10-PCS

499

UPPER JOINTS 0R2-0RW

0   **Medical and Surgical**
R   **Upper Joints**
S   **Reposition:** Moving to its normal location, or other suitable location, all or a portion of a body part

Body Part	Approach	Device	Qualifier
Character 4	Character 5	Character 6	Character 7
0 Occipital-cervical Joint **1** Cervical Vertebral Joint **4** Cervicothoracic Vertebral Joint **6** Thoracic Vertebral Joint **A** Thoracolumbar Vertebral Joint **C** Temporomandibular Joint, Right **D** Temporomandibular Joint, Left **E** Sternoclavicular Joint, Right **F** Sternoclavicular Joint, Left **G** Acromioclavicular Joint, Right **H** Acromioclavicular Joint, Left **J** Shoulder Joint, Right **K** Shoulder Joint, Left	**0** Open **3** Percutaneous **4** Percutaneous Endoscopic **X** External	**4** Internal Fixation Device **Z** No Device	**Z** No Qualifier
L Elbow Joint, Right **M** Elbow Joint, Left **N** Wrist Joint, Right **P** Wrist Joint, Left **Q** Carpal Joint, Right **R** Carpal Joint, Left **S** Carpometacarpal Joint, Right **T** Carpometacarpal Joint, Left **U** Metacarpophalangeal Joint, Right **V** Metacarpophalangeal Joint, Left **W** Finger Phalangeal Joint, Right **X** Finger Phalangeal Joint, Left	**0** Open **3** Percutaneous **4** Percutaneous Endoscopic **X** External	**4** Internal Fixation Device **5** External Fixation Device **Z** No Device	**Z** No Qualifier

LC Limited Coverage   **NC** Noncovered   **HAC** HAC-associated Procedure   **CC** Combination Cluster - See Appendix G for code lists
DRG Non-OR-Affecting MS-DRG Assignment   New/Revised Text in **Orange**   ♂ Male   ♀ Female

500   **2021 ICD-10-PCS**

0 **Medical and Surgical**
R **Upper Joints**
T **Resection:** Cutting out or off, without replacement, all of a body part

Body Part	Approach	Device	Qualifier
Character 4	Character 5	Character 6	Character 7
3 Cervical Vertebral Disc	0 Open	Z No Device	Z No Qualifier
4 Cervicothoracic Vertebral Joint			
5 Cervicothoracic Vertebral Disc			
9 Thoracic Vertebral Disc			
B Thoracolumbar Vertebral Disc			
C Temporomandibular Joint, Right			
D Temporomandibular Joint, Left			
E Sternoclavicular Joint, Right			
F Sternoclavicular Joint, Left			
G Acromioclavicular Joint, Right			
H Acromioclavicular Joint, Left			
J Shoulder Joint, Right			
K Shoulder Joint, Left			
L Elbow Joint, Right			
M Elbow Joint, Left			
N Wrist Joint, Right			
P Wrist Joint, Left			
Q Carpal Joint, Right			
R Carpal Joint, Left			
S Carpometacarpal Joint, Right			
T Carpometacarpal Joint, Left			
U Metacarpophalangeal Joint, Right			
V Metacarpophalangeal Joint, Left			
W Finger Phalangeal Joint, Right			
X Finger Phalangeal Joint, Left			

LC Limited Coverage   **NC** Noncovered   **HAC** HAC-associated Procedure   **CC** Combination Cluster - See Appendix G for code lists
⊗ Non-OR-Affecting MS-DRG Assignment   New/Revised Text in **Orange**   ♂ Male   ♀ Female

2021 ICD-10-PCS

501

ORT

UPPER JOINTS 0R2–0RW

0 **Medical and Surgical**
R **Upper Joints**
U **Supplement:** Putting in or on biological or synthetic material that physically reinforces and/or augments the function of a portion of a body part

Body Part	Approach	Device	Qualifier
Character 4	Character 5	Character 6	Character 7
0 Occipital-cervical Joint 1 Cervical Vertebral Joint 3 Cervical Vertebral Disc 4 Cervicothoracic Vertebral Joint 5 Cervicothoracic Vertebral Disc 6 Thoracic Vertebral Joint 9 Thoracic Vertebral Disc A Thoracolumbar Vertebral Joint B Thoracolumbar Vertebral Disc C Temporomandibular Joint, Right D Temporomandibular Joint, Left E Sternoclavicular Joint, Right `HAC` F Sternoclavicular Joint, Left `HAC` G Acromioclavicular Joint, Right `HAC` H Acromioclavicular Joint, Left `HAC` J Shoulder Joint, Right `HAC` K Shoulder Joint, Left `HAC` L Elbow Joint, Right `HAC` M Elbow Joint, Left `HAC` N Wrist Joint, Right P Wrist Joint, Left Q Carpal Joint, Right R Carpal Joint, Left S Carpometacarpal Joint, Right T Carpometacarpal Joint, Left U Metacarpophalangeal Joint, Right V Metacarpophalangeal Joint, Left W Finger Phalangeal Joint, Right X Finger Phalangeal Joint, Left	0 Open 3 Percutaneous 4 Percutaneous Endoscopic	7 Autologous Tissue Substitute J Synthetic Substitute K Nonautologous Tissue Substitute	Z No Qualifier

`HAC` 0RUE07Z 0RUE0JZ 0RUE0KZ 0RUE37Z 0RUE3JZ 0RUE3KZ 0RUE47Z 0RUE4JZ 0RUE4KZ 0RUF07Z 0RUF0JZ 0RUF0KZ 0RUF37Z
 0RUF3JZ 0RUF3KZ 0RUF47Z 0RUF4JZ 0RUF4KZ 0RUG07Z 0RUG0JZ 0RUG0KZ 0RUG37Z 0RUG3JZ 0RUG3KZ 0RUG47Z 0RUG4JZ
 0RUG4KZ 0RUH07Z 0RUH0JZ 0RUH0KZ 0RUH37Z 0RUH3JZ 0RUH3KZ 0RUH47Z 0RUH4JZ 0RUH4KZ 0RUJ07Z 0RUJ0JZ 0RUJ0KZ
 0RUJ37Z 0RUJ3JZ 0RUJ3KZ 0RUJ47Z 0RUJ4JZ 0RUJ4KZ 0RUK07Z 0RUK0JZ 0RUK0KZ 0RUK37Z 0RUK3JZ 0RUK3KZ 0RUK47Z
 0RUK4JZ 0RUK4KZ 0RUL07Z 0RUL0JZ 0RUL0KZ 0RUL37Z 0RUL3JZ 0RUL3KZ 0RUL47Z 0RUL4JZ 0RUL4KZ 0RUM07Z 0RUM0JZ
 0RUM0KZ 0RUM37Z 0RUM3JZ 0RUM3KZ 0RUM47Z 0RUM4JZ 0RUM4KZ

Surgical site infection following certain orthopedic procedures of spine, shoulder and elbow procedures and secondary diagnosis K68.11, T81.40XA, T81.41XA, T81.42XA, T81.43XA, T81.44XA, T81.49XA, T84.60XA, T84.610A, T84.611A, T84.612A, T84.613A, T84.614A, T84.615A, T84.619A, T84.63XA, T84.69XA, T84.7XXA.

`LC` Limited Coverage   `NC` Noncovered   `HAC` HAC-associated Procedure   `CC` Combination Cluster - See Appendix G for code lists
`DRG` Non-OR-Affecting MS-DRG Assignment   New/Revised Text in **Orange**   ♂ Male   ♀ Female

0 **Medical and Surgical**
R **Upper Joints**
W **Revision:** Correcting, to the extent possible, a portion of a malfunctioning device or the position of a displaced device

Body Part	Approach	Device	Qualifier
Character 4	Character 5	Character 6	Character 7
0 Occipital-cervical Joint 1 Cervical Vertebral Joint 4 Cervicothoracic Vertebral Joint 6 Thoracic Vertebral Joint A Thoracolumbar Vertebral Joint	0 Open 3 Percutaneous 4 Percutaneous Endoscopic X External	0 Drainage Device 3 Infusion Device 4 Internal Fixation Device 7 Autologous Tissue Substitute 8 Spacer A Interbody Fusion Device J Synthetic Substitute K Nonautologous Tissue Substitute	Z No Qualifier
3 Cervical Vertebral Disc 5 Cervicothoracic Vertebral Disc 9 Thoracic Vertebral Disc B Thoracolumbar Vertebral Disc	0 Open 3 Percutaneous 4 Percutaneous Endoscopic X External	0 Drainage Device 3 Infusion Device 7 Autologous Tissue Substitute J Synthetic Substitute K Nonautologous Tissue Substitute	Z No Qualifier
C Temporomandibular Joint, Right D Temporomandibular Joint, Left E Sternoclavicular Joint, Right F Sternoclavicular Joint, Left G Acromioclavicular Joint, Right H Acromioclavicular Joint, Left J Shoulder Joint, Right K Shoulder Joint, Left	0 Open 3 Percutaneous 4 Percutaneous Endoscopic X External	0 Drainage Device 3 Infusion Device 4 Internal Fixation Device 7 Autologous Tissue Substitute 8 Spacer J Synthetic Substitute K Nonautologous Tissue Substitute	Z No Qualifier
L Elbow Joint, Right M Elbow Joint, Left N Wrist Joint, Right P Wrist Joint, Left Q Carpal Joint, Right R Carpal Joint, Left S Carpometacarpal Joint, Right T Carpometacarpal Joint, Left U Metacarpophalangeal Joint, Right V Metacarpophalangeal Joint, Left W Finger Phalangeal Joint, Right X Finger Phalangeal Joint, Left	0 Open 3 Percutaneous 4 Percutaneous Endoscopic X External	0 Drainage Device 3 Infusion Device 4 Internal Fixation Device 5 External Fixation Device 7 Autologous Tissue Substitute 8 Spacer J Synthetic Substitute K Nonautologous Tissue Substitute	Z No Qualifier

LC Limited Coverage   NC Noncovered   HAC HAC-associated Procedure   CC Combination Cluster - See Appendix G for code lists
ORG Non-OR-Affecting MS-DRG Assignment   New/Revised Text in Orange   ♂ Male   ♀ Female

2021 ICD-10-PCS

503

UPPER JOINTS 0R2-0RW

NOTES

Lower Joints 0S2-0SW

0 Medical and Surgical
S Lower Joints
2 Change: Taking out or off a device from a body part and putting back an identical or similar device in or on the same body part without cutting or puncturing the skin or a mucous membrane

Body Part	Approach	Device	Qualifier
Character 4	Character 5	Character 6	Character 7
Y Lower Joint	**X** External	**0** Drainage Device **Y** Other Device	**Z** No Qualifier

0 Medical and Surgical
S Lower Joints
5 Destruction: Physical eradication of all or a portion of a body part by the direct use of energy, force, or a destructive agent

Body Part	Approach	Device	Qualifier
Character 4	Character 5	Character 6	Character 7
0 Lumbar Vertebral Joint **2** Lumbar Vertebral Disc **3** Lumbosacral Joint **4** Lumbosacral Disc **5** Sacrococcygeal Joint **6** Coccygeal Joint **7** Sacroiliac Joint, Right **8** Sacroiliac Joint, Left **9** Hip Joint, Right **B** Hip Joint, Left **C** Knee Joint, Right **D** Knee Joint, Left **F** Ankle Joint, Right **G** Ankle Joint, Left **H** Tarsal Joint, Right **J** Tarsal Joint, Left **K** Tarsometatarsal Joint, Right **L** Tarsometatarsal Joint, Left **M** Metatarsal-Phalangeal Joint, Right **N** Metatarsal-Phalangeal Joint, Left **P** Toe Phalangeal Joint, Right **Q** Toe Phalangeal Joint, Left	**0** Open **3** Percutaneous **4** Percutaneous Endoscopic	**Z** No Device	**Z** No Qualifier

0   Medical and Surgical
S   Lower Joints
9   Drainage: Taking or letting out fluids and/or gases from a body part

Body Part	Approach	Device	Qualifier
Character 4	**Character 5**	**Character 6**	**Character 7**
0 Lumbar Vertebral Joint **2** Lumbar Vertebral Disc **3** Lumbosacral Joint **4** Lumbosacral Disc **5** Sacrococcygeal Joint **6** Coccygeal Joint **7** Sacroiliac Joint, Right **8** Sacroiliac Joint, Left **9** Hip Joint, Right **B** Hip Joint, Left **C** Knee Joint, Right **D** Knee Joint, Left **F** Ankle Joint, Right **G** Ankle Joint, Left **H** Tarsal Joint, Right **J** Tarsal Joint, Left **K** Tarsometatarsal Joint, Right **L** Tarsometatarsal Joint, Left **M** Metatarsal-Phalangeal Joint, Right **N** Metatarsal-Phalangeal Joint, Left **P** Toe Phalangeal Joint, Right **Q** Toe Phalangeal Joint, Left	**0** Open **3** Percutaneous **4** Percutaneous Endoscopic	**0** Drainage Device	**Z** No Qualifier
0 Lumbar Vertebral Joint **2** Lumbar Vertebral Disc **3** Lumbosacral Joint **4** Lumbosacral Disc **5** Sacrococcygeal Joint **6** Coccygeal Joint **7** Sacroiliac Joint, Right **8** Sacroiliac Joint, Left **9** Hip Joint, Right **B** Hip Joint, Left **C** Knee Joint, Right **D** Knee Joint, Left **F** Ankle Joint, Right **G** Ankle Joint, Left **H** Tarsal Joint, Right **J** Tarsal Joint, Left **K** Tarsometatarsal Joint, Right **L** Tarsometatarsal Joint, Left **M** Metatarsal-Phalangeal Joint, Right **N** Metatarsal-Phalangeal Joint, Left **P** Toe Phalangeal Joint, Right **Q** Toe Phalangeal Joint, Left	**0** Open **3** Percutaneous **4** Percutaneous Endoscopic	**Z** No Device	**X** Diagnostic **Z** No Qualifier

LC Limited Coverage   **NC** Noncovered   **HAC** HAC-associated Procedure   **CC** Combination Cluster - See Appendix G for code lists
DRG Non-OR-Affecting MS-DRG Assignment   New/Revised Text in **Orange**   ♂ Male   ♀ Female

506

2021 ICD-10-PCS

0 Medical and Surgical

S Lower Joints

B Excision: Cutting out or off, without replacement, a portion of a body part

Body Part	Approach	Device	Qualifier
Character 4	Character 5	Character 6	Character 7
0 Lumbar Vertebral Joint **2** Lumbar Vertebral Disc **3** Lumbosacral Joint **4** Lumbosacral Disc **5** Sacrococcygeal Joint **6** Coccygeal Joint **7** Sacroiliac Joint, Right **8** Sacroiliac Joint, Left **9** Hip Joint, Right **B** Hip Joint, Left **C** Knee Joint, Right **D** Knee Joint, Left **F** Ankle Joint, Right **G** Ankle Joint, Left **H** Tarsal Joint, Right **J** Tarsal Joint, Left **K** Tarsometatarsal Joint, Right **L** Tarsometatarsal Joint, Left **M** Metatarsal-Phalangeal Joint, Right **N** Metatarsal-Phalangeal Joint, Left **P** Toe Phalangeal Joint, Right **Q** Toe Phalangeal Joint, Left	**0** Open **3** Percutaneous **4** Percutaneous Endoscopic	**Z** No Device	**X** Diagnostic **Z** No Qualifier

0 Medical and Surgical

S Lower Joints

C Extirpation: Taking or cutting out solid matter from a body part

Body Part	Approach	Device	Qualifier
Character 4	Character 5	Character 6	Character 7
0 Lumbar Vertebral Joint **2** Lumbar Vertebral Disc **3** Lumbosacral Joint **4** Lumbosacral Disc **5** Sacrococcygeal Joint **6** Coccygeal Joint **7** Sacroiliac Joint, Right **8** Sacroiliac Joint, Left **9** Hip Joint, Right **B** Hip Joint, Left **C** Knee Joint, Right **D** Knee Joint, Left **F** Ankle Joint, Right **G** Ankle Joint, Left **H** Tarsal Joint, Right **J** Tarsal Joint, Left **K** Tarsometatarsal Joint, Right **L** Tarsometatarsal Joint, Left **M** Metatarsal-Phalangeal Joint, Right **N** Metatarsal-Phalangeal Joint, Left **P** Toe Phalangeal Joint, Right **Q** Toe Phalangeal Joint, Left	**0** Open **3** Percutaneous **4** Percutaneous Endoscopic	**Z** No Device	**Z** No Qualifier

LC Limited Coverage   **NC** Noncovered   **HAC** HAC-associated Procedure   **CC** Combination Cluster - See Appendix G for code lists

Non-OR-Affecting MS-DRG Assignment   New/Revised Text in Orange   ♂ Male   ♀ Female

2021 ICD-10-PCS

507

0 Medical and Surgical
S Lower Joints
G Fusion: Joining together portions of an articular body part rendering the articular body part immobile

Body Part	Approach	Device	Qualifier
Character 4	**Character 5**	**Character 6**	**Character 7**
0 Lumbar Vertebral Joint HAC **1** Lumbar Vertebral Joints, 2 or more HAC CC **3** Lumbosacral Joint HAC	**0** Open **3** Percutaneous **4** Percutaneous Endoscopic	**7** Autologous Tissue Substitute **J** Synthetic Substitute **K** Nonautologous Tissue Substitute	**0** Anterior Approach, Anterior Column **1** Posterior Approach, Posterior Column **J** Posterior Approach, Anterior Column
0 Lumbar Vertebral Joint HAC **1** Lumbar Vertebral Joints, 2 or more HAC CC **3** Lumbosacral Joint HAC	**0** Open **3** Percutaneous **4** Percutaneous Endoscopic	**A** Interbody Fusion Device	**0** Anterior Approach, Anterior Column **J** Posterior Approach, Anterior Column
5 Sacrococcygeal Joint **6** Coccygeal Joint **7** Sacroiliac Joint, Right HAC **8** Sacroiliac Joint, Left HAC	**0** Open **3** Percutaneous **4** Percutaneous Endoscopic	**4** Internal Fixation Device **7** Autologous Tissue Substitute **J** Synthetic Substitute **K** Nonautologous Tissue Substitute	**Z** No Qualifier
9 Hip Joint, Right **B** Hip Joint, Left **C** Knee Joint, Right **D** Knee Joint, Left **F** Ankle Joint, Right **G** Ankle Joint, Left **H** Tarsal Joint, Right **J** Tarsal Joint, Left **K** Tarsometatarsal Joint, Right **L** Tarsometatarsal Joint, Left **M** Metatarsal-Phalangeal Joint, Right **N** Metatarsal-Phalangeal Joint, Left **P** Toe Phalangeal Joint, Right **Q** Toe Phalangeal Joint, Left	**0** Open **3** Percutaneous **4** Percutaneous Endoscopic	**3** Internal Fixation Device, Sustained Compression **4** Internal Fixation Device **5** External Fixation Device **7** Autologous Tissue Substitute **J** Synthetic Substitute **K** Nonautologous Tissue Substitute	**Z** No Qualifier

HAC

0SG0070	0SG0071	0SG007J	0SG00A0	0SG00AJ	0SG00J0	0SG00J1	0SG00JJ	0SG00K0	0SG00K1	0SG00KJ	0SG0370	0SG0371
0SG037J	0SG03A0	0SG03AJ	0SG03J0	0SG03J1	0SG03JJ	0SG03K0	0SG03K1	0SG03KJ	0SG0470	0SG0471	0SG047J	0SG04A0
0SG04AJ	0SG04J0	0SG04J1	0SG04JJ	0SG04K0	0SG04K1	0SG04KJ	0SG1070	0SG1071	0SG107J	0SG10A0	0SG10AJ	0SG10J0
0SG10J1	0SG10JJ	0SG10K0	0SG10K1	0SG10KJ	0SG1370	0SG1371	0SG137J	0SG13A0	0SG13AJ	0SG13J0	0SG13J1	0SG13JJ
0SG13K0	0SG13K1	0SG13KJ	0SG1470	0SG1471	0SG147J	0SG14A0	0SG14AJ	0SG14J0	0SG14J1	0SG14JJ	0SG14K0	0SG14K1
0SG14KJ	0SG3070	0SG3071	0SG307J	0SG30A0	0SG30AJ	0SG30J0	0SG30J1	0SG30JJ	0SG30K0	0SG30K1	0SG30KJ	0SG3370
0SG3371	0SG337J	0SG33A0	0SG33AJ	0SG33J0	0SG33J1	0SG33JJ	0SG33K0	0SG33K1	0SG33KJ	0SG3470	0SG3471	0SG347J
0SG34A0	0SG34AJ	0SG34J0	0SG34J1	0SG34JJ	0SG34K0	0SG34K1	0SG34KJ	0SG704Z	0SG707Z	0SG70JZ	0SG70KZ	0SG734Z
0SG737Z	0SG73JZ	0SG73KZ	0SG744Z	0SG747Z	0SG74JZ	0SG74KZ	0SG804Z	0SG807Z	0SG80JZ	0SG80KZ	0SG834Z	0SG837Z
0SG83JZ	0SG83KZ	0SG844Z	0SG847Z	0SG84JZ	0SG84KZ							

Surgical site infection following certain orthopedic procedures of spine, shoulder and elbow procedures and secondary diagnosis K68.11, T81.40XA, T81.41XA, T81.42XA, T81.43XA, T81.44XA, T81.49XA, T84.60XA, T84.610A, T84.611A, T84.612A, T84.613A, T84.614A, T84.615A, T84.619A, T84.63XA, T84.69XA, T84.7XXA.

CC

0SG1070	0SG1071	0SG107J	0SG10A0	0SG10AJ	0SG10J0	0SG10J1	0SG10JJ	0SG10K0	0SG10K1	0SG10KJ	0SG1370	0SG1371
0SG137J	0SG13A0	0SG13AJ	0SG13J0	0SG13J1	0SG13JJ	0SG13K0	0SG13K1	0SG13KJ	0SG1470	0SG1471	0SG147J	0SG14A0
0SG14AJ	0SG14J0	0SG14J1	0SG14JJ	0SG14K0	0SG14K1	0SG14KJ						

LC Limited Coverage   **NC** Noncovered   **HAC** HAC-associated Procedure   **CC** Combination Cluster - See Appendix G for code lists

DRG Non-OR-Affecting MS-DRG Assignment   New/Revised Text in **Orange**   ♂ Male   ♀ Female

508

2021 ICD-10-PCS

0 **Medical and Surgical**
S **Lower Joints**
H **Insertion:** Putting in a nonbiological appliance that monitors, assists, performs, or prevents a physiological function but does not physically take the place of a body part

Body Part	Approach	Device	Qualifier
Character 4	Character 5	Character 6	Character 7
0 Lumbar Vertebral Joint **3** Lumbosacral Joint	**0** Open **3** Percutaneous **4** Percutaneous Endoscopic	**3** Infusion Device **4** Internal Fixation Device **8** Spacer **B** Spinal Stabilization Device, Interspinous Process **C** Spinal Stabilization Device, Pedicle-Based **D** Spinal Stabilization Device, Facet Replacement	**Z** No Qualifier
2 Lumbar Vertebral Disc **4** Lumbosacral Disc	**0** Open **3** Percutaneous **4** Percutaneous Endoscopic	**3** Infusion Device **8** Spacer	**Z** No Qualifier
5 Sacrococcygeal Joint **6** Coccygeal Joint **7** Sacroiliac Joint, Right **8** Sacroiliac Joint, Left	**0** Open **3** Percutaneous **4** Percutaneous Endoscopic	**3** Infusion Device **4** Internal Fixation Device **8** Spacer	**Z** No Qualifier
9 Hip Joint, Right **B** Hip Joint, Left **C** Knee Joint, Right **D** Knee Joint, Left **F** Ankle Joint, Right **G** Ankle Joint, Left **H** Tarsal Joint, Right **J** Tarsal Joint, Left **K** Tarsometatarsal Joint, Right **L** Tarsometatarsal Joint, Left **M** Metatarsal-Phalangeal Joint, Right **N** Metatarsal-Phalangeal Joint, Left **P** Toe Phalangeal Joint, Right **Q** Toe Phalangeal Joint, Left	**0** Open **3** Percutaneous **4** Percutaneous Endoscopic	**3** Infusion Device **4** Internal Fixation Device **5** External Fixation Device **8** Spacer	**Z** No Qualifier

0 Medical and Surgical
S Lower Joints
J Inspection: Visually and/or manually exploring a body part

Body Part	Approach	Device	Qualifier
Character 4	Character 5	Character 6	Character 7
0 Lumbar Vertebral Joint 2 Lumbar Vertebral Disc 3 Lumbosacral Joint 4 Lumbosacral Disc 5 Sacrococcygeal Joint 6 Coccygeal Joint 7 Sacroiliac Joint, Right 8 Sacroiliac Joint, Left 9 Hip Joint, Right B Hip Joint, Left C Knee Joint, Right D Knee Joint, Left F Ankle Joint, Right G Ankle Joint, Left H Tarsal Joint, Right J Tarsal Joint, Left K Tarsometatarsal Joint, Right L Tarsometatarsal Joint, Left M Metatarsal-Phalangeal Joint, Right N Metatarsal-Phalangeal Joint, Left P Toe Phalangeal Joint, Right Q Toe Phalangeal Joint, Left	0 Open 3 Percutaneous 4 Percutaneous Endoscopic X External	Z No Device	Z No Qualifier

0 Medical and Surgical
S Lower Joints
N Release: Freeing a body part from an abnormal physical constraint by cutting or by the use of force

Body Part	Approach	Device	Qualifier
Character 4	Character 5	Character 6	Character 7
0 Lumbar Vertebral Joint 2 Lumbar Vertebral Disc 3 Lumbosacral Joint 4 Lumbosacral Disc 5 Sacrococcygeal Joint 6 Coccygeal Joint 7 Sacroiliac Joint, Right 8 Sacroiliac Joint, Left 9 Hip Joint, Right B Hip Joint, Left C Knee Joint, Right D Knee Joint, Left F Ankle Joint, Right G Ankle Joint, Left H Tarsal Joint, Right J Tarsal Joint, Left K Tarsometatarsal Joint, Right L Tarsometatarsal Joint, Left M Metatarsal-Phalangeal Joint, Right N Metatarsal-Phalangeal Joint, Left P Toe Phalangeal Joint, Right Q Toe Phalangeal Joint, Left	0 Open 3 Percutaneous 4 Percutaneous Endoscopic X External	Z No Device	Z No Qualifier

0 Medical and Surgical
S Lower Joints
P Removal: Taking out or off a device from a body part

Body Part	Approach	Device	Qualifier
Character 4	Character 5	Character 6	Character 7
0 Lumbar Vertebral Joint **3** Lumbosacral Joint	**0** Open **3** Percutaneous **4** Percutaneous Endoscopic	**0** Drainage Device **3** Infusion Device **4** Internal Fixation Device **7** Autologous Tissue Substitute **8** Spacer **A** Interbody Fusion Device **J** Synthetic Substitute **K** Nonautologous Tissue Substitute	**Z** No Qualifier
0 Lumbar Vertebral Joint **3** Lumbosacral Joint	**X** External	**0** Drainage Device **3** Infusion Device **4** Internal Fixation Device	**Z** No Qualifier
2 Lumbar Vertebral Disc **4** Lumbosacral Disc	**0** Open **3** Percutaneous **4** Percutaneous Endoscopic	**0** Drainage Device **3** Infusion Device **7** Autologous Tissue Substitute **J** Synthetic Substitute **K** Nonautologous Tissue Substitute	**Z** No Qualifier
2 Lumbar Vertebral Disc **4** Lumbosacral Disc	**X** External	**0** Drainage Device **3** Infusion Device	**Z** No Qualifier
5 Sacrococcygeal Joint **6** Coccygeal Joint **7** Sacroiliac Joint, Right **8** Sacroiliac Joint, Left	**0** Open **3** Percutaneous **4** Percutaneous Endoscopic	**0** Drainage Device **3** Infusion Device **4** Internal Fixation Device **7** Autologous Tissue Substitute **8** Spacer **J** Synthetic Substitute **K** Nonautologous Tissue Substitute	**Z** No Qualifier
5 Sacrococcygeal Joint **6** Coccygeal Joint **7** Sacroiliac Joint, Right **8** Sacroiliac Joint, Left	**X** External	**0** Drainage Device **3** Infusion Device **4** Internal Fixation Device	**Z** No Qualifier
9 Hip Joint, Right [CC] **B** Hip Joint, Left [CC]	**0** Open	**0** Drainage Device **3** Infusion Device **4** Internal Fixation Device **5** External Fixation Device **7** Autologous Tissue Substitute **8** Spacer **9** Liner **B** Resurfacing Device **E** Articulating Spacer **J** Synthetic Substitute **K** Nonautologous Tissue Substitute	**Z** No Qualifier
9 Hip Joint, Right [DRG] [CC] **B** Hip Joint, Left [DRG] [CC]	**3** Percutaneous **4** Percutaneous Endoscopic	**0** Drainage Device **3** Infusion Device **4** Internal Fixation Device **5** External Fixation Device **7** Autologous Tissue Substitute **8** Spacer **J** Synthetic Substitute **K** Nonautologous Tissue Substitute	**Z** No Qualifier
9 Hip Joint, Right **B** Hip Joint, Left	**X** External	**0** Drainage Device **3** Infusion Device **4** Internal Fixation Device **5** External Fixation Device	**Z** No Qualifier

0SP continued on next page

0   Medical and Surgical
S   Lower Joints
P   Removal: Taking out or off a device from a body part

0SP continued from previous page

Body Part	Approach	Device	Qualifier
Character 4	**Character 5**	**Character 6**	**Character 7**
A Hip Joint, Acetabular Surface, Right ⦏	0 Open	J Synthetic Substitute	Z No Qualifier
E Hip Joint, Acetabular Surface, Left ⦏	3 Percutaneous		
R Hip Joint, Femoral Surface, Right ⦏	4 Percutaneous Endoscopic		
S Hip Joint, Femoral Surface, Left ⦏			
T Knee Joint, Femoral Surface, Right ⦏			
U Knee Joint, Femoral Surface, Left ⦏			
V Knee Joint, Tibial Surface, Right ⦏			
W Knee Joint, Tibial Surface, Left ⦏			
C Knee Joint, Right ⦏	0 Open	0 Drainage Device	Z No Qualifier
D Knee Joint, Left ⦏		3 Infusion Device	
		4 Internal Fixation Device	
		5 External Fixation Device	
		7 Autologous Tissue Substitute	
		8 Spacer	
		9 Liner	
		E Articulating Spacer	
		K Nonautologous Tissue Substitute	
		L Synthetic Substitute, Unicondylar Medial	
		M Synthetic Substitute, Unicondylar Lateral	
		N Synthetic Substitute, Patellofemoral	
C Knee Joint, Right ⦏	0 Open	J Synthetic Substitute	C Patellar Surface
D Knee Joint, Left ⦏			Z No Qualifier
C Knee Joint, Right ⓘ ⦏	3 Percutaneous	0 Drainage Device	Z No Qualifier
D Knee Joint, Left ⓘ ⦏	4 Percutaneous Endoscopic	3 Infusion Device	
		4 Internal Fixation Device	
		5 External Fixation Device	
		7 Autologous Tissue Substitute	
		8 Spacer	
		K Nonautologous Tissue Substitute	
		L Synthetic Substitute, Unicondylar Medial	
		M Synthetic Substitute, Unicondylar Lateral	
		N Synthetic Substitute, Patellofemoral	
C Knee Joint, Right ⦏	3 Percutaneous	J Synthetic Substitute	C Patellar Surface
D Knee Joint, Left ⦏	4 Percutaneous Endoscopic		Z No Qualifier
C Knee Joint, Right	X External	0 Drainage Device	Z No Qualifier
D Knee Joint, Left		3 Infusion Device	
		4 Internal Fixation Device	
		5 External Fixation Device	

0SP continued on next page

0   **Medical and Surgical**   0SP continued from previous page
S   **Lower Joints**
P   **Removal:** Taking out or off a device from a body part

Body Part	Approach	Device	Qualifier
Character 4	Character 5	Character 6	Character 7
F Ankle Joint, Right **G** Ankle Joint, Left **H** Tarsal Joint, Right **J** Tarsal Joint, Left **K** Tarsometatarsal Joint, Right **L** Tarsometatarsal Joint, Left **M** Metatarsal-Phalangeal Joint, Right **N** Metatarsal-Phalangeal Joint, Left **P** Toe Phalangeal Joint, Right **Q** Toe Phalangeal Joint, Left	**0** Open **3** Percutaneous **4** Percutaneous Endoscopic	**0** Drainage Device **3** Infusion Device **4** Internal Fixation Device **5** External Fixation Device **7** Autologous Tissue Substitute **8** Spacer **J** Synthetic Substitute **K** Nonautologous Tissue Substitute	**Z** No Qualifier
F Ankle Joint, Right **G** Ankle Joint, Left **H** Tarsal Joint, Right **J** Tarsal Joint, Left **K** Tarsometatarsal Joint, Right **L** Tarsometatarsal Joint, Left **M** Metatarsal-Phalangeal Joint, Right **N** Metatarsal-Phalangeal Joint, Left **P** Toe Phalangeal Joint, Right **Q** Toe Phalangeal Joint, Left	**X** External	**0** Drainage Device **3** Infusion Device **4** Internal Fixation Device **5** External Fixation Device	**Z** No Qualifier

ORG   0SP948Z   0SPB48Z   0SPC38Z   0SPC48Z   0SPD38Z   0SPD48Z
CC   0SP908Z   0SP909Z   0SP90BZ   0SP90EZ   0SP90JZ   0SP948Z   0SP94JZ   0SPA0JZ   0SPA4JZ   0SPB08Z   0SPB09Z   0SPB0BZ   0SPB0EZ
     0SPB0JZ   0SPB48Z   0SPB4JZ   0SPC08Z   0SPC09Z   0SPC0EZ   0SPC0JC   0SPC0JZ   0SPC0LZ   0SPC0MZ   0SPC0NZ   0SPC38Z   0SPC48Z
     0SPC4JC   0SPC4JZ   0SPC4LZ   0SPC4MZ   0SPC4NZ   0SPD08Z   0SPD09Z   0SPD0EZ   0SPD0JC   0SPD0JZ   0SPD0LZ   0SPD0MZ   0SPD0NZ
     0SPD38Z   0SPD48Z   0SPD4JC   0SPD4JZ   0SPD4LZ   0SPD4MZ   0SPD4NZ   0SPE0JZ   0SPE4JZ   0SPR0JZ   0SPR4JZ   0SPS0JZ   0SPS4JZ
     0SPT0JZ   0SPT4JZ   0SPU0JZ   0SPU4JZ   0SPV0JZ   0SPV4JZ   0SPW0JZ   0SPW4JZ

0   **Medical and Surgical**
S   **Lower Joints**
Q   **Repair:** Restoring, to the extent possible, a body part to its normal anatomic structure and function

Body Part	Approach	Device	Qualifier
Character 4	Character 5	Character 6	Character 7
0 Lumbar Vertebral Joint **2** Lumbar Vertebral Disc **3** Lumbosacral Joint **4** Lumbosacral Disc **5** Sacrococcygeal Joint **6** Coccygeal Joint **7** Sacroiliac Joint, Right **8** Sacroiliac Joint, Left **9** Hip Joint, Right **B** Hip Joint, Left **C** Knee Joint, Right **D** Knee Joint, Left **F** Ankle Joint, Right **G** Ankle Joint, Left **H** Tarsal Joint, Right **J** Tarsal Joint, Left **K** Tarsometatarsal Joint, Right **L** Tarsometatarsal Joint, Left **M** Metatarsal-Phalangeal Joint, Right **N** Metatarsal-Phalangeal Joint, Left **P** Toe Phalangeal Joint, Right **Q** Toe Phalangeal Joint, Left	**0** Open **3** Percutaneous **4** Percutaneous Endoscopic **X** External	**Z** No Device	**Z** No Qualifier

---

0 Medical and Surgical
S Lower Joints
R Replacement: Putting in or on biological or synthetic material that physically takes the place and/or function of all or a portion of a body part

Body Part	Approach	Device	Qualifier
Character 4	Character 5	Character 6	Character 7
0 Lumbar Vertebral Joint 2 Lumbar Vertebral Disc 🆖 3 Lumbosacral Joint 4 Lumbosacral Disc 🆖 5 Sacrococcygeal Joint 6 Coccygeal Joint 7 Sacroiliac Joint, Right 8 Sacroiliac Joint, Left H Tarsal Joint, Right J Tarsal Joint, Left K Tarsometatarsal Joint, Right L Tarsometatarsal Joint, Left M Metatarsal-Phalangeal Joint, Right N Metatarsal-Phalangeal Joint, Left P Toe Phalangeal Joint, Right Q Toe Phalangeal Joint, Left	0 Open	7 Autologous Tissue Substitute J Synthetic Substitute K Nonautologous Tissue Substitute	Z No Qualifier
9 Hip Joint, Right 🅷🅐🅒 🅒🅒 B Hip Joint, Left 🅷🅐🅒 🅒🅒	0 Open	1 Synthetic Substitute, Metal 2 Synthetic Substitute, Metal on Polyethylene 3 Synthetic Substitute, Ceramic 4 Synthetic Substitute, Ceramic on Polyethylene 6 Synthetic Substitute, Oxidized Zirconium on Polyethylene J Synthetic Substitute	9 Cemented A Uncemented Z No Qualifier
9 Hip Joint, Right 🅷🅐🅒 🅒🅒 B Hip Joint, Left 🅷🅐🅒 🅒🅒	0 Open	7 Autologous Tissue Substitute E Articulating Spacer K Nonautologous Tissue Substitute	Z No Qualifier
A Hip Joint, Acetabular Surface, Right 🅷🅐🅒 🅒🅒 E Hip Joint, Acetabular Surface, Left 🅷🅐🅒 🅒🅒	0 Open	0 Synthetic Substitute, Polyethylene 1 Synthetic Substitute, Metal 3 Synthetic Substitute, Ceramic J Synthetic Substitute	9 Cemented A Uncemented Z No Qualifier
A Hip Joint, Acetabular Surface, Right 🅷🅐🅒 E Hip Joint, Acetabular Surface, Left 🅷🅐🅒	0 Open	7 Autologous Tissue Substitute K Nonautologous Tissue Substitute	Z No Qualifier
C Knee Joint, Right 🅷🅐🅒 🅒🅒 D Knee Joint, Left 🅷🅐🅒 🅒🅒	0 Open	6 Synthetic Substitute, Oxidized Zirconium on Polyethylene J Synthetic Substitute L Synthetic Substitute, Unicondylar Medial M Synthetic Substitute, Unicondylar Lateral N Synthetic Substitute, Patellofemoral	9 Cemented A Uncemented Z No Qualifier
C Knee Joint, Right 🅷🅐🅒 🅒🅒 D Knee Joint, Left 🅷🅐🅒 🅒🅒	0 Open	7 Autologous Tissue Substitute E Articulating Spacer K Nonautologous Tissue Substitute	Z No Qualifier

0SR continued on next page

🅛🅒 Limited Coverage   🆖 Noncovered   🅷🅐🅒 HAC-associated Procedure   🅒🅒 Combination Cluster - See Appendix G for code lists
🔁 Non-OR-Affecting MS-DRG Assignment   New/Revised Text in **Orange**   ♂ Male   ♀ Female

0 Medical and Surgical
S Lower Joints
R Replacement: Putting in or on biological or synthetic material that physically takes the place and/or function of all or a portion of a body part

0SR continued from previous page

Body Part	Approach	Device	Qualifier
Character 4	**Character 5**	**Character 6**	**Character 7**
F Ankle Joint, Right **G** Ankle Joint, Left **T** Knee Joint, Femoral Surface, Right [HAC] **U** Knee Joint, Femoral Surface, Left [HAC] **V** Knee Joint, Tibial Surface, Right [HAC] **W** Knee Joint, Tibial Surface, Left [HAC]	**0** Open	**7** Autologous Tissue Substitute **K** Nonautologous Tissue Substitute	**Z** No Qualifier
F Ankle Joint, Right **G** Ankle Joint, Left **T** Knee Joint, Femoral Surface, Right [HAC] [CC] **U** Knee Joint, Femoral Surface, Left [HAC] [CC] **V** Knee Joint, Tibial Surface, Right [HAC] [CC] **W** Knee Joint, Tibial Surface, Left [HAC] [CC]	**0** Open	**J** Synthetic Substitute	**9** Cemented **A** Uncemented **Z** No Qualifier
R Hip Joint, Femoral Surface, Right [HAC] [CC] **S** Hip Joint, Femoral Surface, Left [HAC] [CC]	**0** Open	**1** Synthetic Substitute, Metal **3** Synthetic Substitute, Ceramic **J** Synthetic Substitute	**9** Cemented **A** Uncemented **Z** No Qualifier
R Hip Joint, Femoral Surface, Right [HAC] **S** Hip Joint, Femoral Surface, Left [HAC]	**0** Open	**7** Autologous Tissue Substitute **K** Nonautologous Tissue Substitute	**Z** No Qualifier

[NC] 0SR20JZ   0SR40JZ

When the beneficiary is over age 60.

[HAC] 0SR9019   0SR901A   0SR901Z   0SR9029   0SR902A   0SR902Z   0SR9039   0SR903A   0SR903Z   0SR9049   0SR904A   0SR904Z   0SR9069
0SR906A   0SR906Z   0SR907Z   0SR90EZ   0SR90J9   0SR90JA   0SR90JZ   0SR90KZ   0SRA009   0SRA00A   0SRA00Z   0SRA019   0SRA01A
0SRA01Z   0SRA039   0SRA03A   0SRA03Z   0SRA07Z   0SRA0J9   0SRA0JA   0SRA0JZ   0SRA0KZ   0SRB019   0SRB01A   0SRB01Z   0SRB029
0SRB02A   0SRB02Z   0SRB039   0SRB03A   0SRB03Z   0SRB049   0SRB04A   0SRB04Z   0SRB069   0SRB06A   0SRB06Z   0SRB07Z   0SRB0EZ
0SRB0J9   0SRB0JA   0SRB0JZ   0SRB0KZ   0SRC069   0SRC06A   0SRC06Z   0SRC07Z   0SRC0EZ   0SRC0J9   0SRC0JA   0SRC0JZ   0SRC0KZ
0SRC0L9   0SRC0LA   0SRC0LZ   0SRC0M9   0SRC0MA   0SRC0MZ   0SRC0N9   0SRC0NA   0SRC0NZ   0SRD069   0SRD06A   0SRD06Z   0SRD07Z
0SRD0EZ   0SRD0J9   0SRD0JA   0SRD0JZ   0SRD0KZ   0SRD0L9   0SRD0LA   0SRD0LZ   0SRD0M9   0SRD0MA   0SRD0MZ   0SRD0N9   0SRD0NA
0SRD0NZ   0SRE009   0SRE00A   0SRE00Z   0SRE019   0SRE01A   0SRE01Z   0SRE039   0SRE03A   0SRE03Z   0SRE07Z   0SRE0J9   0SRE0JA
0SRE0JZ   0SRE0KZ   0SRR019   0SRR01A   0SRR01Z   0SRR039   0SRR03A   0SRR03Z   0SRR07Z   0SRR0J9   0SRR0JA   0SRR0JZ   0SRR0KZ
0SRS019   0SRS01A   0SRS01Z   0SRS039   0SRS03A   0SRS03Z   0SRS07Z   0SRS0J9   0SRS0JA   0SRS0JZ   0SRS0KZ   0SRT07Z   0SRT0J9
0SRT0JA   0SRT0JZ   0SRT0KZ   0SRU07Z   0SRU0J9   0SRU0JA   0SRU0JZ   0SRU0KZ   0SRV07Z   0SRV0J9   0SRV0JA   0SRV0JZ   0SRV0KZ
0SRW07Z   0SRW0J9   0SRW0JA   0SRW0JZ   0SRW0KZ

Deep vein thrombosis (DVT) / Pulmonary Embolism (PE) with total knee or hip replacement and secondary diagnosis I26.02, I26.09, I26.92, I26.93, I26.94, I26.99, I82.401, I82.402, I82.403, I82.409, I82.411, I82.412, I82.413, I82.419, I82.421, I82.422, I82.423, I82.429, I82.431, I82.432, I82.433, I82.439, I82.441, I82.442, I82.443, I82.449, I82.451, I82.452, I82.453, I82.459, I82.491, I82.492, I82.493, I82.499, I82.4Y1, I82.4Y2, I82.4Y3, I82.4Y9, I82.4Z1, I82.4Z2, I82.4Z3, I82.4Z9

[CC] 0SR9019   0SR901A   0SR901Z   0SR9029   0SR902A   0SR902Z   0SR9039   0SR903A   0SR903Z   0SR9049   0SR904A   0SR904Z   0SR9069
0SR906A   0SR906Z   0SR90EZ   0SR90J9   0SR90JA   0SR90JZ   0SRA009   0SRA00A   0SRA00Z   0SRA019   0SRA01A   0SRA01Z   0SRA039
0SRA03A   0SRA03Z   0SRA0J9   0SRA0JA   0SRA0JZ   0SRB019   0SRB01A   0SRB01Z   0SRB029   0SRB02A   0SRB02Z   0SRB039   0SRB03A
0SRB03Z   0SRB049   0SRB04A   0SRB04Z   0SRB069   0SRB06A   0SRB06Z   0SRB0EZ   0SRB0J9   0SRB0JA   0SRB0JZ   0SRC069   0SRC06A
0SRC06Z   0SRC0EZ   0SRC0J9   0SRC0JA   0SRC0JZ   0SRC0L9   0SRC0LA   0SRC0LZ   0SRC0M9   0SRC0MA   0SRC0MZ   0SRC0N9   0SRC0NA
0SRC0NZ   0SRD069   0SRD06A   0SRD06Z   0SRD0EZ   0SRD0J9   0SRD0JA   0SRD0JZ   0SRD0L9   0SRD0LA   0SRD0LZ   0SRD0M9   0SRD0MA
0SRD0MZ   0SRD0N9   0SRD0NA   0SRD0NZ   0SRE009   0SRE00A   0SRE00Z   0SRE019   0SRE01A   0SRE01Z   0SRE039   0SRE03A   0SRE03Z
0SRE0J9   0SRE0JA   0SRE0JZ   0SRR019   0SRR01A   0SRR01Z   0SRR039   0SRR03A   0SRR03Z   0SRR0J9   0SRR0JA   0SRR0JZ   0SRS019
0SRS01A   0SRS01Z   0SRS039   0SRS03A   0SRS03Z   0SRS0J9   0SRS0JA   0SRS0JZ   0SRT0J9   0SRT0JA   0SRT0JZ   0SRU0J9   0SRU0JA
0SRU0JZ   0SRV0J9   0SRV0JA   0SRV0JZ   0SRW0J9   0SRW0JA   0SRW0JZ

[LC] Limited Coverage   [NC] Noncovered   [HAC] HAC-associated Procedure   [CC] Combination Cluster - See Appendix G for code lists
[dae] Non-OR-Affecting MS-DRG Assignment   New/Revised Text in **Orange**   ♂ Male   ♀ Female

2021 ICD-10-PCS

515

0   **Medical and Surgical**
S   **Lower Joints**
S   **Reposition:** Moving to its normal location, or other suitable location, all or a portion of a body part

Body Part	Approach	Device	Qualifier
Character 4	Character 5	Character 6	Character 7
0 Lumbar Vertebral Joint **3** Lumbosacral Joint **5** Sacrococcygeal Joint **6** Coccygeal Joint **7** Sacroiliac Joint, Right **8** Sacroiliac Joint, Left	**0** Open **3** Percutaneous **4** Percutaneous Endoscopic **X** External	**4** Internal Fixation Device **Z** No Device	**Z** No Qualifier
9 Hip Joint, Right **B** Hip Joint, Left **C** Knee Joint, Right **D** Knee Joint, Left **F** Ankle Joint, Right **G** Ankle Joint, Left **H** Tarsal Joint, Right **J** Tarsal Joint, Left **K** Tarsometatarsal Joint, Right **L** Tarsometatarsal Joint, Left **M** Metatarsal-Phalangeal Joint, Right **N** Metatarsal-Phalangeal Joint, Left **P** Toe Phalangeal Joint, Right **Q** Toe Phalangeal Joint, Left	**0** Open **3** Percutaneous **4** Percutaneous Endoscopic **X** External	**4** Internal Fixation Device **5** External Fixation Device **Z** No Device	**Z** No Qualifier

0   **Medical and Surgical**
S   **Lower Joints**
T   **Resection:** Cutting out or off, without replacement, all of a body part

Body Part	Approach	Device	Qualifier
Character 4	Character 5	Character 6	Character 7
2 Lumbar Vertebral Disc **4** Lumbosacral Disc **5** Sacrococcygeal Joint **6** Coccygeal Joint **7** Sacroiliac Joint, Right **8** Sacroiliac Joint, Left **9** Hip Joint, Right **B** Hip Joint, Left **C** Knee Joint, Right **D** Knee Joint, Left **F** Ankle Joint, Right **G** Ankle Joint, Left **H** Tarsal Joint, Right **J** Tarsal Joint, Left **K** Tarsometatarsal Joint, Right **L** Tarsometatarsal Joint, Left **M** Metatarsal-Phalangeal Joint, Right **N** Metatarsal-Phalangeal Joint, Left **P** Toe Phalangeal Joint, Right **Q** Toe Phalangeal Joint, Left	**0** Open	**Z** No Device	**Z** No Qualifier

LC Limited Coverage   NC Noncovered   HAC HAC-associated Procedure   CC Combination Cluster - See Appendix G for code lists
 DNR Non-OR-Affecting MS-DRG Assignment   New/Revised Text in **Orange**   ♂ Male   ♀ Female

516   **2021 ICD-10-PCS**

0 Medical and Surgical
S Lower Joints
U Supplement: Putting in or on biological or synthetic material that physically reinforces and/or augments the function of a portion of a body part

Body Part	Approach	Device	Qualifier
Character 4	**Character 5**	**Character 6**	**Character 7**
0 Lumbar Vertebral Joint 2 Lumbar Vertebral Disc 3 Lumbosacral Joint 4 Lumbosacral Disc 5 Sacrococcygeal Joint 6 Coccygeal Joint 7 Sacroiliac Joint, Right 8 Sacroiliac Joint, Left F Ankle Joint, Right G Ankle Joint, Left H Tarsal Joint, Right J Tarsal Joint, Left K Tarsometatarsal Joint, Right L Tarsometatarsal Joint, Left M Metatarsal-Phalangeal Joint, Right N Metatarsal-Phalangeal Joint, Left P Toe Phalangeal Joint, Right Q Toe Phalangeal Joint, Left	0 Open 3 Percutaneous 4 Percutaneous Endoscopic	7 Autologous Tissue Substitute J Synthetic Substitute K Nonautologous Tissue Substitute	Z No Qualifier
9 Hip Joint, Right ᴴᴬᶜ ᶜᶜ B Hip Joint, Left ᴴᴬᶜ ᶜᶜ	0 Open	7 Autologous Tissue Substitute 9 Liner B Resurfacing Device J Synthetic Substitute K Nonautologous Tissue Substitute	Z No Qualifier
9 Hip Joint, Right B Hip Joint, Left	3 Percutaneous 4 Percutaneous Endoscopic	7 Autologous Tissue Substitute J Synthetic Substitute K Nonautologous Tissue Substitute	Z No Qualifier
A Hip Joint, Acetabular Surface, Right ᴴᴬᶜ ᶜᶜ E Hip Joint, Acetabular Surface, Left ᴴᴬᶜ ᶜᶜ R Hip Joint, Femoral Surface, Right ᴴᴬᶜ ᶜᶜ S Hip Joint, Femoral Surface, Left ᴴᴬᶜ ᶜᶜ	0 Open	9 Liner B Resurfacing Device	Z No Qualifier
C Knee Joint, Right D Knee Joint, Left	0 Open	7 Autologous Tissue Substitute J Synthetic Substitute K Nonautologous Tissue Substitute	Z No Qualifier
C Knee Joint, Right D Knee Joint, Left	0 Open	9 Liner	C Patellar Surface Z No Qualifier
C Knee Joint, Right D Knee Joint, Left	3 Percutaneous 4 Percutaneous Endoscopic	7 Autologous Tissue Substitute J Synthetic Substitute K Nonautologous Tissue Substitute	Z No Qualifier
T Knee Joint, Femoral Surface, Right U Knee Joint, Femoral Surface, Left V Knee Joint, Tibial Surface, Right ᶜᶜ W Knee Joint, Tibial Surface, Left ᶜᶜ	0 Open	9 Liner	Z No Qualifier

ᴴᴬᶜ 0SU90BZ   0SUA0BZ   0SUB0BZ   0SUE0BZ   0SUR0BZ   0SUS0BZ
Deep vein thrombosis (DVT) / Pulmonary Embolism (PE) with total knee or hip replacement and secondary diagnosis I26.02, I26.09, I26.92, I26.93, I26.94, I26.99, I82.401, I82.402, I82.403, I82.409, I82.411, I82.412, I82.413, I82.419, I82.421, I82.422, I82.423, I82.429, I82.431, I82.432, I82.433, I82.439, I82.441, I82.442, I82.443, I82.449, I82.451, I82.452, I82.453, I82.459, I82.491, I82.492, I82.493, I82.499, I82.4Y1, I82.4Y2, I82.4Y3, I82.4Y9, I82.4Z1, I82.4Z2, I82.4Z3, I82.4Z9

ᶜᶜ 0SU909Z   0SUA09Z   0SUB09Z   0SUE09Z   0SUR09Z   0SUS09Z   0SUV09Z   0SUW09Z

ᴸᶜ Limited Coverage   ᴺᶜ Noncovered   ᴴᴬᶜ HAC-associated Procedure   ᶜᶜ Combination Cluster - See Appendix G for code lists
ᴰᴿᴳ Non-OR-Affecting MS-DRG Assignment   New/Revised Text in **Orange**   ♂ Male   ♀ Female

0 Medical and Surgical
S Lower Joints
W Revision: Correcting, to the extent possible, a portion of a malfunctioning device or the position of a displaced device

Body Part	Approach	Device	Qualifier
Character 4	**Character 5**	**Character 6**	**Character 7**
0 Lumbar Vertebral Joint 3 Lumbosacral Joint	0 Open 3 Percutaneous 4 Percutaneous Endoscopic X External	0 Drainage Device 3 Infusion Device 4 Internal Fixation Device 7 Autologous Tissue Substitute 8 Spacer A Interbody Fusion Device J Synthetic Substitute K Nonautologous Tissue Substitute	Z No Qualifier
2 Lumbar Vertebral Disc 4 Lumbosacral Disc	0 Open 3 Percutaneous 4 Percutaneous Endoscopic X External	0 Drainage Device 3 Infusion Device 7 Autologous Tissue Substitute J Synthetic Substitute K Nonautologous Tissue Substitute	Z No Qualifier
5 Sacrococcygeal Joint 6 Coccygeal Joint 7 Sacroiliac Joint, Right 8 Sacroiliac Joint, Left	0 Open 3 Percutaneous 4 Percutaneous Endoscopic X External	0 Drainage Device 3 Infusion Device 4 Internal Fixation Device 7 Autologous Tissue Substitute 8 Spacer J Synthetic Substitute K Nonautologous Tissue Substitute	Z No Qualifier
9 Hip Joint, Right B Hip Joint, Left	0 Open	0 Drainage Device 3 Infusion Device 4 Internal Fixation Device 5 External Fixation Device 7 Autologous Tissue Substitute 8 Spacer 9 Liner B Resurfacing Device J Synthetic Substitute K Nonautologous Tissue Substitute	Z No Qualifier
9 Hip Joint, Right B Hip Joint, Left	3 Percutaneous 4 Percutaneous Endoscopic X External	0 Drainage Device 3 Infusion Device 4 Internal Fixation Device 5 External Fixation Device 7 Autologous Tissue Substitute 8 Spacer J Synthetic Substitute K Nonautologous Tissue Substitute	Z No Qualifier

A Hip Joint, Acetabular Surface,
   Right
E Hip Joint, Acetabular Surface,
   Left
R Hip Joint, Femoral Surface, Right
S Hip Joint, Femoral Surface, Left
T Knee Joint, Femoral Surface,
   Right
U Knee Joint, Femoral Surface, Left
V Knee Joint, Tibial Surface, Right
W Knee Joint, Tibial Surface, Left
	0 Open
	3 Percutaneous
	4 Percutaneous Endoscopic
	X External
		J Synthetic Substitute	Z No Qualifier

0SW continued on next page

LC Limited Coverage   NC Noncovered   HAC HAC-associated Procedure   CC Combination Cluster - See Appendix G for code lists
    ⓝ Non-OR-Affecting MS-DRG Assignment   New/Revised Text in **Orange**   ♂ Male   ♀ Female

518   **2021 ICD-10-PCS**

0   **Medical and Surgical**   0SW continued from previous page
S   **Lower Joints**
W   **Revision:** Correcting, to the extent possible, a portion of a malfunctioning device or the position of a displaced device

Body Part	Approach	Device	Qualifier
Character 4	**Character 5**	**Character 6**	**Character 7**
C Knee Joint, Right D Knee Joint, Left	0 Open	0 Drainage Device 3 Infusion Device 4 Internal Fixation Device 5 External Fixation Device 7 Autologous Tissue Substitute 8 Spacer 9 Liner K Nonautologous Tissue Substitute	Z No Qualifier
C Knee Joint, Right D Knee Joint, Left	0 Open	J Synthetic Substitute	C Patellar Surface Z No Qualifier
C Knee Joint, Right D Knee Joint, Left	3 Percutaneous 4 Percutaneous Endoscopic X External	0 Drainage Device 3 Infusion Device 4 Internal Fixation Device 5 External Fixation Device 7 Autologous Tissue Substitute 8 Spacer K Nonautologous Tissue Substitute	Z No Qualifier
C Knee Joint, Right D Knee Joint, Left	3 Percutaneous 4 Percutaneous Endoscopic X External	J Synthetic Substitute	C Patellar Surface Z No Qualifier

F Ankle Joint, Right
G Ankle Joint, Left
H Tarsal Joint, Right
J Tarsal Joint, Left
K Tarsometatarsal Joint, Right
L Tarsometatarsal Joint, Left
M Metatarsal-Phalangeal Joint,
     Right
N Metatarsal-Phalangeal Joint,
     Left
P Toe Phalangeal Joint, Right
Q Toe Phalangeal Joint, Left
	0 Open
	3 Percutaneous
	4 Percutaneous Endoscopic
	X External
		0 Drainage Device
		3 Infusion Device
		4 Internal Fixation Device
		5 External Fixation Device
		7 Autologous Tissue Substitute
		8 Spacer
		J Synthetic Substitute
		K Nonautologous Tissue
		     Substitute
			Z No Qualifier

NOTES

Urinary System 0T1-0TY

0 **Medical and Surgical**
T **Urinary System**
1 **Bypass:** Altering the route of passage of the contents of a tubular body part

Body Part	Approach	Device	Qualifier
Character 4	**Character 5**	**Character 6**	**Character 7**
3 Kidney Pelvis, Right 4 Kidney Pelvis, Left	0 Open 4 Percutaneous Endoscopic	7 Autologous Tissue Substitute J Synthetic Substitute K Nonautologous Tissue Substitute Z No Device	3 Kidney Pelvis, Right 4 Kidney Pelvis, Left 6 Ureter, Right 7 Ureter, Left 8 Colon 9 Colocutaneous A Ileum B Bladder C Ileocutaneous D Cutaneous
3 Kidney Pelvis, Right 4 Kidney Pelvis, Left	3 Percutaneous	J Synthetic Substitute	D Cutaneous
6 Ureter, Right 7 Ureter, Left 8 Ureters, Bilateral	0 Open 4 Percutaneous Endoscopic	7 Autologous Tissue Substitute J Synthetic Substitute K Nonautologous Tissue Substitute Z No Device	6 Ureter, Right 7 Ureter, Left 8 Colon 9 Colocutaneous A Ileum B Bladder C Ileocutaneous D Cutaneous
6 Ureter, Right 7 Ureter, Left 8 Ureters, Bilateral	3 Percutaneous	J Synthetic Substitute	D Cutaneous
B Bladder	0 Open 4 Percutaneous Endoscopic	7 Autologous Tissue Substitute J Synthetic Substitute K Nonautologous Tissue Substitute Z No Device	9 Colocutaneous C Ileocutaneous D Cutaneous
B Bladder	3 Percutaneous	J Synthetic Substitute	D Cutaneous

0 **Medical and Surgical**
T **Urinary System**
2 **Change:** Taking out or off a device from a body part and putting back an identical or similar device in or on the same body part without cutting or puncturing the skin or a mucous membrane

Body Part	Approach	Device	Qualifier
Character 4	**Character 5**	**Character 6**	**Character 7**
5 Kidney 9 Ureter B Bladder D Urethra	X External	0 Drainage Device Y Other Device	Z No Qualifier

0 Medical and Surgical

T Urinary System

5 Destruction: Physical eradication of all or a portion of a body part by the direct use of energy, force, or a destructive agent

Body Part	Approach	Device	Qualifier
Character 4	Character 5	Character 6	Character 7
0 Kidney, Right **1** Kidney, Left **3** Kidney Pelvis, Right **4** Kidney Pelvis, Left **6** Ureter, Right **7** Ureter, Left **B** Bladder **C** Bladder Neck	**0** Open **3** Percutaneous **4** Percutaneous Endoscopic **7** Via Natural or Artificial Opening **8** Via Natural or Artificial Opening Endoscopic	**Z** No Device	**Z** No Qualifier
D Urethra	**0** Open **3** Percutaneous **4** Percutaneous Endoscopic **7** Via Natural or Artificial Opening **8** Via Natural or Artificial Opening Endoscopic **X** External	**Z** No Device	**Z** No Qualifier

0 Medical and Surgical

T Urinary System

7 Dilation: Expanding an orifice or the lumen of a tubular body part

Body Part	Approach	Device	Qualifier
Character 4	Character 5	Character 6	Character 7
3 Kidney Pelvis, Right **4** Kidney Pelvis, Left **6** Ureter, Right **7** Ureter, Left **8** Ureters, Bilateral **B** Bladder **C** Bladder Neck **D** Urethra	**0** Open **3** Percutaneous **4** Percutaneous Endoscopic **7** Via Natural or Artificial Opening **8** Via Natural or Artificial Opening Endoscopic	**D** Intraluminal Device **Z** No Device	**Z** No Qualifier

0 Medical and Surgical

T Urinary System

8 Division: Cutting into a body part, without draining fluids and/or gases from the body part, in order to separate or transect a body part

Body Part	Approach	Device	Qualifier
Character 4	Character 5	Character 6	Character 7
2 Kidneys, Bilateral **C** Bladder Neck	**0** Open **3** Percutaneous **4** Percutaneous Endoscopic	**Z** No Device	**Z** No Qualifier

LC Limited Coverage   **NC** Noncovered   **HAC** HAC-associated Procedure   **CC** Combination Cluster - See Appendix G for code lists

⊶ Non-OR-Affecting MS-DRG Assignment   New/Revised Text in **Orange**   ♂ Male   ♀ Female

522

2021 ICD-10-PCS

0 **Medical and Surgical**
T **Urinary System**
9 **Drainage:** Taking or letting out fluids and/or gases from a body part

Body Part	Approach	Device	Qualifier
Character 4	Character 5	Character 6	Character 7
0 Kidney, Right **1** Kidney, Left **3** Kidney Pelvis, Right **4** Kidney Pelvis, Left **6** Ureter, Right **7** Ureter, Left **8** Ureters, Bilateral **B** Bladder **C** Bladder Neck	**0** Open **3** Percutaneous **4** Percutaneous Endoscopic **7** Via Natural or Artificial Opening **8** Via Natural or Artificial Opening Endoscopic	**0** Drainage Device	**Z** No Qualifier
0 Kidney, Right **1** Kidney, Left **3** Kidney Pelvis, Right **4** Kidney Pelvis, Left **6** Ureter, Right **7** Ureter, Left **8** Ureters, Bilateral **B** Bladder **C** Bladder Neck	**0** Open **3** Percutaneous **4** Percutaneous Endoscopic **7** Via Natural or Artificial Opening **8** Via Natural or Artificial Opening Endoscopic	**Z** No Device	**X** Diagnostic **Z** No Qualifier
D Urethra	**0** Open **3** Percutaneous **4** Percutaneous Endoscopic **7** Via Natural or Artificial Opening **8** Via Natural or Artificial Opening Endoscopic **X** External	**0** Drainage Device	**Z** No Qualifier
D Urethra	**0** Open **3** Percutaneous **4** Percutaneous Endoscopic **7** Via Natural or Artificial Opening **8** Via Natural or Artificial Opening Endoscopic **X** External	**Z** No Device	**X** Diagnostic **Z** No Qualifier

0 **Medical and Surgical**
T **Urinary System**
B **Excision:** Cutting out or off, without replacement, a portion of a body part

Body Part	Approach	Device	Qualifier
Character 4	Character 5	Character 6	Character 7
0 Kidney, Right **1** Kidney, Left **3** Kidney Pelvis, Right **4** Kidney Pelvis, Left **6** Ureter, Right **7** Ureter, Left **B** Bladder **C** Bladder Neck	**0** Open **3** Percutaneous **4** Percutaneous Endoscopic **7** Via Natural or Artificial Opening **8** Via Natural or Artificial Opening Endoscopic	**Z** No Device	**X** Diagnostic **Z** No Qualifier
D Urethra	**0** Open **3** Percutaneous **4** Percutaneous Endoscopic **7** Via Natural or Artificial Opening **8** Via Natural or Artificial Opening Endoscopic **X** External	**Z** No Device	**X** Diagnostic **Z** No Qualifier

0 Medical and Surgical
T Urinary System
C Extirpation: Taking or cutting out solid matter from a body part

Body Part	Approach	Device	Qualifier
Character 4	Character 5	Character 6	Character 7
0 Kidney, Right **1** Kidney, Left **3** Kidney Pelvis, Right **4** Kidney Pelvis, Left **6** Ureter, Right **7** Ureter, Left **B** Bladder **C** Bladder Neck	**0** Open **3** Percutaneous **4** Percutaneous Endoscopic **7** Via Natural or Artificial Opening **8** Via Natural or Artificial Opening Endoscopic	**Z** No Device	**Z** No Qualifier
D Urethra	**0** Open **3** Percutaneous **4** Percutaneous Endoscopic **7** Via Natural or Artificial Opening **8** Via Natural or Artificial Opening Endoscopic **X** External	**Z** No Device	**Z** No Qualifier

0 Medical and Surgical
T Urinary System
D Extraction: Pulling or stripping out or off all or a portion of a body part by the use of force

Body Part	Approach	Device	Qualifier
Character 4	Character 5	Character 6	Character 7
0 Kidney, Right **1** Kidney, Left	**0** Open **3** Percutaneous **4** Percutaneous Endoscopic	**Z** No Device	**Z** No Qualifier

0 Medical and Surgical
T Urinary System
F Fragmentation: Breaking solid matter in a body part into pieces

Body Part	Approach	Device	Qualifier
Character 4	Character 5	Character 6	Character 7
3 Kidney Pelvis, Right **4** Kidney Pelvis, Left **6** Ureter, Right **7** Ureter, Left **B** Bladder **C** Bladder Neck **D** Urethra NC	**0** Open **3** Percutaneous **4** Percutaneous Endoscopic **7** Via Natural or Artificial Opening **8** Via Natural or Artificial Opening Endoscopic **X** External	**Z** No Device	**Z** No Qualifier

NC 0TFDXZZ

LC Limited Coverage   NC Noncovered   HAC HAC-associated Procedure   CC Combination Cluster - See Appendix G for code lists
DRG Non-OR-Affecting MS-DRG Assignment   New/Revised Text in **Orange**   ♂ Male   ♀ Female

524

2021 ICD-10-PCS

0 **Medical and Surgical**
T **Urinary System**
H **Insertion:** Putting in a nonbiological appliance that monitors, assists, performs, or prevents a physiological function but does not physically take the place of a body part

Body Part	Approach	Device	Qualifier
Character 4	Character 5	Character 6	Character 7
5 Kidney	0 Open 3 Percutaneous 4 Percutaneous Endoscopic 7 Via Natural or Artificial Opening 8 Via Natural or Artificial Opening Endoscopic	1 Radioactive Element 2 Monitoring Device 3 Infusion Device Y Other Device	Z No Qualifier
9 Ureter	0 Open 3 Percutaneous 4 Percutaneous Endoscopic 7 Via Natural or Artificial Opening 8 Via Natural or Artificial Opening Endoscopic	1 Radioactive Element 2 Monitoring Device 3 Infusion Device M Stimulator Lead Y Other Device	Z No Qualifier
B Bladder ☒	0 Open 3 Percutaneous 4 Percutaneous Endoscopic 7 Via Natural or Artificial Opening 8 Via Natural or Artificial Opening Endoscopic	1 Radioactive Element 2 Monitoring Device 3 Infusion Device L Artificial Sphincter M Stimulator Lead Y Other Device	Z No Qualifier
C Bladder Neck	0 Open 3 Percutaneous 4 Percutaneous Endoscopic 7 Via Natural or Artificial Opening 8 Via Natural or Artificial Opening Endoscopic	L Artificial Sphincter	Z No Qualifier
D Urethra	0 Open 3 Percutaneous 4 Percutaneous Endoscopic 7 Via Natural or Artificial Opening 8 Via Natural or Artificial Opening Endoscopic	1 Radioactive Element 2 Monitoring Device 3 Infusion Device L Artificial Sphincter Y Other Device	Z No Qualifier
D Urethra	X External	2 Monitoring Device 3 Infusion Device L Artificial Sphincter	Z No Qualifier

☒ 0THB0MZ   0THB3MZ   0THB4MZ   0THB7MZ   0THB8MZ

0 **Medical and Surgical**
T **Urinary System**
J **Inspection:** Visually and/or manually exploring a body part

Body Part	Approach	Device	Qualifier
Character 4	Character 5	Character 6	Character 7
5 Kidney 9 Ureter B Bladder D Urethra	0 Open 3 Percutaneous 4 Percutaneous Endoscopic 7 Via Natural or Artificial Opening 8 Via Natural or Artificial Opening Endoscopic X External	Z No Device	Z No Qualifier

☒ Limited Coverage   ☒ Noncovered   ☒ HAC-associated Procedure   ☒ Combination Cluster - See Appendix G for code lists
☒ Non-OR-Affecting MS-DRG Assignment   New/Revised Text in **Orange**   ♂ Male   ♀ Female

2021 ICD-10-PCS

525

URINARY SYSTEM 0T1-0TY

0 Medical and Surgical
T Urinary System
L Occlusion: Completely closing an orifice or the lumen of a tubular body part

Body Part	Approach	Device	Qualifier
Character 4	Character 5	Character 6	Character 7
3 Kidney Pelvis, Right 4 Kidney Pelvis, Left 6 Ureter, Right 7 Ureter, Left B Bladder C Bladder Neck	0 Open 3 Percutaneous 4 Percutaneous Endoscopic	C Extraluminal Device D Intraluminal Device Z No Device	Z No Qualifier
3 Kidney Pelvis, Right 4 Kidney Pelvis, Left 6 Ureter, Right 7 Ureter, Left B Bladder C Bladder Neck	7 Via Natural or Artificial Opening 8 Via Natural or Artificial Opening Endoscopic	D Intraluminal Device Z No Device	Z No Qualifier
D Urethra	0 Open 3 Percutaneous 4 Percutaneous Endoscopic X External	C Extraluminal Device D Intraluminal Device Z No Device	Z No Qualifier
D Urethra	7 Via Natural or Artificial Opening 8 Via Natural or Artificial Opening Endoscopic	D Intraluminal Device Z No Device	Z No Qualifier

0 Medical and Surgical
T Urinary System
M Reattachment: Putting back in or on all or a portion of a separated body part to its normal location or other suitable location

Body Part	Approach	Device	Qualifier
Character 4	Character 5	Character 6	Character 7
0 Kidney, Right 1 Kidney, Left 2 Kidneys, Bilateral 3 Kidney Pelvis, Right 4 Kidney Pelvis, Left 6 Ureter, Right 7 Ureter, Left 8 Ureters, Bilateral B Bladder C Bladder Neck D Urethra	0 Open 4 Percutaneous Endoscopic	Z No Device	Z No Qualifier

0 Medical and Surgical
T Urinary System
N Release: Freeing a body part from an abnormal physical constraint by cutting or by the use of force

Body Part	Approach	Device	Qualifier
Character 4	Character 5	Character 6	Character 7
0 Kidney, Right 1 Kidney, Left 3 Kidney Pelvis, Right 4 Kidney Pelvis, Left 6 Ureter, Right 7 Ureter, Left B Bladder C Bladder Neck	0 Open 3 Percutaneous 4 Percutaneous Endoscopic 7 Via Natural or Artificial Opening 8 Via Natural or Artificial Opening Endoscopic	Z No Device	Z No Qualifier
D Urethra	0 Open 3 Percutaneous 4 Percutaneous Endoscopic 7 Via Natural or Artificial Opening 8 Via Natural or Artificial Opening Endoscopic X External	Z No Device	Z No Qualifier

LC Limited Coverage   **NC** Noncovered   **HAC** HAC-associated Procedure   **CC** Combination Cluster - See Appendix G for code lists
DRG Non-OR-Affecting MS-DRG Assignment   New/Revised Text in Orange   ♂ Male   ♀ Female

526   2021 ICD-10-PCS

0 Medical and Surgical
T Urinary System
P Removal: Taking out or off a device from a body part

Body Part	Approach	Device	Qualifier
Character 4	**Character 5**	**Character 6**	**Character 7**
5 Kidney	**0** Open **3** Percutaneous **4** Percutaneous Endoscopic **7** Via Natural or Artificial Opening **8** Via Natural or Artificial Opening Endoscopic	**0** Drainage Device **2** Monitoring Device **3** Infusion Device **7** Autologous Tissue Substitute **C** Extraluminal Device **D** Intraluminal Device **J** Synthetic Substitute **K** Nonautologous Tissue Substitute **Y** Other Device	**Z** No Qualifier
5 Kidney	**X** External	**0** Drainage Device **2** Monitoring Device **3** Infusion Device **D** Intraluminal Device	**Z** No Qualifier
9 Ureter	**0** Open **3** Percutaneous **4** Percutaneous Endoscopic **7** Via Natural or Artificial Opening **8** Via Natural or Artificial Opening Endoscopic	**0** Drainage Device **2** Monitoring Device **3** Infusion Device **7** Autologous Tissue Substitute **C** Extraluminal Device **D** Intraluminal Device **J** Synthetic Substitute **K** Nonautologous Tissue Substitute **M** Stimulator Lead **Y** Other Device	**Z** No Qualifier
9 Ureter	**X** External	**0** Drainage Device **2** Monitoring Device **3** Infusion Device **D** Intraluminal Device **M** Stimulator Lead	**Z** No Qualifier
B Bladder 🅽🅲	**0** Open **3** Percutaneous **4** Percutaneous Endoscopic **7** Via Natural or Artificial Opening **8** Via Natural or Artificial Opening Endoscopic	**0** Drainage Device **2** Monitoring Device **3** Infusion Device **7** Autologous Tissue Substitute **C** Extraluminal Device **D** Intraluminal Device **J** Synthetic Substitute **K** Nonautologous Tissue Substitute **L** Artificial Sphincter **M** Stimulator Lead **Y** Other Device	**Z** No Qualifier
B Bladder	**X** External	**0** Drainage Device **2** Monitoring Device **3** Infusion Device **D** Intraluminal Device **L** Artificial Sphincter **M** Stimulator Lead	**Z** No Qualifier
D Urethra	**0** Open **3** Percutaneous **4** Percutaneous Endoscopic **7** Via Natural or Artificial Opening **8** Via Natural or Artificial Opening Endoscopic	**0** Drainage Device **2** Monitoring Device **3** Infusion Device **7** Autologous Tissue Substitute **C** Extraluminal Device **D** Intraluminal Device **J** Synthetic Substitute **K** Nonautologous Tissue Substitute **L** Artificial Sphincter **Y** Other Device	**Z** No Qualifier

0TP continued on next page

🅛🅒 Limited Coverage   🅝🅒 Noncovered   🅗🅐🅒 HAC-associated Procedure   🅒🅒 Combination Cluster - See Appendix G for code lists
🅓🅡🅖 Non-OR-Affecting MS-DRG Assignment   New/Revised Text in Orange   ♂ Male   ♀ Female

0   Medical and Surgical
T   Urinary System
P   Removal: Taking out or off a device from a body part

0TP continued from previous page

Body Part	Approach	Device	Qualifier
Character 4	Character 5	Character 6	Character 7
D Urethra	**X** External	**0** Drainage Device **2** Monitoring Device **3** Infusion Device **D** Intraluminal Device **L** Artificial Sphincter	**Z** No Qualifier

NC 0TPB0MZ   0TPB3MZ   0TPB4MZ   0TPB7MZ   0TPB8MZ

0   Medical and Surgical
T   Urinary System
Q   Repair: Restoring, to the extent possible, a body part to its normal anatomic structure and function

Body Part	Approach	Device	Qualifier
Character 4	Character 5	Character 6	Character 7
0 Kidney, Right **1** Kidney, Left **3** Kidney Pelvis, Right **4** Kidney Pelvis, Left **6** Ureter, Right **7** Ureter, Left **B** Bladder CC **C** Bladder Neck	**0** Open **3** Percutaneous **4** Percutaneous Endoscopic **7** Via Natural or Artificial Opening **8** Via Natural or Artificial Opening Endoscopic	**Z** No Device	**Z** No Qualifier
D Urethra	**0** Open **3** Percutaneous **4** Percutaneous Endoscopic **7** Via Natural or Artificial Opening **8** Via Natural or Artificial Opening Endoscopic **X** External	**Z** No Device	**Z** No Qualifier

CC 0TQB0ZZ   0TQB3ZZ   0TQB4ZZ

0   Medical and Surgical
T   Urinary System
R   Replacement: Putting in or on biological or synthetic material that physically takes the place and/or function of all or a portion of a body part

Body Part	Approach	Device	Qualifier
Character 4	Character 5	Character 6	Character 7
3 Kidney Pelvis, Right **4** Kidney Pelvis, Left **6** Ureter, Right **7** Ureter, Left **B** Bladder **C** Bladder Neck	**0** Open **4** Percutaneous Endoscopic **7** Via Natural or Artificial Opening **8** Via Natural or Artificial Opening Endoscopic	**7** Autologous Tissue Substitute **J** Synthetic Substitute **K** Nonautologous Tissue Substitute	**Z** No Qualifier
D Urethra	**0** Open **4** Percutaneous Endoscopic **7** Via Natural or Artificial Opening **8** Via Natural or Artificial Opening Endoscopic **X** External	**7** Autologous Tissue Substitute **J** Synthetic Substitute **K** Nonautologous Tissue Substitute	**Z** No Qualifier

LC Limited Coverage   NC Noncovered   HAC HAC-associated Procedure   CC Combination Cluster - See Appendix G for code lists
Non-OR-Affecting MS-DRG Assignment   New/Revised Text in **Orange**   ♂ Male   ♀ Female

528   **2021 ICD-10-PCS**

0 Medical and Surgical
T Urinary System
S **Reposition:** Moving to its normal location, or other suitable location, all or a portion of a body part

Body Part	Approach	Device	Qualifier
Character 4	Character 5	Character 6	Character 7
0 Kidney, Right **1** Kidney, Left **2** Kidneys, Bilateral **3** Kidney Pelvis, Right **4** Kidney Pelvis, Left **6** Ureter, Right **7** Ureter, Left **8** Ureters, Bilateral **B** Bladder **C** Bladder Neck **D** Urethra	**0** Open **4** Percutaneous Endoscopic	**Z** No Device	**Z** No Qualifier

0 Medical and Surgical
T Urinary System
T **Resection:** Cutting out or off, without replacement, all of a body part

Body Part	Approach	Device	Qualifier
Character 4	Character 5	Character 6	Character 7
0 Kidney, Right **1** Kidney, Left **2** Kidneys, Bilateral	**0** Open **4** Percutaneous Endoscopic	**Z** No Device	**Z** No Qualifier
3 Kidney Pelvis, Right **4** Kidney Pelvis, Left **6** Ureter, Right **7** Ureter, Left **B** Bladder **CC** **C** Bladder Neck **D** Urethra **CC** **ORG**	**0** Open **4** Percutaneous Endoscopic **7** Via Natural or Artificial Opening **8** Via Natural or Artificial Opening Endoscopic	**Z** No Device	**Z** No Qualifier

ORG 0TTD0ZZ
CC 0TTB0ZZ   0TTD0ZZ

0 Medical and Surgical
T Urinary System
U **Supplement:** Putting in or on biological or synthetic material that physically reinforces and/or augments the function of a portion of a body part

Body Part	Approach	Device	Qualifier
Character 4	Character 5	Character 6	Character 7
3 Kidney Pelvis, Right **4** Kidney Pelvis, Left **6** Ureter, Right **7** Ureter, Left **B** Bladder **C** Bladder Neck	**0** Open **4** Percutaneous Endoscopic **7** Via Natural or Artificial Opening **8** Via Natural or Artificial Opening Endoscopic	**7** Autologous Tissue Substitute **J** Synthetic Substitute **K** Nonautologous Tissue Substitute	**Z** No Qualifier
D Urethra	**0** Open **4** Percutaneous Endoscopic **7** Via Natural or Artificial Opening **8** Via Natural or Artificial Opening Endoscopic **X** External	**7** Autologous Tissue Substitute **J** Synthetic Substitute **K** Nonautologous Tissue Substitute	**Z** No Qualifier

LC Limited Coverage   **NC** Noncovered   **HAC** HAC-associated Procedure   **CC** Combination Cluster - See Appendix G for code lists
ORG Non-OR-Affecting MS-DRG Assignment   New/Revised Text in **Orange**   ♂ Male   ♀ Female

2021 ICD-10-PCS

529

0 Medical and Surgical
T Urinary System
V Restriction: Partially closing an orifice or the lumen of a tubular body part

Body Part	Approach	Device	Qualifier
Character 4	Character 5	Character 6	Character 7
3 Kidney Pelvis, Right 4 Kidney Pelvis, Left 6 Ureter, Right 7 Ureter, Left B Bladder C Bladder Neck	0 Open 3 Percutaneous 4 Percutaneous Endoscopic	C Extraluminal Device D Intraluminal Device Z No Device	Z No Qualifier
3 Kidney Pelvis, Right 4 Kidney Pelvis, Left 6 Ureter, Right 7 Ureter, Left B Bladder C Bladder Neck	7 Via Natural or Artificial Opening 8 Via Natural or Artificial Opening Endoscopic	D Intraluminal Device Z No Device	Z No Qualifier
D Urethra	0 Open 3 Percutaneous 4 Percutaneous Endoscopic	C Extraluminal Device D Intraluminal Device Z No Device	Z No Qualifier
D Urethra	7 Via Natural or Artificial Opening 8 Via Natural or Artificial Opening Endoscopic	D Intraluminal Device Z No Device	Z No Qualifier
D Urethra	X External	Z No Device	Z No Qualifier

0 Medical and Surgical
T Urinary System
W Revision: Correcting, to the extent possible, a portion of a malfunctioning device or the position of a displaced device

Body Part	Approach	Device	Qualifier
Character 4	Character 5	Character 6	Character 7
5 Kidney	0 Open 3 Percutaneous 4 Percutaneous Endoscopic 7 Via Natural or Artificial Opening 8 Via Natural or Artificial Opening Endoscopic	0 Drainage Device 2 Monitoring Device 3 Infusion Device 7 Autologous Tissue Substitute C Extraluminal Device D Intraluminal Device J Synthetic Substitute K Nonautologous Tissue Substitute Y Other Device	Z No Qualifier
5 Kidney	X External	0 Drainage Device 2 Monitoring Device 3 Infusion Device 7 Autologous Tissue Substitute C Extraluminal Device D Intraluminal Device J Synthetic Substitute K Nonautologous Tissue Substitute	Z No Qualifier
9 Ureter	0 Open 3 Percutaneous 4 Percutaneous Endoscopic 7 Via Natural or Artificial Opening 8 Via Natural or Artificial Opening Endoscopic	0 Drainage Device 2 Monitoring Device 3 Infusion Device 7 Autologous Tissue Substitute C Extraluminal Device D Intraluminal Device J Synthetic Substitute K Nonautologous Tissue Substitute M Stimulator Lead Y Other Device	Z No Qualifier
9 Ureter	X External	0 Drainage Device 2 Monitoring Device 3 Infusion Device 7 Autologous Tissue Substitute C Extraluminal Device D Intraluminal Device J Synthetic Substitute K Nonautologous Tissue Substitute M Stimulator Lead	Z No Qualifier

0TW continued on next page

LC Limited Coverage   NC Noncovered   HAC HAC-associated Procedure   CC Combination Cluster - See Appendix G for code lists
Non-OR-Affecting MS-DRG Assignment   New/Revised Text in Orange   ♂ Male   ♀ Female

0 Medical and Surgical
T Urinary System
W Revision: Correcting, to the extent possible, a portion of a malfunctioning device or the position of a displaced device

0TW continued from previous page

Body Part	Approach	Device	Qualifier
Character 4	Character 5	Character 6	Character 7
B Bladder	**0** Open **3** Percutaneous **4** Percutaneous Endoscopic **7** Via Natural or Artificial Opening **8** Via Natural or Artificial Opening Endoscopic	**0** Drainage Device **2** Monitoring Device **3** Infusion Device **7** Autologous Tissue Substitute **C** Extraluminal Device **D** Intraluminal Device **J** Synthetic Substitute **K** Nonautologous Tissue Substitute **L** Artificial Sphincter **M** Stimulator Lead **Y** Other Device	**Z** No Qualifier
B Bladder	**X** External	**0** Drainage Device **2** Monitoring Device **3** Infusion Device **7** Autologous Tissue Substitute **C** Extraluminal Device **D** Intraluminal Device **J** Synthetic Substitute **K** Nonautologous Tissue Substitute **L** Artificial Sphincter **M** Stimulator Lead	**Z** No Qualifier
D Urethra	**0** Open **3** Percutaneous **4** Percutaneous Endoscopic **7** Via Natural or Artificial Opening **8** Via Natural or Artificial Opening Endoscopic	**0** Drainage Device **2** Monitoring Device **3** Infusion Device **7** Autologous Tissue Substitute **C** Extraluminal Device **D** Intraluminal Device **J** Synthetic Substitute **K** Nonautologous Tissue Substitute **L** Artificial Sphincter **Y** Other Device	**Z** No Qualifier
D Urethra	**X** External	**0** Drainage Device **2** Monitoring Device **3** Infusion Device **7** Autologous Tissue Substitute **C** Extraluminal Device **D** Intraluminal Device **J** Synthetic Substitute **K** Nonautologous Tissue Substitute **L** Artificial Sphincter	**Z** No Qualifier

0 Medical and Surgical
T Urinary System
Y Transplantation: Putting in or on all or a portion of a living body part taken from another individual or animal to physically take the place and/or function of all or a portion of a similar body part

Body Part	Approach	Device	Qualifier
Character 4	Character 5	Character 6	Character 7
0 Kidney, Right ᴸᶜ ᶜᶜ **1** Kidney, Left ᴸᶜ ᶜᶜ	**0** Open	**Z** No Device	**0** Allogeneic **1** Syngeneic **2** Zooplastic

ᴸᶜ 0TY00Z0   0TY00Z1   0TY00Z2   0TY10Z0   0TY10Z1   0TY10Z2
ᶜᶜ 0TY00Z0   0TY00Z1   0TY00Z2   0TY10Z0   0TY10Z1   0TY10Z2

ᴸᶜ Limited Coverage   ᴺᶜ Noncovered   ᴴᴬᶜ HAC-associated Procedure   ᶜᶜ Combination Cluster - See Appendix G for code lists
ᴰᴿᴳ Non-OR-Affecting MS-DRG Assignment   New/Revised Text in **Orange**   ♂ Male   ♀ Female

2021 ICD-10-PCS

531

NOTES

Female Reproductive System 0U1-0UY

0 **Medical and Surgical**
U **Female Reproductive System**
1 **Bypass:** Altering the route of passage of the contents of a tubular body part

Body Part	Approach	Device	Qualifier
Character 4	Character 5	Character 6	Character 7
5 Fallopian Tube, Right ♀ **6** Fallopian Tube, Left ♀	**0** Open **4** Percutaneous Endoscopic	**7** Autologous Tissue Substitute **J** Synthetic Substitute **K** Nonautologous Tissue Substitute **Z** No Device	**5** Fallopian Tube, Right **6** Fallopian Tube, Left **9** Uterus

♀ 0U15075 0U15076 0U15079 0U150J5 0U150J6 0U150J9 0U150K5 0U150K6 0U150K9 0U150Z5 0U150Z6 0U150Z9 0U15475
0U15476 0U15479 0U154J5 0U154J6 0U154J9 0U154K5 0U154K6 0U154K9 0U154Z5 0U154Z6 0U154Z9 0U16075 0U16076
0U16079 0U160J5 0U160J6 0U160J9 0U160K5 0U160K6 0U160K9 0U160Z5 0U160Z6 0U160Z9 0U16475 0U16476 0U16479
0U164J5 0U164J6 0U164J9 0U164K5 0U164K6 0U164K9 0U164Z5 0U164Z6 0U164Z9

0 **Medical and Surgical**
U **Female Reproductive System**
2 **Change:** Taking out or off a device from a body part and putting back an identical or similar device in or on the same body part without cutting or puncturing the skin or a mucous membrane

Body Part	Approach	Device	Qualifier
Character 4	Character 5	Character 6	Character 7
3 Ovary ♀ **8** Fallopian Tube ♀ **M** Vulva ♀	**X** External	**0** Drainage Device **Y** Other Device	**Z** No Qualifier
D Uterus and Cervix ♀	**X** External	**0** Drainage Device **H** Contraceptive Device **Y** Other Device	**Z** No Qualifier
H Vagina and Cul-de-sac ♀	**X** External	**0** Drainage Device **G** Intraluminal Device, Pessary **Y** Other Device	**Z** No Qualifier

♀ 0U23X0Z 0U23XYZ 0U28X0Z 0U28XYZ 0U2DX0Z 0U2DXHZ 0U2DXYZ 0U2HX0Z 0U2HXGZ 0U2HXYZ 0U2MX0Z 0U2MXYZ

0 **Medical and Surgical**
U **Female Reproductive System**
5 **Destruction:** Physical eradication of all or a portion of a body part by the direct use of energy, force, or a destructive agent

Body Part	Approach	Device	Qualifier
Character 4	Character 5	Character 6	Character 7
0 Ovary, Right ♀ **1** Ovary, Left ♀ **2** Ovaries, Bilateral ♀ **4** Uterine Supporting Structure ♀	**0** Open **3** Percutaneous **4** Percutaneous Endoscopic **8** Via Natural or Artificial Opening Endoscopic	**Z** No Device	**Z** No Qualifier
5 Fallopian Tube, Right ♀ **6** Fallopian Tube, Left ♀ **7** Fallopian Tubes, Bilateral ♀ NC **9** Uterus ♀ **B** Endometrium ♀ **C** Cervix ♀ **F** Cul-de-sac ♀	**0** Open **3** Percutaneous **4** Percutaneous Endoscopic **7** Via Natural or Artificial Opening **8** Via Natural or Artificial Opening Endoscopic	**Z** No Device	**Z** No Qualifier
G Vagina ♀ **K** Hymen ♀	**0** Open **3** Percutaneous **4** Percutaneous Endoscopic **7** Via Natural or Artificial Opening **8** Via Natural or Artificial Opening Endoscopic **X** External	**Z** No Device	**Z** No Qualifier

0U5 continued on next page

LC Limited Coverage   NC Noncovered   HAC HAC-associated Procedure   CC Combination Cluster - See Appendix G for code lists
DRG Non-OR-Affecting MS-DRG Assignment   New/Revised Text in **Orange**   ♂ Male   ♀ Female

0 Medical and Surgical
U Female Reproductive System

0U5 continued from previous page

5 Destruction: Physical eradication of all or a portion of a body part by the direct use of energy, force, or a destructive agent

Body Part	Approach	Device	Qualifier
Character 4	Character 5	Character 6	Character 7
J Clitoris ♀ **L** Vestibular Gland ♀ **M** Vulva ♀	**0** Open **X** External	**Z** No Device	**Z** No Qualifier

♀ 0U500ZZ 0U503ZZ 0U504ZZ 0U508ZZ 0U510ZZ 0U513ZZ 0U514ZZ 0U518ZZ 0U520ZZ 0U523ZZ 0U524ZZ 0U528ZZ 0U540ZZ
0U543ZZ 0U544ZZ 0U548ZZ 0U550ZZ 0U553ZZ 0U554ZZ 0U557ZZ 0U558ZZ 0U560ZZ 0U563ZZ 0U564ZZ 0U567ZZ 0U568ZZ
0U570ZZ 0U573ZZ 0U574ZZ 0U577ZZ 0U578ZZ 0U590ZZ 0U593ZZ 0U594ZZ 0U597ZZ 0U598ZZ 0U5B0ZZ 0U5B3ZZ 0U5B4ZZ
0U5B7ZZ 0U5B8ZZ 0U5C0ZZ 0U5C3ZZ 0U5C4ZZ 0U5C7ZZ 0U5C8ZZ 0U5F0ZZ 0U5F3ZZ 0U5F4ZZ 0U5F7ZZ 0U5F8ZZ 0U5G0ZZ
0U5G3ZZ 0U5G4ZZ 0U5G7ZZ 0U5G8ZZ 0U5GXZZ 0U5J0ZZ 0U5JXZZ 0U5K0ZZ 0U5K3ZZ 0U5K4ZZ 0U5K7ZZ 0U5K8ZZ 0U5KXZZ
0U5L0ZZ 0U5LXZZ 0U5M0ZZ 0U5MXZZ
NC 0U570ZZ 0U573ZZ 0U574ZZ 0U577ZZ 0U578ZZ

Codes in this list are noncovered procedures only when reported with Z30.2 as either a principal or secondary diagnosis.

0 Medical and Surgical
U Female Reproductive System
7 Dilation: Expanding an orifice or the lumen of a tubular body part

Body Part	Approach	Device	Qualifier
Character 4	Character 5	Character 6	Character 7
5 Fallopian Tube, Right ♀ **6** Fallopian Tube, Left ♀ **7** Fallopian Tubes, Bilateral ♀ **9** Uterus ♀ **C** Cervix ♀ **G** Vagina ♀	**0** Open **3** Percutaneous **4** Percutaneous Endoscopic **7** Via Natural or Artificial Opening **8** Via Natural or Artificial Opening Endoscopic	**D** Intraluminal Device **Z** No Device	**Z** No Qualifier
K Hymen ♀	**0** Open **3** Percutaneous **4** Percutaneous Endoscopic **7** Via Natural or Artificial Opening **8** Via Natural or Artificial Opening Endoscopic **X** External	**D** Intraluminal Device **Z** No Device	**Z** No Qualifier

♀ 0U750DZ 0U750ZZ 0U753DZ 0U753ZZ 0U754DZ 0U754ZZ 0U757DZ 0U757ZZ 0U758DZ 0U758ZZ 0U760DZ 0U760ZZ 0U763DZ
0U763ZZ 0U764DZ 0U764ZZ 0U767DZ 0U767ZZ 0U768DZ 0U768ZZ 0U770DZ 0U770ZZ 0U773DZ 0U773ZZ 0U774DZ 0U774ZZ
0U777DZ 0U777ZZ 0U778DZ 0U778ZZ 0U790DZ 0U790ZZ 0U793DZ 0U793ZZ 0U794DZ 0U794ZZ 0U797DZ 0U797ZZ 0U798DZ
0U798ZZ 0U7C0DZ 0U7C0ZZ 0U7C3DZ 0U7C3ZZ 0U7C4DZ 0U7C4ZZ 0U7C7DZ 0U7C7ZZ 0U7C8DZ 0U7C8ZZ 0U7G0DZ 0U7G0ZZ
0U7G3DZ 0U7G3ZZ 0U7G4DZ 0U7G4ZZ 0U7G7DZ 0U7G7ZZ 0U7G8DZ 0U7G8ZZ 0U7K0DZ 0U7K0ZZ 0U7K3DZ 0U7K3ZZ 0U7K4DZ
0U7K4ZZ 0U7K7DZ 0U7K7ZZ 0U7K8DZ 0U7K8ZZ 0U7KXDZ 0U7KXZZ

0 Medical and Surgical
U Female Reproductive System
8 Division: Cutting into a body part, without draining fluids and/or gases from the body part, in order to separate or transect a body part

Body Part	Approach	Device	Qualifier
Character 4	Character 5	Character 6	Character 7
0 Ovary, Right ♀ **1** Ovary, Left ♀ **2** Ovaries, Bilateral ♀ **4** Uterine Supporting Structure ♀	**0** Open **3** Percutaneous **4** Percutaneous Endoscopic	**Z** No Device	**Z** No Qualifier
K Hymen ♀	**7** Via Natural or Artificial Opening **8** Via Natural or Artificial Opening Endoscopic **X** External	**Z** No Device	**Z** No Qualifier

♀ 0U800ZZ 0U803ZZ 0U804ZZ 0U810ZZ 0U813ZZ 0U814ZZ 0U820ZZ 0U823ZZ 0U824ZZ 0U840ZZ 0U843ZZ 0U844ZZ 0U8K7ZZ
0U8K8ZZ 0U8KXZZ

LC Limited Coverage **NC** Noncovered **HAC** HAC-associated Procedure **CC** Combination Cluster - See Appendix G for code lists
DRG Non-OR-Affecting MS-DRG Assignment New/Revised Text in **Orange** ♂ Male ♀ Female

534 **2021 ICD-10-PCS**

FEMALE REPRODUCTIVE SYSTEM 0U1-0UY

0 Medical and Surgical
U Female Reproductive System
9 Drainage: Taking or letting out fluids and/or gases from a body part

Body Part	Approach	Device	Qualifier
Character 4	Character 5	Character 6	Character 7
0 Ovary, Right ♀ 1 Ovary, Left ♀ 2 Ovaries, Bilateral ♀	0 Open 3 Percutaneous 4 Percutaneous Endoscopic 8 Via Natural or Artificial Opening Endoscopic	0 Drainage Device	Z No Qualifier
0 Ovary, Right ♀ 1 Ovary, Left ♀ 2 Ovaries, Bilateral ♀	0 Open 3 Percutaneous 4 Percutaneous Endoscopic 8 Via Natural or Artificial Opening Endoscopic	Z No Device	X Diagnostic Z No Qualifier
0 Ovary, Right ♀ 1 Ovary, Left ♀ 2 Ovaries, Bilateral ♀	X External	Z No Device	Z No Qualifier
4 Uterine Supporting Structure ♀	0 Open 3 Percutaneous 4 Percutaneous Endoscopic 8 Via Natural or Artificial Opening Endoscopic	0 Drainage Device	Z No Qualifier
4 Uterine Supporting Structure ♀	0 Open 3 Percutaneous 4 Percutaneous Endoscopic 8 Via Natural or Artificial Opening Endoscopic	Z No Device	X Diagnostic Z No Qualifier
5 Fallopian Tube, Right ♀ 6 Fallopian Tube, Left ♀ 7 Fallopian Tubes, Bilateral ♀ 9 Uterus ♀ C Cervix ♀ F Cul-de-sac ♀	0 Open 3 Percutaneous 4 Percutaneous Endoscopic 7 Via Natural or Artificial Opening 8 Via Natural or Artificial Opening Endoscopic	0 Drainage Device	Z No Qualifier
5 Fallopian Tube, Right ♀ 6 Fallopian Tube, Left ♀ 7 Fallopian Tubes, Bilateral ♀ 9 Uterus ♀ C Cervix ♀ F Cul-de-sac ♀	0 Open 3 Percutaneous 4 Percutaneous Endoscopic 7 Via Natural or Artificial Opening 8 Via Natural or Artificial Opening Endoscopic	Z No Device	X Diagnostic Z No Qualifier
G Vagina ♀ K Hymen ♀	0 Open 3 Percutaneous 4 Percutaneous Endoscopic 7 Via Natural or Artificial Opening 8 Via Natural or Artificial Opening Endoscopic X External	0 Drainage Device	Z No Qualifier
G Vagina ♀ K Hymen ♀	0 Open 3 Percutaneous 4 Percutaneous Endoscopic 7 Via Natural or Artificial Opening 8 Via Natural or Artificial Opening Endoscopic X External	Z No Device	X Diagnostic Z No Qualifier
J Clitoris ♀ L Vestibular Gland ♀ M Vulva ♀	0 Open X External	0 Drainage Device	Z No Qualifier

0U9 continued on next page

0 Medical and Surgical
U Female Reproductive System
9 Drainage: Taking or letting out fluids and/or gases from a body part

0U9 continued from previous page

Body Part	Approach	Device	Qualifier
Character 4	Character 5	Character 6	Character 7
J Clitoris ♀ L Vestibular Gland ♀ M Vulva ♀	0 Open X External	Z No Device	X Diagnostic Z No Qualifier

♀
0U9000Z	0U900ZX	0U900ZZ	0U9030Z	0U903ZX	0U903ZZ	0U9040Z	0U904ZX	0U904ZZ	0U9080Z	0U908ZX	0U908ZZ	0U90XZZ
0U9100Z	0U910ZX	0U910ZZ	0U9130Z	0U913ZX	0U913ZZ	0U9140Z	0U914ZX	0U914ZZ	0U9180Z	0U918ZX	0U918ZZ	0U91XZZ
0U9200Z	0U920ZX	0U920ZZ	0U9230Z	0U923ZX	0U923ZZ	0U9240Z	0U924ZX	0U924ZZ	0U9280Z	0U928ZX	0U928ZZ	0U92XZZ
0U9400Z	0U940ZX	0U940ZZ	0U9430Z	0U943ZX	0U943ZZ	0U9440Z	0U944ZX	0U944ZZ	0U9480Z	0U948ZX	0U948ZZ	0U9500Z
0U950ZX	0U950ZZ	0U9530Z	0U953ZX	0U953ZZ	0U9540Z	0U954ZX	0U954ZZ	0U9570Z	0U957ZX	0U957ZZ	0U9580Z	0U958ZX
0U958ZZ	0U9600Z	0U960ZX	0U960ZZ	0U9630Z	0U963ZX	0U963ZZ	0U9640Z	0U964ZX	0U964ZZ	0U9670Z	0U967ZX	0U967ZZ
0U9680Z	0U968ZX	0U968ZZ	0U9700Z	0U970ZX	0U970ZZ	0U9730Z	0U973ZX	0U973ZZ	0U9740Z	0U974ZX	0U974ZZ	0U9770Z
0U977ZX	0U977ZZ	0U9780Z	0U978ZX	0U978ZZ	0U9900Z	0U990ZX	0U990ZZ	0U9930Z	0U993ZX	0U993ZZ	0U9940Z	0U994ZX
0U994ZZ	0U9970Z	0U997ZX	0U997ZZ	0U9980Z	0U998ZX	0U998ZZ	0U9C00Z	0U9C0ZX	0U9C0ZZ	0U9C30Z	0U9C3ZX	0U9C3ZZ
0U9C40Z	0U9C4ZX	0U9C4ZZ	0U9C70Z	0U9C7ZX	0U9C7ZZ	0U9C80Z	0U9C8ZX	0U9C8ZZ	0U9F00Z	0U9F0ZX	0U9F0ZZ	0U9F30Z
0U9F3ZX	0U9F3ZZ	0U9F40Z	0U9F4ZX	0U9F4ZZ	0U9F70Z	0U9F7ZX	0U9F7ZZ	0U9F80Z	0U9F8ZX	0U9F8ZZ	0U9G00Z	0U9G0ZX
0U9G0ZZ	0U9G30Z	0U9G3ZX	0U9G3ZZ	0U9G40Z	0U9G4ZX	0U9G4ZZ	0U9G70Z	0U9G7ZX	0U9G7ZZ	0U9G80Z	0U9G8ZX	0U9G8ZZ
0U9GX0Z	0U9GXZX	0U9GXZZ	0U9J00Z	0U9J0ZX	0U9J0ZZ	0U9JX0Z	0U9JXZX	0U9JXZZ	0U9K00Z	0U9K0ZX	0U9K0ZZ	0U9K30Z
0U9K3ZX	0U9K3ZZ	0U9K40Z	0U9K4ZX	0U9K4ZZ	0U9K70Z	0U9K7ZX	0U9K7ZZ	0U9K80Z	0U9K8ZX	0U9K8ZZ	0U9KX0Z	0U9KXZX
0U9KXZZ	0U9L00Z	0U9L0ZZ	0U9LX0Z	0U9LXZX	0U9LXZZ	0U9M00Z	0U9M0ZX	0U9M0ZZ	0U9MX0Z	0U9MXZX	0U9MXZZ	

0 Medical and Surgical
U Female Reproductive System
B Excision: Cutting out or off, without replacement, a portion of a body part

Body Part	Approach	Device	Qualifier
Character 4	Character 5	Character 6	Character 7
0 Ovary, Right ♀ 1 Ovary, Left ♀ 2 Ovaries, Bilateral ♀ 4 Uterine Supporting Structure ♀ 5 Fallopian Tube, Right ♀ 6 Fallopian Tube, Left ♀ 7 Fallopian Tubes, Bilateral ♀ 9 Uterus ♀ C Cervix ♀ F Cul-de-sac ♀	0 Open 3 Percutaneous 4 Percutaneous Endoscopic 7 Via Natural or Artificial Opening 8 Via Natural or Artificial Opening Endoscopic	Z No Device	X Diagnostic Z No Qualifier
G Vagina ♀ K Hymen ♀	0 Open 3 Percutaneous 4 Percutaneous Endoscopic 7 Via Natural or Artificial Opening 8 Via Natural or Artificial Opening Endoscopic X External	Z No Device	X Diagnostic Z No Qualifier
J Clitoris ♀ L Vestibular Gland ♀ M Vulva ♀	0 Open X External	Z No Device	X Diagnostic Z No Qualifier

♀
0UB00ZX	0UB00ZZ	0UB03ZX	0UB03ZZ	0UB04ZX	0UB04ZZ	0UB07ZX	0UB07ZZ	0UB08ZX	0UB08ZZ	0UB10ZX	0UB10ZZ	0UB13ZX
0UB13ZZ	0UB14ZX	0UB14ZZ	0UB17ZX	0UB17ZZ	0UB18ZX	0UB18ZZ	0UB20ZX	0UB20ZZ	0UB23ZX	0UB23ZZ	0UB24ZX	0UB24ZZ
0UB27ZX	0UB27ZZ	0UB28ZX	0UB28ZZ	0UB40ZX	0UB40ZZ	0UB43ZX	0UB43ZZ	0UB44ZX	0UB44ZZ	0UB47ZX	0UB47ZZ	0UB48ZX
0UB48ZZ	0UB50ZX	0UB50ZZ	0UB53ZX	0UB53ZZ	0UB54ZX	0UB54ZZ	0UB57ZX	0UB57ZZ	0UB58ZX	0UB58ZZ	0UB60ZX	0UB60ZZ
0UB63ZX	0UB63ZZ	0UB64ZX	0UB64ZZ	0UB67ZX	0UB67ZZ	0UB68ZX	0UB68ZZ	0UB70ZX	0UB70ZZ	0UB73ZX	0UB73ZZ	0UB74ZX
0UB74ZZ	0UB77ZX	0UB77ZZ	0UB78ZX	0UB78ZZ	0UB90ZX	0UB90ZZ	0UB93ZX	0UB93ZZ	0UB94ZX	0UB94ZZ	0UB97ZX	0UB97ZZ
0UB98ZX	0UB98ZZ	0UBC0ZX	0UBC0ZZ	0UBC3ZX	0UBC3ZZ	0UBC4ZX	0UBC4ZZ	0UBC7ZX	0UBC7ZZ	0UBC8ZX	0UBC8ZZ	0UBF0ZX
0UBF0ZZ	0UBF3ZX	0UBF3ZZ	0UBF4ZX	0UBF4ZZ	0UBF7ZX	0UBF7ZZ	0UBF8ZX	0UBF8ZZ	0UBG0ZX	0UBG0ZZ	0UBG3ZX	0UBG3ZZ
0UBG4ZX	0UBG4ZZ	0UBG7ZX	0UBG7ZZ	0UBG8ZX	0UBG8ZZ	0UBGXZX	0UBGXZZ	0UBJ0ZX	0UBJ0ZZ	0UBJXZX	0UBJXZZ	0UBK0ZX
0UBK0ZZ	0UBK3ZX	0UBK3ZZ	0UBK4ZX	0UBK4ZZ	0UBK7ZX	0UBK7ZZ	0UBK8ZX	0UBK8ZZ	0UBKXZX	0UBKXZZ	0UBL0ZX	0UBL0ZZ
0UBLXZX	0UBLXZZ	0UBM0ZX	0UBM0ZZ	0UBMXZX	0UBMXZZ							

LC Limited Coverage   NC Noncovered   HAC HAC-associated Procedure   CC Combination Cluster - See Appendix G for code lists
DRG Non-OR-Affecting MS-DRG Assignment   New/Revised Text in Orange   ♂ Male   ♀ Female

536

2021 ICD-10-PCS

0 Medical and Surgical
U Female Reproductive System
C Extirpation: Taking or cutting out solid matter from a body part

Body Part	Approach	Device	Qualifier
Character 4	Character 5	Character 6	Character 7
0 Ovary, Right ♀ **1** Ovary, Left ♀ **2** Ovaries, Bilateral ♀ **4** Uterine Supporting Structure ♀	**0** Open **3** Percutaneous **4** Percutaneous Endoscopic **8** Via Natural or Artificial Opening Endoscopic	**Z** No Device	**Z** No Qualifier
5 Fallopian Tube, Right ♀ **6** Fallopian Tube, Left ♀ **7** Fallopian Tubes, Bilateral ♀ **9** Uterus ♀ **B** Endometrium ♀ **C** Cervix ♀ **F** Cul-de-sac ♀	**0** Open **3** Percutaneous **4** Percutaneous Endoscopic **7** Via Natural or Artificial Opening **8** Via Natural or Artificial Opening Endoscopic	**Z** No Device	**Z** No Qualifier
G Vagina ♀ **K** Hymen ♀	**0** Open **3** Percutaneous **4** Percutaneous Endoscopic **7** Via Natural or Artificial Opening **8** Via Natural or Artificial Opening Endoscopic **X** External	**Z** No Device	**Z** No Qualifier
J Clitoris ♀ **L** Vestibular Gland ♀ **M** Vulva ♀	**0** Open **X** External	**Z** No Device	**Z** No Qualifier

♀ 0UC00ZZ 0UC03ZZ 0UC04ZZ 0UC08ZZ 0UC10ZZ 0UC13ZZ 0UC14ZZ 0UC18ZZ 0UC20ZZ 0UC23ZZ 0UC24ZZ 0UC28ZZ 0UC40ZZ
0UC43ZZ 0UC44ZZ 0UC48ZZ 0UC50ZZ 0UC53ZZ 0UC54ZZ 0UC57ZZ 0UC58ZZ 0UC60ZZ 0UC63ZZ 0UC64ZZ 0UC67ZZ 0UC68ZZ
0UC70ZZ 0UC73ZZ 0UC74ZZ 0UC77ZZ 0UC78ZZ 0UC90ZZ 0UC93ZZ 0UC94ZZ 0UC97ZZ 0UC98ZZ 0UCB0ZZ 0UCB3ZZ 0UCB4ZZ
0UCB7ZZ 0UCB8ZZ 0UCC0ZZ 0UCC3ZZ 0UCC4ZZ 0UCC7ZZ 0UCC8ZZ 0UCF0ZZ 0UCF3ZZ 0UCF4ZZ 0UCF7ZZ 0UCF8ZZ 0UCG0ZZ
0UCG3ZZ 0UCG4ZZ 0UCG7ZZ 0UCG8ZZ 0UCGXZZ 0UCJ0ZZ 0UCJXZZ 0UCK0ZZ 0UCK3ZZ 0UCK4ZZ 0UCK7ZZ 0UCK8ZZ 0UCKXZZ
0UCL0ZZ 0UCLXZZ 0UCM0ZZ 0UCMXZZ

0 Medical and Surgical
U Female Reproductive System
D Extraction: Pulling or stripping out or off all or a portion of a body part by the use of force

Body Part	Approach	Device	Qualifier
Character 4	Character 5	Character 6	Character 7
B Endometrium ♀	**7** Via Natural or Artificial Opening **8** Via Natural or Artificial Opening Endoscopic	**Z** No Device	**X** Diagnostic **Z** No Qualifier
N Ova ♀	**0** Open **3** Percutaneous **4** Percutaneous Endoscopic	**Z** No Device	**Z** No Qualifier

♀ 0UDB7ZX 0UDB7ZZ 0UDB8ZX 0UDB8ZZ 0UDN0ZZ 0UDN3ZZ 0UDN4ZZ

0 Medical and Surgical
U Female Reproductive System
F Fragmentation: Breaking solid matter in a body part into pieces

Body Part	Approach	Device	Qualifier
Character 4	Character 5	Character 6	Character 7
5 Fallopian Tube, Right ♀ NC **6** Fallopian Tube, Left ♀ NC **7** Fallopian Tubes, Bilateral ♀ NC **9** Uterus ♀ NC	**0** Open **3** Percutaneous **4** Percutaneous Endoscopic **7** Via Natural or Artificial Opening **8** Via Natural or Artificial Opening Endoscopic **X** External	**Z** No Device	**Z** No Qualifier

♀ 0UF50ZZ 0UF53ZZ 0UF54ZZ 0UF57ZZ 0UF58ZZ 0UF5XZZ 0UF60ZZ 0UF63ZZ 0UF64ZZ 0UF67ZZ 0UF68ZZ 0UF6XZZ 0UF70ZZ
0UF73ZZ 0UF74ZZ 0UF77ZZ 0UF78ZZ 0UF7XZZ 0UF90ZZ 0UF93ZZ 0UF94ZZ 0UF97ZZ 0UF98ZZ 0UF9XZZ

NC 0UF5XZZ 0UF6XZZ 0UF7XZZ 0UF9XZZ

LC Limited Coverage   NC Noncovered   HAC HAC-associated Procedure   CC Combination Cluster - See Appendix G for code lists
DRG Non-OR-Affecting MS-DRG Assignment   New/Revised Text in Orange   ♂ Male   ♀ Female

0 **Medical and Surgical**
U **Female Reproductive System**
H **Insertion:** Putting in a nonbiological appliance that monitors, assists, performs, or prevents a physiological function but does not physically take the place of a body part

Body Part	Approach	Device	Qualifier
Character 4	Character 5	Character 6	Character 7
3 Ovary ♀	0 Open 3 Percutaneous 4 Percutaneous Endoscopic	1 Radioactive Element 3 Infusion Device Y Other Device	Z No Qualifier
3 Ovary ♀	7 Via Natural or Artificial Opening 8 Via Natural or Artificial Opening Endoscopic	1 Radioactive Element Y Other Device	Z No Qualifier
8 Fallopian Tube ♀ D Uterus and Cervix ♀ H Vagina and Cul-de-sac ♀	0 Open 3 Percutaneous 4 Percutaneous Endoscopic 7 Via Natural or Artificial Opening 8 Via Natural or Artificial Opening Endoscopic	3 Infusion Device Y Other Device	Z No Qualifier
9 Uterus ♀	0 Open 7 Via Natural or Artificial Opening 8 Via Natural or Artificial Opening Endoscopic	1 Radioactive Element H Contraceptive Device	Z No Qualifier
C Cervix ♀	0 Open 3 Percutaneous 4 Percutaneous Endoscopic	1 Radioactive Element	Z No Qualifier
C Cervix ♀	7 Via Natural or Artificial Opening 8 Via Natural or Artificial Opening Endoscopic	1 Radioactive Element H Contraceptive Device	Z No Qualifier
F Cul-de-sac ♀	7 Via Natural or Artificial Opening 8 Via Natural or Artificial Opening Endoscopic	G Intraluminal Device, Pessary	Z No Qualifier
G Vagina ♀	0 Open 3 Percutaneous 4 Percutaneous Endoscopic X External	1 Radioactive Element	Z No Qualifier
G Vagina ♀	7 Via Natural or Artificial Opening 8 Via Natural or Artificial Opening Endoscopic	1 Radioactive Element G Intraluminal Device, Pessary	Z No Qualifier

♀ 0UH303Z   0UH30YZ   0UH333Z   0UH33YZ   0UH343Z   0UH34YZ   0UH37YZ   0UH38YZ   0UH803Z   0UH80YZ   0UH833Z   0UH83YZ   0UH843Z
0UH84YZ   0UH873Z   0UH87YZ   0UH883Z   0UH88YZ   0UH90HZ   0UH97HZ   0UH98HZ   0UHC01Z   0UHC31Z   0UHC41Z   0UHC71Z   0UHC7HZ
0UHC81Z   0UHC8HZ   0UHD03Z   0UHD0YZ   0UHD33Z   0UHD3YZ   0UHD43Z   0UHD4YZ   0UHD73Z   0UHD7YZ   0UHD83Z   0UHD8YZ   0UHF7GZ
0UHF8GZ   0UHG01Z   0UHG31Z   0UHG41Z   0UHG71Z   0UHG7GZ   0UHG81Z   0UHG8GZ   0UHGX1Z   0UHH03Z   0UHH0YZ   0UHH33Z   0UHH3YZ
0UHH43Z   0UHH4YZ   0UHH73Z   0UHH7YZ   0UHH83Z   0UHH8YZ

0 **Medical and Surgical**
U **Female Reproductive System**
J **Inspection:** Visually and/or manually exploring a body part

Body Part	Approach	Device	Qualifier
Character 4	Character 5	Character 6	Character 7
3 Ovary ♀	0 Open 3 Percutaneous 4 Percutaneous Endoscopic 8 Via Natural or Artificial Opening Endoscopic X External	Z No Device	Z No Qualifier

0UJ continued on next page

0 Medical and Surgical
U Female Reproductive System
J Inspection: Visually and/or manually exploring a body part

0UJ continued from previous page

Body Part	Approach	Device	Qualifier
Character 4	Character 5	Character 6	Character 7
8 Fallopian Tube ♀ **D** Uterus and Cervix ♀ **H** Vagina and Cul-de-sac ♀	**0** Open **3** Percutaneous **4** Percutaneous Endoscopic **7** Via Natural or Artificial Opening **8** Via Natural or Artificial Opening Endoscopic **X** External	**Z** No Device	**Z** No Qualifier
M Vulva ♀	**0** Open **X** External	**Z** No Device	**Z** No Qualifier

♀ 0UJ30ZZ 0UJ33ZZ 0UJ34ZZ 0UJ38ZZ 0UJ3XZZ 0UJ80ZZ 0UJ83ZZ 0UJ84ZZ 0UJ87ZZ 0UJ88ZZ 0UJ8XZZ 0UJD0ZZ 0UJD3ZZ
0UJD4ZZ 0UJD7ZZ 0UJD8ZZ 0UJDXZZ 0UJH0ZZ 0UJH3ZZ 0UJH4ZZ 0UJH7ZZ 0UJH8ZZ 0UJHXZZ 0UJM0ZZ 0UJMXZZ

0 Medical and Surgical
U Female Reproductive System
L Occlusion: Completely closing an orifice or the lumen of a tubular body part

Body Part	Approach	Device	Qualifier
Character 4	Character 5	Character 6	Character 7
5 Fallopian Tube, Right ♀ **6** Fallopian Tube, Left ♀ **7** Fallopian Tubes, Bilateral ♀ NC	**0** Open **3** Percutaneous **4** Percutaneous Endoscopic	**C** Extraluminal Device **D** Intraluminal Device **Z** No Device	**Z** No Qualifier
5 Fallopian Tube, Right ♀ **6** Fallopian Tube, Left ♀ **7** Fallopian Tubes, Bilateral ♀ NC	**7** Via Natural or Artificial Opening **8** Via Natural or Artificial Opening Endoscopic	**D** Intraluminal Device **Z** No Device	**Z** No Qualifier
F Cul-de-sac ♀ **G** Vagina ♀	**7** Via Natural or Artificial Opening **8** Via Natural or Artificial Opening Endoscopic	**D** Intraluminal Device **Z** No Device	**Z** No Qualifier

♀ 0UL50CZ 0UL50DZ 0UL50ZZ 0UL53CZ 0UL53DZ 0UL53ZZ 0UL54CZ 0UL54DZ 0UL54ZZ 0UL57DZ 0UL57ZZ 0UL58DZ 0UL58ZZ
0UL60CZ 0UL60DZ 0UL60ZZ 0UL63CZ 0UL63DZ 0UL63ZZ 0UL64CZ 0UL64DZ 0UL64ZZ 0UL67DZ 0UL67ZZ 0UL68DZ 0UL68ZZ
0UL70CZ 0UL70DZ 0UL70ZZ 0UL73CZ 0UL73DZ 0UL73ZZ 0UL74CZ 0UL74DZ 0UL74ZZ 0UL77DZ 0UL77ZZ 0UL78DZ 0UL78ZZ
0ULF7DZ 0ULF7ZZ 0ULF8DZ 0ULF8ZZ 0ULG7DZ 0ULG7ZZ 0ULG8DZ 0ULG8ZZ
NC 0UL70CZ 0UL70DZ 0UL70ZZ 0UL73CZ 0UL73DZ 0UL73ZZ 0UL74CZ 0UL74DZ 0UL74ZZ 0UL77DZ 0UL77ZZ 0UL78DZ 0UL78ZZ
Codes in this list are noncovered procedures only when reported with Z30.2 as either a principal or secondary diagnosis.

0 Medical and Surgical
U Female Reproductive System
M Reattachment: Putting back in or on all or a portion of a separated body part to its normal location or other suitable location

Body Part	Approach	Device	Qualifier
Character 4	Character 5	Character 6	Character 7
0 Ovary, Right ♀ **1** Ovary, Left ♀ **2** Ovaries, Bilateral ♀ **4** Uterine Supporting Structure ♀ **5** Fallopian Tube, Right ♀ **6** Fallopian Tube, Left ♀ **7** Fallopian Tubes, Bilateral ♀ **9** Uterus ♀ **C** Cervix ♀ **F** Cul-de-sac ♀ **G** Vagina ♀	**0** Open **4** Percutaneous Endoscopic	**Z** No Device	**Z** No Qualifier
J Clitoris ♀ **M** Vulva ♀	**X** External	**Z** No Device	**Z** No Qualifier
K Hymen ♀	**0** Open **4** Percutaneous Endoscopic **X** External	**Z** No Device	**Z** No Qualifier

♀ 0UM00ZZ 0UM04ZZ 0UM10ZZ 0UM14ZZ 0UM20ZZ 0UM24ZZ 0UM40ZZ 0UM44ZZ 0UM50ZZ 0UM54ZZ 0UM60ZZ 0UM64ZZ 0UM70ZZ
0UM74ZZ 0UM90ZZ 0UM94ZZ 0UMC0ZZ 0UMC4ZZ 0UMF0ZZ 0UMF4ZZ 0UMG0ZZ 0UMG4ZZ 0UMJXZZ 0UMK0ZZ 0UMK4ZZ 0UMKXZZ
0UMMXZZ

LC Limited Coverage NC Noncovered HAC HAC-associated Procedure CC Combination Cluster - See Appendix G for code lists
ONI Non-OR-Affecting MS-DRG Assignment New/Revised Text in Orange ♂ Male ♀ Female

0 Medical and Surgical
U Female Reproductive System
N Release: Freeing a body part from an abnormal physical constraint by cutting or by the use of force

Body Part	Approach	Device	Qualifier
Character 4	**Character 5**	**Character 6**	**Character 7**
0 Ovary, Right ♀ **1** Ovary, Left ♀ **2** Ovaries, Bilateral ♀ **4** Uterine Supporting Structure ♀	**0** Open **3** Percutaneous **4** Percutaneous Endoscopic **8** Via Natural or Artificial Opening Endoscopic	**Z** No Device	**Z** No Qualifier
5 Fallopian Tube, Right ♀ **6** Fallopian Tube, Left ♀ **7** Fallopian Tubes, Bilateral ♀ **9** Uterus ♀ **C** Cervix ♀ **F** Cul-de-sac ♀	**0** Open **3** Percutaneous **4** Percutaneous Endoscopic **7** Via Natural or Artificial Opening **8** Via Natural or Artificial Opening Endoscopic	**Z** No Device	**Z** No Qualifier
G Vagina ♀ **K** Hymen ♀	**0** Open **3** Percutaneous **4** Percutaneous Endoscopic **7** Via Natural or Artificial Opening **8** Via Natural or Artificial Opening Endoscopic **X** External	**Z** No Device	**Z** No Qualifier
J Clitoris ♀ **L** Vestibular Gland ♀ **M** Vulva ♀	**0** Open **X** External	**Z** No Device	**Z** No Qualifier

♀ 0UN00ZZ 0UN03ZZ 0UN04ZZ 0UN08ZZ 0UN10ZZ 0UN13ZZ 0UN14ZZ 0UN18ZZ 0UN20ZZ 0UN23ZZ 0UN24ZZ 0UN28ZZ 0UN40ZZ
0UN43ZZ 0UN44ZZ 0UN48ZZ 0UN50ZZ 0UN53ZZ 0UN54ZZ 0UN57ZZ 0UN58ZZ 0UN60ZZ 0UN63ZZ 0UN64ZZ 0UN67ZZ 0UN68ZZ
0UN70ZZ 0UN73ZZ 0UN74ZZ 0UN77ZZ 0UN78ZZ 0UN90ZZ 0UN93ZZ 0UN94ZZ 0UN97ZZ 0UN98ZZ 0UNC0ZZ 0UNC3ZZ 0UNC4ZZ
0UNC7ZZ 0UNC8ZZ 0UNF0ZZ 0UNF3ZZ 0UNF4ZZ 0UNF7ZZ 0UNF8ZZ 0UNG0ZZ 0UNG3ZZ 0UNG4ZZ 0UNG7ZZ 0UNG8ZZ 0UNGXZZ
0UNJ0ZZ 0UNJXZZ 0UNK0ZZ 0UNK3ZZ 0UNK4ZZ 0UNK7ZZ 0UNK8ZZ 0UNKXZZ 0UNL0ZZ 0UNLXZZ 0UNM0ZZ 0UNMXZZ

0 Medical and Surgical
U Female Reproductive System
P Removal: Taking out or off a device from a body part

Body Part	Approach	Device	Qualifier
Character 4	**Character 5**	**Character 6**	**Character 7**
3 Ovary ♀	**0** Open **3** Percutaneous **4** Percutaneous Endoscopic	**0** Drainage Device **3** Infusion Device **Y** Other Device	**Z** No Qualifier
3 Ovary ♀	**7** Via Natural or Artificial Opening **8** Via Natural or Artificial Opening Endoscopic	**Y** Other Device	**Z** No Qualifier
3 Ovary ♀	**X** External	**0** Drainage Device **3** Infusion Device	**Z** No Qualifier
8 Fallopian Tube ♀	**0** Open **3** Percutaneous **4** Percutaneous Endoscopic **7** Via Natural or Artificial Opening **8** Via Natural or Artificial Opening Endoscopic	**0** Drainage Device **3** Infusion Device **7** Autologous Tissue Substitute **C** Extraluminal Device **D** Intraluminal Device **J** Synthetic Substitute **K** Nonautologous Tissue Substitute **Y** Other Device	**Z** No Qualifier
8 Fallopian Tube ♀	**X** External	**0** Drainage Device **3** Infusion Device **D** Intraluminal Device	**Z** No Qualifier

0UP continued on next page

0   Medical and Surgical
U   Female Reproductive System
P   Removal: Taking out or off a device from a body part

0UP continued from previous page

Body Part	Approach	Device	Qualifier
Character 4	Character 5	Character 6	Character 7
D Uterus and Cervix ♀	**0** Open **3** Percutaneous **4** Percutaneous Endoscopic **7** Via Natural or Artificial Opening **8** Via Natural or Artificial Opening Endoscopic	**0** Drainage Device **1** Radioactive Element **3** Infusion Device **7** Autologous Tissue Substitute **C** Extraluminal Device **D** Intraluminal Device **H** Contraceptive Device **J** Synthetic Substitute **K** Nonautologous Tissue Substitute **Y** Other Device	**Z** No Qualifier
D Uterus and Cervix ♀	**X** External	**0** Drainage Device **3** Infusion Device **D** Intraluminal Device **H** Contraceptive Device	**Z** No Qualifier

H Vagina and Cul-de-sac ♀	**0** Open
	3 Percutaneous
	4 Percutaneous Endoscopic
	7 Via Natural or Artificial Opening
	8 Via Natural or Artificial Opening
	     Endoscopic
		0 Drainage Device
		1 Radioactive Element
		3 Infusion Device
		7 Autologous Tissue Substitute
		D Intraluminal Device
		J Synthetic Substitute
		K Nonautologous Tissue
		     Substitute
		Y Other Device
			Z No Qualifier

H Vagina and Cul-de-sac ♀	**X** External	**0** Drainage Device **1** Radioactive Element **3** Infusion Device **D** Intraluminal Device	**Z** No Qualifier
M Vulva ♀	**0** Open	**0** Drainage Device **7** Autologous Tissue Substitute **J** Synthetic Substitute **K** Nonautologous Tissue Substitute	**Z** No Qualifier
M Vulva ♀	**X** External	**0** Drainage Device	**Z** No Qualifier

♀ 0UP300Z 0UP303Z 0UP30YZ 0UP330Z 0UP333Z 0UP33YZ 0UP340Z 0UP343Z 0UP34YZ 0UP37YZ 0UP38YZ 0UP3X0Z 0UP3X3Z
0UP800Z 0UP803Z 0UP807Z 0UP80CZ 0UP80DZ 0UP80JZ 0UP80KZ 0UP80YZ 0UP830Z 0UP833Z 0UP837Z 0UP83CZ 0UP83DZ
0UP83JZ 0UP83KZ 0UP83YZ 0UP840Z 0UP843Z 0UP847Z 0UP84CZ 0UP84DZ 0UP84JZ 0UP84KZ 0UP84YZ 0UP870Z 0UP873Z
0UP877Z 0UP87CZ 0UP87DZ 0UP87JZ 0UP87KZ 0UP87YZ 0UP880Z 0UP883Z 0UP887Z 0UP88CZ 0UP88DZ 0UP88JZ 0UP88KZ
0UP88YZ 0UP8X0Z 0UP8X3Z 0UP8XDZ 0UPD00Z 0UPD01Z 0UPD03Z 0UPD07Z 0UPD0CZ 0UPD0DZ 0UPD0HZ 0UPD0JZ 0UPD0KZ
0UPD0YZ 0UPD30Z 0UPD31Z 0UPD33Z 0UPD37Z 0UPD3CZ 0UPD3DZ 0UPD3HZ 0UPD3JZ 0UPD3KZ 0UPD3YZ 0UPD40Z 0UPD41Z
0UPD43Z 0UPD47Z 0UPD4CZ 0UPD4DZ 0UPD4HZ 0UPD4JZ 0UPD4KZ 0UPD4YZ 0UPD70Z 0UPD71Z 0UPD73Z 0UPD77Z 0UPD7CZ
0UPD7DZ 0UPD7HZ 0UPD7JZ 0UPD7KZ 0UPD7YZ 0UPD80Z 0UPD81Z 0UPD83Z 0UPD87Z 0UPD8CZ 0UPD8DZ 0UPD8HZ 0UPD8JZ
0UPD8KZ 0UPD8YZ 0UPDX0Z 0UPDX3Z 0UPDXDZ 0UPDXHZ 0UPH00Z 0UPH01Z 0UPH03Z 0UPH07Z 0UPH0DZ 0UPH0JZ 0UPH0KZ
0UPH0YZ 0UPH30Z 0UPH31Z 0UPH33Z 0UPH37Z 0UPH3DZ 0UPH3JZ 0UPH3KZ 0UPH3YZ 0UPH40Z 0UPH41Z 0UPH43Z 0UPH47Z
0UPH4DZ 0UPH4JZ 0UPH4KZ 0UPH4YZ 0UPH70Z 0UPH71Z 0UPH73Z 0UPH77Z 0UPH7DZ 0UPH7JZ 0UPH7KZ 0UPH7YZ 0UPH80Z
0UPH81Z 0UPH83Z 0UPH87Z 0UPH8DZ 0UPH8JZ 0UPH8KZ 0UPH8YZ 0UPHX0Z 0UPHX1Z 0UPHX3Z 0UPHXDZ 0UPM00Z 0UPM07Z
0UPM0JZ 0UPM0KZ 0UPMX0Z

LC Limited Coverage   **NC** Noncovered   **HAC** HAC-associated Procedure   **CC** Combination Cluster - See Appendix G for code lists
⊕ Non-OR-Affecting MS-DRG Assignment   New/Revised Text in **Orange**   ♂ Male   ♀ Female

2021 ICD-10-PCS   541

0   Medical and Surgical
U   Female Reproductive System
Q   Repair: Restoring, to the extent possible, a body part to its normal anatomic structure and function

Body Part	Approach	Device	Qualifier
Character 4	Character 5	Character 6	Character 7
0 Ovary, Right ♀ 1 Ovary, Left ♀ 2 Ovaries, Bilateral ♀ 4 Uterine Supporting Structure ♀	0 Open 3 Percutaneous 4 Percutaneous Endoscopic 8 Via Natural or Artificial Opening Endoscopic	Z No Device	Z No Qualifier
5 Fallopian Tube, Right ♀ 6 Fallopian Tube, Left ♀ 7 Fallopian Tubes, Bilateral ♀ 9 Uterus ♀ C Cervix ♀ F Cul-de-sac ♀	0 Open 3 Percutaneous 4 Percutaneous Endoscopic 7 Via Natural or Artificial Opening 8 Via Natural or Artificial Opening Endoscopic	Z No Device	Z No Qualifier
G Vagina ♀ K Hymen ♀	0 Open 3 Percutaneous 4 Percutaneous Endoscopic 7 Via Natural or Artificial Opening 8 Via Natural or Artificial Opening Endoscopic X External	Z No Device	Z No Qualifier
J Clitoris ♀ L Vestibular Gland ♀ M Vulva ♀	0 Open X External	Z No Device	Z No Qualifier

♀ 0UQ00ZZ 0UQ03ZZ 0UQ04ZZ 0UQ08ZZ 0UQ10ZZ 0UQ13ZZ 0UQ14ZZ 0UQ18ZZ 0UQ20ZZ 0UQ23ZZ 0UQ24ZZ 0UQ28ZZ 0UQ40ZZ
0UQ43ZZ 0UQ44ZZ 0UQ48ZZ 0UQ50ZZ 0UQ53ZZ 0UQ54ZZ 0UQ57ZZ 0UQ58ZZ 0UQ60ZZ 0UQ63ZZ 0UQ64ZZ 0UQ67ZZ 0UQ68ZZ
0UQ70ZZ 0UQ73ZZ 0UQ74ZZ 0UQ77ZZ 0UQ78ZZ 0UQ90ZZ 0UQ93ZZ 0UQ94ZZ 0UQ97ZZ 0UQ98ZZ 0UQC0ZZ 0UQC3ZZ 0UQC4ZZ
0UQC7ZZ 0UQC8ZZ 0UQF0ZZ 0UQF3ZZ 0UQF4ZZ 0UQF7ZZ 0UQF8ZZ 0UQG0ZZ 0UQG3ZZ 0UQG4ZZ 0UQG7ZZ 0UQG8ZZ 0UQGXZZ
0UQJ0ZZ 0UQJXZZ 0UQK0ZZ 0UQK3ZZ 0UQK4ZZ 0UQK7ZZ 0UQK8ZZ 0UQKXZZ 0UQL0ZZ 0UQLXZZ 0UQM0ZZ 0UQMXZZ

0   Medical and Surgical
U   Female Reproductive System
S   Reposition: Moving to its normal location, or other suitable location, all or a portion of a body part

Body Part	Approach	Device	Qualifier
Character 4	Character 5	Character 6	Character 7
0 Ovary, Right ♀ 1 Ovary, Left ♀ 2 Ovaries, Bilateral ♀ 4 Uterine Supporting Structure ♀ 5 Fallopian Tube, Right ♀ 6 Fallopian Tube, Left ♀ 7 Fallopian Tubes, Bilateral ♀ C Cervix ♀ F Cul-de-sac ♀	0 Open 4 Percutaneous Endoscopic 8 Via Natural or Artificial Opening Endoscopic	Z No Device	Z No Qualifier
9 Uterus ♀ G Vagina ♀	0 Open 4 Percutaneous Endoscopic 7 Via Natural or Artificial Opening 8 Via Natural or Artificial Opening Endoscopic X External	Z No Device	Z No Qualifier

♀ 0US00ZZ 0US04ZZ 0US08ZZ 0US10ZZ 0US14ZZ 0US18ZZ 0US20ZZ 0US24ZZ 0US28ZZ 0US40ZZ 0US44ZZ 0US48ZZ 0US50ZZ
0US54ZZ 0US58ZZ 0US60ZZ 0US64ZZ 0US68ZZ 0US70ZZ 0US74ZZ 0US78ZZ 0US90ZZ 0US94ZZ 0US97ZZ 0US98ZZ 0US9XZZ
0USC0ZZ 0USC4ZZ 0USC8ZZ 0USF0ZZ 0USF4ZZ 0USF8ZZ 0USG0ZZ 0USG4ZZ 0USG7ZZ 0USG8ZZ 0USGXZZ

LC Limited Coverage   NC Noncovered   HAC HAC-associated Procedure   CC Combination Cluster - See Appendix G for code lists
⬛ Non-OR-Affecting MS-DRG Assignment   New/Revised Text in **Orange**   ♂ Male   ♀ Female

0   Medical and Surgical
U   Female Reproductive System
T   Resection: Cutting out or off, without replacement, all of a body part

Body Part	Approach	Device	Qualifier
Character 4	Character 5	Character 6	Character 7
0 Ovary, Right ♀ **1** Ovary, Left ♀ **2** Ovaries, Bilateral ♀ CC **5** Fallopian Tube, Right ♀ **6** Fallopian Tube, Left ♀ **7** Fallopian Tubes, Bilateral ♀ CC	**0** Open **4** Percutaneous Endoscopic **7** Via Natural or Artificial Opening **8** Via Natural or Artificial Opening Endoscopic **F** Via Natural or Artificial Opening With Percutaneous Endoscopic Assistance	**Z** No Device	**Z** No Qualifier
4 Uterine Supporting Structure ♀ CC **C** Cervix ♀ CC **F** Cul-de-sac ♀ **G** Vagina ♀ CC	**0** Open **4** Percutaneous Endoscopic **7** Via Natural or Artificial Opening **8** Via Natural or Artificial Opening Endoscopic	**Z** No Device	**Z** No Qualifier
9 Uterus ♀ CC	**0** Open **4** Percutaneous Endoscopic **7** Via Natural or Artificial Opening **8** Via Natural or Artificial Opening Endoscopic **F** Via Natural or Artificial Opening With Percutaneous Endoscopic Assistance	**Z** No Device	**L** Supracervical **Z** No Qualifier
J Clitoris ♀ **L** Vestibular Gland ♀ **M** Vulva ♀ CC	**0** Open **X** External	**Z** No Device	**Z** No Qualifier
K Hymen ♀	**0** Open **4** Percutaneous Endoscopic **7** Via Natural or Artificial Opening **8** Via Natural or Artificial Opening Endoscopic **X** External	**Z** No Device	**Z** No Qualifier

♀   0UT00ZZ   0UT04ZZ   0UT07ZZ   0UT08ZZ   0UT0FZZ   0UT10ZZ   0UT14ZZ   0UT17ZZ   0UT18ZZ   0UT1FZZ   0UT20ZZ   0UT24ZZ   0UT27ZZ
     0UT28ZZ   0UT2FZZ   0UT40ZZ   0UT44ZZ   0UT47ZZ   0UT48ZZ   0UT50ZZ   0UT54ZZ   0UT57ZZ   0UT58ZZ   0UT5FZZ   0UT60ZZ   0UT64ZZ
     0UT67ZZ   0UT68ZZ   0UT6FZZ   0UT70ZZ   0UT74ZZ   0UT77ZZ   0UT78ZZ   0UT7FZZ   0UT90ZL   0UT90ZZ   0UT94ZZ   0UT94ZZ   0UT97ZL
     0UT97ZZ   0UT98ZL   0UT98ZZ   0UT9FZL   0UT9FZZ   0UTC0ZZ   0UTC4ZZ   0UTC7ZZ   0UTC8ZZ   0UTF0ZZ   0UTF4ZZ   0UTF7ZZ   0UTF8ZZ
     0UTG0ZZ   0UTG4ZZ   0UTG7ZZ   0UTG8ZZ   0UTJ0ZZ   0UTJXZZ   0UTK0ZZ   0UTK4ZZ   0UTK7ZZ   0UTK8ZZ   0UTKXZZ   0UTL0ZZ   0UTLXZZ
     0UTM0ZZ   0UTMXZZ

CC   0UT20ZZ   0UT40ZZ   0UT44ZZ   0UT47ZZ   0UT48ZZ   0UT70ZZ   0UT90ZZ   0UT94ZZ   0UT97ZZ   0UT98ZZ   0UT9FZZ   0UTC0ZZ   0UTC4ZZ
     0UTC7ZZ   0UTC8ZZ   0UTG0ZZ   0UTM0ZZ   0UTMXZZ

0   Medical and Surgical
U   Female Reproductive System
U   Supplement: Putting in or on biological or synthetic material that physically reinforces and/or augments the function of a portion of a body part

Body Part	Approach	Device	Qualifier
Character 4	Character 5	Character 6	Character 7
4 Uterine Supporting Structure ♀	**0** Open **4** Percutaneous Endoscopic	**7** Autologous Tissue Substitute **J** Synthetic Substitute **K** Nonautologous Tissue Substitute	**Z** No Qualifier
5 Fallopian Tube, Right ♀ **6** Fallopian Tube, Left ♀ **7** Fallopian Tubes, Bilateral ♀ **F** Cul-de-sac ♀	**0** Open **4** Percutaneous Endoscopic **7** Via Natural or Artificial Opening **8** Via Natural or Artificial Opening Endoscopic	**7** Autologous Tissue Substitute **J** Synthetic Substitute **K** Nonautologous Tissue Substitute	**Z** No Qualifier

0UU continued on next page

---

0 Medical and Surgical
U Female Reproductive System
U Supplement: Putting in or on biological or synthetic material that physically reinforces and/or augments the function of a portion of a body part

0UU continued from previous page

Body Part	Approach	Device	Qualifier
Character 4	Character 5	Character 6	Character 7
G Vagina ♀ **K** Hymen ♀	**0** Open **4** Percutaneous Endoscopic **7** Via Natural or Artificial Opening **8** Via Natural or Artificial Opening Endoscopic **X** External	**7** Autologous Tissue Substitute **J** Synthetic Substitute **K** Nonautologous Tissue Substitute	**Z** No Qualifier
J Clitoris ♀ **M** Vulva ♀	**0** Open **X** External	**7** Autologous Tissue Substitute **J** Synthetic Substitute **K** Nonautologous Tissue Substitute	**Z** No Qualifier

♀ 0UU407Z 0UU40JZ 0UU40KZ 0UU447Z 0UU44JZ 0UU44KZ 0UU507Z 0UU50JZ 0UU50KZ 0UU547Z 0UU54JZ 0UU54KZ 0UU577Z
0UU57JZ 0UU57KZ 0UU587Z 0UU58JZ 0UU58KZ 0UU607Z 0UU60JZ 0UU60KZ 0UU647Z 0UU64JZ 0UU64KZ 0UU677Z 0UU67JZ
0UU67KZ 0UU687Z 0UU68JZ 0UU68KZ 0UU707Z 0UU70JZ 0UU70KZ 0UU747Z 0UU74JZ 0UU74KZ 0UU777Z 0UU77JZ 0UU77KZ
0UU787Z 0UU78JZ 0UU78KZ 0UUF07Z 0UUF0JZ 0UUF0KZ 0UUF47Z 0UUF4JZ 0UUF4KZ 0UUF77Z 0UUF7JZ 0UUF7KZ 0UUF87Z
0UUF8JZ 0UUF8KZ 0UUG07Z 0UUG0JZ 0UUG0KZ 0UUG47Z 0UUG4JZ 0UUG4KZ 0UUG77Z 0UUG7JZ 0UUG7KZ 0UUG87Z 0UUG8JZ
0UUG8KZ 0UUGX7Z 0UUGXJZ 0UUGXKZ 0UUJ07Z 0UUJ0JZ 0UUJ0KZ 0UUJX7Z 0UUJXJZ 0UUJXKZ 0UUK07Z 0UUK0JZ 0UUK0KZ
0UUK47Z 0UUK4JZ 0UUK4KZ 0UUK77Z 0UUK7JZ 0UUK7KZ 0UUK87Z 0UUK8JZ 0UUK8KZ 0UUKX7Z 0UUKXJZ 0UUKXKZ 0UUM07Z
0UUM0JZ 0UUM0KZ 0UUMX7Z 0UUMXJZ 0UUMXKZ

0 Medical and Surgical
U Female Reproductive System
V Restriction: Partially closing an orifice or the lumen of a tubular body part

Body Part	Approach	Device	Qualifier
Character 4	Character 5	Character 6	Character 7
C Cervix ♀	**0** Open **3** Percutaneous **4** Percutaneous Endoscopic	**C** Extraluminal Device **D** Intraluminal Device **Z** No Device	**Z** No Qualifier
C Cervix ♀	**7** Via Natural or Artificial Opening **8** Via Natural or Artificial Opening Endoscopic	**D** Intraluminal Device **Z** No Device	**Z** No Qualifier

♀ 0UVC0CZ 0UVC0DZ 0UVC0ZZ 0UVC3CZ 0UVC3DZ 0UVC3ZZ 0UVC4CZ 0UVC4DZ 0UVC4ZZ 0UVC7DZ 0UVC7ZZ 0UVC8DZ 0UVC8ZZ

0 Medical and Surgical
U Female Reproductive System
W Revision: Correcting, to the extent possible, a portion of a malfunctioning device or the position of a displaced device

Body Part	Approach	Device	Qualifier
Character 4	Character 5	Character 6	Character 7
3 Ovary ♀	**0** Open **3** Percutaneous **4** Percutaneous Endoscopic	**0** Drainage Device **3** Infusion Device **Y** Other Device	**Z** No Qualifier
3 Ovary ♀	**7** Via Natural or Artificial Opening **8** Via Natural or Artificial Opening Endoscopic	**Y** Other Device	**Z** No Qualifier
3 Ovary ♀	**X** External	**0** Drainage Device **3** Infusion Device	**Z** No Qualifier
8 Fallopian Tube ♀	**0** Open **3** Percutaneous **4** Percutaneous Endoscopic **7** Via Natural or Artificial Opening **8** Via Natural or Artificial Opening Endoscopic	**0** Drainage Device **3** Infusion Device **7** Autologous Tissue Substitute **C** Extraluminal Device **D** Intraluminal Device **J** Synthetic Substitute **K** Nonautologous Tissue Substitute **Y** Other Device	**Z** No Qualifier

0UW continued on next page

LC Limited Coverage NC Noncovered HAC HAC-associated Procedure CC Combination Cluster - See Appendix G for code lists
DRG Non-OR-Affecting MS-DRG Assignment New/Revised Text in Orange ♂ Male ♀ Female

544

2021 ICD-10-PCS

0 **Medical and Surgical**
U **Female Reproductive System**
W **Revision:** Correcting, to the extent possible, a portion of a malfunctioning device or the position of a displaced device

0UW continued from previous page

Body Part	Approach	Device	Qualifier
Character 4	Character 5	Character 6	Character 7
8 Fallopian Tube ♀	**X** External	**0** Drainage Device **3** Infusion Device **7** Autologous Tissue Substitute **C** Extraluminal Device **D** Intraluminal Device **J** Synthetic Substitute **K** Nonautologous Tissue Substitute	**Z** No Qualifier
D Uterus and Cervix ♀	**0** Open **3** Percutaneous **4** Percutaneous Endoscopic **7** Via Natural or Artificial Opening **8** Via Natural or Artificial Opening Endoscopic	**0** Drainage Device **1** Radioactive Element **3** Infusion Device **7** Autologous Tissue Substitute **C** Extraluminal Device **D** Intraluminal Device **H** Contraceptive Device **J** Synthetic Substitute **K** Nonautologous Tissue Substitute **Y** Other Device	**Z** No Qualifier
D Uterus and Cervix ♀	**X** External	**0** Drainage Device **3** Infusion Device **7** Autologous Tissue Substitute **C** Extraluminal Device **D** Intraluminal Device **H** Contraceptive Device **J** Synthetic Substitute **K** Nonautologous Tissue Substitute	**Z** No Qualifier
H Vagina and Cul-de-sac ♀	**0** Open **3** Percutaneous **4** Percutaneous Endoscopic **7** Via Natural or Artificial Opening **8** Via Natural or Artificial Opening Endoscopic	**0** Drainage Device **1** Radioactive Element **3** Infusion Device **7** Autologous Tissue Substitute **D** Intraluminal Device **J** Synthetic Substitute **K** Nonautologous Tissue Substitute **Y** Other Device	**Z** No Qualifier
H Vagina and Cul-de-sac ♀	**X** External	**0** Drainage Device **3** Infusion Device **7** Autologous Tissue Substitute **D** Intraluminal Device **J** Synthetic Substitute **K** Nonautologous Tissue Substitute	**Z** No Qualifier
M Vulva ♀	**0** Open **X** External	**0** Drainage Device **7** Autologous Tissue Substitute **J** Synthetic Substitute **K** Nonautologous Tissue Substitute	**Z** No Qualifier

♀ 0UW300Z 0UW303Z 0UW30YZ 0UW330Z 0UW333Z 0UW33YZ 0UW340Z 0UW343Z 0UW34YZ 0UW37YZ 0UW38YZ 0UW3X0Z 0UW3X3Z
0UW800Z 0UW803Z 0UW807Z 0UW80CZ 0UW80DZ 0UW80JZ 0UW80KZ 0UW80YZ 0UW830Z 0UW833Z 0UW837Z 0UW83CZ 0UW83DZ
0UW83JZ 0UW83KZ 0UW83YZ 0UW840Z 0UW843Z 0UW847Z 0UW84CZ 0UW84DZ 0UW84JZ 0UW84KZ 0UW84YZ 0UW870Z 0UW873Z
0UW877Z 0UW87CZ 0UW87DZ 0UW87JZ 0UW87KZ 0UW87YZ 0UW880Z 0UW883Z 0UW887Z 0UW88CZ 0UW88DZ 0UW88JZ 0UW88KZ
0UW88YZ 0UW8X0Z 0UW8X3Z 0UW8X7Z 0UW8XCZ 0UW8XDZ 0UW8XJZ 0UW8XKZ 0UWD00Z 0UWD01Z 0UWD03Z 0UWD07Z 0UWD0CZ
0UWD0DZ 0UWD0HZ 0UWD0JZ 0UWD0KZ 0UWD0YZ 0UWD30Z 0UWD31Z 0UWD33Z 0UWD37Z 0UWD3CZ 0UWD3DZ 0UWD3HZ 0UWD3JZ
0UWD3KZ 0UWD3YZ 0UWD40Z 0UWD41Z 0UWD43Z 0UWD47Z 0UWD4CZ 0UWD4DZ 0UWD4HZ 0UWD4JZ 0UWD4KZ 0UWD4YZ 0UWD70Z
0UWD71Z 0UWD73Z 0UWD77Z 0UWD7CZ 0UWD7DZ 0UWD7HZ 0UWD7JZ 0UWD7KZ 0UWD7YZ 0UWD80Z 0UWD81Z 0UWD83Z 0UWD87Z
0UWD8CZ 0UWD8DZ 0UWD8HZ 0UWD8JZ 0UWD8KZ 0UWD8YZ 0UWDX0Z 0UWDX3Z 0UWDX7Z 0UWDXCZ 0UWDXDZ 0UWDXHZ 0UWDXJZ
0UWDXKZ 0UWH00Z 0UWH01Z 0UWH03Z 0UWH07Z 0UWH0DZ 0UWH0JZ 0UWH0KZ 0UWH0YZ 0UWH30Z 0UWH31Z 0UWH33Z 0UWH37Z
0UWH3DZ 0UWH3JZ 0UWH3KZ 0UWH3YZ 0UWH40Z 0UWH41Z 0UWH43Z 0UWH47Z 0UWH4DZ 0UWH4JZ 0UWH4KZ 0UWH4YZ 0UWH70Z
0UWH71Z 0UWH73Z 0UWH77Z 0UWH7DZ 0UWH7JZ 0UWH7KZ 0UWH7YZ 0UWH80Z 0UWH81Z 0UWH83Z 0UWH87Z 0UWH8DZ 0UWH8JZ
0UWH8KZ 0UWH8YZ 0UWHX0Z 0UWHX3Z 0UWHX7Z 0UWHXDZ 0UWHXJZ 0UWHXKZ 0UWM00Z 0UWM07Z 0UWM0JZ 0UWM0KZ 0UWMX0Z
0UWMX7Z 0UWMXJZ 0UWMXKZ

0 **Medical and Surgical**
U **Female Reproductive System**
Y **Transplantation:** Putting in or on all or a portion of a living body part taken from another individual or animal to physically take the place and/or function of all or a portion of a similar body part

Body Part	Approach	Device	Qualifier
Character 4	Character 5	Character 6	Character 7
0 Ovary, Right ♀	**0** Open	**Z** No Device	**0** Allogeneic
1 Ovary, Left ♀			**1** Syngeneic
9 Uterus ♀			**2** Zooplastic

♀   0UY00Z0   0UY00Z1   0UY00Z2   0UY10Z0   0UY10Z1   0UY10Z2   0UY90Z0   0UY90Z1   0UY90Z2

LC Limited Coverage   **NC** Noncovered   **HAC** HAC-associated Procedure   **CC** Combination Cluster - See Appendix G for code lists
⊕ Non-OR-Affecting MS-DRG Assignment   New/Revised Text in **Orange**   ♂ Male   ♀ Female

546

2021 ICD-10-PCS

NOTES

NOTES

Male Reproductive System 0V1-0VY

0 Medical and Surgical
V Male Reproductive System
1 **Bypass:** Altering the route of passage of the contents of a tubular body part

Body Part	Approach	Device	Qualifier
Character 4	Character 5	Character 6	Character 7
N Vas Deferens, Right ♂ **P** Vas Deferens, Left ♂ **Q** Vas Deferens, Bilateral ♂	**0** Open **4** Percutaneous Endoscopic	**7** Autologous Tissue Substitute **J** Synthetic Substitute **K** Nonautologous Tissue Substitute **Z** No Device	**J** Epididymis, Right **K** Epididymis, Left **N** Vas Deferens, Right **P** Vas Deferens, Left

♂   0V1N07J   0V1N07K   0V1N07N   0V1N07P   0V1N0JJ   0V1N0JK   0V1N0JN   0V1N0JP   0V1N0KJ   0V1N0KK   0V1N0KN   0V1N0KP   0V1N0ZJ
0V1N0ZK   0V1N0ZN   0V1N0ZP   0V1N47J   0V1N47K   0V1N47N   0V1N47P   0V1N4JJ   0V1N4JK   0V1N4JN   0V1N4JP   0V1N4KJ   0V1N4KK
0V1N4KN   0V1N4KP   0V1N4ZJ   0V1N4ZK   0V1N4ZN   0V1N4ZP   0V1P07J   0V1P07K   0V1P07N   0V1P07P   0V1P0JJ   0V1P0JK   0V1P0JN
0V1P0JP   0V1P0KJ   0V1P0KK   0V1P0KN   0V1P0KP   0V1P0ZJ   0V1P0ZK   0V1P0ZN   0V1P0ZP   0V1P47J   0V1P47K   0V1P47N   0V1P47P
0V1P4JJ   0V1P4JK   0V1P4JN   0V1P4JP   0V1P4KJ   0V1P4KK   0V1P4KN   0V1P4KP   0V1P4ZJ   0V1P4ZK   0V1P4ZN   0V1P4ZP   0V1Q07J
0V1Q07K   0V1Q07N   0V1Q07P   0V1Q0JJ   0V1Q0JK   0V1Q0JN   0V1Q0JP   0V1Q0KJ   0V1Q0KK   0V1Q0KN   0V1Q0KP   0V1Q0ZJ   0V1Q0ZK
0V1Q0ZN   0V1Q0ZP   0V1Q47J   0V1Q47K   0V1Q47N   0V1Q47P   0V1Q4JJ   0V1Q4JK   0V1Q4JN   0V1Q4JP   0V1Q4KJ   0V1Q4KK   0V1Q4KN
0V1Q4KP   0V1Q4ZJ   0V1Q4ZK   0V1Q4ZN   0V1Q4ZP

0 Medical and Surgical
V Male Reproductive System
2 **Change:** Taking out or off a device from a body part and putting back an identical or similar device in or on the same body part without cutting or puncturing the skin or a mucous membrane

Body Part	Approach	Device	Qualifier
Character 4	Character 5	Character 6	Character 7
4 Prostate and Seminal Vesicles ♂ **8** Scrotum and Tunica Vaginalis ♂ **D** Testis ♂ **M** Epididymis and Spermatic Cord ♂ **R** Vas Deferens ♂ **S** Penis ♂	**X** External	**0** Drainage Device **Y** Other Device	**Z** No Qualifier

♂   0V24X0Z   0V24XYZ   0V28X0Z   0V28XYZ   0V2DX0Z   0V2DXYZ   0V2MX0Z   0V2MXYZ   0V2RX0Z   0V2RXYZ   0V2SX0Z   0V2SXYZ

0 Medical and Surgical
V Male Reproductive System
5 Destruction: Physical eradication of all or a portion of a body part by the direct use of energy, force, or a destructive agent

Body Part	Approach	Device	Qualifier
Character 4	Character 5	Character 6	Character 7
0 Prostate ♂	**0** Open **3** Percutaneous **4** Percutaneous Endoscopic **7** Via Natural or Artificial Opening **8** Via Natural or Artificial Opening Endoscopic	**Z** No Device	**Z** No Qualifier
1 Seminal Vesicle, Right ♂ **2** Seminal Vesicle, Left ♂ **3** Seminal Vesicles, Bilateral ♂ **6** Tunica Vaginalis, Right ♂ **7** Tunica Vaginalis, Left ♂ **9** Testis, Right ♂ **B** Testis, Left ♂ **C** Testes, Bilateral ♂	**0** Open **3** Percutaneous **4** Percutaneous Endoscopic	**Z** No Device	**Z** No Qualifier
5 Scrotum ♂ **S** Penis ♂ **T** Prepuce ♂	**0** Open **3** Percutaneous **4** Percutaneous Endoscopic **X** External	**Z** No Device	**Z** No Qualifier
F Spermatic Cord, Right ♂ **G** Spermatic Cord, Left ♂ **H** Spermatic Cords, Bilateral ♂ **J** Epididymis, Right ♂ **K** Epididymis, Left ♂ **L** Epididymis, Bilateral ♂ **N** Vas Deferens, Right ♂ NC **P** Vas Deferens, Left ♂ NC **Q** Vas Deferens, Bilateral ♂ NC	**0** Open **3** Percutaneous **4** Percutaneous Endoscopic **8** Via Natural or Artificial Opening Endoscopic	**Z** No Device	**Z** No Qualifier

♂   0V500ZZ   0V503ZZ   0V504ZZ   0V507ZZ   0V508ZZ   0V510ZZ   0V513ZZ   0V514ZZ   0V520ZZ   0V523ZZ   0V524ZZ   0V530ZZ   0V533ZZ
    0V534ZZ   0V550ZZ   0V553ZZ   0V554ZZ   0V55XZZ   0V560ZZ   0V563ZZ   0V564ZZ   0V570ZZ   0V573ZZ   0V574ZZ   0V590ZZ   0V593ZZ
    0V594ZZ   0V5B0ZZ   0V5B3ZZ   0V5B4ZZ   0V5C0ZZ   0V5C3ZZ   0V5C4ZZ   0V5F0ZZ   0V5F3ZZ   0V5F4ZZ   0V5F8ZZ   0V5G0ZZ   0V5G3ZZ
    0V5G4ZZ   0V5G8ZZ   0V5H0ZZ   0V5H3ZZ   0V5H4ZZ   0V5H8ZZ   0V5J0ZZ   0V5J3ZZ   0V5J4ZZ   0V5J8ZZ   0V5K0ZZ   0V5K3ZZ   0V5K4ZZ
    0V5K8ZZ   0V5L0ZZ   0V5L3ZZ   0V5L4ZZ   0V5L8ZZ   0V5N0ZZ   0V5N3ZZ   0V5N4ZZ   0V5N8ZZ   0V5P0ZZ   0V5P3ZZ   0V5P4ZZ   0V5P8ZZ
    0V5Q0ZZ   0V5Q3ZZ   0V5Q4ZZ   0V5Q8ZZ   0V5S0ZZ   0V5S3ZZ   0V5S4ZZ   0V5SXZZ   0V5T0ZZ   0V5T3ZZ   0V5T4ZZ   0V5TXZZ
NC   0V5N0ZZ   0V5N3ZZ   0V5N4ZZ   0V5P0ZZ   0V5P3ZZ   0V5P4ZZ   0V5Q0ZZ   0V5Q3ZZ   0V5Q4ZZ
    Codes in this list are noncovered procedures only when reported with Z30.2 as either a principal or secondary diagnosis.

0 Medical and Surgical
V Male Reproductive System
7 Dilation: Expanding an orifice or the lumen of a tubular body part

Body Part	Approach	Device	Qualifier
Character 4	Character 5	Character 6	Character 7
N Vas Deferens, Right ♂ **P** Vas Deferens, Left ♂ **Q** Vas Deferens, Bilateral ♂	**0** Open **3** Percutaneous **4** Percutaneous Endoscopic	**D** Intraluminal Device **Z** No Device	**Z** No Qualifier

♂   0V7N0DZ   0V7N0ZZ   0V7N3DZ   0V7N3ZZ   0V7N4DZ   0V7N4ZZ   0V7P0DZ   0V7P0ZZ   0V7P3DZ   0V7P3ZZ   0V7P4DZ   0V7P4ZZ   0V7Q0DZ
    0V7Q0ZZ   0V7Q3DZ   0V7Q3ZZ   0V7Q4DZ   0V7Q4ZZ

LC Limited Coverage   NC Noncovered   HAC HAC-associated Procedure   CC Combination Cluster - See Appendix G for code lists
DRG Non-OR-Affecting MS-DRG Assignment   New/Revised Text in **Orange**   ♂ Male   ♀ Female

550   2021 ICD-10-PCS

0 Medical and Surgical
V Male Reproductive System
9 Drainage: Taking or letting out fluids and/or gases from a body part

Body Part	Approach	Device	Qualifier
Character 4	**Character 5**	**Character 6**	**Character 7**
0 Prostate ♂	**0** Open **3** Percutaneous **4** Percutaneous Endoscopic **7** Via Natural or Artificial Opening **8** Via Natural or Artificial Opening Endoscopic	**0** Drainage Device	**Z** No Qualifier
0 Prostate ♂	**0** Open **3** Percutaneous **4** Percutaneous Endoscopic **7** Via Natural or Artificial Opening **8** Via Natural or Artificial Opening Endoscopic	**Z** No Device	**X** Diagnostic **Z** No Qualifier
1 Seminal Vesicle, Right ♂ **2** Seminal Vesicle, Left ♂ **3** Seminal Vesicles, Bilateral ♂ **6** Tunica Vaginalis, Right ♂ **7** Tunica Vaginalis, Left ♂ **9** Testis, Right ♂ **B** Testis, Left ♂ **C** Testes, Bilateral ♂ **F** Spermatic Cord, Right ♂ **G** Spermatic Cord, Left ♂ **H** Spermatic Cords, Bilateral ♂ **J** Epididymis, Right ♂ **K** Epididymis, Left ♂ **L** Epididymis, Bilateral ♂ **N** Vas Deferens, Right ♂ **P** Vas Deferens, Left ♂ **Q** Vas Deferens, Bilateral ♂	**0** Open **3** Percutaneous **4** Percutaneous Endoscopic	**0** Drainage Device	**Z** No Qualifier
1 Seminal Vesicle, Right ♂ **2** Seminal Vesicle, Left ♂ **3** Seminal Vesicles, Bilateral ♂ **6** Tunica Vaginalis, Right ♂ **7** Tunica Vaginalis, Left ♂ **9** Testis, Right ♂ **B** Testis, Left ♂ **C** Testes, Bilateral ♂ **F** Spermatic Cord, Right ♂ **G** Spermatic Cord, Left ♂ **H** Spermatic Cords, Bilateral ♂ **J** Epididymis, Right ♂ **K** Epididymis, Left ♂ **L** Epididymis, Bilateral ♂ **N** Vas Deferens, Right ♂ **P** Vas Deferens, Left ♂ **Q** Vas Deferens, Bilateral ♂	**0** Open **3** Percutaneous **4** Percutaneous Endoscopic	**Z** No Device	**X** Diagnostic **Z** No Qualifier
5 Scrotum ♂ **S** Penis ♂ **T** Prepuce ♂	**0** Open **3** Percutaneous **4** Percutaneous Endoscopic **X** External	**0** Drainage Device	**Z** No Qualifier
5 Scrotum ♂ **S** Penis ♂ **T** Prepuce ♂	**0** Open **3** Percutaneous **4** Percutaneous Endoscopic **X** External	**Z** No Device	**X** Diagnostic **Z** No Qualifier

♂ 0V9000Z 0V900ZX 0V900ZZ 0V9030Z 0V903ZX 0V903ZZ 0V9040Z 0V904ZX 0V904ZZ 0V9070Z 0V907ZX 0V907ZZ 0V9080Z
0V908ZX 0V908ZZ 0V9100Z 0V910ZX 0V910ZZ 0V9130Z 0V913ZX 0V913ZZ 0V9140Z 0V914ZX 0V914ZZ 0V9200Z 0V920ZX
0V920ZZ 0V9230Z 0V923ZX 0V923ZZ 0V9240Z 0V924ZX 0V924ZZ 0V9300Z 0V930ZX 0V930ZZ 0V9330Z 0V933ZX 0V933ZZ
0V9340Z 0V934ZX 0V934ZZ 0V9500Z 0V950ZX 0V950ZZ 0V9530Z 0V953ZX 0V953ZZ 0V9540Z 0V954ZX 0V954ZZ 0V95X0Z

0V9 continued on next page

LC Limited Coverage **NC** Noncovered **HAC** HAC-associated Procedure **CC** Combination Cluster - See Appendix G for code lists
Non-OR-Affecting MS-DRG Assignment New/Revised Text in **Orange** ♂ Male ♀ Female

0V9 continued from previous page

0V95XZX	0V95XZZ	0V9600Z	0V960ZX	0V960ZZ	0V9630Z	0V963ZX	0V963ZZ	0V9640Z	0V964ZX	0V964ZZ	0V9700Z	0V970ZX
0V970ZZ	0V9730Z	0V973ZX	0V973ZZ	0V9740Z	0V974ZX	0V974ZZ	0V9900Z	0V990ZX	0V990ZZ	0V9930Z	0V993ZX	0V993ZZ
0V9940Z	0V994ZX	0V994ZZ	0V9B00Z	0V9B0ZX	0V9B0ZZ	0V9B30Z	0V9B3ZX	0V9B3ZZ	0V9B40Z	0V9B4ZX	0V9B4ZZ	0V9C00Z
0V9C0ZX	0V9C0ZZ	0V9C30Z	0V9C3ZX	0V9C3ZZ	0V9C40Z	0V9C4ZX	0V9C4ZZ	0V9F00Z	0V9F0ZX	0V9F0ZZ	0V9F30Z	0V9F3ZX
0V9F3ZZ	0V9F40Z	0V9F4ZX	0V9F4ZZ	0V9G00Z	0V9G0ZX	0V9G0ZZ	0V9G30Z	0V9G3ZX	0V9G3ZZ	0V9G40Z	0V9G4ZX	0V9G4ZZ
0V9H00Z	0V9H0ZX	0V9H0ZZ	0V9H30Z	0V9H3ZX	0V9H3ZZ	0V9H40Z	0V9H4ZX	0V9H4ZZ	0V9J00Z	0V9J0ZX	0V9J0ZZ	0V9J30Z
0V9J3ZX	0V9J3ZZ	0V9J40Z	0V9J4ZX	0V9J4ZZ	0V9K00Z	0V9K0ZX	0V9K0ZZ	0V9K30Z	0V9K3ZX	0V9K3ZZ	0V9K40Z	0V9K4ZX
0V9K4ZZ	0V9L00Z	0V9L0ZX	0V9L0ZZ	0V9L30Z	0V9L3ZX	0V9L3ZZ	0V9L40Z	0V9L4ZX	0V9L4ZZ	0V9N00Z	0V9N0ZX	0V9N0ZZ
0V9N30Z	0V9N3ZX	0V9N3ZZ	0V9N40Z	0V9N4ZX	0V9N4ZZ	0V9P00Z	0V9P0ZX	0V9P0ZZ	0V9P30Z	0V9P3ZX	0V9P3ZZ	0V9P40Z
0V9P4ZX	0V9P4ZZ	0V9Q00Z	0V9Q0ZX	0V9Q0ZZ	0V9Q30Z	0V9Q3ZX	0V9Q3ZZ	0V9Q40Z	0V9Q4ZX	0V9Q4ZZ	0V9S00Z	0V9S0ZX
0V9S0ZZ	0V9S30Z	0V9S3ZX	0V9S3ZZ	0V9S40Z	0V9S4ZX	0V9S4ZZ	0V9SX0Z	0V9SXZX	0V9SXZZ	0V9T00Z	0V9T0ZX	0V9T0ZZ
0V9T30Z	0V9T3ZX	0V9T3ZZ	0V9T40Z	0V9T4ZX	0V9T4ZZ	0V9TX0Z	0V9TXZX	0V9TXZZ				

0 Medical and Surgical
V Male Reproductive System
B Excision: Cutting out or off, without replacement, a portion of a body part

Body Part	Approach	Device	Qualifier
Character 4	Character 5	Character 6	Character 7
0 Prostate ♂	**0** Open **3** Percutaneous **4** Percutaneous Endoscopic **7** Via Natural or Artificial Opening **8** Via Natural or Artificial Opening Endoscopic	**Z** No Device	**X** Diagnostic **Z** No Qualifier
1 Seminal Vesicle, Right ♂ **2** Seminal Vesicle, Left ♂ **3** Seminal Vesicles, Bilateral ♂ **6** Tunica Vaginalis, Right ♂ **7** Tunica Vaginalis, Left ♂ **9** Testis, Right ♂ **B** Testis, Left ♂ **C** Testes, Bilateral ♂	**0** Open **3** Percutaneous **4** Percutaneous Endoscopic	**Z** No Device	**X** Diagnostic **Z** No Qualifier
5 Scrotum ♂ **S** Penis ♂ **T** Prepuce ♂	**0** Open **3** Percutaneous **4** Percutaneous Endoscopic **X** External	**Z** No Device	**X** Diagnostic **Z** No Qualifier
F Spermatic Cord, Right ♂ **G** Spermatic Cord, Left ♂ **H** Spermatic Cords, Bilateral ♂ **J** Epididymis, Right ♂ **K** Epididymis, Left ♂ **L** Epididymis, Bilateral ♂ **N** Vas Deferens, Right ♂ NC **P** Vas Deferens, Left ♂ NC **Q** Vas Deferens, Bilateral ♂ NC	**0** Open **3** Percutaneous **4** Percutaneous Endoscopic **8** Via Natural or Artificial Opening Endoscopic	**Z** No Device	**X** Diagnostic **Z** No Qualifier

♂
0VB00ZX	0VB00ZZ	0VB03ZX	0VB03ZZ	0VB04ZX	0VB04ZZ	0VB07ZX	0VB07ZZ	0VB08ZX	0VB08ZZ	0VB10ZX	0VB10ZZ	0VB13ZX
0VB13ZZ	0VB14ZX	0VB14ZZ	0VB20ZX	0VB20ZZ	0VB23ZX	0VB23ZZ	0VB24ZX	0VB24ZZ	0VB30ZX	0VB30ZZ	0VB33ZX	0VB33ZZ
0VB34ZX	0VB34ZZ	0VB50ZX	0VB50ZZ	0VB53ZX	0VB53ZZ	0VB54ZX	0VB54ZZ	0VB5XZX	0VB5XZZ	0VB60ZX	0VB60ZZ	0VB63ZX
0VB63ZZ	0VB64ZX	0VB64ZZ	0VB70ZX	0VB70ZZ	0VB73ZX	0VB73ZZ	0VB74ZX	0VB74ZZ	0VB90ZX	0VB90ZZ	0VB93ZX	0VB93ZZ
0VB94ZX	0VB94ZZ	0VBB0ZX	0VBB0ZZ	0VBB3ZX	0VBB3ZZ	0VBB4ZX	0VBB4ZZ	0VBC0ZX	0VBC0ZZ	0VBC3ZX	0VBC3ZZ	0VBC4ZX
0VBC4ZZ	0VBF0ZX	0VBF0ZZ	0VBF3ZX	0VBF3ZZ	0VBF4ZX	0VBF4ZZ	0VBF8ZX	0VBF8ZZ	0VBG0ZX	0VBG0ZZ	0VBG3ZX	0VBG3ZZ
0VBG4ZX	0VBG4ZZ	0VBG8ZX	0VBG8ZZ	0VBH0ZX	0VBH0ZZ	0VBH3ZX	0VBH3ZZ	0VBH4ZX	0VBH4ZZ	0VBH8ZX	0VBH8ZZ	0VBJ0ZX
0VBJ0ZZ	0VBJ3ZX	0VBJ3ZZ	0VBJ4ZX	0VBJ4ZZ	0VBJ8ZX	0VBJ8ZZ	0VBK0ZX	0VBK0ZZ	0VBK3ZX	0VBK3ZZ	0VBK4ZX	0VBK4ZZ
0VBK8ZX	0VBK8ZZ	0VBL0ZX	0VBL0ZZ	0VBL3ZX	0VBL3ZZ	0VBL4ZX	0VBL4ZZ	0VBL8ZX	0VBL8ZZ	0VBN0ZX	0VBN0ZZ	0VBN3ZX
0VBN3ZZ	0VBN4ZX	0VBN4ZZ	0VBN8ZX	0VBN8ZZ	0VBP0ZX	0VBP0ZZ	0VBP3ZX	0VBP3ZZ	0VBP4ZX	0VBP4ZZ	0VBP8ZX	0VBP8ZZ
0VBQ0ZX	0VBQ0ZZ	0VBQ3ZX	0VBQ3ZZ	0VBQ4ZX	0VBQ4ZZ	0VBQ8ZX	0VBQ8ZZ	0VBS0ZX	0VBS0ZZ	0VBS3ZX	0VBS3ZZ	0VBS4ZX
0VBS4ZZ	0VBSXZX	0VBSXZZ	0VBT0ZX	0VBT0ZZ	0VBT3ZX	0VBT3ZZ	0VBT4ZX	0VBT4ZZ	0VBTXZX	0VBTXZZ		

NC
0VBN0ZZ	0VBN3ZZ	0VBN4ZZ	0VBP0ZZ	0VBP3ZZ	0VBP4ZZ	0VBQ0ZZ	0VBQ3ZZ	0VBQ4ZZ

Codes in this list are noncovered procedures only when reported with Z30.2 as either a principal or secondary diagnosis.

LC Limited Coverage   NC Noncovered   HAC HAC-associated Procedure   CC Combination Cluster - See Appendix G for code lists
Non-OR-Affecting MS-DRG Assignment   New/Revised Text in **Orange**   ♂ Male   ♀ Female

552

2021 ICD-10-PCS

0   Medical and Surgical
V   Male Reproductive System
C   Extirpation: Taking or cutting out solid matter from a body part

Body Part	Approach	Device	Qualifier
Character 4	Character 5	Character 6	Character 7
0 Prostate ♂	**0** Open **3** Percutaneous **4** Percutaneous Endoscopic **7** Via Natural or Artificial Opening **8** Via Natural or Artificial Opening Endoscopic	**Z** No Device	**Z** No Qualifier
1 Seminal Vesicle, Right ♂ **2** Seminal Vesicle, Left ♂ **3** Seminal Vesicles, Bilateral ♂ **6** Tunica Vaginalis, Right ♂ **7** Tunica Vaginalis, Left ♂ **9** Testis, Right ♂ **B** Testis, Left ♂ **C** Testes, Bilateral ♂ **F** Spermatic Cord, Right ♂ **G** Spermatic Cord, Left ♂ **H** Spermatic Cords, Bilateral ♂ **J** Epididymis, Right ♂ **K** Epididymis, Left ♂ **L** Epididymis, Bilateral ♂ **N** Vas Deferens, Right ♂ **P** Vas Deferens, Left ♂ **Q** Vas Deferens, Bilateral ♂	**0** Open **3** Percutaneous **4** Percutaneous Endoscopic	**Z** No Device	**Z** No Qualifier
5 Scrotum ♂ **S** Penis ♂ **T** Prepuce ♂	**0** Open **3** Percutaneous **4** Percutaneous Endoscopic **X** External	**Z** No Device	**Z** No Qualifier

♂ 0VC00ZZ 0VC03ZZ 0VC04ZZ 0VC07ZZ 0VC08ZZ 0VC10ZZ 0VC13ZZ 0VC14ZZ 0VC20ZZ 0VC23ZZ 0VC24ZZ 0VC30ZZ 0VC33ZZ
   0VC34ZZ 0VC50ZZ 0VC53ZZ 0VC54ZZ 0VC5XZZ 0VC60ZZ 0VC63ZZ 0VC64ZZ 0VC70ZZ 0VC73ZZ 0VC74ZZ 0VC90ZZ 0VC93ZZ
   0VC94ZZ 0VCB0ZZ 0VCB3ZZ 0VCB4ZZ 0VCC0ZZ 0VCC3ZZ 0VCC4ZZ 0VCF0ZZ 0VCF3ZZ 0VCF4ZZ 0VCG0ZZ 0VCG3ZZ 0VCG4ZZ
   0VCH0ZZ 0VCH3ZZ 0VCH4ZZ 0VCJ0ZZ 0VCJ3ZZ 0VCJ4ZZ 0VCK0ZZ 0VCK3ZZ 0VCK4ZZ 0VCL0ZZ 0VCL3ZZ 0VCL4ZZ 0VCN0ZZ
   0VCN3ZZ 0VCN4ZZ 0VCP0ZZ 0VCP3ZZ 0VCP4ZZ 0VCQ0ZZ 0VCQ3ZZ 0VCQ4ZZ 0VCS0ZZ 0VCS3ZZ 0VCS4ZZ 0VCSXZZ 0VCT0ZZ
   0VCT3ZZ 0VCT4ZZ 0VCTXZZ

0   Medical and Surgical
V   Male Reproductive System
H   Insertion: Putting in a nonbiological appliance that monitors, assists, performs, or prevents a physiological function but does not physically take the place of a body part

Body Part	Approach	Device	Qualifier
Character 4	**Character 5**	**Character 6**	**Character 7**
0 Prostate ♂	**0** Open **3** Percutaneous **4** Percutaneous Endoscopic **7** Via Natural or Artificial Opening **8** Via Natural or Artificial Opening Endoscopic	**1** Radioactive Element	**Z** No Qualifier
4 Prostate and Seminal Vesicles ♂ **8** Scrotum and Tunica Vaginalis ♂ **M** Epididymis and Spermatic Cord ♂ **R** Vas Deferens ♂	**0** Open **3** Percutaneous **4** Percutaneous Endoscopic **7** Via Natural or Artificial Opening **8** Via Natural or Artificial Opening Endoscopic	**3** Infusion Device **Y** Other Device	**Z** No Qualifier
D Testis ♂	**0** Open **3** Percutaneous **4** Percutaneous Endoscopic **7** Via Natural or Artificial Opening **8** Via Natural or Artificial Opening Endoscopic	**1** Radioactive Element **3** Infusion Device **Y** Other Device	**Z** No Qualifier
S Penis ♂	**0** Open **3** Percutaneous **4** Percutaneous Endoscopic	**3** Infusion Device **Y** Other Device	**Z** No Qualifier
S Penis ♂	**7** Via Natural or Artificial Opening **8** Via Natural or Artificial Opening Endoscopic	**Y** Other Device	**Z** No Qualifier
S Penis ♂	**X** External	**3** Infusion Device	**Z** No Qualifier

♂ 0VH001Z   0VH031Z   0VH041Z   0VH071Z   0VH081Z   0VH403Z   0VH40YZ   0VH433Z   0VH43YZ   0VH443Z   0VH44YZ   0VH473Z   0VH47YZ
0VH483Z   0VH48YZ   0VH803Z   0VH80YZ   0VH833Z   0VH83YZ   0VH843Z   0VH84YZ   0VH873Z   0VH87YZ   0VH883Z   0VH88YZ   0VHD03Z
0VHD0YZ   0VHD33Z   0VHD3YZ   0VHD43Z   0VHD4YZ   0VHD73Z   0VHD7YZ   0VHD83Z   0VHD8YZ   0VHM03Z   0VHM0YZ   0VHM33Z   0VHM3YZ
0VHM43Z   0VHM4YZ   0VHM73Z   0VHM7YZ   0VHM83Z   0VHM8YZ   0VHR03Z   0VHR0YZ   0VHR33Z   0VHR3YZ   0VHR43Z   0VHR4YZ   0VHR73Z
0VHR7YZ   0VHR83Z   0VHR8YZ   0VHS03Z   0VHS0YZ   0VHS33Z   0VHS3YZ   0VHS43Z   0VHS4YZ   0VHS7YZ   0VHS8YZ   0VHSX3Z

0   Medical and Surgical
V   Male Reproductive System
J   Inspection: Visually and/or manually exploring a body part

Body Part	Approach	Device	Qualifier
Character 4	**Character 5**	**Character 6**	**Character 7**
4 Prostate and Seminal Vesicles ♂ **8** Scrotum and Tunica Vaginalis ♂ **D** Testis ♂ **M** Epididymis and Spermatic Cord ♂ **R** Vas Deferens ♂ **S** Penis ♂	**0** Open **3** Percutaneous **4** Percutaneous Endoscopic **X** External	**Z** No Device	**Z** No Qualifier

♂ 0VJ40ZZ   0VJ43ZZ   0VJ44ZZ   0VJ4XZZ   0VJ80ZZ   0VJ83ZZ   0VJ84ZZ   0VJ8XZZ   0VJD0ZZ   0VJD3ZZ   0VJD4ZZ   0VJDXZZ   0VJM0ZZ
0VJM3ZZ   0VJM4ZZ   0VJMXZZ   0VJR0ZZ   0VJR3ZZ   0VJR4ZZ   0VJRXZZ   0VJS0ZZ   0VJS3ZZ   0VJS4ZZ   0VJSXZZ

LC Limited Coverage   **NC** Noncovered   **HAC** HAC-associated Procedure   **CC** Combination Cluster - See Appendix G for code lists
DRG Non-OR-Affecting MS-DRG Assignment   New/Revised Text in **Orange**   ♂ Male   ♀ Female

554   2021 ICD-10-PCS

0 Medical and Surgical
V Male Reproductive System
L Occlusion: Completely closing an orifice or the lumen of a tubular body part

Body Part			Approach			Device			Qualifier		
Character 4			**Character 5**			**Character 6**			**Character 7**		
F Spermatic Cord, Right ♂ NC			**0** Open			**C** Extraluminal Device			**Z** No Qualifier		
G Spermatic Cord, Left ♂ NC			**3** Percutaneous			**D** Intraluminal Device					
H Spermatic Cords, Bilateral ♂ NC			**4** Percutaneous Endoscopic			**Z** No Device					
N Vas Deferens, Right ♂ NC			**8** Via Natural or Artificial Opening								
P Vas Deferens, Left ♂ NC			Endoscopic								
Q Vas Deferens, Bilateral ♂ NC											

♂
OVLF0CZ	OVLF0DZ	OVLF0ZZ	OVLF3CZ	OVLF3DZ	OVLF3ZZ	OVLF4CZ	OVLF4DZ	OVLF4ZZ	OVLF8CZ	OVLF8DZ	OVLF8ZZ	OVLG0CZ
OVLG0DZ	OVLG0ZZ	OVLG3CZ	OVLG3DZ	OVLG3ZZ	OVLG4CZ	OVLG4DZ	OVLG4ZZ	OVLG8CZ	OVLG8DZ	OVLG8ZZ	OVLH0CZ	OVLH0DZ
OVLH0ZZ	OVLH3CZ	OVLH3DZ	OVLH3ZZ	OVLH4CZ	OVLH4DZ	OVLH4ZZ	OVLH8CZ	OVLH8DZ	OVLH8ZZ	OVLN0CZ	OVLN0DZ	OVLN0ZZ
OVLN3CZ	OVLN3DZ	OVLN3ZZ	OVLN4CZ	OVLN4DZ	OVLN4ZZ	OVLN8CZ	OVLN8DZ	OVLN8ZZ	OVLP0CZ	OVLP0DZ	OVLP0ZZ	OVLP3CZ
OVLP3DZ	OVLP3ZZ	OVLP4CZ	OVLP4DZ	OVLP4ZZ	OVLP8CZ	OVLP8DZ	OVLP8ZZ	OVLQ0CZ	OVLQ0DZ	OVLQ0ZZ	OVLQ3CZ	OVLQ3DZ
OVLQ3ZZ	OVLQ4CZ	OVLQ4DZ	OVLQ4ZZ	OVLQ8CZ	OVLQ8DZ	OVLQ8ZZ						

NC
OVLF0CZ	OVLF0DZ	OVLF0ZZ	OVLF3CZ	OVLF3DZ	OVLF3ZZ	OVLF4CZ	OVLF4DZ	OVLF4ZZ	OVLG0CZ	OVLG0DZ	OVLG0ZZ	OVLG3CZ
OVLG3DZ	OVLG3ZZ	OVLG4CZ	OVLG4DZ	OVLG4ZZ	OVLH0CZ	OVLH0DZ	OVLH0ZZ	OVLH3CZ	OVLH3DZ	OVLH3ZZ	OVLH4CZ	OVLH4DZ
OVLH4ZZ	OVLN0CZ	OVLN0ZZ	OVLN3CZ	OVLN3ZZ	OVLN4CZ	OVLN4ZZ	OVLP0CZ	OVLP0ZZ	OVLP3CZ	OVLP3ZZ	OVLP4CZ	OVLP4ZZ
OVLQ0CZ	OVLQ0ZZ	OVLQ3CZ	OVLQ3ZZ	OVLQ4CZ	OVLQ4ZZ							

Codes in this list are noncovered procedures only when reported with Z30.2 as either a principal or secondary diagnosis.

0 Medical and Surgical
V Male Reproductive System
M Reattachment: Putting back in or on all or a portion of a separated body part to its normal location or other suitable location

Body Part			Approach			Device			Qualifier		
Character 4			**Character 5**			**Character 6**			**Character 7**		
5 Scrotum ♂			**X** External			**Z** No Device			**Z** No Qualifier		
S Penis ♂											
6 Tunica Vaginalis, Right ♂			**0** Open			**Z** No Device			**Z** No Qualifier		
7 Tunica Vaginalis, Left ♂			**4** Percutaneous Endoscopic								
9 Testis, Right ♂											
B Testis, Left ♂											
C Testes, Bilateral ♂											
F Spermatic Cord, Right ♂											
G Spermatic Cord, Left ♂											
H Spermatic Cords, Bilateral ♂											

♂
0VM5XZZ	0VM60ZZ	0VM64ZZ	0VM70ZZ	0VM74ZZ	0VM90ZZ	0VM94ZZ	0VMB0ZZ	0VMB4ZZ	0VMC0ZZ	0VMC4ZZ	0VMF0ZZ	0VMF4ZZ
0VMG0ZZ	0VMG4ZZ	0VMH0ZZ	0VMH4ZZ	0VMSXZZ								

LC Limited Coverage **NC** Noncovered **HAC** HAC-associated Procedure **CC** Combination Cluster - See Appendix G for code lists
DRG Non-OR-Affecting MS-DRG Assignment New/Revised Text in **Orange** ♂ Male ♀ Female

2021 ICD-10-PCS   **555**

0   Medical and Surgical
V   Male Reproductive System
N   Release: Freeing a body part from an abnormal physical constraint by cutting or by the use of force

Body Part			Approach		Device	Qualifier
Character 4			**Character 5**		**Character 6**	**Character 7**
0	Prostate ♂		**0** Open **3** Percutaneous **4** Percutaneous Endoscopic **7** Via Natural or Artificial Opening **8** Via Natural or Artificial Opening Endoscopic		**Z** No Device	**Z** No Qualifier
1 **2** **3** **6** **7** **9** **B** **C**	Seminal Vesicle, Right ♂ Seminal Vesicle, Left ♂ Seminal Vesicles, Bilateral ♂ Tunica Vaginalis, Right ♂ Tunica Vaginalis, Left ♂ Testis, Right ♂ Testis, Left ♂ Testes, Bilateral ♂		**0** Open **3** Percutaneous **4** Percutaneous Endoscopic		**Z** No Device	**Z** No Qualifier
5 **S** **T**	Scrotum ♂ Penis ♂ Prepuce ♂		**0** Open **3** Percutaneous **4** Percutaneous Endoscopic **X** External		**Z** No Device	**Z** No Qualifier
F **G** **H** **J** **K** **L** **N** **P** **Q**	Spermatic Cord, Right ♂ Spermatic Cord, Left ♂ Spermatic Cords, Bilateral ♂ Epididymis, Right ♂ Epididymis, Left ♂ Epididymis, Bilateral ♂ Vas Deferens, Right ♂ Vas Deferens, Left ♂ Vas Deferens, Bilateral ♂		**0** Open **3** Percutaneous **4** Percutaneous Endoscopic **8** Via Natural or Artificial Opening Endoscopic		**Z** No Device	**Z** No Qualifier

♂   0VN00ZZ   0VN03ZZ   0VN04ZZ   0VN07ZZ   0VN08ZZ   0VN10ZZ   0VN13ZZ   0VN14ZZ   0VN20ZZ   0VN23ZZ   0VN24ZZ   0VN30ZZ   0VN33ZZ
    0VN34ZZ   0VN50ZZ   0VN53ZZ   0VN54ZZ   0VN5XZZ   0VN60ZZ   0VN63ZZ   0VN64ZZ   0VN70ZZ   0VN73ZZ   0VN74ZZ   0VN90ZZ   0VN93ZZ
    0VN94ZZ   0VNB0ZZ   0VNB3ZZ   0VNB4ZZ   0VNC0ZZ   0VNC3ZZ   0VNC4ZZ   0VNF0ZZ   0VNF3ZZ   0VNF4ZZ   0VNF8ZZ   0VNG0ZZ   0VNG3ZZ
    0VNG4ZZ   0VNG8ZZ   0VNH0ZZ   0VNH3ZZ   0VNH4ZZ   0VNH8ZZ   0VNJ0ZZ   0VNJ3ZZ   0VNJ4ZZ   0VNJ8ZZ   0VNK0ZZ   0VNK3ZZ   0VNK4ZZ
    0VNK8ZZ   0VNL0ZZ   0VNL3ZZ   0VNL4ZZ   0VNL8ZZ   0VNN0ZZ   0VNN3ZZ   0VNN4ZZ   0VNN8ZZ   0VNP0ZZ   0VNP3ZZ   0VNP4ZZ   0VNP8ZZ
    0VNQ0ZZ   0VNQ3ZZ   0VNQ4ZZ   0VNQ8ZZ   0VNS0ZZ   0VNS3ZZ   0VNS4ZZ   0VNSXZZ   0VNT0ZZ   0VNT3ZZ   0VNT4ZZ   0VNTXZZ

LC Limited Coverage   NC Noncovered   HAC HAC-associated Procedure   CC Combination Cluster - See Appendix G for code lists
DRG Non-OR-Affecting MS-DRG Assignment   New/Revised Text in **Orange**   ♂ Male   ♀ Female

556   **2021 ICD-10-PCS**

0 Medical and Surgical
V Male Reproductive System
P Removal: Taking out or off a device from a body part

Body Part	Approach	Device	Qualifier
Character 4	Character 5	Character 6	Character 7
4 Prostate and Seminal Vesicles ♂	**0** Open **3** Percutaneous **4** Percutaneous Endoscopic **7** Via Natural or Artificial Opening **8** Via Natural or Artificial Opening Endoscopic	**0** Drainage Device **1** Radioactive Element **3** Infusion Device **7** Autologous Tissue Substitute **J** Synthetic Substitute **K** Nonautologous Tissue Substitute **Y** Other Device	**Z** No Qualifier
4 Prostate and Seminal Vesicles ♂	**X** External	**0** Drainage Device **1** Radioactive Element **3** Infusion Device	**Z** No Qualifier
8 Scrotum and Tunica Vaginalis ♂ **D** Testis ♂ **S** Penis ♂	**0** Open **3** Percutaneous **4** Percutaneous Endoscopic **7** Via Natural or Artificial Opening **8** Via Natural or Artificial Opening Endoscopic	**0** Drainage Device **3** Infusion Device **7** Autologous Tissue Substitute **J** Synthetic Substitute **K** Nonautologous Tissue Substitute **Y** Other Device	**Z** No Qualifier
8 Scrotum and Tunica Vaginalis ♂ **D** Testis ♂ **S** Penis ♂	**X** External	**0** Drainage Device **3** Infusion Device	**Z** No Qualifier
M Epididymis and Spermatic Cord ♂	**0** Open **3** Percutaneous **4** Percutaneous Endoscopic **7** Via Natural or Artificial Opening **8** Via Natural or Artificial Opening Endoscopic	**0** Drainage Device **3** Infusion Device **7** Autologous Tissue Substitute **C** Extraluminal Device **J** Synthetic Substitute **K** Nonautologous Tissue Substitute **Y** Other Device	**Z** No Qualifier
M Epididymis and Spermatic Cord ♂	**X** External	**0** Drainage Device **3** Infusion Device	**Z** No Qualifier
R Vas Deferens ♂	**0** Open **3** Percutaneous **4** Percutaneous Endoscopic **7** Via Natural or Artificial Opening **8** Via Natural or Artificial Opening Endoscopic	**0** Drainage Device **3** Infusion Device **7** Autologous Tissue Substitute **C** Extraluminal Device **D** Intraluminal Device **J** Synthetic Substitute **K** Nonautologous Tissue Substitute **Y** Other Device	**Z** No Qualifier
R Vas Deferens ♂	**X** External	**0** Drainage Device **3** Infusion Device **D** Intraluminal Device	**Z** No Qualifier

♂ 0VP400Z 0VP401Z 0VP403Z 0VP407Z 0VP40JZ 0VP40KZ 0VP40YZ 0VP430Z 0VP431Z 0VP433Z 0VP437Z 0VP43JZ 0VP43KZ
0VP43YZ 0VP440Z 0VP441Z 0VP443Z 0VP447Z 0VP44JZ 0VP44KZ 0VP44YZ 0VP470Z 0VP471Z 0VP473Z 0VP477Z 0VP47JZ
0VP47KZ 0VP47YZ 0VP480Z 0VP481Z 0VP483Z 0VP487Z 0VP48JZ 0VP48KZ 0VP48YZ 0VP4X0Z 0VP4X1Z 0VP4X3Z 0VP800Z
0VP803Z 0VP807Z 0VP80JZ 0VP80KZ 0VP80YZ 0VP830Z 0VP833Z 0VP837Z 0VP83JZ 0VP83KZ 0VP83YZ 0VP840Z 0VP843Z
0VP847Z 0VP84JZ 0VP84KZ 0VP84YZ 0VP870Z 0VP873Z 0VP877Z 0VP87JZ 0VP87KZ 0VP87YZ 0VP880Z 0VP883Z 0VP887Z
0VP88JZ 0VP88KZ 0VP88YZ 0VP8X0Z 0VP8X3Z 0VPD00Z 0VPD03Z 0VPD07Z 0VPD0JZ 0VPD0KZ 0VPD0YZ 0VPD30Z 0VPD33Z
0VPD37Z 0VPD3JZ 0VPD3KZ 0VPD3YZ 0VPD40Z 0VPD43Z 0VPD47Z 0VPD4JZ 0VPD4KZ 0VPD4YZ 0VPD70Z 0VPD73Z 0VPD77Z
0VPD7JZ 0VPD7KZ 0VPD7YZ 0VPD80Z 0VPD83Z 0VPD87Z 0VPD8JZ 0VPD8KZ 0VPD8YZ 0VPDX0Z 0VPDX3Z 0VPM00Z 0VPM03Z
0VPM07Z 0VPM0CZ 0VPM0JZ 0VPM0KZ 0VPM0YZ 0VPM30Z 0VPM33Z 0VPM37Z 0VPM3CZ 0VPM3JZ 0VPM3KZ 0VPM3YZ 0VPM40Z
0VPM43Z 0VPM47Z 0VPM4CZ 0VPM4JZ 0VPM4KZ 0VPM4YZ 0VPM70Z 0VPM73Z 0VPM77Z 0VPM7CZ 0VPM7JZ 0VPM7KZ 0VPM7YZ
0VPM80Z 0VPM83Z 0VPM87Z 0VPM8CZ 0VPM8JZ 0VPM8KZ 0VPM8YZ 0VPMX0Z 0VPMX3Z 0VPR00Z 0VPR03Z 0VPR07Z 0VPR0CZ
0VPR0DZ 0VPR0JZ 0VPR0KZ 0VPR0YZ 0VPR30Z 0VPR33Z 0VPR37Z 0VPR3CZ 0VPR3DZ 0VPR3JZ 0VPR3KZ 0VPR3YZ 0VPR40Z
0VPR43Z 0VPR47Z 0VPR4CZ 0VPR4DZ 0VPR4JZ 0VPR4KZ 0VPR4YZ 0VPR70Z 0VPR73Z 0VPR77Z 0VPR7CZ 0VPR7DZ 0VPR7JZ
0VPR7KZ 0VPR7YZ 0VPR80Z 0VPR83Z 0VPR87Z 0VPR8CZ 0VPR8DZ 0VPR8JZ 0VPR8KZ 0VPR8YZ 0VPRX0Z 0VPRX3Z 0VPRXDZ
0VPS00Z 0VPS03Z 0VPS07Z 0VPS0JZ 0VPS0KZ 0VPS0YZ 0VPS30Z 0VPS33Z 0VPS37Z 0VPS3JZ 0VPS3KZ 0VPS3YZ 0VPS40Z
0VPS43Z 0VPS47Z 0VPS4JZ 0VPS4KZ 0VPS4YZ 0VPS70Z 0VPS73Z 0VPS77Z 0VPS7JZ 0VPS7KZ 0VPS7YZ 0VPS80Z 0VPS83Z
0VPS87Z 0VPS8JZ 0VPS8KZ 0VPS8YZ 0VPSX0Z 0VPSX3Z

0   Medical and Surgical
V   Male Reproductive System
Q   Repair: Restoring, to the extent possible, a body part to its normal anatomic structure and function

Body Part	Approach	Device	Qualifier
Character 4	Character 5	Character 6	Character 7
0 Prostate ♂	**0** Open **3** Percutaneous **4** Percutaneous Endoscopic **7** Via Natural or Artificial Opening **8** Via Natural or Artificial Opening Endoscopic	**Z** No Device	**Z** No Qualifier
1 Seminal Vesicle, Right ♂ **2** Seminal Vesicle, Left ♂ **3** Seminal Vesicles, Bilateral ♂ **6** Tunica Vaginalis, Right ♂ **7** Tunica Vaginalis, Left ♂ **9** Testis, Right ♂ **B** Testis, Left ♂ **C** Testes, Bilateral ♂	**0** Open **3** Percutaneous **4** Percutaneous Endoscopic	**Z** No Device	**Z** No Qualifier
5 Scrotum ♂ **S** Penis ♂ **T** Prepuce ♂	**0** Open **3** Percutaneous **4** Percutaneous Endoscopic **X** External	**Z** No Device	**Z** No Qualifier
F Spermatic Cord, Right ♂ **G** Spermatic Cord, Left ♂ **H** Spermatic Cords, Bilateral ♂ **J** Epididymis, Right ♂ **K** Epididymis, Left ♂ **L** Epididymis, Bilateral ♂ **N** Vas Deferens, Right ♂ **P** Vas Deferens, Left ♂ **Q** Vas Deferens, Bilateral ♂	**0** Open **3** Percutaneous **4** Percutaneous Endoscopic **8** Via Natural or Artificial Opening Endoscopic	**Z** No Device	**Z** No Qualifier

♂   0VQ00ZZ   0VQ03ZZ   0VQ04ZZ   0VQ07ZZ   0VQ08ZZ   0VQ10ZZ   0VQ13ZZ   0VQ14ZZ   0VQ20ZZ   0VQ23ZZ   0VQ24ZZ   0VQ30ZZ   0VQ33ZZ
    0VQ34ZZ   0VQ50ZZ   0VQ53ZZ   0VQ54ZZ   0VQ5XZZ   0VQ60ZZ   0VQ63ZZ   0VQ64ZZ   0VQ70ZZ   0VQ73ZZ   0VQ74ZZ   0VQ90ZZ   0VQ93ZZ
    0VQ94ZZ   0VQB0ZZ   0VQB3ZZ   0VQB4ZZ   0VQC0ZZ   0VQC3ZZ   0VQC4ZZ   0VQF0ZZ   0VQF3ZZ   0VQF4ZZ   0VQF8ZZ   0VQG0ZZ   0VQG3ZZ
    0VQG4ZZ   0VQG8ZZ   0VQH0ZZ   0VQH3ZZ   0VQH4ZZ   0VQH8ZZ   0VQJ0ZZ   0VQJ3ZZ   0VQJ4ZZ   0VQJ8ZZ   0VQK0ZZ   0VQK3ZZ   0VQK4ZZ
    0VQK8ZZ   0VQL0ZZ   0VQL3ZZ   0VQL4ZZ   0VQL8ZZ   0VQN0ZZ   0VQN3ZZ   0VQN4ZZ   0VQN8ZZ   0VQP0ZZ   0VQP3ZZ   0VQP4ZZ   0VQP8ZZ
    0VQQ0ZZ   0VQQ3ZZ   0VQQ4ZZ   0VQQ8ZZ   0VQS0ZZ   0VQS3ZZ   0VQS4ZZ   0VQSXZZ   0VQT0ZZ   0VQT3ZZ   0VQT4ZZ   0VQTXZZ

0   Medical and Surgical
V   Male Reproductive System
R   Replacement: Putting in or on biological or synthetic material that physically takes the place and/or function of all or a portion of a body part

Body Part	Approach	Device	Qualifier
Character 4	Character 5	Character 6	Character 7
9 Testis, Right ♂ **B** Testis, Left ♂ **C** Testes, Bilateral ♂	**0** Open	**J** Synthetic Substitute	**Z** No Qualifier

♂   0VR90JZ   0VRB0JZ   0VRC0JZ

LC Limited Coverage   **NC** Noncovered   **HAC** HAC-associated Procedure   **CC** Combination Cluster - See Appendix G for code lists
⊕ Non-OR-Affecting MS-DRG Assignment   New/Revised Text in **Orange**   ♂ Male   ♀ Female

558   **2021 ICD-10-PCS**

0 **Medical and Surgical**
V **Male Reproductive System**
S **Reposition:** Moving to its normal location, or other suitable location, all or a portion of a body part

Body Part	Approach	Device	Qualifier
Character 4	Character 5	Character 6	Character 7
9 Testis, Right ♂ **B** Testis, Left ♂ **C** Testes, Bilateral ♂ **F** Spermatic Cord, Right ♂ **G** Spermatic Cord, Left ♂ **H** Spermatic Cords, Bilateral ♂	**0** Open **3** Percutaneous **4** Percutaneous Endoscopic **8** Via Natural or Artificial Opening Endoscopic	**Z** No Device	**Z** No Qualifier

♂ 0VS90ZZ 0VS93ZZ 0VS94ZZ 0VS98ZZ 0VSB0ZZ 0VSB3ZZ 0VSB4ZZ 0VSB8ZZ 0VSC0ZZ 0VSC3ZZ 0VSC4ZZ 0VSC8ZZ 0VSF0ZZ
0VSF3ZZ 0VSF4ZZ 0VSF8ZZ 0VSG0ZZ 0VSG3ZZ 0VSG4ZZ 0VSG8ZZ 0VSH0ZZ 0VSH3ZZ 0VSH4ZZ 0VSH8ZZ

0 **Medical and Surgical**
V **Male Reproductive System**
T **Resection:** Cutting out or off, without replacement, all of a body part

Body Part	Approach	Device	Qualifier
Character 4	Character 5	Character 6	Character 7
0 Prostate ♂ 🆔	**0** Open **4** Percutaneous Endoscopic **7** Via Natural or Artificial Opening **8** Via Natural or Artificial Opening Endoscopic	**Z** No Device	**Z** No Qualifier
1 Seminal Vesicle, Right ♂ **2** Seminal Vesicle, Left ♂ **3** Seminal Vesicles, Bilateral ♂ 🆔 **6** Tunica Vaginalis, Right ♂ **7** Tunica Vaginalis, Left ♂ **9** Testis, Right ♂ **B** Testis, Left ♂ **C** Testes, Bilateral ♂ **F** Spermatic Cord, Right ♂ **G** Spermatic Cord, Left ♂ **H** Spermatic Cords, Bilateral ♂ **J** Epididymis, Right ♂ **K** Epididymis, Left ♂ **L** Epididymis, Bilateral ♂ **N** Vas Deferens, Right ♂ 🆔 **P** Vas Deferens, Left ♂ 🆔 **Q** Vas Deferens, Bilateral ♂ 🆔	**0** Open **4** Percutaneous Endoscopic	**Z** No Device	**Z** No Qualifier
5 Scrotum ♂ **S** Penis ♂ **T** Prepuce ♂	**0** Open **4** Percutaneous Endoscopic **X** External	**Z** No Device	**Z** No Qualifier

♂ 0VT00ZZ 0VT04ZZ 0VT07ZZ 0VT08ZZ 0VT10ZZ 0VT14ZZ 0VT20ZZ 0VT24ZZ 0VT30ZZ 0VT34ZZ 0VT50ZZ 0VT54ZZ 0VT5XZZ
0VT60ZZ 0VT64ZZ 0VT70ZZ 0VT74ZZ 0VT90ZZ 0VT94ZZ 0VTB0ZZ 0VTB4ZZ 0VTC0ZZ 0VTC4ZZ 0VTF0ZZ 0VTF4ZZ 0VTG0ZZ
0VTG4ZZ 0VTH0ZZ 0VTH4ZZ 0VTJ0ZZ 0VTJ4ZZ 0VTK0ZZ 0VTK4ZZ 0VTL0ZZ 0VTL4ZZ 0VTN0ZZ 0VTN4ZZ 0VTP0ZZ 0VTP4ZZ
0VTQ0ZZ 0VTQ4ZZ 0VTS0ZZ 0VTS4ZZ 0VTSXZZ 0VTT0ZZ 0VTT4ZZ 0VTTXZZ

🆖 0VTN0ZZ 0VTN4ZZ 0VTP0ZZ 0VTP4ZZ 0VTQ0ZZ 0VTQ4ZZ
Codes in this list are noncovered procedures only when reported with Z30.2 as either a principal or secondary diagnosis.
🆔 0VT00ZZ 0VT04ZZ 0VT07ZZ 0VT08ZZ 0VT30ZZ 0VT34ZZ

🆔 Limited Coverage 🆖 Noncovered HAC HAC-associated Procedure 🆔 Combination Cluster - See Appendix G for code lists
DRG Non-OR-Affecting MS-DRG Assignment New/Revised Text in **Orange** ♂ Male ♀ Female

0 **Medical and Surgical**
V **Male Reproductive System**
U **Supplement:** Putting in or on biological or synthetic material that physically reinforces and/or augments the function of a portion of a body part

Body Part		Approach		Device		Qualifier	
Character 4		**Character 5**		**Character 6**		**Character 7**	
1 Seminal Vesicle, Right ♂ 2 Seminal Vesicle, Left ♂ 3 Seminal Vesicles, Bilateral ♂ 6 Tunica Vaginalis, Right ♂ 7 Tunica Vaginalis, Left ♂ F Spermatic Cord, Right ♂ G Spermatic Cord, Left ♂ H Spermatic Cords, Bilateral ♂ J Epididymis, Right ♂ K Epididymis, Left ♂ L Epididymis, Bilateral ♂ N Vas Deferens, Right ♂ P Vas Deferens, Left ♂ Q Vas Deferens, Bilateral ♂		0 Open 4 Percutaneous Endoscopic 8 Via Natural or Artificial Opening Endoscopic		7 Autologous Tissue Substitute J Synthetic Substitute K Nonautologous Tissue Substitute		Z No Qualifier	
5 Scrotum ♂ S Penis ♂ T Prepuce ♂		0 Open 4 Percutaneous Endoscopic X External		7 Autologous Tissue Substitute J Synthetic Substitute K Nonautologous Tissue Substitute		Z No Qualifier	
9 Testis, Right ♂ B Testis, Left ♂ C Testes, Bilateral ♂		0 Open		7 Autologous Tissue Substitute J Synthetic Substitute K Nonautologous Tissue Substitute		Z No Qualifier	

♂ 0VU107Z 0VU10JZ 0VU10KZ 0VU147Z 0VU14JZ 0VU14KZ 0VU187Z 0VU18JZ 0VU18KZ 0VU207Z 0VU20JZ 0VU20KZ 0VU247Z
0VU24JZ 0VU24KZ 0VU287Z 0VU28JZ 0VU28KZ 0VU307Z 0VU30JZ 0VU30KZ 0VU347Z 0VU34JZ 0VU34KZ 0VU387Z 0VU38JZ
0VU38KZ 0VU507Z 0VU50JZ 0VU50KZ 0VU547Z 0VU54JZ 0VU54KZ 0VU5X7Z 0VU5XJZ 0VU5XKZ 0VU607Z 0VU60JZ 0VU60KZ
0VU647Z 0VU64JZ 0VU64KZ 0VU687Z 0VU68JZ 0VU68KZ 0VU707Z 0VU70JZ 0VU70KZ 0VU747Z 0VU74JZ 0VU74KZ 0VU787Z
0VU78JZ 0VU78KZ 0VU907Z 0VU90JZ 0VU90KZ 0VUB07Z 0VUB0JZ 0VUB0KZ 0VUC07Z 0VUC0JZ 0VUC0KZ 0VUF07Z 0VUF0JZ
0VUF0KZ 0VUF47Z 0VUF4JZ 0VUF4KZ 0VUF87Z 0VUF8JZ 0VUF8KZ 0VUG07Z 0VUG0JZ 0VUG0KZ 0VUG47Z 0VUG4JZ 0VUG4KZ
0VUG87Z 0VUG8JZ 0VUG8KZ 0VUH07Z 0VUH0JZ 0VUH0KZ 0VUH47Z 0VUH4JZ 0VUH4KZ 0VUH87Z 0VUH8JZ 0VUH8KZ 0VUJ07Z
0VUJ0JZ 0VUJ0KZ 0VUJ47Z 0VUJ4JZ 0VUJ4KZ 0VUJ87Z 0VUJ8JZ 0VUJ8KZ 0VUK07Z 0VUK0JZ 0VUK0KZ 0VUK47Z 0VUK4JZ
0VUK4KZ 0VUK87Z 0VUK8JZ 0VUK8KZ 0VUL07Z 0VUL0JZ 0VUL0KZ 0VUL47Z 0VUL4JZ 0VUL4KZ 0VUL87Z 0VUL8JZ 0VUL8KZ
0VUN07Z 0VUN0JZ 0VUN0KZ 0VUN47Z 0VUN4JZ 0VUN4KZ 0VUN87Z 0VUN8JZ 0VUN8KZ 0VUP07Z 0VUP0JZ 0VUP0KZ 0VUP47Z
0VUP4JZ 0VUP4KZ 0VUP87Z 0VUP8JZ 0VUP8KZ 0VUQ07Z 0VUQ0JZ 0VUQ0KZ 0VUQ47Z 0VUQ4JZ 0VUQ4KZ 0VUQ87Z 0VUQ8JZ
0VUQ8KZ 0VUS07Z 0VUS0JZ 0VUS0KZ 0VUS47Z 0VUS4JZ 0VUS4KZ 0VUSX7Z 0VUSXJZ 0VUSXKZ 0VUT07Z 0VUT0JZ 0VUT0KZ
0VUT47Z 0VUT4JZ 0VUT4KZ 0VUTX7Z 0VUTXJZ 0VUTXKZ

LC Limited Coverage   **NC** Noncovered   **HAC** HAC-associated Procedure   **CC** Combination Cluster - See Appendix G for code lists
NMR Non-OR-Affecting MS-DRG Assignment   New/Revised Text in **Orange**   ♂ Male   ♀ Female

560

2021 ICD-10-PCS

0 Medical and Surgical
V Male Reproductive System
W Revision: Correcting, to the extent possible, a portion of a malfunctioning device or the position of a displaced device

Body Part	Approach	Device	Qualifier
Character 4	Character 5	Character 6	Character 7
4 Prostate and Seminal Vesicles ♂ 8 Scrotum and Tunica Vaginalis ♂ D Testis ♂ S Penis ♂	0 Open 3 Percutaneous 4 Percutaneous Endoscopic 7 Via Natural or Artificial Opening 8 Via Natural or Artificial Opening Endoscopic	0 Drainage Device 3 Infusion Device 7 Autologous Tissue Substitute J Synthetic Substitute K Nonautologous Tissue Substitute Y Other Device	Z No Qualifier
4 Prostate and Seminal Vesicles ♂ 8 Scrotum and Tunica Vaginalis ♂ D Testis ♂ S Penis ♂	X External	0 Drainage Device 3 Infusion Device 7 Autologous Tissue Substitute J Synthetic Substitute K Nonautologous Tissue Substitute	Z No Qualifier

M Epididymis and Spermatic
   Cord ♂
	0 Open
	3 Percutaneous
	4 Percutaneous Endoscopic
	7 Via Natural or Artificial Opening
	8 Via Natural or Artificial Opening
	   Endoscopic
		0 Drainage Device
		3 Infusion Device
		7 Autologous Tissue Substitute
		C Extraluminal Device
		J Synthetic Substitute
		K Nonautologous Tissue Substitute
		Y Other Device
			Z No Qualifier

M Epididymis and Spermatic Cord ♂	X External	0 Drainage Device 3 Infusion Device 7 Autologous Tissue Substitute C Extraluminal Device J Synthetic Substitute K Nonautologous Tissue Substitute	Z No Qualifier
R Vas Deferens ♂	0 Open 3 Percutaneous 4 Percutaneous Endoscopic 7 Via Natural or Artificial Opening 8 Via Natural or Artificial Opening Endoscopic	0 Drainage Device 3 Infusion Device 7 Autologous Tissue Substitute C Extraluminal Device D Intraluminal Device J Synthetic Substitute K Nonautologous Tissue Substitute Y Other Device	Z No Qualifier
R Vas Deferens ♂	X External	0 Drainage Device 3 Infusion Device 7 Autologous Tissue Substitute C Extraluminal Device D Intraluminal Device J Synthetic Substitute K Nonautologous Tissue Substitute	Z No Qualifier

♂ 0VW400Z 0VW403Z 0VW407Z 0VW40JZ 0VW40KZ 0VW40YZ 0VW430Z 0VW433Z 0VW437Z 0VW43JZ 0VW43KZ 0VW43YZ 0VW440Z
0VW443Z 0VW447Z 0VW44JZ 0VW44KZ 0VW44YZ 0VW470Z 0VW473Z 0VW477Z 0VW47JZ 0VW47KZ 0VW47YZ 0VW480Z 0VW483Z
0VW487Z 0VW48JZ 0VW48KZ 0VW48YZ 0VW4X0Z 0VW4X3Z 0VW4X7Z 0VW4XJZ 0VW4XKZ 0VW800Z 0VW803Z 0VW807Z 0VW80JZ
0VW80KZ 0VW80YZ 0VW830Z 0VW833Z 0VW837Z 0VW83JZ 0VW83KZ 0VW83YZ 0VW840Z 0VW843Z 0VW847Z 0VW84JZ 0VW84KZ
0VW84YZ 0VW870Z 0VW873Z 0VW877Z 0VW87JZ 0VW87KZ 0VW87YZ 0VW880Z 0VW883Z 0VW887Z 0VW88JZ 0VW88KZ 0VW88YZ
0VW8X0Z 0VW8X3Z 0VW8X7Z 0VW8XJZ 0VW8XKZ 0VWD00Z 0VWD03Z 0VWD07Z 0VWD0JZ 0VWD0KZ 0VWD0YZ 0VWD30Z 0VWD33Z
0VWD37Z 0VWD3JZ 0VWD3KZ 0VWD3YZ 0VWD40Z 0VWD43Z 0VWD47Z 0VWD4JZ 0VWD4KZ 0VWD4YZ 0VWD70Z 0VWD73Z 0VWD77Z
0VWD7JZ 0VWD7KZ 0VWD7YZ 0VWD80Z 0VWD83Z 0VWD87Z 0VWD8JZ 0VWD8KZ 0VWD8YZ 0VWDX0Z 0VWDX3Z 0VWDX7Z 0VWDXJZ
0VWDXKZ 0VWM00Z 0VWM03Z 0VWM07Z 0VWM0CZ 0VWM0JZ 0VWM0KZ 0VWM0YZ 0VWM30Z 0VWM33Z 0VWM37Z 0VWM3CZ 0VWM3JZ
0VWM3KZ 0VWM3YZ 0VWM40Z 0VWM43Z 0VWM47Z 0VWM4CZ 0VWM4JZ 0VWM4KZ 0VWM4YZ 0VWM70Z 0VWM73Z 0VWM77Z 0VWM7CZ
0VWM7JZ 0VWM7KZ 0VWM7YZ 0VWM80Z 0VWM83Z 0VWM87Z 0VWM8CZ 0VWM8JZ 0VWM8KZ 0VWM8YZ 0VWMX0Z 0VWMX3Z 0VWMX7Z
0VWMXCZ 0VWMXJZ 0VWMXKZ 0VWR00Z 0VWR03Z 0VWR07Z 0VWR0CZ 0VWR0DZ 0VWR0JZ 0VWR0KZ 0VWR0YZ 0VWR30Z 0VWR33Z
0VWR37Z 0VWR3CZ 0VWR3DZ 0VWR3JZ 0VWR3KZ 0VWR3YZ 0VWR40Z 0VWR43Z 0VWR47Z 0VWR4CZ 0VWR4DZ 0VWR4JZ 0VWR4KZ
0VWR4YZ 0VWR70Z 0VWR73Z 0VWR77Z 0VWR7CZ 0VWR7DZ 0VWR7JZ 0VWR7KZ 0VWR7YZ 0VWR80Z 0VWR83Z 0VWR87Z 0VWR8CZ
0VWR8DZ 0VWR8JZ 0VWR8KZ 0VWR8YZ 0VWRX0Z 0VWRX3Z 0VWRX7Z 0VWRXCZ 0VWRXDZ 0VWRXJZ 0VWRXKZ 0VWS00Z 0VWS03Z
0VWS07Z 0VWS0JZ 0VWS0KZ 0VWS0YZ 0VWS30Z 0VWS33Z 0VWS37Z 0VWS3JZ 0VWS3KZ 0VWS3YZ 0VWS40Z 0VWS43Z 0VWS47Z
0VWS4JZ 0VWS4KZ 0VWS4YZ 0VWS70Z 0VWS73Z 0VWS77Z 0VWS7JZ 0VWS7KZ 0VWS7YZ 0VWS80Z 0VWS83Z 0VWS87Z 0VWS8JZ
0VWS8KZ 0VWS8YZ 0VWSX0Z 0VWSX3Z 0VWSX7Z 0VWSXJZ 0VWSXKZ

LC Limited Coverage   NC Noncovered   HAC HAC-associated Procedure   CC Combination Cluster - See Appendix G for code lists
Non-OR-Affecting MS-DRG Assignment   New/Revised Text in Orange   ♂ Male   ♀ Female

2021 ICD-10-PCS   561

0 Medical and Surgical
V Male Reproductive System
X Transfer: Moving, without taking out, all or a portion of a body part to another location to take over the function of all or a portion of a body part

Body Part	Approach	Device	Qualifier
Character 4	Character 5	Character 6	Character 7
T Prepuce	**0** Open **X** External	**Z** No Device	**D** Urethra **S** Penis

0 Medical and Surgical
V Male Reproductive System
Y Transplantation: Putting in or on all or a portion of a living body part taken from another individual or animal to physically take the place and/or function of all or a portion of a similar body part

Body Part	Approach	Device	Qualifier
Character 4	Character 5	Character 6	Character 7
5 Scrotum **S** Penis	**0** Open	**Z** No Device	**0** Allogeneic **1** Syngeneic **2** Zooplastic

LC Limited Coverage   **NC** Noncovered   **HAC** HAC-associated Procedure   **CC** Combination Cluster - See Appendix G for code lists
Non-OR-Affecting MS-DRG Assignment   New/Revised Text in **Orange**   ♂ Male   ♀ Female

562

2021 ICD-10-PCS

NOTES

NOTES

Anatomical Regions, General 0W0-0WY

0 Medical and Surgical
W Anatomical Regions, General
0 **Alteration:** Modifying the anatomic structure of a body part without affecting the function of the body part

Body Part	Approach	Device	Qualifier
Character 4	Character 5	Character 6	Character 7
0 Head **2** Face **4** Upper Jaw **5** Lower Jaw **6** Neck **8** Chest Wall **F** Abdominal Wall **K** Upper Back **L** Lower Back **M** Perineum, Male ♂ **N** Perineum, Female ♀	**0** Open **3** Percutaneous **4** Percutaneous Endoscopic	**7** Autologous Tissue Substitute **J** Synthetic Substitute **K** Nonautologous Tissue Substitute **Z** No Device	**Z** No Qualifier

♂ 0W0M07Z 0W0M0JZ 0W0M0KZ 0W0M0ZZ 0W0M37Z 0W0M3JZ 0W0M3KZ 0W0M3ZZ 0W0M47Z 0W0M4JZ 0W0M4KZ 0W0M4ZZ
♀ 0W0N07Z 0W0N0JZ 0W0N0KZ 0W0N0ZZ 0W0N37Z 0W0N3JZ 0W0N3KZ 0W0N3ZZ 0W0N47Z 0W0N4JZ 0W0N4KZ 0W0N4ZZ

0 Medical and Surgical
W Anatomical Regions, General
1 **Bypass:** Altering the route of passage of the contents of a tubular body part

Body Part	Approach	Device	Qualifier
Character 4	Character 5	Character 6	Character 7
1 Cranial Cavity	**0** Open	**J** Synthetic Substitute	**9** Pleural Cavity, Right **B** Pleural Cavity, Left **G** Peritoneal Cavity **J** Pelvic Cavity
9 Pleural Cavity, Right **B** Pleural Cavity, Left **J** Pelvic Cavity	**0** Open **3** Percutaneous **4** Percutaneous Endoscopic	**J** Synthetic Substitute	**4** Cutaneous **9** Pleural Cavity, Right **B** Pleural Cavity, Left **G** Peritoneal Cavity **J** Pelvic Cavity **W** Upper Vein **Y** Lower Vein
G Peritoneal Cavity	**0** Open **3** Percutaneous **4** Percutaneous Endoscopic	**J** Synthetic Substitute	**4** Cutaneous **6** Bladder **9** Pleural Cavity, Right **B** Pleural Cavity, Left **G** Peritoneal Cavity **J** Pelvic Cavity **W** Upper Vein **Y** Lower Vein

LC Limited Coverage **NC** Noncovered **HAC** HAC-associated Procedure **CC** Combination Cluster - See Appendix G for code lists
DRG Non-OR-Affecting MS-DRG Assignment New/Revised Text in Orange ♂ Male ♀ Female

2021 ICD-10-PCS 565

0 Medical and Surgical
W Anatomical Regions, General
2 Change: Taking out or off a device from a body part and putting back an identical or similar device in or on the same body part without cutting or puncturing the skin or a mucous membrane

Body Part	Approach	Device	Qualifier
Character 4	Character 5	Character 6	Character 7
0 Head	X External	0 Drainage Device	Z No Qualifier
1 Cranial Cavity		Y Other Device	
2 Face			
4 Upper Jaw			
5 Lower Jaw			
6 Neck			
8 Chest Wall			
9 Pleural Cavity, Right			
B Pleural Cavity, Left			
C Mediastinum			
D Pericardial Cavity			
F Abdominal Wall			
G Peritoneal Cavity			
H Retroperitoneum			
J Pelvic Cavity			
K Upper Back			
L Lower Back			
M Perineum, Male ♂			
N Perineum, Female ♀			

♂ 0W2MX0Z 0W2MXYZ
♀ 0W2NX0Z 0W2NXYZ

0 Medical and Surgical
W Anatomical Regions, General
3 Control: Stopping, or attempting to stop, postprocedural or other acute bleeding

Body Part	Approach	Device	Qualifier
Character 4	Character 5	Character 6	Character 7
0 Head	0 Open	Z No Device	Z No Qualifier
1 Cranial Cavity	3 Percutaneous		
2 Face	4 Percutaneous Endoscopic		
4 Upper Jaw			
5 Lower Jaw			
6 Neck			
8 Chest Wall			
9 Pleural Cavity, Right			
B Pleural Cavity, Left			
C Mediastinum			
D Pericardial Cavity			
F Abdominal Wall			
G Peritoneal Cavity			
H Retroperitoneum			
J Pelvic Cavity			
K Upper Back			
L Lower Back			
M Perineum, Male ♂			
N Perineum, Female ♀			
3 Oral Cavity and Throat	0 Open	Z No Device	Z No Qualifier
	3 Percutaneous		
	4 Percutaneous Endoscopic		
	7 Via Natural or Artificial Opening		
	8 Via Natural or Artificial Opening Endoscopic		
	X External		
P Gastrointestinal Tract	0 Open	Z No Device	Z No Qualifier
Q Respiratory Tract	3 Percutaneous		
R Genitourinary Tract	4 Percutaneous Endoscopic		
	7 Via Natural or Artificial Opening		
	8 Via Natural or Artificial Opening Endoscopic		

♂ 0W3M0ZZ 0W3M3ZZ 0W3M4ZZ
♀ 0W3N0ZZ 0W3N3ZZ 0W3N4ZZ

LC Limited Coverage **NC** Noncovered **HAC** HAC-associated Procedure **CC** Combination Cluster - See Appendix G for code lists
DRG Non-OR-Affecting MS-DRG Assignment New/Revised Text in **Orange** ♂ Male ♀ Female

566

2021 ICD-10-PCS

0 Medical and Surgical
W Anatomical Regions, General
4 Creation: Putting in or on biological or synthetic material to form a new body part that to the extent possible replicates the anatomic structure or function of an absent body part

Body Part	Approach	Device	Qualifier
Character 4	Character 5	Character 6	Character 7
M Perineum, Male ♂	**0** Open	**7** Autologous Tissue Substitute **J** Synthetic Substitute **K** Nonautologous Tissue Substitute	**0** Vagina
N Perineum, Female ♀	**0** Open	**7** Autologous Tissue Substitute **J** Synthetic Substitute **K** Nonautologous Tissue Substitute	**1** Penis

♂ 0W4M070 0W4M0J0 0W4M0K0
♀ 0W4N071 0W4N0J1 0W4N0K1

0 Medical and Surgical
W Anatomical Regions, General
8 Division: Cutting into a body part, without draining fluids and/or gases from the body part, in order to separate or transect a body part

Body Part	Approach	Device	Qualifier
Character 4	Character 5	Character 6	Character 7
N Perineum, Female ♀	**X** External	**Z** No Device	**Z** No Qualifier

♀ 0W8NXZZ

0 Medical and Surgical
W Anatomical Regions, General
9 Drainage: Taking or letting out fluids and/or gases from a body part

Body Part	Approach	Device	Qualifier
Character 4	Character 5	Character 6	Character 7
0 Head **1** Cranial Cavity **2** Face **3** Oral Cavity and Throat **4** Upper Jaw **5** Lower Jaw **6** Neck **8** Chest Wall **9** Pleural Cavity, Right **B** Pleural Cavity, Left **C** Mediastinum **D** Pericardial Cavity **F** Abdominal Wall **G** Peritoneal Cavity **H** Retroperitoneum **K** Upper Back **L** Lower Back **M** Perineum, Male ♂ **N** Perineum, Female ♀	**0** Open **3** Percutaneous **4** Percutaneous Endoscopic	**0** Drainage Device	**Z** No Qualifier

0W9 continued on next page

0W9-0WB

ANATOMICAL REGIONS, GENERAL 0W0-0WY

0 Medical and Surgical
W Anatomical Regions, General
9 Drainage: Taking or letting out fluids and/or gases from a body part

0W9 continued from previous page

Body Part	Approach	Device	Qualifier
Character 4	**Character 5**	**Character 6**	**Character 7**
0 Head 1 Cranial Cavity 2 Face 3 Oral Cavity and Throat 4 Upper Jaw 5 Lower Jaw 6 Neck 8 Chest Wall 9 Pleural Cavity, Right B Pleural Cavity, Left C Mediastinum D Pericardial Cavity F Abdominal Wall G Peritoneal Cavity H Retroperitoneum K Upper Back L Lower Back M Perineum, Male ♂ N Perineum, Female ♀	0 Open 3 Percutaneous 4 Percutaneous Endoscopic	Z No Device	X Diagnostic Z No Qualifier
J Pelvic Cavity	0 Open 3 Percutaneous 4 Percutaneous Endoscopic 7 Via Natural or Artificial Opening 8 Via Natural or Artificial Opening Endoscopic	0 Drainage Device	Z No Qualifier
J Pelvic Cavity	0 Open 3 Percutaneous 4 Percutaneous Endoscopic 7 Via Natural or Artificial Opening 8 Via Natural or Artificial Opening Endoscopic	Z No Device	X Diagnostic Z No Qualifier

♂ 0W9M00Z   0W9M0ZX   0W9M0ZZ   0W9M30Z   0W9M3ZX   0W9M3ZZ   0W9M40Z   0W9M4ZX   0W9M4ZZ
♀ 0W9N00Z   0W9N0ZX   0W9N0ZZ   0W9N30Z   0W9N3ZX   0W9N3ZZ   0W9N40Z   0W9N4ZZ

0 Medical and Surgical
W Anatomical Regions, General
B Excision: Cutting out or off, without replacement, a portion of a body part

Body Part	Approach	Device	Qualifier
Character 4	**Character 5**	**Character 6**	**Character 7**
0 Head 2 Face 3 Oral Cavity and Throat 4 Upper Jaw 5 Lower Jaw 8 Chest Wall K Upper Back L Lower Back M Perineum, Male ♂ N Perineum, Female ♀	0 Open 3 Percutaneous 4 Percutaneous Endoscopic X External	Z No Device	X Diagnostic Z No Qualifier
6 Neck F Abdominal Wall	0 Open 3 Percutaneous 4 Percutaneous Endoscopic	Z No Device	X Diagnostic Z No Qualifier
6 Neck F Abdominal Wall	X External	Z No Device	2 Stoma X Diagnostic Z No Qualifier
C Mediastinum H Retroperitoneum	0 Open 3 Percutaneous 4 Percutaneous Endoscopic	Z No Device	X Diagnostic Z No Qualifier

♂ 0WBM0ZX   0WBM0ZZ   0WBM3ZX   0WBM3ZZ   0WBM4ZX   0WBM4ZZ   0WBMXZX   0WBMXZZ
♀ 0WBN0ZX   0WBN0ZZ   0WBN3ZX   0WBN3ZZ   0WBN4ZX   0WBN4ZZ   0WBNXZX   0WBNXZZ

LC Limited Coverage   NC Noncovered   HAC HAC-associated Procedure   CC Combination Cluster - See Appendix G for code lists
Non-OR-Affecting MS-DRG Assignment   New/Revised Text in **Orange**   ♂ Male   ♀ Female

0 **Medical and Surgical**
W **Anatomical Regions, General**
C **Extirpation:** Taking or cutting out solid matter from a body part

Body Part	Approach	Device	Qualifier
Character 4	Character 5	Character 6	Character 7
1 Cranial Cavity 3 Oral Cavity and Throat 9 Pleural Cavity, Right B Pleural Cavity, Left C Mediastinum D Pericardial Cavity G Peritoneal Cavity H Retroperitoneum J Pelvic Cavity	0 Open 3 Percutaneous 4 Percutaneous Endoscopic X External	Z No Device	Z No Qualifier
4 Upper Jaw 5 Lower Jaw	0 Open 3 Percutaneous 4 Percutaneous Endoscopic	Z No Device	Z No Qualifier
P Gastrointestinal Tract Q Respiratory Tract R Genitourinary Tract	0 Open 3 Percutaneous 4 Percutaneous Endoscopic 7 Via Natural or Artificial Opening 8 Via Natural or Artificial Opening Endoscopic X External	Z No Device	Z No Qualifier

0 **Medical and Surgical**
W **Anatomical Regions, General**
F **Fragmentation:** Breaking solid matter in a body part into pieces

Body Part	Approach	Device	Qualifier
Character 4	Character 5	Character 6	Character 7
1 Cranial Cavity NC 3 Oral Cavity and Throat NC 9 Pleural Cavity, Right NC B Pleural Cavity, Left NC C Mediastinum NC D Pericardial Cavity G Peritoneal Cavity NC J Pelvic Cavity NC	0 Open 3 Percutaneous 4 Percutaneous Endoscopic X External	Z No Device	Z No Qualifier
P Gastrointestinal Tract NC Q Respiratory Tract NC R Genitourinary Tract	0 Open 3 Percutaneous 4 Percutaneous Endoscopic 7 Via Natural or Artificial Opening 8 Via Natural or Artificial Opening Endoscopic X External	Z No Device	Z No Qualifier

NC 0WF1XZZ   0WF3XZZ   0WF9XZZ   0WFBXZZ   0WFCXZZ   0WFGXZZ   0WFJXZZ   0WFPXZZ   0WFQXZZ

LC Limited Coverage   NC Noncovered   HAC HAC-associated Procedure   CC Combination Cluster - See Appendix G for code lists
ORG Non-OR-Affecting MS-DRG Assignment   New/Revised Text in **Orange**   ♂ Male   ♀ Female

2021 ICD-10-PCS 569

0 Medical and Surgical
W Anatomical Regions, General
H Insertion: Putting in a nonbiological appliance that monitors, assists, performs, or prevents a physiological function but does not physically take the place of a body part

Body Part	Approach	Device	Qualifier
Character 4	**Character 5**	**Character 6**	**Character 7**
0 Head ᴰᴿᴳ 1 Cranial Cavity 2 Face ᴰᴿᴳ 3 Oral Cavity and Throat 4 Upper Jaw ᴰᴿᴳ 5 Lower Jaw ᴰᴿᴳ 6 Neck ᴰᴿᴳ 8 Chest Wall 9 Pleural Cavity, Right B Pleural Cavity, Left C Mediastinum D Pericardial Cavity F Abdominal Wall G Peritoneal Cavity H Retroperitoneum J Pelvic Cavity K Upper Back ᴰᴿᴳ L Lower Back ᴰᴿᴳ M Perineum, Male ᴰᴿᴳ N Perineum, Female ♀	0 Open 3 Percutaneous 4 Percutaneous Endoscopic	1 Radioactive Element 3 Infusion Device Y Other Device	Z No Qualifier
P Gastrointestinal Tract Q Respiratory Tract R Genitourinary Tract	0 Open 3 Percutaneous 4 Percutaneous Endoscopic 7 Via Natural or Artificial Opening 8 Via Natural or Artificial Opening Endoscopic	1 Radioactive Element 3 Infusion Device Y Other Device	Z No Qualifier

♀ 0WHN03Z 0WHN0YZ 0WHN33Z 0WHN3YZ 0WHN43Z 0WHN4YZ
ᴰᴿᴳ 0WH003Z 0WH00YZ 0WH033Z 0WH03YZ 0WH043Z 0WH04YZ 0WH203Z 0WH20YZ 0WH233Z 0WH23YZ 0WH243Z 0WH24YZ 0WH403Z
0WH40YZ 0WH433Z 0WH43YZ 0WH443Z 0WH44YZ 0WH503Z 0WH50YZ 0WH533Z 0WH53YZ 0WH543Z 0WH54YZ 0WH603Z 0WH60YZ
0WH633Z 0WH63YZ 0WH643Z 0WH64YZ 0WHK03Z 0WHK0YZ 0WHK33Z 0WHK3YZ 0WHK43Z 0WHK4YZ 0WHL03Z 0WHL0YZ 0WHL33Z
0WHL3YZ 0WHL43Z 0WHL4YZ 0WHM03Z 0WHM0YZ 0WHM33Z 0WHM3YZ 0WHM43Z 0WHM4YZ

0 **Medical and Surgical**
W **Anatomical Regions, General**
J **Inspection:** Visually and/or manually exploring a body part

Body Part	Approach	Device	Qualifier
Character 4	Character 5	Character 6	Character 7
0 Head ᴰᴿᴳ 2 Face ᴰᴿᴳ 3 Oral Cavity and Throat 4 Upper Jaw ᴰᴿᴳ 5 Lower Jaw ᴰᴿᴳ 6 Neck 8 Chest Wall F Abdominal Wall K Upper Back ᴰᴿᴳ L Lower Back ᴰᴿᴳ M Perineum, Male ♂ ᴰᴿᴳ N Perineum, Female ♀	0 Open 3 Percutaneous 4 Percutaneous Endoscopic X External	Z No Device	Z No Qualifier
1 Cranial Cavity 9 Pleural Cavity, Right B Pleural Cavity, Left C Mediastinum D Pericardial Cavity G Peritoneal Cavity H Retroperitoneum J Pelvic Cavity	0 Open 3 Percutaneous 4 Percutaneous Endoscopic	Z No Device	Z No Qualifier
P Gastrointestinal Tract Q Respiratory Tract R Genitourinary Tract	0 Open 3 Percutaneous 4 Percutaneous Endoscopic 7 Via Natural or Artificial Opening 8 Via Natural or Artificial Opening Endoscopic	Z No Device	Z No Qualifier

♂ 0WJM0ZZ 0WJM3ZZ 0WJM4ZZ 0WJMXZZ
♀ 0WJN0ZZ 0WJN3ZZ 0WJN4ZZ 0WJNXZZ
ᴰᴿᴳ 0WJ00ZZ 0WJ20ZZ 0WJ40ZZ 0WJ50ZZ 0WJK0ZZ 0WJL0ZZ 0WJM0ZZ 0WJM4ZZ

0 **Medical and Surgical**
W **Anatomical Regions, General**
M **Reattachment:** Putting back in or on all or a portion of a separated body part to its normal location or other suitable location

Body Part	Approach	Device	Qualifier
Character 4	Character 5	Character 6	Character 7
2 Face 4 Upper Jaw 5 Lower Jaw 6 Neck 8 Chest Wall F Abdominal Wall K Upper Back L Lower Back M Perineum, Male ♂ N Perineum, Female ♀	0 Open	Z No Device	Z No Qualifier

♂ 0WMM0ZZ
♀ 0WMN0ZZ

0 Medical and Surgical
W Anatomical Regions, General
P **Removal:** Taking out or off a device from a body part

Body Part	Approach	Device	Qualifier
Character 4	Character 5	Character 6	Character 7
0 Head **2** Face **4** Upper Jaw **5** Lower Jaw **6** Neck **8** Chest Wall **C** Mediastinum **F** Abdominal Wall **K** Upper Back **L** Lower Back **M** Perineum, Male ♂ **N** Perineum, Female ♀	**0** Open **3** Percutaneous **4** Percutaneous Endoscopic **X** External	**0** Drainage Device **1** Radioactive Element **3** Infusion Device **7** Autologous Tissue Substitute **J** Synthetic Substitute **K** Nonautologous Tissue Substitute **Y** Other Device	**Z** No Qualifier
1 Cranial Cavity **9** Pleural Cavity, Right **B** Pleural Cavity, Left **G** Peritoneal Cavity **J** Pelvic Cavity	**0** Open **3** Percutaneous **4** Percutaneous Endoscopic	**0** Drainage Device **1** Radioactive Element **3** Infusion Device **J** Synthetic Substitute **Y** Other Device	**Z** No Qualifier
1 Cranial Cavity **9** Pleural Cavity, Right **B** Pleural Cavity, Left **G** Peritoneal Cavity **J** Pelvic Cavity	**X** External	**0** Drainage Device **1** Radioactive Element **3** Infusion Device	**Z** No Qualifier
D Pericardial Cavity **H** Retroperitoneum	**0** Open **3** Percutaneous **4** Percutaneous Endoscopic	**0** Drainage Device **1** Radioactive Element **3** Infusion Device **Y** Other Device	**Z** No Qualifier
D Pericardial Cavity **H** Retroperitoneum	**X** External	**0** Drainage Device **1** Radioactive Element **3** Infusion Device	**Z** No Qualifier
P Gastrointestinal Tract **Q** Respiratory Tract **R** Genitourinary Tract	**0** Open **3** Percutaneous **4** Percutaneous Endoscopic **7** Via Natural or Artificial Opening **8** Via Natural or Artificial Opening Endoscopic **X** External	**1** Radioactive Element **3** Infusion Device **Y** Other Device	**Z** No Qualifier

♂ 0WPM00Z 0WPM01Z 0WPM03Z 0WPM07Z 0WPM0JZ 0WPM0KZ 0WPM0YZ 0WPM30Z 0WPM31Z 0WPM33Z 0WPM37Z 0WPM3JZ 0WPM3KZ
0WPM3YZ 0WPM40Z 0WPM41Z 0WPM43Z 0WPM47Z 0WPM4JZ 0WPM4KZ 0WPM4YZ 0WPMX0Z 0WPMX1Z 0WPMX3Z 0WPMX7Z 0WPMXJZ
0WPMXKZ 0WPMXYZ

♀ 0WPN00Z 0WPN01Z 0WPN03Z 0WPN07Z 0WPN0JZ 0WPN0KZ 0WPN0YZ 0WPN30Z 0WPN31Z 0WPN33Z 0WPN37Z 0WPN3JZ 0WPN3KZ
0WPN3YZ 0WPN40Z 0WPN41Z 0WPN43Z 0WPN47Z 0WPN4JZ 0WPN4KZ 0WPN4YZ 0WPNX0Z 0WPNX1Z 0WPNX3Z 0WPNX7Z 0WPNXJZ
0WPNXKZ 0WPNXYZ

LC Limited Coverage **NC** Noncovered **HAC** HAC-associated Procedure **CC** Combination Cluster - See Appendix G for code lists
DRG Non-OR-Affecting MS-DRG Assignment New/Revised Text in **Orange** ♂ Male ♀ Female

572

2021 ICD-10-PCS

0   **Medical and Surgical**
W   **Anatomical Regions, General**
Q   **Repair:** Restoring, to the extent possible, a body part to its normal anatomic structure and function

Body Part	Approach	Device	Qualifier
Character 4	Character 5	Character 6	Character 7
0 Head 2 Face 3 Oral Cavity and Throat 4 Upper Jaw 5 Lower Jaw 8 Chest Wall K Upper Back L Lower Back M Perineum, Male ♂ N Perineum, Female ♀	0 Open 3 Percutaneous 4 Percutaneous Endoscopic X External	Z No Device	Z No Qualifier
6 Neck F Abdominal Wall	0 Open 3 Percutaneous 4 Percutaneous Endoscopic	Z No Device	Z No Qualifier
6 Neck F Abdominal Wall CC	X External	Z No Device	2 Stoma Z No Qualifier
C Mediastinum	0 Open 3 Percutaneous 4 Percutaneous Endoscopic	Z No Device	Z No Qualifier

♂   0WQM0ZZ   0WQM3ZZ   0WQM4ZZ   0WQMXZZ
♀   0WQN0ZZ   0WQN3ZZ   0WQN4ZZ   0WQNXZZ
CC 0WQFXZ2   0WQFXZZ

0   **Medical and Surgical**
W   **Anatomical Regions, General**
U   **Supplement:** Putting in or on biological or synthetic material that physically reinforces and/or augments the function of a portion of a body part

Body Part	Approach	Device	Qualifier
Character 4	Character 5	Character 6	Character 7
0 Head 2 Face 4 Upper Jaw 5 Lower Jaw 6 Neck 8 Chest Wall C Mediastinum F Abdominal Wall K Upper Back L Lower Back M Perineum, Male ♂ N Perineum, Female ♀	0 Open 4 Percutaneous Endoscopic	7 Autologous Tissue Substitute J Synthetic Substitute K Nonautologous Tissue Substitute	Z No Qualifier

♂   0WUM07Z   0WUM0JZ   0WUM0KZ   0WUM47Z   0WUM4JZ   0WUM4KZ
♀   0WUN07Z   0WUN0JZ   0WUN0KZ   0WUN47Z   0WUN4JZ   0WUN4KZ

0 Medical and Surgical
W Anatomical Regions, General
W Revision: Correcting, to the extent possible, a portion of a malfunctioning device or the position of a displaced device

Body Part	Approach	Device	Qualifier
Character 4	**Character 5**	**Character 6**	**Character 7**
0 Head ☻ 2 Face ☻ 4 Upper Jaw ☻ 5 Lower Jaw ☻ 6 Neck ☻ 8 Chest Wall C Mediastinum F Abdominal Wall K Upper Back ☻ L Lower Back ☻ M Perineum, Male ♂ ☻ N Perineum, Female ♀	0 Open 3 Percutaneous 4 Percutaneous Endoscopic X External	0 Drainage Device 1 Radioactive Element 3 Infusion Device 7 Autologous Tissue Substitute J Synthetic Substitute K Nonautologous Tissue Substitute Y Other Device	Z No Qualifier
1 Cranial Cavity 9 Pleural Cavity, Right B Pleural Cavity, Left G Peritoneal Cavity J Pelvic Cavity	0 Open 3 Percutaneous 4 Percutaneous Endoscopic X External	0 Drainage Device 1 Radioactive Element 3 Infusion Device J Synthetic Substitute Y Other Device	Z No Qualifier
D Pericardial Cavity H Retroperitoneum	0 Open 3 Percutaneous 4 Percutaneous Endoscopic X External	0 Drainage Device 1 Radioactive Element 3 Infusion Device Y Other Device	Z No Qualifier
P Gastrointestinal Tract Q Respiratory Tract R Genitourinary Tract	0 Open 3 Percutaneous 4 Percutaneous Endoscopic 7 Via Natural or Artificial Opening 8 Via Natural or Artificial Opening Endoscopic X External	1 Radioactive Element 3 Infusion Device Y Other Device	Z No Qualifier

♂ 0WWM00Z 0WWM01Z 0WWM03Z 0WWM07Z 0WWM0JZ 0WWM0KZ 0WWM0YZ 0WWM30Z 0WWM31Z 0WWM33Z 0WWM37Z 0WWM3JZ 0WWM3KZ
0WWM3YZ 0WWM40Z 0WWM41Z 0WWM43Z 0WWM47Z 0WWM4JZ 0WWM4KZ 0WWM4YZ 0WWMX0Z 0WWMX1Z 0WWMX3Z 0WWMX7Z 0WWMXJZ
0WWMXKZ 0WWMXYZ

♀ 0WWN00Z 0WWN01Z 0WWN03Z 0WWN07Z 0WWN0JZ 0WWN0KZ 0WWN0YZ 0WWN30Z 0WWN31Z 0WWN33Z 0WWN37Z 0WWN3JZ 0WWN3KZ
0WWN3YZ 0WWN40Z 0WWN41Z 0WWN43Z 0WWN47Z 0WWN4JZ 0WWN4KZ 0WWN4YZ 0WWNX0Z 0WWNX1Z 0WWNX3Z 0WWNX7Z 0WWNXJZ
0WWNXKZ 0WWNXYZ

☻ 0WW000Z 0WW001Z 0WW003Z 0WW007Z 0WW00JZ 0WW00KZ 0WW00YZ 0WW030Z 0WW031Z 0WW033Z 0WW037Z 0WW03JZ 0WW03KZ
0WW03YZ 0WW040Z 0WW041Z 0WW043Z 0WW047Z 0WW04JZ 0WW04KZ 0WW04YZ 0WW200Z 0WW201Z 0WW203Z 0WW207Z 0WW20JZ
0WW20KZ 0WW20YZ 0WW230Z 0WW231Z 0WW233Z 0WW237Z 0WW23JZ 0WW23KZ 0WW23YZ 0WW240Z 0WW241Z 0WW243Z 0WW247Z
0WW24JZ 0WW24KZ 0WW24YZ 0WW400Z 0WW401Z 0WW403Z 0WW407Z 0WW40JZ 0WW40KZ 0WW40YZ 0WW430Z 0WW431Z 0WW433Z
0WW437Z 0WW43JZ 0WW43KZ 0WW43YZ 0WW440Z 0WW441Z 0WW443Z 0WW447Z 0WW44JZ 0WW44KZ 0WW500Z 0WW501Z
0WW503Z 0WW507Z 0WW50JZ 0WW50KZ 0WW50YZ 0WW530Z 0WW531Z 0WW533Z 0WW537Z 0WW53JZ 0WW53KZ 0WW53YZ 0WW540Z
0WW541Z 0WW543Z 0WW547Z 0WW54JZ 0WW54KZ 0WW54YZ 0WW600Z 0WW601Z 0WW603Z 0WW607Z 0WW60JZ 0WW60KZ 0WW60YZ
0WW630Z 0WW631Z 0WW633Z 0WW637Z 0WW63JZ 0WW63KZ 0WW63YZ 0WW640Z 0WW641Z 0WW643Z 0WW647Z 0WW64JZ 0WW64KZ
0WW64YZ 0WWK00Z 0WWK01Z 0WWK03Z 0WWK07Z 0WWK0JZ 0WWK0KZ 0WWK0YZ 0WWK30Z 0WWK31Z 0WWK33Z 0WWK37Z 0WWK3JZ
0WWK3KZ 0WWK3YZ 0WWK40Z 0WWK41Z 0WWK43Z 0WWK47Z 0WWK4JZ 0WWK4KZ 0WWK4YZ 0WWL00Z 0WWL01Z 0WWL03Z 0WWL07Z
0WWL0JZ 0WWL0KZ 0WWL0YZ 0WWL30Z 0WWL31Z 0WWL33Z 0WWL37Z 0WWL3JZ 0WWL3KZ 0WWL3YZ 0WWL40Z 0WWL41Z 0WWL43Z
0WWL47Z 0WWL4JZ 0WWL4KZ 0WWL4YZ 0WWM00Z 0WWM01Z 0WWM03Z 0WWM0JZ 0WWM0YZ 0WWM30Z 0WWM31Z 0WWM33Z 0WWM3JZ
0WWM3YZ 0WWM40Z 0WWM41Z 0WWM43Z 0WWM4JZ 0WWM4YZ

0 Medical and Surgical
W Anatomical Regions, General
Y Transplantation: Putting in or on all or a portion of a living body part taken from another individual or animal to physically take the place and/or function of all or a portion of a similar body part

Body Part	Approach	Device	Qualifier
Character 4	**Character 5**	**Character 6**	**Character 7**
2 Face	0 Open	Z No Device	0 Allogeneic 1 Syngeneic

NOTES

NOTES

Anatomical Regions, Upper Extremities 0X0-0XY

0 Medical and Surgical
X Anatomical Regions, Upper Extremities
0 Alteration: Modifying the anatomic structure of a body part without affecting the function of the body part

Body Part	Approach	Device	Qualifier
Character 4	Character 5	Character 6	Character 7
2 Shoulder Region, Right **3** Shoulder Region, Left **4** Axilla, Right **5** Axilla, Left **6** Upper Extremity, Right **7** Upper Extremity, Left **8** Upper Arm, Right **9** Upper Arm, Left **B** Elbow Region, Right **C** Elbow Region, Left **D** Lower Arm, Right **F** Lower Arm, Left **G** Wrist Region, Right **H** Wrist Region, Left	**0** Open **3** Percutaneous **4** Percutaneous Endoscopic	**7** Autologous Tissue Substitute **J** Synthetic Substitute **K** Nonautologous Tissue Substitute **Z** No Device	**Z** No Qualifier

0 Medical and Surgical
X Anatomical Regions, Upper Extremities
2 Change: Taking out or off a device from a body part and putting back an identical or similar device in or on the same body part without cutting or puncturing the skin or a mucous membrane

Body Part	Approach	Device	Qualifier
Character 4	Character 5	Character 6	Character 7
6 Upper Extremity, Right **7** Upper Extremity, Left	**X** External	**0** Drainage Device **Y** Other Device	**Z** No Qualifier

0 Medical and Surgical
X Anatomical Regions, Upper Extremities
3 Control: Stopping, or attempting to stop, postprocedural or other acute bleeding

Body Part	Approach	Device	Qualifier
Character 4	Character 5	Character 6	Character 7
2 Shoulder Region, Right **3** Shoulder Region, Left **4** Axilla, Right **5** Axilla, Left **6** Upper Extremity, Right **7** Upper Extremity, Left **8** Upper Arm, Right **9** Upper Arm, Left **B** Elbow Region, Right **C** Elbow Region, Left **D** Lower Arm, Right **F** Lower Arm, Left **G** Wrist Region, Right **H** Wrist Region, Left **J** Hand, Right **K** Hand, Left	**0** Open **3** Percutaneous **4** Percutaneous Endoscopic	**Z** No Device	**Z** No Qualifier

LC Limited Coverage   **NC** Noncovered   **HAC** HAC-associated Procedure   **CC** Combination Cluster - See Appendix G for code lists
DRG Non-OR-Affecting MS-DRG Assignment   New/Revised Text in Orange   ♂ Male   ♀ Female

2021 ICD-10-PCS   577

0 **Medical and Surgical**
X **Anatomical Regions, Upper Extremities**
6 **Detachment:** Cutting off all or a portion of the upper or lower extremities

Body Part	Approach	Device	Qualifier
Character 4	**Character 5**	**Character 6**	**Character 7**
0 Forequarter, Right **1** Forequarter, Left **2** Shoulder Region, Right **3** Shoulder Region, Left **B** Elbow Region, Right **C** Elbow Region, Left	**0** Open	**Z** No Device	**Z** No Qualifier
8 Upper Arm, Right **9** Upper Arm, Left **D** Lower Arm, Right **F** Lower Arm, Left	**0** Open	**Z** No Device	**1** High **2** Mid **3** Low
J Hand, Right **K** Hand, Left	**0** Open	**Z** No Device	**0** Complete **4** Complete 1st Ray **5** Complete 2nd Ray **6** Complete 3rd Ray **7** Complete 4th Ray **8** Complete 5th Ray **9** Partial 1st Ray **B** Partial 2nd Ray **C** Partial 3rd Ray **D** Partial 4th Ray **F** Partial 5th Ray
L Thumb, Right **M** Thumb, Left **N** Index Finger, Right **P** Index Finger, Left **Q** Middle Finger, Right **R** Middle Finger, Left **S** Ring Finger, Right **T** Ring Finger, Left **V** Little Finger, Right **W** Little Finger, Left	**0** Open	**Z** No Device	**0** Complete **1** High **2** Mid **3** Low

LC Limited Coverage   **NC** Noncovered   **HAC** HAC-associated Procedure   **CC** Combination Cluster - See Appendix G for code lists
DRG Non-OR-Affecting MS-DRG Assignment   New/Revised Text in **Orange** ♂ Male ♀ Female

578   **2021 ICD-10-PCS**

0 Medical and Surgical
X Anatomical Regions, Upper Extremities
9 Drainage: Taking or letting out fluids and/or gases from a body part

Body Part	Approach	Device	Qualifier
Character 4	Character 5	Character 6	Character 7
2 Shoulder Region, Right **3** Shoulder Region, Left **4** Axilla, Right **5** Axilla, Left **6** Upper Extremity, Right **7** Upper Extremity, Left **8** Upper Arm, Right **9** Upper Arm, Left **B** Elbow Region, Right **C** Elbow Region, Left **D** Lower Arm, Right **F** Lower Arm, Left **G** Wrist Region, Right **H** Wrist Region, Left **J** Hand, Right **K** Hand, Left	**0** Open **3** Percutaneous **4** Percutaneous Endoscopic	**0** Drainage Device	**Z** No Qualifier
2 Shoulder Region, Right **3** Shoulder Region, Left **4** Axilla, Right **5** Axilla, Left **6** Upper Extremity, Right **7** Upper Extremity, Left **8** Upper Arm, Right **9** Upper Arm, Left **B** Elbow Region, Right **C** Elbow Region, Left **D** Lower Arm, Right **F** Lower Arm, Left **G** Wrist Region, Right **H** Wrist Region, Left **J** Hand, Right **K** Hand, Left	**0** Open **3** Percutaneous **4** Percutaneous Endoscopic	**Z** No Device	**X** Diagnostic **Z** No Qualifier

0   **Medical and Surgical**
X   **Anatomical Regions, Upper Extremities**
B   **Excision:** Cutting out or off, without replacement, a portion of a body part

Body Part	Approach	Device	Qualifier
Character 4	Character 5	Character 6	Character 7
2 Shoulder Region, Right **3** Shoulder Region, Left **4** Axilla, Right **5** Axilla, Left **6** Upper Extremity, Right **7** Upper Extremity, Left **8** Upper Arm, Right **9** Upper Arm, Left **B** Elbow Region, Right **C** Elbow Region, Left **D** Lower Arm, Right **F** Lower Arm, Left **G** Wrist Region, Right **H** Wrist Region, Left **J** Hand, Right **K** Hand, Left	**0** Open **3** Percutaneous **4** Percutaneous Endoscopic	**Z** No Device	**X** Diagnostic **Z** No Qualifier

0   **Medical and Surgical**
X   **Anatomical Regions, Upper Extremities**
H   **Insertion:** Putting in a nonbiological appliance that monitors, assists, performs, or prevents a physiological function but does not physically take the place of a body part

Body Part	Approach	Device	Qualifier
Character 4	Character 5	Character 6	Character 7
2 Shoulder Region, Right ᴰᴿᴳ **3** Shoulder Region, Left ᴰᴿᴳ **4** Axilla, Right ᴰᴿᴳ **5** Axilla, Left ᴰᴿᴳ **6** Upper Extremity, Right ᴰᴿᴳ **7** Upper Extremity, Left ᴰᴿᴳ **8** Upper Arm, Right ᴰᴿᴳ **9** Upper Arm, Left ᴰᴿᴳ **B** Elbow Region, Right ᴰᴿᴳ **C** Elbow Region, Left ᴰᴿᴳ **D** Lower Arm, Right ᴰᴿᴳ **F** Lower Arm, Left ᴰᴿᴳ **G** Wrist Region, Right ᴰᴿᴳ **H** Wrist Region, Left ᴰᴿᴳ **J** Hand, Right ᴰᴿᴳ **K** Hand, Left ᴰᴿᴳ	**0** Open **3** Percutaneous **4** Percutaneous Endoscopic	**1** Radioactive Element **3** Infusion Device **Y** Other Device	**Z** No Qualifier

ᴰᴿᴳ
0XH203Z	0XH20YZ	0XH233Z	0XH23YZ	0XH243Z	0XH24YZ	0XH303Z	0XH30YZ	0XH333Z	0XH33YZ	0XH343Z	0XH34YZ	0XH403Z
0XH40YZ	0XH433Z	0XH43YZ	0XH443Z	0XH44YZ	0XH503Z	0XH50YZ	0XH533Z	0XH53YZ	0XH543Z	0XH54YZ	0XH603Z	0XH60YZ
0XH633Z	0XH63YZ	0XH643Z	0XH64YZ	0XH703Z	0XH70YZ	0XH733Z	0XH73YZ	0XH743Z	0XH74YZ	0XH803Z	0XH80YZ	0XH833Z
0XH83YZ	0XH843Z	0XH84YZ	0XH903Z	0XH90YZ	0XH933Z	0XH93YZ	0XH943Z	0XH94YZ	0XHB03Z	0XHB0YZ	0XHB33Z	0XHB3YZ
0XHB43Z	0XHB4YZ	0XHC03Z	0XHC0YZ	0XHC33Z	0XHC3YZ	0XHC43Z	0XHC4YZ	0XHD03Z	0XHD0YZ	0XHD33Z	0XHD3YZ	0XHD43Z
0XHD4YZ	0XHF03Z	0XHF0YZ	0XHF33Z	0XHF3YZ	0XHF43Z	0XHF4YZ	0XHG03Z	0XHG0YZ	0XHG33Z	0XHG3YZ	0XHG43Z	0XHG4YZ
0XHH03Z	0XHH0YZ	0XHH33Z	0XHH3YZ	0XHH43Z	0XHH4YZ	0XHJ03Z	0XHJ0YZ	0XHJ33Z	0XHJ3YZ	0XHJ43Z	0XHJ4YZ	0XHK03Z
0XHK0YZ	0XHK33Z	0XHK3YZ	0XHK43Z	0XHK4YZ							

ᴸᶜ Limited Coverage   ᴺᶜ Noncovered   ᴴᴬᶜ HAC-associated Procedure   ᶜᶜ Combination Cluster - See Appendix G for code lists
ᴰᴿᴳ Non-OR-Affecting MS-DRG Assignment   New/Revised Text in **Orange**   ♂ Male   ♀ Female

0 Medical and Surgical
X Anatomical Regions, Upper Extremities
J Inspection: Visually and/or manually exploring a body part

Body Part	Approach	Device	Qualifier
Character 4	Character 5	Character 6	Character 7
2 Shoulder Region, Right ᴼᴿᴳ **3** Shoulder Region, Left ᴼᴿᴳ **4** Axilla, Right ᴼᴿᴳ **5** Axilla, Left ᴼᴿᴳ **6** Upper Extremity, Right ᴼᴿᴳ **7** Upper Extremity, Left ᴼᴿᴳ **8** Upper Arm, Right ᴼᴿᴳ **9** Upper Arm, Left ᴼᴿᴳ **B** Elbow Region, Right ᴼᴿᴳ **C** Elbow Region, Left ᴼᴿᴳ **D** Lower Arm, Right ᴼᴿᴳ **F** Lower Arm, Left ᴼᴿᴳ **G** Wrist Region, Right ᴼᴿᴳ **H** Wrist Region, Left ᴼᴿᴳ **J** Hand, Right ᴼᴿᴳ **K** Hand, Left ᴼᴿᴳ	**0** Open **3** Percutaneous **4** Percutaneous Endoscopic **X** External	**Z** No Device	**Z** No Qualifier

ᴼᴿᴳ 0XJ20ZZ   0XJ30ZZ   0XJ40ZZ   0XJ50ZZ   0XJ60ZZ   0XJ70ZZ   0XJ80ZZ   0XJ90ZZ   0XJB0ZZ   0XJC0ZZ   0XJD0ZZ   0XJF0ZZ   0XJG0ZZ
0XJH0ZZ   0XJJ0ZZ   0XJK0ZZ

0 Medical and Surgical
X Anatomical Regions, Upper Extremities
M Reattachment: Putting back in or on all or a portion of a separated body part to its normal location or other suitable location

Body Part	Approach	Device	Qualifier
Character 4	Character 5	Character 6	Character 7
0 Forequarter, Right **1** Forequarter, Left **2** Shoulder Region, Right **3** Shoulder Region, Left **4** Axilla, Right **5** Axilla, Left **6** Upper Extremity, Right **7** Upper Extremity, Left **8** Upper Arm, Right **9** Upper Arm, Left **B** Elbow Region, Right **C** Elbow Region, Left **D** Lower Arm, Right **F** Lower Arm, Left **G** Wrist Region, Right **H** Wrist Region, Left **J** Hand, Right **K** Hand, Left **L** Thumb, Right **M** Thumb, Left **N** Index Finger, Right **P** Index Finger, Left **Q** Middle Finger, Right **R** Middle Finger, Left **S** Ring Finger, Right **T** Ring Finger, Left **V** Little Finger, Right **W** Little Finger, Left	**0** Open	**Z** No Device	**Z** No Qualifier

0 Medical and Surgical
X Anatomical Regions, Upper Extremities
P Removal: Taking out or off a device from a body part

Body Part	Approach	Device	Qualifier
Character 4	Character 5	Character 6	Character 7
6 Upper Extremity, Right 7 Upper Extremity, Left	0 Open 3 Percutaneous 4 Percutaneous Endoscopic X External	0 Drainage Device 1 Radioactive Element 3 Infusion Device 7 Autologous Tissue Substitute J Synthetic Substitute K Nonautologous Tissue Substitute Y Other Device	Z No Qualifier

0 Medical and Surgical
X Anatomical Regions, Upper Extremities
Q Repair: Restoring, to the extent possible, a body part to its normal anatomic structure and function

Body Part	Approach	Device	Qualifier
Character 4	Character 5	Character 6	Character 7
2 Shoulder Region, Right 3 Shoulder Region, Left 4 Axilla, Right 5 Axilla, Left 6 Upper Extremity, Right 7 Upper Extremity, Left 8 Upper Arm, Right 9 Upper Arm, Left B Elbow Region, Right C Elbow Region, Left D Lower Arm, Right F Lower Arm, Left G Wrist Region, Right H Wrist Region, Left J Hand, Right K Hand, Left L Thumb, Right M Thumb, Left N Index Finger, Right P Index Finger, Left Q Middle Finger, Right R Middle Finger, Left S Ring Finger, Right T Ring Finger, Left V Little Finger, Right W Little Finger, Left	0 Open 3 Percutaneous 4 Percutaneous Endoscopic X External	Z No Device	Z No Qualifier

0 Medical and Surgical
X Anatomical Regions, Upper Extremities
R Replacement: Putting in or on biological or synthetic material that physically takes the place and/or function of all or a portion of a body part

Body Part	Approach	Device	Qualifier
Character 4	Character 5	Character 6	Character 7
L Thumb, Right M Thumb, Left	0 Open 4 Percutaneous Endoscopic	7 Autologous Tissue Substitute	N Toe, Right P Toe, Left

        🄻🄲 Limited Coverage   🄽🄲 Noncovered   🄷🄰🄲 HAC-associated Procedure   🄲🄲 Combination Cluster - See Appendix G for code lists
           🄳🅁🄶 Non-OR-Affecting MS-DRG Assignment   New/Revised Text in **Orange**   ♂ Male   ♀ Female

582   **2021 ICD-10-PCS**

0 Medical and Surgical
X Anatomical Regions, Upper Extremities
U Supplement: Putting in or on biological or synthetic material that physically reinforces and/or augments the function of a portion of a body part

Body Part	Approach	Device	Qualifier
Character 4	**Character 5**	**Character 6**	**Character 7**
2 Shoulder Region, Right **3** Shoulder Region, Left **4** Axilla, Right **5** Axilla, Left **6** Upper Extremity, Right **7** Upper Extremity, Left **8** Upper Arm, Right **9** Upper Arm, Left **B** Elbow Region, Right **C** Elbow Region, Left **D** Lower Arm, Right **F** Lower Arm, Left **G** Wrist Region, Right **H** Wrist Region, Left **J** Hand, Right **K** Hand, Left **L** Thumb, Right **M** Thumb, Left **N** Index Finger, Right **P** Index Finger, Left **Q** Middle Finger, Right **R** Middle Finger, Left **S** Ring Finger, Right **T** Ring Finger, Left **V** Little Finger, Right **W** Little Finger, Left	**0** Open **4** Percutaneous Endoscopic	**7** Autologous Tissue Substitute **J** Synthetic Substitute **K** Nonautologous Tissue Substitute	**Z** No Qualifier

0 Medical and Surgical
X Anatomical Regions, Upper Extremities
W Revision: Correcting, to the extent possible, a portion of a malfunctioning device or the position of a displaced device

Body Part	Approach	Device	Qualifier
Character 4	**Character 5**	**Character 6**	**Character 7**
6 Upper Extremity, Right 🐾 **7** Upper Extremity, Left 🐾	**0** Open **3** Percutaneous **4** Percutaneous Endoscopic **X** External	**0** Drainage Device **3** Infusion Device **7** Autologous Tissue Substitute **J** Synthetic Substitute **K** Nonautologous Tissue Substitute **Y** Other Device	**Z** No Qualifier

🐾   0XW600Z   0XW603Z   0XW607Z   0XW60JZ   0XW60KZ   0XW60YZ   0XW630Z   0XW633Z   0XW637Z   0XW63JZ   0XW63KZ   0XW63YZ   0XW640Z
    0XW643Z   0XW647Z   0XW64JZ   0XW64KZ   0XW64YZ   0XW700Z   0XW703Z   0XW707Z   0XW70JZ   0XW70KZ   0XW70YZ   0XW730Z   0XW733Z
    0XW737Z   0XW73JZ   0XW73KZ   0XW73YZ   0XW740Z   0XW743Z   0XW747Z   0XW74JZ   0XW74KZ   0XW74YZ

0 Medical and Surgical
X Anatomical Regions, Upper Extremities
X Transfer: Moving, without taking out, all or a portion of a body part to another location to take over the function of all or a portion of a body part

Body Part	Approach	Device	Qualifier
Character 4	**Character 5**	**Character 6**	**Character 7**
N Index Finger, Right	**0** Open	**Z** No Device	**L** Thumb, Right
P Index Finger, Left	**0** Open	**Z** No Device	**M** Thumb, Left

0 Medical and Surgical
X Anatomical Regions, Upper Extremities
Y Transplantation: Putting in or on all or a portion of a living body part taken from another individual or animal to physically take the place and/or function of all or a portion of a similar body part

Body Part	Approach	Device	Qualifier
Character 4	**Character 5**	**Character 6**	**Character 7**
J Hand, Right **K** Hand, Left	**0** Open	**Z** No Device	**0** Allogeneic **1** Syngeneic

NOTES

Anatomical Regions, Lower Extremities 0Y0–0YW

0 Medical and Surgical
Y Anatomical Regions, Lower Extremities
0 Alteration: Modifying the anatomic structure of a body part without affecting the function of the body part

Body Part	Approach	Device	Qualifier
Character 4	**Character 5**	**Character 6**	**Character 7**
0 Buttock, Right 1 Buttock, Left 9 Lower Extremity, Right B Lower Extremity, Left C Upper Leg, Right D Upper Leg, Left F Knee Region, Right G Knee Region, Left H Lower Leg, Right J Lower Leg, Left K Ankle Region, Right L Ankle Region, Left	0 Open 3 Percutaneous 4 Percutaneous Endoscopic	7 Autologous Tissue Substitute J Synthetic Substitute K Nonautologous Tissue Substitute Z No Device	Z No Qualifier

0 Medical and Surgical
Y Anatomical Regions, Lower Extremities
2 Change: Taking out or off a device from a body part and putting back an identical or similar device in or on the same body part without cutting or puncturing the skin or a mucous membrane

Body Part	Approach	Device	Qualifier
Character 4	**Character 5**	**Character 6**	**Character 7**
9 Lower Extremity, Right B Lower Extremity, Left	X External	0 Drainage Device Y Other Device	Z No Qualifier

0 Medical and Surgical
Y Anatomical Regions, Lower Extremities
3 Control: Stopping, or attempting to stop, postprocedural or other acute bleeding

Body Part	Approach	Device	Qualifier
Character 4	**Character 5**	**Character 6**	**Character 7**
0 Buttock, Right 1 Buttock, Left 5 Inguinal Region, Right 6 Inguinal Region, Left 7 Femoral Region, Right 8 Femoral Region, Left 9 Lower Extremity, Right B Lower Extremity, Left C Upper Leg, Right D Upper Leg, Left F Knee Region, Right G Knee Region, Left H Lower Leg, Right J Lower Leg, Left K Ankle Region, Right L Ankle Region, Left M Foot, Right N Foot, Left	0 Open 3 Percutaneous 4 Percutaneous Endoscopic	Z No Device	Z No Qualifier

LC Limited Coverage   NC Noncovered   HAC HAC-associated Procedure   CC Combination Cluster - See Appendix G for code lists
DRG Non-OR-Affecting MS-DRG Assignment   New/Revised Text in **Orange**   ♂ Male   ♀ Female

2021 ICD-10-PCS   585

0 **Medical and Surgical**
Y **Anatomical Regions, Lower Extremities**
6 **Detachment:** Cutting off all or a portion of the upper or lower extremities

Body Part	Approach	Device	Qualifier
Character 4	Character 5	Character 6	Character 7
2 Hindquarter, Right **3** Hindquarter, Left **4** Hindquarter, Bilateral **7** Femoral Region, Right **8** Femoral Region, Left **F** Knee Region, Right **G** Knee Region, Left	**0** Open	**Z** No Device	**Z** No Qualifier
C Upper Leg, Right **D** Upper Leg, Left **H** Lower Leg, Right **J** Lower Leg, Left	**0** Open	**Z** No Device	**1** High **2** Mid **3** Low
M Foot, Right **N** Foot, Left	**0** Open	**Z** No Device	**0** Complete **4** Complete 1st Ray **5** Complete 2nd Ray **6** Complete 3rd Ray **7** Complete 4th Ray **8** Complete 5th Ray **9** Partial 1st Ray **B** Partial 2nd Ray **C** Partial 3rd Ray **D** Partial 4th Ray **F** Partial 5th Ray
P 1st Toe, Right **Q** 1st Toe, Left **R** 2nd Toe, Right **S** 2nd Toe, Left **T** 3rd Toe, Right **U** 3rd Toe, Left **V** 4th Toe, Right **W** 4th Toe, Left **X** 5th Toe, Right **Y** 5th Toe, Left	**0** Open	**Z** No Device	**0** Complete **1** High **2** Mid **3** Low

0 **Medical and Surgical**
Y **Anatomical Regions, Lower Extremities**
9 **Drainage:** Taking or letting out fluids and/or gases from a body part

Body Part	Approach	Device	Qualifier
Character 4	**Character 5**	**Character 6**	**Character 7**
0 Buttock, Right 1 Buttock, Left 5 Inguinal Region, Right 6 Inguinal Region, Left 7 Femoral Region, Right 8 Femoral Region, Left 9 Lower Extremity, Right B Lower Extremity, Left C Upper Leg, Right D Upper Leg, Left F Knee Region, Right G Knee Region, Left H Lower Leg, Right J Lower Leg, Left K Ankle Region, Right L Ankle Region, Left M Foot, Right N Foot, Left	0 Open 3 Percutaneous 4 Percutaneous Endoscopic	0 Drainage Device	Z No Qualifier
0 Buttock, Right 1 Buttock, Left 5 Inguinal Region, Right 6 Inguinal Region, Left 7 Femoral Region, Right 8 Femoral Region, Left 9 Lower Extremity, Right B Lower Extremity, Left C Upper Leg, Right D Upper Leg, Left F Knee Region, Right G Knee Region, Left H Lower Leg, Right J Lower Leg, Left K Ankle Region, Right L Ankle Region, Left M Foot, Right N Foot, Left	0 Open 3 Percutaneous 4 Percutaneous Endoscopic	Z No Device	X Diagnostic Z No Qualifier

0 **Medical and Surgical**
Y **Anatomical Regions, Lower Extremities**
B **Excision:** Cutting out or off, without replacement, a portion of a body part

Body Part	Approach	Device	Qualifier
Character 4	**Character 5**	**Character 6**	**Character 7**
0 Buttock, Right 1 Buttock, Left 5 Inguinal Region, Right 6 Inguinal Region, Left 7 Femoral Region, Right 8 Femoral Region, Left 9 Lower Extremity, Right B Lower Extremity, Left C Upper Leg, Right D Upper Leg, Left F Knee Region, Right G Knee Region, Left H Lower Leg, Right J Lower Leg, Left K Ankle Region, Right L Ankle Region, Left M Foot, Right N Foot, Left	0 Open 3 Percutaneous 4 Percutaneous Endoscopic	Z No Device	X Diagnostic Z No Qualifier

LC Limited Coverage NC Noncovered HAC HAC-associated Procedure CC Combination Cluster - See Appendix G for code lists
DRG Non-OR-Affecting MS-DRG Assignment New/Revised Text in **Orange** ♂ Male ♀ Female

0 **Medical and Surgical**
Y **Anatomical Regions, Lower Extremities**
H **Insertion:** Putting in a nonbiological appliance that monitors, assists, performs, or prevents a physiological function but does not physically take the place of a body part

Body Part	Approach	Device	Qualifier
Character 4	**Character 5**	**Character 6**	**Character 7**

Body Part	Approach	Device	Qualifier
0 Buttock, Right ᴰᴿᴳ	**0** Open	**1** Radioactive Element	**Z** No Qualifier
1 Buttock, Left ᴰᴿᴳ	**3** Percutaneous	**3** Infusion Device	
5 Inguinal Region, Right ᴰᴿᴳ	**4** Percutaneous Endoscopic	**Y** Other Device	
6 Inguinal Region, Left ᴰᴿᴳ			
7 Femoral Region, Right ᴰᴿᴳ			
8 Femoral Region, Left ᴰᴿᴳ			
9 Lower Extremity, Right ᴰᴿᴳ			
B Lower Extremity, Left ᴰᴿᴳ			
C Upper Leg, Right ᴰᴿᴳ			
D Upper Leg, Left ᴰᴿᴳ			
F Knee Region, Right ᴰᴿᴳ			
G Knee Region, Left ᴰᴿᴳ			
H Lower Leg, Right ᴰᴿᴳ			
J Lower Leg, Left ᴰᴿᴳ			
K Ankle Region, Right ᴰᴿᴳ			
L Ankle Region, Left ᴰᴿᴳ			
M Foot, Right ᴰᴿᴳ			
N Foot, Left ᴰᴿᴳ			

ᴰᴿᴳ 0YH003Z 0YH00YZ 0YH033Z 0YH03YZ 0YH043Z 0YH04YZ 0YH103Z 0YH10YZ 0YH133Z 0YH13YZ 0YH143Z 0YH14YZ 0YH503Z
0YH50YZ 0YH533Z 0YH53YZ 0YH543Z 0YH54YZ 0YH603Z 0YH60YZ 0YH633Z 0YH63YZ 0YH643Z 0YH64YZ 0YH703Z 0YH70YZ
0YH733Z 0YH73YZ 0YH743Z 0YH74YZ 0YH803Z 0YH80YZ 0YH833Z 0YH83YZ 0YH843Z 0YH84YZ 0YH903Z 0YH90YZ 0YH933Z
0YH93YZ 0YH943Z 0YH94YZ 0YHB03Z 0YHB0YZ 0YHB33Z 0YHB3YZ 0YHB43Z 0YHB4YZ 0YHC03Z 0YHC0YZ 0YHC33Z 0YHC3YZ
0YHC43Z 0YHC4YZ 0YHD03Z 0YHD0YZ 0YHD33Z 0YHD3YZ 0YHD43Z 0YHD4YZ 0YHF03Z 0YHF0YZ 0YHF33Z 0YHF3YZ 0YHF43Z
0YHF4YZ 0YHG03Z 0YHG0YZ 0YHG33Z 0YHG3YZ 0YHG43Z 0YHG4YZ 0YHH03Z 0YHH0YZ 0YHH33Z 0YHH3YZ 0YHH43Z 0YHH4YZ
0YHJ03Z 0YHJ0YZ 0YHJ33Z 0YHJ3YZ 0YHJ43Z 0YHJ4YZ 0YHK03Z 0YHK0YZ 0YHK33Z 0YHK3YZ 0YHK43Z 0YHK4YZ 0YHL03Z
0YHL0YZ 0YHL33Z 0YHL3YZ 0YHL43Z 0YHL4YZ 0YHM03Z 0YHM0YZ 0YHM33Z 0YHM3YZ 0YHM43Z 0YHM4YZ 0YHN03Z 0YHN0YZ
0YHN33Z 0YHN3YZ 0YHN43Z 0YHN4YZ

0 **Medical and Surgical**
Y **Anatomical Regions, Lower Extremities**
J **Inspection:** Visually and/or manually exploring a body part

Body Part	Approach	Device	Qualifier
Character 4	**Character 5**	**Character 6**	**Character 7**

Body Part	Approach	Device	Qualifier
0 Buttock, Right ᴰᴿᴳ	**0** Open	**Z** No Device	**Z** No Qualifier
1 Buttock, Left ᴰᴿᴳ	**3** Percutaneous		
5 Inguinal Region, Right	**4** Percutaneous Endoscopic		
6 Inguinal Region, Left	**X** External		
7 Femoral Region, Right			
8 Femoral Region, Left ᴰᴿᴳ			
9 Lower Extremity, Right ᴰᴿᴳ			
A Inguinal Region, Bilateral			
B Lower Extremity, Left ᴰᴿᴳ			
C Upper Leg, Right ᴰᴿᴳ			
D Upper Leg, Left ᴰᴿᴳ			
E Femoral Region, Bilateral ᴰᴿᴳ			
F Knee Region, Right ᴰᴿᴳ			
G Knee Region, Left ᴰᴿᴳ			
H Lower Leg, Right ᴰᴿᴳ			
J Lower Leg, Left ᴰᴿᴳ			
K Ankle Region, Right ᴰᴿᴳ			
L Ankle Region, Left ᴰᴿᴳ			
M Foot, Right ᴰᴿᴳ			
N Foot, Left ᴰᴿᴳ			

ᴰᴿᴳ 0YJ00ZZ 0YJ10ZZ 0YJ80ZZ 0YJ90ZZ 0YJB0ZZ 0YJC0ZZ 0YJD0ZZ 0YJE0ZZ 0YJF0ZZ 0YJG0ZZ 0YJH0ZZ 0YJJ0ZZ 0YJK0ZZ
0YJL0ZZ 0YJM0ZZ 0YJN0ZZ

ᴸᶜ Limited Coverage ᴺᶜ Noncovered ᴴᴬᶜ HAC-associated Procedure ᶜᶜ Combination Cluster - See Appendix G for code lists
ᴰᴿᴳ Non-OR-Affecting MS-DRG Assignment New/Revised Text in **Orange** ♂ Male ♀ Female

0 **Medical and Surgical**
Y **Anatomical Regions, Lower Extremities**
M **Reattachment:** Putting back in or on all or a portion of a separated body part to its normal location or other suitable location

Body Part	Approach	Device	Qualifier
Character 4	**Character 5**	**Character 6**	**Character 7**
0 Buttock, Right	0 Open	Z No Device	Z No Qualifier
1 Buttock, Left			
2 Hindquarter, Right			
3 Hindquarter, Left			
4 Hindquarter, Bilateral			
5 Inguinal Region, Right			
6 Inguinal Region, Left			
7 Femoral Region, Right			
8 Femoral Region, Left			
9 Lower Extremity, Right			
B Lower Extremity, Left			
C Upper Leg, Right			
D Upper Leg, Left			
F Knee Region, Right			
G Knee Region, Left			
H Lower Leg, Right			
J Lower Leg, Left			
K Ankle Region, Right			
L Ankle Region, Left			
M Foot, Right			
N Foot, Left			
P 1st Toe, Right			
Q 1st Toe, Left			
R 2nd Toe, Right			
S 2nd Toe, Left			
T 3rd Toe, Right			
U 3rd Toe, Left			
V 4th Toe, Right			
W 4th Toe, Left			
X 5th Toe, Right			
Y 5th Toe, Left			

0 **Medical and Surgical**
Y **Anatomical Regions, Lower Extremities**
P **Removal:** Taking out or off a device from a body part

Body Part	Approach	Device	Qualifier
Character 4	**Character 5**	**Character 6**	**Character 7**
9 Lower Extremity, Right	0 Open	0 Drainage Device	Z No Qualifier
B Lower Extremity, Left	3 Percutaneous	1 Radioactive Element	
	4 Percutaneous Endoscopic	3 Infusion Device	
	X External	7 Autologous Tissue Substitute	
		J Synthetic Substitute	
		K Nonautologous Tissue Substitute	
		Y Other Device	

0   **Medical and Surgical**
Y   **Anatomical Regions, Lower Extremities**
Q   **Repair:** Restoring, to the extent possible, a body part to its normal anatomic structure and function

Body Part	Approach	Device	Qualifier
Character 4	**Character 5**	**Character 6**	**Character 7**
0 Buttock, Right **1** Buttock, Left **5** Inguinal Region, Right **6** Inguinal Region, Left **7** Femoral Region, Right **8** Femoral Region, Left **9** Lower Extremity, Right **A** Inguinal Region, Bilateral **B** Lower Extremity, Left **C** Upper Leg, Right **D** Upper Leg, Left **E** Femoral Region, Bilateral **F** Knee Region, Right **G** Knee Region, Left **H** Lower Leg, Right **J** Lower Leg, Left **K** Ankle Region, Right **L** Ankle Region, Left **M** Foot, Right **N** Foot, Left **P** 1st Toe, Right **Q** 1st Toe, Left **R** 2nd Toe, Right **S** 2nd Toe, Left **T** 3rd Toe, Right **U** 3rd Toe, Left **V** 4th Toe, Right **W** 4th Toe, Left **X** 5th Toe, Right **Y** 5th Toe, Left	**0** Open **3** Percutaneous **4** Percutaneous Endoscopic **X** External	**Z** No Device	**Z** No Qualifier

LC Limited Coverage   **NC** Noncovered   **HAC** HAC-associated Procedure   **CC** Combination Cluster - See Appendix G for code lists

DRG Non-OR-Affecting MS-DRG Assignment   New/Revised Text in **Orange**   ♂ Male   ♀ Female

590

2021 ICD-10-PCS

0 Medical and Surgical
Y Anatomical Regions, Lower Extremities
U **Supplement:** Putting in or on biological or synthetic material that physically reinforces and/or augments the function of a portion of a body part

Body Part	Approach	Device	Qualifier
Character 4	**Character 5**	**Character 6**	**Character 7**
0 Buttock, Right	**0** Open	**7** Autologous Tissue Substitute	**Z** No Qualifier
1 Buttock, Left	**4** Percutaneous Endoscopic	**J** Synthetic Substitute	
5 Inguinal Region, Right		**K** Nonautologous Tissue	
6 Inguinal Region, Left		Substitute	
7 Femoral Region, Right			
8 Femoral Region, Left			
9 Lower Extremity, Right			
A Inguinal Region, Bilateral			
B Lower Extremity, Left			
C Upper Leg, Right			
D Upper Leg, Left			
E Femoral Region, Bilateral			
F Knee Region, Right			
G Knee Region, Left			
H Lower Leg, Right			
J Lower Leg, Left			
K Ankle Region, Right			
L Ankle Region, Left			
M Foot, Right			
N Foot, Left			
P 1st Toe, Right			
Q 1st Toe, Left			
R 2nd Toe, Right			
S 2nd Toe, Left			
T 3rd Toe, Right			
U 3rd Toe, Left			
V 4th Toe, Right			
W 4th Toe, Left			
X 5th Toe, Right			
Y 5th Toe, Left			

0 Medical and Surgical
Y Anatomical Regions, Lower Extremities
W **Revision:** Correcting, to the extent possible, a portion of a malfunctioning device or the position of a displaced device

Body Part	Approach	Device	Qualifier
Character 4	**Character 5**	**Character 6**	**Character 7**
9 Lower Extremity, Right ᴅʀɢ	**0** Open	**0** Drainage Device	**Z** No Qualifier
B Lower Extremity, Left ᴅʀɢ	**3** Percutaneous	**3** Infusion Device	
	4 Percutaneous Endoscopic	**7** Autologous Tissue Substitute	
	X External	**J** Synthetic Substitute	
		K Nonautologous Tissue Substitute	
		Y Other Device	

ᴅʀɢ 0YW900Z 0YW903Z 0YW907Z 0YW90JZ 0YW90KZ 0YW90YZ 0YW930Z 0YW933Z 0YW937Z 0YW93JZ 0YW93KZ 0YW93YZ 0YW940Z
0YW943Z 0YW947Z 0YW94JZ 0YW94KZ 0YW94YZ 0YWB00Z 0YWB03Z 0YWB07Z 0YWB0JZ 0YWB0KZ 0YWB0YZ 0YWB30Z 0YWB33Z
0YWB37Z 0YWB3JZ 0YWB3KZ 0YWB3YZ 0YWB40Z 0YWB43Z 0YWB47Z 0YWB4JZ 0YWB4KZ 0YWB4YZ

ɪᴄ Limited Coverage ɴᴄ Noncovered ʜᴀᴄ HAC-associated Procedure ᴄᴄ Combination Cluster - See Appendix G for code lists
ᴅʀɢ Non-OR-Affecting MS-DRG Assignment New/Revised Text in **Orange** ♂ Male ♀ Female

2021 ICD-10-PCS 591

NOTES

1 Obstetrics
0 Pregnancy
2 Change: Taking out or off a device from a body part and putting back an identical or similar device in or on the same body part without cutting or puncturing the skin or a mucous membrane

Body Part	Approach	Device	Qualifier
Character 4	Character 5	Character 6	Character 7
0 Products of Conception ♀	**7** Via Natural or Artificial Opening	**3** Monitoring Electrode **Y** Other Device	**Z** No Qualifier

♀ 102073Z 10207YZ

1 Obstetrics
0 Pregnancy
9 Drainage: Taking or letting out fluids and/or gases from a body part

Body Part	Approach	Device	Qualifier
Character 4	Character 5	Character 6	Character 7
0 Products of Conception ♀	**0** Open **3** Percutaneous **4** Percutaneous Endoscopic **7** Via Natural or Artificial Opening **8** Via Natural or Artificial Opening Endoscopic	**Z** No Device	**9** Fetal Blood **A** Fetal Cerebrospinal Fluid **B** Fetal Fluid, Other **C** Amniotic Fluid, Therapeutic **D** Fluid, Other **U** Amniotic Fluid, Diagnostic

♀ 10900Z9 10900ZA 10900ZB 10900ZC 10900ZD 10900ZU 10903Z9 10903ZA 10903ZB 10903ZC 10903ZD 10903ZU 10904Z9
10904ZA 10904ZB 10904ZC 10904ZD 10904ZU 10907Z9 10907ZA 10907ZB 10907ZC 10907ZD 10907ZU 10908Z9 10908ZA
10908ZB 10908ZC 10908ZD 10908ZU

1 Obstetrics
0 Pregnancy
A Abortion: Artificially terminating a pregnancy

Body Part	Approach	Device	Qualifier
Character 4	Character 5	Character 6	Character 7
0 Products of Conception ♀	**0** Open **3** Percutaneous **4** Percutaneous Endoscopic **8** Via Natural or Artificial Opening Endoscopic	**Z** No Device	**Z** No Qualifier
0 Products of Conception ♀	**7** Via Natural or Artificial Opening	**Z** No Device	**6** Vacuum **W** Laminaria **X** Abortifacient **Z** No Qualifier

♀ 10A00ZZ 10A03ZZ 10A04ZZ 10A07Z6 10A07ZW 10A07ZX 10A07ZZ 10A08ZZ

1 Obstetrics
0 Pregnancy
D Extraction: Pulling or stripping out or off all or a portion of a body part by the use of force

Body Part	Approach	Device	Qualifier
Character 4	Character 5	Character 6	Character 7
0 Products of Conception ♀ QOA	**0** Open	**Z** No Device	**0** High **1** Low **2** Extraperitoneal
0 Products of Conception ♀ DRG QOA	**7** Via Natural or Artificial Opening	**Z** No Device	**3** Low Forceps **4** Mid Forceps **5** High Forceps **6** Vacuum **7** Internal Version **8** Other
1 Products of Conception, Retained ♀	**7** Via Natural or Artificial Opening **8** Via Natural or Artificial Opening Endoscopic	**Z** No Device	**9** Manual **Z** No Qualifier
2 Products of Conception, Ectopic ♀	**0** Open **4** Percutaneous Endoscopic **7** Via Natural or Artificial Opening **8** Via Natural or Artificial Opening Endoscopic	**Z** No Device	**Z** No Qualifier

♀ 10D00Z0   10D00Z1   10D00Z2   10D07Z3   10D07Z4   10D07Z5   10D07Z6   10D07Z7   10D07Z8   10D17Z9   10D17ZZ   10D18Z9   10D18ZZ
  10D27ZZ   10D28ZZ
DRG 10D07Z3   10D07Z4   10D07Z5   10D07Z6   10D07Z7   10D07Z8
QOA 10D00Z0   10D00Z1   10D00Z2   10D07Z3   10D07Z4   10D07Z5   10D07Z7
The list of codes is a questionable admission except when reported with a corresponding secondary diagnosis
Z37.0, Z37.1, Z37.2, Z37.3, Z37.4, Z37.50, Z37.51, Z37.52, Z37.53, Z37.54, Z37.59, Z37.60, Z37.61, Z37.62, Z37.63, Z37.64, Z37.69, Z37.7, Z37.9

1 Obstetrics
0 Pregnancy
E Delivery: Assisting the passage of the products of conception from the genital canal

Body Part	Approach	Device	Qualifier
Character 4	Character 5	Character 6	Character 7
0 Products of Conception ♀ DRG QOA	**X** External	**Z** No Device	**Z** No Qualifier

♀ 10E0XZZ
DRG 10E0XZZ
QOA 10E0XZZ
The list of codes is a questionable admission except when reported with a corresponding secondary diagnosis
Z37.0, Z37.1, Z37.2, Z37.3, Z37.4, Z37.50, Z37.51, Z37.52, Z37.53, Z37.54, Z37.59, Z37.60, Z37.61, Z37.62, Z37.63, Z37.64, Z37.69, Z37.7, Z37.9

1 Obstetrics
0 Pregnancy
H Insertion: Putting in a nonbiological appliance that monitors, assists, performs, or prevents a physiological function but does not physically take the place of a body part

Body Part	Approach	Device	Qualifier
Character 4	Character 5	Character 6	Character 7
0 Products of Conception ♀	**0** Open **7** Via Natural or Artificial Opening	**3** Monitoring Electrode **Y** Other Device	**Z** No Qualifier

♀ 10H003Z   10H00YZ   10H073Z   10H07YZ

LC Limited Coverage   NC Noncovered   HAC HAC-associated Procedure   CC Combination Cluster - See Appendix G for code lists
DRG Non-OR-Affecting MS-DRG Assignment   QOA Questionable Obstetric Admission   New/Revised Text in Orange   ♂ Male   ♀ Female

594

2021 ICD-10-PCS

1 Obstetrics
0 Pregnancy
J Inspection: Visually and/or manually exploring a body part

Body Part	Approach	Device	Qualifier
Character 4	**Character 5**	**Character 6**	**Character 7**
0 Products of Conception ♀ **1** Products of Conception, Retained ♀ **2** Products of Conception, Ectopic ♀	**0** Open **3** Percutaneous **4** Percutaneous Endoscopic **7** Via Natural or Artificial Opening **8** Via Natural or Artificial Opening Endoscopic **X** External	**Z** No Device	**Z** No Qualifier

♀   10J00ZZ   10J03ZZ   10J04ZZ   10J07ZZ   10J08ZZ   10J0XZZ   10J10ZZ   10J13ZZ   10J14ZZ   10J17ZZ   10J18ZZ   10J1XZZ   10J20ZZ
   10J23ZZ   10J24ZZ   10J27ZZ   10J28ZZ   10J2XZZ

1 Obstetrics
0 Pregnancy
P Removal: Taking out or off a device from a body part, region, or orifice

Body Part	Approach	Device	Qualifier
Character 4	**Character 5**	**Character 6**	**Character 7**
0 Products of Conception ♀	**0** Open **7** Via Natural or Artificial Opening	**3** Monitoring Electrode **Y** Other Device	**Z** No Qualifier

♀   10P003Z   10P00YZ   10P073Z   10P07YZ

1 Obstetrics
0 Pregnancy
Q Repair: Restoring, to the extent possible, a body part to its normal anatomic structure and function

Body Part	Approach	Device	Qualifier
Character 4	**Character 5**	**Character 6**	**Character 7**
0 Products of Conception ♀	**0** Open **3** Percutaneous **4** Percutaneous Endoscopic **7** Via Natural or Artificial Opening **8** Via Natural or Artificial Opening Endoscopic	**Y** Other Device **Z** No Device	**E** Nervous System **F** Cardiovascular System **G** Lymphatics and Hemic **H** Eye **J** Ear, Nose and Sinus **K** Respiratory System **L** Mouth and Throat **M** Gastrointestinal System **N** Hepatobiliary and Pancreas **P** Endocrine System **Q** Skin **R** Musculoskeletal System **S** Urinary System **T** Female Reproductive System **V** Male Reproductive System **Y** Other Body System

♀   10Q00YE   10Q00YF   10Q00YG   10Q00YH   10Q00YJ   10Q00YK   10Q00YL   10Q00YM   10Q00YN   10Q00YP   10Q00YQ   10Q00YR   10Q00YS
   10Q00YT   10Q00YV   10Q00YY   10Q00ZE   10Q00ZF   10Q00ZG   10Q00ZH   10Q00ZJ   10Q00ZK   10Q00ZL   10Q00ZM   10Q00ZN   10Q00ZP
   10Q00ZQ   10Q00ZR   10Q00ZS   10Q00ZT   10Q00ZV   10Q00ZY   10Q03YE   10Q03YF   10Q03YG   10Q03YH   10Q03YJ   10Q03YK   10Q03YL
   10Q03YM   10Q03YN   10Q03YP   10Q03YQ   10Q03YR   10Q03YS   10Q03YT   10Q03YV   10Q03YY   10Q03ZE   10Q03ZF   10Q03ZG   10Q03ZH
   10Q03ZJ   10Q03ZK   10Q03ZL   10Q03ZM   10Q03ZN   10Q03ZP   10Q03ZQ   10Q03ZR   10Q03ZS   10Q03ZT   10Q03ZV   10Q03ZY   10Q04YE
   10Q04YF   10Q04YG   10Q04YH   10Q04YJ   10Q04YK   10Q04YL   10Q04YM   10Q04YN   10Q04YP   10Q04YQ   10Q04YR   10Q04YS   10Q04YT
   10Q04YV   10Q04YY   10Q04ZE   10Q04ZF   10Q04ZG   10Q04ZH   10Q04ZJ   10Q04ZK   10Q04ZL   10Q04ZM   10Q04ZN   10Q04ZP   10Q04ZQ
   10Q04ZR   10Q04ZS   10Q04ZT   10Q04ZV   10Q04ZY   10Q07YE   10Q07YF   10Q07YG   10Q07YH   10Q07YJ   10Q07YK   10Q07YL   10Q07YM
   10Q07YN   10Q07YP   10Q07YQ   10Q07YR   10Q07YS   10Q07YT   10Q07YV   10Q07YY   10Q07ZE   10Q07ZF   10Q07ZG   10Q07ZH   10Q07ZJ
   10Q07ZK   10Q07ZL   10Q07ZM   10Q07ZP   10Q07ZQ   10Q07ZR   10Q07ZS   10Q07ZT   10Q07ZV   10Q07ZY   10Q08YE   10Q08YF
   10Q08YG   10Q08YH   10Q08YJ   10Q08YK   10Q08YL   10Q08YM   10Q08YN   10Q08YP   10Q08YQ   10Q08YR   10Q08YS   10Q08YT   10Q08YV
   10Q08YY   10Q08ZE   10Q08ZF   10Q08ZG   10Q08ZH   10Q08ZJ   10Q08ZK   10Q08ZL   10Q08ZM   10Q08ZN   10Q08ZP   10Q08ZQ   10Q08ZR
   10Q08ZS   10Q08ZT   10Q08ZV   10Q08ZY

LC Limited Coverage   **NC** Noncovered   **HAC** HAC-associated Procedure   **CC** Combination Cluster - See Appendix G for code lists
DRG Non-OR-Affecting MS-DRG Assignment   **QOA** Questionable Obstetric Admission   New/Revised Text in **Orange**   ♂ Male   ♀ Female

2021 ICD-10-PCS

595

OBSTETRICS 102-10Y

1 Obstetrics
0 Pregnancy
S Reposition: Moving to its normal location, or other suitable location, all or a portion of a body part

Body Part	Approach	Device	Qualifier
Character 4	Character 5	Character 6	Character 7
0 Products of Conception ♀	**7** Via Natural or Artificial Opening **X** External	**Z** No Device	**Z** No Qualifier
2 Products of Conception, Ectopic ♀	**0** Open **3** Percutaneous **4** Percutaneous Endoscopic **7** Via Natural or Artificial Opening **8** Via Natural or Artificial Opening Endoscopic	**Z** No Device	**Z** No Qualifier

♀ 10S07ZZ   10S0XZZ   10S20ZZ   10S23ZZ   10S24ZZ   10S27ZZ   10S28ZZ

1 Obstetrics
0 Pregnancy
T Resection: Cutting out or off, without replacement, all of a body part

Body Part	Approach	Device	Qualifier
Character 4	Character 5	Character 6	Character 7
2 Products of Conception, Ectopic ♀	**0** Open **3** Percutaneous **4** Percutaneous Endoscopic **7** Via Natural or Artificial Opening **8** Via Natural or Artificial Opening Endoscopic	**Z** No Device	**Z** No Qualifier

♀ 10T20ZZ   10T23ZZ   10T24ZZ   10T27ZZ   10T28ZZ

1 Obstetrics
0 Pregnancy
Y Transplantation: Putting in or on all or a portion of a living body part taken from another individual or animal to physically take the place and/or function of all or a portion of a similar body part

Body Part	Approach	Device	Qualifier
Character 4	Character 5	Character 6	Character 7
0 Products of Conception ♀	**3** Percutaneous **4** Percutaneous Endoscopic **7** Via Natural or Artificial Opening	**Z** No Device	**E** Nervous System **F** Cardiovascular System **G** Lymphatics and Hemic **H** Eye **J** Ear, Nose and Sinus **K** Respiratory System **L** Mouth and Throat **M** Gastrointestinal System **N** Hepatobiliary and Pancreas **P** Endocrine System **Q** Skin **R** Musculoskeletal System **S** Urinary System **T** Female Reproductive System **V** Male Reproductive System **Y** Other Body System

♀ 10Y03ZE   10Y03ZF   10Y03ZG   10Y03ZH   10Y03ZJ   10Y03ZK   10Y03ZL   10Y03ZM   10Y03ZN   10Y03ZP   10Y03ZQ   10Y03ZR   10Y03ZS
  10Y03ZT   10Y03ZV   10Y03ZY   10Y04ZE   10Y04ZF   10Y04ZG   10Y04ZH   10Y04ZJ   10Y04ZK   10Y04ZL   10Y04ZM   10Y04ZN   10Y04ZP
  10Y04ZQ   10Y04ZR   10Y04ZS   10Y04ZT   10Y04ZV   10Y04ZY   10Y07ZE   10Y07ZF   10Y07ZG   10Y07ZH   10Y07ZJ   10Y07ZK   10Y07ZL
  10Y07ZM   10Y07ZN   10Y07ZP   10Y07ZQ   10Y07ZR   10Y07ZS   10Y07ZT   10Y07ZV   10Y07ZY

NOTES

NOTES

Placement-Anatomical Regions 2W0-2W6

2 Placement
W Anatomical Regions
0 Change: Taking out or off a device from a body part and putting back an identical or similar device in or on the same body part without cutting or puncturing the skin or a mucous membrane

Body Region	Approach	Device	Qualifier
Character 4	**Character 5**	**Character 6**	**Character 7**
0 Head **2** Neck **3** Abdominal Wall **4** Chest Wall **5** Back **6** Inguinal Region, Right **7** Inguinal Region, Left **8** Upper Extremity, Right **9** Upper Extremity, Left **A** Upper Arm, Right **B** Upper Arm, Left **C** Lower Arm, Right **D** Lower Arm, Left **E** Hand, Right **F** Hand, Left **G** Thumb, Right **H** Thumb, Left **J** Finger, Right **K** Finger, Left **L** Lower Extremity, Right **M** Lower Extremity, Left **N** Upper Leg, Right **P** Upper Leg, Left **Q** Lower Leg, Right **R** Lower Leg, Left **S** Foot, Right **T** Foot, Left **U** Toe, Right **V** Toe, Left	**X** External	**0** Traction Apparatus **1** Splint **2** Cast **3** Brace **4** Bandage **5** Packing Material **6** Pressure Dressing **7** Intermittent Pressure Device **Y** Other Device	**Z** No Qualifier
1 Face	**X** External	**0** Traction Apparatus **1** Splint **2** Cast **3** Brace **4** Bandage **5** Packing Material **6** Pressure Dressing **7** Intermittent Pressure Device **9** Wire **Y** Other Device	**Z** No Qualifier

LC Limited Coverage   NC Noncovered   HAC HAC-associated Procedure   CC Combination Cluster - See Appendix G for code lists
Non-OR-Affecting MS-DRG Assignment   New/Revised Text in Orange   ♂ Male   ♀ Female

2 **Placement**
W **Anatomical Regions**
1 **Compression:** Putting pressure on a body region

Body Region	Approach	Device	Qualifier
Character 4	Character 5	Character 6	Character 7
0 Head	X External	6 Pressure Dressing	Z No Qualifier
1 Face		7 Intermittent Pressure Device	
2 Neck			
3 Abdominal Wall			
4 Chest Wall			
5 Back			
6 Inguinal Region, Right			
7 Inguinal Region, Left			
8 Upper Extremity, Right			
9 Upper Extremity, Left			
A Upper Arm, Right			
B Upper Arm, Left			
C Lower Arm, Right			
D Lower Arm, Left			
E Hand, Right			
F Hand, Left			
G Thumb, Right			
H Thumb, Left			
J Finger, Right			
K Finger, Left			
L Lower Extremity, Right			
M Lower Extremity, Left			
N Upper Leg, Right			
P Upper Leg, Left			
Q Lower Leg, Right			
R Lower Leg, Left			
S Foot, Right			
T Foot, Left			
U Toe, Right			
V Toe, Left			

LC Limited Coverage **NC** Noncovered **HAC** HAC-associated Procedure **CC** Combination Cluster - See Appendix G for code lists
DRG Non-OR-Affecting MS-DRG Assignment New/Revised Text in **Orange** ♂ Male ♀ Female

600

2021 ICD-10-PCS

2 Placement
W Anatomical Regions
2 Dressing: Putting material on a body region for protection

Body Region	Approach	Device	Qualifier
Character 4	Character 5	Character 6	Character 7
0 Head	X External	4 Bandage	Z No Qualifier
1 Face			
2 Neck			
3 Abdominal Wall			
4 Chest Wall			
5 Back			
6 Inguinal Region, Right			
7 Inguinal Region, Left			
8 Upper Extremity, Right			
9 Upper Extremity, Left			
A Upper Arm, Right			
B Upper Arm, Left			
C Lower Arm, Right			
D Lower Arm, Left			
E Hand, Right			
F Hand, Left			
G Thumb, Right			
H Thumb, Left			
J Finger, Right			
K Finger, Left			
L Lower Extremity, Right			
M Lower Extremity, Left			
N Upper Leg, Right			
P Upper Leg, Left			
Q Lower Leg, Right			
R Lower Leg, Left			
S Foot, Right			
T Foot, Left			
U Toe, Right			
V Toe, Left			

LC Limited Coverage   **NC** Noncovered   **HAC** HAC-associated Procedure   **CC** Combination Cluster - See Appendix G for code lists
DRG Non-OR-Affecting MS-DRG Assignment   New/Revised Text in **Orange**   ♂ Male   ♀ Female

2021 ICD-10-PCS   601

PLACEMENT-ANATOMICAL REGIONS 2W0-2W6

2 **Placement**
W **Anatomical Regions**
3 **Immobilization:** Limiting or preventing motion of a body region

Body Region	Approach	Device	Qualifier
Character 4	**Character 5**	**Character 6**	**Character 7**
0 Head 2 Neck 3 Abdominal Wall 4 Chest Wall 5 Back 6 Inguinal Region, Right 7 Inguinal Region, Left 8 Upper Extremity, Right 9 Upper Extremity, Left A Upper Arm, Right B Upper Arm, Left C Lower Arm, Right D Lower Arm, Left E Hand, Right F Hand, Left G Thumb, Right H Thumb, Left J Finger, Right K Finger, Left L Lower Extremity, Right M Lower Extremity, Left N Upper Leg, Right P Upper Leg, Left Q Lower Leg, Right R Lower Leg, Left S Foot, Right T Foot, Left U Toe, Right V Toe, Left	**X** External	1 Splint 2 Cast 3 Brace Y Other Device	**Z** No Qualifier
1 Face	**X** External	1 Splint 2 Cast 3 Brace 9 Wire Y Other Device	**Z** No Qualifier

2 Placement
W Anatomical Regions
4 Packing: Putting material in a body region or orifice

Body Region	Approach	Device	Qualifier
Character 4	Character 5	Character 6	Character 7
0 Head	**X** External	**5** Packing Material	**Z** No Qualifier
1 Face			
2 Neck			
3 Abdominal Wall			
4 Chest Wall			
5 Back			
6 Inguinal Region, Right			
7 Inguinal Region, Left			
8 Upper Extremity, Right			
9 Upper Extremity, Left			
A Upper Arm, Right			
B Upper Arm, Left			
C Lower Arm, Right			
D Lower Arm, Left			
E Hand, Right			
F Hand, Left			
G Thumb, Right			
H Thumb, Left			
J Finger, Right			
K Finger, Left			
L Lower Extremity, Right			
M Lower Extremity, Left			
N Upper Leg, Right			
P Upper Leg, Left			
Q Lower Leg, Right			
R Lower Leg, Left			
S Foot, Right			
T Foot, Left			
U Toe, Right			
V Toe, Left			

LC Limited Coverage   **NC** Noncovered   **HAC** HAC-associated Procedure   **CC** Combination Cluster - See Appendix G for code lists
DRG Non-OR-Affecting MS-DRG Assignment   New/Revised Text in **Orange**   ♂ Male   ♀ Female

2021 ICD-10-PCS

603

2 Placement
W Anatomical Regions
5 Removal: Taking out or off a device from a body part

Body Region	Approach	Device	Qualifier
Character 4	**Character 5**	**Character 6**	**Character 7**
0 Head 2 Neck 3 Abdominal Wall 4 Chest Wall 5 Back 6 Inguinal Region, Right 7 Inguinal Region, Left 8 Upper Extremity, Right 9 Upper Extremity, Left A Upper Arm, Right B Upper Arm, Left C Lower Arm, Right D Lower Arm, Left E Hand, Right F Hand, Left G Thumb, Right H Thumb, Left J Finger, Right K Finger, Left L Lower Extremity, Right M Lower Extremity, Left N Upper Leg, Right P Upper Leg, Left Q Lower Leg, Right R Lower Leg, Left S Foot, Right T Foot, Left U Toe, Right V Toe, Left	X External	0 Traction Apparatus 1 Splint 2 Cast 3 Brace 4 Bandage 5 Packing Material 6 Pressure Dressing 7 Intermittent Pressure Device Y Other Device	Z No Qualifier
1 Face	X External	0 Traction Apparatus 1 Splint 2 Cast 3 Brace 4 Bandage 5 Packing Material 6 Pressure Dressing 7 Intermittent Pressure Device 9 Wire Y Other Device	Z No Qualifier

IC Limited Coverage   **NC** Noncovered   **HAC** HAC-associated Procedure   **CC** Combination Cluster - See Appendix G for code lists
DRG Non-OR-Affecting MS-DRG Assignment   New/Revised Text in **Orange**   ♂ Male   ♀ Female

2 Placement
W Anatomical Regions
6 Traction: Exerting a pulling force on a body region in a distal direction

Body Region	Approach	Device	Qualifier
Character 4	Character 5	Character 6	Character 7
0 Head	X External	0 Traction Apparatus	Z No Qualifier
1 Face		Z No Device	
2 Neck			
3 Abdominal Wall			
4 Chest Wall			
5 Back			
6 Inguinal Region, Right			
7 Inguinal Region, Left			
8 Upper Extremity, Right			
9 Upper Extremity, Left			
A Upper Arm, Right			
B Upper Arm, Left			
C Lower Arm, Right			
D Lower Arm, Left			
E Hand, Right			
F Hand, Left			
G Thumb, Right			
H Thumb, Left			
J Finger, Right			
K Finger, Left			
L Lower Extremity, Right			
M Lower Extremity, Left			
N Upper Leg, Right			
P Upper Leg, Left			
Q Lower Leg, Right			
R Lower Leg, Left			
S Foot, Right			
T Foot, Left			
U Toe, Right			
V Toe, Left			

NOTES

Placement-Anatomical Orifices 2Y0-2Y5

2 Placement
Y Anatomical Orifices
0 Change: Taking out or off a device from a body part and putting back an identical or similar device in or on the same body part without cutting or puncturing the skin or a mucous membrane

Body Region	Approach	Device	Qualifier
Character 4	Character 5	Character 6	Character 7
0 Mouth and Pharynx **1** Nasal **2** Ear **3** Anorectal **4** Female Genital Tract ♀ **5** Urethra	**X** External	**5** Packing Material	**Z** No Qualifier

♀ 2Y04X5Z

2 Placement
Y Anatomical Orifices
4 Packing: Putting material in a body region or orifice

Body Region	Approach	Device	Qualifier
Character 4	Character 5	Character 6	Character 7
0 Mouth and Pharynx **1** Nasal **2** Ear **3** Anorectal **4** Female Genital Tract ♀ **5** Urethra	**X** External	**5** Packing Material	**Z** No Qualifier

♀ 2Y44X5Z

2 Placement
Y Anatomical Orifices
5 Removal: Taking out or off a device from a body part

Body Region	Approach	Device	Qualifier
Character 4	Character 5	Character 6	Character 7
0 Mouth and Pharynx **1** Nasal **2** Ear **3** Anorectal **4** Female Genital Tract ♀ **5** Urethra	**X** External	**5** Packing Material	**Z** No Qualifier

♀ 2Y54X5Z

NOTES

Administration 302-3E1

3 **Administration**
0 **Circulatory**
2 **Transfusion:** Putting in blood or blood products

Body System / Region	Approach	Substance	Qualifier
Character 4	**Character 5**	**Character 6**	**Character 7**
3 Peripheral Vein 🔲🔲 4 Central Vein 🔲🔲	0 Open 3 Percutaneous	A Stem Cells, Embryonic	Z No Qualifier
3 Peripheral Vein 🔲 4 Central Vein 🔲	0 Open 3 Percutaneous	C Hematopoietic Stem/Progenitor Cells, Genetically Modified	0 Autologous
3 Peripheral Vein 🔲🔲 4 Central Vein 🔲🔲	0 Open 3 Percutaneous	G Bone Marrow X Stem Cells, Cord Blood Y Stem Cells, Hematopoietic	0 Autologous 2 Allogeneic, Related 3 Allogeneic, Unrelated 4 Allogeneic, Unspecified
3 Peripheral Vein 4 Central Vein	0 Open 3 Percutaneous	H Whole Blood J Serum Albumin K Frozen Plasma L Fresh Plasma M Plasma Cryoprecipitate N Red Blood Cells P Frozen Red Cells Q White Cells R Platelets S Globulin T Fibrinogen V Antihemophilic Factors W Factor IX	0 Autologous 1 Nonautologous
3 Peripheral Vein 🔲 4 Central Vein 🔲	0 Open 3 Percutaneous	U Stem Cells, T-cell Depleted Hematopoietic	2 Allogeneic, Related 3 Allogeneic, Unrelated 4 Allogeneic, Unspecified
7 Products of Conception, Circulatory ♀	3 Percutaneous 7 Via Natural or Artificial Opening	H Whole Blood J Serum Albumin K Frozen Plasma L Fresh Plasma M Plasma Cryoprecipitate N Red Blood Cells P Frozen Red Cells Q White Cells R Platelets S Globulin T Fibrinogen V Antihemophilic Factors W Factor IX	1 Nonautologous
8 Vein	0 Open 3 Percutaneous	B 4-Factor Prothrombin Complex Concentrate	1 Nonautologous

♀ 30273H1 30273J1 30273K1 30273L1 30273M1 30273N1 30273P1 30273Q1 30273R1 30273S1 30273T1 30273V1 30273W1
  30277H1 30277J1 30277K1 30277L1 30277M1 30277N1 30277P1 30277Q1 30277R1 30277S1 30277T1 30277V1 30277W1

🔲 30230AZ 30230G0 30230Y0 30233AZ 30233G0 30233Y0 30240AZ 30240G0 30240Y0 30243AZ 30243G0 30243Y0
Codes in this list are noncovered procedures only when reported with C91.00, C92.00, C92.10, C92.11, C92.40, C92.50, C92.60, C92.A0, C93.00, C94.00, C95.00 as either a principal or secondary diagnosis.

🔲 30230AZ 30230G0 30230G2 30230G3 30230G4 30230U2 30230U3 30230U4 30230X0 30230X2 30230X3 30230X4 30230Y0
  30230Y2 30230Y3 30230Y4 30233AZ 30233G0 30233G2 30233G3 30233U2 30233U3 30233U4 30233X0 30233X2
  30233X3 30233X4 30233Y0 30233Y2 30233Y3 30233Y4 30240AZ 30240G0 30240G2 30240G3 30240G4 30240U2 30240U3
  30240U4 30240X0 30240X2 30240X3 30240X4 30240Y0 30240Y2 30240Y3 30240Y4 30243AZ 30243G0 30243G2 30243G3
  30243G4 30243U2 30243U3 30243U4 30243X0 30243X2 30243X3 30243X4 30243Y0 30243Y2 30243Y3 30243Y4

3 **Administration**
C **Indwelling Device**
1 **Irrigation:** Putting in or on a cleansing substance

Body System / Region	Approach	Substance	Qualifier
Character 4	**Character 5**	**Character 6**	**Character 7**
Z None	X External	8 Irrigating Substance	Z No Qualifier

🔲 Limited Coverage 🔲 Noncovered 🔲 HAC-associated Procedure 🔲 Combination Cluster - See Appendix G for code lists
🔲 Non-OR-Affecting MS-DRG Assignment New/Revised Text in **Orange** ♂ Male ♀ Female

3 **Administration**
E **Physiological Systems and Anatomical Regions**
0 **Introduction:** Putting in or on a therapeutic, diagnostic, nutritional, physiological, or prophylactic substance except blood or blood products

Body System / Region		Approach		Substance		Qualifier	
Character 4		**Character 5**		**Character 6**		**Character 7**	
0	Skin and Mucous Membranes	X	External	0	Antineoplastic	5	Other Antineoplastic
						M	Monoclonal Antibody
0	Skin and Mucous Membranes	X	External	2	Anti-infective	8	Oxazolidinones
						9	Other Anti-infective
0	Skin and Mucous Membranes	X	External	3	Anti-inflammatory	Z	No Qualifier
				4	Serum, Toxoid and Vaccine		
				B	Anesthetic Agent		
				K	Other Diagnostic Substance		
				M	Pigment		
				N	Analgesics, Hypnotics, Sedatives		
				T	Destructive Agent		
0	Skin and Mucous Membranes	X	External	G	Other Therapeutic Substance	C	Other Substance
1	Subcutaneous Tissue	0	Open	2	Anti-infective	A	Anti-Infective Envelope
1	Subcutaneous Tissue	3	Percutaneous	0	Antineoplastic	5	Other Antineoplastic
						M	Monoclonal Antibody
1	Subcutaneous Tissue	3	Percutaneous	2	Anti-infective	8	Oxazolidinones
						9	Other Anti-infective
						A	Anti-Infective Envelope
1	Subcutaneous Tissue	3	Percutaneous	3	Anti-inflammatory	Z	No Qualifier
				6	Nutritional Substance		
				7	Electrolytic and Water Balance Substance		
				B	Anesthetic Agent		
				H	Radioactive Substance		
				K	Other Diagnostic Substance		
				N	Analgesics, Hypnotics, Sedatives		
				T	Destructive Agent		
1	Subcutaneous Tissue	3	Percutaneous	4	Serum, Toxoid and Vaccine	0	Influenza Vaccine
						Z	No Qualifier
1	Subcutaneous Tissue	3	Percutaneous	G	Other Therapeutic Substance	C	Other Substance
1	Subcutaneous Tissue	3	Percutaneous	V	Hormone	G	Insulin
						J	Other Hormone
2	Muscle	3	Percutaneous	0	Antineoplastic	5	Other Antineoplastic
						M	Monoclonal Antibody
2	Muscle	3	Percutaneous	2	Anti-infective	8	Oxazolidinones
						9	Other Anti-infective
2	Muscle	3	Percutaneous	3	Anti-inflammatory	Z	No Qualifier
				6	Nutritional Substance		
				7	Electrolytic and Water Balance Substance		
				B	Anesthetic Agent		
				H	Radioactive Substance		
				K	Other Diagnostic Substance		
				N	Analgesics, Hypnotics, Sedatives		
				T	Destructive Agent		
2	Muscle	3	Percutaneous	4	Serum, Toxoid and Vaccine	0	Influenza Vaccine
						Z	No Qualifier
2	Muscle	3	Percutaneous	G	Other Therapeutic Substance	C	Other Substance
3	Peripheral Vein ᴅʀɢ	0	Open	0	Antineoplastic	2	High-dose Interleukin-2
						3	Low-dose Interleukin-2
						5	Other Antineoplastic
						M	Monoclonal Antibody
						P	Clofarabine

3E0 continued on next page

LC Limited Coverage **NC** Noncovered **HAC** HAC-associated Procedure **CC** Combination Cluster - See Appendix G for code lists
ᴅʀɢ Non-OR-Affecting MS-DRG Assignment New/Revised Text in **Orange** ♂ Male ♀ Female

610

2021 ICD-10-PCS

3 Administration
E Physiological Systems and Anatomical Regions
0 Introduction: Putting in or on a therapeutic, diagnostic, nutritional, physiological, or prophylactic substance except blood or blood products

Body System / Region	Approach	Substance	Qualifier
Character 4	Character 5	Character 6	Character 7
3 Peripheral Vein 🅡🅖	0 Open	1 Thrombolytic	6 Recombinant Human-activated Protein C 7 Other Thrombolytic
3 Peripheral Vein	0 Open	2 Anti-infective	8 Oxazolidinones 9 Other Anti-infective
3 Peripheral Vein	0 Open	3 Anti-inflammatory 4 Serum, Toxoid and Vaccine 6 Nutritional Substance 7 Electrolytic and Water Balance Substance F Intracirculatory Anesthetic H Radioactive Substance K Other Diagnostic Substance N Analgesics, Hypnotics, Sedatives P Platelet Inhibitor R Antiarrhythmic T Destructive Agent X Vasopressor	Z No Qualifier
3 Peripheral Vein	0 Open	G Other Therapeutic Substance	C Other Substance N Blood Brain Barrier Disruption
3 Peripheral Vein 🅡🅖	0 Open	U Pancreatic Islet Cells	0 Autologous 1 Nonautologous
3 Peripheral Vein	0 Open	V Hormone	G Insulin H Human B -type Natriuretic Peptide J Other Hormone
3 Peripheral Vein	0 Open	W Immunotherapeutic	K Immunostimulator L Immunosuppressive
3 Peripheral Vein 🅡🅖	3 Percutaneous	0 Antineoplastic	2 High-dose Interleukin-2 3 Low-dose Interleukin-2 5 Other Antineoplastic M Monoclonal Antibody P Clofarabine
3 Peripheral Vein 🅡🅖	3 Percutaneous	1 Thrombolytic	6 Recombinant Human-activated Protein C 7 Other Thrombolytic
3 Peripheral Vein	3 Percutaneous	2 Anti-infective	8 Oxazolidinones 9 Other Anti-infective
3 Peripheral Vein	3 Percutaneous	3 Anti-inflammatory 4 Serum, Toxoid and Vaccine 6 Nutritional Substance 7 Electrolytic and Water Balance Substance F Intracirculatory Anesthetic H Radioactive Substance K Other Diagnostic Substance N Analgesics, Hypnotics, Sedatives P Platelet Inhibitor R Antiarrhythmic T Destructive Agent X Vasopressor	Z No Qualifier
3 Peripheral Vein	3 Percutaneous	G Other Therapeutic Substance	C Other Substance N Blood Brain Barrier Disruption Q Glucarpidase

3E0 continued on next page

3 Administration
E Physiological Systems and Anatomical Regions
0 Introduction: Putting in or on a therapeutic, diagnostic, nutritional, physiological, or prophylactic substance except blood or blood products

3E0 continued from previous page

Body System / Region	Approach	Substance	Qualifier
Character 4	**Character 5**	**Character 6**	**Character 7**
3 Peripheral Vein DRG	3 Percutaneous	U Pancreatic Islet Cells	0 Autologous 1 Nonautologous
3 Peripheral Vein	3 Percutaneous	V Hormone	G Insulin H Human B-type Natriuretic Peptide J Other Hormone
3 Peripheral Vein	3 Percutaneous	W Immunotherapeutic	K Immunostimulator L Immunosuppressive
4 Central Vein DRG	0 Open	0 Antineoplastic	2 High-dose Interleukin-2 3 Low-dose Interleukin-2 5 Other Antineoplastic M Monoclonal Antibody P Clofarabine
4 Central Vein DRG	0 Open	1 Thrombolytic	6 Recombinant Human-activated Protein C 7 Other Thrombolytic
4 Central Vein	0 Open	2 Anti-infective	8 Oxazolidinones 9 Other Anti-infective
4 Central Vein	0 Open	3 Anti-inflammatory 4 Serum, Toxoid and Vaccine 6 Nutritional Substance 7 Electrolytic and Water Balance Substance F Intracirculatory Anesthetic H Radioactive Substance K Other Diagnostic Substance N Analgesics, Hypnotics, Sedatives P Platelet Inhibitor R Antiarrhythmic T Destructive Agent X Vasopressor	Z No Qualifier
4 Central Vein	0 Open	G Other Therapeutic Substance	C Other Substance N Blood Brain Barrier Disruption
4 Central Vein	0 Open	V Hormone	G Insulin H Human B-type Natriuretic Peptide J Other Hormone
4 Central Vein	0 Open	W Immunotherapeutic	K Immunostimulator L Immunosuppressive
4 Central Vein DRG	3 Percutaneous	0 Antineoplastic	2 High-dose Interleukin-2 3 Low-dose Interleukin-2 5 Other Antineoplastic M Monoclonal Antibody P Clofarabine
4 Central Vein DRG	3 Percutaneous	1 Thrombolytic	6 Recombinant Human-activated Protein C 7 Other Thrombolytic
4 Central Vein	3 Percutaneous	2 Anti-infective	8 Oxazolidinones 9 Other Anti-infective

3E0 continued on next page

LC Limited Coverage   NC Noncovered   HAC HAC-associated Procedure   CC Combination Cluster - See Appendix G for code lists
DRG Non-OR-Affecting MS-DRG Assignment   New/Revised Text in **Orange**   ♂ Male   ♀ Female

3 Administration
E Physiological Systems and Anatomical Regions
0 Introduction: Putting in or on a therapeutic, diagnostic, nutritional, physiological, or prophylactic substance except blood or blood products

3E0 continued from previous page

Body System / Region	Approach	Substance	Qualifier
Character 4	**Character 5**	**Character 6**	**Character 7**
4 Central Vein	**3** Percutaneous	**3** Anti-inflammatory **4** Serum, Toxoid and Vaccine **6** Nutritional Substance **7** Electrolytic and Water Balance Substance **F** Intracirculatory Anesthetic **H** Radioactive Substance **K** Other Diagnostic Substance **N** Analgesics, Hypnotics, Sedatives **P** Platelet Inhibitor **R** Antiarrhythmic **T** Destructive Agent **X** Vasopressor	**Z** No Qualifier
4 Central Vein	**3** Percutaneous	**G** Other Therapeutic Substance	**C** Other Substance **N** Blood Brain Barrier Disruption **Q** Glucarpidase
4 Central Vein	**3** Percutaneous	**V** Hormone	**G** Insulin **H** Human B-type Natriuretic Peptide **J** Other Hormone
4 Central Vein	**3** Percutaneous	**W** Immunotherapeutic	**K** Immunostimulator **L** Immunosuppressive
5 Peripheral Artery ᴰᴿᴳ **6** Central Artery ᴰᴿᴳ	**0** Open **3** Percutaneous	**0** Antineoplastic	**2** High-dose Interleukin-2 **3** Low-dose Interleukin-2 **5** Other Antineoplastic **M** Monoclonal Antibody **P** Clofarabine
5 Peripheral Artery ᴰᴿᴳ **6** Central Artery ᴰᴿᴳ	**0** Open **3** Percutaneous	**1** Thrombolytic	**6** Recombinant Human-activated Protein C **7** Other Thrombolytic
5 Peripheral Artery **6** Central Artery	**0** Open **3** Percutaneous	**2** Anti-infective	**8** Oxazolidinones **9** Other Anti-infective
5 Peripheral Artery **6** Central Artery	**0** Open **3** Percutaneous	**3** Anti-inflammatory **4** Serum, Toxoid and Vaccine **6** Nutritional Substance **7** Electrolytic and Water Balance Substance **F** Intracirculatory Anesthetic **H** Radioactive Substance **K** Other Diagnostic Substance **N** Analgesics, Hypnotics, Sedatives **P** Platelet Inhibitor **R** Antiarrhythmic **T** Destructive Agent **X** Vasopressor	**Z** No Qualifier
5 Peripheral Artery **6** Central Artery	**0** Open **3** Percutaneous	**G** Other Therapeutic Substance	**C** Other Substance **N** Blood Brain Barrier Disruption
5 Peripheral Artery **6** Central Artery	**0** Open **3** Percutaneous	**V** Hormone	**G** Insulin **H** Human B-type Natriuretic Peptide **J** Other Hormone
5 Peripheral Artery **6** Central Artery	**0** Open **3** Percutaneous	**W** Immunotherapeutic	**K** Immunostimulator **L** Immunosuppressive

3E0 continued on next page

3 Administration   **3E0 continued from previous page**

E Physiological Systems and Anatomical Regions

0 **Introduction:** Putting in or on a therapeutic, diagnostic, nutritional, physiological, or prophylactic substance except blood or blood products

Body System / Region	Approach	Substance	Qualifier
Character 4	**Character 5**	**Character 6**	**Character 7**
7 Coronary Artery 8 Heart ᴼᴿᴳ	0 Open 3 Percutaneous	1 Thrombolytic	6 Recombinant Human-activated Protein C 7 Other Thrombolytic
7 Coronary Artery 8 Heart	0 Open 3 Percutaneous	G Other Therapeutic Substance	C Other Substance
7 Coronary Artery 8 Heart	0 Open 3 Percutaneous	K Other Diagnostic Substance P Platelet Inhibitor	Z No Qualifier
7 Coronary Artery 8 Heart	4 Percutaneous Endoscopic	G Other Therapeutic Substance	C Other Substance
9 Nose	3 Percutaneous 7 Via Natural or Artificial Opening X External	0 Antineoplastic	5 Other Antineoplastic M Monoclonal Antibody
9 Nose	3 Percutaneous 7 Via Natural or Artificial Opening X External	2 Anti-infective	8 Oxazolidinones 9 Other Anti-infective
9 Nose	3 Percutaneous 7 Via Natural or Artificial Opening X External	3 Anti-inflammatory 4 Serum, Toxoid and Vaccine B Anesthetic Agent H Radioactive Substance K Other Diagnostic Substance N Analgesics, Hypnotics, Sedatives T Destructive Agent	Z No Qualifier
9 Nose	3 Percutaneous 7 Via Natural or Artificial Opening X External	G Other Therapeutic Substance	C Other Substance
A Bone Marrow	3 Percutaneous	0 Antineoplastic	5 Other Antineoplastic M Monoclonal Antibody
A Bone Marrow	3 Percutaneous	G Other Therapeutic Substance	C Other Substance
B Ear	3 Percutaneous 7 Via Natural or Artificial Opening X External	0 Antineoplastic	4 Liquid Brachytherapy Radioisotope 5 Other Antineoplastic M Monoclonal Antibody
B Ear	3 Percutaneous 7 Via Natural or Artificial Opening X External	2 Anti-infective	8 Oxazolidinones 9 Other Anti-infective
B Ear	3 Percutaneous 7 Via Natural or Artificial Opening X External	3 Anti-inflammatory B Anesthetic Agent H Radioactive Substance K Other Diagnostic Substance N Analgesics, Hypnotics, Sedatives T Destructive Agent	Z No Qualifier
B Ear	3 Percutaneous 7 Via Natural or Artificial Opening X External	G Other Therapeutic Substance	C Other Substance
C Eye	3 Percutaneous 7 Via Natural or Artificial Opening X External	0 Antineoplastic	4 Liquid Brachytherapy Radioisotope 5 Other Antineoplastic M Monoclonal Antibody
C Eye	3 Percutaneous 7 Via Natural or Artificial Opening X External	2 Anti-infective	8 Oxazolidinones 9 Other Anti-infective

3E0 continued on next page

3 **Administration**
E **Physiological Systems and Anatomical Regions**
0 **Introduction:** Putting in or on a therapeutic, diagnostic, nutritional, physiological, or prophylactic substance except blood or blood products

Body System / Region	Approach	Substance	Qualifier
Character 4	Character 5	Character 6	Character 7
C Eye	**3** Percutaneous **7** Via Natural or Artificial Opening **X** External	**3** Anti-inflammatory **B** Anesthetic Agent **H** Radioactive Substance **K** Other Diagnostic Substance **M** Pigment **N** Analgesics, Hypnotics, Sedatives **T** Destructive Agent	**Z** No Qualifier
C Eye	**3** Percutaneous **7** Via Natural or Artificial Opening **X** External	**G** Other Therapeutic Substance	**C** Other Substance
C Eye	**3** Percutaneous **7** Via Natural or Artificial Opening **X** External	**S** Gas	**F** Other Gas
D Mouth and Pharynx	**3** Percutaneous **7** Via Natural or Artificial Opening **X** External	**0** Antineoplastic	**4** Liquid Brachytherapy Radioisotope **5** Other Antineoplastic **M** Monoclonal Antibody
D Mouth and Pharynx	**3** Percutaneous **7** Via Natural or Artificial Opening **X** External	**2** Anti-infective	**8** Oxazolidinones **9** Other Anti-infective
D Mouth and Pharynx	**3** Percutaneous **7** Via Natural or Artificial Opening **X** External	**3** Anti-inflammatory **4** Serum, Toxoid and Vaccine **6** Nutritional Substance **7** Electrolytic and Water Balance Substance **B** Anesthetic Agent **H** Radioactive Substance **K** Other Diagnostic Substance **N** Analgesics, Hypnotics, Sedatives **R** Antiarrhythmic **T** Destructive Agent	**Z** No Qualifier
D Mouth and Pharynx	**3** Percutaneous **7** Via Natural or Artificial Opening **X** External	**G** Other Therapeutic Substance	**C** Other Substance
E Products of Conception ♀ **G** Upper GI **H** Lower GI **K** Genitourinary Tract **N** Male Reproductive ♂	**3** Percutaneous **7** Via Natural or Artificial Opening **8** Via Natural or Artificial Opening Endoscopic	**0** Antineoplastic	**4** Liquid Brachytherapy Radioisotope **5** Other Antineoplastic **M** Monoclonal Antibody
E Products of Conception ♀ **G** Upper GI **H** Lower GI **K** Genitourinary Tract **N** Male Reproductive ♂	**3** Percutaneous **7** Via Natural or Artificial Opening **8** Via Natural or Artificial Opening Endoscopic	**2** Anti-infective	**8** Oxazolidinones **9** Other Anti-infective
E Products of Conception ♀ **G** Upper GI **H** Lower GI **K** Genitourinary Tract **N** Male Reproductive ♂	**3** Percutaneous **7** Via Natural or Artificial Opening **8** Via Natural or Artificial Opening Endoscopic	**3** Anti-inflammatory **6** Nutritional Substance **7** Electrolytic and Water Balance Substance **B** Anesthetic Agent **H** Radioactive Substance **K** Other Diagnostic Substance **N** Analgesics, Hypnotics, Sedatives **T** Destructive Agent	**Z** No Qualifier

3E0 continued on next page

3 **Administration**
E **Physiological Systems and Anatomical Regions**
0 **Introduction:** Putting in or on a therapeutic, diagnostic, nutritional, physiological, or prophylactic substance except blood or blood products

3E0 continued from previous page

Body System / Region	Approach	Substance	Qualifier
Character 4	Character 5	Character 6	Character 7
E Products of Conception ♀ G Upper GI H Lower GI K Genitourinary Tract N Male Reproductive ♂	3 Percutaneous 7 Via Natural or Artificial Opening 8 Via Natural or Artificial Opening Endoscopic	G Other Therapeutic Substance	C Other Substance
E Products of Conception ♀ G Upper GI H Lower GI K Genitourinary Tract N Male Reproductive ♂	3 Percutaneous 7 Via Natural or Artificial Opening 8 Via Natural or Artificial Opening Endoscopic	S Gas	F Other Gas
E Products of Conception ♀ G Upper GI H Lower GI K Genitourinary Tract N Male Reproductive ♂	4 Percutaneous Endoscopic	G Other Therapeutic Substance	C Other Substance
F Respiratory Tract	3 Percutaneous 7 Via Natural or Artificial Opening 8 Via Natural or Artificial Opening Endoscopic	0 Antineoplastic	4 Liquid Brachytherapy Radioisotope 5 Other Antineoplastic M Monoclonal Antibody
F Respiratory Tract	3 Percutaneous 7 Via Natural or Artificial Opening 8 Via Natural or Artificial Opening Endoscopic	2 Anti-infective	8 Oxazolidinones 9 Other Anti-infective
F Respiratory Tract	3 Percutaneous 7 Via Natural or Artificial Opening 8 Via Natural or Artificial Opening Endoscopic	3 Anti-inflammatory 6 Nutritional Substance 7 Electrolytic and Water Balance Substance B Anesthetic Agent H Radioactive Substance K Other Diagnostic Substance N Analgesics, Hypnotics, Sedatives T Destructive Agent	Z No Qualifier
F Respiratory Tract	3 Percutaneous 7 Via Natural or Artificial Opening 8 Via Natural or Artificial Opening Endoscopic	G Other Therapeutic Substance	C Other Substance
F Respiratory Tract	3 Percutaneous 7 Via Natural or Artificial Opening 8 Via Natural or Artificial Opening Endoscopic	S Gas	D Nitric Oxide F Other Gas
F Respiratory Tract	4 Percutaneous Endoscopic	G Other Therapeutic Substance	C Other Substance
J Biliary and Pancreatic Tract	3 Percutaneous 7 Via Natural or Artificial Opening 8 Via Natural or Artificial Opening Endoscopic	0 Antineoplastic	4 Liquid Brachytherapy Radioisotope 5 Other Antineoplastic M Monoclonal Antibody
J Biliary and Pancreatic Tract	3 Percutaneous 7 Via Natural or Artificial Opening 8 Via Natural or Artificial Opening Endoscopic	2 Anti-infective	8 Oxazolidinones 9 Other Anti-infective

3E0 continued on next page

3 Administration

3E0 continued from previous page

E Physiological Systems and Anatomical Regions

0 Introduction: Putting in or on a therapeutic, diagnostic, nutritional, physiological, or prophylactic substance except blood or blood products

Body System / Region	Approach	Substance	Qualifier
Character 4	**Character 5**	**Character 6**	**Character 7**
J Biliary and Pancreatic Tract	**3** Percutaneous **7** Via Natural or Artificial Opening **8** Via Natural or Artificial Opening Endoscopic	**3** Anti-inflammatory **6** Nutritional Substance **7** Electrolytic and Water Balance Substance **B** Anesthetic Agent **H** Radioactive Substance **K** Other Diagnostic Substance **N** Analgesics, Hypnotics, Sedatives **T** Destructive Agent	**Z** No Qualifier
J Biliary and Pancreatic Tract	**3** Percutaneous **7** Via Natural or Artificial Opening **8** Via Natural or Artificial Opening Endoscopic	**G** Other Therapeutic Substance	**C** Other Substance
J Biliary and Pancreatic Tract	**3** Percutaneous **7** Via Natural or Artificial Opening **8** Via Natural or Artificial Opening Endoscopic	**S** Gas	**F** Other Gas
J Biliary and Pancreatic Tract ᴰᴿᴳ	**3** Percutaneous **7** Via Natural or Artificial Opening **8** Via Natural or Artificial Opening Endoscopic	**U** Pancreatic Islet Cells	**0** Autologous **1** Nonautologous
J Biliary and Pancreatic Tract	**4** Percutaneous Endoscopic	**G** Other Therapeutic Substance	**C** Other Substance
L Pleural Cavity	**0** Open	**5** Adhesion Barrier	**Z** No Qualifier
L Pleural Cavity	**3** Percutaneous	**0** Antineoplastic	**4** Liquid Brachytherapy Radioisotope **5** Other Antineoplastic **M** Monoclonal Antibody
L Pleural Cavity	**3** Percutaneous	**2** Anti-infective	**8** Oxazolidinones **9** Other Anti-infective
L Pleural Cavity	**3** Percutaneous	**3** Anti-inflammatory **5** Adhesion Barrier **6** Nutritional Substance **7** Electrolytic and Water Balance Substance **B** Anesthetic Agent **H** Radioactive Substance **K** Other Diagnostic Substance **N** Analgesics, Hypnotics, Sedatives **T** Destructive Agent	**Z** No Qualifier
L Pleural Cavity	**3** Percutaneous	**G** Other Therapeutic Substance	**C** Other Substance
L Pleural Cavity	**3** Percutaneous	**S** Gas	**F** Other Gas
L Pleural Cavity	**4** Percutaneous Endoscopic	**5** Adhesion Barrier	**Z** No Qualifier
L Pleural Cavity	**4** Percutaneous Endoscopic	**G** Other Therapeutic Substance	**C** Other Substance
L Pleural Cavity	**7** Via Natural or Artificial Opening	**0** Antineoplastic	**4** Liquid Brachytherapy Radioisotope **5** Other Antineoplastic **M** Monoclonal Antibody
L Pleural Cavity	**7** Via Natural or Artificial Opening	**S** Gas	**F** Other Gas
M Peritoneal Cavity	**0** Open	**5** Adhesion Barrier	**Z** No Qualifier

3E0 continued on next page

3 **Administration**
E **Physiological Systems and Anatomical Regions**
0 **Introduction:** Putting in or on a therapeutic, diagnostic, nutritional, physiological, or prophylactic substance except blood or blood products

3E0 continued from previous page

Body System / Region	Approach	Substance	Qualifier
Character 4	**Character 5**	**Character 6**	**Character 7**
M Peritoneal Cavity	**3** Percutaneous	**0** Antineoplastic	**4** Liquid Brachytherapy Radioisotope **5** Other Antineoplastic **M** Monoclonal Antibody **Y** Hyperthermic
M Peritoneal Cavity	**3** Percutaneous	**2** Anti-infective	**8** Oxazolidinones **9** Other Anti-infective
M Peritoneal Cavity	**3** Percutaneous	**3** Anti-inflammatory **5** Adhesion Barrier **6** Nutritional Substance **7** Electrolytic and Water Balance Substance **B** Anesthetic Agent **H** Radioactive Substance **K** Other Diagnostic Substance **N** Analgesics, Hypnotics, Sedatives **T** Destructive Agent	**Z** No Qualifier
M Peritoneal Cavity	**3** Percutaneous	**G** Other Therapeutic Substance	**C** Other Substance
M Peritoneal Cavity	**3** Percutaneous	**S** Gas	**F** Other Gas
M Peritoneal Cavity	**4** Percutaneous Endoscopic	**5** Adhesion Barrier	**Z** No Qualifier
M Peritoneal Cavity	**4** Percutaneous Endoscopic	**G** Other Therapeutic Substance	**C** Other Substance
M Peritoneal Cavity	**7** Via Natural or Artificial Opening	**0** Antineoplastic	**4** Liquid Brachytherapy Radioisotope **5** Other Antineoplastic **M** Monoclonal Antibody
M Peritoneal Cavity	**7** Via Natural or Artificial Opening	**S** Gas	**F** Other Gas
P Female Reproductive ♀	**0** Open	**5** Adhesion Barrier	**Z** No Qualifier
P Female Reproductive ♀	**3** Percutaneous	**0** Antineoplastic	**4** Liquid Brachytherapy Radioisotope **5** Other Antineoplastic **M** Monoclonal Antibody
P Female Reproductive ♀	**3** Percutaneous	**2** Anti-infective	**8** Oxazolidinones **9** Other Anti-infective
P Female Reproductive ♀	**3** Percutaneous	**3** Anti-inflammatory **5** Adhesion Barrier **6** Nutritional Substance **7** Electrolytic and Water Balance Substance **B** Anesthetic Agent **H** Radioactive Substance **K** Other Diagnostic Substance **L** Sperm **N** Analgesics, Hypnotics, Sedatives **T** Destructive Agent **V** Hormone	**Z** No Qualifier
P Female Reproductive ♀	**3** Percutaneous	**G** Other Therapeutic Substance	**C** Other Substance
P Female Reproductive ♀	**3** Percutaneous	**Q** Fertilized Ovum	**0** Autologous **1** Nonautologous
P Female Reproductive ♀	**3** Percutaneous	**S** Gas	**F** Other Gas
P Female Reproductive ♀	**4** Percutaneous Endoscopic	**5** Adhesion Barrier	**Z** No Qualifier
P Female Reproductive ♀	**4** Percutaneous Endoscopic	**G** Other Therapeutic Substance	**C** Other Substance

3E0 continued on next page

LC Limited Coverage   NC Noncovered   HAC HAC-associated Procedure   CC Combination Cluster - See Appendix G for code lists
DRG Non-OR-Affecting MS-DRG Assignment   New/Revised Text in Orange   ♂ Male   ♀ Female

3 Administration
E Physiological Systems and Anatomical Regions
0 Introduction: Putting in or on a therapeutic, diagnostic, nutritional, physiological, or prophylactic substance except blood or blood products

3E0 continued from previous page

Body System / Region	Approach	Substance	Qualifier
Character 4	Character 5	Character 6	Character 7
P Female Reproductive ♀	**7** Via Natural or Artificial Opening	**0** Antineoplastic	**4** Liquid Brachytherapy Radioisotope **5** Other Antineoplastic **M** Monoclonal Antibody
P Female Reproductive ♀	**7** Via Natural or Artificial Opening	**2** Anti-infective	**8** Oxazolidinones **9** Other Anti-infective
P Female Reproductive ♀	**7** Via Natural or Artificial Opening	**3** Anti-inflammatory **6** Nutritional Substance **7** Electrolytic and Water Balance Substance **B** Anesthetic Agent **H** Radioactive Substance **K** Other Diagnostic Substance **L** Sperm **N** Analgesics, Hypnotics, Sedatives **T** Destructive Agent **V** Hormone	**Z** No Qualifier
P Female Reproductive ♀	**7** Via Natural or Artificial Opening	**G** Other Therapeutic Substance	**C** Other Substance
P Female Reproductive ♀	**7** Via Natural or Artificial Opening	**Q** Fertilized Ovum	**0** Autologous **1** Nonautologous
P Female Reproductive ♀	**7** Via Natural or Artificial Opening	**S** Gas	**F** Other Gas
P Female Reproductive ♀	**8** Via Natural or Artificial Opening Endoscopic	**0** Antineoplastic	**4** Liquid Brachytherapy Radioisotope **5** Other Antineoplastic **M** Monoclonal Antibody
P Female Reproductive ♀	**8** Via Natural or Artificial Opening Endoscopic	**2** Anti-infective	**8** Oxazolidinones **9** Other Anti-infective
P Female Reproductive ♀	**8** Via Natural or Artificial Opening Endoscopic	**3** Anti-inflammatory **6** Nutritional Substance **7** Electrolytic and Water Balance Substance **B** Anesthetic Agent **H** Radioactive Substance **K** Other Diagnostic Substance **N** Analgesics, Hypnotics, Sedatives **T** Destructive Agent	**Z** No Qualifier
P Female Reproductive ♀	**8** Via Natural or Artificial Opening Endoscopic	**G** Other Therapeutic Substance	**C** Other Substance
P Female Reproductive ♀	**8** Via Natural or Artificial Opening Endoscopic	**S** Gas	**F** Other Gas
Q Cranial Cavity and Brain ᴰᴿᴳ	**0** Open **3** Percutaneous	**0** Antineoplastic	**4** Liquid Brachytherapy Radioisotope **5** Other Antineoplastic **M** Monoclonal Antibody
Q Cranial Cavity and Brain	**0** Open **3** Percutaneous	**2** Anti-infective	**8** Oxazolidinones **9** Other Anti-infective
Q Cranial Cavity and Brain	**0** Open **3** Percutaneous	**3** Anti-inflammatory **6** Nutritional Substance **7** Electrolytic and Water Balance Substance **A** Stem Cells, Embryonic **B** Anesthetic Agent **H** Radioactive Substance **K** Other Diagnostic Substance **N** Analgesics, Hypnotics, Sedatives **T** Destructive Agent	**Z** No Qualifier

3E0 continued on next page

3 Administration
E Physiological Systems and Anatomical Regions
0 Introduction: Putting in or on a therapeutic, diagnostic, nutritional, physiological, or prophylactic substance except blood or blood products

3E0 continued from previous page

Body System / Region	Approach	Substance	Qualifier
Character 4	**Character 5**	**Character 6**	**Character 7**
Q Cranial Cavity and Brain	**0** Open **3** Percutaneous	**E** Stem Cells, Somatic	**0** Autologous **1** Nonautologous
Q Cranial Cavity and Brain	**0** Open **3** Percutaneous	**G** Other Therapeutic Substance	**C** Other Substance
Q Cranial Cavity and Brain	**0** Open **3** Percutaneous	**S** Gas	**F** Other Gas
Q Cranial Cavity and Brain ᴰᴿᴳ	**7** Via Natural or Artificial Opening	**0** Antineoplastic	**4** Liquid Brachytherapy Radioisotope **5** Other Antineoplastic **M** Monoclonal Antibody
Q Cranial Cavity and Brain	**7** Via Natural or Artificial Opening	**S** Gas	**F** Other Gas
R Spinal Canal	**0** Open	**A** Stem Cells, Embryonic	**Z** No Qualifier
R Spinal Canal	**0** Open	**E** Stem Cells, Somatic	**0** Autologous **1** Nonautologous
R Spinal Canal ᴰᴿᴳ	**3** Percutaneous	**0** Antineoplastic	**2** High-dose Interleukin-2 **3** Low-dose Interleukin-2 **4** Liquid Brachytherapy Radioisotope **5** Other Antineoplastic **M** Monoclonal Antibody
R Spinal Canal	**3** Percutaneous	**2** Anti-infective	**8** Oxazolidinones **9** Other Anti-infective
R Spinal Canal	**3** Percutaneous	**3** Anti-inflammatory **6** Nutritional Substance **7** Electrolytic and Water Balance Substance **A** Stem Cells, Embryonic **B** Anesthetic Agent **H** Radioactive Substance **K** Other Diagnostic Substance **N** Analgesics, Hypnotics, Sedatives **T** Destructive Agent	**Z** No Qualifier
R Spinal Canal	**3** Percutaneous	**E** Stem Cells, Somatic	**0** Autologous **1** Nonautologous
R Spinal Canal	**3** Percutaneous	**G** Other Therapeutic Substance	**C** Other Substance
R Spinal Canal	**3** Percutaneous	**S** Gas	**F** Other Gas
R Spinal Canal	**7** Via Natural or Artificial Opening	**S** Gas	**F** Other Gas
S Epidural Space ᴰᴿᴳ	**3** Percutaneous	**0** Antineoplastic	**2** High-dose Interleukin-2 **3** Low-dose Interleukin-2 **4** Liquid Brachytherapy Radioisotope **5** Other Antineoplastic **M** Monoclonal Antibody
S Epidural Space	**3** Percutaneous	**2** Anti-infective	**8** Oxazolidinones **9** Other Anti-infective
S Epidural Space	**3** Percutaneous	**3** Anti-inflammatory **6** Nutritional Substance **7** Electrolytic and Water Balance Substance **B** Anesthetic Agent **H** Radioactive Substance **K** Other Diagnostic Substance **N** Analgesics, Hypnotics, Sedatives **T** Destructive Agent	**Z** No Qualifier
S Epidural Space	**3** Percutaneous	**G** Other Therapeutic Substance	**C** Other Substance

3E0 continued on next page

LC Limited Coverage NC Noncovered HAC HAC-associated Procedure CC Combination Cluster - See Appendix G for code lists
ᴰᴿᴳ Non-OR-Affecting MS-DRG Assignment New/Revised Text in Orange ♂ Male ♀ Female

3 **Administration**
E **Physiological Systems and Anatomical Regions**
0 **Introduction:** Putting in or on a therapeutic, diagnostic, nutritional, physiological, or prophylactic substance except blood or blood products

3E0 continued from previous page

Body System / Region	Approach	Substance	Qualifier
Character 4	Character 5	Character 6	Character 7
S Epidural Space	**3** Percutaneous	**S** Gas	**F** Other Gas
S Epidural Space	**7** Via Natural or Artificial Opening	**S** Gas	**F** Other Gas
T Peripheral Nerves and Plexi **X** Cranial Nerves	**3** Percutaneous	**3** Anti-inflammatory **B** Anesthetic Agent **T** Destructive Agent	**Z** No Qualifier
T Peripheral Nerves and Plexi **X** Cranial Nerves	**3** Percutaneous	**G** Other Therapeutic Substance	**C** Other Substance
U Joints	**0** Open	**2** Anti-infective	**8** Oxazolidinones **9** Other Anti-infective
U Joints	**0** Open	**G** Other Therapeutic Substance	**B** Recombinant Bone Morphogenetic Protein
U Joints	**3** Percutaneous	**0** Antineoplastic	**4** Liquid Brachytherapy Radioisotope **5** Other Antineoplastic **M** Monoclonal Antibody
U Joints	**3** Percutaneous	**2** Anti-infective	**8** Oxazolidinones **9** Other Anti-infective
U Joints	**3** Percutaneous	**3** Anti-inflammatory **6** Nutritional Substance **7** Electrolytic and Water Balance Substance **B** Anesthetic Agent **H** Radioactive Substance **K** Other Diagnostic Substance **N** Analgesics, Hypnotics, Sedatives **T** Destructive Agent	**Z** No Qualifier
U Joints	**3** Percutaneous	**G** Other Therapeutic Substance	**B** Recombinant Bone Morphogenetic Protein **C** Other Substance
U Joints	**3** Percutaneous	**S** Gas	**F** Other Gas
U Joints	**4** Percutaneous Endoscopic	**G** Other Therapeutic Substance	**C** Other Substance
V Bones	**0** Open	**G** Other Therapeutic Substance	**B** Recombinant Bone Morphogenetic Protein
V Bones	**3** Percutaneous	**0** Antineoplastic	**5** Other Antineoplastic **M** Monoclonal Antibody
V Bones	**3** Percutaneous	**2** Anti-infective	**8** Oxazolidinones **9** Other Anti-infective
V Bones	**3** Percutaneous	**3** Anti-inflammatory **6** Nutritional Substance **7** Electrolytic and Water Balance Substance **B** Anesthetic Agent **H** Radioactive Substance **K** Other Diagnostic Substance **N** Analgesics, Hypnotics, Sedatives **T** Destructive Agent	**Z** No Qualifier
V Bones	**3** Percutaneous	**G** Other Therapeutic Substance	**B** Recombinant Bone Morphogenetic Protein **C** Other Substance
W Lymphatics	**3** Percutaneous	**0** Antineoplastic	**5** Other Antineoplastic **M** Monoclonal Antibody
W Lymphatics	**3** Percutaneous	**2** Anti-infective	**8** Oxazolidinones **9** Other Anti-infective

3E0 continued on next page

3 Administration
E Physiological Systems and Anatomical Regions

3E0 continued from previous page

0 Introduction: Putting in or on a therapeutic, diagnostic, nutritional, physiological, or prophylactic substance except blood or blood products

Body System / Region	Approach	Substance	Qualifier
Character 4	**Character 5**	**Character 6**	**Character 7**
W Lymphatics	**3** Percutaneous	**3** Anti-inflammatory **6** Nutritional Substance **7** Electrolytic and Water Balance Substance **B** Anesthetic Agent **H** Radioactive Substance **K** Other Diagnostic Substance **N** Analgesics, Hypnotics, Sedatives **T** Destructive Agent	**Z** No Qualifier
W Lymphatics	**3** Percutaneous	**G** Other Therapeutic Substance	**C** Other Substance
Y Pericardial Cavity	**3** Percutaneous	**0** Antineoplastic	**4** Liquid Brachytherapy Radioisotope **5** Other Antineoplastic **M** Monoclonal Antibody
Y Pericardial Cavity	**3** Percutaneous	**2** Anti-infective	**8** Oxazolidinones **9** Other Anti-infective
Y Pericardial Cavity	**3** Percutaneous	**3** Anti-inflammatory **6** Nutritional Substance **7** Electrolytic and Water Balance Substance **B** Anesthetic Agent **H** Radioactive Substance **K** Other Diagnostic Substance **N** Analgesics, Hypnotics, Sedatives **T** Destructive Agent	**Z** No Qualifier
Y Pericardial Cavity	**3** Percutaneous	**G** Other Therapeutic Substance	**C** Other Substance
Y Pericardial Cavity	**3** Percutaneous	**S** Gas	**F** Other Gas
Y Pericardial Cavity	**4** Percutaneous Endoscopic	**G** Other Therapeutic Substance	**C** Other Substance
Y Pericardial Cavity	**7** Via Natural or Artificial Opening	**0** Antineoplastic	**4** Liquid Brachytherapy Radioisotope **5** Other Antineoplastic **M** Monoclonal Antibody
Y Pericardial Cavity	**7** Via Natural or Artificial Opening	**S** Gas	**F** Other Gas

♀ 3E0E304 3E0E305 3E0E30M 3E0E328 3E0E329 3E0E33Z 3E0E36Z 3E0E37Z 3E0E3BZ 3E0E3GC 3E0E3HZ 3E0E3KZ 3E0E3NZ
  3E0E3SF 3E0E3TZ 3E0E4GC 3E0E704 3E0E705 3E0E70M 3E0E728 3E0E729 3E0E73Z 3E0E76Z 3E0E77Z 3E0E7BZ 3E0E7GC
  3E0E7HZ 3E0E7KZ 3E0E7NZ 3E0E7SF 3E0E7TZ 3E0E804 3E0E805 3E0E80M 3E0E828 3E0E829 3E0E83Z 3E0E86Z 3E0E87Z
  3E0E8BZ 3E0E8GC 3E0E8HZ 3E0E8KZ 3E0E8NZ 3E0E8SF 3E0E8TZ 3E0P05Z 3E0P304 3E0P305 3E0P30M 3E0P328 3E0P329
  3E0P33Z 3E0P35Z 3E0P36Z 3E0P37Z 3E0P3BZ 3E0P3GC 3E0P3HZ 3E0P3KZ 3E0P3LZ 3E0P3NZ 3E0P3Q0 3E0P3Q1 3E0P3SF
  3E0P3TZ 3E0P3VZ 3E0P45Z 3E0P4GC 3E0P704 3E0P705 3E0P70M 3E0P728 3E0P729 3E0P73Z 3E0P76Z 3E0P77Z 3E0P7BZ
  3E0P7GC 3E0P7HZ 3E0P7KZ 3E0P7LZ 3E0P7NZ 3E0P7Q0 3E0P7Q1 3E0P7SF 3E0P7TZ 3E0P7VZ 3E0P804 3E0P805 3E0P80M
  3E0P828 3E0P829 3E0P83Z 3E0P86Z 3E0P87Z 3E0P8BZ 3E0P8GC 3E0P8HZ 3E0P8KZ 3E0P8NZ 3E0P8SF 3E0P8TZ

♂ 3E0N304 3E0N305 3E0N30M 3E0N328 3E0N329 3E0N33Z 3E0N36Z 3E0N37Z 3E0N3BZ 3E0N3GC 3E0N3HZ 3E0N3KZ 3E0N3NZ
  3E0N3SF 3E0N3TZ 3E0N4GC 3E0N704 3E0N705 3E0N70M 3E0N728 3E0N729 3E0N73Z 3E0N76Z 3E0N77Z 3E0N7BZ 3E0N7GC
  3E0N7HZ 3E0N7KZ 3E0N7NZ 3E0N7SF 3E0N7TZ 3E0N804 3E0N805 3E0N80M 3E0N828 3E0N829 3E0N83Z 3E0N86Z 3E0N87Z
  3E0N8BZ 3E0N8GC 3E0N8HZ 3E0N8KZ 3E0N8NZ 3E0N8SF 3E0N8TZ

🄳🅁🄶 3E03002 3E03017 3E030U0 3E030U1 3E03302 3E03317 3E033U0 3E033U1 3E04002 3E04017 3E04302 3E04317 3E05002
  3E05017 3E05302 3E05317 3E06002 3E06017 3E06302 3E06317 3E08017 3E08317 3E0J3U0 3E0J3U1 3E0J7U0 3E0J7U1
  3E0J8U0 3E0J8U1 3E0Q005 3E0Q305 3E0Q705 3E0R302 3E0S302

3 Administration
E Physiological Systems and Anatomical Regions
1 Irrigation: Putting in or on a cleansing substance

Body System / Region	Approach	Substance	Qualifier
Character 4	**Character 5**	**Character 6**	**Character 7**
0 Skin and Mucous Membranes **C** Eye	**3** Percutaneous **X** External	**8** Irrigating Substance	**X** Diagnostic **Z** No Qualifier
9 Nose **B** Ear **F** Respiratory Tract **G** Upper GI **H** Lower GI **J** Biliary and Pancreatic Tract **K** Genitourinary Tract **N** Male Reproductive ♂ **P** Female Reproductive ♀	**3** Percutaneous **7** Via Natural or Artificial Opening **8** Via Natural or Artificial Opening Endoscopic	**8** Irrigating Substance	**X** Diagnostic **Z** No Qualifier
L Pleural Cavity **Q** Cranial Cavity and Brain **R** Spinal Canal **S** Epidural Space **Y** Pericardial Cavity	**3** Percutaneous	**8** Irrigating Substance	**X** Diagnostic **Z** No Qualifier
M Peritoneal Cavity	**3** Percutaneous	**8** Irrigating Substance	**X** Diagnostic **Z** No Qualifier
M Peritoneal Cavity	**3** Percutaneous	**9** Dialysate	**Z** No Qualifier
U Joints	**3** Percutaneous **4** Percutaneous Endoscopic	**8** Irrigating Substance	**X** Diagnostic **Z** No Qualifier

♀ 3E1P38X　3E1P38Z　3E1P78X　3E1P78Z　3E1P88X　3E1P88Z
♂ 3E1N38X　3E1N38Z　3E1N78X　3E1N78Z　3E1N88X　3E1N88Z

LC Limited Coverage　**NC** Noncovered　**HAC** HAC-associated Procedure　**CC** Combination Cluster - See Appendix G for code lists
DRG Non-OR-Affecting MS-DRG Assignment　New/Revised Text in **Orange**　♂ Male　♀ Female

2021 ICD-10-PCS　　　　　　　　　　　　　　　　　　　　　　　　　　　　　　　　**623**

ADMINISTRATION 302-3E1

NOTES

Measurement and Monitoring 4A0-4B0

4 **Measurement and Monitoring**
A **Physiological Systems**
0 **Measurement:** Determining the level of a physiological or physical function at a point in time

Body System	Approach	Function/Device	Qualifier
Character 4	**Character 5**	**Character 6**	**Character 7**
0 Central Nervous	**0** Open	**2** Conductivity **4** Electrical Activity **B** Pressure	**Z** No Qualifier
0 Central Nervous	**3** Percutaneous **7** Via Natural or Artificial Opening **8** Via Natural or Artificial Opening Endoscopic	**4** Electrical Activity	**Z** No Qualifier
0 Central Nervous	**3** Percutaneous **7** Via Natural or Artificial Opening **8** Via Natural or Artificial Opening Endoscopic	**B** Pressure **K** Temperature **R** Saturation	**D** Intracranial
0 Central Nervous	**X** External	**2** Conductivity **4** Electrical Activity	**Z** No Qualifier
1 Peripheral Nervous	**0** Open **3** Percutaneous **7** Via Natural or Artificial Opening **8** Via Natural or Artificial Opening Endoscopic **X** External	**2** Conductivity	**9** Sensory **B** Motor
1 Peripheral Nervous	**0** Open **3** Percutaneous **7** Via Natural or Artificial Opening **8** Via Natural or Artificial Opening Endoscopic **X** External	**4** Electrical Activity	**Z** No Qualifier
2 Cardiac ᴅʀɢ	**0** Open **3** Percutaneous **7** Via Natural or Artificial Opening **8** Via Natural or Artificial Opening Endoscopic	**4** Electrical Activity **9** Output **C** Rate **F** Rhythm **H** Sound **P** Action Currents	**Z** No Qualifier
2 Cardiac ᴅʀɢ	**0** Open **3** Percutaneous **7** Via Natural or Artificial Opening **8** Via Natural or Artificial Opening Endoscopic	**N** Sampling and Pressure	**6** Right Heart **7** Left Heart **8** Bilateral
2 Cardiac	**X** External	**4** Electrical Activity	**A** Guidance **Z** No Qualifier
2 Cardiac	**X** External	**9** Output **C** Rate **F** Rhythm **H** Sound **P** Action Currents	**Z** No Qualifier
2 Cardiac	**X** External	**M** Total Activity	**4** Stress
3 Arterial	**0** Open **3** Percutaneous	**5** Flow **J** Pulse	**1** Peripheral **3** Pulmonary **C** Coronary
3 Arterial	**0** Open **3** Percutaneous	**B** Pressure	**1** Peripheral **3** Pulmonary **C** Coronary **F** Other Thoracic

4A0 continued on next page

ʟᴄ Limited Coverage   ɴᴄ Noncovered   ʜᴀᴄ HAC-associated Procedure   ᴄᴄ Combination Cluster - See Appendix G for code lists
ᴅʀɢ Non-OR-Affecting MS-DRG Assignment   New/Revised Text in **Orange**   ♂ Male   ♀ Female

4 Measurement and Monitoring
A Physiological Systems
0 Measurement: Determining the level of a physiological or physical function at a point in time

4A0 continued from previous page

Body System	Approach	Function/Device	Qualifier
Character 4	Character 5	Character 6	Character 7
3 Arterial	**0** Open **3** Percutaneous	**H** Sound **R** Saturation	**1** Peripheral
3 Arterial	**X** External	**5** Flow	**1** Peripheral **D** Intracranial
3 Arterial	**X** External	**B** Pressure **H** Sound **J** Pulse **R** Saturation	**1** Peripheral
4 Venous	**0** Open **3** Percutaneous	**5** Flow **B** Pressure **J** Pulse	**0** Central **1** Peripheral **2** Portal **3** Pulmonary
4 Venous	**0** Open **3** Percutaneous	**R** Saturation	**1** Peripheral
4 Venous	**4** Percutaneous Endoscopic	**B** Pressure	**2** Portal
4 Venous	**X** External	**5** Flow **B** Pressure **J** Pulse **R** Saturation	**1** Peripheral
5 Circulatory	**X** External	**L** Volume	**Z** No Qualifier
6 Lymphatic	**0** Open **3** Percutaneous **7** Via Natural or Artificial Opening **8** Via Natural or Artificial Opening Endoscopic	**5** Flow **B** Pressure	**Z** No Qualifier
7 Visual	**X** External	**0** Acuity **7** Mobility **B** Pressure	**Z** No Qualifier
8 Olfactory	**X** External	**0** Acuity	**Z** No Qualifier
9 Respiratory	**7** Via Natural or Artificial Opening **8** Via Natural or Artificial Opening Endoscopic **X** External	**1** Capacity **5** Flow **C** Rate **D** Resistance **L** Volume **M** Total Activity	**Z** No Qualifier
B Gastrointestinal	**7** Via Natural or Artificial Opening **8** Via Natural or Artificial Opening Endoscopic	**8** Motility **B** Pressure **G** Secretion	**Z** No Qualifier
C Biliary	**3** Percutaneous **4** Percutaneous Endoscopic **7** Via Natural or Artificial Opening **8** Via Natural or Artificial Opening Endoscopic	**5** Flow **B** Pressure	**Z** No Qualifier
D Urinary	**7** Via Natural or Artificial Opening **8** Via Natural or Artificial Opening Endoscopic	**3** Contractility **5** Flow **B** Pressure **D** Resistance **L** Volume	**Z** No Qualifier
F Musculoskeletal	**3** Percutaneous	**3** Contractility	**Z** No Qualifier
F Musculoskeletal	**3** Percutaneous	**B** Pressure	**E** Compartment
F Musculoskeletal	**X** External	**3** Contractility	**Z** No Qualifier

4A0 continued on next page

4 Measurement and Monitoring
A Physiological Systems
0 Measurement: Determining the level of a physiological or physical function at a point in time

4A0 continued from previous page

Body System	Approach	Function/Device	Qualifier
Character 4	Character 5	Character 6	Character 7
H Products of Conception, Cardiac ♀	**7** Via Natural or Artificial Opening **8** Via Natural or Artificial Opening Endoscopic **X** External	**4** Electrical Activity **C** Rate **F** Rhythm **H** Sound	**Z** No Qualifier
J Products of Conception, Nervous ♀	**7** Via Natural or Artificial Opening **8** Via Natural or Artificial Opening Endoscopic **X** External	**2** Conductivity **4** Electrical Activity **B** Pressure	**Z** No Qualifier
Z None	**7** Via Natural or Artificial Opening	**6** Metabolism **K** Temperature	**Z** No Qualifier
Z None	**X** External	**6** Metabolism **K** Temperature **Q** Sleep	**Z** No Qualifier

♀ 4A0H74Z 4A0H7CZ 4A0H7FZ 4A0H7HZ 4A0H84Z 4A0H8CZ 4A0H8FZ 4A0H8HZ 4A0HX4Z 4A0HXCZ 4A0HXFZ 4A0HXHZ 4A0J72Z
  4A0J74Z 4A0J7BZ 4A0J82Z 4A0J84Z 4A0J8BZ 4A0JX2Z 4A0JX4Z 4A0JXBZ

ᴅᴿɢ 4A020N6 4A020N7 4A020N8 4A023FZ 4A023N6 4A023N7 4A023N8 4A027FZ 4A027N6 4A027N7 4A027N8 4A028FZ 4A028N6
  4A028N7 4A028N8

4 Measurement and Monitoring
A Physiological Systems
1 Monitoring: Determining the level of a physiological or physical function repetitively over a period of time

Body System	Approach	Function/Device	Qualifier
Character 4	Character 5	Character 6	Character 7
0 Central Nervous	**0** Open	**2** Conductivity **B** Pressure	**Z** No Qualifier
0 Central Nervous	**0** Open	**4** Electrical Activity	**G** Intraoperative **Z** No Qualifier
0 Central Nervous	**3** Percutaneous **7** Via Natural or Artificial Opening **8** Via Natural or Artificial Opening Endoscopic	**4** Electrical Activity	**G** Intraoperative **Z** No Qualifier
0 Central Nervous	**3** Percutaneous **7** Via Natural or Artificial Opening **8** Via Natural or Artificial Opening Endoscopic	**B** Pressure **K** Temperature **R** Saturation	**D** Intracranial
0 Central Nervous	**X** External	**2** Conductivity	**Z** No Qualifier
0 Central Nervous	**X** External	**4** Electrical Activity	**G** Intraoperative **Z** No Qualifier
1 Peripheral Nervous	**0** Open **3** Percutaneous **7** Via Natural or Artificial Opening **8** Via Natural or Artificial Opening Endoscopic **X** External	**2** Conductivity	**9** Sensory **B** Motor
1 Peripheral Nervous	**0** Open **3** Percutaneous **7** Via Natural or Artificial Opening **8** Via Natural or Artificial Opening Endoscopic **X** External	**4** Electrical Activity	**G** Intraoperative **Z** No Qualifier

4A1 continued on next page

4 Measurement and Monitoring
A Physiological Systems
1 Monitoring: Determining the level of a physiological or physical function repetitively over a period of time

4A1 continued from previous page

Body System	Approach	Function/Device	Qualifier
Character 4	**Character 5**	**Character 6**	**Character 7**
2 Cardiac	**0** Open **3** Percutaneous **7** Via Natural or Artificial Opening **8** Via Natural or Artificial Opening Endoscopic	**4** Electrical Activity **9** Output **C** Rate **F** Rhythm **H** Sound	**Z** No Qualifier
2 Cardiac	**X** External	**4** Electrical Activity	**5** Ambulatory **Z** No Qualifier
2 Cardiac	**X** External	**9** Output **C** Rate **F** Rhythm **H** Sound	**Z** No Qualifier
2 Cardiac	**X** External	**M** Total Activity	**4** Stress
2 Cardiac	**X** External	**S** Vascular Perfusion	**H** Indocyanine Green Dye
3 Arterial	**0** Open **3** Percutaneous	**5** Flow **B** Pressure **J** Pulse	**1** Peripheral **3** Pulmonary **C** Coronary
3 Arterial	**0** Open **3** Percutaneous	**H** Sound **R** Saturation	**1** Peripheral
3 Arterial	**X** External	**5** Flow **B** Pressure **H** Sound **J** Pulse **R** Saturation	**1** Peripheral
4 Venous	**0** Open **3** Percutaneous	**5** Flow **B** Pressure **J** Pulse	**0** Central **1** Peripheral **2** Portal **3** Pulmonary
4 Venous	**0** Open **3** Percutaneous	**R** Saturation	**0** Central **2** Portal **3** Pulmonary
4 Venous	**X** External	**5** Flow **B** Pressure **J** Pulse	**1** Peripheral
6 Lymphatic	**0** Open **3** Percutaneous **7** Via Natural or Artificial Opening **8** Via Natural or Artificial Opening Endoscopic	**5** Flow	**H** Indocyanine Green Dye **Z** No Qualifier
6 Lymphatic	**0** Open **3** Percutaneous **7** Via Natural or Artificial Opening **8** Via Natural or Artificial Opening Endoscopic	**B** Pressure	**Z** No Qualifier
9 Respiratory	**7** Via Natural or Artificial Opening **X** External	**1** Capacity **5** Flow **C** Rate **D** Resistance **L** Volume	**Z** No Qualifier
B Gastrointestinal	**7** Via Natural or Artificial Opening **8** Via Natural or Artificial Opening Endoscopic	**8** Motility **B** Pressure **G** Secretion	**Z** No Qualifier
B Gastrointestinal	**X** External	**S** Vascular Perfusion	**H** Indocyanine Green Dye

4A1 continued on next page

4 **Measurement and Monitoring**
A **Physiological Systems**
1 **Monitoring:** Determining the level of a physiological or physical function repetitively over a period of time

4A1 continued from previous page

Body System	Approach	Function/Device	Qualifier
Character 4	Character 5	Character 6	Character 7
D Urinary	**7** Via Natural or Artificial Opening **8** Via Natural or Artificial Opening Endoscopic	**3** Contractility **5** Flow **B** Pressure **D** Resistance **L** Volume	**Z** No Qualifier
G Skin and Breast	**X** External	**S** Vascular Perfusion	**H** Indocyanine Green Dye
H Products of Conception, Cardiac ♀	**7** Via Natural or Artificial Opening **8** Via Natural or Artificial Opening Endoscopic **X** External	**4** Electrical Activity **C** Rate **F** Rhythm **H** Sound	**Z** No Qualifier
J Products of Conception, Nervous ♀	**7** Via Natural or Artificial Opening **8** Via Natural or Artificial Opening Endoscopic **X** External	**2** Conductivity **4** Electrical Activity **B** Pressure	**Z** No Qualifier
Z None	**7** Via Natural or Artificial Opening	**K** Temperature	**Z** No Qualifier
Z None	**X** External	**K** Temperature **Q** Sleep	**Z** No Qualifier

♀   4A1H74Z   4A1H7CZ   4A1H7FZ   4A1H7HZ   4A1H84Z   4A1H8CZ   4A1H8FZ   4A1H8HZ   4A1HX4Z   4A1HXCZ   4A1HXFZ   4A1HXHZ   4A1J72Z
    4A1J74Z   4A1J7BZ   4A1J82Z   4A1J84Z   4A1J8BZ   4A1JX2Z   4A1JX4Z   4A1JXBZ

4 **Measurement and Monitoring**
B **Physiological Devices**
0 **Measurement:** Determining the level of a physiological or physical function at a point in time

Body System	Approach	Function/Device	Qualifier
Character 4	Character 5	Character 6	Character 7
0 Central Nervous **1** Peripheral Nervous **F** Musculoskeletal	**X** External	**V** Stimulator	**Z** No Qualifier
2 Cardiac	**X** External	**S** Pacemaker **T** Defibrillator	**Z** No Qualifier
9 Respiratory	**X** External	**S** Pacemaker	**Z** No Qualifier

NOTES

Extracorporeal or Systemic Assistance and Performance 5A0-5A2

5 Extracorporeal or Systemic Assistance and Performance
A Physiological Systems
0 **Assistance:** Taking over a portion of a physiological function by extracorporeal means

Body System	Duration	Function	Qualifier
Character 4	**Character 5**	**Character 6**	**Character 7**
2 Cardiac	**1** Intermittent **2** Continuous	**1** Output	**0** Balloon Pump **5** Pulsatile Compression **6** Other Pump **D** Impeller Pump
5 Circulatory	**1** Intermittent **2** Continuous	**2** Oxygenation	**1** Hyperbaric **C** Supersaturated
9 Respiratory	**2** Continuous	**0** Filtration	**Z** No Qualifier
9 Respiratory	**3** Less than 24 Consecutive Hours **4** 24-96 Consecutive Hours **5** Greater than 96 Consecutive Hours	**5** Ventilation	**7** Continuous Positive Airway Pressure **8** Intermittent Positive Airway Pressure **9** Continuous Negative Airway Pressure **A** High Nasal Flow/Velocity **B** Intermittent Negative Airway Pressure **Z** No Qualifier

5 Extracorporeal or Systemic Assistance and Performance
A Physiological Systems
1 **Performance:** Completely taking over a physiological function by extracorporeal means

Body System	Duration	Function	Qualifier
Character 4	**Character 5**	**Character 6**	**Character 7**
2 Cardiac	**0** Single	**1** Output	**2** Manual
2 Cardiac	**1** Intermittent	**3** Pacing	**Z** No Qualifier
2 Cardiac	**2** Continuous	**1** Output **3** Pacing	**Z** No Qualifier
5 Circulatory ᴼᴿᴳ	**2** Continuous **A** Intraoperative	**2** Oxygenation	**F** Membrane, Central **G** Membrane, Peripheral Veno-arterial **H** Membrane, Peripheral Veno-venous
9 Respiratory	**0** Single	**5** Ventilation	**4** Nonmechanical
9 Respiratory ᴼᴿᴳ	**3** Less than 24 Consecutive Hours **4** 24-96 Consecutive Hours **5** Greater than 96 Consecutive Hours	**5** Ventilation	**Z** No Qualifier
C Biliary	**0** Single **6** Multiple	**0** Filtration	**Z** No Qualifier
D Urinary ᴼᴿᴳ	**7** Intermittent, Less than 6 Hours Per Day **8** Prolonged Intermittent, 6-18 hours Per Day **9** Continuous, Greater than 18 hours Per Day	**0** Filtration	**Z** No Qualifier

ᴼᴿᴳ 5A1522G   5A1522H   5A1935Z   5A1945Z   5A1955Z   5A1D70Z   5A1D80Z   5A1D90Z

5 Extracorporeal or Systemic Assistance and Performance
A Physiological Systems
2 **Restoration:** Returning, or attempting to return, a physiological function to its original state by extracorporeal means.

Body System	Duration	Function	Qualifier
Character 4	**Character 5**	**Character 6**	**Character 7**
2 Cardiac	**0** Single	**4** Rhythm	**Z** No Qualifier

NOTES

Extracorporeal or Systemic Therapies 6A0-6AB

6 Extracorporeal or Systemic Therapies
A Physiological Systems
0 Atmospheric Control: Extracorporeal control of atmospheric pressure and composition

Body System	Duration	Qualifier	Qualifier
Character 4	Character 5	Character 6	Character 7
Z None	**0** Single **1** Multiple	**Z** No Qualifier	**Z** No Qualifier

6 Extracorporeal or Systemic Therapies
A Physiological Systems
1 Decompression: Extracorporeal elimination of undissolved gas from body fluids

Body System	Duration	Qualifier	Qualifier
Character 4	Character 5	Character 6	Character 7
5 Circulatory	**0** Single **1** Multiple	**Z** No Qualifier	**Z** No Qualifier

6 Extracorporeal or Systemic Therapies
A Physiological Systems
2 Electromagnetic Therapy: Extracorporeal treatment by electromagnetic rays

Body System	Duration	Qualifier	Qualifier
Character 4	Character 5	Character 6	Character 7
1 Urinary **2** Central Nervous	**0** Single **1** Multiple	**Z** No Qualifier	**Z** No Qualifier

6 Extracorporeal or Systemic Therapies
A Physiological Systems
3 Hyperthermia: Extracorporeal raising of body temperature

Body System	Duration	Qualifier	Qualifier
Character 4	Character 5	Character 6	Character 7
Z None	**0** Single **1** Multiple	**Z** No Qualifier	**Z** No Qualifier

6 Extracorporeal or Systemic Therapies
A Physiological Systems
4 Hypothermia: Extracorporeal lowering of body temperature

Body System	Duration	Qualifier	Qualifier
Character 4	Character 5	Character 6	Character 7
Z None	**0** Single **1** Multiple	**Z** No Qualifier	**Z** No Qualifier

6 Extracorporeal or Systemic Therapies
A Physiological Systems
5 Pheresis: Extracorporeal separation of blood products

Body System	Duration	Qualifier	Qualifier
Character 4	Character 5	Character 6	Character 7
5 Circulatory	**0** Single **1** Multiple	**Z** No Qualifier	**0** Erythrocytes **1** Leukocytes **2** Platelets **3** Plasma **T** Stem Cells, Cord Blood **V** Stem Cells, Hematopoietic

6 Extracorporeal or Systemic Therapies
A Physiological Systems
6 Phototherapy: Extracorporeal treatment by light rays

Body System	Duration	Qualifier	Qualifier
Character 4	Character 5	Character 6	Character 7
0 Skin **5** Circulatory	**0** Single **1** Multiple	**Z** No Qualifier	**Z** No Qualifier

6 Extracorporeal or Systemic Therapies
A Physiological Systems
7 Ultrasound Therapy: Extracorporeal treatment by ultrasound

Body System Character 4	Duration Character 5	Qualifier Character 6	Qualifier Character 7
5 Circulatory	**0** Single **1** Multiple	**Z** No Qualifier	**4** Head and Neck Vessels **5** Heart **6** Peripheral Vessels **7** Other Vessels **Z** No Qualifier

6 Extracorporeal or Systemic Therapies
A Physiological Systems
8 Ultraviolet Light Therapy: Extracorporeal treatment by ultraviolet light

Body System	Duration	Qualifier	Qualifier
Character 4	Character 5	Character 6	Character 7
0 Skin	**0** Single **1** Multiple	**Z** No Qualifier	**Z** No Qualifier

6 Extracorporeal or Systemic Therapies
A Physiological Systems
9 Shock Wave Therapy: Extracorporeal treatment by shock waves

Body System	Duration	Qualifier	Qualifier
Character 4	Character 5	Character 6	Character 7
3 Musculoskeletal	**0** Single **1** Multiple	**Z** No Qualifier	**Z** No Qualifier

6 Extracorporeal or Systemic Therapies
A Physiological Systems
B Perfusion: Extracorporeal treatment by diffusion of therapeutic fluid

Body System	Duration	Qualifier	Qualifier
Character 4	Character 5	Character 6	Character 7
5 Circulatory **B** Respiratory System **F** Hepatobiliary System and Pancreas **T** Urinary System	**0** Single	**B** Donor Organ	**Z** No Qualifier

---

🄛🄒 Limited Coverage   🄝🄒 Noncovered   🄗🄐🄒 HAC-associated Procedure   🄒🄒 Combination Cluster - See Appendix G for code lists
🄓🄡🄖 Non-OR-Affecting MS-DRG Assignment   New/Revised Text in **Orange**   ♂ Male   ♀ Female

634   **2021 ICD-10-PCS**

NOTES

NOTES

Osteopathic 7W0

7 Osteopathic
W Anatomical Regions
0 Treatment: Manual treatment to eliminate or alleviate somatic dysfunction and related disorders

Body Region	Approach	Method	Qualifier
Character 4	Character 5	Character 6	Character 7
0 Head	X External	0 Articulatory-Raising	Z None
1 Cervical		1 Fascial Release	
2 Thoracic		2 General Mobilization	
3 Lumbar		3 High Velocity-Low Amplitude	
4 Sacrum		4 Indirect	
5 Pelvis		5 Low Velocity-High Amplitude	
6 Lower Extremities		6 Lymphatic Pump	
7 Upper Extremities		7 Muscle Energy-Isometric	
8 Rib Cage		8 Muscle Energy-Isotonic	
9 Abdomen		9 Other Method	

NOTES

Other Procedures 8C0-8E0

8 Other Procedures
C Indwelling Device
0 Other Procedures: Methodologies which attempt to remediate or cure a disorder or disease

Body Region	Approach	Method	Qualifier
Character 4	Character 5	Character 6	Character 7
1 Nervous System	**X** External	**6** Collection	**J** Cerebrospinal Fluid **L** Other Fluid
2 Circulatory System	**X** External	**6** Collection	**K** Blood **L** Other Fluid

8 Other Procedures
E Physiological Systems and Anatomical Regions
0 Other Procedures: Methodologies which attempt to remediate or cure a disorder or disease

Body Region	Approach	Method	Qualifier
Character 4	Character 5	Character 6	Character 7
1 Nervous System **U** Female Reproductive System ♀	**X** External	**Y** Other Method	**7** Examination
2 Circulatory System	**3** Percutaneous **X** External	**D** Near Infrared Spectroscopy	**Z** No Qualifier
9 Head and Neck Region	**0** Open	**C** Robotic Assisted Procedure	**Z** No Qualifier
9 Head and Neck Region	**0** Open	**E** Fluorescence Guided Procedure	**M** Aminolevulinic Acid **Z** No Qualifier
9 Head and Neck Region	**3** Percutaneous **4** Percutaneous Endoscopic **7** Via Natural or Artificial Opening **8** Via Natural or Artificial Opening Endoscopic	**C** Robotic Assisted Procedure **E** Fluorescence Guided Procedure	**Z** No Qualifier
9 Head and Neck Region	**X** External	**B** Computer Assisted Procedure	**F** With Fluoroscopy **G** With Computerized Tomography **H** With Magnetic Resonance Imaging **Z** No Qualifier
9 Head and Neck Region	**X** External	**C** Robotic Assisted Procedure	**Z** No Qualifier
9 Head and Neck Region	**X** External	**Y** Other Method	**8** Suture Removal
H Integumentary System and Breast ♀	**3** Percutaneous	**0** Acupuncture	**0** Anesthesia **Z** No Qualifier
H Integumentary System and Breast	**X** External	**6** Collection	**2** Breast Milk
H Integumentary System and Breast	**X** External	**Y** Other Method	**9** Piercing
K Musculoskeletal System	**X** External	**1** Therapeutic Massage	**Z** No Qualifier
K Musculoskeletal System	**X** External	**Y** Other Method	**7** Examination
V Male Reproductive System ♂	**X** External	**1** Therapeutic Massage	**C** Prostate **D** Rectum
V Male Reproductive System ♂	**X** External	**6** Collection	**3** Sperm
W Trunk Region	**0** Open **3** Percutaneous **4** Percutaneous Endoscopic **7** Via Natural or Artificial Opening **8** Via Natural or Artificial Opening Endoscopic	**C** Robotic Assisted Procedure **E** Fluorescence Guided Procedure	**Z** No Qualifier

8E0 continued on next page

LC Limited Coverage   **NC** Noncovered   **HAC** HAC-associated Procedure   **CC** Combination Cluster - See Appendix G for code lists
DRG Non-OR-Affecting MS-DRG Assignment   New/Revised Text in **Orange**   ♂ Male   ♀ Female

2021 ICD-10-PCS

639

OTHER PROCEDURES 8C0-8E0

8 **Other Procedures**
E **Physiological Systems and Anatomical Regions**

8E0 continued from previous page

0 **Other Procedures:** Methodologies which attempt to remediate or cure a disorder or disease

Body Region	Approach	Method	Qualifier
Character 4	Character 5	Character 6	Character 7
W Trunk Region	**X** External	**B** Computer Assisted Procedure	**F** With Fluoroscopy **G** With Computerized Tomography **H** With Magnetic Resonance Imaging **Z** No Qualifier
W Trunk Region	**X** External	**C** Robotic Assisted Procedure	**Z** No Qualifier
W Trunk Region	**X** External	**Y** Other Method	**8** Suture Removal
X Upper Extremity **Y** Lower Extremity	**0** Open **3** Percutaneous **4** Percutaneous Endoscopic	**C** Robotic Assisted Procedure **E** Fluorescence Guided Procedure	**Z** No Qualifier
X Upper Extremity **Y** Lower Extremity	**X** External	**B** Computer Assisted Procedure	**F** With Fluoroscopy **G** With Computerized Tomography **H** With Magnetic Resonance Imaging **Z** No Qualifier
X Upper Extremity **Y** Lower Extremity	**X** External	**C** Robotic Assisted Procedure	**Z** No Qualifier
X Upper Extremity **Y** Lower Extremity	**X** External	**Y** Other Method	**8** Suture Removal
Z None	**X** External	**Y** Other Method	**1** In Vitro Fertilization **4** Yoga Therapy **5** Meditation **6** Isolation

♀ 8E0HX62   8E0UXY7
♂ 8E0VX1C   8E0VX63

LC Limited Coverage   **NC** Noncovered   **HAC** HAC-associated Procedure   **CC** Combination Cluster - See Appendix G for code lists
DRG Non-OR-Affecting MS-DRG Assignment   New/Revised Text in **Orange**   ♂ Male   ♀ Female

640

2021 ICD-10-PCS

NOTES

NOTES

9 Chiropractic
W Anatomical Regions
B **Manipulation:** Manual procedure that involves a directed thrust to move a joint past the physiological range of motion, without exceeding the anatomical limit

Body Region	Approach	Method	Qualifier
Character 4	Character 5	Character 6	Character 7
0 Head	**X** External	**B** Non-Manual	**Z** None
1 Cervical		**C** Indirect Visceral	
2 Thoracic		**D** Extra-Articular	
3 Lumbar		**F** Direct Visceral	
4 Sacrum		**G** Long Lever Specific Contact	
5 Pelvis		**H** Short Lever Specific Contact	
6 Lower Extremities		**J** Long and Short Lever Specific	
7 Upper Extremities		Contact	
8 Rib Cage		**K** Mechanically Assisted	
9 Abdomen		**L** Other Method	

NOTES

B Imaging
0 Central Nervous System
0 Plain Radiography: Planar display of an image developed from the capture of external ionizing radiation on photographic or photoconductive plate

Body Part	Contrast	Qualifier	Qualifier
Character 4	Character 5	Character 6	Character 7
B Spinal Cord	**0** High Osmolar **1** Low Osmolar **Y** Other Contrast **Z** None	**Z** None	**Z** None

B Imaging
0 Central Nervous System
1 Fluoroscopy: Single plane or bi-plane real time display of an image developed from the capture of external ionizing radiation on a fluorescent screen. The image may also be stored by either digital or analog means

Body Part	Contrast	Qualifier	Qualifier
Character 4	Character 5	Character 6	Character 7
B Spinal Cord	**0** High Osmolar **1** Low Osmolar **Y** Other Contrast **Z** None	**Z** None	**Z** None

B Imaging
0 Central Nervous System
2 Computerized Tomography (CT Scan): Computer reformatted digital display of multiplanar images developed from the capture of multiple exposures of external ionizing radiation

Body Part	Contrast	Qualifier	Qualifier
Character 4	Character 5	Character 6	Character 7
0 Brain **7** Cisterna **8** Cerebral Ventricle(s) **9** Sella Turcica/Pituitary Gland **B** Spinal Cord	**0** High Osmolar **1** Low Osmolar **Y** Other Contrast	**0** Unenhanced and Enhanced **Z** None	**Z** None
0 Brain **7** Cisterna **8** Cerebral Ventricle(s) **9** Sella Turcica/Pituitary Gland **B** Spinal Cord	**Z** None	**Z** None	**Z** None

B Imaging
0 Central Nervous System
3 Magnetic Resonance Imaging (MRI): Computer reformatted digital display of multiplanar images developed from the capture of radiofrequency signals emitted by nuclei in a body site excited within a magnetic field

Body Part	Contrast	Qualifier	Qualifier
Character 4	Character 5	Character 6	Character 7
0 Brain **9** Sella Turcica/Pituitary Gland **B** Spinal Cord **C** Acoustic Nerves	**Y** Other Contrast	**0** Unenhanced and Enhanced **Z** None	**Z** None
0 Brain **9** Sella Turcica/Pituitary Gland **B** Spinal Cord **C** Acoustic Nerves	**Z** None	**Z** None	**Z** None

LC Limited Coverage **NC** Noncovered **HAC** HAC-associated Procedure **CC** Combination Cluster - See Appendix G for code lists
DRG Non-OR-Affecting MS-DRG Assignment New/Revised Text in Orange ♂ Male ♀ Female

2021 ICD-10-PCS　　　　　　　　　　　　　　　　　　　　　　　　　　　　　　　　　　**645**

B **Imaging**
0 **Central Nervous System**
4 **Ultrasonography:** Real time display of images of anatomy or flow information developed from the capture of reflected and attenuated high frequency sound waves

Body Part	Contrast	Qualifier	Qualifier
Character 4	Character 5	Character 6	Character 7
0 Brain **B** Spinal Cord	**Z** None	**Z** None	**Z** None

B **Imaging**
2 **Heart**
0 **Plain Radiography:** Planar display of an image developed from the capture of external ionizing radiation on photographic or photoconductive plate

Body Part	Contrast	Qualifier	Qualifier
Character 4	Character 5	Character 6	Character 7
0 Coronary Artery, Single ᴼᴿᴳ **1** Coronary Arteries, Multiple ᴼᴿᴳ **2** Coronary Artery Bypass Graft, Single ᴼᴿᴳ **3** Coronary Artery Bypass Grafts, Multiple ᴼᴿᴳ **4** Heart, Right ᴼᴿᴳ **5** Heart, Left ᴼᴿᴳ **6** Heart, Right and Left ᴼᴿᴳ **7** Internal Mammary Bypass Graft, Right ᴼᴿᴳ **8** Internal Mammary Bypass Graft, Left ᴼᴿᴳ **F** Bypass Graft, Other ᴼᴿᴳ	**0** High Osmolar **1** Low Osmolar **Y** Other Contrast	**Z** None	**Z** None

ᴼᴿᴳ B2000ZZ   B2001ZZ   B200YZZ   B2010ZZ   B2011ZZ   B201YZZ   B2020ZZ   B2021ZZ   B202YZZ   B2030ZZ   B2031ZZ   B203YZZ   B2040ZZ
B2041ZZ   B204YZZ   B2050ZZ   B2051ZZ   B205YZZ   B2060ZZ   B2061ZZ   B206YZZ   B2070ZZ   B2071ZZ   B207YZZ   B2080ZZ   B2081ZZ
B208YZZ   B20F0ZZ   B20F1ZZ   B20FYZZ

B **Imaging**
2 **Heart**
1 **Fluoroscopy:** Single plane or bi-plane real time display of an image developed from the capture of external ionizing radiation on a fluorescent screen. The image may also be stored by either digital or analog means

Body Part	Contrast	Qualifier	Qualifier
Character 4	Character 5	Character 6	Character 7
0 Coronary Artery, Single **1** Coronary Arteries, Multiple **2** Coronary Artery Bypass Graft, Single **3** Coronary Artery Bypass Grafts, Multiple	**0** High Osmolar **1** Low Osmolar **Y** Other Contrast	**1** Laser	**0** Intraoperative
0 Coronary Artery, Single ᴼᴿᴳ **1** Coronary Arteries, Multiple ᴼᴿᴳ **2** Coronary Artery Bypass Graft, Single ᴼᴿᴳ **3** Coronary Artery Bypass Grafts, Multiple ᴼᴿᴳ	**0** High Osmolar **1** Low Osmolar **Y** Other Contrast	**Z** None	**Z** None
4 Heart, Right ᴼᴿᴳ **5** Heart, Left ᴼᴿᴳ **6** Heart, Right and Left ᴼᴿᴳ **7** Internal Mammary Bypass Graft, Right ᴼᴿᴳ **8** Internal Mammary Bypass Graft, Left ᴼᴿᴳ **F** Bypass Graft, Other ᴼᴿᴳ	**0** High Osmolar **1** Low Osmolar **Y** Other Contrast	**Z** None	**Z** None

ᴼᴿᴳ B2100ZZ   B2101ZZ   B210YZZ   B2110ZZ   B2111ZZ   B211YZZ   B2120ZZ   B2121ZZ   B212YZZ   B2130ZZ   B2131ZZ   B213YZZ   B2140ZZ
B2141ZZ   B214YZZ   B2150ZZ   B2151ZZ   B215YZZ   B2160ZZ   B2161ZZ   B216YZZ   B2170ZZ   B2171ZZ   B217YZZ   B2180ZZ   B2181ZZ
B218YZZ   B21F0ZZ   B21F1ZZ   B21FYZZ

ᴸᶜ Limited Coverage   ᴺᶜ Noncovered   ᴴᴬᶜ HAC-associated Procedure   ᶜᶜ Combination Cluster - See Appendix G for code lists
ᴼᴿᴳ Non-OR-Affecting MS-DRG Assignment   New/Revised Text in **Orange**   ♂ Male   ♀ Female

646   **2021 ICD-10-PCS**

B Imaging
2 Heart
2 Computerized Tomography (CT Scan): Computer reformatted digital display of multiplanar images developed from the capture of multiple exposures of external ionizing radiation

Body Part	Contrast	Qualifier	Qualifier
Character 4	Character 5	Character 6	Character 7
1 Coronary Arteries, Multiple **3** Coronary Artery Bypass Grafts, Multiple **6** Heart, Right and Left	**0** High Osmolar **1** Low Osmolar **Y** Other Contrast	**0** Unenhanced and Enhanced **Z** None	**Z** None
1 Coronary Arteries, Multiple **3** Coronary Artery Bypass Grafts, Multiple **6** Heart, Right and Left	**Z** None	**2** Intravascular Optical Coherence **Z** None	**Z** None

B Imaging
2 Heart
3 Magnetic Resonance Imaging (MRI): Computer reformatted digital display of multiplanar images developed from the capture of radiofrequency signals emitted by nuclei in a body site excited within a magnetic field

Body Part	Contrast	Qualifier	Qualifier
Character 4	Character 5	Character 6	Character 7
1 Coronary Arteries, Multiple **3** Coronary Artery Bypass Grafts, Multiple **6** Heart, Right and Left	**Y** Other Contrast	**0** Unenhanced and Enhanced **Z** None	**Z** None
1 Coronary Arteries, Multiple **3** Coronary Artery Bypass Grafts, Multiple **6** Heart, Right and Left	**Z** None	**Z** None	**Z** None

B Imaging
2 Heart
4 Ultrasonography: Real time display of images of anatomy or flow information developed from the capture of reflected and attenuated high frequency sound waves

Body Part	Contrast	Qualifier	Qualifier
Character 4	Character 5	Character 6	Character 7
0 Coronary Artery, Single **1** Coronary Arteries, Multiple **4** Heart, Right **5** Heart, Left **6** Heart, Right and Left **B** Heart with Aorta **C** Pericardium **D** Pediatric Heart	**Y** Other Contrast	**Z** None	**Z** None
0 Coronary Artery, Single **1** Coronary Arteries, Multiple **4** Heart, Right **5** Heart, Left **6** Heart, Right and Left **B** Heart with Aorta **C** Pericardium **D** Pediatric Heart	**Z** None	**Z** None	**3** Intravascular **4** Transesophageal **Z** None

LC Limited Coverage **NC** Noncovered **HAC** HAC-associated Procedure **CC** Combination Cluster - See Appendix G for code lists
⊘ Non-OR-Affecting MS-DRG Assignment New/Revised Text in **Orange** ♂ Male ♀ Female

2021 ICD-10-PCS

647

IMAGING B00-BY4

B **Imaging**
3 **Upper Arteries**
0 **Plain Radiography:** Planar display of an image developed from the capture of external ionizing radiation on photographic or photoconductive plate

Body Part	Contrast	Qualifier	Qualifier
Character 4	Character 5	Character 6	Character 7
0 Thoracic Aorta **1** Brachiocephalic-Subclavian Artery, Right **2** Subclavian Artery, Left **3** Common Carotid Artery, Right **4** Common Carotid Artery, Left **5** Common Carotid Arteries, Bilateral **6** Internal Carotid Artery, Right **7** Internal Carotid Artery, Left **8** Internal Carotid Arteries, Bilateral **9** External Carotid Artery, Right **B** External Carotid Artery, Left **C** External Carotid Arteries, Bilateral **D** Vertebral Artery, Right **F** Vertebral Artery, Left **G** Vertebral Arteries, Bilateral **H** Upper Extremity Arteries, Right **J** Upper Extremity Arteries, Left **K** Upper Extremity Arteries, Bilateral **L** Intercostal and Bronchial Arteries **M** Spinal Arteries **N** Upper Arteries, Other **P** Thoraco-Abdominal Aorta **Q** Cervico-Cerebral Arch **R** Intracranial Arteries **S** Pulmonary Artery, Right **T** Pulmonary Artery, Left	**0** High Osmolar **1** Low Osmolar **Y** Other Contrast **Z** None	**Z** None	**Z** None

B Imaging
3 Upper Arteries
1 Fluoroscopy: Single plane or bi-plane real time display of an image developed from the capture of external ionizing radiation on a fluorescent screen. The image may also be stored by either digital or analog means

Body Part	Contrast	Qualifier	Qualifier
Character 4	Character 5	Character 6	Character 7
0 Thoracic Aorta 1 Brachiocephalic-Subclavian Artery, Right 2 Subclavian Artery, Left 3 Common Carotid Artery, Right 4 Common Carotid Artery, Left 5 Common Carotid Arteries, Bilateral 6 Internal Carotid Artery, Right 7 Internal Carotid Artery, Left 8 Internal Carotid Arteries, Bilateral 9 External Carotid Artery, Right B External Carotid Artery, Left C External Carotid Arteries, Bilateral D Vertebral Artery, Right F Vertebral Artery, Left G Vertebral Arteries, Bilateral H Upper Extremity Arteries, Right J Upper Extremity Arteries, Left K Upper Extremity Arteries, Bilateral L Intercostal and Bronchial Arteries M Spinal Arteries N Upper Arteries, Other P Thoraco-Abdominal Aorta Q Cervico-Cerebral Arch R Intracranial Arteries S Pulmonary Artery, Right T Pulmonary Artery, Left U Pulmonary Trunk	0 High Osmolar 1 Low Osmolar Y Other Contrast	1 Laser	0 Intraoperative

B31 continued on next page

B Imaging

B31 continued from previous page

3 Upper Arteries

1 Fluoroscopy: Single plane or bi-plane real time display of an image developed from the capture of external ionizing radiation on a fluorescent screen. The image may also be stored by either digital or analog means

Body Part	Contrast	Qualifier	Qualifier
Character 4	Character 5	Character 6	Character 7
0 Thoracic Aorta	0 High Osmolar	Z None	Z None
1 Brachiocephalic-Subclavian Artery, Right	1 Low Osmolar		
2 Subclavian Artery, Left	Y Other Contrast		
3 Common Carotid Artery, Right			
4 Common Carotid Artery, Left			
5 Common Carotid Arteries, Bilateral			
6 Internal Carotid Artery, Right			
7 Internal Carotid Artery, Left			
8 Internal Carotid Arteries, Bilateral			
9 External Carotid Artery, Right			
B External Carotid Artery, Left			
C External Carotid Arteries, Bilateral			
D Vertebral Artery, Right			
F Vertebral Artery, Left			
G Vertebral Arteries, Bilateral			
H Upper Extremity Arteries, Right			
J Upper Extremity Arteries, Left			
K Upper Extremity Arteries, Bilateral			
L Intercostal and Bronchial Arteries			
M Spinal Arteries			
N Upper Arteries, Other			
P Thoraco-Abdominal Aorta			
Q Cervico-Cerebral Arch			
R Intracranial Arteries			
S Pulmonary Artery, Right			
T Pulmonary Artery, Left			
U Pulmonary Trunk			

B31 continued on next page

B Imaging
3 Upper Arteries
1 Fluoroscopy: Single plane or bi-plane real time display of an image developed from the capture of external ionizing radiation on a fluorescent screen. The image may also be stored by either digital or analog means

Body Part	Contrast	Qualifier	Qualifier
Character 4	Character 5	Character 6	Character 7
0 Thoracic Aorta 1 Brachiocephalic-Subclavian Artery, Right 2 Subclavian Artery, Left 3 Common Carotid Artery, Right 4 Common Carotid Artery, Left 5 Common Carotid Arteries, Bilateral 6 Internal Carotid Artery, Right 7 Internal Carotid Artery, Left 8 Internal Carotid Arteries, Bilateral 9 External Carotid Artery, Right B External Carotid Artery, Left C External Carotid Arteries, Bilateral D Vertebral Artery, Right F Vertebral Artery, Left G Vertebral Arteries, Bilateral H Upper Extremity Arteries, Right J Upper Extremity Arteries, Left K Upper Extremity Arteries, Bilateral L Intercostal and Bronchial Arteries M Spinal Arteries N Upper Arteries, Other P Thoraco-Abdominal Aorta Q Cervico-Cerebral Arch R Intracranial Arteries S Pulmonary Artery, Right T Pulmonary Artery, Left U Pulmonary Trunk	Z None	Z None	Z None

B Imaging
3 Upper Arteries
2 Computerized Tomography (CT Scan): Computer reformatted digital display of multiplanar images developed from the capture of multiple exposures of external ionizing radiation

Body Part	Contrast	Qualifier	Qualifier
Character 4	Character 5	Character 6	Character 7
0 Thoracic Aorta 5 Common Carotid Arteries, Bilateral 8 Internal Carotid Arteries, Bilateral G Vertebral Arteries, Bilateral R Intracranial Arteries S Pulmonary Artery, Right T Pulmonary Artery, Left	0 High Osmolar 1 Low Osmolar Y Other Contrast	Z None	Z None
0 Thoracic Aorta 5 Common Carotid Arteries, Bilateral 8 Internal Carotid Arteries, Bilateral G Vertebral Arteries, Bilateral R Intracranial Arteries S Pulmonary Artery, Right T Pulmonary Artery, Left	Z None	2 Intravascular Optical Coherence Z None	Z None

B31 continued from previous page

B Imaging
3 Upper Arteries
3 Magnetic Resonance Imaging (MRI): Computer reformatted digital display of multiplanar images developed from the capture of radiofrequency signals emitted by nuclei in a body site excited within a magnetic field

Body Part	Contrast	Qualifier	Qualifier
Character 4	Character 5	Character 6	Character 7
0 Thoracic Aorta 5 Common Carotid Arteries, Bilateral 8 Internal Carotid Arteries, Bilateral G Vertebral Arteries, Bilateral H Upper Extremity Arteries, Right J Upper Extremity Arteries, Left K Upper Extremity Arteries, Bilateral M Spinal Arteries Q Cervico-Cerebral Arch R Intracranial Arteries	Y Other Contrast	0 Unenhanced and Enhanced Z None	Z None
0 Thoracic Aorta 5 Common Carotid Arteries, Bilateral 8 Internal Carotid Arteries, Bilateral G Vertebral Arteries, Bilateral H Upper Extremity Arteries, Right J Upper Extremity Arteries, Left K Upper Extremity Arteries, Bilateral M Spinal Arteries Q Cervico-Cerebral Arch R Intracranial Arteries	Z None	Z None	Z None

B Imaging
3 Upper Arteries
4 Ultrasonography: Real time display of images of anatomy or flow information developed from the capture of reflected and attenuated high frequency sound waves

Body Part	Contrast	Qualifier	Qualifier
Character 4	Character 5	Character 6	Character 7
0 Thoracic Aorta 1 Brachiocephalic-Subclavian Artery, Right 2 Subclavian Artery, Left 3 Common Carotid Artery, Right 4 Common Carotid Artery, Left 5 Common Carotid Arteries, Bilateral 6 Internal Carotid Artery, Right 7 Internal Carotid Artery, Left 8 Internal Carotid Arteries, Bilateral H Upper Extremity Arteries, Right J Upper Extremity Arteries, Left K Upper Extremity Arteries, Bilateral R Intracranial Arteries S Pulmonary Artery, Right T Pulmonary Artery, Left V Ophthalmic Arteries	Z None	Z None	3 Intravascular Z None

LC Limited Coverage **NC** Noncovered **HAC** HAC-associated Procedure **CC** Combination Cluster - See Appendix G for code lists
DRG Non-OR-Affecting MS-DRG Assignment New/Revised Text in **Orange** ♂ Male ♀ Female

652

2021 ICD-10-PCS

B   Imaging
4   **Lower Arteries**
0   **Plain Radiography:** Planar display of an image developed from the capture of external ionizing radiation on photographic or photoconductive plate

Body Part	Contrast	Qualifier	Qualifier
Character 4	Character 5	Character 6	Character 7
0 Abdominal Aorta 2 Hepatic Artery 3 Splenic Arteries 4 Superior Mesenteric Artery 5 Inferior Mesenteric Artery 6 Renal Artery, Right 7 Renal Artery, Left 8 Renal Arteries, Bilateral 9 Lumbar Arteries B Intra-Abdominal Arteries, Other C Pelvic Arteries D Aorta and Bilateral Lower Extremity Arteries F Lower Extremity Arteries, Right G Lower Extremity Arteries, Left J Lower Arteries, Other M Renal Artery Transplant	0 High Osmolar 1 Low Osmolar Y Other Contrast	Z None	Z None

LC Limited Coverage   **NC** Noncovered   **HAC** HAC-associated Procedure   **CC** Combination Cluster - See Appendix G for code lists
DRG Non-OR-Affecting MS-DRG Assignment   New/Revised Text in **Orange**   ♂ Male   ♀ Female

2021 ICD-10-PCS

653

B   Imaging
4   Lower Arteries
1   Fluoroscopy: Single plane or bi-plane real time display of an image developed from the capture of external ionizing radiation on a fluorescent screen. The image may also be stored by either digital or analog means

Body Part	Contrast	Qualifier	Qualifier
Character 4	Character 5	Character 6	Character 7
0 Abdominal Aorta 2 Hepatic Artery 3 Splenic Arteries 4 Superior Mesenteric Artery 5 Inferior Mesenteric Artery 6 Renal Artery, Right 7 Renal Artery, Left 8 Renal Arteries, Bilateral 9 Lumbar Arteries B Intra-Abdominal Arteries, Other C Pelvic Arteries D Aorta and Bilateral Lower Extremity Arteries F Lower Extremity Arteries, Right G Lower Extremity Arteries, Left J Lower Arteries, Other	0 High Osmolar 1 Low Osmolar Y Other Contrast	1 Laser	0 Intraoperative
0 Abdominal Aorta 2 Hepatic Artery 3 Splenic Arteries 4 Superior Mesenteric Artery 5 Inferior Mesenteric Artery 6 Renal Artery, Right 7 Renal Artery, Left 8 Renal Arteries, Bilateral 9 Lumbar Arteries B Intra-Abdominal Arteries, Other C Pelvic Arteries D Aorta and Bilateral Lower Extremity Arteries F Lower Extremity Arteries, Right G Lower Extremity Arteries, Left J Lower Arteries, Other	0 High Osmolar 1 Low Osmolar Y Other Contrast	Z None	Z None
0 Abdominal Aorta 2 Hepatic Artery 3 Splenic Arteries 4 Superior Mesenteric Artery 5 Inferior Mesenteric Artery 6 Renal Artery, Right 7 Renal Artery, Left 8 Renal Arteries, Bilateral 9 Lumbar Arteries B Intra-Abdominal Arteries, Other C Pelvic Arteries D Aorta and Bilateral Lower Extremity Arteries F Lower Extremity Arteries, Right G Lower Extremity Arteries, Left J Lower Arteries, Other	Z None	Z None	Z None

LC Limited Coverage   **NC** Noncovered   **HAC** HAC-associated Procedure   **CC** Combination Cluster - See Appendix G for code lists
DRG Non-OR-Affecting MS-DRG Assignment   New/Revised Text in **Orange**   ♂ Male   ♀ Female

654

2021 ICD-10-PCS

B   **Imaging**
4   **Lower Arteries**
2   **Computerized Tomography (CT Scan):** Computer reformatted digital display of multiplanar images developed from the capture of multiple exposures of external ionizing radiation

Body Part	Contrast	Qualifier	Qualifier
Character 4	Character 5	Character 6	Character 7
0 Abdominal Aorta **1** Celiac Artery **4** Superior Mesenteric Artery **8** Renal Arteries, Bilateral **C** Pelvic Arteries **F** Lower Extremity Arteries, Right **G** Lower Extremity Arteries, Left **H** Lower Extremity Arteries, Bilateral **M** Renal Artery Transplant	**0** High Osmolar **1** Low Osmolar **Y** Other Contrast	**Z** None	**Z** None
0 Abdominal Aorta **1** Celiac Artery **4** Superior Mesenteric Artery **8** Renal Arteries, Bilateral **C** Pelvic Arteries **F** Lower Extremity Arteries, Right **G** Lower Extremity Arteries, Left **H** Lower Extremity Arteries, Bilateral **M** Renal Artery Transplant	**Z** None	**2** Intravascular Optical Coherence **Z** None	**Z** None

B   **Imaging**
4   **Lower Arteries**
3   **Magnetic Resonance Imaging (MRI):** Computer reformatted digital display of multiplanar images developed from the capture of radiofrequency signals emitted by nuclei in a body site excited within a magnetic field

Body Part	Contrast	Qualifier	Qualifier
Character 4	Character 5	Character 6	Character 7
0 Abdominal Aorta **1** Celiac Artery **4** Superior Mesenteric Artery **8** Renal Arteries, Bilateral **C** Pelvic Arteries **F** Lower Extremity Arteries, Right **G** Lower Extremity Arteries, Left **H** Lower Extremity Arteries, Bilateral	**Y** Other Contrast	**0** Unenhanced and Enhanced **Z** None	**Z** None
0 Abdominal Aorta **1** Celiac Artery **4** Superior Mesenteric Artery **8** Renal Arteries, Bilateral **C** Pelvic Arteries **F** Lower Extremity Arteries, Right **G** Lower Extremity Arteries, Left **H** Lower Extremity Arteries, Bilateral	**Z** None	**Z** None	**Z** None

B **Imaging**
4 **Lower Arteries**
4 **Ultrasonography:** Real time display of images of anatomy or flow information developed from the capture of reflected and attenuated high frequency sound waves

Body Part	Contrast	Qualifier	Qualifier
Character 4	Character 5	Character 6	Character 7
0 Abdominal Aorta **4** Superior Mesenteric Artery **5** Inferior Mesenteric Artery **6** Renal Artery, Right **7** Renal Artery, Left **8** Renal Arteries, Bilateral **B** Intra-Abdominal Arteries, Other **F** Lower Extremity Arteries, Right **G** Lower Extremity Arteries, Left **H** Lower Extremity Arteries, Bilateral **K** Celiac and Mesenteric Arteries **L** Femoral Artery **N** Penile Arteries	**Z** None	**Z** None	**3** Intravascular **Z** None

B **Imaging**
5 **Veins**
0 **Plain Radiography:** Planar display of an image developed from the capture of external ionizing radiation on photographic or photoconductive plate

Body Part	Contrast	Qualifier	Qualifier
Character 4	Character 5	Character 6	Character 7
0 Epidural Veins **1** Cerebral and Cerebellar Veins **2** Intracranial Sinuses **3** Jugular Veins, Right **4** Jugular Veins, Left **5** Jugular Veins, Bilateral **6** Subclavian Vein, Right **7** Subclavian Vein, Left **8** Superior Vena Cava **9** Inferior Vena Cava **B** Lower Extremity Veins, Right **C** Lower Extremity Veins, Left **D** Lower Extremity Veins, Bilateral **F** Pelvic (Iliac) Veins, Right **G** Pelvic (Iliac) Veins, Left **H** Pelvic (Iliac) Veins, Bilateral **J** Renal Vein, Right **K** Renal Vein, Left **L** Renal Veins, Bilateral **M** Upper Extremity Veins, Right **N** Upper Extremity Veins, Left **P** Upper Extremity Veins, Bilateral **Q** Pulmonary Vein, Right **R** Pulmonary Vein, Left **S** Pulmonary Veins, Bilateral **T** Portal and Splanchnic Veins **V** Veins, Other **W** Dialysis Shunt/Fistula	**0** High Osmolar **1** Low Osmolar **Y** Other Contrast	**Z** None	**Z** None

LC Limited Coverage   **NC** Noncovered   **HAC** HAC-associated Procedure   **CC** Combination Cluster - See Appendix G for code lists
DRG Non-OR-Affecting MS-DRG Assignment   New/Revised Text in **Orange**   ♂ Male   ♀ Female

656   **2021 ICD-10-PCS**

B Imaging
5 Veins
1 Fluoroscopy: Single plane or bi-plane real time display of an image developed from the capture of external ionizing radiation on a fluorescent screen. The image may also be stored by either digital or analog means

Body Part	Contrast	Qualifier	Qualifier
Character 4	Character 5	Character 6	Character 7
0 Epidural Veins 1 Cerebral and Cerebellar Veins 2 Intracranial Sinuses 3 Jugular Veins, Right 4 Jugular Veins, Left 5 Jugular Veins, Bilateral 6 Subclavian Vein, Right 7 Subclavian Vein, Left 8 Superior Vena Cava 9 Inferior Vena Cava B Lower Extremity Veins, Right C Lower Extremity Veins, Left D Lower Extremity Veins, Bilateral F Pelvic (Iliac) Veins, Right G Pelvic (Iliac) Veins, Left H Pelvic (Iliac) Veins, Bilateral J Renal Vein, Right K Renal Vein, Left L Renal Veins, Bilateral M Upper Extremity Veins, Right N Upper Extremity Veins, Left P Upper Extremity Veins, Bilateral Q Pulmonary Vein, Right R Pulmonary Vein, Left S Pulmonary Veins, Bilateral T Portal and Splanchnic Veins V Veins, Other W Dialysis Shunt/Fistula	0 High Osmolar 1 Low Osmolar Y Other Contrast Z None	Z None	A Guidance Z None

LC Limited Coverage   **NC** Noncovered   **HAC** HAC-associated Procedure   **CC** Combination Cluster - See Appendix G for code lists
Non-OR-Affecting MS-DRG Assignment   New/Revised Text in **Orange**   ♂ Male   ♀ Female

2021 ICD-10-PCS   **657**

B Imaging
5 Veins
2 **Computerized Tomography (CT Scan):** Computer reformatted digital display of multiplanar images developed from the capture of multiple exposures of external ionizing radiation

Body Part	Contrast	Qualifier	Qualifier
Character 4	Character 5	Character 6	Character 7
2 Intracranial Sinuses **8** Superior Vena Cava **9** Inferior Vena Cava **F** Pelvic (Iliac) Veins, Right **G** Pelvic (Iliac) Veins, Left **H** Pelvic (Iliac) Veins, Bilateral **J** Renal Vein, Right **K** Renal Vein, Left **L** Renal Veins, Bilateral **Q** Pulmonary Vein, Right **R** Pulmonary Vein, Left **S** Pulmonary Veins, Bilateral **T** Portal and Splanchnic Veins	**0** High Osmolar **1** Low Osmolar **Y** Other Contrast	**0** Unenhanced and Enhanced **Z** None	**Z** None
2 Intracranial Sinuses **8** Superior Vena Cava **9** Inferior Vena Cava **F** Pelvic (Iliac) Veins, Right **G** Pelvic (Iliac) Veins, Left **H** Pelvic (Iliac) Veins, Bilateral **J** Renal Vein, Right **K** Renal Vein, Left **L** Renal Veins, Bilateral **Q** Pulmonary Vein, Right **R** Pulmonary Vein, Left **S** Pulmonary Veins, Bilateral **T** Portal and Splanchnic Veins	**Z** None	**2** Intravascular Optical Coherence **Z** None	**Z** None

LC Limited Coverage   **NC** Noncovered   **HAC** HAC-associated Procedure   **CC** Combination Cluster - See Appendix G for code lists
NA Non-OR-Affecting MS-DRG Assignment   New/Revised Text in **Orange**   ♂ Male   ♀ Female

658

2021 ICD-10-PCS

B Imaging

5 Veins

3 Magnetic Resonance Imaging (MRI): Computer reformatted digital display of multiplanar images developed from the capture of radiofrequency signals emitted by nuclei in a body site excited within a magnetic field

Body Part	Contrast	Qualifier	Qualifier
Character 4	Character 5	Character 6	Character 7
1 Cerebral and Cerebellar Veins **2** Intracranial Sinuses **5** Jugular Veins, Bilateral **8** Superior Vena Cava **9** Inferior Vena Cava **B** Lower Extremity Veins, Right **C** Lower Extremity Veins, Left **D** Lower Extremity Veins, Bilateral **H** Pelvic (Iliac) Veins, Bilateral **L** Renal Veins, Bilateral **M** Upper Extremity Veins, Right **N** Upper Extremity Veins, Left **P** Upper Extremity Veins, Bilateral **S** Pulmonary Veins, Bilateral **T** Portal and Splanchnic Veins **V** Veins, Other	**Y** Other Contrast	**0** Unenhanced and Enhanced **Z** None	**Z** None
1 Cerebral and Cerebellar Veins **2** Intracranial Sinuses **5** Jugular Veins, Bilateral **8** Superior Vena Cava **9** Inferior Vena Cava **B** Lower Extremity Veins, Right **C** Lower Extremity Veins, Left **D** Lower Extremity Veins, Bilateral **H** Pelvic (Iliac) Veins, Bilateral **L** Renal Veins, Bilateral **M** Upper Extremity Veins, Right **N** Upper Extremity Veins, Left **P** Upper Extremity Veins, Bilateral **S** Pulmonary Veins, Bilateral **T** Portal and Splanchnic Veins **V** Veins, Other	**Z** None	**Z** None	**Z** None

LC Limited Coverage **NC** Noncovered **HAC** HAC-associated Procedure **CC** Combination Cluster - See Appendix G for code lists
DRG Non-OR-Affecting MS-DRG Assignment New/Revised Text in **Orange** ♂ Male ♀ Female

2021 ICD-10-PCS 659

B Imaging
5 Veins
4 Ultrasonography: Real time display of images of anatomy or flow information developed from the capture of reflected and attenuated high frequency sound waves

Body Part	Contrast	Qualifier	Qualifier
Character 4	Character 5	Character 6	Character 7
3 Jugular Veins, Right **4** Jugular Veins, Left **6** Subclavian Vein, Right **7** Subclavian Vein, Left **8** Superior Vena Cava **9** Inferior Vena Cava **B** Lower Extremity Veins, Right **C** Lower Extremity Veins, Left **D** Lower Extremity Veins, Bilateral **J** Renal Vein, Right **K** Renal Vein, Left **L** Renal Veins, Bilateral **M** Upper Extremity Veins, Right **N** Upper Extremity Veins, Left **P** Upper Extremity Veins, Bilateral **T** Portal and Splanchnic Veins	**Z** None	**Z** None	**3** Intravascular **A** Guidance **Z** None

B Imaging
7 Lymphatic System
0 Plain Radiography: Planar display of an image developed from the capture of external ionizing radiation on photographic or photoconductive plate

Body Part	Contrast	Qualifier	Qualifier
Character 4	Character 5	Character 6	Character 7
0 Abdominal/Retroperitoneal Lymphatics, Unilateral **1** Abdominal/Retroperitoneal Lymphatics, Bilateral **4** Lymphatics, Head and Neck **5** Upper Extremity Lymphatics, Right **6** Upper Extremity Lymphatics, Left **7** Upper Extremity Lymphatics, Bilateral **8** Lower Extremity Lymphatics, Right **9** Lower Extremity Lymphatics, Left **B** Lower Extremity Lymphatics, Bilateral **C** Lymphatics, Pelvic	**0** High Osmolar **1** Low Osmolar **Y** Other Contrast	**Z** None	**Z** None

LC Limited Coverage   NC Noncovered   HAC HAC-associated Procedure   CC Combination Cluster - See Appendix G for code lists
 Non-OR-Affecting MS-DRG Assignment   New/Revised Text in **Orange**   ♂ Male   ♀ Female

660   **2021 ICD-10-PCS**

B   Imaging
8   Eye
0   Plain Radiography: Planar display of an image developed from the capture of external ionizing radiation on photographic or photoconductive plate

Body Part	Contrast	Qualifier	Qualifier
Character 4	Character 5	Character 6	Character 7
0 Lacrimal Duct, Right 1 Lacrimal Duct, Left 2 Lacrimal Ducts, Bilateral	0 High Osmolar 1 Low Osmolar Y Other Contrast	Z None	Z None
3 Optic Foramina, Right 4 Optic Foramina, Left 5 Eye, Right 6 Eye, Left 7 Eyes, Bilateral	Z None	Z None	Z None

B   Imaging
8   Eye
2   Computerized Tomography (CT Scan): Computer reformatted digital display of multiplanar images developed from the capture of multiple exposures of external ionizing radiation

Body Part	Contrast	Qualifier	Qualifier
Character 4	Character 5	Character 6	Character 7
5 Eye, Right 6 Eye, Left 7 Eyes, Bilateral	0 High Osmolar 1 Low Osmolar Y Other Contrast	0 Unenhanced and Enhanced Z None	Z None
5 Eye, Right 6 Eye, Left 7 Eyes, Bilateral	Z None	Z None	Z None

B   Imaging
8   Eye
3   Magnetic Resonance Imaging (MRI): Computer reformatted digital display of multiplanar images developed from the capture of radiofrequency signals emitted by nuclei in a body site excited within a magnetic field

Body Part	Contrast	Qualifier	Qualifier
Character 4	Character 5	Character 6	Character 7
5 Eye, Right 6 Eye, Left 7 Eyes, Bilateral	Y Other Contrast	0 Unenhanced and Enhanced Z None	Z None
5 Eye, Right 6 Eye, Left 7 Eyes, Bilateral	Z None	Z None	Z None

B   Imaging
8   Eye
4   Ultrasonography: Real time display of images of anatomy or flow information developed from the capture of reflected and attenuated high frequency sound waves

Body Part	Contrast	Qualifier	Qualifier
Character 4	Character 5	Character 6	Character 7
5 Eye, Right 6 Eye, Left 7 Eyes, Bilateral	Z None	Z None	Z None

B **Imaging**
9 **Ear, Nose, Mouth and Throat**
0 **Plain Radiography:** Planar display of an image developed from the capture of external ionizing radiation on photographic or photoconductive plate

Body Part	Contrast	Qualifier	Qualifier
Character 4	Character 5	Character 6	Character 7
2 Paranasal Sinuses **F** Nasopharynx/Oropharynx **H** Mastoids	**Z** None	**Z** None	**Z** None
4 Parotid Gland, Right **5** Parotid Gland, Left **6** Parotid Glands, Bilateral **7** Submandibular Gland, Right **8** Submandibular Gland, Left **9** Submandibular Glands, Bilateral **B** Salivary Gland, Right **C** Salivary Gland, Left **D** Salivary Glands, Bilateral	**0** High Osmolar **1** Low Osmolar **Y** Other Contrast	**Z** None	**Z** None

B **Imaging**
9 **Ear, Nose, Mouth and Throat**
1 **Fluoroscopy:** Single plane or bi-plane real time display of an image developed from the capture of external ionizing radiation on a fluorescent screen. The image may also be stored by either digital or analog means

Body Part	Contrast	Qualifier	Qualifier
Character 4	Character 5	Character 6	Character 7
G Pharynx and Epiglottis **J** Larynx	**Y** Other Contrast **Z** None	**Z** None	**Z** None

B **Imaging**
9 **Ear, Nose, Mouth and Throat**
2 **Computerized Tomography (CT Scan):** Computer reformatted digital display of multiplanar images developed from the capture of multiple exposures of external ionizing radiation

Body Part	Contrast	Qualifier	Qualifier
Character 4	Character 5	Character 6	Character 7
0 Ear **2** Paranasal Sinuses **6** Parotid Glands, Bilateral **9** Submandibular Glands, Bilateral **D** Salivary Glands, Bilateral **F** Nasopharynx/Oropharynx **J** Larynx	**0** High Osmolar **1** Low Osmolar **Y** Other Contrast	**0** Unenhanced and Enhanced **Z** None	**Z** None
0 Ear **2** Paranasal Sinuses **6** Parotid Glands, Bilateral **9** Submandibular Glands, Bilateral **D** Salivary Glands, Bilateral **F** Nasopharynx/Oropharynx **J** Larynx	**Z** None	**Z** None	**Z** None

---

B Imaging
9 Ear, Nose, Mouth and Throat
3 Magnetic Resonance Imaging (MRI): Computer reformatted digital display of multiplanar images developed from the capture of radiofrequency signals emitted by nuclei in a body site excited within a magnetic field

Body Part	Contrast	Qualifier	Qualifier
Character 4	Character 5	Character 6	Character 7
0 Ear **2** Paranasal Sinuses **6** Parotid Glands, Bilateral **9** Submandibular Glands, Bilateral **D** Salivary Glands, Bilateral **F** Nasopharynx/Oropharynx **J** Larynx	**Y** Other Contrast	**0** Unenhanced and Enhanced **Z** None	**Z** None
0 Ear **2** Paranasal Sinuses **6** Parotid Glands, Bilateral **9** Submandibular Glands, Bilateral **D** Salivary Glands, Bilateral **F** Nasopharynx/Oropharynx **J** Larynx	**Z** None	**Z** None	**Z** None

B Imaging
B Respiratory System
0 Plain Radiography: Planar display of an image developed from the capture of external ionizing radiation on photographic or photoconductive plate

Body Part	Contrast	Qualifier	Qualifier
Character 4	Character 5	Character 6	Character 7
7 Tracheobronchial Tree, Right **8** Tracheobronchial Tree, Left **9** Tracheobronchial Trees, Bilateral	**Y** Other Contrast	**Z** None	**Z** None
D Upper Airways	**Z** None	**Z** None	**Z** None

B Imaging
B Respiratory System
1 Fluoroscopy: Single plane or bi-plane real time display of an image developed from the capture of external ionizing radiation on a fluorescent screen. The image may also be stored by either digital or analog means

Body Part	Contrast	Qualifier	Qualifier
Character 4	Character 5	Character 6	Character 7
2 Lung, Right **3** Lung, Left **4** Lungs, Bilateral **6** Diaphragm **C** Mediastinum **D** Upper Airways	**Z** None	**Z** None	**Z** None
7 Tracheobronchial Tree, Right **8** Tracheobronchial Tree, Left **9** Tracheobronchial Trees, Bilateral	**Y** Other Contrast	**Z** None	**Z** None

B   **Imaging**
B   **Respiratory System**
2   **Computerized Tomography (CT Scan):** Computer reformatted digital display of multiplanar images developed from the capture of multiple exposures of external ionizing radiation

Body Part	Contrast	Qualifier	Qualifier
Character 4	Character 5	Character 6	Character 7
4 Lungs, Bilateral **7** Tracheobronchial Tree, Right **8** Tracheobronchial Tree, Left **9** Tracheobronchial Trees, Bilateral **F** Trachea/Airways	**0** High Osmolar **1** Low Osmolar **Y** Other Contrast	**0** Unenhanced and Enhanced **Z** None	**Z** None
4 Lungs, Bilateral **7** Tracheobronchial Tree, Right **8** Tracheobronchial Tree, Left **9** Tracheobronchial Trees, Bilateral **F** Trachea/Airways	**Z** None	**Z** None	**Z** None

B   **Imaging**
B   **Respiratory System**
3   **Magnetic Resonance Imaging (MRI):** Computer reformatted digital display of multiplanar images developed from the capture of radiofrequency signals emitted by nuclei in a body site excited within a magnetic field

Body Part	Contrast	Qualifier	Qualifier
Character 4	Character 5	Character 6	Character 7
G Lung Apices	**Y** Other Contrast	**0** Unenhanced and Enhanced **Z** None	**Z** None
G Lung Apices	**Z** None	**Z** None	**Z** None

B   **Imaging**
B   **Respiratory System**
4   **Ultrasonography:** Real time display of images of anatomy or flow information developed from the capture of reflected and attenuated high frequency sound waves

Body Part	Contrast	Qualifier	Qualifier
Character 4	Character 5	Character 6	Character 7
B Pleura **C** Mediastinum	**Z** None	**Z** None	**Z** None

B   **Imaging**
D   **Gastrointestinal System**
1   **Fluoroscopy:** Single plane or bi-plane real time display of an image developed from the capture of external ionizing radiation on a fluorescent screen. The image may also be stored by either digital or analog means

Body Part	Contrast	Qualifier	Qualifier
Character 4	Character 5	Character 6	Character 7
1 Esophagus **2** Stomach **3** Small Bowel **4** Colon **5** Upper GI **6** Upper GI and Small Bowel **9** Duodenum **B** Mouth/Oropharynx	**Y** Other Contrast **Z** None	**Z** None	**Z** None

Limited Coverage   **Noncovered**   **HAC-associated Procedure**   **Combination Cluster - See Appendix G for code lists**
Non-OR-Affecting MS-DRG Assignment   New/Revised Text in **Orange**   ♂ Male   ♀ Female

664   **2021 ICD-10-PCS**

B **Imaging**
D **Gastrointestinal System**
2 **Computerized Tomography (CT Scan):** Computer reformatted digital display of multiplanar images developed from the capture of multiple exposures of external ionizing radiation

Body Part	Contrast	Qualifier	Qualifier
Character 4	Character 5	Character 6	Character 7
4 Colon	**0** High Osmolar **1** Low Osmolar **Y** Other Contrast	**0** Unenhanced and Enhanced **Z** None	**Z** None
4 Colon	**Z** None	**Z** None	**Z** None

B **Imaging**
D **Gastrointestinal System**
4 **Ultrasonography:** Real time display of images of anatomy or flow information developed from the capture of reflected and attenuated high frequency sound waves

Body Part	Contrast	Qualifier	Qualifier
Character 4	Character 5	Character 6	Character 7
1 Esophagus **2** Stomach **7** Gastrointestinal Tract **8** Appendix **9** Duodenum **C** Rectum	**Z** None	**Z** None	**Z** None

B **Imaging**
F **Hepatobiliary System and Pancreas**
0 **Plain Radiography:** Planar display of an image developed from the capture of external ionizing radiation on photographic or photoconductive plate

Body Part	Contrast	Qualifier	Qualifier
Character 4	Character 5	Character 6	Character 7
0 Bile Ducts **3** Gallbladder and Bile Ducts **C** Hepatobiliary System, All	**0** High Osmolar **1** Low Osmolar **Y** Other Contrast	**Z** None	**Z** None

B **Imaging**
F **Hepatobiliary System and Pancreas**
1 **Fluoroscopy:** Single plane or bi-plane real time display of an image developed from the capture of external ionizing radiation on a fluorescent screen. The image may also be stored by either digital or analog means

Body Part	Contrast	Qualifier	Qualifier
Character 4	Character 5	Character 6	Character 7
0 Bile Ducts **1** Biliary and Pancreatic Ducts **2** Gallbladder **3** Gallbladder and Bile Ducts **4** Gallbladder, Bile Ducts and Pancreatic Ducts **8** Pancreatic Ducts	**0** High Osmolar **1** Low Osmolar **Y** Other Contrast	**Z** None	**Z** None

B **Imaging**
F **Hepatobiliary System and Pancreas**
2 **Computerized Tomography (CT Scan):** Computer reformatted digital display of multiplanar images developed from the capture of multiple exposures of external ionizing radiation

Body Part	Contrast	Qualifier	Qualifier
Character 4	Character 5	Character 6	Character 7
5 Liver **6** Liver and Spleen **7** Pancreas **C** Hepatobiliary System, All	**0** High Osmolar **1** Low Osmolar **Y** Other Contrast	**0** Unenhanced and Enhanced **Z** None	**Z** None
5 Liver **6** Liver and Spleen **7** Pancreas **C** Hepatobiliary System, All	**Z** None	**Z** None	**Z** None

B Imaging
F Hepatobiliary System and Pancreas
3 Magnetic Resonance Imaging (MRI): Computer reformatted digital display of multiplanar images developed from the capture of radiofrequency signals emitted by nuclei in a body site excited within a magnetic field

Body Part	Contrast	Qualifier	Qualifier
Character 4	Character 5	Character 6	Character 7
5 Liver 6 Liver and Spleen 7 Pancreas	Y Other Contrast	0 Unenhanced and Enhanced Z None	Z None
5 Liver 6 Liver and Spleen 7 Pancreas	Z None	Z None	Z None

B Imaging
F Hepatobiliary System and Pancreas
4 Ultrasonography: Real time display of images of anatomy or flow information developed from the capture of reflected and attenuated high frequency sound waves

Body Part	Contrast	Qualifier	Qualifier
Character 4	Character 5	Character 6	Character 7
0 Bile Ducts 2 Gallbladder 3 Gallbladder and Bile Ducts 5 Liver 6 Liver and Spleen 7 Pancreas C Hepatobiliary System, All	Z None	Z None	Z None

B Imaging
F Hepatobiliary System and Pancreas
5 Other Imaging: Other specified modality for visualizing a body part

Body Part	Contrast	Qualifier	Qualifier
Character 4	Character 5	Character 6	Character 7
0 Bile Ducts 2 Gallbladder 3 Gallbladder and Bile Ducts 5 Liver 6 Liver and Spleen 7 Pancreas C Hepatobiliary System, All	2 Fluorescing Agent	0 Indocyanine Green Dye Z None	0 Intraoperative Z None

B Imaging
G Endocrine System
2 Computerized Tomography (CT Scan): Computer reformatted digital display of multiplanar images developed from the capture of multiple exposures of external ionizing radiation

Body Part	Contrast	Qualifier	Qualifier
Character 4	Character 5	Character 6	Character 7
2 Adrenal Glands, Bilateral 3 Parathyroid Glands 4 Thyroid Gland	0 High Osmolar 1 Low Osmolar Y Other Contrast	0 Unenhanced and Enhanced Z None	Z None
2 Adrenal Glands, Bilateral 3 Parathyroid Glands 4 Thyroid Gland	Z None	Z None	Z None

B Imaging
G Endocrine System
3 **Magnetic Resonance Imaging (MRI):** Computer reformatted digital display of multiplanar images developed from the capture of radiofrequency signals emitted by nuclei in a body site excited within a magnetic field

Body Part	Contrast	Qualifier	Qualifier
Character 4	Character 5	Character 6	Character 7
2 Adrenal Glands, Bilateral **3** Parathyroid Glands **4** Thyroid Gland	**Y** Other Contrast	**0** Unenhanced and Enhanced **Z** None	**Z** None
2 Adrenal Glands, Bilateral **3** Parathyroid Glands **4** Thyroid Gland	**Z** None	**Z** None	**Z** None

B Imaging
G Endocrine System
4 **Ultrasonography:** Real time display of images of anatomy or flow information developed from the capture of reflected and attenuated high frequency sound waves

Body Part	Contrast	Qualifier	Qualifier
Character 4	Character 5	Character 6	Character 7
0 Adrenal Gland, Right **1** Adrenal Gland, Left **2** Adrenal Glands, Bilateral **3** Parathyroid Glands **4** Thyroid Gland	**Z** None	**Z** None	**Z** None

B Imaging
H Skin, Subcutaneous Tissue and Breast
0 **Plain Radiography:** Planar display of an image developed from the capture of external ionizing radiation on photographic or photoconductive plate

Body Part	Contrast	Qualifier	Qualifier
Character 4	Character 5	Character 6	Character 7
0 Breast, Right **1** Breast, Left **2** Breasts, Bilateral	**Z** None	**Z** None	**Z** None
3 Single Mammary Duct, Right **4** Single Mammary Duct, Left **5** Multiple Mammary Ducts, Right **6** Multiple Mammary Ducts, Left	**0** High Osmolar **1** Low Osmolar **Y** Other Contrast **Z** None	**Z** None	**Z** None

B Imaging
H Skin, Subcutaneous Tissue and Breast
3 **Magnetic Resonance Imaging (MRI):** Computer reformatted digital display of multiplanar images developed from the capture of radiofrequency signals emitted by nuclei in a body site excited within a magnetic field

Body Part	Contrast	Qualifier	Qualifier
Character 4	Character 5	Character 6	Character 7
0 Breast, Right **1** Breast, Left **2** Breasts, Bilateral **D** Subcutaneous Tissue, Head/Neck **F** Subcutaneous Tissue, Upper Extremity **G** Subcutaneous Tissue, Thorax **H** Subcutaneous Tissue, Abdomen and Pelvis **J** Subcutaneous Tissue, Lower Extremity	**Y** Other Contrast	**0** Unenhanced and Enhanced **Z** None	**Z** None
0 Breast, Right **1** Breast, Left **2** Breasts, Bilateral **D** Subcutaneous Tissue, Head/Neck **F** Subcutaneous Tissue, Upper Extremity **G** Subcutaneous Tissue, Thorax **H** Subcutaneous Tissue, Abdomen and Pelvis **J** Subcutaneous Tissue, Lower Extremity	**Z** None	**Z** None	**Z** None

B Imaging
H Skin, Subcutaneous Tissue and Breast
4 **Ultrasonography:** Real time display of images of anatomy or flow information developed from the capture of reflected and attenuated high frequency sound waves

Body Part	Contrast	Qualifier	Qualifier
Character 4	Character 5	Character 6	Character 7
0 Breast, Right **1** Breast, Left **2** Breasts, Bilateral **7** Extremity, Upper **8** Extremity, Lower **9** Abdominal Wall **B** Chest Wall **C** Head and Neck	**Z** None	**Z** None	**Z** None

B **Imaging**
L **Connective Tissue**
3 **Magnetic Resonance Imaging (MRI):** Computer reformatted digital display of multiplanar images developed from the capture of radiofrequency signals emitted by nuclei in a body site excited within a magnetic field

Body Part	Contrast	Qualifier	Qualifier
Character 4	Character 5	Character 6	Character 7
0 Connective Tissue, Upper Extremity **1** Connective Tissue, Lower Extremity **2** Tendons, Upper Extremity **3** Tendons, Lower Extremity	**Y** Other Contrast	**0** Unenhanced and Enhanced **Z** None	**Z** None
0 Connective Tissue, Upper Extremity **1** Connective Tissue, Lower Extremity **2** Tendons, Upper Extremity **3** Tendons, Lower Extremity	**Z** None	**Z** None	**Z** None

B **Imaging**
L **Connective Tissue**
4 **Ultrasonography:** Real time display of images of anatomy or flow information developed from the capture of reflected and attenuated high frequency sound waves

Body Part	Contrast	Qualifier	Qualifier
Character 4	Character 5	Character 6	Character 7
0 Connective Tissue, Upper Extremity **1** Connective Tissue, Lower Extremity **2** Tendons, Upper Extremity **3** Tendons, Lower Extremity	**Z** None	**Z** None	**Z** None

B **Imaging**
N **Skull and Facial Bones**
0 **Plain Radiography:** Planar display of an image developed from the capture of external ionizing radiation on photographic or photoconductive plate

Body Part	Contrast	Qualifier	Qualifier
Character 4	Character 5	Character 6	Character 7
0 Skull **1** Orbit, Right **2** Orbit, Left **3** Orbits, Bilateral **4** Nasal Bones **5** Facial Bones **6** Mandible **B** Zygomatic Arch, Right **C** Zygomatic Arch, Left **D** Zygomatic Arches, Bilateral **G** Tooth, Single **H** Teeth, Multiple **J** Teeth, All	**Z** None	**Z** None	**Z** None
7 Temporomandibular Joint, Right **8** Temporomandibular Joint, Left **9** Temporomandibular Joints, Bilateral	**0** High Osmolar **1** Low Osmolar **Y** Other Contrast **Z** None	**Z** None	**Z** None

---

LC Limited Coverage   **NC** Noncovered   **HAC** HAC-associated Procedure   **CC** Combination Cluster - See Appendix G for code lists
DRG Non-OR-Affecting MS-DRG Assignment   New/Revised Text in **Orange**   ♂ Male   ♀ Female

2021 ICD-10-PCS   **669**

B Imaging
N Skull and Facial Bones
1 Fluoroscopy: Single plane or bi-plane real time display of an image developed from the capture of external ionizing radiation on a fluorescent screen. The image may also be stored by either digital or analog means

Body Part	Contrast	Qualifier	Qualifier
Character 4	Character 5	Character 6	Character 7
7 Temporomandibular Joint, Right 8 Temporomandibular Joint, Left 9 Temporomandibular Joints, Bilateral	0 High Osmolar 1 Low Osmolar Y Other Contrast Z None	Z None	Z None

B Imaging
N Skull and Facial Bones
2 Computerized Tomography (CT Scan): Computer reformatted digital display of multiplanar images developed from the capture of multiple exposures of external ionizing radiation

Body Part	Contrast	Qualifier	Qualifier
Character 4	Character 5	Character 6	Character 7
0 Skull 3 Orbits, Bilateral 5 Facial Bones 6 Mandible 9 Temporomandibular Joints, Bilateral F Temporal Bones	0 High Osmolar 1 Low Osmolar Y Other Contrast Z None	Z None	Z None

B Imaging
N Skull and Facial Bones
3 Magnetic Resonance Imaging (MRI): Computer reformatted digital display of multiplanar images developed from the capture of radiofrequency signals emitted by nuclei in a body site excited within a magnetic field

Body Part	Contrast	Qualifier	Qualifier
Character 4	Character 5	Character 6	Character 7
9 Temporomandibular Joints, Bilateral	Y Other Contrast Z None	Z None	Z None

B Imaging
P Non-Axial Upper Bones
0 Plain Radiography: Planar display of an image developed from the capture of external ionizing radiation on photographic or photoconductive plate

Body Part	Contrast	Qualifier	Qualifier
Character 4	Character 5	Character 6	Character 7
0 Sternoclavicular Joint, Right 1 Sternoclavicular Joint, Left 2 Sternoclavicular Joints, Bilateral 3 Acromioclavicular Joints, Bilateral 4 Clavicle, Right 5 Clavicle, Left 6 Scapula, Right 7 Scapula, Left A Humerus, Right B Humerus, Left E Upper Arm, Right F Upper Arm, Left J Forearm, Right K Forearm, Left N Hand, Right P Hand, Left R Finger(s), Right S Finger(s), Left X Ribs, Right Y Ribs, Left	Z None	Z None	Z None

BP0 continued on next page

B Imaging
P Non-Axial Upper Bones
0 Plain Radiography: Planar display of an image developed from the capture of external ionizing radiation on photographic or photoconductive plate

BP0 continued from previous page

Body Part	Contrast	Qualifier	Qualifier
Character 4	Character 5	Character 6	Character 7
8 Shoulder, Right 9 Shoulder, Left C Hand/Finger Joint, Right D Hand/Finger Joint, Left G Elbow, Right H Elbow, Left L Wrist, Right M Wrist, Left	0 High Osmolar 1 Low Osmolar Y Other Contrast Z None	Z None	Z None

B Imaging
P Non-Axial Upper Bones
1 Fluoroscopy: Single plane or bi-plane real time display of an image developed from the capture of external ionizing radiation on a fluorescent screen. The image may also be stored by either digital or analog means

Body Part	Contrast	Qualifier	Qualifier
Character 4	Character 5	Character 6	Character 7
0 Sternoclavicular Joint, Right 1 Sternoclavicular Joint, Left 2 Sternoclavicular Joints, Bilateral 3 Acromioclavicular Joints, Bilateral 4 Clavicle, Right 5 Clavicle, Left 6 Scapula, Right 7 Scapula, Left A Humerus, Right B Humerus, Left E Upper Arm, Right F Upper Arm, Left J Forearm, Right K Forearm, Left N Hand, Right P Hand, Left R Finger(s), Right S Finger(s), Left X Ribs, Right Y Ribs, Left	Z None	Z None	Z None
8 Shoulder, Right 9 Shoulder, Left L Wrist, Right M Wrist, Left	0 High Osmolar 1 Low Osmolar Y Other Contrast Z None	Z None	Z None
C Hand/Finger Joint, Right D Hand/Finger Joint, Left G Elbow, Right H Elbow, Left	0 High Osmolar 1 Low Osmolar Y Other Contrast	Z None	Z None

B   Imaging
P   Non-Axial Upper Bones
2   Computerized Tomography (CT Scan): Computer reformatted digital display of multiplanar images developed from the capture of multiple exposures of external ionizing radiation

Body Part	Contrast	Qualifier	Qualifier
Character 4	Character 5	Character 6	Character 7
0 Sternoclavicular Joint, Right **1** Sternoclavicular Joint, Left **W** Thorax	**0** High Osmolar **1** Low Osmolar **Y** Other Contrast	**Z** None	**Z** None
2 Sternoclavicular Joints, Bilateral **3** Acromioclavicular Joints, Bilateral **4** Clavicle, Right **5** Clavicle, Left **6** Scapula, Right **7** Scapula, Left **8** Shoulder, Right **9** Shoulder, Left **A** Humerus, Right **B** Humerus, Left **E** Upper Arm, Right **F** Upper Arm, Left **G** Elbow, Right **H** Elbow, Left **J** Forearm, Right **K** Forearm, Left **L** Wrist, Right **M** Wrist, Left **N** Hand, Right **P** Hand, Left **Q** Hands and Wrists, Bilateral **R** Finger(s), Right **S** Finger(s), Left **T** Upper Extremity, Right **U** Upper Extremity, Left **V** Upper Extremities, Bilateral **X** Ribs, Right **Y** Ribs, Left	**0** High Osmolar **1** Low Osmolar **Y** Other Contrast **Z** None	**Z** None	**Z** None
C Hand/Finger Joint, Right **D** Hand/Finger Joint, Left	**Z** None	**Z** None	**Z** None

B   Imaging
P   Non-Axial Upper Bones
3   Magnetic Resonance Imaging (MRI): Computer reformatted digital display of multiplanar images developed from the capture of radiofrequency signals emitted by nuclei in a body site excited within a magnetic field

Body Part	Contrast	Qualifier	Qualifier
Character 4	Character 5	Character 6	Character 7
8 Shoulder, Right **9** Shoulder, Left **C** Hand/Finger Joint, Right **D** Hand/Finger Joint, Left **E** Upper Arm, Right **F** Upper Arm, Left **G** Elbow, Right **H** Elbow, Left **J** Forearm, Right **K** Forearm, Left **L** Wrist, Right **M** Wrist, Left	**Y** Other Contrast	**0** Unenhanced and Enhanced **Z** None	**Z** None

BP3 continued on next page

B Imaging
P Non-Axial Upper Bones

BP3 continued from previous page

3 Magnetic Resonance Imaging (MRI): Computer reformatted digital display of multiplanar images developed from the capture of radiofrequency signals emitted by nuclei in a body site excited within a magnetic field

Body Part	Contrast	Qualifier	Qualifier
Character 4	Character 5	Character 6	Character 7
8 Shoulder, Right 9 Shoulder, Left C Hand/Finger Joint, Right D Hand/Finger Joint, Left E Upper Arm, Right F Upper Arm, Left G Elbow, Right H Elbow, Left J Forearm, Right K Forearm, Left L Wrist, Right M Wrist, Left	Z None	Z None	Z None

B Imaging
P Non-Axial Upper Bones
4 Ultrasonography: Real time display of images of anatomy or flow information developed from the capture of reflected and attenuated high frequency sound waves

Body Part	Contrast	Qualifier	Qualifier
Character 4	Character 5	Character 6	Character 7
8 Shoulder, Right 9 Shoulder, Left G Elbow, Right H Elbow, Left L Wrist, Right M Wrist, Left N Hand, Right P Hand, Left	Z None	Z None	1 Densitometry Z None

B Imaging
Q Non-Axial Lower Bones
0 Plain Radiography: Planar display of an image developed from the capture of external ionizing radiation on photographic or photoconductive plate

Body Part	Contrast	Qualifier	Qualifier
Character 4	Character 5	Character 6	Character 7
0 Hip, Right 1 Hip, Left	0 High Osmolar 1 Low Osmolar Y Other Contrast	Z None	Z None
0 Hip, Right 1 Hip, Left	Z None	Z None	1 Densitometry Z None
3 Femur, Right 4 Femur, Left	Z None	Z None	1 Densitometry Z None
7 Knee, Right 8 Knee, Left G Ankle, Right H Ankle, Left	0 High Osmolar 1 Low Osmolar Y Other Contrast Z None	Z None	Z None
D Lower Leg, Right F Lower Leg, Left J Calcaneus, Right K Calcaneus, Left L Foot, Right M Foot, Left P Toe(s), Right Q Toe(s), Left V Patella, Right W Patella, Left	Z None	Z None	Z None
X Foot/Toe Joint, Right Y Foot/Toe Joint, Left	0 High Osmolar 1 Low Osmolar Y Other Contrast	Z None	Z None

B Imaging
Q Non-Axial Lower Bones
1 Fluoroscopy: Single plane or bi-plane real time display of an image developed from the capture of external ionizing radiation on a fluorescent screen. The image may also be stored by either digital or analog means

Body Part	Contrast	Qualifier	Qualifier
Character 4	Character 5	Character 6	Character 7
0 Hip, Right 1 Hip, Left 7 Knee, Right 8 Knee, Left G Ankle, Right H Ankle, Left X Foot/Toe Joint, Right Y Foot/Toe Joint, Left	0 High Osmolar 1 Low Osmolar Y Other Contrast Z None	Z None	Z None
3 Femur, Right 4 Femur, Left D Lower Leg, Right F Lower Leg, Left J Calcaneus, Right K Calcaneus, Left L Foot, Right M Foot, Left P Toe(s), Right Q Toe(s), Left V Patella, Right W Patella, Left	Z None	Z None	Z None

B Imaging
Q Non-Axial Lower Bones
2 Computerized Tomography (CT Scan): Computer reformatted digital display of multiplanar images developed from the capture of multiple exposures of external ionizing radiation

Body Part	Contrast	Qualifier	Qualifier
Character 4	Character 5	Character 6	Character 7
0 Hip, Right 1 Hip, Left 3 Femur, Right 4 Femur, Left 7 Knee, Right 8 Knee, Left D Lower Leg, Right F Lower Leg, Left G Ankle, Right H Ankle, Left J Calcaneus, Right K Calcaneus, Left L Foot, Right M Foot, Left P Toe(s), Right Q Toe(s), Left R Lower Extremity, Right S Lower Extremity, Left V Patella, Right W Patella, Left X Foot/Toe Joint, Right Y Foot/Toe Joint, Left	0 High Osmolar 1 Low Osmolar Y Other Contrast Z None	Z None	Z None
B Tibia/Fibula, Right C Tibia/Fibula, Left	0 High Osmolar 1 Low Osmolar Y Other Contrast	Z None	Z None

LC Limited Coverage   **NC** Noncovered   **HAC** HAC-associated Procedure   **CC** Combination Cluster - See Appendix G for code lists
DRG Non-OR-Affecting MS-DRG Assignment   New/Revised Text in **Orange**   ♂ Male   ♀ Female

674   **2021 ICD-10-PCS**

B Imaging
Q Non-Axial Lower Bones
3 Magnetic Resonance Imaging (MRI): Computer reformatted digital display of multiplanar images developed from the capture of radiofrequency signals emitted by nuclei in a body site excited within a magnetic field

Body Part	Contrast	Qualifier	Qualifier
Character 4	Character 5	Character 6	Character 7
0 Hip, Right 1 Hip, Left 3 Femur, Right 4 Femur, Left 7 Knee, Right 8 Knee, Left D Lower Leg, Right F Lower Leg, Left G Ankle, Right H Ankle, Left J Calcaneus, Right K Calcaneus, Left L Foot, Right M Foot, Left P Toe(s), Right Q Toe(s), Left V Patella, Right W Patella, Left	Y Other Contrast	0 Unenhanced and Enhanced Z None	Z None
0 Hip, Right 1 Hip, Left 3 Femur, Right 4 Femur, Left 7 Knee, Right 8 Knee, Left D Lower Leg, Right F Lower Leg, Left G Ankle, Right H Ankle, Left J Calcaneus, Right K Calcaneus, Left L Foot, Right M Foot, Left P Toe(s), Right Q Toe(s), Left V Patella, Right W Patella, Left	Z None	Z None	Z None

B Imaging
Q Non-Axial Lower Bones
4 Ultrasonography: Real time display of images of anatomy or flow information developed from the capture of reflected and attenuated high frequency sound waves

Body Part	Contrast	Qualifier	Qualifier
Character 4	Character 5	Character 6	Character 7
0 Hip, Right 1 Hip, Left 2 Hips, Bilateral 7 Knee, Right 8 Knee, Left 9 Knees, Bilateral	Z None	Z None	Z None

LC Limited Coverage   **NC** Noncovered   **HAC** HAC-associated Procedure   **CC** Combination Cluster - See Appendix G for code lists

DRG Non-OR-Affecting MS-DRG Assignment   New/Revised Text in **Orange**   ♂ Male   ♀ Female

2021 ICD-10-PCS

675

B   Imaging
R   Axial Skeleton, Except Skull and Facial Bones
0   Plain Radiography: Planar display of an image developed from the capture of external ionizing radiation on photographic or photoconductive plate

Body Part	Contrast	Qualifier	Qualifier
Character 4	Character 5	Character 6	Character 7
0 Cervical Spine **7** Thoracic Spine **9** Lumbar Spine **G** Whole Spine	**Z** None	**Z** None	**1** Densitometry **Z** None
1 Cervical Disc(s) **2** Thoracic Disc(s) **3** Lumbar Disc(s) **4** Cervical Facet Joint(s) **5** Thoracic Facet Joint(s) **6** Lumbar Facet Joint(s) **D** Sacroiliac Joints	**0** High Osmolar **1** Low Osmolar **Y** Other Contrast **Z** None	**Z** None	**Z** None
8 Thoracolumbar Joint **B** Lumbosacral Joint **C** Pelvis **F** Sacrum and Coccyx **H** Sternum	**Z** None	**Z** None	**Z** None

B   Imaging
R   Axial Skeleton, Except Skull and Facial Bones
1   Fluoroscopy: Single plane or bi-plane real time display of an image developed from the capture of external ionizing radiation on a fluorescent screen. The image may also be stored by either digital or analog means

Body Part	Contrast	Qualifier	Qualifier
Character 4	Character 5	Character 6	Character 7
0 Cervical Spine **1** Cervical Disc(s) **2** Thoracic Disc(s) **3** Lumbar Disc(s) **4** Cervical Facet Joint(s) **5** Thoracic Facet Joint(s) **6** Lumbar Facet Joint(s) **7** Thoracic Spine **8** Thoracolumbar Joint **9** Lumbar Spine **B** Lumbosacral Joint **C** Pelvis **D** Sacroiliac Joints **F** Sacrum and Coccyx **G** Whole Spine **H** Sternum	**0** High Osmolar **1** Low Osmolar **Y** Other Contrast **Z** None	**Z** None	**Z** None

B   Imaging
R   Axial Skeleton, Except Skull and Facial Bones
2   Computerized Tomography (CT Scan): Computer reformatted digital display of multiplanar images developed from the capture of multiple exposures of external ionizing radiation

Body Part	Contrast	Qualifier	Qualifier
Character 4	Character 5	Character 6	Character 7
0 Cervical Spine **7** Thoracic Spine **9** Lumbar Spine **C** Pelvis **D** Sacroiliac Joints **F** Sacrum and Coccyx	**0** High Osmolar **1** Low Osmolar **Y** Other Contrast **Z** None	**Z** None	**Z** None

LC Limited Coverage   **NC** Noncovered   **HAC** HAC-associated Procedure   **CC** Combination Cluster - See Appendix G for code lists
DRG Non-OR-Affecting MS-DRG Assignment   New/Revised Text in **Orange**   ♂ Male   ♀ Female

676   **2021 ICD-10-PCS**

B Imaging
R Axial Skeleton, Except Skull and Facial Bones
3 Magnetic Resonance Imaging (MRI): Computer reformatted digital display of multiplanar images developed from the capture of radiofrequency signals emitted by nuclei in a body site excited within a magnetic field

Body Part	Contrast	Qualifier	Qualifier
Character 4	Character 5	Character 6	Character 7
0 Cervical Spine 1 Cervical Disc(s) 2 Thoracic Disc(s) 3 Lumbar Disc(s) 7 Thoracic Spine 9 Lumbar Spine C Pelvis F Sacrum and Coccyx	Y Other Contrast	0 Unenhanced and Enhanced Z None	Z None
0 Cervical Spine 1 Cervical Disc(s) 2 Thoracic Disc(s) 3 Lumbar Disc(s) 7 Thoracic Spine 9 Lumbar Spine C Pelvis F Sacrum and Coccyx	Z None	Z None	Z None

B Imaging
R Axial Skeleton, Except Skull and Facial Bones
4 Ultrasonography: Real time display of images of anatomy or flow information developed from the capture of reflected and attenuated high frequency sound waves

Body Part	Contrast	Qualifier	Qualifier
Character 4	Character 5	Character 6	Character 7
0 Cervical Spine 7 Thoracic Spine 9 Lumbar Spine F Sacrum and Coccyx	Z None	Z None	Z None

B Imaging
T Urinary System
0 Plain Radiography: Planar display of an image developed from the capture of external ionizing radiation on photographic or photoconductive plate

Body Part	Contrast	Qualifier	Qualifier
Character 4	Character 5	Character 6	Character 7
0 Bladder 1 Kidney, Right 2 Kidney, Left 3 Kidneys, Bilateral 4 Kidneys, Ureters and Bladder 5 Urethra 6 Ureter, Right 7 Ureter, Left 8 Ureters, Bilateral B Bladder and Urethra C Ileal Diversion Loop	0 High Osmolar 1 Low Osmolar Y Other Contrast Z None	Z None	Z None

LC Limited Coverage   NC Noncovered   HAC HAC-associated Procedure   CC Combination Cluster - See Appendix G for code lists
DRG Non-OR-Affecting MS-DRG Assignment   New/Revised Text in Orange   ♂ Male   ♀ Female

2021 ICD-10-PCS   677

IMAGING B00-BY4

B Imaging
T Urinary System
1 Fluoroscopy: Single plane or bi-plane real time display of an image developed from the capture of external ionizing radiation on a fluorescent screen. The image may also be stored by either digital or analog means

Body Part	Contrast	Qualifier	Qualifier
Character 4	Character 5	Character 6	Character 7
0 Bladder 1 Kidney, Right 2 Kidney, Left 3 Kidneys, Bilateral 4 Kidneys, Ureters and Bladder 5 Urethra 6 Ureter, Right 7 Ureter, Left B Bladder and Urethra C Ileal Diversion Loop D Kidney, Ureter and Bladder, Right F Kidney, Ureter and Bladder, Left G Ileal Loop, Ureters and Kidneys	0 High Osmolar 1 Low Osmolar Y Other Contrast Z None	Z None	Z None

B Imaging
T Urinary System
2 Computerized Tomography (CT Scan): Computer reformatted digital display of multiplanar images developed from the capture of multiple exposures of external ionizing radiation

Body Part	Contrast	Qualifier	Qualifier
Character 4	Character 5	Character 6	Character 7
0 Bladder 1 Kidney, Right 2 Kidney, Left 3 Kidneys, Bilateral 9 Kidney Transplant	0 High Osmolar 1 Low Osmolar Y Other Contrast	0 Unenhanced and Enhanced Z None	Z None
0 Bladder 1 Kidney, Right 2 Kidney, Left 3 Kidneys, Bilateral 9 Kidney Transplant	Z None	Z None	Z None

B Imaging
T Urinary System
3 Magnetic Resonance Imaging (MRI): Computer reformatted digital display of multiplanar images developed from the capture of radiofrequency signals emitted by nuclei in a body site excited within a magnetic field

Body Part	Contrast	Qualifier	Qualifier
Character 4	Character 5	Character 6	Character 7
0 Bladder 1 Kidney, Right 2 Kidney, Left 3 Kidneys, Bilateral 9 Kidney Transplant	Y Other Contrast	0 Unenhanced and Enhanced Z None	Z None
0 Bladder 1 Kidney, Right 2 Kidney, Left 3 Kidneys, Bilateral 9 Kidney Transplant	Z None	Z None	Z None

LC Limited Coverage   **NC** Noncovered   **HAC** HAC-associated Procedure   **CC** Combination Cluster - See Appendix G for code lists
DRG Non-OR-Affecting MS-DRG Assignment   New/Revised Text in **Orange**   ♂ Male   ♀ Female

678

2021 ICD-10-PCS

B Imaging
T Urinary System
4 Ultrasonography: Real time display of images of anatomy or flow information developed from the capture of reflected and attenuated high frequency sound waves

Body Part	Contrast	Qualifier	Qualifier
Character 4	Character 5	Character 6	Character 7
0 Bladder **1** Kidney, Right **2** Kidney, Left **3** Kidneys, Bilateral **5** Urethra **6** Ureter, Right **7** Ureter, Left **8** Ureters, Bilateral **9** Kidney Transplant **J** Kidneys and Bladder	**Z** None	**Z** None	**Z** None

B Imaging
U Female Reproductive System
0 Plain Radiography: Planar display of an image developed from the capture of external ionizing radiation on photographic or photoconductive plate

Body Part	Contrast	Qualifier	Qualifier
Character 4	Character 5	Character 6	Character 7
0 Fallopian Tube, Right ♀ **1** Fallopian Tube, Left ♀ **2** Fallopian Tubes, Bilateral ♀ **6** Uterus ♀ **8** Uterus and Fallopian Tubes ♀ **9** Vagina ♀	**0** High Osmolar **1** Low Osmolar **Y** Other Contrast	**Z** None	**Z** None

♀   BU000ZZ   BU001ZZ   BU00YZZ   BU010ZZ   BU011ZZ   BU01YZZ   BU020ZZ   BU021ZZ   BU02YZZ   BU060ZZ   BU061ZZ   BU06YZZ   BU080ZZ
   BU081ZZ   BU08YZZ   BU090ZZ   BU091ZZ   BU09YZZ

B Imaging
U Female Reproductive System
1 Fluoroscopy: Single plane or bi-plane real time display of an image developed from the capture of external ionizing radiation on a fluorescent screen. The image may also be stored by either digital or analog means

Body Part	Contrast	Qualifier	Qualifier
Character 4	Character 5	Character 6	Character 7
0 Fallopian Tube, Right ♀ **1** Fallopian Tube, Left ♀ **2** Fallopian Tubes, Bilateral ♀ **6** Uterus ♀ **8** Uterus and Fallopian Tubes ♀ **9** Vagina ♀	**0** High Osmolar **1** Low Osmolar **Y** Other Contrast **Z** None	**Z** None	**Z** None

♀   BU100ZZ   BU101ZZ   BU10YZZ   BU10ZZZ   BU110ZZ   BU111ZZ   BU11YZZ   BU11ZZZ   BU120ZZ   BU121ZZ   BU12YZZ   BU12ZZZ   BU160ZZ
   BU161ZZ   BU16YZZ   BU16ZZZ   BU180ZZ   BU181ZZ   BU18YZZ   BU18ZZZ   BU190ZZ   BU191ZZ   BU19YZZ   BU19ZZZ

B Imaging
U Female Reproductive System
3 Magnetic Resonance Imaging (MRI): Computer reformatted digital display of multiplanar images developed from the capture of radiofrequency signals emitted by nuclei in a body site excited within a magnetic field

Body Part	Contrast	Qualifier	Qualifier
Character 4	Character 5	Character 6	Character 7
3 Ovary, Right ♀ **4** Ovary, Left ♀ **5** Ovaries, Bilateral ♀ **6** Uterus ♀ **9** Vagina ♀ **B** Pregnant Uterus ♀ **C** Uterus and Ovaries ♀	**Y** Other Contrast	**0** Unenhanced and Enhanced **Z** None	**Z** None
3 Ovary, Right ♀ **4** Ovary, Left ♀ **5** Ovaries, Bilateral ♀ **6** Uterus ♀ **9** Vagina ♀ **B** Pregnant Uterus ♀ **C** Uterus and Ovaries ♀	**Z** None	**Z** None	**Z** None

♀ BU33Y0Z BU33YZZ BU33ZZZ BU34Y0Z BU34YZZ BU34ZZZ BU35Y0Z BU35YZZ BU35ZZZ BU36Y0Z BU36YZZ BU36ZZZ BU39Y0Z
BU39YZZ BU39ZZZ BU3BY0Z BU3BYZZ BU3BZZZ BU3CY0Z BU3CYZZ BU3CZZZ

B Imaging
U Female Reproductive System
4 Ultrasonography: Real time display of images of anatomy or flow information developed from the capture of reflected and attenuated high frequency sound waves

Body Part	Contrast	Qualifier	Qualifier
Character 4	Character 5	Character 6	Character 7
0 Fallopian Tube, Right ♀ **1** Fallopian Tube, Left ♀ **2** Fallopian Tubes, Bilateral ♀ **3** Ovary, Right ♀ **4** Ovary, Left ♀ **5** Ovaries, Bilateral ♀ **6** Uterus ♀ **C** Uterus and Ovaries ♀	**Y** Other Contrast **Z** None	**Z** None	**Z** None

♀ BU40YZZ BU40ZZZ BU41YZZ BU41ZZZ BU42YZZ BU42ZZZ BU43YZZ BU43ZZZ BU44YZZ BU44ZZZ BU45YZZ BU45ZZZ BU46YZZ
BU46ZZZ BU4CYZZ BU4CZZZ

B Imaging
V Male Reproductive System
0 Plain Radiography: Planar display of an image developed from the capture of external ionizing radiation on photographic or photoconductive plate

Body Part	Contrast	Qualifier	Qualifier
Character 4	Character 5	Character 6	Character 7
0 Corpora Cavernosa ♂ **1** Epididymis, Right ♂ **2** Epididymis, Left ♂ **3** Prostate ♂ **5** Testicle, Right ♂ **6** Testicle, Left ♂ **8** Vasa Vasorum ♂	**0** High Osmolar **1** Low Osmolar **Y** Other Contrast	**Z** None	**Z** None

♂ BV000ZZ BV001ZZ BV00YZZ BV010ZZ BV011ZZ BV01YZZ BV020ZZ BV021ZZ BV02YZZ BV030ZZ BV031ZZ BV03YZZ BV050ZZ
BV051ZZ BV05YZZ BV060ZZ BV061ZZ BV06YZZ BV080ZZ BV081ZZ BV08YZZ

B Imaging
V Male Reproductive System
1 Fluoroscopy: Single plane or bi-plane real time display of an image developed from the capture of external ionizing radiation on a fluorescent screen. The image may also be stored by either digital or analog means

Body Part	Contrast	Qualifier	Qualifier
Character 4	Character 5	Character 6	Character 7
0 Corpora Cavernosa ♂ **8** Vasa Vasorum ♂	**0** High Osmolar **1** Low Osmolar **Y** Other Contrast **Z** None	**Z** None	**Z** None

♂ BV100ZZ   BV101ZZ   BV10YZZ   BV10ZZZ   BV180ZZ   BV181ZZ   BV18YZZ   BV18ZZZ

B Imaging
V Male Reproductive System
2 Computerized Tomography (CT Scan): Computer reformatted digital display of multiplanar images developed from the capture of multiple exposures of external ionizing radiation

Body Part	Contrast	Qualifier	Qualifier
Character 4	Character 5	Character 6	Character 7
3 Prostate ♂	**0** High Osmolar **1** Low Osmolar **Y** Other Contrast	**0** Unenhanced and Enhanced **Z** None	**Z** None
3 Prostate ♂	**Z** None	**Z** None	**Z** None

♂ BV2300Z   BV230ZZ   BV2310Z   BV23Y0Z   BV23YZZ   BV23ZZZ

B Imaging
V Male Reproductive System
3 Magnetic Resonance Imaging (MRI): Computer reformatted digital display of multiplanar images developed from the capture of radiofrequency signals emitted by nuclei in a body site excited within a magnetic field

Body Part	Contrast	Qualifier	Qualifier
Character 4	Character 5	Character 6	Character 7
0 Corpora Cavernosa ♂ **3** Prostate ♂ **4** Scrotum ♂ **5** Testicle, Right ♂ **6** Testicle, Left ♂ **7** Testicles, Bilateral ♂	**Y** Other Contrast	**0** Unenhanced and Enhanced **Z** None	**Z** None
0 Corpora Cavernosa ♂ **3** Prostate ♂ **4** Scrotum ♂ **5** Testicle, Right ♂ **6** Testicle, Left ♂ **7** Testicles, Bilateral ♂	**Z** None	**Z** None	**Z** None

♂ BV30Y0Z   BV30YZZ   BV30ZZZ   BV33Y0Z   BV33YZZ   BV33ZZZ   BV34Y0Z   BV34YZZ   BV34ZZZ   BV35Y0Z   BV35YZZ   BV35ZZZ   BV36Y0Z
    BV36YZZ   BV36ZZZ   BV37Y0Z   BV37YZZ   BV37ZZZ

B Imaging
V Male Reproductive System
4 Ultrasonography: Real time display of images of anatomy or flow information developed from the capture of reflected and attenuated high frequency sound waves

Body Part	Contrast	Qualifier	Qualifier
Character 4	Character 5	Character 6	Character 7
4 Scrotum ♂ **9** Prostate and Seminal Vesicles ♂ **B** Penis ♂	**Z** None	**Z** None	**Z** None

♂ BV44ZZZ   BV49ZZZ   BV4BZZZ

B Imaging
W Anatomical Regions
0 Plain Radiography: Planar display of an image developed from the capture of external ionizing radiation on photographic or photoconductive plate

Body Part	Contrast	Qualifier	Qualifier
Character 4	Character 5	Character 6	Character 7
0 Abdomen **1** Abdomen and Pelvis **3** Chest **B** Long Bones, All **C** Lower Extremity **J** Upper Extremity **K** Whole Body **L** Whole Skeleton **M** Whole Body, Infant	**Z** None	**Z** None	**Z** None

B Imaging
W Anatomical Regions
1 Fluoroscopy: Single plane or bi-plane real time display of an image developed from the capture of external ionizing radiation on a fluorescent screen. The image may also be stored by either digital or analog means

Body Part	Contrast	Qualifier	Qualifier
Character 4	Character 5	Character 6	Character 7
1 Abdomen and Pelvis **9** Head and Neck **C** Lower Extremity **J** Upper Extremity	**0** High Osmolar **1** Low Osmolar **Y** Other Contrast **Z** None	**Z** None	**Z** None

B Imaging
W Anatomical Regions
2 Computerized Tomography (CT Scan): Computer reformatted digital display of multiplanar images developed from the capture of multiple exposures of external ionizing radiation

Body Part	Contrast	Qualifier	Qualifier
Character 4	Character 5	Character 6	Character 7
0 Abdomen **1** Abdomen and Pelvis **4** Chest and Abdomen **5** Chest, Abdomen and Pelvis **8** Head **9** Head and Neck **F** Neck **G** Pelvic Region	**0** High Osmolar **1** Low Osmolar **Y** Other Contrast	**0** Unenhanced and Enhanced **Z** None	**Z** None
0 Abdomen **1** Abdomen and Pelvis **4** Chest and Abdomen **5** Chest, Abdomen and Pelvis **8** Head **9** Head and Neck **F** Neck **G** Pelvic Region	**Z** None	**Z** None	**Z** None

LC Limited Coverage **NC** Noncovered **HAC** HAC-associated Procedure **CC** Combination Cluster - See Appendix G for code lists

DRG Non-OR-Affecting MS-DRG Assignment New/Revised Text in **Orange** ♂ Male ♀ Female

682

2021 ICD-10-PCS

B Imaging
W Anatomical Regions
3 Magnetic Resonance Imaging (MRI): Computer reformatted digital display of multiplanar images developed from the capture of radiofrequency signals emitted by nuclei in a body site excited within a magnetic field

Body Part	Contrast	Qualifier	Qualifier
Character 4	Character 5	Character 6	Character 7
0 Abdomen 8 Head F Neck G Pelvic Region H Retroperitoneum P Brachial Plexus	Y Other Contrast	0 Unenhanced and Enhanced Z None	Z None
0 Abdomen 8 Head F Neck G Pelvic Region H Retroperitoneum P Brachial Plexus	Z None	Z None	Z None
3 Chest	Y Other Contrast	0 Unenhanced and Enhanced Z None	Z None

B Imaging
W Anatomical Regions
4 Ultrasonography: Real time display of images of anatomy or flow information developed from the capture of reflected and attenuated high frequency sound waves

Body Part	Contrast	Qualifier	Qualifier
Character 4	Character 5	Character 6	Character 7
0 Abdomen 1 Abdomen and Pelvis F Neck G Pelvic Region	Z None	Z None	Z None

B Imaging
W Anatomical Regions
5 Other Imaging: Other specified modality for visualizing a body part

Body Part	Contrast	Qualifier	Qualifier
Character 4	Character 5	Character 6	Character 7
2 Trunk 9 Head and Neck C Lower Extremity J Upper Extremity	Z None	1 Bacterial Autofluorescence	Z None

IC Limited Coverage   NC Noncovered   HAC HAC-associated Procedure   CC Combination Cluster - See Appendix G for code lists
DRG Non-OR-Affecting MS-DRG Assignment   New/Revised Text in **Orange**   ♂ Male   ♀ Female

2021 ICD-10-PCS

683

B Imaging
Y Fetus and Obstetrical
3 Magnetic Resonance Imaging (MRI): Computer reformatted digital display of multiplanar images developed from the capture of radiofrequency signals emitted by nuclei in a body site excited within a magnetic field

Body Part	Contrast	Qualifier	Qualifier
Character 4	Character 5	Character 6	Character 7
0 Fetal Head ♀ **1** Fetal Heart ♀ **2** Fetal Thorax ♀ **3** Fetal Abdomen ♀ **4** Fetal Spine ♀ **5** Fetal Extremities ♀ **6** Whole Fetus ♀	**Y** Other Contrast	**0** Unenhanced and Enhanced **Z** None	**Z** None
0 Fetal Head ♀ **1** Fetal Heart ♀ **2** Fetal Thorax ♀ **3** Fetal Abdomen ♀ **4** Fetal Spine ♀ **5** Fetal Extremities ♀ **6** Whole Fetus ♀	**Z** None	**Z** None	**Z** None

♀ BY30Y0Z   BY30YZZ   BY30ZZZ   BY31Y0Z   BY31YZZ   BY31ZZZ   BY32Y0Z   BY32YZZ   BY32ZZZ   BY33Y0Z   BY33YZZ   BY33ZZZ   BY34YZZ
  BY34ZZZ   BY35Y0Z   BY35YZZ   BY35ZZZ   BY36Y0Z   BY36YZZ   BY36ZZZ

B Imaging
Y Fetus and Obstetrical
4 Ultrasonography: Real time display of images of anatomy or flow information developed from the capture of reflected and attenuated high frequency sound waves

Body Part	Contrast	Qualifier	Qualifier
Character 4	Character 5	Character 6	Character 7
7 Fetal Umbilical Cord ♀ **8** Placenta ♀ **9** First Trimester, Single Fetus ♀ **B** First Trimester, Multiple Gestation ♀ **C** Second Trimester, Single Fetus ♀ **D** Second Trimester, Multiple Gestation ♀ **F** Third Trimester, Single Fetus ♀ **G** Third Trimester, Multiple Gestation ♀	**Z** None	**Z** None	**Z** None

♀ BY47ZZZ   BY48ZZZ   BY49ZZZ   BY4BZZZ   BY4CZZZ   BY4DZZZ   BY4FZZZ   BY4GZZZ

IC Limited Coverage   **NC** Noncovered   **HAC** HAC-associated Procedure   **CC** Combination Cluster - See Appendix G for code lists
DRG Non-OR-Affecting MS-DRG Assignment   New/Revised Text in Orange   ♂ Male   ♀ Female

684   **2021 ICD-10-PCS**

NOTES

NOTES

Nuclear Medicine C01-CW7

C Nuclear Medicine
0 Central Nervous System
1 Planar Nuclear Medicine Imaging: Introduction of radioactive materials into the body for single plane display of images developed from the capture of radioactive emissions

Body Part	Radionuclide	Qualifier	Qualifier
Character 4	Character 5	Character 6	Character 7
0 Brain	**1** Technetium 99m (Tc-99m) **Y** Other Radionuclide	**Z** None	**Z** None
5 Cerebrospinal Fluid	**D** Indium 111 (In-111) **Y** Other Radionuclide	**Z** None	**Z** None
Y Central Nervous System	**Y** Other Radionuclide	**Z** None	**Z** None

C Nuclear Medicine
0 Central Nervous System
2 Tomographic (Tomo) Nuclear Medicine Imaging: Introduction of radioactive materials into the body for three dimensional display of images developed from the capture of radioactive emissions

Body Part	Radionuclide	Qualifier	Qualifier
Character 4	Character 5	Character 6	Character 7
0 Brain	**1** Technetium 99m (Tc-99m) **F** Iodine 123 (I-123) **S** Thallium 201 (Tl-201) **Y** Other Radionuclide	**Z** None	**Z** None
5 Cerebrospinal Fluid	**D** Indium 111 (In-111) **Y** Other Radionuclide	**Z** None	**Z** None
Y Central Nervous System	**Y** Other Radionuclide	**Z** None	**Z** None

C Nuclear Medicine
0 Central Nervous System
3 Positron Emission Tomographic (PET) Imaging: Introduction of radioactive materials into the body for three dimensional display of images developed from the simultaneous capture, 180 degrees apart, of radioactive emissions

Body Part	Radionuclide	Qualifier	Qualifier
Character 4	Character 5	Character 6	Character 7
0 Brain	**B** Carbon 11 (C-11) **K** Fluorine 18 (F-18) **M** Oxygen 15 (O-15) **Y** Other Radionuclide	**Z** None	**Z** None
Y Central Nervous System	**Y** Other Radionuclide	**Z** None	**Z** None

C Nuclear Medicine
0 Central Nervous System
5 Nonimaging Nuclear Medicine Probe: Introduction of radioactive materials into the body for the study of distribution and fate of certain substances by the detection of radioactive emissions; or, alternatively, measurement of absorption of radioactive emissions from an external source

Body Part	Radionuclide	Qualifier	Qualifier
Character 4	Character 5	Character 6	Character 7
0 Brain	**V** Xenon 133 (Xe-133) **Y** Other Radionuclide	**Z** None	**Z** None
Y Central Nervous System	**Y** Other Radionuclide	**Z** None	**Z** None

C Nuclear Medicine
2 Heart
1 Planar Nuclear Medicine Imaging: Introduction of radioactive materials into the body for single plane display of images developed from the capture of radioactive emissions

Body Part	Radionuclide	Qualifier	Qualifier
Character 4	Character 5	Character 6	Character 7
6 Heart, Right and Left	**1** Technetium 99m (Tc-99m) **Y** Other Radionuclide	**Z** None	**Z** None
G Myocardium	**1** Technetium 99m (Tc-99m) **D** Indium 111 (In-111) **S** Thallium 201 (Tl-201) **Y** Other Radionuclide **Z** None	**Z** None	**Z** None
Y Heart	**Y** Other Radionuclide	**Z** None	**Z** None

C Nuclear Medicine
2 Heart
2 Tomographic (Tomo) Nuclear Medicine Imaging: Introduction of radioactive materials into the body for three dimensional display of images developed from the capture of radioactive emissions

Body Part	Radionuclide	Qualifier	Qualifier
Character 4	Character 5	Character 6	Character 7
6 Heart, Right and Left	**1** Technetium 99m (Tc-99m) **Y** Other Radionuclide	**Z** None	**Z** None
G Myocardium	**1** Technetium 99m (Tc-99m) **D** Indium 111 (In-111) **K** Fluorine 18 (F-18) **S** Thallium 201 (Tl-201) **Y** Other Radionuclide **Z** None	**Z** None	**Z** None
Y Heart	**Y** Other Radionuclide	**Z** None	**Z** None

C Nuclear Medicine
2 Heart
3 Positron Emission Tomographic (PET) Imaging: Introduction of radioactive materials into the body for three dimensional display of images developed from the simultaneous capture, 180 degrees apart, of radioactive emissions

Body Part	Radionuclide	Qualifier	Qualifier
Character 4	Character 5	Character 6	Character 7
G Myocardium	**K** Fluorine 18 (F-18) **M** Oxygen 15 (O-15) **Q** Rubidium 82 (Rb-82) **R** Nitrogen 13 (N-13) **Y** Other Radionuclide	**Z** None	**Z** None
Y Heart	**Y** Other Radionuclide	**Z** None	**Z** None

C Nuclear Medicine
2 Heart
5 Nonimaging Nuclear Medicine Probe: Introduction of radioactive materials into the body for the study of distribution and fate of certain substances by the detection of radioactive emissions; or, alternatively, measurement of absorption of radioactive emissions from an external source

Body Part	Radionuclide	Qualifier	Qualifier
Character 4	Character 5	Character 6	Character 7
6 Heart, Right and Left	**1** Technetium 99m (Tc-99m) **Y** Other Radionuclide	**Z** None	**Z** None
Y Heart	**Y** Other Radionuclide	**Z** None	**Z** None

C Nuclear Medicine

5 Veins

1 Planar Nuclear Medicine Imaging: Introduction of radioactive materials into the body for single plane display of images developed from the capture of radioactive emissions

Body Part	Radionuclide	Qualifier	Qualifier
Character 4	Character 5	Character 6	Character 7
B Lower Extremity Veins, Right **C** Lower Extremity Veins, Left **D** Lower Extremity Veins, Bilateral **N** Upper Extremity Veins, Right **P** Upper Extremity Veins, Left **Q** Upper Extremity Veins, Bilateral **R** Central Veins	**1** Technetium 99m (Tc-99m) **Y** Other Radionuclide	**Z** None	**Z** None
Y Veins	**Y** Other Radionuclide	**Z** None	**Z** None

C Nuclear Medicine

7 Lymphatic and Hematologic System

1 Planar Nuclear Medicine Imaging: Introduction of radioactive materials into the body for single plane display of images developed from the capture of radioactive emissions

Body Part	Radionuclide	Qualifier	Qualifier
Character 4	Character 5	Character 6	Character 7
0 Bone Marrow	**1** Technetium 99m (Tc-99m) **D** Indium 111 (In-111) **Y** Other Radionuclide	**Z** None	**Z** None
2 Spleen **5** Lymphatics, Head and Neck **D** Lymphatics, Pelvic **J** Lymphatics, Head **K** Lymphatics, Neck **L** Lymphatics, Upper Chest **M** Lymphatics, Trunk **N** Lymphatics, Upper Extremity **P** Lymphatics, Lower Extremity	**1** Technetium 99m (Tc-99m) **Y** Other Radionuclide	**Z** None	**Z** None
3 Blood	**D** Indium 111 (In-111) **Y** Other Radionuclide	**Z** None	**Z** None
Y Lymphatic and Hematologic System	**Y** Other Radionuclide	**Z** None	**Z** None

C Nuclear Medicine

7 Lymphatic and Hematologic System

2 Tomographic (Tomo) Nuclear Medicine Imaging: Introduction of radioactive materials into the body for three dimensional display of images developed from the capture of radioactive emissions

Body Part	Radionuclide	Qualifier	Qualifier
Character 4	Character 5	Character 6	Character 7
2 Spleen	**1** Technetium 99m (Tc-99m) **Y** Other Radionuclide	**Z** None	**Z** None
Y Lymphatic and Hematologic System	**Y** Other Radionuclide	**Z** None	**Z** None

C **Nuclear Medicine**

7 **Lymphatic and Hematologic System**

5 **Nonimaging Nuclear Medicine Probe:** Introduction of radioactive materials into the body for the study of distribution and fate of certain substances by the detection of radioactive emissions; or, alternatively, measurement of absorption of radioactive emissions from an external source

Body Part	Radionuclide	Qualifier	Qualifier
Character 4	Character 5	Character 6	Character 7
5 Lymphatics, Head and Neck **D** Lymphatics, Pelvic **J** Lymphatics, Head **K** Lymphatics, Neck **L** Lymphatics, Upper Chest **M** Lymphatics, Trunk **N** Lymphatics, Upper Extremity **P** Lymphatics, Lower Extremity	**1** Technetium 99m (Tc-99m) **Y** Other Radionuclide	**Z** None	**Z** None
Y Lymphatic and Hematologic System	**Y** Other Radionuclide	**Z** None	**Z** None

C **Nuclear Medicine**

7 **Lymphatic and Hematologic System**

6 **Nonimaging Nuclear Medicine Assay:** Introduction of radioactive materials into the body for the study of body fluids and blood elements, by the detection of radioactive emissions

Body Part	Radionuclide	Qualifier	Qualifier
Character 4	Character 5	Character 6	Character 7
3 Blood	**1** Technetium 99m (Tc-99m) **7** Cobalt 58 (Co-58) **C** Cobalt 57 (Co-57) **D** Indium 111 (In-111) **H** Iodine 125 (I-125) **W** Chromium (Cr-51) **Y** Other Radionuclide	**Z** None	**Z** None
Y Lymphatic and Hematologic System	**Y** Other Radionuclide	**Z** None	**Z** None

C **Nuclear Medicine**

8 **Eye**

1 **Planar Nuclear Medicine Imaging:** Introduction of radioactive materials into the body for single plane display of images developed from the capture of radioactive emissions

Body Part	Radionuclide	Qualifier	Qualifier
Character 4	Character 5	Character 6	Character 7
9 Lacrimal Ducts, Bilateral	**1** Technetium 99m (Tc-99m) **Y** Other Radionuclide	**Z** None	**Z** None
Y Eye	**Y** Other Radionuclide	**Z** None	**Z** None

C **Nuclear Medicine**

9 **Ear, Nose, Mouth and Throat**

1 **Planar Nuclear Medicine Imaging:** Introduction of radioactive materials into the body for single plane display of images developed from the capture of radioactive emissions

Body Part	Radionuclide	Qualifier	Qualifier
Character 4	Character 5	Character 6	Character 7
B Salivary Glands, Bilateral	**1** Technetium 99m (Tc-99m) **Y** Other Radionuclide	**Z** None	**Z** None
Y Ear, Nose, Mouth and Throat	**Y** Other Radionuclide	**Z** None	**Z** None

C Nuclear Medicine
B Respiratory System
1 Planar Nuclear Medicine Imaging: Introduction of radioactive materials into the body for single plane display of images developed from the capture of radioactive emissions

Body Part	Radionuclide	Qualifier	Qualifier
Character 4	Character 5	Character 6	Character 7
2 Lungs and Bronchi	1 Technetium 99m (Tc-99m) 9 Krypton (Kr-81m) T Xenon 127 (Xe-127) V Xenon 133 (Xe-133) Y Other Radionuclide	Z None	Z None
Y Respiratory System	Y Other Radionuclide	Z None	Z None

C Nuclear Medicine
B Respiratory System
2 Tomographic (Tomo) Nuclear Medicine Imaging: Introduction of radioactive materials into the body for three dimensional display of images developed from the capture of radioactive emissions

Body Part	Radionuclide	Qualifier	Qualifier
Character 4	Character 5	Character 6	Character 7
2 Lungs and Bronchi	1 Technetium 99m (Tc-99m) 9 Krypton (Kr-81m) Y Other Radionuclide	Z None	Z None
Y Respiratory System	Y Other Radionuclide	Z None	Z None

C Nuclear Medicine
B Respiratory System
3 Positron Emission Tomographic (PET) Imaging: Introduction of radioactive materials into the body for three dimensional display of images developed from the simultaneous capture, 180 degrees apart, of radioactive emissions

Body Part	Radionuclide	Qualifier	Qualifier
Character 4	Character 5	Character 6	Character 7
2 Lungs and Bronchi	K Fluorine 18 (F-18) Y Other Radionuclide	Z None	Z None
Y Respiratory System	Y Other Radionuclide	Z None	Z None

C Nuclear Medicine
D Gastrointestinal System
1 Planar Nuclear Medicine Imaging: Introduction of radioactive materials into the body for single plane display of images developed from the capture of radioactive emissions

Body Part	Radionuclide	Qualifier	Qualifier
Character 4	Character 5	Character 6	Character 7
5 Upper Gastrointestinal Tract 7 Gastrointestinal Tract	1 Technetium 99m (Tc-99m) D Indium 111 (In-111) Y Other Radionuclide	Z None	Z None
Y Digestive System	Y Other Radionuclide	Z None	Z None

C Nuclear Medicine
D Gastrointestinal System
2 Tomographic (Tomo) Nuclear Medicine Imaging: Introduction of radioactive materials into the body for three dimensional display of images developed from the capture of radioactive emissions

Body Part	Radionuclide	Qualifier	Qualifier
Character 4	Character 5	Character 6	Character 7
7 Gastrointestinal Tract	1 Technetium 99m (Tc-99m) D Indium 111 (In-111) Y Other Radionuclide	Z None	Z None
Y Digestive System	Y Other Radionuclide	Z None	Z None

C **Nuclear Medicine**
F **Hepatobiliary System and Pancreas**
1 **Planar Nuclear Medicine Imaging:** Introduction of radioactive materials into the body for single plane display of images developed from the capture of radioactive emissions

Body Part	Radionuclide	Qualifier	Qualifier
Character 4	Character 5	Character 6	Character 7
4 Gallbladder **5** Liver **6** Liver and Spleen **C** Hepatobiliary System, All	**1** Technetium 99m (Tc-99m) **Y** Other Radionuclide	**Z** None	**Z** None
Y Hepatobiliary System and Pancreas	**Y** Other Radionuclide	**Z** None	**Z** None

C **Nuclear Medicine**
F **Hepatobiliary System and Pancreas**
2 **Tomographic (Tomo) Nuclear Medicine Imaging:** Introduction of radioactive materials into the body for three dimensional display of images developed from the capture of radioactive emissions

Body Part	Radionuclide	Qualifier	Qualifier
Character 4	Character 5	Character 6	Character 7
4 Gallbladder **5** Liver **6** Liver and Spleen	**1** Technetium 99m (Tc-99m) **Y** Other Radionuclide	**Z** None	**Z** None
Y Hepatobiliary System and Pancreas	**Y** Other Radionuclide	**Z** None	**Z** None

C **Nuclear Medicine**
G **Endocrine System**
1 **Planar Nuclear Medicine Imaging:** Introduction of radioactive materials into the body for single plane display of images developed from the capture of radioactive emissions

Body Part	Radionuclide	Qualifier	Qualifier
Character 4	Character 5	Character 6	Character 7
1 Parathyroid Glands	**1** Technetium 99m (Tc-99m) **S** Thallium 201 (Tl-201) **Y** Other Radionuclide	**Z** None	**Z** None
2 Thyroid Gland	**1** Technetium 99m (Tc-99m) **F** Iodine 123 (I-123) **G** Iodine 131 (I-131) **Y** Other Radionuclide	**Z** None	**Z** None
4 Adrenal Glands, Bilateral	**G** Iodine 131 (I-131) **Y** Other Radionuclide	**Z** None	**Z** None
Y Endocrine System	**Y** Other Radionuclide	**Z** None	**Z** None

C **Nuclear Medicine**
G **Endocrine System**
2 **Tomographic (Tomo) Nuclear Medicine Imaging:** Introduction of radioactive materials into the body for three dimensional display of images developed from the capture of radioactive emissions

Body Part	Radionuclide	Qualifier	Qualifier
Character 4	Character 5	Character 6	Character 7
1 Parathyroid Glands	**1** Technetium 99m (Tc-99m) **S** Thallium 201 (Tl-201) **Y** Other Radionuclide	**Z** None	**Z** None
Y Endocrine System	**Y** Other Radionuclide	**Z** None	**Z** None

LC Limited Coverage   NC Noncovered   HAC HAC-associated Procedure   CC Combination Cluster - See Appendix G for code lists
DRG Non-OR-Affecting MS-DRG Assignment   New/Revised Text in **Orange**   ♂ Male   ♀ Female

692

2021 ICD-10-PCS

C **Nuclear Medicine**
G **Endocrine System**
4 **Nonimaging Nuclear Medicine Uptake:** Introduction of radioactive materials into the body for measurements of organ function, from the detection of radioactive emissions

Body Part	Radionuclide	Qualifier	Qualifier
Character 4	Character 5	Character 6	Character 7
2 Thyroid Gland	**1** Technetium 99m (Tc-99m) **F** Iodine 123 (I-123) **G** Iodine 131 (I-131) **Y** Other Radionuclide	**Z** None	**Z** None
Y Endocrine System	**Y** Other Radionuclide	**Z** None	**Z** None

C **Nuclear Medicine**
H **Skin, Subcutaneous Tissue and Breast**
1 **Planar Nuclear Medicine Imaging:** Introduction of radioactive materials into the body for single plane display of images developed from the capture of radioactive emissions

Body Part	Radionuclide	Qualifier	Qualifier
Character 4	Character 5	Character 6	Character 7
0 Breast, Right **1** Breast, Left **2** Breasts, Bilateral	**1** Technetium 99m (Tc-99m) **S** Thallium 201 (Tl-201) **Y** Other Radionuclide	**Z** None	**Z** None
Y Skin, Subcutaneous Tissue and Breast	**Y** Other Radionuclide	**Z** None	**Z** None

C **Nuclear Medicine**
H **Skin, Subcutaneous Tissue and Breast**
2 **Tomographic (Tomo) Nuclear Medicine Imaging:** Introduction of radioactive materials into the body for three dimensional display of images developed from the capture of radioactive emissions

Body Part	Radionuclide	Qualifier	Qualifier
Character 4	Character 5	Character 6	Character 7
0 Breast, Right **1** Breast, Left **2** Breasts, Bilateral	**1** Technetium 99m (Tc-99m) **S** Thallium 201 (Tl-201) **Y** Other Radionuclide	**Z** None	**Z** None
Y Skin, Subcutaneous Tissue and Breast	**Y** Other Radionuclide	**Z** None	**Z** None

C **Nuclear Medicine**
P **Musculoskeletal System**
1 **Planar Nuclear Medicine Imaging:** Introduction of radioactive materials into the body for single plane display of images developed from the capture of radioactive emissions

Body Part	Radionuclide	Qualifier	Qualifier
Character 4	Character 5	Character 6	Character 7
1 Skull **4** Thorax **5** Spine **6** Pelvis **7** Spine and Pelvis **8** Upper Extremity, Right **9** Upper Extremity, Left **B** Upper Extremities, Bilateral **C** Lower Extremity, Right **D** Lower Extremity, Left **F** Lower Extremities, Bilateral **Z** Musculoskeletal System, All	**1** Technetium 99m (Tc-99m) **Y** Other Radionuclide	**Z** None	**Z** None
Y Musculoskeletal System, Other	**Y** Other Radionuclide	**Z** None	**Z** None

C Nuclear Medicine
P Musculoskeletal System
2 Tomographic (Tomo) Nuclear Medicine Imaging: Introduction of radioactive materials into the body for three dimensional display of images developed from the capture of radioactive emissions

Body Part	Radionuclide	Qualifier	Qualifier
Character 4	Character 5	Character 6	Character 7
1 Skull 2 Cervical Spine 3 Skull and Cervical Spine 4 Thorax 6 Pelvis 7 Spine and Pelvis 8 Upper Extremity, Right 9 Upper Extremity, Left B Upper Extremities, Bilateral C Lower Extremity, Right D Lower Extremity, Left F Lower Extremities, Bilateral G Thoracic Spine H Lumbar Spine J Thoracolumbar Spine	1 Technetium 99m (Tc-99m) Y Other Radionuclide	Z None	Z None
Y Musculoskeletal System, Other	Y Other Radionuclide	Z None	Z None

C Nuclear Medicine
P Musculoskeletal System
5 Nonimaging Nuclear Medicine Probe: Introduction of radioactive materials into the body for the study of distribution and fate of certain substances by the detection of radioactive emissions; or, alternatively, measurement of absorption of radioactive emissions from an external source

Body Part	Radionuclide	Qualifier	Qualifier
Character 4	Character 5	Character 6	Character 7
5 Spine N Upper Extremities P Lower Extremities	Z None	Z None	Z None
Y Musculoskeletal System, Other	Y Other Radionuclide	Z None	Z None

C Nuclear Medicine
T Urinary System
1 Planar Nuclear Medicine Imaging: Introduction of radioactive materials into the body for single plane display of images developed from the capture of radioactive emissions

Body Part	Radionuclide	Qualifier	Qualifier
Character 4	Character 5	Character 6	Character 7
3 Kidneys, Ureters and Bladder	1 Technetium 99m (Tc-99m) F Iodine 123 (I-123) G Iodine 131 (I-131) Y Other Radionuclide	Z None	Z None
H Bladder and Ureters	1 Technetium 99m (Tc-99m) Y Other Radionuclide	Z None	Z None
Y Urinary System	Y Other Radionuclide	Z None	Z None

C Nuclear Medicine
T Urinary System
2 Tomographic (Tomo) Nuclear Medicine Imaging: Introduction of radioactive materials into the body for three dimensional display of images developed from the capture of radioactive emissions

Body Part	Radionuclide	Qualifier	Qualifier
Character 4	Character 5	Character 6	Character 7
3 Kidneys, Ureters and Bladder	1 Technetium 99m (Tc-99m) Y Other Radionuclide	Z None	Z None
Y Urinary System	Y Other Radionuclide	Z None	Z None

[LC] Limited Coverage   [NC] Noncovered   [HAC] HAC-associated Procedure   [CC] Combination Cluster - See Appendix G for code lists
[DRG] Non-OR-Affecting MS-DRG Assignment   New/Revised Text in **Orange**   ♂ Male   ♀ Female

694   2021 ICD-10-PCS

C **Nuclear Medicine**
T **Urinary System**
6 **Nonimaging Nuclear Medicine Assay:** Introduction of radioactive materials into the body for the study of body fluids and blood elements, by the detection of radioactive emissions

Body Part	Radionuclide	Qualifier	Qualifier
Character 4	Character 5	Character 6	Character 7
3 Kidneys, Ureters and Bladder	**1** Technetium 99m (Tc-99m) **F** Iodine 123 (I-123) **G** Iodine 131 (I-131) **H** Iodine 125 (I-125) **Y** Other Radionuclide	**Z** None	**Z** None
Y Urinary System	**Y** Other Radionuclide	**Z** None	**Z** None

C **Nuclear Medicine**
V **Male Reproductive System**
1 **Planar Nuclear Medicine Imaging:** Introduction of radioactive materials into the body for single plane display of images developed from the capture of radioactive emissions

Body Part	Radionuclide	Qualifier	Qualifier
Character 4	Character 5	Character 6	Character 7
9 Testicles, Bilateral ♂	**1** Technetium 99m (Tc-99m) **Y** Other Radionuclide	**Z** None	**Z** None
Y Male Reproductive System ♂	**Y** Other Radionuclide	**Z** None	**Z** None

♂ CV191ZZ   CV19YZZ   CV1YYZZ

C **Nuclear Medicine**
W **Anatomical Regions**
1 **Planar Nuclear Medicine Imaging:** Introduction of radioactive materials into the body for single plane display of images developed from the capture of radioactive emissions

Body Part	Radionuclide	Qualifier	Qualifier
Character 4	Character 5	Character 6	Character 7
0 Abdomen **1** Abdomen and Pelvis **4** Chest and Abdomen **6** Chest and Neck **B** Head and Neck **D** Lower Extremity **J** Pelvic Region **M** Upper Extremity **N** Whole Body	**1** Technetium 99m (Tc-99m) **D** Indium 111 (In-111) **F** Iodine 123 (I-123) **G** Iodine 131 (I-131) **L** Gallium 67 (Ga-67) **S** Thallium 201 (Tl-201) **Y** Other Radionuclide	**Z** None	**Z** None
3 Chest	**1** Technetium 99m (Tc-99m) **D** Indium 111 (In-111) **F** Iodine 123 (I-123) **G** Iodine 131 (I-131) **K** Fluorine 18 (F-18) **L** Gallium 67 (Ga-67) **S** Thallium 201 (Tl-201) **Y** Other Radionuclide	**Z** None	**Z** None
Y Anatomical Regions, Multiple	**Y** Other Radionuclide	**Z** None	**Z** None
Z Anatomical Region, Other	**Z** None	**Z** None	**Z** None

C Nuclear Medicine
W Anatomical Regions
2 **Tomographic (Tomo) Nuclear Medicine Imaging:** Introduction of radioactive materials into the body for three dimensional display of images developed from the capture of radioactive emissions

Body Part	Radionuclide	Qualifier	Qualifier
Character 4	Character 5	Character 6	Character 7
0 Abdomen **1** Abdomen and Pelvis **3** Chest **4** Chest and Abdomen **6** Chest and Neck **B** Head and Neck **D** Lower Extremity **J** Pelvic Region **M** Upper Extremity	**1** Technetium 99m (Tc-99m) **D** Indium 111 (In-111) **F** Iodine 123 (I-123) **G** Iodine 131 (I-131) **K** Fluorine 18 (F-18) **L** Gallium 67 (Ga-67) **S** Thallium 201 (Tl-201) **Y** Other Radionuclide	**Z** None	**Z** None
Y Anatomical Regions, Multiple	**Y** Other Radionuclide	**Z** None	**Z** None

C Nuclear Medicine
W Anatomical Regions
3 **Positron Emission Tomographic (PET) Imaging:** Introduction of radioactive materials into the body for three dimensional display of images developed from the simultaneous capture, 180 degrees apart, of radioactive emissions

Body Part	Radionuclide	Qualifier	Qualifier
Character 4	Character 5	Character 6	Character 7
N Whole Body	**Y** Other Radionuclide	**Z** None	**Z** None

C Nuclear Medicine
W Anatomical Regions
5 **Nonimaging Nuclear Medicine Probe:** Introduction of radioactive materials into the body for the study of distribution and fate of certain substances by the detection of radioactive emissions; or, alternatively, measurement of absorption of radioactive emissions from an external source

Body Part	Radionuclide	Qualifier	Qualifier
Character 4	Character 5	Character 6	Character 7
0 Abdomen **1** Abdomen and Pelvis **3** Chest **4** Chest and Abdomen **6** Chest and Neck **B** Head and Neck **D** Lower Extremity **J** Pelvic Region **M** Upper Extremity	**1** Technetium 99m (Tc-99m) **D** Indium 111 (In-111) **Y** Other Radionuclide	**Z** None	**Z** None

C Nuclear Medicine
W Anatomical Regions
7 **Systemic Nuclear Medicine Therapy:** Introduction of unsealed radioactive materials into the body for treatment

Body Part	Radionuclide	Qualifier	Qualifier
Character 4	Character 5	Character 6	Character 7
0 Abdomen **3** Chest	**N** Phosphorus 32 (P-32) **Y** Other Radionuclide	**Z** None	**Z** None
G Thyroid	**G** Iodine 131 (I-131) **Y** Other Radionuclide	**Z** None	**Z** None
N Whole Body	**8** Samarium 153 (Sm-153) **G** Iodine 131 (I-131) **N** Phosphorus 32 (P-32) **P** Strontium 89 (Sr-89) **Y** Other Radionuclide	**Z** None	**Z** None
Y Anatomical Regions, Multiple	**Y** Other Radionuclide	**Z** None	**Z** None

LC Limited Coverage   **NC** Noncovered   **HAC** HAC-associated Procedure   **CC** Combination Cluster - See Appendix G for code lists
DRG Non-OR-Affecting MS-DRG Assignment   New/Revised Text in **Orange**   ♂ Male   ♀ Female

696

2021 ICD-10-PCS

NOTES

NOTES

Radiation Therapy D00-DWY

D Radiation Therapy
0 Central and Peripheral Nervous System
0 Beam Radiation

Treatment Site	Modality Qualifier	Isotope	Qualifier
Character 4	**Character 5**	**Character 6**	**Character 7**
0 Brain **1** Brain Stem **6** Spinal Cord **7** Peripheral Nerve	**0** Photons <1 MeV **1** Photons 1 - 10 MeV **2** Photons >10 MeV **4** Heavy Particles (Protons, Ions) **5** Neutrons **6** Neutron Capture	**Z** None	**Z** None
0 Brain **1** Brain Stem **6** Spinal Cord **7** Peripheral Nerve	**3** Electrons	**Z** None	**0** Intraoperative **Z** None

D Radiation Therapy
0 Central and Peripheral Nervous System
1 Brachytherapy

Treatment Site	Modality Qualifier	Isotope	Qualifier
Character 4	**Character 5**	**Character 6**	**Character 7**
0 Brain **1** Brain Stem **6** Spinal Cord **7** Peripheral Nerve	**9** High Dose Rate (HDR)	**7** Cesium 137 (Cs-137) **8** Iridium 192 (Ir-192) **9** Iodine 125 (I-125) **B** Palladium 103 (Pd-103) **C** Californium 252 (Cf-252) **Y** Other Isotope	**Z** None
0 Brain **1** Brain Stem **6** Spinal Cord **7** Peripheral Nerve	**B** Low Dose Rate (LDR)	**6** Cesium 131 (Cs-131) **7** Cesium 137 (Cs-137) **8** Iridium 192 (Ir-192) **9** Iodine 125 (I-125) **C** Californium 252 (Cf-252) **Y** Other Isotope	**Z** None
0 Brain **1** Brain Stem **6** Spinal Cord **7** Peripheral Nerve	**B** Low Dose Rate (LDR)	**B** Palladium 103 (Pd-103)	**1** Unidirectional Source **Z** None

D Radiation Therapy
0 Central and Peripheral Nervous System
2 Stereotactic Radiosurgery

Treatment Site	Modality Qualifier	Isotope	Qualifier
Character 4	**Character 5**	**Character 6**	**Character 7**
0 Brain ᴰᴿᴳ **1** Brain Stem ᴰᴿᴳ **6** Spinal Cord ᴰᴿᴳ **7** Peripheral Nerve ᴰᴿᴳ	**D** Stereotactic Other Photon Radiosurgery **H** Stereotactic Particulate Radiosurgery **J** Stereotactic Gamma Beam Radiosurgery	**Z** None	**Z** None

ᴰᴿᴳ D020DZZ D020HZZ D020JZZ D021DZZ D021HZZ D021JZZ D026DZZ D026HZZ D026JZZ D027DZZ D027HZZ D027JZZ

D Radiation Therapy
0 Central and Peripheral Nervous System
Y Other Radiation

Treatment Site	Modality Qualifier	Isotope	Qualifier
Character 4	**Character 5**	**Character 6**	**Character 7**
0 Brain	7 Contact Radiation	Z None	Z None
1 Brain Stem	8 Hyperthermia		
6 Spinal Cord	C Intraoperative Radiation Therapy (IORT)		
7 Peripheral Nerve	F Plaque Radiation		
	K Laser Interstitial Thermal Therapy		

D Radiation Therapy
7 Lymphatic and Hematologic System
0 Beam Radiation

Treatment Site	Modality Qualifier	Isotope	Qualifier
Character 4	**Character 5**	**Character 6**	**Character 7**
0 Bone Marrow	0 Photons <1 MeV	Z None	Z None
1 Thymus	1 Photons 1 - 10 MeV		
2 Spleen	2 Photons >10 MeV		
3 Lymphatics, Neck	4 Heavy Particles (Protons, Ions)		
4 Lymphatics, Axillary	5 Neutrons		
5 Lymphatics, Thorax	6 Neutron Capture		
6 Lymphatics, Abdomen			
7 Lymphatics, Pelvis			
8 Lymphatics, Inguinal			
0 Bone Marrow	3 Electrons	Z None	0 Intraoperative
1 Thymus			Z None
2 Spleen			
3 Lymphatics, Neck			
4 Lymphatics, Axillary			
5 Lymphatics, Thorax			
6 Lymphatics, Abdomen			
7 Lymphatics, Pelvis			
8 Lymphatics, Inguinal			

LC Limited Coverage   NC Noncovered   HAC HAC-associated Procedure   CC Combination Cluster - See Appendix G for code lists
DRG Non-OR-Affecting MS-DRG Assignment   New/Revised Text in Orange   ♂ Male   ♀ Female

700   2021 ICD-10-PCS

D Radiation Therapy
7 Lymphatic and Hematologic System
1 Brachytherapy

Treatment Site	Modality Qualifier	Isotope	Qualifier
Character 4	Character 5	Character 6	Character 7
0 Bone Marrow 1 Thymus 2 Spleen 3 Lymphatics, Neck 4 Lymphatics, Axillary 5 Lymphatics, Thorax 6 Lymphatics, Abdomen 7 Lymphatics, Pelvis 8 Lymphatics, Inguinal	9 High Dose Rate (HDR)	7 Cesium 137 (Cs-137) 8 Iridium 192 (Ir-192) 9 Iodine 125 (I-125) B Palladium 103 (Pd-103) C Californium 252 (Cf-252) Y Other Isotope	Z None
0 Bone Marrow 1 Thymus 2 Spleen 3 Lymphatics, Neck 4 Lymphatics, Axillary 5 Lymphatics, Thorax 6 Lymphatics, Abdomen 7 Lymphatics, Pelvis 8 Lymphatics, Inguinal	B Low Dose Rate (LDR)	6 Cesium 131 (Cs-131) 7 Cesium 137 (Cs-137) 8 Iridium 192 (Ir-192) 9 Iodine 125 (I-125) C Californium 252 (Cf-252) Y Other Isotope	Z None
0 Bone Marrow 1 Thymus 2 Spleen 3 Lymphatics, Neck 4 Lymphatics, Axillary 5 Lymphatics, Thorax 6 Lymphatics, Abdomen 7 Lymphatics, Pelvis 8 Lymphatics, Inguinal	B Low Dose Rate (LDR)	B Palladium 103 (Pd-103)	1 Unidirectional Source Z None

D Radiation Therapy
7 Lymphatic and Hematologic System
2 Stereotactic Radiosurgery

Treatment Site	Modality Qualifier	Isotope	Qualifier
Character 4	Character 5	Character 6	Character 7
0 Bone Marrow ᴰᴿᴳ 1 Thymus ᴰᴿᴳ 2 Spleen 3 Lymphatics, Neck ᴰᴿᴳ 4 Lymphatics, Axillary ᴰᴿᴳ 5 Lymphatics, Thorax ᴰᴿᴳ 6 Lymphatics, Abdomen ᴰᴿᴳ 7 Lymphatics, Pelvis ᴰᴿᴳ 8 Lymphatics, Inguinal ᴰᴿᴳ	D Stereotactic Other Photon Radiosurgery H Stereotactic Particulate Radiosurgery J Stereotactic Gamma Beam Radiosurgery	Z None	Z None

ᴰᴿᴳ D720DZZ D720HZZ D720JZZ D721DZZ D721HZZ D721JZZ D722DZZ D722HZZ D722JZZ D723DZZ D723HZZ D723JZZ D724DZZ
D724HZZ D724JZZ D725DZZ D725HZZ D725JZZ D726DZZ D726HZZ D726JZZ D727DZZ D727HZZ D727JZZ D728DZZ D728HZZ
D728JZZ

D **Radiation Therapy**
7 **Lymphatic and Hematologic System**
Y **Other Radiation**

Treatment Site	Modality Qualifier	Isotope	Qualifier
Character 4	Character 5	Character 6	Character 7
0 Bone Marrow 1 Thymus 2 Spleen 3 Lymphatics, Neck 4 Lymphatics, Axillary 5 Lymphatics, Thorax 6 Lymphatics, Abdomen 7 Lymphatics, Pelvis 8 Lymphatics, Inguinal	8 Hyperthermia F Plaque Radiation	Z None	Z None

D **Radiation Therapy**
8 **Eye**
0 **Beam Radiation**

Treatment Site	Modality Qualifier	Isotope	Qualifier
Character 4	Character 5	Character 6	Character 7
0 Eye	0 Photons <1 MeV 1 Photons 1 - 10 MeV 2 Photons >10 MeV 4 Heavy Particles (Protons, Ions) 5 Neutrons 6 Neutron Capture	Z None	Z None
0 Eye	3 Electrons	Z None	0 Intraoperative Z None

D **Radiation Therapy**
8 **Eye**
1 **Brachytherapy**

Treatment Site	Modality Qualifier	Isotope	Qualifier
Character 4	Character 5	Character 6	Character 7
0 Eye	9 High Dose Rate (HDR)	7 Cesium 137 (Cs-137) 8 Iridium 192 (Ir-192) 9 Iodine 125 (I-125) B Palladium 103 (Pd-103) C Californium 252 (Cf-252) Y Other Isotope	Z None
0 Eye	B Low Dose Rate (LDR)	6 Cesium 131 (Cs-131) 7 Cesium 137 (Cs-137) 8 Iridium 192 (Ir-192) 9 Iodine 125 (I-125) C Californium 252 (Cf-252) Y Other Isotope	Z None
0 Eye	B Low Dose Rate (LDR)	B Palladium 103 (Pd-103)	1 Unidirectional Source Z None

D **Radiation Therapy**
8 **Eye**
2 **Stereotactic Radiosurgery**

Treatment Site	Modality Qualifier	Isotope	Qualifier
Character 4	Character 5	Character 6	Character 7
0 Eye ⚕	D Stereotactic Other Photon Radiosurgery H Stereotactic Particulate Radiosurgery J Stereotactic Gamma Beam Radiosurgery	Z None	Z None

⚕ D820DZZ   D820HZZ   D820JZZ

D Radiation Therapy
8 Eye
Y Other Radiation

Treatment Site	Modality Qualifier	Isotope	Qualifier
Character 4	Character 5	Character 6	Character 7
0 Eye	**7** Contact Radiation **8** Hyperthermia **F** Plaque Radiation	**Z** None	**Z** None

D Radiation Therapy
9 Ear, Nose, Mouth and Throat
0 Beam Radiation

Treatment Site	Modality Qualifier	Isotope	Qualifier
Character 4	Character 5	Character 6	Character 7
0 Ear **1** Nose **3** Hypopharynx **4** Mouth **5** Tongue **6** Salivary Glands **7** Sinuses **8** Hard Palate **9** Soft Palate **B** Larynx **D** Nasopharynx **F** Oropharynx	**0** Photons <1 MeV **1** Photons 1 - 10 MeV **2** Photons >10 MeV **4** Heavy Particles (Protons, Ions) **5** Neutrons **6** Neutron Capture	**Z** None	**Z** None
0 Ear **1** Nose **3** Hypopharynx **4** Mouth **5** Tongue **6** Salivary Glands **7** Sinuses **8** Hard Palate **9** Soft Palate **B** Larynx **D** Nasopharynx **F** Oropharynx	**3** Electrons	**Z** None	**0** Intraoperative **Z** None

D Radiation Therapy
9 Ear, Nose, Mouth and Throat
1 Brachytherapy

Treatment Site	Modality Qualifier	Isotope	Qualifier
Character 4	**Character 5**	**Character 6**	**Character 7**
0 Ear 1 Nose 3 Hypopharynx 4 Mouth 5 Tongue 6 Salivary Glands 7 Sinuses 8 Hard Palate 9 Soft Palate B Larynx D Nasopharynx F Oropharynx	9 High Dose Rate (HDR)	7 Cesium 137 (Cs-137) 8 Iridium 192 (Ir-192) 9 Iodine 125 (I-125) B Palladium 103 (Pd-103) C Californium 252 (Cf-252) Y Other Isotope	Z None
0 Ear 1 Nose 3 Hypopharynx 4 Mouth 5 Tongue 6 Salivary Glands 7 Sinuses 8 Hard Palate 9 Soft Palate B Larynx D Nasopharynx F Oropharynx	B Low Dose Rate (LDR)	6 Cesium 131 (Cs-131) 7 Cesium 137 (Cs-137) 8 Iridium 192 (Ir-192) 9 Iodine 125 (I-125) C Californium 252 (Cf-252) Y Other Isotope	Z None
0 Ear 1 Nose 3 Hypopharynx 4 Mouth 5 Tongue 6 Salivary Glands 7 Sinuses 8 Hard Palate 9 Soft Palate B Larynx D Nasopharynx F Oropharynx	B Low Dose Rate (LDR)	B Palladium 103 (Pd-103)	1 Unidirectional Source Z None

D Radiation Therapy
9 Ear, Nose, Mouth and Throat
2 Stereotactic Radiosurgery

Treatment Site	Modality Qualifier	Isotope	Qualifier
Character 4	**Character 5**	**Character 6**	**Character 7**
0 Ear ᴼᴿᴳ 1 Nose ᴼᴿᴳ 4 Mouth ᴼᴿᴳ 5 Tongue ᴼᴿᴳ 6 Salivary Glands ᴼᴿᴳ 7 Sinuses ᴼᴿᴳ 8 Hard Palate ᴼᴿᴳ 9 Soft Palate ᴼᴿᴳ B Larynx ᴼᴿᴳ C Pharynx ᴼᴿᴳ D Nasopharynx ᴼᴿᴳ	D Stereotactic Other Photon Radiosurgery H Stereotactic Particulate Radiosurgery J Stereotactic Gamma Beam Radiosurgery	Z None	Z None

ᴼᴿᴳ D920DZZ D920HZZ D920JZZ D921DZZ D921HZZ D921JZZ D924DZZ D924HZZ D924JZZ D925DZZ D925HZZ D925JZZ D926DZZ
D926HZZ D926JZZ D927DZZ D927HZZ D927JZZ D928DZZ D928HZZ D928JZZ D929DZZ D929HZZ D929JZZ D92BDZZ D92BHZZ
D92BJZZ D92CDZZ D92CHZZ D92CJZZ D92DDZZ D92DHZZ D92DJZZ

ᴸᶜ Limited Coverage   ᴺᶜ Noncovered   ᴴᴬᶜ HAC-associated Procedure   ᶜᶜ Combination Cluster - See Appendix G for code lists
ᴼᴿᴳ Non-OR-Affecting MS-DRG Assignment   New/Revised Text in **Orange**   ♂ Male   ♀ Female

D Radiation Therapy
9 Ear, Nose, Mouth and Throat
Y Other Radiation

Treatment Site	Modality Qualifier	Isotope	Qualifier
Character 4	Character 5	Character 6	Character 7
0 Ear 1 Nose 5 Tongue 6 Salivary Glands 7 Sinuses 8 Hard Palate 9 Soft Palate	7 Contact Radiation 8 Hyperthermia F Plaque Radiation	Z None	Z None
3 Hypopharynx F Oropharynx	7 Contact Radiation 8 Hyperthermia	Z None	Z None
4 Mouth B Larynx D Nasopharynx	7 Contact Radiation 8 Hyperthermia C Intraoperative Radiation Therapy (IORT) F Plaque Radiation	Z None	Z None
C Pharynx	C Intraoperative Radiation Therapy (IORT) F Plaque Radiation	Z None	Z None

D Radiation Therapy
B Respiratory System
0 Beam Radiation

Treatment Site	Modality Qualifier	Isotope	Qualifier
Character 4	Character 5	Character 6	Character 7
0 Trachea 1 Bronchus 2 Lung 5 Pleura 6 Mediastinum 7 Chest Wall 8 Diaphragm	0 Photons <1 MeV 1 Photons 1 - 10 MeV 2 Photons >10 MeV 4 Heavy Particles (Protons, Ions) 5 Neutrons 6 Neutron Capture	Z None	Z None
0 Trachea 1 Bronchus 2 Lung 5 Pleura 6 Mediastinum 7 Chest Wall 8 Diaphragm	3 Electrons	Z None	0 Intraoperative Z None

LC Limited Coverage   NC Noncovered   HAC HAC-associated Procedure   CC Combination Cluster - See Appendix G for code lists
DRG Non-OR-Affecting MS-DRG Assignment   New/Revised Text in Orange   ♂ Male   ♀ Female

2021 ICD-10-PCS

705

RADIATION THERAPY D00-DWY

D Radiation Therapy
B Respiratory System
1 Brachytherapy

Treatment Site	Modality Qualifier	Isotope	Qualifier
Character 4	Character 5	Character 6	Character 7
0 Trachea 1 Bronchus 2 Lung 5 Pleura 6 Mediastinum 7 Chest Wall 8 Diaphragm	9 High Dose Rate (HDR)	7 Cesium 137 (Cs-137) 8 Iridium 192 (Ir-192) 9 Iodine 125 (I-125) B Palladium 103 (Pd-103) C Californium 252 (Cf-252) Y Other Isotope	Z None
0 Trachea 1 Bronchus 2 Lung 5 Pleura 6 Mediastinum 7 Chest Wall 8 Diaphragm	B Low Dose Rate (LDR)	6 Cesium 131 (Cs-131) 7 Cesium 137 (Cs-137) 8 Iridium 192 (Ir-192) 9 Iodine 125 (I-125) C Californium 252 (Cf-252) Y Other Isotope	Z None
0 Trachea 1 Bronchus 2 Lung 5 Pleura 6 Mediastinum 7 Chest Wall 8 Diaphragm	B Low Dose Rate (LDR)	B Palladium 103 (Pd-103)	1 Unidirectional Source Z None

D Radiation Therapy
B Respiratory System
2 Stereotactic Radiosurgery

Treatment Site	Modality Qualifier	Isotope	Qualifier
Character 4	Character 5	Character 6	Character 7

0 Trachea ⓓⓡⓖ
1 Bronchus ⓓⓡⓖ
2 Lung ⓓⓡⓖ
5 Pleura ⓓⓡⓖ
6 Mediastinum ⓓⓡⓖ
7 Chest Wall ⓓⓡⓖ
8 Diaphragm ⓓⓡⓖ
	D Stereotactic Other Photon
	    Radiosurgery
	H Stereotactic Particulate
	    Radiosurgery
	J Stereotactic Gamma Beam
	    Radiosurgery
		Z None	Z None

ⓓⓡⓖ DB20DZZ   DB20HZZ   DB20JZZ   DB21DZZ   DB21HZZ   DB21JZZ   DB22DZZ   DB22HZZ   DB22JZZ   DB25DZZ   DB25HZZ   DB25JZZ   DB26DZZ
       DB26HZZ   DB26JZZ   DB27DZZ   DB27HZZ   DB27JZZ   DB28DZZ   DB28HZZ   DB28JZZ

D Radiation Therapy
B Respiratory System
Y Other Radiation

Treatment Site	Modality Qualifier	Isotope	Qualifier
Character 4	Character 5	Character 6	Character 7
0 Trachea 1 Bronchus 2 Lung 5 Pleura 6 Mediastinum 7 Chest Wall 8 Diaphragm	7 Contact Radiation 8 Hyperthermia F Plaque Radiation K Laser Interstitial Thermal Therapy	Z None	Z None

D Radiation Therapy
D Gastrointestinal System
0 Beam Radiation

Treatment Site	Modality Qualifier	Isotope	Qualifier
Character 4	Character 5	Character 6	Character 7
0 Esophagus 1 Stomach 2 Duodenum 3 Jejunum 4 Ileum 5 Colon 7 Rectum	0 Photons <1 MeV 1 Photons 1 - 10 MeV 2 Photons >10 MeV 4 Heavy Particles (Protons, Ions) 5 Neutrons 6 Neutron Capture	Z None	Z None
0 Esophagus 1 Stomach 2 Duodenum 3 Jejunum 4 Ileum 5 Colon 7 Rectum	3 Electrons	Z None	0 Intraoperative Z None

D Radiation Therapy
D Gastrointestinal System
1 Brachytherapy

Treatment Site	Modality Qualifier	Isotope	Qualifier
Character 4	Character 5	Character 6	Character 7
0 Esophagus 1 Stomach 2 Duodenum 3 Jejunum 4 Ileum 5 Colon 7 Rectum	9 High Dose Rate (HDR)	7 Cesium 137 (Cs-137) 8 Iridium 192 (Ir-192) 9 Iodine 125 (I-125) B Palladium 103 (Pd-103) C Californium 252 (Cf-252) Y Other Isotope	Z None
0 Esophagus 1 Stomach 2 Duodenum 3 Jejunum 4 Ileum 5 Colon 7 Rectum	B Low Dose Rate (LDR)	6 Cesium 131 (Cs-131) 7 Cesium 137 (Cs-137) 8 Iridium 192 (Ir-192) 9 Iodine 125 (I-125) C Californium 252 (Cf-252) Y Other Isotope	Z None
0 Esophagus 1 Stomach 2 Duodenum 3 Jejunum 4 Ileum 5 Colon 7 Rectum	B Low Dose Rate (LDR)	B Palladium 103 (Pd-103)	1 Unidirectional Source Z None

D Radiation Therapy
D Gastrointestinal System
2 Stereotactic Radiosurgery

Treatment Site	Modality Qualifier	Isotope	Qualifier
Character 4	Character 5	Character 6	Character 7
0 Esophagus 🅐 1 Stomach 🅐 2 Duodenum 🅐 3 Jejunum 🅐 4 Ileum 🅐 5 Colon 🅐 7 Rectum 🅐	D Stereotactic Other Photon Radiosurgery H Stereotactic Particulate Radiosurgery J Stereotactic Gamma Beam Radiosurgery	Z None	Z None

🅐 DD20DZZ DD20HZZ DD20JZZ DD21DZZ DD21HZZ DD21JZZ DD22DZZ DD22HZZ DD22JZZ DD23DZZ DD23HZZ DD23JZZ DD24DZZ
DD24HZZ DD24JZZ DD25DZZ DD25HZZ DD25JZZ DD27DZZ DD27HZZ DD27JZZ

LC Limited Coverage   **NC** Noncovered   **HAC** HAC-associated Procedure   **CC** Combination Cluster - See Appendix G for code lists
🅐 Non-OR-Affecting MS-DRG Assignment   New/Revised Text in **Orange**   ♂ Male   ♀ Female

D **Radiation Therapy**
D **Gastrointestinal System**
Y **Other Radiation**

Treatment Site	Modality Qualifier	Isotope	Qualifier
Character 4	Character 5	Character 6	Character 7
0 Esophagus	**7** Contact Radiation **8** Hyperthermia **F** Plaque Radiation **K** Laser Interstitial Thermal Therapy	**Z** None	**Z** None
1 Stomach **2** Duodenum **3** Jejunum **4** Ileum **5** Colon **7** Rectum	**7** Contact Radiation **8** Hyperthermia **C** Intraoperative Radiation Therapy (IORT) **F** Plaque Radiation **K** Laser Interstitial Thermal Therapy	**Z** None	**Z** None
8 Anus	**C** Intraoperative Radiation Therapy (IORT) **F** Plaque Radiation **K** Laser Interstitial Thermal Therapy	**Z** None	**Z** None

D **Radiation Therapy**
F **Hepatobiliary System and Pancreas**
0 **Beam Radiation**

Treatment Site	Modality Qualifier	Isotope	Qualifier
Character 4	Character 5	Character 6	Character 7
0 Liver **1** Gallbladder **2** Bile Ducts **3** Pancreas	**0** Photons <1 MeV **1** Photons 1 - 10 MeV **2** Photons >10 MeV **4** Heavy Particles (Protons, Ions) **5** Neutrons **6** Neutron Capture	**Z** None	**Z** None
0 Liver **1** Gallbladder **2** Bile Ducts **3** Pancreas	**3** Electrons	**Z** None	**0** Intraoperative **Z** None

D **Radiation Therapy**
F **Hepatobiliary System and Pancreas**
1 **Brachytherapy**

Treatment Site	Modality Qualifier	Isotope	Qualifier
Character 4	Character 5	Character 6	Character 7
0 Liver **1** Gallbladder **2** Bile Ducts **3** Pancreas	**9** High Dose Rate (HDR)	**7** Cesium 137 (Cs-137) **8** Iridium 192 (Ir-192) **9** Iodine 125 (I-125) **B** Palladium 103 (Pd-103) **C** Californium 252 (Cf-252) **Y** Other Isotope	**Z** None
0 Liver **1** Gallbladder **2** Bile Ducts **3** Pancreas	**B** Low Dose Rate (LDR)	**6** Cesium 131 (Cs-131) **7** Cesium 137 (Cs-137) **8** Iridium 192 (Ir-192) **9** Iodine 125 (I-125) **C** Californium 252 (Cf-252) **Y** Other Isotope	**Z** None
0 Liver **1** Gallbladder **2** Bile Ducts **3** Pancreas	**B** Low Dose Rate (LDR)	**B** Palladium 103 (Pd-103)	**1** Unidirectional Source **Z** None

D Radiation Therapy
F Hepatobiliary System and Pancreas
2 Stereotactic Radiosurgery

Treatment Site	Modality Qualifier	Isotope	Qualifier
Character 4	Character 5	Character 6	Character 7
0 Liver ᴰᴿᴳ 1 Gallbladder ᴰᴿᴳ 2 Bile Ducts ᴰᴿᴳ 3 Pancreas ᴰᴿᴳ	D Stereotactic Other Photon Radiosurgery H Stereotactic Particulate Radiosurgery J Stereotactic Gamma Beam Radiosurgery	Z None	Z None

ᴰᴿᴳ   DF20DZZ   DF20HZZ   DF20JZZ   DF21DZZ   DF21HZZ   DF21JZZ   DF22DZZ   DF22HZZ   DF22JZZ   DF23DZZ   DF23HZZ   DF23JZZ

D Radiation Therapy
F Hepatobiliary System and Pancreas
Y Other Radiation

Treatment Site	Modality Qualifier	Isotope	Qualifier
Character 4	Character 5	Character 6	Character 7
0 Liver 1 Gallbladder 2 Bile Ducts 3 Pancreas	7 Contact Radiation 8 Hyperthermia C Intraoperative Radiation Therapy (IORT) F Plaque Radiation K Laser Interstitial Thermal Therapy	Z None	Z None

D Radiation Therapy
G Endocrine System
0 Beam Radiation

Treatment Site	Modality Qualifier	Isotope	Qualifier
Character 4	Character 5	Character 6	Character 7
0 Pituitary Gland 1 Pineal Body 2 Adrenal Glands 4 Parathyroid Glands 5 Thyroid	0 Photons <1 MeV 1 Photons 1 - 10 MeV 2 Photons >10 MeV 5 Neutrons 6 Neutron Capture	Z None	Z None
0 Pituitary Gland 1 Pineal Body 2 Adrenal Glands 4 Parathyroid Glands 5 Thyroid	3 Electrons	Z None	0 Intraoperative Z None

D Radiation Therapy
G Endocrine System
1 Brachytherapy

Treatment Site	Modality Qualifier	Isotope	Qualifier
Character 4	Character 5	Character 6	Character 7
0 Pituitary Gland 1 Pineal Body 2 Adrenal Glands 4 Parathyroid Glands 5 Thyroid	9 High Dose Rate (HDR)	7 Cesium 137 (Cs-137) 8 Iridium 192 (Ir-192) 9 Iodine 125 (I-125) B Palladium 103 (Pd-103) C Californium 252 (Cf-252) Y Other Isotope	Z None
0 Pituitary Gland 1 Pineal Body 2 Adrenal Glands 4 Parathyroid Glands 5 Thyroid	B Low Dose Rate (LDR)	6 Cesium 131 (Cs-131) 7 Cesium 137 (Cs-137) 8 Iridium 192 (Ir-192) 9 Iodine 125 (I-125) C Californium 252 (Cf-252) Y Other Isotope	Z None
0 Pituitary Gland 1 Pineal Body 2 Adrenal Glands 4 Parathyroid Glands 5 Thyroid	B Low Dose Rate (LDR)	B Palladium 103 (Pd-103)	1 Unidirectional Source Z None

D Radiation Therapy
G Endocrine System
2 Stereotactic Radiosurgery

Treatment Site	Modality Qualifier	Isotope	Qualifier
Character 4	Character 5	Character 6	Character 7
0 Pituitary Gland ᴰᴿᴳ **1** Pineal Body ᴰᴿᴳ **2** Adrenal Glands ᴰᴿᴳ **4** Parathyroid Glands ᴰᴿᴳ **5** Thyroid ᴰᴿᴳ	**D** Stereotactic Other Photon Radiosurgery **H** Stereotactic Particulate Radiosurgery **J** Stereotactic Gamma Beam Radiosurgery	**Z** None	**Z** None

ᴰᴿᴳ DG20DZZ   DG20HZZ   DG20JZZ   DG21DZZ   DG21HZZ   DG21JZZ   DG22DZZ   DG22HZZ   DG22JZZ   DG24DZZ   DG24HZZ   DG24JZZ   DG25DZZ
DG25HZZ   DG25JZZ

D Radiation Therapy
G Endocrine System
Y Other Radiation

Treatment Site	Modality Qualifier	Isotope	Qualifier
Character 4	Character 5	Character 6	Character 7
0 Pituitary Gland **1** Pineal Body **2** Adrenal Glands **4** Parathyroid Glands **5** Thyroid	**7** Contact Radiation **8** Hyperthermia **F** Plaque Radiation **K** Laser Interstitial Thermal Therapy	**Z** None	**Z** None

D Radiation Therapy
H Skin
0 Beam Radiation

Treatment Site	Modality Qualifier	Isotope	Qualifier
Character 4	Character 5	Character 6	Character 7
2 Skin, Face **3** Skin, Neck **4** Skin, Arm **6** Skin, Chest **7** Skin, Back **8** Skin, Abdomen **9** Skin, Buttock **B** Skin, Leg	**0** Photons <1 MeV **1** Photons 1 - 10 MeV **2** Photons >10 MeV **4** Heavy Particles (Protons, Ions) **5** Neutrons **6** Neutron Capture	**Z** None	**Z** None
2 Skin, Face **3** Skin, Neck **4** Skin, Arm **6** Skin, Chest **7** Skin, Back **8** Skin, Abdomen **9** Skin, Buttock **B** Skin, Leg	**3** Electrons	**Z** None	**0** Intraoperative **Z** None

LC Limited Coverage   **NC** Noncovered   **HAC** HAC-associated Procedure   **CC** Combination Cluster - See Appendix G for code lists
ᴰᴿᴳ Non-OR-Affecting MS-DRG Assignment   New/Revised Text in **Orange**   ♂ Male   ♀ Female

710   **2021 ICD-10-PCS**

D Radiation Therapy
H Skin
Y Other Radiation

Treatment Site	Modality Qualifier	Isotope	Qualifier
Character 4	Character 5	Character 6	Character 7
2 Skin, Face 3 Skin, Neck 4 Skin, Arm 6 Skin, Chest 7 Skin, Back 8 Skin, Abdomen 9 Skin, Buttock B Skin, Leg	7 Contact Radiation 8 Hyperthermia F Plaque Radiation	Z None	Z None
5 Skin, Hand C Skin, Foot	F Plaque Radiation	Z None	Z None

D Radiation Therapy
M Breast
0 Beam Radiation

Treatment Site	Modality Qualifier	Isotope	Qualifier
Character 4	Character 5	Character 6	Character 7
0 Breast, Left 1 Breast, Right	0 Photons <1 MeV 1 Photons 1 - 10 MeV 2 Photons >10 MeV 4 Heavy Particles (Protons, Ions) 5 Neutrons 6 Neutron Capture	Z None	Z None
0 Breast, Left 1 Breast, Right	3 Electrons	Z None	0 Intraoperative Z None

D Radiation Therapy
M Breast
1 Brachytherapy

Treatment Site	Modality Qualifier	Isotope	Qualifier
Character 4	Character 5	Character 6	Character 7
0 Breast, Left 1 Breast, Right	9 High Dose Rate (HDR)	7 Cesium 137 (Cs-137) 8 Iridium 192 (Ir-192) 9 Iodine 125 (I-125) B Palladium 103 (Pd-103) C Californium 252 (Cf-252) Y Other Isotope	Z None
0 Breast, Left 1 Breast, Right	B Low Dose Rate (LDR)	6 Cesium 131 (Cs-131) 7 Cesium 137 (Cs-137) 8 Iridium 192 (Ir-192) 9 Iodine 125 (I-125) C Californium 252 (Cf-252) Y Other Isotope	Z None
0 Breast, Left 1 Breast, Right	B Low Dose Rate (LDR)	B Palladium 103 (Pd-103)	1 Unidirectional Source Z None

LC Limited Coverage   **NC** Noncovered   **HAC** HAC-associated Procedure   **CC** Combination Cluster - See Appendix G for code lists
DRG Non-OR-Affecting MS-DRG Assignment   New/Revised Text in **Orange**   ♂ Male   ♀ Female

2021 ICD-10-PCS

711

D Radiation Therapy
M Breast
2 Stereotactic Radiosurgery

Treatment Site	Modality Qualifier	Isotope	Qualifier
Character 4	Character 5	Character 6	Character 7
0 Breast, Left ᴰᴿᴳ **1** Breast, Right ᴰᴿᴳ	**D** Stereotactic Other Photon Radiosurgery **H** Stereotactic Particulate Radiosurgery **J** Stereotactic Gamma Beam Radiosurgery	**Z** None	**Z** None

ᴰᴿᴳ   DM20DZZ   DM20HZZ   DM20JZZ   DM21DZZ   DM21HZZ   DM21JZZ

D Radiation Therapy
M Breast
Y Other Radiation

Treatment Site	Modality Qualifier	Isotope	Qualifier
Character 4	Character 5	Character 6	Character 7
0 Breast, Left **1** Breast, Right	**7** Contact Radiation **8** Hyperthermia **F** Plaque Radiation **K** Laser Interstitial Thermal Therapy	**Z** None	**Z** None

D Radiation Therapy
P Musculoskeletal System
0 Beam Radiation

Treatment Site	Modality Qualifier	Isotope	Qualifier
Character 4	Character 5	Character 6	Character 7
0 Skull **2** Maxilla **3** Mandible **4** Sternum **5** Rib(s) **6** Humerus **7** Radius/Ulna **8** Pelvic Bones **9** Femur **B** Tibia/Fibula **C** Other Bone	**0** Photons <1 MeV **1** Photons 1 - 10 MeV **2** Photons >10 MeV **4** Heavy Particles (Protons, Ions) **5** Neutrons **6** Neutron Capture	**Z** None	**Z** None
0 Skull **2** Maxilla **3** Mandible **4** Sternum **5** Rib(s) **6** Humerus **7** Radius/Ulna **8** Pelvic Bones **9** Femur **B** Tibia/Fibula **C** Other Bone	**3** Electrons	**Z** None	**0** Intraoperative **Z** None

🅛🅒 Limited Coverage   🅝🅒 Noncovered   🅗🅐🅒 HAC-associated Procedure   🅒🅒 Combination Cluster - See Appendix G for code lists
ᴰᴿᴳ Non-OR-Affecting MS-DRG Assignment   New/Revised Text in **Orange**   ♂ Male   ♀ Female

712

2021 ICD-10-PCS

D Radiation Therapy
P Musculoskeletal System
Y Other Radiation

Treatment Site	Modality Qualifier	Isotope	Qualifier
Character 4	Character 5	Character 6	Character 7
0 Skull 2 Maxilla 3 Mandible 4 Sternum 5 Rib(s) 6 Humerus 7 Radius/Ulna 8 Pelvic Bones 9 Femur B Tibia/Fibula C Other Bone	7 Contact Radiation 8 Hyperthermia F Plaque Radiation	Z None	Z None

D Radiation Therapy
T Urinary System
0 Beam Radiation

Treatment Site	Modality Qualifier	Isotope	Qualifier
Character 4	Character 5	Character 6	Character 7
0 Kidney 1 Ureter 2 Bladder 3 Urethra	0 Photons <1 MeV 1 Photons 1 - 10 MeV 2 Photons >10 MeV 4 Heavy Particles (Protons, Ions) 5 Neutrons 6 Neutron Capture	Z None	Z None
0 Kidney 1 Ureter 2 Bladder 3 Urethra	3 Electrons	Z None	0 Intraoperative Z None

D Radiation Therapy
T Urinary System
1 Brachytherapy

Treatment Site	Modality Qualifier	Isotope	Qualifier
Character 4	Character 5	Character 6	Character 7
0 Kidney 1 Ureter 2 Bladder 3 Urethra	9 High Dose Rate (HDR)	7 Cesium 137 (Cs-137) 8 Iridium 192 (Ir-192) 9 Iodine 125 (I-125) B Palladium 103 (Pd-103) C Californium 252 (Cf-252) Y Other Isotope	Z None
0 Kidney 1 Ureter 2 Bladder 3 Urethra	B Low Dose Rate (LDR)	6 Cesium 131 (Cs-131) 7 Cesium 137 (Cs-137) 8 Iridium 192 (Ir-192) 9 Iodine 125 (I-125) C Californium 252 (Cf-252) Y Other Isotope	Z None
0 Kidney 1 Ureter 2 Bladder 3 Urethra	B Low Dose Rate (LDR)	B Palladium 103 (Pd-103)	1 Unidirectional Source Z None

D Radiation Therapy
T Urinary System
2 Stereotactic Radiosurgery

Treatment Site	Modality Qualifier	Isotope	Qualifier
Character 4	Character 5	Character 6	Character 7
0 Kidney ᴰᴿᴳ **1** Ureter ᴰᴿᴳ **2** Bladder ᴰᴿᴳ **3** Urethra ᴰᴿᴳ	**D** Stereotactic Other Photon Radiosurgery **H** Stereotactic Particulate Radiosurgery **J** Stereotactic Gamma Beam Radiosurgery	**Z** None	**Z** None

ᴰᴿᴳ   DT20DZZ   DT20HZZ   DT20JZZ   DT21DZZ   DT21HZZ   DT21JZZ   DT22DZZ   DT22HZZ   DT22JZZ   DT23DZZ   DT23HZZ   DT23JZZ

D Radiation Therapy
T Urinary System
Y Other Radiation

Treatment Site	Modality Qualifier	Isotope	Qualifier
Character 4	Character 5	Character 6	Character 7
0 Kidney **1** Ureter **2** Bladder **3** Urethra	**7** Contact Radiation **8** Hyperthermia **C** Intraoperative Radiation Therapy (IORT) **F** Plaque Radiation	**Z** None	**Z** None

D Radiation Therapy
U Female Reproductive System
0 Beam Radiation

Treatment Site	Modality Qualifier	Isotope	Qualifier
Character 4	Character 5	Character 6	Character 7
0 Ovary ♀ **1** Cervix ♀ **2** Uterus ♀	**0** Photons <1 MeV **1** Photons 1 - 10 MeV **2** Photons >10 MeV **4** Heavy Particles (Protons, Ions) **5** Neutrons **6** Neutron Capture	**Z** None	**Z** None
0 Ovary ♀ **1** Cervix ♀ **2** Uterus ♀	**3** Electrons	**Z** None	**0** Intraoperative **Z** None

♀   DU000ZZ   DU001ZZ   DU002ZZ   DU003Z0   DU003ZZ   DU004ZZ   DU005ZZ   DU006ZZ   DU010ZZ   DU011ZZ   DU012ZZ   DU013Z0   DU013ZZ
     DU014ZZ   DU015ZZ   DU016ZZ   DU020ZZ   DU021ZZ   DU022ZZ   DU023Z0   DU023ZZ   DU024ZZ   DU025ZZ   DU026ZZ

ᴸᶜ Limited Coverage   ᴺᶜ Noncovered   ᴴᴬᶜ HAC-associated Procedure   ᶜᶜ Combination Cluster - See Appendix G for code lists
ᴰᴿᴳ Non-OR-Affecting MS-DRG Assignment   New/Revised Text in **Orange**   ♂ Male   ♀ Female

714

2021 ICD-10-PCS

D Radiation Therapy
U Female Reproductive System
1 Brachytherapy

Treatment Site	Modality Qualifier	Isotope	Qualifier
Character 4	**Character 5**	**Character 6**	**Character 7**
0 Ovary ♀ **1** Cervix ♀ **2** Uterus ♀	**9** High Dose Rate (HDR)	**7** Cesium 137 (Cs-137) **8** Iridium 192 (Ir-192) **9** Iodine 125 (I-125) **B** Palladium 103 (Pd-103) **C** Californium 252 (Cf-252) **Y** Other Isotope	**Z** None
0 Ovary ♀ **1** Cervix ♀ **2** Uterus	**B** Low Dose Rate (LDR)	**6** Cesium 131 (Cs-131) **7** Cesium 137 (Cs-137) **8** Iridium 192 (Ir-192) **9** Iodine 125 (I-125) **C** Californium 252 (Cf-252) **Y** Other Isotope	**Z** None
0 Ovary ♀ **1** Cervix ♀ **2** Uterus ♀	**B** Low Dose Rate (LDR)	**B** Palladium 103 (Pd-103)	**1** Unidirectional Source **Z** None

♀ DU1097Z   DU1098Z   DU1099Z   DU109BZ   DU109CZ   DU109YZ   DU10B7Z   DU10B8Z   DU10B9Z   DU10BB1   DU10BBZ   DU10BCZ   DU10BYZ
   DU1197Z   DU1198Z   DU1199Z   DU119BZ   DU119CZ   DU119YZ   DU11B7Z   DU11B8Z   DU11B9Z   DU11BB1   DU11BBZ   DU11BCZ   DU11BYZ
   DU1297Z   DU1298Z   DU1299Z   DU129BZ   DU129CZ   DU129YZ   DU12B7Z   DU12B8Z   DU12B9Z   DU12BB1   DU12BBZ   DU12BCZ   DU12BYZ

D Radiation Therapy
U Female Reproductive System
2 Stereotactic Radiosurgery

Treatment Site	Modality Qualifier	Isotope	Qualifier
Character 4	**Character 5**	**Character 6**	**Character 7**
0 Ovary ♀ ᴅʀɢ **1** Cervix ♀ ᴅʀɢ **2** Uterus ♀ ᴅʀɢ	**D** Stereotactic Other Photon Radiosurgery **H** Stereotactic Particulate Radiosurgery **J** Stereotactic Gamma Beam Radiosurgery	**Z** None	**Z** None

♀   DU20DZZ   DU20HZZ   DU20JZZ   DU21DZZ   DU21HZZ   DU21JZZ   DU22DZZ   DU22HZZ   DU22JZZ

ᴅʀɢ DU20DZZ   DU20HZZ   DU20JZZ   DU21DZZ   DU21HZZ   DU21JZZ   DU22DZZ   DU22HZZ   DU22JZZ

D Radiation Therapy
U Female Reproductive System
Y Other Radiation

Treatment Site	Modality Qualifier	Isotope	Qualifier
Character 4	**Character 5**	**Character 6**	**Character 7**
0 Ovary ♀ **1** Cervix ♀ **2** Uterus ♀	**7** Contact Radiation **8** Hyperthermia **C** Intraoperative Radiation Therapy (IORT) **F** Plaque Radiation	**Z** None	**Z** None

♀   DUY07ZZ   DUY08ZZ   DUY0CZZ   DUY0FZZ   DUY17ZZ   DUY18ZZ   DUY1CZZ   DUY1FZZ   DUY27ZZ   DUY28ZZ   DUY2CZZ   DUY2FZZ

ʟᴄ Limited Coverage   ɴᴄ Noncovered   ʜᴀᴄ HAC-associated Procedure   ᴄᴄ Combination Cluster - See Appendix G for code lists
ᴅʀɢ Non-OR-Affecting MS-DRG Assignment   New/Revised Text in **Orange**   ♂ Male   ♀ Female

D Radiation Therapy
V Male Reproductive System
0 Beam Radiation

Treatment Site	Modality Qualifier	Isotope	Qualifier
Character 4	Character 5	Character 6	Character 7
0 Prostate ♂ 1 Testis ♂	0 Photons <1 MeV 1 Photons 1 - 10 MeV 2 Photons >10 MeV 4 Heavy Particles (Protons, Ions) 5 Neutrons 6 Neutron Capture	Z None	Z None
0 Prostate ♂ 1 Testis ♂	3 Electrons	Z None	0 Intraoperative Z None

♂ DV000ZZ   DV001ZZ   DV002ZZ   DV003Z0   DV003ZZ   DV004ZZ   DV005ZZ   DV006ZZ   DV010ZZ   DV011ZZ   DV012ZZ   DV013Z0   DV013ZZ
　 DV014ZZ   DV015ZZ   DV016ZZ

D Radiation Therapy
V Male Reproductive System
1 Brachytherapy

Treatment Site	Modality Qualifier	Isotope	Qualifier
Character 4	Character 5	Character 6	Character 7
0 Prostate ♂ 1 Testis ♂	9 High Dose Rate (HDR)	7 Cesium 137 (Cs-137) 8 Iridium 192 (Ir-192) 9 Iodine 125 (I-125) B Palladium 103 (Pd-103) C Californium 252 (Cf-252) Y Other Isotope	Z None
0 Prostate ♂ 1 Testis ♂	B Low Dose Rate (LDR)	6 Cesium 131 (Cs-131) 7 Cesium 137 (Cs-137) 8 Iridium 192 (Ir-192) 9 Iodine 125 (I-125) C Californium 252 (Cf-252) Y Other Isotope	Z None
0 Prostate ♂ 1 Testis ♂	B Low Dose Rate (LDR)	B Palladium 103 (Pd-103)	1 Unidirectional Source Z None

♂ DV1097Z   DV1098Z   DV1099Z   DV109BZ   DV109CZ   DV109YZ   DV10B7Z   DV10B8Z   DV10B9Z   DV10BB1   DV10BBZ   DV10BCZ   DV10BYZ
　 DV1197Z   DV1198Z   DV1199Z   DV119BZ   DV119CZ   DV119YZ   DV11B7Z   DV11B8Z   DV11B9Z   DV11BB1   DV11BBZ   DV11BCZ   DV11BYZ

D Radiation Therapy
V Male Reproductive System
2 Stereotactic Radiosurgery

Treatment Site	Modality Qualifier	Isotope	Qualifier
Character 4	Character 5	Character 6	Character 7
0 Prostate ♂ ⓓ 1 Testis ♂ ⓓ	D Stereotactic Other Photon 　 Radiosurgery H Stereotactic Particulate 　 Radiosurgery J Stereotactic Gamma Beam 　 Radiosurgery	Z None	Z None

♂ DV20DZZ   DV20HZZ   DV20JZZ   DV21DZZ   DV21HZZ   DV21JZZ
ⓓ DV20DZZ   DV20HZZ   DV20JZZ   DV21DZZ   DV21HZZ   DV21JZZ

ⓛⓒ Limited Coverage   ⓝⓒ Noncovered   ⒽⒶⒸ HAC-associated Procedure   ⓒⓒ Combination Cluster - See Appendix G for code lists
ⓓ Non-OR-Affecting MS-DRG Assignment   New/Revised Text in **Orange**   ♂ Male   ♀ Female

716   2021 ICD-10-PCS

D Radiation Therapy
V Male Reproductive System
Y Other Radiation

Treatment Site	Modality Qualifier	Isotope	Qualifier
Character 4	**Character 5**	**Character 6**	**Character 7**
0 Prostate ♂	**7** Contact Radiation **8** Hyperthermia **C** Intraoperative Radiation Therapy (IORT) **F** Plaque Radiation **K** Laser Interstitial Thermal Therapy	**Z** None	**Z** None
1 Testis ♂	**7** Contact Radiation **8** Hyperthermia **F** Plaque Radiation	**Z** None	**Z** None

♂ DVY07ZZ   DVY08ZZ   DVY0CZZ   DVY0FZZ   DVY0KZZ   DVY17ZZ   DVY18ZZ   DVY1FZZ

D Radiation Therapy
W Anatomical Regions
0 Beam Radiation

Treatment Site	Modality Qualifier	Isotope	Qualifier
Character 4	**Character 5**	**Character 6**	**Character 7**
1 Head and Neck **2** Chest **3** Abdomen **4** Hemibody **5** Whole Body **6** Pelvic Region	**0** Photons <1 MeV **1** Photons 1 - 10 MeV **2** Photons >10 MeV **4** Heavy Particles (Protons, Ions) **5** Neutrons **6** Neutron Capture	**Z** None	**Z** None
1 Head and Neck **2** Chest **3** Abdomen **4** Hemibody **5** Whole Body **6** Pelvic Region	**3** Electrons	**Z** None	**0** Intraoperative **Z** None

D Radiation Therapy
W Anatomical Regions
1 Brachytherapy

Treatment Site	Modality Qualifier	Isotope	Qualifier
Character 4	**Character 5**	**Character 6**	**Character 7**
0 Cranial Cavity **K** Upper Back **L** Lower Back **P** Gastrointestinal Tract **Q** Respiratory Tract **R** Genitourinary Tract **X** Upper Extremity **Y** Lower Extremity	**B** Low Dose Rate (LDR)	**B** Palladium 103 (Pd-103)	**1** Unidirectional Source **Z** None
1 Head and Neck **2** Chest **3** Abdomen **6** Pelvic Region	**9** High Dose Rate (HDR)	**7** Cesium 137 (Cs-137) **8** Iridium 192 (Ir-192) **9** Iodine 125 (I-125) **B** Palladium 103 (Pd-103) **C** Californium 252 (Cf-252) **Y** Other Isotope	**Z** None
1 Head and Neck **2** Chest **3** Abdomen **6** Pelvic Region	**B** Low Dose Rate (LDR)	**6** Cesium 131 (Cs-131) **7** Cesium 137 (Cs-137) **8** Iridium 192 (Ir-192) **9** Iodine 125 (I-125) **C** Californium 252 (Cf-252) **Y** Other Isotope	**Z** None
1 Head and Neck **2** Chest **3** Abdomen **6** Pelvic Region	**B** Low Dose Rate (LDR)	**B** Palladium 103 (Pd-103)	**1** Unidirectional Source **Z** None

D Radiation Therapy
W Anatomical Regions
2 Stereotactic Radiosurgery

Treatment Site	Modality Qualifier	Isotope	Qualifier
Character 4	**Character 5**	**Character 6**	**Character 7**
1 Head and Neck ⒟⒭⒢ **2** Chest ⒟⒭⒢ **3** Abdomen ⒟⒭⒢ **6** Pelvic Region ⒟⒭⒢	**D** Stereotactic Other Photon Radiosurgery **H** Stereotactic Particulate Radiosurgery **J** Stereotactic Gamma Beam Radiosurgery	**Z** None	**Z** None

⒟⒭⒢ DW21DZZ DW21HZZ DW21JZZ DW22DZZ DW22HZZ DW22JZZ DW23DZZ DW23HZZ DW23JZZ DW26DZZ DW26HZZ DW26JZZ

D Radiation Therapy
W Anatomical Regions
Y Other Radiation

Treatment Site	Modality Qualifier	Isotope	Qualifier
Character 4	**Character 5**	**Character 6**	**Character 7**
1 Head and Neck **2** Chest **3** Abdomen **4** Hemibody **6** Pelvic Region	**7** Contact Radiation **8** Hyperthermia **F** Plaque Radiation	**Z** None	**Z** None
5 Whole Body	**7** Contact Radiation **8** Hyperthermia **F** Plaque Radiation	**Z** None	**Z** None
5 Whole Body	**G** Isotope Administration	**D** Iodine 131 (I-131) **F** Phosphorus 32 (P-32) **G** Strontium 89 (Sr-89) **H** Strontium 90 (Sr-90) **Y** Other Isotope	**Z** None

ⓛⓒ Limited Coverage   ⓝⓒ Noncovered   ⒽⒶⒸ HAC-associated Procedure   ⓒⓒ Combination Cluster - See Appendix G for code lists
⒟⒭⒢ Non-OR-Affecting MS-DRG Assignment   New/Revised Text in Orange   ♂ Male   ♀ Female

NOTES

NOTES

Physical Rehabilitation and Diagnostic Audiology F00-F15

F **Physical Rehabilitation and Diagnostic Audiology**
0 **Rehabilitation**
0 **Speech Assessment:** Measurement of speech and related functions

Body system/ Region	Type Qualifier	Equipment	Qualifier
Character 4	**Character 5**	**Character 6**	**Character 7**
3 Neurological System - Whole Body 🔵	**G** Communicative/Cognitive Integration Skills	**K** Audiovisual **M** Augmentative / Alternative Communication **P** Computer **Y** Other Equipment **Z** None	**Z** None
Z None 🔵	**0** Filtered Speech **3** Staggered Spondaic Word **Q** Performance Intensity Phonetically Balanced Speech Discrimination **R** Brief Tone Stimuli **S** Distorted Speech **T** Dichotic Stimuli **V** Temporal Ordering of Stimuli **W** Masking Patterns	**1** Audiometer **2** Sound Field / Booth **K** Audiovisual **Z** None	**Z** None
Z None 🔵	**1** Speech Threshold **2** Speech/Word Recognition	**1** Audiometer **2** Sound Field / Booth **9** Cochlear Implant **K** Audiovisual **Z** None	**Z** None
Z None 🔵	**4** Sensorineural Acuity Level	**1** Audiometer **2** Sound Field / Booth **Z** None	**Z** None
Z None 🔵	**5** Synthetic Sentence Identification	**1** Audiometer **2** Sound Field / Booth **9** Cochlear Implant **K** Audiovisual	**Z** None
Z None 🔵	**6** Speech and/or Language Screening **7** Nonspoken Language **8** Receptive/Expressive Language **C** Aphasia **G** Communicative/Cognitive Integration Skills **L** Augmentative/Alternative Communication System	**K** Audiovisual **M** Augmentative / Alternative Communication **P** Computer **Y** Other Equipment **Z** None	**Z** None
Z None 🔵	**9** Articulation/Phonology	**K** Audiovisual **P** Computer **Q** Speech Analysis **Y** Other Equipment **Z** None	**Z** None
Z None 🔵	**B** Motor Speech	**K** Audiovisual **N** Biosensory Feedback **P** Computer **Q** Speech Analysis **T** Aerodynamic Function **Y** Other Equipment **Z** None	**Z** None

F00 continued on next page

🔵 Limited Coverage 🔵 Noncovered 🔵 HAC-associated Procedure 🔵 Combination Cluster - See Appendix G for code lists
🔵 Non-OR-Affecting MS-DRG Assignment New/Revised Text in Orange ♂ Male ♀ Female

F   Physical Rehabilitation and Diagnostic Audiology
0   Rehabilitation
0   Speech Assessment: Measurement of speech and related functions

F00 continued from previous page

Body system/ Region	Type Qualifier	Equipment	Qualifier
Character 4	Character 5	Character 6	Character 7
Z None ᴰᴿᴳ	**D** Fluency	**K** Audiovisual **N** Biosensory Feedback **P** Computer **Q** Speech Analysis **S** Voice Analysis **T** Aerodynamic Function **Y** Other Equipment **Z** None	**Z** None
Z None ᴰᴿᴳ	**F** Voice	**K** Audiovisual **N** Biosensory Feedback **P** Computer **S** Voice Analysis **T** Aerodynamic Function **Y** Other Equipment **Z** None	**Z** None
Z None ᴰᴿᴳ	**H** Bedside Swallowing and Oral Function **P** Oral Peripheral Mechanism	**Y** Other Equipment **Z** None	**Z** None
Z None ᴰᴿᴳ	**J** Instrumental Swallowing and Oral Function	**T** Aerodynamic Function **W** Swallowing **Y** Other Equipment	**Z** None
Z None ᴰᴿᴳ	**K** Orofacial Myofunctional	**K** Audiovisual **P** Computer **Y** Other Equipment **Z** None	**Z** None
Z None ᴰᴿᴳ	**M** Voice Prosthetic	**K** Audiovisual **P** Computer **S** Voice Analysis **V** Speech Prosthesis **Y** Other Equipment **Z** None	**Z** None
Z None ᴰᴿᴳ	**N** Non-invasive Instrumental Status	**N** Biosensory Feedback **P** Computer **Q** Speech Analysis **S** Voice Analysis **T** Aerodynamic Function **Y** Other Equipment	**Z** None
Z None ᴰᴿᴳ	**X** Other Specified Central Auditory Processing	**Z** None	**Z** None

ᴰᴿᴳ F003GKZ F003GMZ F003GPZ F003GYZ F003GZZ F00Z01Z F00Z02Z F00Z0KZ F00Z0ZZ F00Z11Z F00Z12Z F00Z19Z F00Z1KZ
F00Z1ZZ F00Z21Z F00Z22Z F00Z29Z F00Z2KZ F00Z2ZZ F00Z31Z F00Z32Z F00Z3KZ F00Z3ZZ F00Z41Z F00Z42Z F00Z4ZZ
F00Z51Z F00Z52Z F00Z59Z F00Z5KZ F00Z6KZ F00Z6MZ F00Z6PZ F00Z6YZ F00Z6ZZ F00Z7KZ F00Z7MZ F00Z7PZ F00Z7YZ
F00Z7ZZ F00Z8KZ F00Z8MZ F00Z8PZ F00Z8YZ F00Z8ZZ F00Z9KZ F00Z9PZ F00Z9QZ F00Z9YZ F00Z9ZZ F00ZBKZ F00ZBNZ
F00ZBPZ F00ZBQZ F00ZBTZ F00ZBYZ F00ZBZZ F00ZCKZ F00ZCMZ F00ZCPZ F00ZCYZ F00ZCZZ F00ZDKZ F00ZDNZ F00ZDPZ
F00ZDQZ F00ZDSZ F00ZDTZ F00ZDYZ F00ZDZZ F00ZFKZ F00ZFNZ F00ZFPZ F00ZFSZ F00ZFTZ F00ZFYZ F00ZFZZ F00ZGKZ
F00ZGMZ F00ZGPZ F00ZGYZ F00ZGZZ F00ZHYZ F00ZHZZ F00ZJTZ F00ZJWZ F00ZJYZ F00ZKKZ F00ZKPZ F00ZKYZ F00ZKZZ
F00ZLKZ F00ZLMZ F00ZLPZ F00ZLYZ F00ZLZZ F00ZMKZ F00ZMPZ F00ZMSZ F00ZMVZ F00ZMYZ F00ZMZZ F00ZNNZ F00ZNPZ
F00ZNQZ F00ZNSZ F00ZNTZ F00ZNYZ F00ZPYZ F00ZPZZ F00ZQ1Z F00ZQ2Z F00ZQKZ F00ZQZZ F00ZR1Z F00ZR2Z F00ZRKZ
F00ZRZZ F00ZS1Z F00ZS2Z F00ZSKZ F00ZSZZ F00ZT1Z F00ZT2Z F00ZTKZ F00ZTZZ F00ZV1Z F00ZV2Z F00ZVKZ F00ZVZZ
F00ZW1Z F00ZW2Z F00ZWKZ F00ZWZZ F00ZXZZ

ᴸᶜ Limited Coverage   ᴺᶜ Noncovered   ᴴᴬᶜ HAC-associated Procedure   ᶜᶜ Combination Cluster - See Appendix G for code lists
ᴰᴿᴳ Non-OR-Affecting MS-DRG Assignment   New/Revised Text in **Orange**   ♂ Male   ♀ Female

722

2021 ICD-10-PCS

F Physical Rehabilitation and Diagnostic Audiology
0 Rehabilitation
1 Motor and/or Nerve Function Assessment: Measurement of motor, nerve, and related functions

Body system/ Region	Type Qualifier	Equipment	Qualifier
Character 4	**Character 5**	**Character 6**	**Character 7**
0 Neurological System - Head and Neck ⓓ **1** Neurological System - Upper Back / Upper Extremity ⓓ **2** Neurological System - Lower Back / Lower Extremity ⓓ **3** Neurological System - Whole Body ⓓ	**0** Muscle Performance	**E** Orthosis **F** Assistive, Adaptive, Supportive or Protective **U** Prosthesis **Y** Other Equipment **Z** None	**Z** None
0 Neurological System - Head and Neck ⓓ **1** Neurological System - Upper Back / Upper Extremity ⓓ **2** Neurological System - Lower Back / Lower Extremity ⓓ **3** Neurological System - Whole Body ⓓ	**1** Integumentary Integrity **3** Coordination/Dexterity **4** Motor Function **G** Reflex Integrity	**Z** None	**Z** None
0 Neurological System - Head and Neck ⓓ **1** Neurological System - Upper Back / Upper Extremity ⓓ **2** Neurological System - Lower Back / Lower Extremity ⓓ **3** Neurological System - Whole Body ⓓ	**5** Range of Motion and Joint Integrity **6** Sensory Awareness/Processing/ Integrity	**Y** Other Equipment **Z** None	**Z** None
D Integumentary System - Head and Neck ⓓ **F** Integumentary System - Upper Back / Upper Extremity ⓓ **G** Integumentary System - Lower Back / Lower Extremity ⓓ **H** Integumentary System - Whole Body ⓓ **J** Musculoskeletal System - Head and Neck ⓓ **K** Musculoskeletal System - Upper Back / Upper Extremity ⓓ **L** Musculoskeletal System - Lower Back / Lower Extremity ⓓ **M** Musculoskeletal System - Whole Body ⓓ	**0** Muscle Performance	**E** Orthosis **F** Assistive, Adaptive, Supportive or Protective **U** Prosthesis **Y** Other Equipment **Z** None	**Z** None
D Integumentary System - Head and Neck ⓓ **F** Integumentary System - Upper Back / Upper Extremity ⓓ **G** Integumentary System - Lower Back / Lower Extremity ⓓ **H** Integumentary System - Whole Body ⓓ **J** Musculoskeletal System - Head and Neck ⓓ **K** Musculoskeletal System - Upper Back / Upper Extremity ⓓ **L** Musculoskeletal System - Lower Back / Lower Extremity ⓓ **M** Musculoskeletal System - Whole Body ⓓ	**1** Integumentary Integrity	**Z** None	**Z** None

F01 continued on next page

F Physical Rehabilitation and Diagnostic Audiology
0 Rehabilitation
1 Motor and/or Nerve Function Assessment: Measurement of motor, nerve, and related functions

F01 continued from previous page

Body system/ Region	Type Qualifier	Equipment	Qualifier
Character 4	Character 5	Character 6	Character 7
D Integumentary System - Head and Neck ⒟ⒽⒼ F Integumentary System - Upper Back / Upper Extremity ⒟ⓇⒼ G Integumentary System - Lower Back / Lower Extremity ⒟ⓇⒼ H Integumentary System - Whole Body ⒟ⓇⒼ J Musculoskeletal System - Head and Neck ⒟ⓇⒼ K Musculoskeletal System - Upper Back / Upper Extremity ⒟ⓇⒼ L Musculoskeletal System - Lower Back / Lower Extremity ⒟ⓇⒼ M Musculoskeletal System - Whole Body ⒟ⓇⒼ	5 Range of Motion and Joint Integrity 6 Sensory Awareness/Processing/ Integrity	Y Other Equipment Z None	Z None
N Genitourinary System ⒟ⓇⒼ	0 Muscle Performance	E Orthosis F Assistive, Adaptive, Supportive or Protective U Prosthesis Y Other Equipment Z None	Z None
Z None ⒟ⓇⒼ	2 Visual Motor Integration	K Audiovisual M Augmentative / Alternative Communication N Biosensory Feedback P Computer Q Speech Analysis S Voice Analysis Y Other Equipment Z None	Z None
Z None ⒟ⓇⒼ	7 Facial Nerve Function	7 Electrophysiologic	Z None
Z None ⒟ⓇⒼ	9 Somatosensory Evoked Potentials	J Somatosensory	Z None
Z None ⒟ⓇⒼ	B Bed Mobility C Transfer F Wheelchair Mobility	E Orthosis F Assistive, Adaptive, Supportive or Protective U Prosthesis Z None	Z None
Z None ⒟ⓇⒼ	D Gait and/or Balance	E Orthosis F Assistive, Adaptive, Supportive or Protective U Prosthesis Y Other Equipment Z None	Z None

ⒹⓇⒼ
F0100EZ	F0100FZ	F0100UZ	F0100YZ	F0100ZZ	F0101ZZ	F0103ZZ	F0104ZZ	F0105YZ	F0105ZZ	F0106YZ	F0106ZZ	F010GZZ
F0110EZ	F0110FZ	F0110UZ	F0110YZ	F0110ZZ	F0111ZZ	F0113ZZ	F0114ZZ	F0115YZ	F0115ZZ	F0116YZ	F0116ZZ	F011GZZ
F0120EZ	F0120FZ	F0120UZ	F0120YZ	F0120ZZ	F0121ZZ	F0123ZZ	F0124ZZ	F0125YZ	F0125ZZ	F0126YZ	F0126ZZ	F012GZZ
F0130EZ	F0130FZ	F0130UZ	F0130YZ	F0130ZZ	F0131ZZ	F0133ZZ	F0134ZZ	F0135YZ	F0135ZZ	F0136YZ	F0136ZZ	F013GZZ
F01D0EZ	F01D0FZ	F01D0UZ	F01D0YZ	F01D0ZZ	F01D1ZZ	F01D5YZ	F01D5ZZ	F01D6YZ	F01D6ZZ	F01F0EZ	F01F0FZ	F01F0UZ
F01F0YZ	F01F0ZZ	F01F1ZZ	F01F5YZ	F01F5ZZ	F01F6YZ	F01F6ZZ	F01G0EZ	F01G0FZ	F01G0UZ	F01G0YZ	F01G0ZZ	F01G1ZZ
F01G5YZ	F01G5ZZ	F01G6YZ	F01G6ZZ	F01H0EZ	F01H0FZ	F01H0UZ	F01H0YZ	F01H0ZZ	F01H1ZZ	F01H5YZ	F01H5ZZ	F01H6YZ
F01H6ZZ	F01J0EZ	F01J0FZ	F01J0UZ	F01J0YZ	F01J0ZZ	F01J1ZZ	F01J5YZ	F01J5ZZ	F01J6YZ	F01J6ZZ	F01K0EZ	F01K0FZ
F01K0UZ	F01K0YZ	F01K0ZZ	F01K1ZZ	F01K5YZ	F01K5ZZ	F01K6YZ	F01K6ZZ	F01L0EZ	F01L0FZ	F01L0UZ	F01L0YZ	F01L0ZZ
F01L1ZZ	F01L5YZ	F01L5ZZ	F01L6YZ	F01L6ZZ	F01M0EZ	F01M0FZ	F01M0UZ	F01M0YZ	F01M0ZZ	F01M1ZZ	F01M5YZ	F01M5ZZ
F01M6YZ	F01M6ZZ	F01N0EZ	F01N0FZ	F01N0UZ	F01N0YZ	F01N0ZZ	F01Z2KZ	F01Z2MZ	F01Z2NZ	F01Z2PZ	F01Z2QZ	F01Z2SZ
F01Z2YZ	F01Z2ZZ	F01Z77Z	F01Z9JZ	F01ZBEZ	F01ZBFZ	F01ZBUZ	F01ZBZZ	F01ZCEZ	F01ZCFZ	F01ZCUZ	F01ZCZZ	F01ZDEZ
F01ZDFZ	F01ZDUZ	F01ZDYZ	F01ZDZZ	F01ZFEZ	F01ZFFZ	F01ZFUZ	F01ZFZZ					

ⓁⒸ Limited Coverage   ⓃⒸ Noncovered   ⒽⒶⒸ HAC-associated Procedure   ⒸⒸ Combination Cluster - See Appendix G for code lists
ⒹⓇⒼ Non-OR-Affecting MS-DRG Assignment   New/Revised Text in **Orange**   ♂ Male   ♀ Female

724

2021 ICD-10-PCS

F **Physical Rehabilitation and Diagnostic Audiology**
0 **Rehabilitation**
2 **Activities of Daily Living Assessment:** Measurement of functional level for activities of daily living

Body system/ Region	Type Qualifier	Equipment	Qualifier
Character 4	**Character 5**	**Character 6**	**Character 7**
0 Neurological System - Head and Neck ⓓⓡⓖ	**9** Cranial Nerve Integrity **D** Neuromotor Development	**Y** Other Equipment **Z** None	**Z** None
1 Neurological System - Upper Back / Upper Extremity ⓓⓡⓖ **2** Neurological System - Lower Back / Lower Extremity ⓓⓡⓖ **3** Neurological System - Whole Body ⓓⓡⓖ	**D** Neuromotor Development	**Y** Other Equipment **Z** None	**Z** None
4 Circulatory System - Head and Neck ⓓⓡⓖ **5** Circulatory System - Upper Back / Upper Extremity ⓓⓡⓖ **6** Circulatory System - Lower Back / Lower Extremity ⓓⓡⓖ **8** Respiratory System - Head and Neck ⓓⓡⓖ **9** Respiratory System - Upper Back / Upper Extremity ⓓⓡⓖ **B** Respiratory System - Lower Back / Lower Extremity ⓓⓡⓖ	**G** Ventilation, Respiration and Circulation	**C** Mechanical **G** Aerobic Endurance and Conditioning **Y** Other Equipment **Z** None	**Z** None
7 Circulatory System - Whole Body ⓓⓡⓖ **C** Respiratory System - Whole Body ⓓⓡⓖ	**7** Aerobic Capacity and Endurance	**E** Orthosis **G** Aerobic Endurance and Conditioning **U** Prosthesis **Y** Other Equipment **Z** None	**Z** None
7 Circulatory System - Whole Body ⓓⓡⓖ **C** Respiratory System - Whole Body ⓓⓡⓖ	**G** Ventilation, Respiration and Circulation	**C** Mechanical **G** Aerobic Endurance and Conditioning **Y** Other Equipment **Z** None	**Z** None
Z None ⓓⓡⓖ	**0** Bathing/Showering **1** Dressing **3** Grooming/Personal Hygiene **4** Home Management	**E** Orthosis **F** Assistive, Adaptive, Supportive or Protective **U** Prosthesis **Z** None	**Z** None
Z None ⓓⓡⓖ	**2** Feeding/Eating **8** Anthropometric Characteristics **F** Pain	**Y** Other Equipment **Z** None	**Z** None
Z None ⓓⓡⓖ	**5** Perceptual Processing	**K** Audiovisual **M** Augmentative / Alternative Communication **N** Biosensory Feedback **P** Computer **Q** Speech Analysis **S** Voice Analysis **Y** Other Equipment **Z** None	**Z** None
Z None ⓓⓡⓖ	**6** Psychosocial Skills	**Z** None	**Z** None
Z None ⓓⓡⓖ	**B** Environmental, Home and Work Barriers **C** Ergonomics and Body Mechanics	**E** Orthosis **F** Assistive, Adaptive, Supportive or Protective **U** Prosthesis **Y** Other Equipment **Z** None	**Z** None

F02 continued on next page

ⓛⓒ Limited Coverage ⓝⓒ Noncovered ⓗⓐⓒ HAC-associated Procedure ⓒⓒ Combination Cluster - See Appendix G for code lists
ⓓⓡⓖ Non-OR-Affecting MS-DRG Assignment New/Revised Text in **Orange** ♂ Male ♀ Female

F Physical Rehabilitation and Diagnostic Audiology
0 Rehabilitation
2 Activities of Daily Living Assessment: Measurement of functional level for activities of daily living

F02 continued from previous page

Body system/ Region	Type Qualifier	Equipment	Qualifier
Character 4	Character 5	Character 6	Character 7
Z None ᴰᴿᴳ	H Vocational Activities and Functional Community or Work Reintegration Skills	E Orthosis F Assistive, Adaptive, Supportive or Protective G Aerobic Endurance and Conditioning U Prosthesis Y Other Equipment Z None	Z None

ᴰᴿᴳ
F0209YZ	F0209ZZ	F020DYZ	F020DZZ	F021DYZ	F021DZZ	F022DYZ	F022DZZ	F023DYZ	F023DZZ	F024GCZ	F024GGZ	F024GYZ
F024GZZ	F025GCZ	F025GGZ	F025GYZ	F025GZZ	F026GCZ	F026GGZ	F026GYZ	F026GZZ	F0277EZ	F0277GZ	F0277UZ	F0277YZ
F0277ZZ	F027GCZ	F027GGZ	F027GYZ	F027GZZ	F028GCZ	F028GGZ	F028GYZ	F028GZZ	F029GCZ	F029GGZ	F029GYZ	F029GZZ
F02BGCZ	F02BGGZ	F02BGYZ	F02BGZZ	F02C7EZ	F02C7GZ	F02C7UZ	F02C7YZ	F02C7ZZ	F02CGCZ	F02CGGZ	F02CGYZ	F02CGZZ
F02Z0EZ	F02Z0FZ	F02Z0UZ	F02Z0ZZ	F02Z1EZ	F02Z1FZ	F02Z1UZ	F02Z1ZZ	F02Z2YZ	F02Z2ZZ	F02Z3EZ	F02Z3FZ	F02Z3UZ
F02Z3ZZ	F02Z4EZ	F02Z4FZ	F02Z4UZ	F02Z4ZZ	F02Z5KZ	F02Z5MZ	F02Z5NZ	F02Z5PZ	F02Z5QZ	F02Z5SZ	F02Z5YZ	F02Z5ZZ
F02Z6ZZ	F02Z8YZ	F02Z8ZZ	F02ZBEZ	F02ZBFZ	F02ZBUZ	F02ZBYZ	F02ZBZZ	F02ZCEZ	F02ZCFZ	F02ZCUZ	F02ZCYZ	F02ZCZZ
F02ZFYZ	F02ZFZZ	F02ZHEZ	F02ZHFZ	F02ZHGZ	F02ZHUZ	F02ZHYZ	F02ZHZZ					

F Physical Rehabilitation and Diagnostic Audiology
0 Rehabilitation
6 Speech Treatment: Application of techniques to improve, augment, or compensate for speech and related functional impairment

Body system/ Region	Type Qualifier	Equipment	Qualifier
Character 4	Character 5	Character 6	Character 7
3 Neurological System - Whole Body ᴰᴿᴳ	6 Communicative/Cognitive Integration Skills	K Audiovisual M Augmentative / Alternative Communication P Computer Y Other Equipment Z None	Z None
Z None ᴰᴿᴳ	0 Nonspoken Language 3 Aphasia 6 Communicative/Cognitive Integration Skills	K Audiovisual M Augmentative / Alternative Communication P Computer Y Other Equipment Z None	Z None
Z None ᴰᴿᴳ	1 Speech-Language Pathology and Related Disorders Counseling 2 Speech-Language Pathology and Related Disorders Prevention	K Audiovisual Z None	Z None
Z None ᴰᴿᴳ	4 Articulation/Phonology	K Audiovisual P Computer Q Speech Analysis T Aerodynamic Function Y Other Equipment Z None	Z None
Z None ᴰᴿᴳ	5 Aural Rehabilitation	K Audiovisual L Assistive Listening M Augmentative / Alternative Communication N Biosensory Feedback P Computer Q Speech Analysis S Voice Analysis Y Other Equipment Z None	Z None

F06 continued on next page

ᴸᶜ Limited Coverage ᴺᶜ Noncovered ᴴᴬᶜ HAC-associated Procedure ᶜᶜ Combination Cluster - See Appendix G for code lists
ᴰᴿᴳ Non-OR-Affecting MS-DRG Assignment New/Revised Text in Orange ♂ Male ♀ Female

F Physical Rehabilitation and Diagnostic Audiology
0 Rehabilitation
6 Speech Treatment: Application of techniques to improve, augment, or compensate for speech and related functional impairment

F06 continued from previous page

Body system/ Region	Type Qualifier	Equipment	Qualifier
Character 4	Character 5	Character 6	Character 7
Z None ᴏʀɢ	**7** Fluency	**4** Electroacoustic Immittance / Acoustic Reflex **K** Audiovisual **N** Biosensory Feedback **Q** Speech Analysis **S** Voice Analysis **T** Aerodynamic Function **Y** Other Equipment **Z** None	**Z** None
Z None ᴏʀɢ	**8** Motor Speech	**K** Audiovisual **N** Biosensory Feedback **P** Computer **Q** Speech Analysis **S** Voice Analysis **T** Aerodynamic Function **Y** Other Equipment **Z** None	**Z** None
Z None ᴏʀɢ	**9** Orofacial Myofunctional	**K** Audiovisual **P** Computer **Y** Other Equipment **Z** None	**Z** None
Z None ᴏʀɢ	**B** Receptive/Expressive Language	**K** Audiovisual **L** Assistive Listening **M** Augmentative / Alternative Communication **P** Computer **Y** Other Equipment **Z** None	**Z** None
Z None ᴏʀɢ	**C** Voice	**K** Audiovisual **N** Biosensory Feedback **P** Computer **S** Voice Analysis **T** Aerodynamic Function **V** Speech Prosthesis **Y** Other Equipment **Z** None	**Z** None
Z None ᴏʀɢ	**D** Swallowing Dysfunction	**M** Augmentative / Alternative Communication **T** Aerodynamic Function **V** Speech Prosthesis **Y** Other Equipment **Z** None	**Z** None

ᴏʀɢ   F0636KZ F0636MZ F0636PZ F0636YZ F0636ZZ F06Z0KZ F06Z0MZ F06Z0PZ F06Z0YZ F06Z0ZZ F06Z1KZ F06Z1ZZ F06Z2KZ
F06Z2ZZ F06Z3KZ F06Z3MZ F06Z3PZ F06Z3YZ F06Z3ZZ F06Z4KZ F06Z4PZ F06Z4QZ F06Z4TZ F06Z4YZ F06Z4ZZ F06Z5KZ
F06Z5LZ F06Z5MZ F06Z5NZ F06Z5PZ F06Z5QZ F06Z5SZ F06Z5YZ F06Z5ZZ F06Z6KZ F06Z6MZ F06Z6PZ F06Z6YZ F06Z6ZZ
F06Z74Z F06Z7KZ F06Z7NZ F06Z7QZ F06Z7SZ F06Z7TZ F06Z7YZ F06Z7ZZ F06Z8KZ F06Z8NZ F06Z8PZ F06Z8QZ F06Z8SZ
F06Z8TZ F06Z8YZ F06Z8ZZ F06Z9KZ F06Z9PZ F06Z9YZ F06Z9ZZ F06ZBKZ F06ZBLZ F06ZBMZ F06ZBPZ F06ZBYZ F06ZBZZ
F06ZCKZ F06ZCNZ F06ZCPZ F06ZCSZ F06ZCTZ F06ZCVZ F06ZCYZ F06ZCZZ F06ZDMZ F06ZDTZ F06ZDVZ F06ZDYZ F06ZDZZ

F Physical Rehabilitation and Diagnostic Audiology
0 Rehabilitation
7 Motor Treatment: Exercise or activities to increase or facilitate motor function

Body system/ Region		Type Qualifier		Equipment		Qualifier	
Character 4		**Character 5**		**Character 6**		**Character 7**	
0	Neurological System - Head and Neck ᴰᴿᴳ	0	Range of Motion and Joint Mobility	E	Orthosis	Z	None
1	Neurological System - Upper Back / Upper Extremity ᴰᴿᴳ	1	Muscle Performance	F	Assistive, Adaptive, Supportive or Protective		
2	Neurological System - Lower Back / Lower Extremity ᴰᴿᴳ	2	Coordination/Dexterity	U	Prosthesis		
3	Neurological System - Whole Body ᴰᴿᴳ	3	Motor Function	Y	Other Equipment		
D	Integumentary System - Head and Neck ᴰᴿᴳ			Z	None		
F	Integumentary System - Upper Back / Upper Extremity ᴰᴿᴳ						
G	Integumentary System - Lower Back / Lower Extremity ᴰᴿᴳ						
H	Integumentary System - Whole Body ᴰᴿᴳ						
J	Musculoskeletal System - Head and Neck ᴰᴿᴳ						
K	Musculoskeletal System - Upper Back / Upper Extremity ᴰᴿᴳ						
L	Musculoskeletal System - Lower Back / Lower Extremity ᴰᴿᴳ						
M	Musculoskeletal System - Whole Body ᴰᴿᴳ						
0	Neurological System - Head and Neck ᴰᴿᴳ	6	Therapeutic Exercise	B	Physical Agents	Z	None
1	Neurological System - Upper Back / Upper Extremity ᴰᴿᴳ			C	Mechanical		
2	Neurological System - Lower Back / Lower Extremity ᴰᴿᴳ			D	Electrotherapeutic		
3	Neurological System - Whole Body ᴰᴿᴳ			E	Orthosis		
D	Integumentary System - Head and Neck ᴰᴿᴳ			F	Assistive, Adaptive, Supportive or Protective		
F	Integumentary System - Upper Back / Upper Extremity ᴰᴿᴳ			G	Aerobic Endurance and Conditioning		
G	Integumentary System - Lower Back / Lower Extremity ᴰᴿᴳ			H	Mechanical or Electromechanical		
H	Integumentary System - Whole Body ᴰᴿᴳ			U	Prosthesis		
J	Musculoskeletal System - Head and Neck ᴰᴿᴳ			Y	Other Equipment		
K	Musculoskeletal System - Upper Back / Upper Extremity ᴰᴿᴳ			Z	None		
L	Musculoskeletal System - Lower Back / Lower Extremity ᴰᴿᴳ						
M	Musculoskeletal System - Whole Body ᴰᴿᴳ						

F07 continued on next page

ᴸᶜ Limited Coverage   ᴺᶜ Noncovered   ᴴᴬᶜ HAC-associated Procedure   ᶜᶜ Combination Cluster - See Appendix G for code lists
ᴰᴿᴳ Non-OR-Affecting MS-DRG Assignment   New/Revised Text in **Orange**   ♂ Male   ♀ Female

F **Physical Rehabilitation and Diagnostic Audiology**

0 **Rehabilitation**

7 **Motor Treatment:** Exercise or activities to increase or facilitate motor function

F07 continued from previous page

Body system/ Region	Type Qualifier	Equipment	Qualifier
Character 4	**Character 5**	**Character 6**	**Character 7**
0 Neurological System - Head and Neck ᴼᴿᴳ 1 Neurological System - Upper Back / Upper Extremity ᴼᴿᴳ 2 Neurological System - Lower Back / Lower Extremity ᴼᴿᴳ 3 Neurological System - Whole Body ᴼᴿᴳ D Integumentary System - Head and Neck ᴼᴿᴳ F Integumentary System - Upper Back / Upper Extremity ᴼᴿᴳ G Integumentary System - Lower Back / Lower Extremity ᴼᴿᴳ H Integumentary System - Whole Body ᴼᴿᴳ J Musculoskeletal System - Head and Neck ᴼᴿᴳ K Musculoskeletal System - Upper Back / Upper Extremity ᴼᴿᴳ L Musculoskeletal System - Lower Back / Lower Extremity ᴼᴿᴳ M Musculoskeletal System - Whole Body ᴼᴿᴳ	7 Manual Therapy Techniques	Z None	Z None
4 Circulatory System - Head and Neck ᴼᴿᴳ 5 Circulatory System - Upper Back / Upper Extremity ᴼᴿᴳ 6 Circulatory System - Lower Back / Lower Extremity ᴼᴿᴳ 7 Circulatory System - Whole Body ᴼᴿᴳ 8 Respiratory System - Head and Neck ᴼᴿᴳ 9 Respiratory System - Upper Back / Upper Extremity ᴼᴿᴳ B Respiratory System - Lower Back / Lower Extremity ᴼᴿᴳ C Respiratory System - Whole Body ᴼᴿᴳ	6 Therapeutic Exercise	B Physical Agents C Mechanical D Electrotherapeutic E Orthosis F Assistive, Adaptive, Supportive or Protective G Aerobic Endurance and Conditioning H Mechanical or Electromechanical U Prosthesis Y Other Equipment Z None	Z None
N Genitourinary System ᴼᴿᴳ	1 Muscle Performance	E Orthosis F Assistive, Adaptive, Supportive or Protective U Prosthesis Y Other Equipment Z None	Z None
N Genitourinary System ᴼᴿᴳ	6 Therapeutic Exercise	B Physical Agents C Mechanical D Electrotherapeutic E Orthosis F Assistive, Adaptive, Supportive or Protective G Aerobic Endurance and Conditioning H Mechanical or Electromechanical U Prosthesis Y Other Equipment Z None	Z None

F07 continued on next page

F Physical Rehabilitation and Diagnostic Audiology
0 Rehabilitation
7 Motor Treatment: Exercise or activities to increase or facilitate motor function

F07 continued from previous page

Body system/ Region	Type Qualifier	Equipment	Qualifier
Character 4	Character 5	Character 6	Character 7
Z None 🔘	4 Wheelchair Mobility	D Electrotherapeutic E Orthosis F Assistive, Adaptive, Supportive or Protective U Prosthesis Y Other Equipment Z None	Z None
Z None 🔘	5 Bed Mobility	C Mechanical E Orthosis F Assistive, Adaptive, Supportive or Protective U Prosthesis Y Other Equipment Z None	Z None
Z None 🔘	8 Transfer Training	C Mechanical D Electrotherapeutic E Orthosis F Assistive, Adaptive, Supportive or Protective U Prosthesis Y Other Equipment Z None	Z None
Z None 🔘	9 Gait Training/Functional Ambulation	C Mechanical D Electrotherapeutic E Orthosis F Assistive, Adaptive, Supportive or Protective G Aerobic Endurance and Conditioning U Prosthesis Y Other Equipment Z None	Z None

🔘
F0700EZ	F0700FZ	F0700UZ	F0700YZ	F0700ZZ	F0701EZ	F0701FZ	F0701UZ	F0701YZ	F0701ZZ	F0702EZ	F0702FZ	F0702UZ
F0702YZ	F0702ZZ	F0703EZ	F0703FZ	F0703UZ	F0703YZ	F0703ZZ	F0706BZ	F0706CZ	F0706DZ	F0706EZ	F0706FZ	F0706GZ
F0706HZ	F0706UZ	F0706YZ	F0706ZZ	F0707ZZ	F0710EZ	F0710FZ	F0710UZ	F0710YZ	F0710ZZ	F0711EZ	F0711FZ	F0711UZ
F0711YZ	F0711ZZ	F0712EZ	F0712FZ	F0712UZ	F0712YZ	F0712ZZ	F0713EZ	F0713FZ	F0713UZ	F0713YZ	F0713ZZ	F0716BZ
F0716CZ	F0716DZ	F0716EZ	F0716FZ	F0716GZ	F0716HZ	F0716UZ	F0716YZ	F0716ZZ	F0717ZZ	F0720EZ	F0720FZ	F0720UZ
F0720YZ	F0720ZZ	F0721EZ	F0721FZ	F0721UZ	F0721YZ	F0721ZZ	F0722EZ	F0722FZ	F0722UZ	F0722YZ	F0722ZZ	F0723EZ
F0723FZ	F0723UZ	F0723YZ	F0723ZZ	F0726BZ	F0726CZ	F0726DZ	F0726EZ	F0726FZ	F0726GZ	F0726HZ	F0726UZ	F0726YZ
F0726ZZ	F0727ZZ	F0730EZ	F0730FZ	F0730UZ	F0730YZ	F0730ZZ	F0731EZ	F0731FZ	F0731UZ	F0731YZ	F0731ZZ	F0732EZ
F0732FZ	F0732UZ	F0732YZ	F0732ZZ	F0733EZ	F0733FZ	F0733UZ	F0733YZ	F0733ZZ	F0736BZ	F0736CZ	F0736DZ	F0736EZ
F0736FZ	F0736GZ	F0736HZ	F0736UZ	F0736YZ	F0736ZZ	F0737ZZ	F0746BZ	F0746CZ	F0746DZ	F0746EZ	F0746FZ	F0746GZ
F0746HZ	F0746UZ	F0746YZ	F0746ZZ	F0756BZ	F0756CZ	F0756DZ	F0756EZ	F0756FZ	F0756GZ	F0756HZ	F0756UZ	F0756YZ
F0756ZZ	F0766BZ	F0766CZ	F0766DZ	F0766EZ	F0766FZ	F0766GZ	F0766HZ	F0766UZ	F0766YZ	F0766ZZ	F0776BZ	F0776CZ
F0776DZ	F0776EZ	F0776FZ	F0776GZ	F0776HZ	F0776UZ	F0776YZ	F0776ZZ	F0786BZ	F0786CZ	F0786DZ	F0786EZ	F0786FZ
F0786GZ	F0786HZ	F0786UZ	F0786YZ	F0786ZZ	F0796BZ	F0796CZ	F0796DZ	F0796EZ	F0796FZ	F0796GZ	F0796HZ	F0796UZ
F0796YZ	F0796ZZ	F07B6BZ	F07B6CZ	F07B6DZ	F07B6EZ	F07B6FZ	F07B6GZ	F07B6HZ	F07B6UZ	F07B6YZ	F07B6ZZ	F07C6BZ
F07C6CZ	F07C6DZ	F07C6EZ	F07C6FZ	F07C6GZ	F07C6HZ	F07C6UZ	F07C6YZ	F07C6ZZ	F07D0EZ	F07D0FZ	F07D0UZ	F07D0YZ
F07D0ZZ	F07D1EZ	F07D1FZ	F07D1UZ	F07D1YZ	F07D1ZZ	F07D2EZ	F07D2FZ	F07D2UZ	F07D2YZ	F07D2ZZ	F07D3EZ	F07D3FZ
F07D3UZ	F07D3YZ	F07D3ZZ	F07D6BZ	F07D6CZ	F07D6DZ	F07D6EZ	F07D6FZ	F07D6GZ	F07D6HZ	F07D6UZ	F07D6YZ	F07D6ZZ
F07D7ZZ	F07F0EZ	F07F0FZ	F07F0UZ	F07F0YZ	F07F0ZZ	F07F1EZ	F07F1FZ	F07F1UZ	F07F1YZ	F07F1ZZ	F07F2EZ	F07F2FZ
F07F2UZ	F07F2YZ	F07F2ZZ	F07F3EZ	F07F3FZ	F07F3UZ	F07F3YZ	F07F3ZZ	F07F6BZ	F07F6CZ	F07F6DZ	F07F6EZ	F07F6FZ
F07F6GZ	F07F6HZ	F07F6UZ	F07F6YZ	F07F6ZZ	F07G0EZ	F07G0FZ	F07G0UZ	F07G0YZ	F07G0ZZ	F07G1EZ	F07G1FZ
F07G1UZ	F07G1YZ	F07G1ZZ	F07G2EZ	F07G2FZ	F07G2UZ	F07G2YZ	F07G2ZZ	F07G3EZ	F07G3FZ	F07G3YZ	F07G3ZZ
F07G6BZ	F07G6CZ	F07G6DZ	F07G6EZ	F07G6FZ	F07G6GZ	F07G6HZ	F07G6UZ	F07G6YZ	F07G6ZZ	F07G7ZZ	F07H0EZ	F07H0FZ
F07H0UZ	F07H0YZ	F07H0ZZ	F07H1EZ	F07H1FZ	F07H1UZ	F07H1YZ	F07H1ZZ	F07H2EZ	F07H2FZ	F07H2UZ	F07H2YZ	F07H2ZZ
F07H3EZ	F07H3FZ	F07H3UZ	F07H3YZ	F07H3ZZ	F07H6BZ	F07H6CZ	F07H6DZ	F07H6EZ	F07H6FZ	F07H6GZ	F07H6HZ	F07H6UZ
F07H6YZ	F07H6ZZ	F07H7ZZ	F07J0EZ	F07J0FZ	F07J0UZ	F07J0YZ	F07J0ZZ	F07J1EZ	F07J1FZ	F07J1UZ	F07J1YZ	F07J1ZZ
F07J2EZ	F07J2FZ	F07J2UZ	F07J2YZ	F07J2ZZ	F07J3EZ	F07J3FZ	F07J3UZ	F07J3YZ	F07J3ZZ	F07J6BZ	F07J6CZ	F07J6DZ
F07J6EZ	F07J6FZ	F07J6GZ	F07J6HZ	F07J6UZ	F07J6YZ	F07J6ZZ	F07J7ZZ	F07K0EZ	F07K0FZ	F07K0UZ	F07K0YZ	F07K0ZZ
F07K1EZ	F07K1FZ	F07K1UZ	F07K1YZ	F07K1ZZ	F07K2EZ	F07K2FZ	F07K2UZ	F07K2YZ	F07K2ZZ	F07K3EZ	F07K3FZ	F07K3UZ

F07 continued on next page

🄻🄲 Limited Coverage   🄽🄲 Noncovered   🄷🄰🄲 HAC-associated Procedure   🄲🄲 Combination Cluster - See Appendix G for code lists
🔘 Non-OR-Affecting MS-DRG Assignment   New/Revised Text in **Orange**   ♂ Male   ♀ Female

F07K3YZ	F07K3ZZ	F07K6BZ	F07K6CZ	F07K6DZ	F07K6EZ	F07K6FZ	F07K6GZ	F07K6HZ	F07K6UZ	F07K6YZ	F07K6ZZ	F07K7ZZ
F07L0EZ	F07L0FZ	F07L0UZ	F07L0YZ	F07L0ZZ	F07L1EZ	F07L1FZ	F07L1UZ	F07L1YZ	F07L1ZZ	F07L2EZ	F07L2FZ	F07L2UZ
F07L2YZ	F07L2ZZ	F07L3EZ	F07L3FZ	F07L3UZ	F07L3YZ	F07L3ZZ	F07L6BZ	F07L6CZ	F07L6DZ	F07L6EZ	F07L6FZ	F07L6GZ
F07L6HZ	F07L6UZ	F07L6YZ	F07L6ZZ	F07L7ZZ	F07M0EZ	F07M0FZ	F07M0UZ	F07M0YZ	F07M0ZZ	F07M1EZ	F07M1FZ	F07M1UZ
F07M1YZ	F07M1ZZ	F07M2EZ	F07M2FZ	F07M2UZ	F07M2YZ	F07M2ZZ	F07M3EZ	F07M3FZ	F07M3UZ	F07M3YZ	F07M3ZZ	F07M6BZ
F07M6CZ	F07M6DZ	F07M6EZ	F07M6FZ	F07M6GZ	F07M6HZ	F07M6UZ	F07M6YZ	F07M6ZZ	F07M7ZZ	F07N1EZ	F07N1FZ	F07N1UZ
F07N1YZ	F07N1ZZ	F07N6BZ	F07N6CZ	F07N6DZ	F07N6EZ	F07N6FZ	F07N6GZ	F07N6HZ	F07N6UZ	F07N6YZ	F07N6ZZ	F07Z4DZ
F07Z4EZ	F07Z4FZ	F07Z4UZ	F07Z4YZ	F07Z4ZZ	F07Z5CZ	F07Z5EZ	F07Z5FZ	F07Z5UZ	F07Z5YZ	F07Z5ZZ	F07Z8CZ	F07Z8DZ
F07Z8EZ	F07Z8FZ	F07Z8UZ	F07Z8YZ	F07Z8ZZ	F07Z9CZ	F07Z9DZ	F07Z9EZ	F07Z9FZ	F07Z9GZ	F07Z9UZ	F07Z9YZ	F07Z9ZZ

F   Physical Rehabilitation and Diagnostic Audiology
0   Rehabilitation
8   Activities of Daily Living Treatment: Exercise or activities to facilitate functional competence for activities of daily living

Body system/ Region		Type Qualifier		Equipment		Qualifier	
Character 4		**Character 5**		**Character 6**		**Character 7**	
D Integumentary System - Head and Neck ᴰᴿᴳ **F** Integumentary System - Upper Back / Upper Extremity ᴰᴿᴳ **G** Integumentary System - Lower Back / Lower Extremity ᴰᴿᴳ **H** Integumentary System - Whole Body ᴰᴿᴳ **J** Musculoskeletal System - Head and Neck ᴰᴿᴳ **K** Musculoskeletal System - Upper Back / Upper Extremity ᴰᴿᴳ **L** Musculoskeletal System - Lower Back / Lower Extremity ᴰᴿᴳ **M** Musculoskeletal System - Whole Body ᴰᴿᴳ		**5** Wound Management		**B** Physical Agents **C** Mechanical **D** Electrotherapeutic **E** Orthosis **F** Assistive, Adaptive, Supportive or Protective **U** Prosthesis **Y** Other Equipment **Z** None		**Z** None	
Z None ᴰᴿᴳ		**0** Bathing/Showering Techniques **1** Dressing Techniques **2** Grooming/Personal Hygiene		**E** Orthosis **F** Assistive, Adaptive, Supportive or Protective **U** Prosthesis **Y** Other Equipment **Z** None		**Z** None	
Z None ᴰᴿᴳ		**3** Feeding/Eating		**C** Mechanical **D** Electrotherapeutic **E** Orthosis **F** Assistive, Adaptive, Supportive or Protective **U** Prosthesis **Y** Other Equipment **Z** None		**Z** None	
Z None ᴰᴿᴳ		**4** Home Management		**D** Electrotherapeutic **E** Orthosis **F** Assistive, Adaptive, Supportive or Protective **U** Prosthesis **Y** Other Equipment **Z** None		**Z** None	
Z None ᴰᴿᴳ		**6** Psychosocial Skills		**Z** None		**Z** None	
Z None ᴰᴿᴳ		**7** Vocational Activities and Functional Community or Work Reintegration Skills		**B** Physical Agents **C** Mechanical **D** Electrotherapeutic **E** Orthosis **F** Assistive, Adaptive, Supportive or Protective **G** Aerobic Endurance and Conditioning **U** Prosthesis **Y** Other Equipment **Z** None		**Z** None	

ᴰᴿᴳ F08D5BZ   F08D5CZ   F08D5DZ   F08D5EZ   F08D5FZ   F08D5UZ   F08D5YZ   F08D5ZZ   F08F5BZ   F08F5CZ   F08F5DZ   F08F5EZ   F08F5FZ
F08F5UZ   F08F5YZ   F08F5ZZ   F08G5BZ   F08G5CZ   F08G5DZ   F08G5EZ   F08G5FZ   F08G5UZ   F08G5YZ   F08G5ZZ   F08H5BZ   F08H5CZ

F08 continued on next page

ᴸᶜ Limited Coverage   ᴺᶜ Noncovered   ᴴᴬᶜ HAC-associated Procedure   ᶜᶜ Combination Cluster - See Appendix G for code lists
ᴰᴿᴳ Non-OR-Affecting MS-DRG Assignment   New/Revised Text in Orange   ♂ Male   ♀ Female

F08 continued from previous page

F08H5DZ	F08H5EZ	F08H5FZ	F08H5UZ	F08H5YZ	F08H5ZZ	F08J5BZ	F08J5CZ	F08J5DZ	F08J5EZ	F08J5FZ	F08J5UZ	F08J5YZ
F08J5ZZ	F08K5BZ	F08K5CZ	F08K5DZ	F08K5EZ	F08K5FZ	F08K5UZ	F08K5YZ	F08K5ZZ	F08L5BZ	F08L5CZ	F08L5DZ	F08L5EZ
F08L5FZ	F08L5UZ	F08L5YZ	F08L5ZZ	F08M5BZ	F08M5CZ	F08M5DZ	F08M5EZ	F08M5FZ	F08M5UZ	F08M5YZ	F08M5ZZ	F08Z0EZ
F08Z0FZ	F08Z0UZ	F08Z0YZ	F08Z0ZZ	F08Z1EZ	F08Z1FZ	F08Z1UZ	F08Z1YZ	F08Z1ZZ	F08Z2EZ	F08Z2FZ	F08Z2UZ	F08Z2YZ
F08Z2ZZ	F08Z3CZ	F08Z3DZ	F08Z3EZ	F08Z3FZ	F08Z3UZ	F08Z3YZ	F08Z3ZZ	F08Z4DZ	F08Z4EZ	F08Z4FZ	F08Z4UZ	F08Z4YZ
F08Z4ZZ	F08Z6ZZ	F08Z7BZ	F08Z7CZ	F08Z7DZ	F08Z7EZ	F08Z7FZ	F08Z7GZ	F08Z7UZ	F08Z7YZ	F08Z7ZZ		

F Physical Rehabilitation and Diagnostic Audiology
0 Rehabilitation
9 Hearing Treatment: Application of techniques to improve, augment, or compensate for hearing and related functional impairment

Body system/ Region	Type Qualifier	Equipment	Qualifier
Character 4	**Character 5**	**Character 6**	**Character 7**
Z None ᴼᴿᴳ	**0** Hearing and Related Disorders Counseling **1** Hearing and Related Disorders Prevention	**K** Audiovisual **Z** None	**Z** None
Z None ᴼᴿᴳ	**2** Auditory Processing	**K** Audiovisual **L** Assistive Listening **P** Computer **Y** Other Equipment **Z** None	**Z** None
Z None ᴼᴿᴳ	**3** Cerumen Management	**X** Cerumen Management **Z** None	**Z** None

ᴼᴿᴳ F09Z0KZ   F09Z0ZZ   F09Z1KZ   F09Z1ZZ   F09Z2KZ   F09Z2LZ   F09Z2PZ   F09Z2YZ   F09Z2ZZ   F09Z3XZ   F09Z3ZZ

F Physical Rehabilitation and Diagnostic Audiology
0 Rehabilitation
B Cochlear Implant Treatment: Application of techniques to improve the communication abilities of individuals with cochlear implant

Body system/ Region	Type Qualifier	Equipment	Qualifier
Character 4	**Character 5**	**Character 6**	**Character 7**
Z None ᴼᴿᴳ	**0** Cochlear Implant Rehabilitation	**1** Audiometer **2** Sound Field / Booth **9** Cochlear Implant **K** Audiovisual **P** Computer **Y** Other Equipment	**Z** None

ᴼᴿᴳ F0BZ01Z   F0BZ02Z   F0BZ09Z   F0BZ0KZ   F0BZ0PZ   F0BZ0YZ

F Physical Rehabilitation and Diagnostic Audiology
0 Rehabilitation
C Vestibular Treatment: Application of techniques to improve, augment, or compensate for vestibular and related functional impairment

Body system/ Region	Type Qualifier	Equipment	Qualifier
Character 4	**Character 5**	**Character 6**	**Character 7**
3 Neurological System - Whole Body ᴼᴿᴳ **H** Integumentary System - Whole Body ᴼᴿᴳ **M** Musculoskeletal System - Whole Body ᴼᴿᴳ	**3** Postural Control	**E** Orthosis **F** Assistive, Adaptive, Supportive or Protective **U** Prosthesis **Y** Other Equipment **Z** None	**Z** None
Z None ᴼᴿᴳ	**0** Vestibular	**8** Vestibular / Balance **Z** None	**Z** None
Z None ᴼᴿᴳ	**1** Perceptual Processing **2** Visual Motor Integration	**K** Audiovisual **L** Assistive Listening **N** Biosensory Feedback **P** Computer **Q** Speech Analysis **S** Voice Analysis **T** Aerodynamic Function **Y** Other Equipment **Z** None	**Z** None

ᴼᴿᴳ F0C33EZ   F0C33FZ   F0C33UZ   F0C33YZ   F0C33ZZ   F0CH3EZ   F0CH3FZ   F0CH3UZ   F0CH3YZ   F0CH3ZZ   F0CM3EZ   F0CM3FZ   F0CM3UZ
F0CM3YZ   F0CM3ZZ   F0CZ08Z   F0CZ0ZZ   F0CZ1KZ   F0CZ1LZ   F0CZ1NZ   F0CZ1PZ   F0CZ1QZ   F0CZ1SZ   F0CZ1TZ   F0CZ1YZ   F0CZ1ZZ
F0CZ2KZ   F0CZ2LZ   F0CZ2NZ   F0CZ2PZ   F0CZ2QZ   F0CZ2SZ   F0CZ2TZ   F0CZ2YZ   F0CZ2ZZ

F Physical Rehabilitation and Diagnostic Audiology
0 Rehabilitation
D Device Fitting: Fitting of a device designed to facilitate or support achievement of a higher level of function

Body system/ Region	Type Qualifier	Equipment	Qualifier
Character 4	**Character 5**	**Character 6**	**Character 7**
Z None 🕮	**0** Tinnitus Masker	**5** Hearing Aid Selection / Fitting / Test **Z** None	**Z** None
Z None 🕮	**1** Monaural Hearing Aid **2** Binaural Hearing Aid **5** Assistive Listening Device	**1** Audiometer **2** Sound Field / Booth **5** Hearing Aid Selection / Fitting / Test **K** Audiovisual **L** Assistive Listening **Z** None	**Z** None
Z None 🕮	**3** Augmentative/Alternative Communication System	**M** Augmentative / Alternative Communication	**Z** None
Z None 🕮	**4** Voice Prosthetic	**S** Voice Analysis **V** Speech Prosthesis	**Z** None
Z None 🕮	**6** Dynamic Orthosis **7** Static Orthosis **8** Prosthesis **9** Assistive, Adaptive, Supportive or Protective Devices	**E** Orthosis **F** Assistive, Adaptive, Supportive or Protective **U** Prosthesis **Z** None	**Z** None

🕮 F0DZ05Z　F0DZ0ZZ　F0DZ11Z　F0DZ12Z　F0DZ15Z　F0DZ1KZ　F0DZ1LZ　F0DZ1ZZ　F0DZ21Z　F0DZ22Z　F0DZ25Z　F0DZ2KZ　F0DZ2LZ
F0DZ2ZZ　F0DZ3MZ　F0DZ4SZ　F0DZ4VZ　F0DZ51Z　F0DZ52Z　F0DZ55Z　F0DZ5KZ　F0DZ5LZ　F0DZ5ZZ　F0DZ6EZ　F0DZ6FZ　F0DZ6UZ
F0DZ6ZZ　F0DZ7EZ　F0DZ7FZ　F0DZ7UZ　F0DZ7ZZ　F0DZ8EZ　F0DZ8FZ　F0DZ8UZ

F Physical Rehabilitation and Diagnostic Audiology
0 Rehabilitation
F Caregiver Training: Training in activities to support patient's optimal level of function

Body system/ Region	Type Qualifier	Equipment	Qualifier
Character 4	**Character 5**	**Character 6**	**Character 7**
Z None 🕮	**0** Bathing/Showering Technique **1** Dressing **2** Feeding and Eating **3** Grooming/Personal Hygiene **4** Bed Mobility **5** Transfer **6** Wheelchair Mobility **7** Therapeutic Exercise **8** Airway Clearance Techniques **9** Wound Management **B** Vocational Activities and Functional Community or Work Reintegration Skills **C** Gait Training/Functional Ambulation **D** Application, Proper Use and Care of Devices **F** Application, Proper Use and Care of Orthoses **G** Application, Proper Use and Care of Prosthesis **H** Home Management	**E** Orthosis **F** Assistive, Adaptive, Supportive or Protective **U** Prosthesis **Z** None	**Z** None
Z None 🕮	**J** Communication Skills	**K** Audiovisual **L** Assistive Listening **M** Augmentative / Alternative Communication **P** Computer **Z** None	**Z** None

🕮 F0FZ0EZ　F0FZ0FZ　F0FZ0UZ　F0FZ0ZZ　F0FZ1EZ　F0FZ1FZ　F0FZ1UZ　F0FZ1ZZ　F0FZ2EZ　F0FZ2FZ　F0FZ2UZ　F0FZ2ZZ　F0FZ3EZ
F0FZ3FZ　F0FZ3UZ　F0FZ3ZZ　F0FZ4EZ　F0FZ4FZ　F0FZ4UZ　F0FZ4ZZ　F0FZ5EZ　F0FZ5FZ　F0FZ5UZ　F0FZ5ZZ　F0FZ6EZ　F0FZ6FZ
F0FZ6UZ　F0FZ6ZZ　F0FZ7EZ　F0FZ7FZ　F0FZ7UZ　F0FZ7ZZ　F0FZ8EZ　F0FZ8FZ　F0FZ8UZ　F0FZ8ZZ　F0FZ9EZ　F0FZ9FZ　F0FZ9UZ
F0FZ9ZZ　F0FZBEZ　F0FZBFZ　F0FZBUZ　F0FZBZZ　F0FZCEZ　F0FZCFZ　F0FZCUZ　F0FZCZZ　F0FZDEZ　F0FZDFZ　F0FZDUZ　F0FZDZZ
F0FZFEZ　F0FZFFZ　F0FZFUZ　F0FZFZZ　F0FZGEZ　F0FZGFZ　F0FZGUZ　F0FZGZZ　F0FZHEZ　F0FZHFZ　F0FZHUZ　F0FZHZZ　F0FZJKZ
F0FZJLZ　F0FZJMZ　F0FZJPZ　F0FZJZZ

F Physical Rehabilitation and Diagnostic Audiology
1 Diagnostic Audiology
3 Hearing Assessment: Measurement of hearing and related functions

Body system/ Region	Type Qualifier	Equipment	Qualifier
Character 4	Character 5	Character 6	Character 7
Z None	0 Hearing Screening	0 Occupational Hearing 1 Audiometer 2 Sound Field / Booth 3 Tympanometer 8 Vestibular / Balance 9 Cochlear Implant Z None	Z None
Z None	1 Pure Tone Audiometry, Air 2 Pure Tone Audiometry, Air and Bone	0 Occupational Hearing 1 Audiometer 2 Sound Field / Booth Z None	Z None
Z None	3 Bekesy Audiometry 6 Visual Reinforcement Audiometry 9 Short Increment Sensitivity Index B Stenger C Pure Tone Stenger	1 Audiometer 2 Sound Field / Booth Z None	Z None
Z None	4 Conditioned Play Audiometry 5 Select Picture Audiometry	1 Audiometer 2 Sound Field / Booth K Audiovisual Z None	Z None
Z None	7 Alternate Binaural or Monaural Loudness Balance	1 Audiometer K Audiovisual Z None	Z None
Z None	8 Tone Decay D Tympanometry F Eustachian Tube Function G Acoustic Reflex Patterns H Acoustic Reflex Threshold J Acoustic Reflex Decay	3 Tympanometer 4 Electroacoustic Immittance / Acoustic Reflex Z None	Z None
Z None	K Electrocochleography L Auditory Evoked Potentials	7 Electrophysiologic Z None	Z None
Z None	M Evoked Otoacoustic Emissions, Screening N Evoked Otoacoustic Emissions, Diagnostic	6 Otoacoustic Emission (OAE) Z None	Z None
Z None	P Aural Rehabilitation Status	1 Audiometer 2 Sound Field / Booth 4 Electroacoustic Immittance / Acoustic Reflex 9 Cochlear Implant K Audiovisual L Assistive Listening P Computer Z None	Z None
Z None	Q Auditory Processing	K Audiovisual P Computer Y Other Equipment Z None	Z None

F Physical Rehabilitation and Diagnostic Audiology
1 Diagnostic Audiology
4 Hearing Aid Assessment: Measurement of the appropriateness and/or effectiveness of a hearing device

Body system/ Region	Type Qualifier	Equipment	Qualifier
Character 4	Character 5	Character 6	Character 7
Z None	**0** Cochlear Implant	**1** Audiometer **2** Sound Field / Booth **3** Tympanometer **4** Electroacoustic Immittance / Acoustic Reflex **5** Hearing Aid Selection / Fitting / Test **7** Electrophysiologic **9** Cochlear Implant **K** Audiovisual **L** Assistive Listening **P** Computer **Y** Other Equipment **Z** None	**Z** None
Z None	**1** Ear Canal Probe Microphone **6** Binaural Electroacoustic Hearing Aid Check **8** Monaural Electroacoustic Hearing Aid Check	**5** Hearing Aid Selection / Fitting / Test **Z** None	**Z** None
Z None	**2** Monaural Hearing Aid **3** Binaural Hearing Aid	**1** Audiometer **2** Sound Field / Booth **3** Tympanometer **4** Electroacoustic Immittance / Acoustic Reflex **5** Hearing Aid Selection / Fitting / Test **K** Audiovisual **L** Assistive Listening **P** Computer **Z** None	**Z** None
Z None	**4** Assistive Listening System/ Device Selection	**1** Audiometer **2** Sound Field / Booth **3** Tympanometer **4** Electroacoustic Immittance / Acoustic Reflex **K** Audiovisual **L** Assistive Listening **Z** None	**Z** None
Z None	**5** Sensory Aids	**1** Audiometer **2** Sound Field / Booth **3** Tympanometer **4** Electroacoustic Immittance / Acoustic Reflex **5** Hearing Aid Selection / Fitting / Test **K** Audiovisual **L** Assistive Listening **Z** None	**Z** None
Z None	**7** Ear Protector Attenuation	**0** Occupational Hearing **Z** None	**Z** None

F Physical Rehabilitation and Diagnostic Audiology
1 Diagnostic Audiology
5 Vestibular Assessment: Measurement of the vestibular system and related functions

Body system/ Region	Type Qualifier	Equipment	Qualifier
Character 4	Character 5	Character 6	Character 7
Z None	**0** Bithermal, Binaural Caloric Irrigation **1** Bithermal, Monaural Caloric Irrigation **2** Unithermal Binaural Screen **3** Oscillating Tracking **4** Sinusoidal Vertical Axis Rotational **5** Dix-Hallpike Dynamic **6** Computerized Dynamic Posturography	**8** Vestibular / Balance **Z** None	**Z** None
Z None	**7** Tinnitus Masker	**5** Hearing Aid Selection / Fitting / Test **Z** None	**Z** None

LC Limited Coverage   **NC** Noncovered   **HAC** HAC-associated Procedure   **CC** Combination Cluster - See Appendix G for code lists
ORG Non-OR-Affecting MS-DRG Assignment   New/Revised Text in **Orange**   ♂ Male   ♀ Female

736

2021 ICD-10-PCS

NOTES

NOTES

Mental Health GZ1-GZJ

G Mental Health
Z None
1 Psychological Tests: The administration and interpretation of standardized psychological tests and measurement instruments for the assessment of psychological function

Qualifier	Qualifier	Qualifier	Qualifier
Character 4	Character 5	Character 6	Character 7
0 Developmental 1 Personality and Behavioral 2 Intellectual and Psychoeducational 3 Neuropsychological 4 Neurobehavioral and Cognitive Status	**Z** None	**Z** None	**Z** None

G Mental Health
Z None
2 Crisis Intervention: Treatment of a traumatized, acutely disturbed or distressed individual for the purpose of short-term stabilization

Qualifier	Qualifier	Qualifier	Qualifier
Character 4	Character 5	Character 6	Character 7
Z None	**Z** None	**Z** None	**Z** None

G Mental Health
Z None
3 Medication Management: Monitoring and adjusting the use of medications for the treatment of a mental health disorder

Qualifier	Qualifier	Qualifier	Qualifier
Character 4	Character 5	Character 6	Character 7
Z None	**Z** None	**Z** None	**Z** None

G Mental Health
Z None
5 Individual Psychotherapy: Treatment of an individual with a mental health disorder by behavioral, cognitive, psychoanalytic, psychodynamic or psychophysiological means to improve functioning or well-being

Qualifier	Qualifier	Qualifier	Qualifier
Character 4	Character 5	Character 6	Character 7
0 Interactive 1 Behavioral 2 Cognitive 3 Interpersonal 4 Psychoanalysis 5 Psychodynamic 6 Supportive 8 Cognitive-Behavioral 9 Psychophysiological	**Z** None	**Z** None	**Z** None

G Mental Health
Z None
6 Counseling: The application of psychological methods to treat an individual with normal developmental issues and psychological problems in order to increase function, improve well-being, alleviate distress, maladjustment or resolve crises

Qualifier	Qualifier	Qualifier	Qualifier
Character 4	Character 5	Character 6	Character 7
0 Educational 1 Vocational 3 Other Counseling	**Z** None	**Z** None	**Z** None

LC Limited Coverage **NC** Noncovered **HAC** HAC-associated Procedure **CC** Combination Cluster - See Appendix G for code lists
DRG Non-OR-Affecting MS-DRG Assignment   New/Revised Text in **Orange**   ♂ Male   ♀ Female

2021 ICD-10-PCS

739

MENTAL HEALTH GZ1-GZJ

GZ7-GZJ

MENTAL HEALTH GZ1-GZJ

G Mental Health
Z None
7 Family Psychotherapy: Treatment that includes one or more family members of an individual with a mental health disorder by behavioral, cognitive, psychoanalytic, psychodynamic or psychophysiological means to improve functioning or well-being

Qualifier	Qualifier	Qualifier	Qualifier
Character 4	Character 5	Character 6	Character 7
2 Other Family Psychotherapy	Z None	Z None	Z None

G Mental Health
Z None
B Electroconvulsive Therapy: The application of controlled electrical voltages to treat a mental health disorder

Qualifier	Qualifier	Qualifier	Qualifier
Character 4	Character 5	Character 6	Character 7
0 Unilateral-Single Seizure 1 Unilateral-Multiple Seizure 2 Bilateral-Single Seizure 3 Bilateral-Multiple Seizure 4 Other Electroconvulsive Therapy	Z None	Z None	Z None

G Mental Health
Z None
C Biofeedback: Provision of information from the monitoring and regulating of physiological processes in conjunction with cognitive-behavioral techniques to improve patient functioning or well-being

Qualifier	Qualifier	Qualifier	Qualifier
Character 4	Character 5	Character 6	Character 7
9 Other Biofeedback	Z None	Z None	Z None

G Mental Health
Z None
F Hypnosis: Induction of a state of heightened suggestibility by auditory, visual and tactile techniques to elicit an emotional or behavioral response

Qualifier	Qualifier	Qualifier	Qualifier
Character 4	Character 5	Character 6	Character 7
Z None	Z None	Z None	Z None

G Mental Health
Z None
G Narcosynthesis: Administration of intravenous barbiturates in order to release suppressed or repressed thoughts

Qualifier	Qualifier	Qualifier	Qualifier
Character 4	Character 5	Character 6	Character 7
Z None	Z None	Z None	Z None

G Mental Health
Z None
H Group Psychotherapy: Treatment of two or more individuals with a mental health disorder by behavioral, cognitive, psychoanalytic, psychodynamic or psychophysiological means to improve functioning or well-being

Qualifier	Qualifier	Qualifier	Qualifier
Character 4	Character 5	Character 6	Character 7
Z None	Z None	Z None	Z None

G Mental Health
Z None
J Light Therapy: Application of specialized light treatments to improve functioning or well-being

Qualifier	Qualifier	Qualifier	Qualifier
Character 4	Character 5	Character 6	Character 7
Z None	Z None	Z None	Z None

LC Limited Coverage   NC Noncovered   HAC HAC-associated Procedure   CC Combination Cluster - See Appendix G for code lists
Non-OR-Affecting MS-DRG Assignment   New/Revised Text in **Orange**   ♂ Male   ♀ Female

740

2021 ICD-10-PCS

NOTES

NOTES

Substance Abuse Treatment HZ2-HZ9

H **Substance Abuse Treatment**
Z **None**
2 **Detoxification Services:** Detoxification from alcohol and/or drugs

Qualifier	Qualifier	Qualifier	Qualifier
Character 4	**Character 5**	**Character 6**	**Character 7**
Z None	**Z** None	**Z** None	**Z** None

H **Substance Abuse Treatment**
Z **None**
3 **Individual Counseling:** The application of psychological methods to treat an individual with addictive behavior

Qualifier	Qualifier	Qualifier	Qualifier
Character 4	**Character 5**	**Character 6**	**Character 7**
0 Cognitive ᴰᴿᴳ **1** Behavioral ᴰᴿᴳ **2** Cognitive-Behavioral ᴰᴿᴳ **3** 12-Step ᴰᴿᴳ **4** Interpersonal ᴰᴿᴳ **5** Vocational ᴰᴿᴳ **6** Psychoeducation ᴰᴿᴳ **7** Motivational Enhancement ᴰᴿᴳ **8** Confrontational ᴰᴿᴳ **9** Continuing Care ᴰᴿᴳ **B** Spiritual ᴰᴿᴳ **C** Pre/Post-Test Infectious Disease	**Z** None	**Z** None	**Z** None

ᴰᴿᴳ   HZ30ZZZ   HZ31ZZZ   HZ32ZZZ   HZ33ZZZ   HZ34ZZZ   HZ35ZZZ   HZ36ZZZ   HZ37ZZZ   HZ38ZZZ   HZ39ZZZ   HZ3BZZZ

H **Substance Abuse Treatment**
Z **None**
4 **Group Counseling:** The application of psychological methods to treat two or more individuals with addictive behavior

Qualifier	Qualifier	Qualifier	Qualifier
Character 4	**Character 5**	**Character 6**	**Character 7**
0 Cognitive ᴰᴿᴳ **1** Behavioral ᴰᴿᴳ **2** Cognitive-Behavioral ᴰᴿᴳ **3** 12-Step ᴰᴿᴳ **4** Interpersonal ᴰᴿᴳ **5** Vocational ᴰᴿᴳ **6** Psychoeducation ᴰᴿᴳ **7** Motivational Enhancement ᴰᴿᴳ **8** Confrontational ᴰᴿᴳ **9** Continuing Care ᴰᴿᴳ **B** Spiritual ᴰᴿᴳ **C** Pre/Post-Test Infectious Disease	**Z** None	**Z** None	**Z** None

ᴰᴿᴳ   HZ40ZZZ   HZ41ZZZ   HZ42ZZZ   HZ43ZZZ   HZ44ZZZ   HZ45ZZZ   HZ46ZZZ   HZ47ZZZ   HZ48ZZZ   HZ49ZZZ   HZ4BZZZ

H   Substance Abuse Treatment
Z   None
5   Individual Psychotherapy: Treatment of an individual with addictive behavior by behavioral, cognitive, psychoanalytic, psychodynamic or psychophysiological means

Qualifier	Qualifier	Qualifier	Qualifier
Character 4	Character 5	Character 6	Character 7
0 Cognitive ⚙	Z None	Z None	Z None
1 Behavioral ⚙			
2 Cognitive-Behavioral ⚙			
3 12-Step ⚙			
4 Interpersonal ⚙			
5 Interactive ⚙			
6 Psychoeducation ⚙			
7 Motivational Enhancement ⚙			
8 Confrontational ⚙			
9 Supportive ⚙			
B Psychoanalysis ⚙			
C Psychodynamic ⚙			
D Psychophysiological ⚙			

⚙   HZ50ZZZ   HZ51ZZZ   HZ52ZZZ   HZ53ZZZ   HZ54ZZZ   HZ55ZZZ   HZ56ZZZ   HZ57ZZZ   HZ58ZZZ   HZ59ZZZ   HZ5BZZZ   HZ5CZZZ   HZ5DZZZ

H   Substance Abuse Treatment
Z   None
6   Family Counseling: The application of psychological methods that includes one or more family members to treat an individual with addictive behavior

Qualifier	Qualifier	Qualifier	Qualifier
Character 4	Character 5	Character 6	Character 7
3 Other Family Counseling	Z None	Z None	Z None

H   Substance Abuse Treatment
Z   None
8   Medication Management: Monitoring and adjusting the use of replacement medications for the treatment of addiction

Qualifier	Qualifier	Qualifier	Qualifier
Character 4	Character 5	Character 6	Character 7
0 Nicotine Replacement	Z None	Z None	Z None
1 Methadone Maintenance			
2 Levo-alpha-acetyl-methadol (LAAM)			
3 Antabuse			
4 Naltrexone			
5 Naloxone			
6 Clonidine			
7 Bupropion			
8 Psychiatric Medication			
9 Other Replacement Medication			

🅛🅒 Limited Coverage   🅝🅒 Noncovered   🅗🅐🅒 HAC-associated Procedure   🅒🅒 Combination Cluster - See Appendix G for code lists
⚙ Non-OR-Affecting MS-DRG Assignment   New/Revised Text in **Orange**   ♂ Male   ♀ Female

744   **2021 ICD-10-PCS**

H Substance Abuse Treatment
Z None
9 Pharmacotherapy: The use of replacement medications for the treatment of addiction

Qualifier	Qualifier	Qualifier	Qualifier
Character 4	**Character 5**	**Character 6**	**Character 7**

0 Nicotine Replacement
1 Methadone Maintenance
2 Levo-alpha-acetyl-methadol
     (LAAM)
3 Antabuse
4 Naltrexone
5 Naloxone
6 Clonidine
7 Bupropion
8 Psychiatric Medication
9 Other Replacement
     Medication
	Z None	**Z** None	**Z** None

NOTES

New Technology X27-XY0

Cardiovascular System X27-X2R

X **New Technology**
2 **Cardiovascular System**
7 **Dilation:** Expanding an orifice or the lumen of a tubular body part

Body Part	Approach	Device/Substance/Technology	Qualifier
Character 4	Character 5	Character 6	Character 7
H Femoral Artery, Right J Femoral Artery, Left K Popliteal Artery, Proximal Right L Popliteal Artery, Proximal Left M Popliteal Artery, Distal Right N Popliteal Artery, Distal Left P Anterior Tibial Artery, Right Q Anterior Tibial Artery, Left R Posterior Tibial Artery, Right S Posterior Tibial Artery, Left T Peroneal Artery, Right U Peroneal Artery, Left	3 Percutaneous	8 Intraluminal Device, Sustained Release Drug-eluting 9 Intraluminal Device, Sustained Release Drug-eluting, Two B Intraluminal Device, Sustained Release Drug-eluting, Three C Intraluminal Device, Sustained Release Drug-eluting, Four or More	5 New Technology Group 5

X **New Technology**
2 **Cardiovascular System**
A **Assistance:** Taking over a portion of a physiological function by extracorporeal means

Body Part	Approach	Device/Substance/Technology	Qualifier
Character 4	Character 5	Character 6	Character 7
5 Innominate Artery and Left Common Carotid Artery	3 Percutaneous	1 Cerebral Embolic Filtration, Dual Filter	2 New Technology Group 2
6 Aortic Arch	3 Percutaneous	2 Cerebral Embolic Filtration, Single Deflection Filter	5 New Technology Group 5
H Common Carotid Artery, Right J Common Carotid Artery, Left	3 Percutaneous	3 Cerebral Embolic Filtration, Extracorporeal Flow Reversal Circuit	6 New Technology Group 6

X **New Technology**
2 **Cardiovascular System**
C **Extirpation:** Taking or cutting out solid matter from a body part

Body Part	Approach	Device/Substance/Technology	Qualifier
Character 4	Character 5	Character 6	Character 7
0 Coronary Artery, One Artery 1 Coronary Artery, Two Arteries 2 Coronary Artery, Three Arteries 3 Coronary Artery, Four or More Arteries	3 Percutaneous	6 Orbital Atherectomy Technology	1 New Technology Group 1

X **New Technology**
2 **Cardiovascular System**
R **Replacement:** Putting in or on biological or synthetic material that physically takes the place and/or function of all or a portion of a body part

Body Part	Approach	Device/Substance/Technology	Qualifier
Character 4	Character 5	Character 6	Character 7
F Aortic Valve	0 Open 3 Percutaneous 4 Percutaneous Endoscopic	3 Zooplastic Tissue, Rapid Deployment Technique	2 New Technology Group 2

NOTES

Skin, Subcutaneous Tissue, Fascia, and Breast XHR

X   New Technology
H   Skin, Subcutaneous Tissue, Fascia and Breast
R   Replacement: Putting in or on biological or synthetic material that physically takes the place and/or function of all or a portion of a body part

Body Part	Approach	Device/Substance/Technology	Qualifier
Character 4	Character 5	Character 6	Character 7
P Skin	**X** External	**L** Skin Substitute, Porcine Liver Derived	**2** New Technology Group 2

NOTES

Muscles, Tendons, Bursae, and Ligaments XK0

X New Technology
K Muscles, Tendons, Bursae and Ligaments
0 Introduction: Putting in or on a therapeutic, diagnostic, nutritional, physiological, or prophylactic substance except blood or blood products

Body Part	Approach	Device/Substance/Technology	Qualifier
Character 4	Character 5	Character 6	Character 7
2 Muscle	**3** Percutaneous	**0** Concentrated Bone Marrow Aspirate	**3** New Technology Group 3

NOTES

X **New Technology**
N **Bones**
S **Reposition:** Moving to its normal location, or other suitable location, all or a portion of a body part

Body Part	Approach	Device/Substance/Technology	Qualifier
Character 4	Character 5	Character 6	Character 7
0 Lumbar Vertebra 3 Cervical Vertebra 4 Thoracic Vertebra	0 Open 3 Percutaneous	3 Magnetically Controlled Growth Rod(s)	2 New Technology Group 2

X **New Technology**
N **Bones**
U **Supplement:** Putting in or on biological or synthetic material that physically reinforces and/or augments the function of a portion of a body part

Body Part	Approach	Device/Substance/Technology	Qualifier
Character 4	Character 5	Character 6	Character 7
0 Lumbar Vertebra 4 Thoracic Vertebra	3 Percutaneous	5 Synthetic Substitute, Mechanically Expandable (Paired)	6 New Technology Group 6

LC Limited Coverage   NC Noncovered   HAC HAC-associated Procedure   CC Combination Cluster - See Appendix G for code lists
Non-OR-Affecting MS-DRG Assignment   New/Revised Text in Orange   ♂ Male   ♀ Female

2021 ICD-10-PCS   **753**

NOTES

X New Technology
R Joints
2 Monitoring: Determining the level of a physiological or physical function repetitively over a period of time

Body Part	Approach	Device/Substance/Technology	Qualifier
Character 4	Character 5	Character 6	Character 7
G Knee Joint, Right **H** Knee Joint, Left	**0** Open	**2** Intraoperative Knee Replacement Sensor	**1** New Technology Group 1

X New Technology
R Joints
G Fusion: Joining together portions of an articular body part rendering the articular body part immobile

Body Part	Approach	Device/Substance/Technology	Qualifier
Character 4	Character 5	Character 6	Character 7
0 Occipital-cervical Joint HAC	**0** Open	**9** Interbody Fusion Device, Nanotextured Surface	**2** New Technology Group 2
0 Occipital-cervical Joint HAC	**0** Open	**F** Interbody Fusion Device, Radiolucent Porous	**3** New Technology Group 3
1 Cervical Vertebral Joint HAC	**0** Open	**9** Interbody Fusion Device, Nanotextured Surface	**2** New Technology Group 2
1 Cervical Vertebral Joint HAC	**0** Open	**F** Interbody Fusion Device, Radiolucent Porous	**3** New Technology Group 3
2 Cervical Vertebral Joints, 2 or more HAC	**0** Open	**9** Interbody Fusion Device, Nanotextured Surface	**2** New Technology Group 2
2 Cervical Vertebral Joints, 2 or more HAC	**0** Open	**F** Interbody Fusion Device, Radiolucent Porous	**3** New Technology Group 3
4 Cervicothoracic Vertebral Joint HAC	**0** Open	**9** Interbody Fusion Device, Nanotextured Surface	**2** New Technology Group 2
4 Cervicothoracic Vertebral Joint HAC	**0** Open	**F** Interbody Fusion Device, Radiolucent Porous	**3** New Technology Group 3
6 Thoracic Vertebral Joint HAC	**0** Open	**9** Interbody Fusion Device, Nanotextured Surface	**2** New Technology Group 2
6 Thoracic Vertebral Joint HAC	**0** Open	**F** Interbody Fusion Device, Radiolucent Porous	**3** New Technology Group 3
7 Thoracic Vertebral Joints, 2 to 7 HAC CC	**0** Open	**9** Interbody Fusion Device, Nanotextured Surface	**2** New Technology Group 2
7 Thoracic Vertebral Joints, 2 to 7 HAC CC	**0** Open	**F** Interbody Fusion Device, Radiolucent Porous	**3** New Technology Group 3
8 Thoracic Vertebral Joints, 8 or more HAC	**0** Open	**9** Interbody Fusion Device, Nanotextured Surface	**2** New Technology Group 2
8 Thoracic Vertebral Joints, 8 or more HAC	**0** Open	**F** Interbody Fusion Device, Radiolucent Porous	**3** New Technology Group 3
A Thoracolumbar Vertebral Joint HAC	**0** Open	**9** Interbody Fusion Device, Nanotextured Surface	**2** New Technology Group 2
A Thoracolumbar Vertebral Joint HAC	**0** Open	**F** Interbody Fusion Device, Radiolucent Porous	**3** New Technology Group 3
B Lumbar Vertebral Joint HAC	**0** Open	**9** Interbody Fusion Device, Nanotextured Surface	**2** New Technology Group 2
B Lumbar Vertebral Joint HAC	**0** Open	**F** Interbody Fusion Device, Radiolucent Porous	**3** New Technology Group 3
C Lumbar Vertebral Joints, 2 or more HAC CC	**0** Open	**9** Interbody Fusion Device, Nanotextured Surface	**2** New Technology Group 2

XRG continued on next page

IC Limited Coverage   NC Noncovered   HAC HAC-associated Procedure   CC Combination Cluster - See Appendix G for code lists
DRG Non-OR-Affecting MS-DRG Assignment   New/Revised Text in **Orange**   ♂ Male   ♀ Female

X **New Technology**

XRG continued from previous page

R **Joints**

G **Fusion:** Joining together portions of an articular body part rendering the articular body part immobile

Body Part	Approach	Device/Substance/Technology	Qualifier
Character 4	Character 5	Character 6	Character 7
C Lumbar Vertebral Joints, 2 or more 🅷🅰🅲 🅲🅲	**0** Open	**F** Interbody Fusion Device, Radiolucent Porous	**3** New Technology Group 3
D Lumbosacral Joint 🅷🅰🅲	**0** Open	**9** Interbody Fusion Device, Nanotextured Surface	**2** New Technology Group 2
D Lumbosacral Joint 🅷🅰🅲	**0** Open	**F** Interbody Fusion Device, Radiolucent Porous	**3** New Technology Group 3

🅷🅰🅲 XRG0092   XRG00F3   XRG1092   XRG10F3   XRG2092   XRG20F3   XRG4092   XRG40F3   XRG6092   XRG60F3   XRG7092   XRG70F3   XRG8092
XRG80F3   XRGA092   XRGA0F3   XRGB092   XRGB0F3   XRGC092   XRGC0F3   XRGD092   XRGD0F3

Surgical site infection following certain orthopedic procedures of spine, shoulder and elbow procedures and secondary diagnosis K68.11, T81.40XA, T81.41XA, T81.42XA, T81.43XA, T81.44XA, T81.49XA, T84.60XA, T84.610A, T84.611A, T84.612A, T84.613A, T84.614A, T84.615A, T84.619A, T84.63XA, T84.69XA, T84.7XXA.

🅲🅲 XRG7092   XRG70F3   XRGC092   XRGC0F3

🅻🅲 Limited Coverage   🅽🅲 Noncovered   🅷🅰🅲 HAC-associated Procedure   🅲🅲 Combination Cluster - See Appendix G for code lists

🅝🅞🅡 Non-OR-Affecting MS-DRG Assignment   New/Revised Text in **Orange**   ♂ Male   ♀ Female

NOTES

NOTES

Urinary System XT2

X New Technology
T Urinary System
2 **Monitoring:** Determining the level of a physiological or physical function repetitively over a period of time

Body Part	Approach	Device/Substance/Technology	Qualifier
Character 4	Character 5	Character 6	Character 7
5 Kidney	**X** External	**E** Fluorescent Pyrazine	**5** New Technology Group 5

LC Limited Coverage   **NC** Noncovered   **HAC** HAC-associated Procedure   **CC** Combination Cluster - See Appendix G for code lists
DRG Non-OR-Affecting MS-DRG Assignment   New/Revised Text in **Orange**   ♂ Male   ♀ Female

2021 ICD-10-PCS

URINARY SYSTEM XT2

759

NOTES

Male Reproductive System XV5

X New Technology
V Male Reproductive System
5 **Destruction:** Physical eradication of all or a portion of a body part by the direct use of energy, force, or a destructive agent

Body Part	Approach	Device/Substance/Technology	Qualifier
Character 4	Character 5	Character 6	Character 7
0 Prostate	**8** Via Natural or Artificial Opening Endoscopic	**A** Robotic Waterjet Ablation	**4** New Technology Group 4

LC Limited Coverage   NC Noncovered   HAC HAC-associated Procedure   CC Combination Cluster - See Appendix G for code lists
DRG Non-OR-Affecting MS-DRG Assignment   New/Revised Text in **Orange**   ♂ Male   ♀ Female

2021 ICD-10-PCS   **761**

NOTES

Anatomical Regions XW0-XW2

X New Technology
W Anatomical Regions
0 Introduction: Putting in or on a therapeutic, diagnostic, nutritional, physiological, or prophylactic substance except blood or blood products

Body Part	Approach	Device/Substance/Technology	Qualifier
Character 4	Character 5	Character 6	Character 7
1 Subcutaneous Tissue	3 Percutaneous	F Other New Technology Therapeutic Substance	5 New Technology Group 5
1 Subcutaneous Tissue	3 Percutaneous	H Other New Technology Monoclonal Antibody K Leronlimab Monoclonal Antibody S COVID-19 Vaccine Dose 1 T COVID-19 Vaccine Dose 2 U COVID-19 Vaccine	6 New Technology Group 6
1 Subcutaneous Tissue	**3 Percutaneous**	**W Caplacizumab**	**5 New Technology Group 5**
2 Muscle	3 Percutaneous	S COVID-19 Vaccine Dose 1 T COVID-19 Vaccine Dose 2 U COVID-19 Vaccine	6 New Technology Group 6
3 Peripheral Vein	3 Percutaneous	0 Brexanolone	6 New Technology Group 6
3 Peripheral Vein	3 Percutaneous	2 Ceftazidime-Avibactam Anti-infective	1 New Technology Group 1
3 Peripheral Vein	3 Percutaneous	2 Nerinitide	6 New Technology Group 6
3 Peripheral Vein	3 Percutaneous	3 Idarucizumab, Dabigatran Reversal Agent	1 New Technology Group 1
3 Peripheral Vein	3 Percutaneous	3 Durvalumab Antineoplastic	6 New Technology Group 6
3 Peripheral Vein	3 Percutaneous	4 Isavuconazole Anti-infective 5 Blinatumomab Antineoplastic Immunotherapy	1 New Technology Group 1
3 Peripheral Vein	3 Percutaneous	6 Lefamulin Anti-infective	6 New Technology Group 6
3 Peripheral Vein	**3 Percutaneous**	**7 Coagulation Factor Xa, Inactivated** **9 Defibrotide Sodium Anticoagulant**	**2 New Technology Group 2**
3 Peripheral Vein	3 Percutaneous	9 Ceftolozane/Tazobactam Anti-infective	6 New Technology Group 6
3 Peripheral Vein	3 Percutaneous	A Bezlotoxumab Monoclonal Antibody	3 New Technology Group 3
3 Peripheral Vein	3 Percutaneous	A Cefiderocol Anti-infective	6 New Technology Group 6
3 Peripheral Vein	3 Percutaneous	B Cytarabine and Daunorubicin Liposome Antineoplastic	3 New Technology Group 3
3 Peripheral Vein	3 Percutaneous	B Omadacycline Anti-infective	6 New Technology Group 6
3 Peripheral Vein ᴰᴿᴳ	3 Percutaneous	C Engineered Autologous Chimeric Antigen Receptor T-cell Immunotherapy	3 New Technology Group 3
3 Peripheral Vein	3 Percutaneous	C Eculizumab D Atezolizumab Antineoplastic	6 New Technology Group 6
3 Peripheral Vein	3 Percutaneous	E Remdesivir Anti-infective	5 New Technology Group 5
3 Peripheral Vein	3 Percutaneous	E Etesevimab Monoclonal Antibody	6 New Technology Group 6
3 Peripheral Vein	3 Percutaneous	F Other New Technology Therapeutic Substance	3 New Technology Group 3
3 Peripheral Vein	3 Percutaneous	F Other New Technology Therapeutic Substance	5 New Technology Group 5
3 Peripheral Vein	3 Percutaneous	F Bamlanivimab Monoclonal Antibody	6 New Technology Group 6
3 Peripheral Vein	3 Percutaneous	G Plazomicin Anti-infective	4 New Technology Group 4

XW0 continued on next page

ᴸᶜ Limited Coverage   ᴺᶜ Noncovered   ᴴᴬᶜ HAC-associated Procedure   ᶜᶜ Combination Cluster - See Appendix G for code lists
ᴰᴿᴳ Non-OR-Affecting MS-DRG Assignment   New/Revised Text in **Orange**   ♂ Male   ♀ Female

X New Technology
W Anatomical Regions
0 Introduction: Putting in or on a therapeutic, diagnostic, nutritional, physiological, or prophylactic substance except blood or blood products

XW0 continued from previous page

Body Part	Approach	Device/Substance/Technology	Qualifier
Character 4	Character 5	Character 6	Character 7
3 Peripheral Vein	3 Percutaneous	G Sarilumab	5 New Technology Group 5
3 Peripheral Vein	3 Percutaneous	G REGN-COV2 Monoclonal Antibody	6 New Technology Group 6
3 Peripheral Vein	3 Percutaneous	H Synthetic Human Angiotensin II	4 New Technology Group 4
3 Peripheral Vein	3 Percutaneous	H Tocilizumab	5 New Technology Group 5
3 Peripheral Vein	3 Percutaneous	H Other New Technology Monoclonal Antibody	6 New Technology Group 6
3 Peripheral Vein	3 Percutaneous	K Fosfomycin Anti-infective	5 New Technology Group 5
3 Peripheral Vein	3 Percutaneous	L CD24Fc Immunomodulator	6 New Technology Group 6
3 Peripheral Vein	3 Percutaneous	N Meropenem-vaborbactam Anti-infective Q Tagraxofusp-erzs Antineoplastic S Iobenguane I-131 Antineoplastic U Imipenem-cilastatin- relebactam Anti-infective W Caplacizumab	5 New Technology Group 5
4 Central Vein	3 Percutaneous	0 Brexanolone	6 New Technology Group 6
4 Central Vein	3 Percutaneous	2 Ceftazidime-Avibactam Anti-infective	1 New Technology Group 1
4 Central Vein	3 Percutaneous	2 Nerinitide	6 New Technology Group 6
4 Central Vein	3 Percutaneous	3 Idarucizumab, Dabigatran Reversal Agent	1 New Technology Group 1
4 Central Vein	3 Percutaneous	3 Durvalumab Antineoplastic	6 New Technology Group 6
4 Central Vein	3 Percutaneous	4 Isavuconazole Anti- infective 5 Blinatumomab Antineoplastic Immunotherapy	1 New Technology Group 1
4 Central Vein	3 Percutaneous	6 Lefamulin Anti-infective	6 New Technology Group 6
4 Central Vein	3 Percutaneous	7 Coagulation Factor Xa, Inactivated 9 Defibrotide Sodium Anticoagulant	2 New Technology Group 2
4 Central Vein	3 Percutaneous	9 Ceftolozane/Tazobactam Anti-infective	6 New Technology Group 6
4 Central Vein	3 Percutaneous	A Bezlotoxumab Monoclonal Antibody	3 New Technology Group 3
4 Central Vein	3 Percutaneous	A Cefiderocol Anti-infective	6 New Technology Group 6
4 Central Vein	3 Percutaneous	B Cytarabine and Daunorubicin Liposome Antineoplastic	3 New Technology Group 3
4 Central Vein	3 Percutaneous	B Omadacycline Anti- infective	6 New Technology Group 6
4 Central Vein ⒹⓇⒼ	3 Percutaneous	C Engineered Autologous Chimeric Antigen Receptor T-cell Immunotherapy	3 New Technology Group 3
4 Central Vein	3 Percutaneous	C Eculizumab D Atezolizumab Antineoplastic	6 New Technology Group 6
4 Central Vein	3 Percutaneous	E Remdesivir Anti-infective	5 New Technology Group 5
4 Central Vein	3 Percutaneous	E Etesevimab Monoclonal Antibody	6 New Technology Group 6
4 Central Vein	3 Percutaneous	F Other New Technology Therapeutic Substance	3 New Technology Group 3
4 Central Vein	3 Percutaneous	F Other New Technology Therapeutic Substance	5 New Technology Group 5
4 Central Vein	3 Percutaneous	F Bamlanivimab Monoclonal Antibody	6 New Technology Group 6

XW0 continued on next page

LC Limited Coverage   NC Noncovered   HAC HAC-associated Procedure   CC Combination Cluster - See Appendix G for code lists
ⒹⓇⒼ Non-OR-Affecting MS-DRG Assignment   New/Revised Text in **Orange**   ♂ Male   ♀ Female

X New Technology
W Anatomical Regions
0 Introduction: Putting in or on a therapeutic, diagnostic, nutritional, physiological, or prophylactic substance except blood or blood products

XW0 continued from previous page

Body Part	Approach	Device/Substance/Technology	Qualifier
Character 4	Character 5	Character 6	Character 7
4 Central Vein	3 Percutaneous	G Plazomicin Anti-infective	4 New Technology Group 4
4 Central Vein	3 Percutaneous	G Sarilumab	5 New Technology Group 5
4 Central Vein	3 Percutaneous	G REGN-COV2 Monoclonal Antibody	6 New Technology Group 6
4 Central Vein	3 Percutaneous	H Synthetic Human Angiotensin II	4 New Technology Group 4
4 Central Vein	3 Percutaneous	H Tocilizumab	5 New Technology Group 5
4 Central Vein	3 Percutaneous	H Other New Technology Monoclonal Antibody	6 New Technology Group 6
4 Central Vein	3 Percutaneous	K Fosfomycin Anti-infective	5 New Technology Group 5
4 Central Vein	3 Percutaneous	L CD24Fc Immunomodulator	6 New Technology Group 6
4 Central Vein	3 Percutaneous	N Meropenem-vaborbactam Anti-infective Q Tagraxofusp-erzs Antineoplastic S Iobenguane I-131 Antineoplastic U Imipenem-cilastatin- relebactam Anti-infective W Caplacizumab	5 New Technology Group 5
9 Nose	7 Via Natural or Artificial Opening	M Esketamine Hydrochloride	5 New Technology Group 5
D Mouth and Pharynx	X External	6 Lefamulin Anti-infective	6 New Technology Group 6
D Mouth and Pharynx	X External	8 Uridine Triacetate	2 New Technology Group 2
D Mouth and Pharynx	X External	F Other New Technology Therapeutic Substance J Apalutamide Antineoplastic L Erdafitinib Antineoplastic	5 New Technology Group 5
D Mouth and Pharynx	X External	M Baricitinib	6 New Technology Group 6
D Mouth and Pharynx	X External	R Venetoclax Antineoplastic T Ruxolitinib V Gilteritinib Antineoplastic	5 New Technology Group 5
G Upper GI H Lower GI	7 Via Natural or Artificial Opening	M Baricitinib	6 New Technology Group 6
G Upper GI H Lower GI	8 Via Natural or Artificial Opening Endoscopic	8 Mineral-based Topical Hemostatic Agent	6 New Technology Group 6
Q Cranial Cavity and Brain	3 Percutaneous	1 Eladocagene exuparvovec	6 New Technology Group 6

DRG XW033C3   XW043C3

X New Technology
W Anatomical Regions
1 Transfusion: Putting in blood or blood products

Body Part	Approach	Device/Substance/Technology	Qualifier
Character 4	Character 5	Character 6	Character 7
3 Peripheral Vein 4 Central Vein	3 Percutaneous	2 Plasma, Convalescent (Nonautologous)	5 New Technology Group 5

X New Technology
W Anatomical Regions
2 Transfusion: Putting in blood or blood products

Body Part	Approach	Device/Substance/Technology	Qualifier
Character 4	Character 5	Character 6	Character 7
3 Peripheral Vein 4 Central Vein	3 Percutaneous	4 Brexucabtagene Autoleucel Immunotherapy 7 Lisocabtagene Maraleucel Immunotherapy	6 New Technology Group 6

NOTES

Physiological Systems XXE

X **New Technology**
X **Physiological Systems**
E **Measurement:** Determining the level of a physiological or physical function at a point in time

Body Part	Approach	Device/Substance/Technology	Qualifier
Character 4	**Character 5**	**Character 6**	**Character 7**
5 Circulatory	**X** External	**M** Infection, Whole Blood Nucleic Acid-base Microbial Detection	**5** New Technology Group 5
5 Circulatory	**X** External	**N** Infection, Positive Blood Culture Fluorescence Hybridization for Organism Identification, Concentration and Susceptibility	**6** New Technology Group 6
B Respiratory	**X** External	**Q** Infection, Lower Respiratory Fluid Nucleic Acid-base Microbial Detection	**6** New Technology Group 6

NOTES

Extracorporeal XY0

X **New Technology**
Y **Extracorporeal**
0 **Introduction:** Putting in or on a therapeutic, diagnostic, nutritional, physiological, or prophylactic substance except blood or blood products

Body Part	Approach	Device/Substance/Technology	Qualifier
Character 4	Character 5	Character 6	Character 7
V Vein Graft	**X** External	**8** Endothelial Damage Inhibitor	**3** New Technology Group 3

NOTES

Appendix A: Root Operations Definitions

0 - Medical and Surgical

Value	Root Operation	Definition/Explanation
0	Alteration	**Definition:** Modifying the anatomic structure of a body part without affecting the function of the body part **Explanation:** Principal purpose is to improve appearance **Includes/Examples:** Face lift, breast augmentation
1	Bypass	**Definition:** Altering the route of passage of the contents of a tubular body part **Explanation:** Rerouting contents of a body part to a downstream area of the normal route, to a similar route and body part, or to an abnormal route and dissimilar body part. Includes one or more anastomoses, with or without the use of a device. **Includes/Examples:** Coronary artery bypass, colostomy formation
2	Change	**Definition:** Taking out or off a device from a body part and putting back an identical or similar device in or on the same body part without cutting or puncturing the skin or a mucous membrane **Explanation:** All CHANGE procedures are coded using the approach EXTERNAL **Includes/Examples:** Urinary catheter change, gastrostomy tube change
3	Control	**Definition:** Stopping, or attempting to stop, postprocedural or other acute bleeding **Includes/Examples:** Control of post-prostatectomy hemorrhage, control of intracranial subdural hemorrhage, control of bleeding duodenal ulcer, control of retroperitoneal hemorrhage
4	Creation	**Definition:** Putting in or on biological or synthetic material to form a new body part that to the extent possible replicates the anatomic structure or function of an absent body part **Explanation:** Used for gender reassignment surgery and corrective procedures in individuals with congenital anomalies **Includes/Examples:** Creation of vagina in a male, creation of right and left atrioventricular valve from common atrioventricular valve
5	Destruction	**Definition:** Physical eradication of all or a portion of a body part by the direct use of energy, force, or a destructive agent **Explanation:** None of the body part is physically taken out **Includes/Examples:** Fulguration of rectal polyp, cautery of skin lesion
6	Detachment	**Definition:** Cutting off all or a portion of the upper or lower extremities **Explanation:** The body part value is the site of the detachment, with a qualifier if applicable to further specify the level where the extremity was detached **Includes/Examples:** Below knee amputation, disarticulation of shoulder
7	Dilation	**Definition:** Expanding an orifice or the lumen of a tubular body part **Explanation:** The orifice can be a natural orifice or an artificially created orifice. Accomplished by stretching a tubular body part using intraluminal pressure or by cutting part of the orifice or wall of the tubular body part **Includes/Examples:** Percutaneous transluminal angioplasty, internal urethrotomy
8	Division	**Definition:** Cutting into a body part, without draining fluids and/or gases from the body part, in order to separate or transect a body part **Explanation:** All or a portion of the body part is separated into two or more portions **Includes/Examples:** Spinal cordotomy, osteotomy
9	Drainage	**Definition:** Taking or letting out fluids and/or gases from a body part **Explanation:** The qualifier DIAGNOSTIC is used to identify drainage procedures that are biopsies **Includes/Examples:** Thoracentesis, incision and drainage
B	Excision	**Definition:** Cutting out or off, without replacement, a portion of a body part **Explanation:** The qualifier DIAGNOSTIC is used to identify excision procedures that are biopsies **Includes/Examples:** Partial nephrectomy, liver biopsy

0 - Medical and Surgical continued on next page

0 - Medical and Surgical continued from previous page

	0 - Medical and Surgical	
Value	**Root Operation**	**Definition/Explanation**
C	Extirpation	**Definition:** Taking or cutting out solid matter from a body part
		Explanation: The solid matter may be an abnormal byproduct of a biological function or a foreign body; it may be imbedded in a body part or in the lumen of a tubular body part. The solid matter may or may not have been previously broken into pieces.
		Includes/Examples: Thrombectomy, choledocholithotomy
D	Extraction	**Definition:** Pulling or stripping out or off all or a portion of a body part by the use of force
		Explanation: The qualifier DIAGNOSTIC is used to identify extraction procedures that are biopsies
		Includes/Examples: Dilation and curettage, vein stripping
F	Fragmentation	**Definition:** Breaking solid matter in a body part into pieces
		Explanation: Physical force (e.g., manual, ultrasonic) applied directly or indirectly is used to break the solid matter into pieces. The solid matter may be an abnormal byproduct of a biological function or a foreign body. The pieces of solid matter are not taken out.
		Includes/Examples: Extracorporeal shockwave lithotripsy, transurethral lithotripsy
G	Fusion	**Definition:** Joining together portions of an articular body part rendering the articular body part immobile
		Explanation: The body part is joined together by fixation device, bone graft, or other means
		Includes/Examples: Spinal fusion, ankle arthrodesis
H	Insertion	**Definition:** Putting in a nonbiological appliance that monitors, assists, performs, or prevents a physiological function but does not physically take the place of a body part
		Includes/Examples: Insertion of radioactive implant, insertion of central venous catheter
J	Inspection	**Definition:** Visually and/or manually exploring a body part
		Explanation: Visual exploration may be performed with or without optical instrumentation. Manual exploration may be performed directly or through intervening body layers.
		Includes/Examples: Diagnostic arthroscopy, exploratory laparotomy
K	Map	**Definition:** Locating the route of passage of electrical impulses and/or locating functional areas in a body part
		Explanation: Applicable only to the cardiac conduction mechanism and the central nervous system
		Includes/Examples: Cardiac mapping, cortical mapping
L	Occlusion	**Definition:** Completely closing an orifice or the lumen of a tubular body part
		Explanation: The orifice can be a natural orifice or an artificially created orifice
		Includes/Examples: Fallopian tube ligation, ligation of inferior vena cava
M	Reattachment	**Definition:** Putting back in or on all or a portion of a separated body part to its normal location or other suitable location
		Explanation: Vascular circulation and nervous pathways may or may not be reestablished
		Includes/Examples: Reattachment of hand, reattachment of avulsed kidney
N	Release	**Definition:** Freeing a body part from an abnormal physical constraint by cutting or by the use of force
		Explanation: Some of the restraining tissue may be taken out but none of the body part is taken out
		Includes/Examples: Adhesiolysis, carpal tunnel release
P	Removal	**Definition:** Taking out or off a device from a body part
		Explanation: If a device is taken out and a similar device put in without cutting or puncturing the skin or mucous membrane, the procedure is coded to the root operation CHANGE. Otherwise, the procedure for taking out a device is coded to the root operation REMOVAL.
		Includes/Examples: Drainage tube removal, cardiac pacemaker removal
Q	Repair	**Definition:** Restoring, to the extent possible, a body part to its normal anatomic structure and function
		Explanation: Used only when the method to accomplish the repair is not one of the other root operations
		Includes/Examples: Colostomy takedown, suture of laceration

0 - Medical and Surgical continued on next page

0 - Medical and Surgical continued from previous page

0 - Medical and Surgical

Value	Root Operation	Definition/Explanation
R	Replacement	**Definition:** Putting in or on biological or synthetic material that physically takes the place and/or function of all or a portion of a body part **Explanation:** The body part may have been taken out or replaced, or may be taken out, physically eradicated, or rendered nonfunctional during the Replacement procedure. A Removal procedure is coded for taking out the device used in a previous replacement procedure. **Includes/Examples:** Total hip replacement, bone graft, free skin graft
S	Reposition	**Definition:** Moving to its normal location, or other suitable location, all or a portion of a body part **Explanation:** The body part is moved to a new location from an abnormal location, or from a normal location where it is not functioning correctly. The body part may or may not be cut out or off to be moved to the new location. **Includes/Examples:** Reposition of undescended testicle, fracture reduction
T	Resection	**Definition:** Cutting out or off, without replacement, all of a body part **Includes/Examples:** Total nephrectomy, total lobectomy of lung
V	Restriction	**Definition:** Partially closing an orifice or the lumen of a tubular body part **Explanation:** The orifice can be a natural orifice or an artificially created orifice **Includes/Examples:** Esophagogastric fundoplication, cervical cerclage
W	Revision	**Definition:** Correcting, to the extent possible, a portion of a malfunctioning device or the position of a displaced device **Explanation:** Revision can include correcting a malfunctioning or displaced device by taking out or putting in components of the device such as a screw or pin **Includes/Examples:** Adjustment of position of pacemaker lead, recementing of hip prosthesis
U	Supplement	**Definition:** Putting in or on biological or synthetic material that physically reinforces and/or augments the function of a portion of a body part **Explanation:** The biological material is non-living, or is living and from the same individual. The body part may have been previously replaced, and the Supplement procedure is performed to physically reinforce and/or augment the function of the replaced body part. **Includes/Examples:** Herniorrhaphy using mesh, mitral valve ring annuloplasty, put a new acetabular liner in a previous hip replacement
X	Transfer	**Definition:** Moving, without taking out, all or a portion of a body part to another location to take over the function of all or a portion of a body part **Explanation:** The body part transferred remains connected to its vascular and nervous supply **Includes/Examples:** Tendon transfer, skin pedicle flap transfer
Y	Transplantation	**Definition:** Putting in or on all or a portion of a living body part taken from another individual or animal to physically take the place and/or function of all or a portion of a similar body part **Explanation:** The native body part may or may not be taken out, and the transplanted body part may take over all or a portion of its function **Includes/Examples:** Kidney transplant, heart transplant

1 - Obstetrics

Value	Root Operation	Definition/Explanation
A	Abortion	**Definition:** Artificially terminating a pregnancy
2	Change	**Definition:** Taking out or off a device from a body part and putting back an identical or similar device in or on the same body part without cutting or puncturing the skin or a mucous membrane
E	Delivery	**Definition:** Assisting the passage of the products of conception from the genital canal
9	Drainage	**Definition:** Taking or letting out fluids and/or gases from a body part
D	Extraction	**Definition:** Pulling or stripping out or off all or a portion of a body part by the use of force

1 - Obstetrics continued on next page

1 - Obstetrics continued from previous page

1 - Obstetrics

Value	Root Operation	Definition/Explanation
H	Insertion	**Definition:** Putting in a nonbiological appliance that monitors, assists, performs, or prevents a physiological function but does not physically take the place of a body part
J	Inspection	**Definition:** Visually and/or manually exploring a body part
		Explanation: Visual exploration may be performed with or without optical instrumentation. Manual exploration may be performed directly or through intervening body layers
P	Removal	**Definition:** Taking out or off a device from a body part, region or orifice
		Explanation: If a device is taken out and a similar device put in without cutting or puncturing the skin or mucous membrane, the procedure is coded to the root operation CHANGE. Otherwise, the procedure for taking out a device is coded to the root operation REMOVAL.
Q	Repair	**Definition:** Restoring, to the extent possible, a body part to its normal anatomic structure and function
		Explanation: Used only when the method to accomplish the repair is not one of the other root operations
S	Reposition	**Definition:** Moving to its normal location, or other suitable location, all or a portion of a body part
		Explanation: The body part is moved to a new location from an abnormal location, or from a normal location where it is not functioning correctly. The body part may or may not be cut out or off to be moved to the new location.
T	Resection	**Definition:** Cutting out or off, without replacement, all of a body part
Y	Transplantation	**Definition:** Putting in or on all or a portion of a living body part taken from another individual or animal to physically take the place and/or function of all or a portion of a similar body part
		Explanation: The native body part may or may not be taken out, and the transplanted body part may take over all or a portion of its function

2 - Placement

Value	Root Operation	Definition/Explanation
0	Change	**Definition:** Taking out or off a device from a body part and putting back an identical or similar device in or on the same body part without cutting or puncturing the skin or a mucous membrane
1	Compression	**Definition:** Putting pressure on a body region
2	Dressing	**Definition:** Putting material on a body region for protection
3	Immobilization	**Definition:** Limiting or preventing motion of a body region
4	Packing	**Definition:** Putting material in a body region or orifice
5	Removal	**Definition:** Taking out or off a device from a body part
6	Traction	**Definition:** Exerting a pulling force on a body region in a distal direction

3 - Administration

Value	Root Operation	Definition/Explanation
0	Introduction	**Definition:** Putting in or on a therapeutic, diagnostic, nutritional, physiological, or prophylactic substance except blood or blood products
1	Irrigation	**Definition:** Putting in or on a cleansing substance
2	Transfusion	**Definition:** Putting in blood or blood products

4 - Measurement and Monitoring

Value	Root Operation	Definition/Explanation
0	Measurement	**Definition:** Determining the level of a physiological or physical function at a point in time
1	Monitoring	**Definition:** Determining the level of a physiological or physical function repetitively over a period of time

5 - Extracorporeal or Systemic Assistance and Performance

Value	Root Operation	Definition/Explanation
0	Assistance	**Definition:** Taking over a portion of a physiological function by extracorporeal means
1	Performance	**Definition:** Completely taking over a physiological function by extracorporeal means
2	Restoration	**Definition:** Returning, or attempting to return, a physiological function to its original state by extracorporeal means.

6 - Extracorporeal or Systemic Therapies

Value	Root Operation	Definition/Explanation
0	Atmospheric Control	**Definition:** Extracorporeal control of atmospheric pressure and composition
1	Decompression	**Definition:** Extracorporeal elimination of undissolved gas from body fluids
2	Electromagnetic Therapy	**Definition:** Extracorporeal treatment by electromagnetic rays
3	Hyperthermia	**Definition:** Extracorporeal raising of body temperature
4	Hypothermia	**Definition:** Extracorporeal lowering of body temperature
B	Perfusion	**Definition:** Extracorporeal treatment by diffusion of therapeutic fluid
5	Pheresis	**Definition:** Extracorporeal separation of blood products
6	Phototherapy	**Definition:** Extracorporeal treatment by light rays
9	Shock Wave Therapy	**Definition:** Extracorporeal treatment by shock waves
7	Ultrasound Therapy	**Definition:** Extracorporeal treatment by ultrasound
8	Ultraviolet Light Therapy	**Definition:** Extracorporeal treatment by ultraviolet light

7 - Osteopathic

Value	Root Operation	Definition/Explanation
0	Treatment	**Definition:** Manual treatment to eliminate or alleviate somatic dysfunction and related disorders

8 - Other Procedures

Value	Root Operation	Definition/Explanation
0	Other Procedures	**Definition:** Methodologies which attempt to remediate or cure a disorder or disease

9 - Chiropractic

Value	Root Operation	Definition/Explanation
B	Manipulation	**Definition:** Manual procedure that involves a directed thrust to move a joint past the physiological range of motion, without exceeding the anatomical limit

X - New Technology

Value	Root Operation	Definition/Explanation
A	Assistance	**Definition:** Taking over a portion of a physiological function by extracorporeal means
5	Destruction	**Definition:** Physical eradication of all or a portion of a body part by the direct use of energy, force, or a destructive agent **Explanation:** None of the body part is physically taken out **Includes/Examples:** Fulguration of rectal polyp, cautery of skin lesion
7	Dilation	**Definition:** Expanding an orifice or the lumen of a tubular body part **Explanation:** The orifice can be a natural orifice or an artificially created orifice. Accomplished by stretching a tubular body part using intraluminal pressure or by cutting part of the orifice or wall of the tubular body part
C	Extirpation	**Definition:** Taking or cutting out solid matter from a body part **Explanation:** The solid matter may be an abnormal byproduct of a biological function or a foreign body; it may be imbedded in a body part or in the lumen of a tubular body part. The solid matter may or may not have been previously broken into pieces. **Includes/Examples:** Thrombectomy, choledocholithotomy
G	Fusion	**Definition:** Joining together portions of an articular body part rendering the articular body part immobile **Explanation:** The body part is joined together by fixation device, bone graft, or other means **Includes/Examples:** Spinal fusion, ankle arthrodesis
0	Introduction	**Definition:** Putting in or on a therapeutic, diagnostic, nutritional, physiological, or prophylactic substance except blood or blood products
E	Measurement	**Definition:** Determining the level of a physiological or physical function at a point in time
2	Monitoring	**Definition:** Determining the level of a physiological or physical function repetitively over a period of time
1	Transfusion	**Definition:** Putting in blood or blood products
2	Transfusion	**Definition:** Putting in blood or blood products
R	Replacement	**Definition:** Putting in or on biological or synthetic material that physically takes the place and/or function of all or a portion of a body part **Explanation:** The body part may have been taken out or replaced, or may be taken out, physically eradicated, or rendered nonfunctional during the Replacement procedure. A Removal procedure is coded for taking out the device used in a previous replacement procedure. **Includes/Examples:** Total hip replacement, bone graft, free skin graft
S	Reposition	**Definition:** Moving to its normal location, or other suitable location, all or a portion of a body part **Explanation:** The body part is moved to a new location from an abnormal location, or from a normal location where it is not functioning correctly. The body part may or may not be cut out or off to be moved to the new location. **Includes/Examples:** Reposition of undescended testicle, fracture reduction
U	Supplement	**Definition:** Putting in or on biological or synthetic material that physically reinforces and/or augments the function of a portion of a body part

Appendix B: Body Part Key

Anatomical Term	ICD-10-PCS Value	Anatomical Term	ICD-10-PCS Value
Abdominal aortic plexus	Abdominal Sympathetic Nerve	Anterior (pectoral) lymph node	Lymphatic, Right Axillary
Abdominal esophagus	Esophagus, Lower		Lymphatic, Left Axillary
Abductor hallucis muscle	Foot Muscle, Right	Anterior cerebral artery	Intracranial Artery
	Foot Muscle, Left	Anterior cerebral vein	Intracranial Vein
Accessory cephalic vein	Cephalic Vein, Right	Anterior choroidal artery	Intracranial Artery
	Cephalic Vein, Left	Anterior circumflex humeral artery	Axillary Artery, Right
Accessory obturator nerve	Lumbar Plexus		Axillary Artery, Left
Accessory phrenic nerve	Phrenic Nerve	Anterior communicating artery	Intracranial Artery
Accessory spleen	Spleen	Anterior cruciate ligament (ACL)	Knee Bursa and Ligament, Right
Acetabulofemoral joint	Hip Joint, Right		Knee Bursa and Ligament, Left
	Hip Joint, Left	Anterior crural nerve	Femoral Nerve
Achilles tendon	Lower Leg Tendon, Right	Anterior facial vein	Face Vein, Right
	Lower Leg Tendon, Left		Face Vein, Left
Acromioclavicular ligament	Shoulder Bursa and Ligament, Right	Anterior intercostal artery	Internal Mammary Artery, Right
	Shoulder Bursa and Ligament, Left		Internal Mammary Artery, Left
Acromion (process)	Scapula, Right	Anterior interosseous nerve	Median Nerve
	Scapula, Left	Anterior lateral malleolar artery	Anterior Tibial Artery, Right
Adductor brevis muscle	Upper Leg Muscle, Right		Anterior Tibial Artery, Left
	Upper Leg Muscle, Left	Anterior lingual gland	Minor Salivary Gland
Adductor hallucis muscle	Foot Muscle, Right	Anterior medial malleolar artery	Anterior Tibial Artery, Right
	Foot Muscle, Left		Anterior Tibial Artery, Left
Adductor longus muscle	Upper Leg Muscle, Right	Anterior spinal artery	Vertebral Artery, Right
	Upper Leg Muscle, Left		Vertebral Artery, Left
Adductor magnus muscle	Upper Leg Muscle, Right	Anterior tibial recurrent artery	Anterior Tibial Artery, Right
	Upper Leg Muscle, Left		Anterior Tibial Artery, Left
Adenohypophysis	Pituitary Gland	Anterior ulnar recurrent artery	Ulnar Artery, Right
Alar ligament of axis	Head and Neck Bursa and Ligament		Ulnar Artery, Left
Alveolar process of mandible	Mandible, Right	Anterior vagal trunk	Vagus Nerve
	Mandible, Left	Anterior vertebral muscle	Neck Muscle, Right
Alveolar process of maxilla	Maxilla		Neck Muscle, Left
Anal orifice	Anus	Antihelix	External Ear, Right
Anatomical snuffbox	Lower Arm and Wrist Muscle, Right		External Ear, Left
	Lower Arm and Wrist Muscle, Left		External Ear, Bilateral
Angular artery	Face Artery	Antitragus	External Ear, Right
Angular vein	Face Vein, Right		External Ear, Left
	Face Vein, Left		External Ear, Bilateral
Annular ligament	Elbow Bursa and Ligament, Right	Antrum of Highmore	Maxillary Sinus, Right
	Elbow Bursa and Ligament, Left		Maxillary Sinus, Left
Anorectal junction	Rectum	Aortic annulus	Aortic Valve
Ansa cervicalis	Cervical Plexus	Aortic arch	Thoracic Aorta, Ascending/Arch
Antebrachial fascia	Subcutaneous Tissue and Fascia, Right Lower Arm	Aortic intercostal artery	Upper Artery
		Apical (subclavicular) lymph node	Lymphatic, Right Axillary
	Subcutaneous Tissue and Fascia, Left Lower Arm		Lymphatic, Left Axillary
		Apneustic center	Pons
		Aqueduct of Sylvius	Cerebral Ventricle

Anatomical Term	ICD-10-PCS Value
Aqueous humour	Anterior Chamber, Right
	Anterior Chamber, Left
Arachnoid mater, intracranial	Cerebral Meninges
Arachnoid mater, spinal	Spinal Meninges
Arcuate artery	Foot Artery, Right
	Foot Artery, Left
Areola	Nipple, Right
	Nipple, Left
Arterial canal (duct)	Pulmonary Artery, Left
Aryepiglottic fold	Larynx
Arytenoid cartilage	Larynx
Arytenoid muscle	Neck Muscle, Right
	Neck Muscle, Left
Ascending aorta	Thoracic Aorta, Ascending/Arch
Ascending palatine artery	Face Artery
Ascending pharyngeal artery	External Carotid Artery, Right
	External Carotid Artery, Left
Atlantoaxial joint	Cervical Vertebral Joint
Atrioventricular node	Conduction Mechanism
Atrium dextrum cordis	Atrium, Right
Atrium pulmonale	Atrium, Left
Auditory tube	Eustachian Tube, Right
	Eustachian Tube, Left
Auerbach's (myenteric) plexus	Abdominal Sympathetic Nerve
Auricle	External Ear, Right
	External Ear, Left
	External Ear, Bilateral
Auricularis muscle	Head Muscle
Axillary fascia	Subcutaneous Tissue and Fascia, Right Upper Arm
	Subcutaneous Tissue and Fascia, Left Upper Arm
Axillary nerve	Brachial Plexus
Bartholin's (greater vestibular) gland	Vestibular Gland
Basal (internal) cerebral vein	Intracranial Vein
Basal nuclei	Basal Ganglia
Base of tongue	Pharynx
Basilar artery	Intracranial Artery
Basis pontis	Pons
Biceps brachii muscle	Upper Arm Muscle, Right
	Upper Arm Muscle, Left
Biceps femoris muscle	Upper Leg Muscle, Right
	Upper Leg Muscle, Left
Bicipital aponeurosis	Subcutaneous Tissue and Fascia, Right Lower Arm
	Subcutaneous Tissue and Fascia, Left Lower Arm

Anatomical Term	ICD-10-PCS Value
Bicuspid valve	Mitral Valve
Body of femur	Femoral Shaft, Right
	Femoral Shaft, Left
Body of fibula	Fibula, Right
	Fibula, Left
Bony labyrinth	Inner Ear, Right
	Inner Ear, Left
Bony orbit	Orbit, Right
	Orbit, Left
Bony vestibule	Inner Ear, Right
	Inner Ear, Left
Botallo's duct	Pulmonary Artery, Left
Brachial (lateral) lymph node	Lymphatic, Right Axillary
	Lymphatic, Left Axillary
Brachialis muscle	Upper Arm Muscle, Right
	Upper Arm Muscle, Left
Brachiocephalic artery	Innominate Artery
Brachiocephalic trunk	Innominate Artery
Brachiocephalic vein	Innominate Vein, Right
	Innominate Vein, Left
Brachioradialis muscle	Lower Arm and Wrist Muscle, Right
	Lower Arm and Wrist Muscle, Left
Breast procedures, skin only	Skin, Chest
Broad ligament	Uterine Supporting Structure
Bronchial artery	Upper Artery
Bronchus intermedius	Main Bronchus, Right
Buccal gland	Buccal Mucosa
Buccinator lymph node	Lymphatic, Head
Buccinator muscle	Facial Muscle
Bulbospongiosus muscle	Perineum Muscle
Bulbourethral (Cowper's) gland	Urethra
Bundle of His	Conduction Mechanism
Bundle of Kent	Conduction Mechanism
Calcaneocuboid joint	Tarsal Joint, Right
	Tarsal Joint, Left
Calcaneocuboid ligament	Foot Bursa and Ligament, Right
	Foot Bursa and Ligament, Left
Calcaneofibular ligament	Ankle Bursa and Ligament, Right
	Ankle Bursa and Ligament, Left
Calcaneus	Tarsal, Right
	Tarsal, Left
Capitate bone	Carpal, Right
	Carpal, Left
Cardia	Esophagogastric Junction
Cardiac plexus	Thoracic Sympathetic Nerve
Cardioesophageal junction	Esophagogastric Junction
Caroticotympanic artery	Internal Carotid Artery, Right
	Internal Carotid Artery, Left

Anatomical Term	ICD-10-PCS Value
Carotid glomus	Carotid Body, Left
	Carotid Body, Right
	Carotid Bodies, Bilateral
Carotid sinus	Internal Carotid Artery, Right
	Internal Carotid Artery, Left
Carotid sinus nerve	Glossopharyngeal Nerve
Carpometacarpal ligament	Hand Bursa and Ligament, Right
	Hand Bursa and Ligament, Left
Cauda equina	Lumbar Spinal Cord
Cavernous plexus	Head and Neck Sympathetic Nerve
Celiac (solar) plexus	Abdominal Sympathetic Nerve
Celiac ganglion	Abdominal Sympathetic Nerve
Celiac lymph node	Lymphatic, Aortic
Celiac trunk	Celiac Artery
Central axillary lymph node	Lymphatic, Right Axillary
	Lymphatic, Left Axillary
Cerebral aqueduct (Sylvius)	Cerebral Ventricle
Cerebrum	Brain
Cervical esophagus	Esophagus, Upper
Cervical facet joint	Cervical Vertebral Joint
	Cervical Vertebral Joints, 2 or more
Cervical ganglion	Head and Neck Sympathetic Nerve
Cervical interspinous ligament	Head and Neck Bursa and Ligament
Cervical intertransverse ligament	Head and Neck Bursa and Ligament
Cervical ligamentum flavum	Head and Neck Bursa and Ligament
Cervical lymph node	Lymphatic, Right Neck
	Lymphatic, Left Neck
Cervicothoracic facet joint	Cervicothoracic Vertebral Joint
Choana	Nasopharynx
Chondroglossus muscle	Tongue, Palate, Pharynx Muscle
Chorda tympani	Facial Nerve
Choroid plexus	Cerebral Ventricle
Ciliary body	Eye, Right
	Eye, Left
Ciliary ganglion	Head and Neck Sympathetic Nerve
Circle of Willis	Intracranial Artery
Circumflex iliac artery	Femoral Artery, Right
	Femoral Artery, Left
Claustrum	Basal Ganglia
Coccygeal body	Coccygeal Glomus
Coccygeus muscle	Trunk Muscle, Right
	Trunk Muscle, Left
Cochlea	Inner Ear, Right
	Inner Ear, Left
Cochlear nerve	Acoustic Nerve

Anatomical Term	ICD-10-PCS Value
Columella	Nasal Mucosa and Soft Tissue
Common digital vein	Foot Vein, Right
	Foot Vein, Left
Common facial vein	Face Vein, Right
	Face Vein, Left
Common fibular nerve	Peroneal Nerve
Common hepatic artery	Hepatic Artery
Common iliac (subaortic) lymph node	Lymphatic, Pelvis
Common interosseous artery	Ulnar Artery, Right
	Ulnar Artery, Left
Common peroneal nerve	Peroneal Nerve
Condyloid process	Mandible, Right
	Mandible, Left
Conus arteriosus	Ventricle, Right
Conus medullaris	Lumbar Spinal Cord
Coracoacromial ligament	Shoulder Bursa and Ligament, Right
	Shoulder Bursa and Ligament, Left
Coracobrachialis muscle	Upper Arm Muscle, Right
	Upper Arm Muscle, Left
Coracoclavicular ligament	Shoulder Bursa and Ligament, Right
	Shoulder Bursa and Ligament, Left
Coracohumeral ligament	Shoulder Bursa and Ligament, Right
	Shoulder Bursa and Ligament, Left
Coracoid process	Scapula, Right
	Scapula, Left
Corniculate cartilage	Larynx
Corpus callosum	Brain
Corpus cavernosum	Penis
Corpus spongiosum	Penis
Corpus striatum	Basal Ganglia
Corrugator supercilii muscle	Facial Muscle
Costocervical trunk	Subclavian Artery, Right
	Subclavian Artery, Left
Costoclavicular ligament	Shoulder Bursa and Ligament, Right
	Shoulder Bursa and Ligament, Left
Costotransverse joint	Thoracic Vertebral Joint
Costotransverse ligament	Rib(s) Bursa and Ligament
Costovertebral joint	Thoracic Vertebral Joint
Costoxiphoid ligament	Sternum Bursa and Ligament
Cowper's (bulbourethral) gland	Urethra
Cremaster muscle	Perineum Muscle
Cribriform plate	Ethmoid Bone, Right
	Ethmoid Bone, Left

Anatomical Term	ICD-10-PCS Value
Cricoid cartilage	Trachea
Cricothyroid artery	Thyroid Artery, Right
	Thyroid Artery, Left
Cricothyroid muscle	Neck Muscle, Right
	Neck Muscle, Left
Crural fascia	Subcutaneous Tissue and Fascia, Right Upper Leg
	Subcutaneous Tissue and Fascia, Left Upper Leg
Cubital lymph node	Lymphatic, Right Upper Extremity
	Lymphatic, Left Upper Extremity
Cubital nerve	Ulnar Nerve
Cuboid bone	Tarsal, Right
	Tarsal, Left
Cuboideonavicular joint	Tarsal Joint, Right
	Tarsal Joint, Left
Culmen	Cerebellum
Cuneiform cartilage	Larynx
Cuneonavicular joint	Tarsal Joint, Right
	Tarsal Joint, Left
Cuneonavicular ligament	Foot Bursa and Ligament, Right
	Foot Bursa and Ligament, Left
Cutaneous (transverse) cervical nerve	Cervical Plexus
Deep cervical fascia	Subcutaneous Tissue and Fascia, Right Neck
	Subcutaneous Tissue and Fascia, Left Neck
Deep cervical vein	Vertebral Vein, Right
	Vertebral Vein, Left
Deep circumflex iliac artery	External Iliac Artery, Right
	External Iliac Artery, Left
Deep facial vein	Face Vein, Right
	Face Vein, Left
Deep femoral (profunda femoris) vein	Femoral Vein, Right
	Femoral Vein, Left
Deep femoral artery	Femoral Artery, Right
	Femoral Artery, Left
Deep palmar arch	Hand Artery, Right
	Hand Artery, Left
Deep transverse perineal muscle	Perineum Muscle
Deferential artery	Internal Iliac Artery, Right
	Internal Iliac Artery, Left
Deltoid fascia	Subcutaneous Tissue and Fascia, Right Upper Arm
	Subcutaneous Tissue and Fascia, Left Upper Arm
Deltoid ligament	Ankle Bursa and Ligament, Right
	Ankle Bursa and Ligament, Left

Anatomical Term	ICD-10-PCS Value
Deltoid muscle	Shoulder Muscle, Right
	Shoulder Muscle, Left
Deltopectoral (infraclavicular) lymph node	Lymphatic, Right Upper Extremity
	Lymphatic, Left Upper Extremity
Dens	Cervical Vertebra
Denticulate (dentate) ligament	Spinal Meninges
Depressor anguli oris muscle	Facial Muscle
Depressor labii inferioris muscle	Facial Muscle
Depressor septi nasi muscle	Facial Muscle
Depressor supercilii muscle	Facial Muscle
Dermis	Skin
Descending genicular artery	Femoral Artery, Right
	Femoral Artery, Left
Diaphragma sellae	Dura Mater
Distal humerus	Humeral Shaft, Right
	Humeral Shaft, Left
Distal humerus, involving joint	Elbow Joint, Right
	Elbow Joint, Left
Distal radioulnar joint	Wrist Joint, Right
	Wrist Joint, Left
Dorsal digital nerve	Radial Nerve
Dorsal metacarpal vein	Hand Vein, Right
	Hand Vein, Left
Dorsal metatarsal artery	Foot Artery, Right
	Foot Artery, Left
Dorsal metatarsal vein	Foot Vein, Right
	Foot Vein, Left
Dorsal scapular artery	Subclavian Artery, Right
	Subclavian Artery, Left
Dorsal scapular nerve	Brachial Plexus
Dorsal venous arch	Foot Vein, Right
	Foot Vein, Left
Dorsalis pedis artery	Anterior Tibial Artery, Right
	Anterior Tibial Artery, Left
Duct of Santorini	Pancreatic Duct, Accessory
Duct of Wirsung	Pancreatic Duct
Ductus deferens	Vas Deferens, Right
	Vas Deferens, Left
	Vas Deferens, Bilateral
	Vas Deferens
Duodenal ampulla	Ampulla of Vater
Duodenojejunal flexure	Jejunum
Dura mater, intracranial	Dura Mater
Dura mater, spinal	Spinal Meninges
Dural venous sinus	Intracranial Vein

Anatomical Term	ICD-10-PCS Value
Earlobe	External Ear, Right
	External Ear, Left
	External Ear, Bilateral
Eighth cranial nerve	Acoustic Nerve
Ejaculatory duct	Vas Deferens, Right
	Vas Deferens, Left
	Vas Deferens, Bilateral
	Vas Deferens
Eleventh cranial nerve	Accessory Nerve
Encephalon	Brain
Ependyma	Cerebral Ventricle
Epidermis	Skin
Epidural space, spinal	Spinal Canal
Epiploic foramen	Peritoneum
Epithalamus	Thalamus
Epitrochlear lymph node	Lymphatic, Right Upper Extremity
	Lymphatic, Left Upper Extremity
Erector spinae muscle	Trunk Muscle, Right
	Trunk Muscle, Left
Esophageal artery	Upper Artery
Esophageal plexus	Thoracic Sympathetic Nerve
Ethmoidal air cell	Ethmoid Sinus, Right
	Ethmoid Sinus, Left
Extensor carpi radialis muscle	Lower Arm and Wrist Muscle, Right
	Lower Arm and Wrist Muscle, Left
Extensor carpi ulnaris muscle	Lower Arm and Wrist Muscle, Right
	Lower Arm and Wrist Muscle, Left
Extensor digitorum brevis muscle	Foot Muscle, Right
	Foot Muscle, Left
Extensor digitorum longus muscle	Lower Leg Muscle, Right
	Lower Leg Muscle, Left
Extensor hallucis brevis muscle	Foot Muscle, Right
	Foot Muscle, Left
Extensor hallucis longus muscle	Lower Leg Muscle, Right
	Lower Leg Muscle, Left
External anal sphincter	Anal Sphincter
External auditory meatus	External Auditory Canal, Right
	External Auditory Canal, Left
External maxillary artery	Face Artery
External naris	Nasal Mucosa and Soft Tissue
External oblique aponeurosis	Subcutaneous Tissue and Fascia, Trunk
External oblique muscle	Abdomen Muscle, Right
	Abdomen Muscle, Left
External popliteal nerve	Peroneal Nerve
External pudendal artery	Femoral Artery, Right
	Femoral Artery, Left

Anatomical Term	ICD-10-PCS Value
External pudendal vein	Saphenous Vein, Right
	Saphenous Vein, Left
External urethral sphincter	Urethra
Extradural space, intracranial	Epidural Space, Intracranial
Extradural space, spinal	Spinal Canal
Facial artery	Face Artery
False vocal cord	Larynx
Falx cerebri	Dura Mater
Fascia lata	Subcutaneous Tissue and Fascia, Right Upper Leg
	Subcutaneous Tissue and Fascia, Left Upper Leg
Femoral head	Upper Femur, Right
	Upper Femur, Left
Femoral lymph node	Lymphatic, Right Lower Extremity
	Lymphatic, Left Lower Extremity
Femoropatellar joint	Knee Joint, Right
	Knee Joint, Left
	Knee Joint, Femoral Surface, Right
	Knee Joint, Femoral Surface, Left
Femorotibial joint	Knee Joint, Right
	Knee Joint, Left
	Knee Joint, Tibial Surface, Right
	Knee Joint, Tibial Surface, Left
Fibular artery	Peroneal Artery, Right
	Peroneal Artery, Left
Fibularis brevis muscle	Lower Leg Muscle, Right
	Lower Leg Muscle, Left
Fibularis longus muscle	Lower Leg Muscle, Right
	Lower Leg Muscle, Left
Fifth cranial nerve	Trigeminal Nerve
Filum terminale	Spinal Meninges
First cranial nerve	Olfactory Nerve
First intercostal nerve	Brachial Plexus
Flexor carpi radialis muscle	Lower Arm and Wrist Muscle, Right
	Lower Arm and Wrist Muscle, Left
Flexor carpi ulnaris muscle	Lower Arm and Wrist Muscle, Right
	Lower Arm and Wrist Muscle, Left
Flexor digitorum brevis muscle	Foot Muscle, Right
	Foot Muscle, Left
Flexor digitorum longus muscle	Lower Leg Muscle, Right
	Lower Leg Muscle, Left
Flexor hallucis brevis muscle	Foot Muscle, Right
	Foot Muscle, Left
Flexor hallucis longus muscle	Lower Leg Muscle, Right
	Lower Leg Muscle, Left
Flexor pollicis longus muscle	Lower Arm and Wrist Muscle, Right
	Lower Arm and Wrist Muscle, Left

Anatomical Term	ICD-10-PCS Value
Foramen magnum	Occipital Bone
Foramen of Monro (intraventricular)	Cerebral Ventricle
Foreskin	Prepuce
Fossa of Rosenmuller	Nasopharynx
Fourth cranial nerve	Trochlear Nerve
Fourth ventricle	Cerebral Ventricle
Fovea	Retina, Right
	Retina, Left
Frenulum labii inferioris	Lower Lip
Frenulum labii superioris	Upper Lip
Frenulum linguae	Tongue
Frontal lobe	Cerebral Hemisphere
Frontal vein	Face Vein, Right
	Face Vein, Left
Fundus uteri	Uterus
Galea aponeurotica	Subcutaneous Tissue and Fascia, Scalp
Ganglion impar (ganglion of Walther)	Sacral Sympathetic Nerve
Gasserian ganglion	Trigeminal Nerve
Gastric lymph node	Lymphatic, Aortic
Gastric plexus	Abdominal Sympathetic Nerve
Gastrocnemius muscle	Lower Leg Muscle, Right
	Lower Leg Muscle, Left
Gastrocolic ligament	Omentum
Gastrocolic omentum	Omentum
Gastroduodenal artery	Hepatic Artery
Gastroesophageal (GE) junction	Esophagogastric Junction
Gastrohepatic omentum	Omentum
Gastrophrenic ligament	Omentum
Gastrosplenic ligament	Omentum
Gemellus muscle	Hip Muscle, Right
	Hip Muscle, Left
Geniculate ganglion	Facial Nerve
Geniculate nucleus	Thalamus
Genioglossus muscle	Tongue, Palate, Pharynx Muscle
Genitofemoral nerve	Lumbar Plexus
Glans penis	Prepuce
Glenohumeral joint	Shoulder Joint, Right
	Shoulder Joint, Left
Glenohumeral ligament	Shoulder Bursa and Ligament, Right
	Shoulder Bursa and Ligament, Left
Glenoid fossa (of scapula)	Glenoid Cavity, Right
	Glenoid Cavity, Left
Glenoid ligament (labrum)	Shoulder Joint, Right
	Shoulder Joint, Left

Anatomical Term	ICD-10-PCS Value
Globus pallidus	Basal Ganglia
Glossoepiglottic fold	Epiglottis
Glottis	Larynx
Gluteal lymph node	Lymphatic, Pelvis
Gluteal vein	Hypogastric Vein, Right
	Hypogastric Vein, Left
Gluteus maximus muscle	Hip Muscle, Right
	Hip Muscle, Left
Gluteus medius muscle	Hip Muscle, Right
	Hip Muscle, Left
Gluteus minimus muscle	Hip Muscle, Right
	Hip Muscle, Left
Gracilis muscle	Upper Leg Muscle, Right
	Upper Leg Muscle, Left
Great auricular nerve	Cervical Plexus
Great cerebral vein	Intracranial Vein
Great(er) saphenous vein	Saphenous Vein, Right
	Saphenous Vein, Left
Greater alar cartilage	Nasal Mucosa and Soft Tissue
Greater occipital nerve	Cervical Nerve
Greater omentum	Omentum
Greater splanchnic nerve	Thoracic Sympathetic Nerve
Greater superficial petrosal nerve	Facial Nerve
Greater trochanter	Upper Femur, Right
	Upper Femur, Left
Greater tuberosity	Humeral Head, Right
	Humeral Head, Left
Greater vestibular (Bartholin's) gland	Vestibular Gland
Greater wing	Sphenoid Bone
Hallux	1st Toe, Right
	1st Toe, Left
Hamate bone	Carpal, Right
	Carpal, Left
Head of fibula	Fibula, Right
	Fibula, Left
Helix	External Ear, Right
	External Ear, Left
	External Ear, Bilateral
Hepatic artery proper	Hepatic Artery
Hepatic flexure	Transverse Colon
Hepatic lymph node	Lymphatic, Aortic
Hepatic plexus	Abdominal Sympathetic Nerve
Hepatic portal vein	Portal Vein
Hepatogastric ligament	Omentum
Hepatopancreatic ampulla	Ampulla of Vater

Anatomical Term	ICD-10-PCS Value
Humeroradial joint	Elbow Joint, Right
	Elbow Joint, Left
Humeroulnar joint	Elbow Joint, Right
	Elbow Joint, Left
Humerus, distal	Humeral Shaft, Right
	Humeral Shaft, Left
Hyoglossus muscle	Tongue, Palate, Pharynx Muscle
Hyoid artery	Thyroid Artery, Right
	Thyroid Artery, Left
Hypogastric artery	Internal Iliac Artery, Right
	Internal Iliac Artery, Left
Hypopharynx	Pharynx
Hypophysis	Pituitary Gland
Hypothenar muscle	Hand Muscle, Right
	Hand Muscle, Left
Ileal artery	Superior Mesenteric Artery
Ileocolic artery	Superior Mesenteric Artery
Ileocolic vein	Colic Vein
Iliac crest	Pelvic Bone, Right
	Pelvic Bone, Left
Iliac fascia	Subcutaneous Tissue and Fascia, Right Upper Leg
	Subcutaneous Tissue and Fascia, Left Upper Leg
Iliac lymph node	Lymphatic, Pelvis
Iliacus muscle	Hip Muscle, Right
	Hip Muscle, Left
Iliofemoral ligament	Hip Bursa and Ligament, Right
	Hip Bursa and Ligament, Left
Iliohypogastric nerve	Lumbar Plexus
Ilioinguinal nerve	Lumbar Plexus
Iliolumbar artery	Internal Iliac Artery, Right
	Internal Iliac Artery, Left
Iliolumbar ligament	Lower Spine Bursa and Ligament
Iliotibial tract (band)	Subcutaneous Tissue and Fascia, Right Upper Leg
	Subcutaneous Tissue and Fascia, Left Upper Leg
Ilium	Pelvic Bone, Right
	Pelvic Bone, Left
Incus	Auditory Ossicle, Right
	Auditory Ossicle, Left
Inferior cardiac nerve	Thoracic Sympathetic Nerve
Inferior cerebellar vein	Intracranial Vein
Inferior cerebral vein	Intracranial Vein
Inferior epigastric artery	External Iliac Artery, Right
	External Iliac Artery, Left
Inferior epigastric lymph node	Lymphatic, Pelvis

Anatomical Term	ICD-10-PCS Value
Inferior genicular artery	Popliteal Artery, Right
	Popliteal Artery, Left
Inferior gluteal artery	Internal Iliac Artery, Right
	Internal Iliac Artery, Left
Inferior gluteal nerve	Sacral Plexus
Inferior hypogastric plexus	Abdominal Sympathetic Nerve
Inferior labial artery	Face Artery
Inferior longitudinal muscle	Tongue, Palate, Pharynx Muscle
Inferior mesenteric ganglion	Abdominal Sympathetic Nerve
Inferior mesenteric lymph node	Lymphatic, Mesenteric
Inferior mesenteric plexus	Abdominal Sympathetic Nerve
Inferior oblique muscle	Extraocular Muscle, Right
	Extraocular Muscle, Left
Inferior pancreaticoduodenal artery	Superior Mesenteric Artery
Inferior phrenic artery	Abdominal Aorta
Inferior rectus muscle	Extraocular Muscle, Right
	Extraocular Muscle, Left
Inferior suprarenal artery	Renal Artery, Right
	Renal Artery, Left
Inferior tarsal plate	Lower Eyelid, Right
	Lower Eyelid, Left
Inferior thyroid vein	Innominate Vein, Right
	Innominate Vein, Left
Inferior tibiofibular joint	Ankle Joint, Right
	Ankle Joint, Left
Inferior turbinate	Nasal Turbinate
Inferior ulnar collateral artery	Brachial Artery, Right
	Brachial Artery, Left
Inferior vesical artery	Internal Iliac Artery, Right
	Internal Iliac Artery, Left
Infraauricular lymph node	Lymphatic, Head
Infraclavicular (deltopectoral) lymph node	Lymphatic, Right Upper Extremity
	Lymphatic, Left Upper Extremity
Infrahyoid muscle	Neck Muscle, Right
	Neck Muscle, Left
Infraparotid lymph node	Lymphatic, Head
Infraspinatus fascia	Subcutaneous Tissue and Fascia, Right Upper Arm
	Subcutaneous Tissue and Fascia, Left Upper Arm
Infraspinatus muscle	Shoulder Muscle, Right
	Shoulder Muscle, Left
Infundibulopelvic ligament	Uterine Supporting Structure
Inguinal canal	Inguinal Region, Right
	Inguinal Region, Left
	Inguinal Region, Bilateral

Anatomical Term	ICD-10-PCS Value
Inguinal triangle	Inguinal Region, Right
	Inguinal Region, Left
	Inguinal Region, Bilateral
Interatrial septum	Atrial Septum
Intercarpal joint	Carpal Joint, Right
	Carpal Joint, Left
Intercarpal ligament	Hand Bursa and Ligament, Right
	Hand Bursa and Ligament, Left
Interclavicular ligament	Shoulder Bursa and Ligament, Right
	Shoulder Bursa and Ligament, Left
Intercostal lymph node	Lymphatic, Thorax
Intercostal muscle	Thorax Muscle, Right
	Thorax Muscle, Left
Intercostal nerve	Thoracic Nerve
Intercostobrachial nerve	Thoracic Nerve
Intercuneiform joint	Tarsal Joint, Right
	Tarsal Joint, Left
Intercuneiform ligament	Foot Bursa and Ligament, Right
	Foot Bursa and Ligament, Left
Intermediate bronchus	Main Bronchus, Right
Intermediate cuneiform bone	Tarsal, Right
	Tarsal, Left
Internal (basal) cerebral vein	Intracranial Vein
Internal anal sphincter	Anal Sphincter
Internal carotid artery, intracranial portion	Intracranial Artery
Internal carotid plexus	Head and Neck Sympathetic Nerve
Internal iliac vein	Hypogastric Vein, Right
	Hypogastric Vein, Left
Internal maxillary artery	External Carotid Artery, Right
	External Carotid Artery, Left
Internal naris	Nasal Mucosa and Soft Tissue
Internal oblique muscle	Abdomen Muscle, Right
	Abdomen Muscle, Left
Internal pudendal artery	Internal Iliac Artery, Right
	Internal Iliac Artery, Left
Internal pudendal vein	Hypogastric Vein, Right
	Hypogastric Vein, Left
Internal thoracic artery	Internal Mammary Artery, Right
	Internal Mammary Artery, Left
	Subclavian Artery, Right
	Subclavian Artery, Left
Internal urethral sphincter	Urethra
Interphalangeal (IP) joint	Finger Phalangeal Joint, Right
	Finger Phalangeal Joint, Left
	Toe Phalangeal Joint, Right
	Toe Phalangeal Joint, Left

Anatomical Term	ICD-10-PCS Value
Interphalangeal ligament	Hand Bursa and Ligament, Right
	Hand Bursa and Ligament, Left
	Foot Bursa and Ligament, Right
	Foot Bursa and Ligament, Left
Interspinalis muscle	Trunk Muscle, Right
	Trunk Muscle, Left
Interspinous ligament, cervical	Head and Neck Bursa and Ligament
Interspinous ligament, lumbar	Lower Spine Bursa and Ligament
Interspinous ligament, thoracic	Upper Spine Bursa and Ligament
Intertransversarius muscle	Trunk Muscle, Right
	Trunk Muscle, Left
Intertransverse ligament, cervical	Head and Neck Bursa and Ligament
Intertransverse ligament, lumbar	Lower Spine Bursa and Ligament
Intertransverse ligament, thoracic	Upper Spine Bursa and Ligament
Interventricular foramen (Monro)	Cerebral Ventricle
Interventricular septum	Ventricular Septum
Intestinal lymphatic trunk	Cisterna Chyli
Ischiatic nerve	Sciatic Nerve
Ischiocavernosus muscle	Perineum Muscle
Ischiofemoral ligament	Hip Bursa and Ligament, Right
	Hip Bursa and Ligament, Left
Ischium	Pelvic Bone, Right
	Pelvic Bone, Left
Jejunal artery	Superior Mesenteric Artery
Jugular body	Glomus Jugulare
Jugular lymph node	Lymphatic, Right Neck
	Lymphatic, Left Neck
Labia majora	Vulva
Labia minora	Vulva
Labial gland	Upper Lip
	Lower Lip
Lacrimal canaliculus	Lacrimal Duct, Right
	Lacrimal Duct, Left
Lacrimal punctum	Lacrimal Duct, Right
	Lacrimal Duct, Left
Lacrimal sac	Lacrimal Duct, Right
	Lacrimal Duct, Left
Laryngopharynx	Pharynx
Lateral (brachial) lymph node	Lymphatic, Right Axillary
	Lymphatic, Left Axillary
Lateral canthus	Upper Eyelid, Right
	Upper Eyelid, Left

Anatomical Term	ICD-10-PCS Value
Lateral collateral ligament (LCL)	Knee Bursa and Ligament, Right
	Knee Bursa and Ligament, Left
Lateral condyle of femur	Lower Femur, Right
	Lower Femur, Left
Lateral condyle of tibia	Tibia, Right
	Tibia, Left
Lateral cuneiform bone	Tarsal, Right
	Tarsal, Left
Lateral epicondyle of femur	Lower Femur, Right
	Lower Femur, Left
Lateral epicondyle of humerus	Humeral Shaft, Right
	Humeral Shaft, Left
Lateral femoral cutaneous nerve	Lumbar Plexus
Lateral malleolus	Fibula, Right
	Fibula, Left
Lateral meniscus	Knee Joint, Right
	Knee Joint, Left
Lateral nasal cartilage	Nasal Mucosa and Soft Tissue
Lateral plantar artery	Foot Artery, Right
	Foot Artery, Left
Lateral plantar nerve	Tibial Nerve
Lateral rectus muscle	Extraocular Muscle, Right
	Extraocular Muscle, Left
Lateral sacral artery	Internal Iliac Artery, Right
	Internal Iliac Artery, Left
Lateral sacral vein	Hypogastric Vein, Right
	Hypogastric Vein, Left
Lateral sural cutaneous nerve	Peroneal Nerve
Lateral tarsal artery	Foot Artery, Right
	Foot Artery, Left
Lateral temporomandibular ligament	Head and Neck Bursa and Ligament
Lateral thoracic artery	Axillary Artery, Right
	Axillary Artery, Left
Latissimus dorsi muscle	Trunk Muscle, Right
	Trunk Muscle, Left
Least splanchnic nerve	Thoracic Sympathetic Nerve
Left ascending lumbar vein	Hemiazygos Vein
Left atrioventricular valve	Mitral Valve
Left auricular appendix	Atrium, Left
Left colic vein	Colic Vein
Left coronary sulcus	Heart, Left
Left gastric artery	Gastric Artery
Left gastroepiploic artery	Splenic Artery
Left gastroepiploic vein	Splenic Vein
Left inferior phrenic vein	Renal Vein, Left

Anatomical Term	ICD-10-PCS Value
Left inferior pulmonary vein	Pulmonary Vein, Left
Left jugular trunk	Thoracic Duct
Left lateral ventricle	Cerebral Ventricle
Left ovarian vein	Renal Vein, Left
Left second lumbar vein	Renal Vein, Left
Left subclavian trunk	Thoracic Duct
Left subcostal vein	Hemiazygos Vein
Left superior pulmonary vein	Pulmonary Vein, Left
Left suprarenal vein	Renal Vein, Left
Left testicular vein	Renal Vein, Left
Leptomeninges, intracranial	Cerebral Meninges
Leptomeninges, spinal	Spinal Meninges
Lesser alar cartilage	Nasal Mucosa and Soft Tissue
Lesser occipital nerve	Cervical Plexus
Lesser omentum	Omentum
Lesser saphenous vein	Saphenous Vein, Right
	Saphenous Vein, Left
Lesser splanchnic nerve	Thoracic Sympathetic Nerve
Lesser trochanter	Upper Femur, Right
	Upper Femur, Left
Lesser tuberosity	Humeral Head, Right
	Humeral Head, Left
Lesser wing	Sphenoid Bone
Levator anguli oris muscle	Facial Muscle
Levator ani muscle	Perineum Muscle
Levator labii superioris alaeque nasi muscle	Facial Muscle
Levator labii superioris muscle	Facial Muscle
Levator palpebrae superioris muscle	Upper Eyelid, Right
	Upper Eyelid, Left
Levator scapulae muscle	Neck Muscle, Right
	Neck Muscle, Left
Levator veli palatini muscle	Tongue, Palate, Pharynx Muscle
Levatores costarum muscle	Thorax Muscle, Right
	Thorax Muscle, Left
Ligament of head of fibula	Knee Bursa and Ligament, Right
	Knee Bursa and Ligament, Left
Ligament of the lateral malleolus	Ankle Bursa and Ligament, Right
	Ankle Bursa and Ligament, Left
Ligamentum flavum, cervical	Head and Neck Bursa and Ligament
Ligamentum flavum, lumbar	Lower Spine Bursa and Ligament
Ligamentum flavum, thoracic	Upper Spine Bursa and Ligament
Lingual artery	External Carotid Artery, Right
	External Carotid Artery, Left
Lingual tonsil	Pharynx
Locus ceruleus	Pons
Long thoracic nerve	Brachial Plexus

Anatomical Term	ICD-10-PCS Value
Lumbar artery	Abdominal Aorta
Lumbar facet joint	Lumbar Vertebral Joint
Lumbar ganglion	Lumbar Sympathetic Nerve
Lumbar lymph node	Lymphatic, Aortic
Lumbar lymphatic trunk	Cisterna Chyli
Lumbar splanchnic nerve	Lumbar Sympathetic Nerve
Lumbosacral facet joint	Lumbosacral Joint
Lumbosacral trunk	Lumbar Nerve
Lunate bone	Carpal, Right
	Carpal, Left
Lunotriquetral ligament	Hand Bursa and Ligament, Right
	Hand Bursa and Ligament, Left
Macula	Retina, Right
	Retina, Left
Malleus	Auditory Ossicle, Right
	Auditory Ossicle, Left
Mammary duct	Breast, Right
	Breast, Left
	Breast, Bilateral
Mammary gland	Breast, Right
	Breast, Left
	Breast, Bilateral
Mammillary body	Hypothalamus
Mandibular nerve	Trigeminal Nerve
Mandibular notch	Mandible, Right
	Mandible, Left
Manubrium	Sternum
Masseter muscle	Head Muscle
Masseteric fascia	Subcutaneous Tissue and Fascia, Face
Mastoid (postauricular) lymph node	Lymphatic, Right Neck
	Lymphatic, Left Neck
Mastoid air cells	Mastoid Sinus, Right
	Mastoid Sinus, Left
Mastoid process	Temporal Bone, Right
	Temporal Bone, Left
Maxillary artery	External Carotid Artery, Right
	External Carotid Artery, Left
Maxillary nerve	Trigeminal Nerve
Medial canthus	Lower Eyelid, Right
	Lower Eyelid, Left
Medial collateral ligament (MCL)	Knee Bursa and Ligament, Right
	Knee Bursa and Ligament, Left
Medial condyle of femur	Lower Femur, Right
	Lower Femur, Left
Medial condyle of tibia	Tibia, Right
	Tibia, Left

Anatomical Term	ICD-10-PCS Value
Medial cuneiform bone	Tarsal, Right
	Tarsal, Left
Medial epicondyle of femur	Lower Femur, Right
	Lower Femur, Left
Medial epicondyle of humerus	Humeral Shaft, Right
	Humeral Shaft, Left
Medial malleolus	Tibia, Right
	Tibia, Left
Medial meniscus	Knee Joint, Right
	Knee Joint, Left
Medial plantar artery	Foot Artery, Right
	Foot Artery, Left
Medial plantar nerve	Tibial Nerve
Medial popliteal nerve	Tibial Nerve
Medial rectus muscle	Extraocular Muscle, Right
	Extraocular Muscle, Left
Medial sural cutaneous nerve	Tibial Nerve
Median antebrachial vein	Basilic Vein, Right
	Basilic Vein, Left
Median cubital vein	Basilic Vein, Right
	Basilic Vein, Left
Median sacral artery	Abdominal Aorta
Mediastinal cavity	Mediastinum
Mediastinal lymph node	Lymphatic, Thorax
Mediastinal space	Mediastinum
Meissner's (submucous) plexus	Abdominal Sympathetic Nerve
Membranous urethra	Urethra
Mental foramen	Mandible, Right
	Mandible, Left
Mentalis muscle	Facial Muscle
Mesoappendix	Mesentery
Mesocolon	Mesentery
Metacarpal ligament	Hand Bursa and Ligament, Right
	Hand Bursa and Ligament, Left
Metacarpophalangeal ligament	Hand Bursa and Ligament, Right
	Hand Bursa and Ligament, Left
Metatarsal ligament	Foot Bursa and Ligament, Right
	Foot Bursa and Ligament, Left
Metatarsophalangeal (MTP) joint	Metatarsal-Phalangeal Joint, Right
	Metatarsal-Phalangeal Joint, Left
Metatarsophalangeal ligament	Foot Bursa and Ligament, Right
	Foot Bursa and Ligament, Left
Metathalamus	Thalamus
Midcarpal joint	Carpal Joint, Right
	Carpal Joint, Left
Middle cardiac nerve	Thoracic Sympathetic Nerve
Middle cerebral artery	Intracranial Artery

Anatomical Term	ICD-10-PCS Value
Middle cerebral vein	Intracranial Vein
Middle colic vein	Colic Vein
Middle genicular artery	Popliteal Artery, Right
	Popliteal Artery, Left
Middle hemorrhoidal vein	Hypogastric Vein, Right
	Hypogastric Vein, Left
Middle rectal artery	Internal Iliac Artery, Right
	Internal Iliac Artery, Left
Middle suprarenal artery	Abdominal Aorta
Middle temporal artery	Temporal Artery, Right
	Temporal Artery, Left
Middle turbinate	Nasal Turbinate
Mitral annulus	Mitral Valve
Molar gland	Buccal Mucosa
Musculocutaneous nerve	Brachial Plexus
Musculophrenic artery	Internal Mammary Artery, Right
	Internal Mammary Artery, Left
Musculospinal nerve	Radial Nerve
Myelencephalon	Medulla Oblongata
Myenteric (Auerbach's) plexus	Abdominal Sympathetic Nerve
Myometrium	Uterus
Nail bed	Finger Nail
	Toe Nail
Nail plate	Finger Nail
	Toe Nail
Nasal cavity	Nasal Mucosa and Soft Tissue
Nasal concha	Nasal Turbinate
Nasalis muscle	Facial Muscle
Nasolacrimal duct	Lacrimal Duct, Right
	Lacrimal Duct, Left
Navicular bone	Tarsal, Right
	Tarsal, Left
Neck of femur	Upper Femur, Right
	Upper Femur, Left
Neck of humerus (anatomical) (surgical)	Humeral Head, Right
	Humeral Head, Left
Nerve to the stapedius	Facial Nerve
Neurohypophysis	Pituitary Gland
Ninth cranial nerve	Glossopharyngeal Nerve
Nostril	Nasal Mucosa and Soft Tissue
Obturator artery	Internal Iliac Artery, Right
	Internal Iliac Artery, Left
Obturator lymph node	Lymphatic, Pelvis
Obturator muscle	Hip Muscle, Right
	Hip Muscle, Left
Obturator nerve	Lumbar Plexus

Anatomical Term	ICD-10-PCS Value
Obturator vein	Hypogastric Vein, Right
	Hypogastric Vein, Left
Obtuse margin	Heart, Left
Occipital artery	External Carotid Artery, Right
	External Carotid Artery, Left
Occipital lobe	Cerebral Hemisphere
Occipital lymph node	Lymphatic, Right Neck
	Lymphatic, Left Neck
Occipitofrontalis muscle	Facial Muscle
Odontoid process	Cervical Vertebra
Olecranon bursa	Elbow Bursa and Ligament, Right
	Elbow Bursa and Ligament, Left
Olecranon process	Ulna, Right
	Ulna, Left
Olfactory bulb	Olfactory Nerve
Ophthalmic artery	Intracranial Artery
Ophthalmic nerve	Trigeminal Nerve
Ophthalmic vein	Intracranial Vein
Optic chiasma	Optic Nerve
Optic disc	Retina, Right
	Retina, Left
Optic foramen	Sphenoid Bone
Orbicularis oculi muscle	Upper Eyelid, Right
	Upper Eyelid, Left
Orbicularis oris muscle	Facial Muscle
Orbital fascia	Subcutaneous Tissue and Fascia, Face
Orbital portion of ethmoid bone	Orbit, Right
	Orbit, Left
Orbital portion of frontal bone	Orbit, Right
	Orbit, Left
Orbital portion of lacrimal bone	Orbit, Right
	Orbit, Left
Orbital portion of maxilla	Orbit, Right
	Orbit, Left
Orbital portion of palatine bone	Orbit, Right
	Orbit, Left
Orbital portion of sphenoid bone	Orbit, Right
	Orbit, Left
Orbital portion of zygomatic bone	Orbit, Right
	Orbit, Left
Oropharynx	Pharynx
Otic ganglion	Head and Neck Sympathetic Nerve
Oval window	Middle Ear, Right
	Middle Ear, Left
Ovarian artery	Abdominal Aorta
Ovarian ligament	Uterine Supporting Structure

Anatomical Term	ICD-10-PCS Value	Anatomical Term	ICD-10-PCS Value
Oviduct	Fallopian Tube, Right	Pectoral (anterior) lymph node	Lymphatic, Right Axillary
	Fallopian Tube, Left		Lymphatic, Left Axillary
Palatine gland	Buccal Mucosa	Pectoral fascia	Subcutaneous Tissue and Fascia, Chest
Palatine tonsil	Tonsils	Pectoralis major muscle	Thorax Muscle, Right
Palatine uvula	Uvula		Thorax Muscle, Left
Palatoglossal muscle	Tongue, Palate, Pharynx Muscle	Pectoralis minor muscle	Thorax Muscle, Right
Palatopharyngeal muscle	Tongue, Palate, Pharynx Muscle		Thorax Muscle, Left
Palmar (volar) digital vein	Hand Vein, Right	Pelvic splanchnic nerve	Abdominal Sympathetic Nerve
	Hand Vein, Left		Sacral Sympathetic Nerve
Palmar (volar) metacarpal vein	Hand Vein, Right	Penile urethra	Urethra
	Hand Vein, Left	Pericardiophrenic artery	Internal Mammary Artery, Right
Palmar cutaneous nerve	Median Nerve		Internal Mammary Artery, Left
	Radial Nerve	Perimetrium	Uterus
Palmar fascia (aponeurosis)	Subcutaneous Tissue and Fascia, Right Hand	Peroneus brevis muscle	Lower Leg Muscle, Right
	Subcutaneous Tissue and Fascia, Left Hand		Lower Leg Muscle, Left
Palmar interosseous muscle	Hand Muscle, Right	Peroneus longus muscle	Lower Leg Muscle, Right
	Hand Muscle, Left		Lower Leg Muscle, Left
Palmar ulnocarpal ligament	Wrist Bursa and Ligament, Right	Petrous part of temporal bone	Temporal Bone, Right
	Wrist Bursa and Ligament, Left		Temporal Bone, Left
Palmaris longus muscle	Lower Arm and Wrist Muscle, Right	Pharyngeal constrictor muscle	Tongue, Palate, Pharynx Muscle
	Lower Arm and Wrist Muscle, Left	Pharyngeal plexus	Vagus Nerve
Pancreatic artery	Splenic Artery	Pharyngeal recess	Nasopharynx
Pancreatic plexus	Abdominal Sympathetic Nerve	Pharyngeal tonsil	Adenoids
Pancreatic vein	Splenic Vein	Pharyngotympanic tube	Eustachian Tube, Right
Pancreaticosplenic lymph node	Lymphatic, Aortic		Eustachian Tube, Left
Paraaortic lymph node	Lymphatic, Aortic	Pia mater, intracranial	Cerebral Meninges
Pararectal lymph node	Lymphatic, Mesenteric	Pia mater, spinal	Spinal Meninges
Parasternal lymph node	Lymphatic, Thorax	Pinna	External Ear, Right
Paratracheal lymph node	Lymphatic, Thorax		External Ear, Left
Paraurethral (Skene's) gland	Vestibular Gland		External Ear, Bilateral
Parietal lobe	Cerebral Hemisphere	Piriform recess (sinus)	Pharynx
Parotid lymph node	Lymphatic, Head	Piriformis muscle	Hip Muscle, Right
Parotid plexus	Facial Nerve		Hip Muscle, Left
Pars flaccida	Tympanic Membrane, Right	Pisiform bone	Carpal, Right
	Tympanic Membrane, Left		Carpal, Left
Patellar ligament	Knee Bursa and Ligament, Right	Pisohamate ligament	Hand Bursa and Ligament, Right
	Knee Bursa and Ligament, Left		Hand Bursa and Ligament, Left
Patellar tendon	Knee Tendon, Right	Pisometacarpal ligament	Hand Bursa and Ligament, Right
	Knee Tendon, Left		Hand Bursa and Ligament, Left
Patellofemoral joint	Knee Joint, Right	Plantar digital vein	Foot Vein, Right
	Knee Joint, Left		Foot Vein, Left
	Knee Joint, Femoral Surface, Right	Plantar fascia (aponeurosis)	Subcutaneous Tissue and Fascia, Right Foot
	Knee Joint, Femoral Surface, Left		Subcutaneous Tissue and Fascia, Left Foot
Pectineus muscle	Upper Leg Muscle, Right		
	Upper Leg Muscle, Left		

Anatomical Term	ICD-10-PCS Value
Plantar metatarsal vein	Foot Vein, Right
	Foot Vein, Left
Plantar venous arch	Foot Vein, Right
	Foot Vein, Left
Platysma muscle	Neck Muscle, Right
	Neck Muscle, Left
Plica semilunaris	Conjunctiva, Right
	Conjunctiva, Left
Pneumogastric nerve	Vagus Nerve
Pneumotaxic center	Pons
Pontine tegmentum	Pons
Popliteal ligament	Knee Bursa and Ligament, Right
	Knee Bursa and Ligament, Left
Popliteal lymph node	Lymphatic, Right Lower Extremity
	Lymphatic, Left Lower Extremity
Popliteal vein	Femoral Vein, Right
	Femoral Vein, Left
Popliteus muscle	Lower Leg Muscle, Right
	Lower Leg Muscle, Left
Postauricular (mastoid) lymph node	Lymphatic, Right Neck
	Lymphatic, Left Neck
Postcava	Inferior Vena Cava
Posterior (subscapular) lymph node	Lymphatic, Right Axillary
	Lymphatic, Left Axillary
Posterior auricular artery	External Carotid Artery, Right
	External Carotid Artery, Left
Posterior auricular nerve	Facial Nerve
Posterior auricular vein	External Jugular Vein, Right
	External Jugular Vein, Left
Posterior cerebral artery	Intracranial Artery
Posterior chamber	Eye, Right
	Eye, Left
Posterior circumflex humeral artery	Axillary Artery, Right
	Axillary Artery, Left
Posterior communicating artery	Intracranial Artery
Posterior cruciate ligament (PCL)	Knee Bursa and Ligament, Right
	Knee Bursa and Ligament, Left
Posterior facial (retromandibular) vein	Face Vein, Right
	Face Vein, Left
Posterior femoral cutaneous nerve	Sacral Plexus
Posterior inferior cerebellar artery (PICA)	Intracranial Artery
Posterior interosseous nerve	Radial Nerve
Posterior labial nerve	Pudendal Nerve
Posterior scrotal nerve	Pudendal Nerve

Anatomical Term	ICD-10-PCS Value
Posterior spinal artery	Vertebral Artery, Right
	Vertebral Artery, Left
Posterior tibial recurrent artery	Anterior Tibial Artery, Right
	Anterior Tibial Artery, Left
Posterior ulnar recurrent artery	Ulnar Artery, Right
	Ulnar Artery, Left
Posterior vagal trunk	Vagus Nerve
Preauricular lymph node	Lymphatic, Head
Precava	Superior Vena Cava
Prepatellar bursa	Knee Bursa and Ligament, Right
	Knee Bursa and Ligament, Left
Pretracheal fascia	Subcutaneous Tissue and Fascia, Right Neck
	Subcutaneous Tissue and Fascia, Left Neck
Prevertebral fascia	Subcutaneous Tissue and Fascia, Right Neck
	Subcutaneous Tissue and Fascia, Left Neck
Princeps pollicis artery	Hand Artery, Right
	Hand Artery, Left
Procerus muscle	Facial Muscle
Profunda brachii	Brachial Artery, Right
	Brachial Artery, Left
Profunda femoris (deep femoral) vein	Femoral Vein, Right
	Femoral Vein, Left
Pronator quadratus muscle	Lower Arm and Wrist Muscle, Right
	Lower Arm and Wrist Muscle, Left
Pronator teres muscle	Lower Arm and Wrist Muscle, Right
	Lower Arm and Wrist Muscle, Left
Prostatic urethra	Urethra
Proximal radioulnar joint	Elbow Joint, Right
	Elbow Joint, Left
Psoas muscle	Hip Muscle, Right
	Hip Muscle, Left
Pterygoid muscle	Head Muscle
Pterygoid process	Sphenoid Bone
Pterygopalatine (sphenopalatine) ganglion	Head and Neck Sympathetic Nerve
Pubis	Pelvic Bone, Right
	Pelvic Bone, Left
Pubofemoral ligament	Hip Bursa and Ligament, Right
	Hip Bursa and Ligament, Left
Pudendal nerve	Sacral Plexus
Pulmoaortic canal	Pulmonary Artery, Left
Pulmonary annulus	Pulmonary Valve
Pulmonary plexus	Vagus Nerve
	Thoracic Sympathetic Nerve

Anatomical Term	ICD-10-PCS Value
Pulmonic valve	Pulmonary Valve
Pulvinar	Thalamus
Pyloric antrum	Stomach, Pylorus
Pyloric canal	Stomach, Pylorus
Pyloric sphincter	Stomach, Pylorus
Pyramidalis muscle	Abdomen Muscle, Right
	Abdomen Muscle, Left
Quadrangular cartilage	Nasal Septum
Quadrate lobe	Liver
Quadratus femoris muscle	Hip Muscle, Right
	Hip Muscle, Left
Quadratus lumborum muscle	Trunk Muscle, Right
	Trunk Muscle, Left
Quadratus plantae muscle	Foot Muscle, Right
	Foot Muscle, Left
Quadriceps (femoris)	Upper Leg Muscle, Right
	Upper Leg Muscle, Left
Radial collateral carpal ligament	Wrist Bursa and Ligament, Right
	Wrist Bursa and Ligament, Left
Radial collateral ligament	Elbow Bursa and Ligament, Right
	Elbow Bursa and Ligament, Left
Radial notch	Ulna, Right
	Ulna, Left
Radial recurrent artery	Radial Artery, Right
	Radial Artery, Left
Radial vein	Brachial Vein, Right
	Brachial Vein, Left
Radialis indicis	Hand Artery, Right
	Hand Artery, Left
Radiocarpal joint	Wrist Joint, Right
	Wrist Joint, Left
Radiocarpal ligament	Wrist Bursa and Ligament, Right
	Wrist Bursa and Ligament, Left
Radioulnar ligament	Wrist Bursa and Ligament, Right
	Wrist Bursa and Ligament, Left
Rectosigmoid junction	Sigmoid Colon
Rectus abdominis muscle	Abdomen Muscle, Right
	Abdomen Muscle, Left
Rectus femoris muscle	Upper Leg Muscle, Right
	Upper Leg Muscle, Left
Recurrent laryngeal nerve	Vagus Nerve
Renal calyx	Kidney, Right
	Kidney, Left
	Kidneys, Bilateral
	Kidney

Anatomical Term	ICD-10-PCS Value
Renal capsule	Kidney, Right
	Kidney, Left
	Kidneys, Bilateral
	Kidney
Renal cortex	Kidney, Right
	Kidney, Left
	Kidneys, Bilateral
	Kidney
Renal nerve	Abdominal Sympathetic Nerve
Renal plexus	Abdominal Sympathetic Nerve
Renal segment	Kidney, Right
	Kidney, Left
	Kidneys, Bilateral
	Kidney
Renal segmental artery	Renal Artery, Right
	Renal Artery, Left
Retroperitoneal cavity	Retroperitoneum
Retroperitoneal lymph node	Lymphatic, Aortic
Retroperitoneal space	Retroperitoneum
Retropharyngeal lymph node	Lymphatic, Right Neck
	Lymphatic, Left Neck
Retropubic space	Pelvic Cavity
Rhinopharynx	Nasopharynx
Rhomboid major muscle	Trunk Muscle, Right
	Trunk Muscle, Left
Rhomboid minor muscle	Trunk Muscle, Right
	Trunk Muscle, Left
Right ascending lumbar vein	Azygos Vein
Right atrioventricular valve	Tricuspid Valve
Right auricular appendix	Atrium, Right
Right colic vein	Colic Vein
Right coronary sulcus	Heart, Right
Right gastric artery	Gastric Artery
Right gastroepiploic vein	Superior Mesenteric Vein
Right inferior phrenic vein	Inferior Vena Cava
Right inferior pulmonary vein	Pulmonary Vein, Right
Right jugular trunk	Lymphatic, Right Neck
Right lateral ventricle	Cerebral Ventricle
Right lymphatic duct	Lymphatic, Right Neck
Right ovarian vein	Inferior Vena Cava
Right second lumbar vein	Inferior Vena Cava
Right subclavian trunk	Lymphatic, Right Neck
Right subcostal vein	Azygos Vein
Right superior pulmonary vein	Pulmonary Vein, Right
Right suprarenal vein	Inferior Vena Cava
Right testicular vein	Inferior Vena Cava
Rima glottidis	Larynx
Risorius muscle	Facial Muscle

Anatomical Term	ICD-10-PCS Value
Round ligament of uterus	Uterine Supporting Structure
Round window	Inner Ear, Right
	Inner Ear, Left
Sacral ganglion	Sacral Sympathetic Nerve
Sacral lymph node	Lymphatic, Pelvis
Sacral splanchnic nerve	Sacral Sympathetic Nerve
Sacrococcygeal ligament	Lower Spine Bursa and Ligament
Sacrococcygeal symphysis	Sacrococcygeal Joint
Sacroiliac ligament	Lower Spine Bursa and Ligament
Sacrospinous ligament	Lower Spine Bursa and Ligament
Sacrotuberous ligament	Lower Spine Bursa and Ligament
Salpingopharyngeus muscle	Tongue, Palate, Pharynx Muscle
Salpinx	Fallopian Tube, Right
	Fallopian Tube, Left
Saphenous nerve	Femoral Nerve
Sartorius muscle	Upper Leg Muscle, Right
	Upper Leg Muscle, Left
Scalene muscle	Neck Muscle, Right
	Neck Muscle, Left
Scaphoid bone	Carpal, Right
	Carpal, Left
Scapholunate ligament	Wrist Bursa and Ligament, Right
	Wrist Bursa and Ligament, Left
Scaphotrapezium ligament	Hand Bursa and Ligament, Right
	Hand Bursa and Ligament, Left
Scarpa's (vestibular) ganglion	Acoustic Nerve
Sebaceous gland	Skin
Second cranial nerve	Optic Nerve
Sella turcica	Sphenoid Bone
Semicircular canal	Inner Ear, Right
	Inner Ear, Left
Semimembranosus muscle	Upper Leg Muscle, Right
	Upper Leg Muscle, Left
Semitendinosus muscle	Upper Leg Muscle, Right
	Upper Leg Muscle, Left
Septal cartilage	Nasal Septum
Serratus anterior muscle	Thorax Muscle, Right
	Thorax Muscle, Left
Serratus posterior muscle	Trunk Muscle, Right
	Trunk Muscle, Left
Seventh cranial nerve	Facial Nerve
Short gastric artery	Splenic Artery
Sigmoid artery	Inferior Mesenteric Artery
Sigmoid flexure	Sigmoid Colon
Sigmoid vein	Inferior Mesenteric Vein
Sinoatrial node	Conduction Mechanism
Sinus venosus	Atrium, Right
Sixth cranial nerve	Abducens Nerve

Anatomical Term	ICD-10-PCS Value
Skene's (paraurethral) gland	Vestibular Gland
Small saphenous vein	Saphenous Vein, Right
	Saphenous Vein, Left
Solar (celiac) plexus	Abdominal Sympathetic Nerve
Soleus muscle	Lower Leg Muscle, Right
	Lower Leg Muscle, Left
Sphenomandibular ligament	Head and Neck Bursa and Ligament
Sphenopalatine (pterygopalatine) ganglion	Head and Neck Sympathetic Nerve
Spinal nerve, cervical	Cervical Nerve
Spinal nerve, lumbar	Lumbar Nerve
Spinal nerve, sacral	Sacral Nerve
Spinal nerve, thoracic	Thoracic Nerve
Spinous process	Cervical Vertebra
	Thoracic Vertebra
	Lumbar Vertebra
Spiral ganglion	Acoustic Nerve
Splenic flexure	Transverse Colon
Splenic plexus	Abdominal Sympathetic Nerve
Splenius capitis muscle	Head Muscle
Splenius cervicis muscle	Neck Muscle, Right
	Neck Muscle, Left
Stapes	Auditory Ossicle, Right
	Auditory Ossicle, Left
Stellate ganglion	Head and Neck Sympathetic Nerve
Stensen's duct	Parotid Duct, Right
	Parotid Duct, Left
Sternoclavicular ligament	Shoulder Bursa and Ligament, Right
	Shoulder Bursa and Ligament, Left
Sternocleidomastoid artery	Thyroid Artery, Right
	Thyroid Artery, Left
Sternocleidomastoid muscle	Neck Muscle, Right
	Neck Muscle, Left
Sternocostal ligament	Sternum Bursa and Ligament
Styloglossus muscle	Tongue, Palate, Pharynx Muscle
Stylomandibular ligament	Head and Neck Bursa and Ligament
Stylopharyngeus muscle	Tongue, Palate, Pharynx Muscle
Subacromial bursa	Shoulder Bursa and Ligament, Right
	Shoulder Bursa and Ligament, Left
Subaortic (common iliac) lymph node	Lymphatic, Pelvis
Subarachnoid space, spinal	Spinal Canal
Subclavicular (apical) lymph node	Lymphatic, Right Axillary
	Lymphatic, Left Axillary
Subclavius muscle	Thorax Muscle, Right
	Thorax Muscle, Left

Anatomical Term	ICD-10-PCS Value
Subclavius nerve	Brachial Plexus
Subcostal artery	Upper Artery
Subcostal muscle	Thorax Muscle, Right
	Thorax Muscle, Left
Subcostal nerve	Thoracic Nerve
Subdural space, spinal	Spinal Canal
Submandibular ganglion	Facial Nerve
	Head and Neck Sympathetic Nerve
Submandibular gland	Submaxillary Gland, Right
	Submaxillary Gland, Left
Submandibular lymph node	Lymphatic, Head
Submandibular space	Subcutaneous Tissue and Fascia, Face
Submaxillary ganglion	Head and Neck Sympathetic Nerve
Submaxillary lymph node	Lymphatic, Head
Submental artery	Face Artery
Submental lymph node	Lymphatic, Head
Submucous (Meissner's) plexus	Abdominal Sympathetic Nerve
Suboccipital nerve	Cervical Nerve
Suboccipital venous plexus	Vertebral Vein, Right
	Vertebral Vein, Left
Subparotid lymph node	Lymphatic, Head
Subscapular (posterior) lymph node	Lymphatic, Right Axillary
	Lymphatic, Left Axillary
Subscapular aponeurosis	Subcutaneous Tissue and Fascia, Right Upper Arm
	Subcutaneous Tissue and Fascia, Left Upper Arm
Subscapular artery	Axillary Artery, Right
	Axillary Artery, Left
Subscapularis muscle	Shoulder Muscle, Right
	Shoulder Muscle, Left
Substantia nigra	Basal Ganglia
Subtalar (talocalcaneal) joint	Tarsal Joint, Right
	Tarsal Joint, Left
Subtalar ligament	Foot Bursa and Ligament, Right
	Foot Bursa and Ligament, Left
Subthalamic nucleus	Basal Ganglia
Superficial circumflex iliac vein	Saphenous Vein, Right
	Saphenous Vein, Left
Superficial epigastric artery	Femoral Artery, Right
	Femoral Artery, Left
Superficial epigastric vein	Saphenous Vein, Right
	Saphenous Vein, Left
Superficial palmar arch	Hand Artery, Right
	Hand Artery, Left

Anatomical Term	ICD-10-PCS Value
Superficial palmar venous arch	Hand Vein, Right
	Hand Vein, Left
Superficial temporal artery	Temporal Artery, Right
	Temporal Artery, Left
Superficial transverse perineal muscle	Perineum Muscle
Superior cardiac nerve	Thoracic Sympathetic Nerve
Superior cerebellar vein	Intracranial Vein
Superior cerebral vein	Intracranial Vein
Superior clunic (cluneal) nerve	Lumbar Nerve
Superior epigastric artery	Internal Mammary Artery, Right
	Internal Mammary Artery, Left
Superior genicular artery	Popliteal Artery, Right
	Popliteal Artery, Left
Superior gluteal artery	Internal Iliac Artery, Right
	Internal Iliac Artery, Left
Superior gluteal nerve	Lumbar Plexus
Superior hypogastric plexus	Abdominal Sympathetic Nerve
Superior labial artery	Face Artery
Superior laryngeal artery	Thyroid Artery, Right
	Thyroid Artery, Left
Superior laryngeal nerve	Vagus Nerve
Superior longitudinal muscle	Tongue, Palate, Pharynx Muscle
Superior mesenteric ganglion	Abdominal Sympathetic Nerve
Superior mesenteric lymph node	Lymphatic, Mesenteric
Superior mesenteric plexus	Abdominal Sympathetic Nerve
Superior oblique muscle	Extraocular Muscle, Right
	Extraocular Muscle, Left
Superior olivary nucleus	Pons
Superior rectal artery	Inferior Mesenteric Artery
Superior rectal vein	Inferior Mesenteric Vein
Superior rectus muscle	Extraocular Muscle, Right
	Extraocular Muscle, Left
Superior tarsal plate	Upper Eyelid, Right
	Upper Eyelid, Left
Superior thoracic artery	Axillary Artery, Right
	Axillary Artery, Left
Superior thyroid artery	External Carotid Artery, Right
	External Carotid Artery, Left
	Thyroid Artery, Right
	Thyroid Artery, Left
Superior turbinate	Nasal Turbinate
Superior ulnar collateral artery	Brachial Artery, Right
	Brachial Artery, Left
Supraclavicular (Virchow's) lymph node	Lymphatic, Right Neck
	Lymphatic, Left Neck

Anatomical Term	ICD-10-PCS Value	Anatomical Term	ICD-10-PCS Value
Supraclavicular nerve	Cervical Plexus	Tensor fasciae latae muscle	Hip Muscle, Right
Suprahyoid lymph node	Lymphatic, Head		Hip Muscle, Left
Suprahyoid muscle	Neck Muscle, Right	Tensor veli palatini muscle	Tongue, Palate, Pharynx Muscle
	Neck Muscle, Left	Tenth cranial nerve	Vagus Nerve
Suprainguinal lymph node	Lymphatic, Pelvis	Tentorium cerebelli	Dura Mater
Supraorbital vein	Face Vein, Right	Teres major muscle	Shoulder Muscle, Right
	Face Vein, Left		Shoulder Muscle, Left
Suprarenal gland	Adrenal Gland, Left	Teres minor muscle	Shoulder Muscle, Right
	Adrenal Gland, Right		Shoulder Muscle, Left
	Adrenal Glands, Bilateral	Testicular artery	Abdominal Aorta
	Adrenal Gland	Thenar muscle	Hand Muscle, Right
Suprarenal plexus	Abdominal Sympathetic Nerve		Hand Muscle, Left
Suprascapular nerve	Brachial Plexus	Third cranial nerve	Oculomotor Nerve
Supraspinatus fascia	Subcutaneous Tissue and Fascia, Right Upper Arm	Third occipital nerve	Cervical Nerve
	Subcutaneous Tissue and Fascia, Left Upper Arm	Third ventricle	Cerebral Ventricle
Supraspinatus muscle	Shoulder Muscle, Right	Thoracic aortic plexus	Thoracic Sympathetic Nerve
	Shoulder Muscle, Left	Thoracic esophagus	Esophagus, Middle
Supraspinous ligament	Upper Spine Bursa and Ligament	Thoracic facet joint	Thoracic Vertebral Joint
	Lower Spine Bursa and Ligament	Thoracic ganglion	Thoracic Sympathetic Nerve
Suprasternal notch	Sternum	Thoracoacromial artery	Axillary Artery, Right
Supratrochlear lymph node	Lymphatic, Right Upper Extremity		Axillary Artery, Left
	Lymphatic, Left Upper Extremity	Thoracolumbar facet joint	Thoracolumbar Vertebral Joint
Sural artery	Popliteal Artery, Right	Thymus gland	Thymus
	Popliteal Artery, Left	Thyroarytenoid muscle	Neck Muscle, Right
Sweat gland	Skin		Neck Muscle, Left
Talocalcaneal (subtalar) joint	Tarsal Joint, Right	Thyrocervical trunk	Thyroid Artery, Right
	Tarsal Joint, Left		Thyroid Artery, Left
Talocalcaneal ligament	Foot Bursa and Ligament, Right	Thyroid cartilage	Larynx
	Foot Bursa and Ligament, Left	Tibialis anterior muscle	Lower Leg Muscle, Right
Talocalcaneonavicular joint	Tarsal Joint, Right		Lower Leg Muscle, Left
	Tarsal Joint, Left	Tibialis posterior muscle	Lower Leg Muscle, Right
Talocalcaneonavicular ligament	Foot Bursa and Ligament, Right		Lower Leg Muscle, Left
	Foot Bursa and Ligament, Left	Tibiofemoral joint	Knee Joint, Right
Talocrural joint	Ankle Joint, Right		Knee Joint, Left
	Ankle Joint, Left		Knee Joint, Tibial Surface, Right
Talofibular ligament	Ankle Bursa and Ligament, Right		Knee Joint, Tibial Surface, Left
	Ankle Bursa and Ligament, Left	Tibioperoneal trunk	Popliteal Artery, Right
Talus bone	Tarsal, Right		Popliteal Artery, Left
	Tarsal, Left	Tongue, base of	Pharynx
Tarsometatarsal ligament	Foot Bursa and Ligament, Right	Tracheobronchial lymph node	Lymphatic, Thorax
	Foot Bursa and Ligament, Left	Tragus	External Ear, Right
Temporal lobe	Cerebral Hemisphere		External Ear, Left
Temporalis muscle	Head Muscle		External Ear, Bilateral
Temporoparietalis muscle	Head Muscle	Transversalis fascia	Subcutaneous Tissue and Fascia, Trunk
		Transverse (cutaneous) cervical nerve	Cervical Plexus

Anatomical Term	ICD-10-PCS Value
Transverse acetabular ligament	Hip Bursa and Ligament, Right
	Hip Bursa and Ligament, Left
Transverse facial artery	Temporal Artery, Right
	Temporal Artery, Left
Transverse foramen	Cervical Vertebra
Transverse humeral ligament	Shoulder Bursa and Ligament, Right
	Shoulder Bursa and Ligament, Left
Transverse ligament of atlas	Head and Neck Bursa and Ligament
Transverse process	Cervical Vertebra
	Thoracic Vertebra
	Lumbar Vertebra
Transverse scapular ligament	Shoulder Bursa and Ligament, Right
	Shoulder Bursa and Ligament, Left
Transverse thoracis muscle	Thorax Muscle, Right
	Thorax Muscle, Left
Transversospinalis muscle	Trunk Muscle, Right
	Trunk Muscle, Left
Transversus abdominis muscle	Abdomen Muscle, Right
	Abdomen Muscle, Left
Trapezium bone	Carpal, Right
	Carpal, Left
Trapezius muscle	Trunk Muscle, Right
	Trunk Muscle, Left
Trapezoid bone	Carpal, Right
	Carpal, Left
Triceps brachii muscle	Upper Arm Muscle, Right
	Upper Arm Muscle, Left
Tricuspid annulus	Tricuspid Valve
Trifacial nerve	Trigeminal Nerve
Trigone of bladder	Bladder
Triquetral bone	Carpal, Right
	Carpal, Left
Trochanteric bursa	Hip Bursa and Ligament, Right
	Hip Bursa and Ligament, Left
Twelfth cranial nerve	Hypoglossal Nerve
Tympanic cavity	Middle Ear, Right
	Middle Ear, Left
Tympanic nerve	Glossopharyngeal Nerve
Tympanic part of temporal bone	Temporal Bone, Right
	Temporal Bone, Left
Ulnar collateral carpal ligament	Wrist Bursa and Ligament, Right
	Wrist Bursa and Ligament, Left
Ulnar collateral ligament	Elbow Bursa and Ligament, Right
	Elbow Bursa and Ligament, Left
Ulnar notch	Radius, Right
	Radius, Left

Anatomical Term	ICD-10-PCS Value
Ulnar vein	Brachial Vein, Right
	Brachial Vein, Left
Umbilical artery	Internal Iliac Artery, Right
	Internal Iliac Artery, Left
	Lower Artery
Ureteral orifice	Ureter, Right
	Ureter, Left
	Ureters, Bilateral
	Ureter
Ureteropelvic junction (UPJ)	Kidney Pelvis, Right
	Kidney Pelvis, Left
Ureterovesical orifice	Ureter, Right
	Ureter, Left
	Ureters, Bilateral
	Ureter
Uterine artery	Internal Iliac Artery, Right
	Internal Iliac Artery, Left
Uterine cornu	Uterus
Uterine tube	Fallopian Tube, Right
	Fallopian Tube, Left
Uterine vein	Hypogastric Vein, Right
	Hypogastric Vein, Left
Vaginal artery	Internal Iliac Artery, Right
	Internal Iliac Artery, Left
Vaginal vein	Hypogastric Vein, Right
	Hypogastric Vein, Left
Vastus intermedius muscle	Upper Leg Muscle, Right
	Upper Leg Muscle, Left
Vastus lateralis muscle	Upper Leg Muscle, Right
	Upper Leg Muscle, Left
Vastus medialis muscle	Upper Leg Muscle, Right
	Upper Leg Muscle, Left
Ventricular fold	Larynx
Vermiform appendix	Appendix
Vermilion border	Upper Lip
	Lower Lip
Vertebral arch	Cervical Vertebra
	Thoracic Vertebra
	Lumbar Vertebra
Vertebral body	Cervical Vertebra
	Thoracic Vertebra
	Lumbar Vertebra
Vertebral canal	Spinal Canal
Vertebral foramen	Cervical Vertebra
	Thoracic Vertebra
	Lumbar Vertebra

Anatomical Term	ICD-10-PCS Value
Vertebral lamina	Cervical Vertebra
	Thoracic Vertebra
	Lumbar Vertebra
Vertebral pedicle	Cervical Vertebra
	Thoracic Vertebra
	Lumbar Vertebra
Vesical vein	Hypogastric Vein, Right
	Hypogastric Vein, Left
Vestibular (Scarpa's) ganglion	Acoustic Nerve
Vestibular nerve	Acoustic Nerve
Vestibulocochlear nerve	Acoustic Nerve
Virchow's (supraclavicular) lymph node	Lymphatic, Right Neck
	Lymphatic, Left Neck
Vitreous body	Vitreous, Right
	Vitreous, Left
Vocal fold	Vocal Cord, Right
	Vocal Cord, Left
Volar (palmar) digital vein	Hand Vein, Right
	Hand Vein, Left
Volar (palmar) metacarpal vein	Hand Vein, Right
	Hand Vein, Left
Vomer bone	Nasal Septum
Vomer of nasal septum	Nasal Bone
Xiphoid process	Sternum
Zonule of Zinn	Lens, Right
	Lens, Left
Zygomatic process of frontal bone	Frontal Bone
Zygomatic process of temporal bone	Temporal Bone, Right
	Temporal Bone, Left
Zygomaticus muscle	Facial Muscle

This page intentionally left blank

Appendix C: Device Key

Device Term	ICD-10-PCS Value
3f® (Aortic) Bioprosthesis valve	Zooplastic Tissue in Heart and Great Vessels
AbioCor® Total Replacement Heart	Synthetic Substitute
Absolute Pro® Vascular (OTW) Self-Expanding Stent System	Intraluminal Device
Acculink™ (RX) Carotid Stent System	Intraluminal Device
Acellular Hydrated Dermis	Nonautologous Tissue Substitute
Acetabular cup	Liner in Lower Joints
Activa PC® neurostimulator	Stimulator Generator, Multiple Array for Insertion in Subcutaneous Tissue and Fascia
Activa RC® neurostimulator	Stimulator Generator, Multiple Array Rechargeable for Insertion in Subcutaneous Tissue and Fascia
Activa SC® neurostimulator	Stimulator Generator, Single Array for Insertion in Subcutaneous Tissue and Fascia
ACUITY™ Steerable Lead	Cardiac Lead, Pacemaker for Insertion in Heart and Great Vessels
	Cardiac Lead, Defibrillator for Insertion in Heart and Great Vessels
Advisa MRI™	Pacemaker, Dual Chamber for Insertion in Subcutaneous Tissue and Fascia
AFX® Endovascular AAA System	Intraluminal Device
AMPLATZER® Muscular VSD Occluder	Synthetic Substitute
AMS 800® Urinary Control System	Artificial Sphincter in Urinary System
AneuRx® AAA Advantage®	Intraluminal Device
Annuloplasty ring	Synthetic Substitute
Articulating Spacer (Antibiotic)	Articulating Spacer in Lower Joints
Artificial anal sphincter (AAS)	Artificial Sphincter in Gastrointestinal System
Artificial bowel sphincter (neosphincter)	Artificial Sphincter in Gastrointestinal System
Artificial urinary sphincter (AUS)	Artificial Sphincter in Urinary System
Ascenda® Intrathecal Catheter	Infusion Device
Assurant (Cobalt)® stent	Intraluminal Device
AtriClip® LAA Exclusion System	Extraluminal Device
Attain Ability® lead	Cardiac Lead, Pacemaker for Insertion in Heart and Great Vessels
	Cardiac Lead, Defibrillator for Insertion in Heart and Great Vessels
Attain StarFix® (OTW) lead	Cardiac Lead, Pacemaker for Insertion in Heart and Great Vessels
	Cardiac Lead, Defibrillator for Insertion in Heart and Great Vessels
Autograft	Autologous Tissue Substitute

Device Term	ICD-10-PCS Value
Autologous artery graft	Autologous Arterial Tissue in Heart and Great Vessels
	Autologous Arterial Tissue in Upper Arteries
	Autologous Arterial Tissue in Lower Arteries
	Autologous Arterial Tissue in Upper Veins
	Autologous Arterial Tissue in Lower Veins
Autologous vein graft	Autologous Venous Tissue in Heart and Great Vessels
	Autologous Venous Tissue in Upper Arteries
	Autologous Venous Tissue in Lower Arteries
	Autologous Venous Tissue in Upper Veins
	Autologous Venous Tissue in Lower Veins
Axial Lumbar Interbody Fusion System	Interbody Fusion Device in Lower Joints
AxiaLIF® System	Interbody Fusion Device in Lower Joints
BAK/C® Interbody Cervical Fusion System	Interbody Fusion Device in Upper Joints
Bard® Composix® (E/X) (LP) mesh	Synthetic Substitute
Bard® Composix® Kugel® patch	Synthetic Substitute
Bard® Dulex™ mesh	Synthetic Substitute
Bard® Ventralex™ hernia patch	Synthetic Substitute
Baroreflex Activation Therapy®(BAT®)	Stimulator Lead in Upper Arteries
	Stimulator Generator in Subcutaneous Tissue and Fascia
Barricaid® Annular Closure Device (ACD)	Synthetic Substitute
Berlin Heart® Ventricular Assist Device	Implantable Heart Assist System in Heart and Great Vessels
Bioactive embolization coil(s)	Intraluminal Device, Bioactive in Upper Arteries
Biventricular external heart assist system	Short-term External Heart Assist System in Heart and Great Vessels
Blood glucose monitoring system	Monitoring Device
Bone anchored hearing device	Hearing Device, Bone Conduction for Insertion in Ear, Nose, Sinus
	Hearing Device in Head and Facial Bones
Bone bank bone graft	Nonautologous Tissue Substitute
Bone screw (interlocking) (lag) (pedicle) (recessed)	Internal Fixation Device in Head and Facial Bones
	Internal Fixation Device in Upper Bones
	Internal Fixation Device in Lower Bones
Bovine pericardial valve	Zooplastic Tissue in Heart and Great Vessels

Device Term	ICD-10-PCS Value
Bovine pericardium graft	Zooplastic Tissue in Heart and Great Vessels
Brachytherapy seeds	Radioactive Element
BRYAN® Cervical Disc System	Synthetic Substitute
BVS 5000® Ventricular Assist Device	Short-term External Heart Assist System in Heart and Great Vessels
Cardiac contractility modulation lead	Cardiac Lead in Heart and Great Vessels
Cardiac event recorder	Monitoring Device
Cardiac resynchronization therapy (CRT) lead	Cardiac Lead, Pacemaker for Insertion in Heart and Great Vessels
	Cardiac Lead, Defibrillator for Insertion in Heart and Great Vessels
CardioMEMS® pressure sensor	Monitoring Device, Pressure Sensor for Insertion in Heart and Great Vessels
Carotid (artery) sinus (baroreceptor) lead	Stimulator Lead in Upper Arteries
Carotid WALLSTENT® Monorail® Endoprosthesis	Intraluminal Device
Centrimag® Blood Pump	Short-term External Heart Assist System in Heart and Great Vessels
Ceramic on ceramic bearing surface	Synthetic Substitute, Ceramic for Replacement in Lower Joints
Cesium-131 Collagen Implant	Radioactive Element, Cesium-131 Collagen Implant for Insertion in Central Nervous System and Cranial Nerves
CivaSheet®	Radioactive Element
Clamp and rod internal fixation system (CRIF)	Internal Fixation Device in Upper Bones
	Internal Fixation Device in Lower Bones
COALESCE® radiolucent interbody fusion device	Interbody Fusion Device, Radiolucent Porous in New Technology
CoAxia NeuroFlo™ catheter	Intraluminal Device
Cobalt/chromium head and polyethylene socket	Synthetic Substitute, Metal on Polyethylene for Replacement in Lower Joints
Cobalt/chromium head and socket	Synthetic Substitute, Metal for Replacement in Lower Joints
Cochlear implant (CI), multiple channel (electrode)	Hearing Device, Multiple Channel Cochlear Prosthesis for Insertion in Ear, Nose, Sinus
Cochlear implant (CI), single channel (electrode)	Hearing Device, Single Channel Cochlear Prosthesis for Insertion in Ear, Nose, Sinus
COGNIS® CRT-D	Cardiac Resynchronization Defibrillator Pulse Generator for Insertion in Subcutaneous Tissue and Fascia
COHERE® radiolucent interbody fusion device	Interbody Fusion Device, Radiolucent Porous in New Technology

Device Term	ICD-10-PCS Value
Colonic Z-Stent®	Intraluminal Device
Complete® (SE) stent	Intraluminal Device
Concerto® II CRT-D	Cardiac Resynchronization Defibrillator Pulse Generator for Insertion in Subcutaneous Tissue and Fascia
CONSERVE® PLUS Total Resurfacing Hip System	Resurfacing Device in Lower Joints
Consulta® CRT-D	Cardiac Resynchronization Defibrillator Pulse Generator for Insertion in Subcutaneous Tissue and Fascia
Consulta® CRT-P	Cardiac Resynchronization Pacemaker Pulse Generator for Insertion in Subcutaneous Tissue and Fascia
CONTAK RENEWAL® 3 RF (HE) CRT-D	Cardiac Resynchronization Defibrillator Pulse Generator for Insertion in Subcutaneous Tissue and Fascia
Contegra® Pulmonary Valved Conduit	Zooplastic Tissue in Heart and Great Vessels
Continuous Glucose Monitoring (CGM) device	Monitoring Device
Cook Biodesign® Fistula Plug(s)	Nonautologous Tissue Substitute
Cook Biodesign® Hernia Graft(s)	Nonautologous Tissue Substitute
Cook Biodesign® Layered Graft(s)	Nonautologous Tissue Substitute
Cook Zenapro™ Layered Graft(s)	Nonautologous Tissue Substitute
Cook Zenith® AAA Endovascular Graft	Intraluminal Device
Cook Zenith® Fenestrated AAA Endovascular Graft	Intraluminal Device, Branched or Fenestrated, One or Two Arteries for Restriction in Lower Arteries
	Intraluminal Device, Branched or Fenestrated, Three or More Arteries for Restriction in Lower Arteries
CoreValve™ transcatheter aortic valve	Zooplastic Tissue in Heart and Great Vessels
Cormet™ Hip Resurfacing System	Resurfacing Device in Lower Joints
CoRoent® XL	Interbody Fusion Device in Lower Joints
Corox® (OTW) Bipolar Lead	Cardiac Lead, Pacemaker for Insertion in Heart and Great Vessels
	Cardiac Lead, Defibrillator for Insertion in Heart and Great Vessels
Cortical strip neurostimulator lead	Neurostimulator Lead in Central Nervous System and Cranial Nerves
Corvia IASD®	Synthetic Substitute
Cultured epidermal cell autograft	Autologous Tissue Substitute
CYPHER® Stent	Intraluminal Device, Drug-eluting in Heart and Great Vessels
Cystostomy tube	Drainage Device

Device Term	ICD-10-PCS Value
DBS™ lead	Neurostimulator Lead in Central Nervous System and Cranial Nerves
DeBakey® Left Ventricular Assist Device	Implantable Heart Assist System in Heart and Great Vessels
Deep brain neurostimulator lead	Neurostimulator Lead in Central Nervous System and Cranial Nerves
Delta frame external fixator	External Fixation Device, Hybrid for Insertion in Upper Bones
	External Fixation Device, Hybrid for Reposition in Upper Bones
	External Fixation Device, Hybrid for Insertion in Lower Bones
	External Fixation Device, Hybrid for Reposition in Lower Bones
Delta III™ Reverse shoulder prosthesis	Synthetic Substitute, Reverse Ball and Socket for Replacement in Upper Joints
Diaphragmatic pacemaker generator	Stimulator Generator in Subcutaneous Tissue and Fascia
Direct Lateral Interbody Fusion (DLIF) device	Interbody Fusion Device in Lower Joints
Driver® stent (RX) (OTW)	Intraluminal Device
DuraHeart® Left Ventricular Assist System	Implantable Heart Assist System in Heart and Great Vessels
Durata® Defibrillation Lead	Cardiac Lead, Defibrillator for Insertion in Heart and Great Vessels
DynaNail Mini®	Internal Fixation Device, Sustained Compression for Fusion in Upper Joints
	Internal Fixation Device, Sustained Compression for Fusion in Lower Joints
DynaNail®	Internal Fixation Device, Sustained Compression for Fusion in Upper Joints
	Internal Fixation Device, Sustained Compression for Fusion in Lower Joints
Dynesys® Dynamic Stabilization System	Spinal Stabilization Device, Pedicle-Based for Insertion in Upper Joints
	Spinal Stabilization Device, Pedicle-Based for Insertion in Lower Joints
E-Luminexx™ (Biliary) (Vascular) Stent	Intraluminal Device
EDWARDS INTUITY Elite™ valve system	Zooplastic Tissue, Rapid Deployment Technique in New Technology
Electrical bone growth stimulator (EBGS)	Bone Growth Stimulator in Head and Facial Bones
	Bone Growth Stimulator in Upper Bones
	Bone Growth Stimulator in Lower Bones
Electrical muscle stimulation (EMS) lead	Stimulator Lead in Muscles

Device Term	ICD-10-PCS Value
Electronic muscle stimulator lead	Stimulator Lead in Muscles
Eluvia™ Drug-Eluting Vascular Stent System	Intraluminal Device, Sustained Release Drug-eluting in New Technology
	Intraluminal Device, Sustained Release Drug-eluting, Two in New Technology
	Intraluminal Device, Sustained Release Drug-eluting, Three in New Technology
	Intraluminal Device, Sustained Release Drug-eluting, Four or More in New Technology
Embolization coil(s)	Intraluminal Device
Endeavor® (III) (IV) (Sprint) Zotarolimus-eluting Coronary Stent System	Intraluminal Device, Drug-eluting in Heart and Great Vessels
Endologix AFX® Endovascular AAA System	Intraluminal Device
EndoSure® sensor	Monitoring Device, Pressure Sensor for Insertion in Heart and Great Vessels
ENDOTAK RELIANCE® (G) Defibrillation Lead	Cardiac Lead, Defibrillator for Insertion in Heart and Great Vessels
Endotracheal tube (cuffed) (double-lumen)	Intraluminal Device, Endotracheal Airway in Respiratory System
Endurant® Endovascular Stent Graft	Intraluminal Device
Endurant® II AAA stent graft system	Intraluminal Device
EnRhythm®	Pacemaker, Dual Chamber for Insertion in Subcutaneous Tissue and Fascia
Enterra® gastric neurostimulator	Stimulator Generator, Multiple Array for Insertion in Subcutaneous Tissue and Fascia
Epic™ Stented Tissue Valve (aortic)	Zooplastic Tissue in Heart and Great Vessels
Epicel® cultured epidermal autograft	Autologous Tissue Substitute
Esophageal obturator airway (EOA)	Intraluminal Device, Airway in Gastrointestinal System
Esteem® implantable hearing system	Hearing Device in Ear, Nose, Sinus
Evera™ (XT) (S) (DR/VR)	Defibrillator Generator for Insertion in Subcutaneous Tissue and Fascia
Everolimus-eluting coronary stent	Intraluminal Device, Drug-eluting in Heart and Great Vessels
Ex-PRESS™ mini glaucoma shunt	Synthetic Substitute
EXCLUDER® AAA Endoprosthesis	Intraluminal Device, Branched or Fenestrated, One or Two Arteries for Restriction in Lower Arteries
	Intraluminal Device, Branched or Fenestrated, Three or More Arteries for Restriction in Lower Arteries
	Intraluminal Device
EXCLUDER® IBE Endoprosthesis	Intraluminal Device, Branched or Fenestrated, One or Two Arteries for Restriction in Lower Arteries

Device Term	ICD-10-PCS Value	Device Term	ICD-10-PCS Value
Express® (LD) Premounted Stent System	Intraluminal Device	GORE® DUALMESH®	Synthetic Substitute
Express® Biliary SD Monorail® Premounted Stent System	Intraluminal Device	Guedel airway	Intraluminal Device, Airway in Mouth and Throat
Express® SD Renal Monorail® Premounted Stent System	Intraluminal Device	Hancock® Bioprosthesis (aortic) (mitral) valve	Zooplastic Tissue in Heart and Great Vessels
External fixator	External Fixation Device in Head and Facial Bones	Hancock® Bioprosthetic Valved Conduit	Zooplastic Tissue in Heart and Great Vessels
	External Fixation Device in Upper Bones	HeartMate 3™ LVAS	Implantable Heart Assist System in Heart and Great Vessels
	External Fixation Device in Lower Bones	HeartMate II® Left Ventricular Assist Device (LVAD)	Implantable Heart Assist System in Heart and Great Vessels
	External Fixation Device in Upper Joints	HeartMate XVE® Left Ventricular Assist Device (LVAD)	Implantable Heart Assist System in Heart and Great Vessels
	External Fixation Device in Lower Joints	Herculink® (RX) Elite Renal Stent System	Intraluminal Device
EXtreme Lateral Interbody Fusion(XLIF) device	Interbody Fusion Device in Lower Joints	Hip (joint) liner	Liner in Lower Joints
Facet replacement spinal stabilization device	Spinal Stabilization Device, Facet Replacement for Insertion in Upper Joints	Holter valve ventricular shunt	Synthetic Substitute
		IASD® (InterAtrial Shunt Device), Corvia	Synthetic Substitute
	Spinal Stabilization Device, Facet Replacement for Insertion in Lower Joints	Ilizarov external fixator	External Fixation Device, Ring for Insertion in Upper Bones
FLAIR® Endovascular Stent Graft	Intraluminal Device		External Fixation Device, Ring for Reposition in Upper Bones
Flexible Composite Mesh	Synthetic Substitute		External Fixation Device, Ring for Insertion in Lower Bones
Flow Diverter embolization device	Intraluminal Device, Flow Diverter for Restriction in Upper Arteries		External Fixation Device, Ring for Reposition in Lower Bones
Foley catheter	Drainage Device	Ilizarov-Vecklich device	External Fixation Device, Limb Lengthening for Insertion in Upper Bones
Formula™ Balloon-Expandable Renal Stent System	Intraluminal Device		
Freestyle® (Stentless) Aortic Root Bioprosthesis	Zooplastic Tissue in Heart and Great Vessels		External Fixation Device, Limb Lengthening for Insertion in Lower Bones
Fusion screw (compression) (lag) (locking)	Internal Fixation Device in Upper Joints	Impella® heart pump	Short-term External Heart Assist System in Heart and Great Vessels
	Internal Fixation Device in Lower Joints	Implantable cardioverter-defibrillator (ICD)	Defibrillator Generator for Insertion in Subcutaneous Tissue and Fascia
GammaTile™	Radioactive Element, Cesium-131 Collagen Implant for Insertion in Central Nervous System and Cranial Nerves	Implantable drug infusion pump (anti-spasmodic) (chemotherapy) (pain)	Infusion Device, Pump in Subcutaneous Tissue and Fascia
Gastric electrical stimulation (GES) lead	Stimulator Lead in Gastrointestinal System	Implantable glucose monitoring device	Monitoring Device
Gastric pacemaker lead	Stimulator Lead in Gastrointestinal System	Implantable hemodynamic monitor (IHM)	Monitoring Device, Hemodynamic for Insertion in Subcutaneous Tissue and Fascia
GORE EXCLUDER® AAA Endoprosthesis	Intraluminal Device, Branched or Fenestrated, One or Two Arteries for Restriction in Lower Arteries	Implantable hemodynamic monitoring system (IHMS)	Monitoring Device, Hemodynamic for Insertion in Subcutaneous Tissue and Fascia
	Intraluminal Device, Branched or Fenestrated, Three or More Arteries for Restriction in Lower Arteries	Implantable Miniature Telescope™(IMT)	Synthetic Substitute, Intraocular Telescope for Replacement in Eye
	Intraluminal Device	Implanted (venous) (access) port	Vascular Access Device, Totally Implantable in Subcutaneous Tissue and Fascia
GORE EXCLUDER® IBE Endoprosthesis	Intraluminal Device, Branched or Fenestrated, One or Two Arteries for Restriction in Lower Arteries		
GORE TAG® Thoracic Endoprosthesis	Intraluminal Device	InDura®, intrathecal catheter (1P) (spinal)	Infusion Device

Device Term	ICD-10-PCS Value
Injection reservoir, port	Vascular Access Device, Totally Implantable in Subcutaneous Tissue and Fascia
Injection reservoir, pump	Infusion Device, Pump in Subcutaneous Tissue and Fascia
InterAtrial Shunt Device IASD®, Corvia	Synthetic Substitute
Interbody fusion (spine) cage	Interbody Fusion Device in Upper Joints
	Interbody Fusion Device in Lower Joints
Interspinous process spinal stabilization device	Spinal Stabilization Device, Interspinous Process for Insertion in Upper Joints
	Spinal Stabilization Device, Interspinous Process for Insertion in Lower Joints
InterStim® Therapy lead	Neurostimulator Lead in Peripheral Nervous System
InterStim® Therapy neurostimulator	Stimulator Generator, Single Array for Insertion in Subcutaneous Tissue and Fascia
Intramedullary (IM) rod (nail)	Internal Fixation Device, Intramedullary in Upper Bones
	Internal Fixation Device, Intramedullary in Lower Bones
Intramedullary skeletal kinetic distractor (ISKD)	Internal Fixation Device, Intramedullary in Upper Bones
	Internal Fixation Device, Intramedullary in Lower Bones
Intrauterine device (IUD)	Contraceptive Device in Female Reproductive System
INTUITY Elite® valve system, EDWARDS	Zooplastic Tissue, Rapid Deployment Technique in New Technology
Itrel® (3) (4) neurostimulator	Stimulator Generator, Single Array for Insertion in Subcutaneous Tissue and Fascia
Joint fixation plate	Internal Fixation Device in Upper Joints
	Internal Fixation Device in Lower Joints
Joint liner (insert)	Liner in Lower Joints
Joint spacer (antibiotic)	Spacer in Upper Joints
	Spacer in Lower Joints
Kappa®	Pacemaker, Dual Chamber for Insertion in Subcutaneous Tissue and Fascia
Kirschner wire (K-wire)	Internal Fixation Device in Head and Facial Bones
	Internal Fixation Device in Upper Bones
	Internal Fixation Device in Lower Bones
	Internal Fixation Device in Upper Joints
	Internal Fixation Device in Lower Joints

Device Term	ICD-10-PCS Value
Knee (implant) insert	Liner in Lower Joints
Kuntscher nail	Internal Fixation Device, Intramedullary in Upper Bones
	Internal Fixation Device, Intramedullary in Lower Bones
LAP-BAND® adjustable gastric banding system	Extraluminal Device
LifeStent® (Flexstar) (XL) Vascular Stent System	Intraluminal Device
LIVIAN™ CRT-D	Cardiac Resynchronization Defibrillator Pulse Generator for Insertion in Subcutaneous Tissue and Fascia
Loop recorder, implantable	Monitoring Device
MAGEC® Spinal Bracing and Distraction System	Magnetically Controlled Growth Rod(s) in New Technology
Mark IV™ Breathing Pacemaker System	Stimulator Generator in Subcutaneous Tissue and Fascia
Maximo® II DR (VR)	Defibrillator Generator for Insertion in Subcutaneous Tissue and Fascia
Maximo® II DR CRT-D	Cardiac Resynchronization Defibrillator Pulse Generator for Insertion in Subcutaneous Tissue and Fascia
Medtronic Endurant® II AAA stent graft system	Intraluminal Device
Melody® transcatheter pulmonary valve	Zooplastic Tissue in Heart and Great Vessels
Metal on metal bearing surface	Synthetic Substitute, Metal for Replacement in Lower Joints
Micro-Driver® stent (RX) (OTW)	Intraluminal Device
MicroMed HeartAssist™	Implantable Heart Assist System in Heart and Great Vessels
Micrus CERECYTE® microcoil	Intraluminal Device, Bioactive in Upper Arteries
MIRODERM™ Biologic Wound Matrix	Skin Substitute, Porcine Liver Derived in New Technology
MitraClip® valve repair system	Synthetic Substitute
Mitroflow® Aortic Pericardial Heart Valve	Zooplastic Tissue in Heart and Great Vessels
Mosaic® Bioprosthesis (aortic) (mitral) valve	Zooplastic Tissue in Heart and Great Vessels
MULTI-LINK (VISION®) (MINI-VISION VISION®) (ULTRA™) Coronary Stent System	Intraluminal Device
nanoLOCK™ interbody fusion device	Interbody Fusion Device, Nanotextured Surface in New Technology
Nasopharyngeal airway (NPA)	Intraluminal Device, Airway in Ear, Nose, Sinus
Neuromuscular electrical stimulation (NEMS) lead	Stimulator Lead in Muscles
Neurostimulator generator, multiple channel	Stimulator Generator, Multiple Array for Insertion in Subcutaneous Tissue and Fascia

Device Term	ICD-10-PCS Value	Device Term	ICD-10-PCS Value
Neurostimulator generator, multiple channel rechargeable	Stimulator Generator, Multiple Array Rechargeable for Insertion in Subcutaneous Tissue and Fascia	Percutaneous endoscopic gastrostomy (PEG) tube	Feeding Device in Gastrointestinal System
Neurostimulator generator, single channel	Stimulator Generator, Single Array for Insertion in Subcutaneous Tissue and Fascia	Percutaneous nephrostomy catheter	Drainage Device
Neurostimulator generator, single channel rechargeable	Stimulator Generator, Single Array Rechargeable for Insertion in Subcutaneous Tissue and Fascia	Peripherally inserted central catheter (PICC)	Infusion Device
Neutralization plate	Internal Fixation Device in Head and Facial Bones	Pessary ring	Intraluminal Device, Pessary in Female Reproductive System
	Internal Fixation Device in Upper Bones	Phrenic nerve stimulator generator	Stimulator Generator in Subcutaneous Tissue and Fascia
	Internal Fixation Device in Lower Bones	Phrenic nerve stimulator lead	Diaphragmatic Pacemaker Lead in Respiratory System
Nitinol framed polymer mesh	Synthetic Substitute	PHYSIOMESH™ Flexible Composite Mesh	Synthetic Substitute
Non-tunneled central venous catheter	Infusion Device	Pipeline™ (Flex) embolization device	Intraluminal Device, Flow Diverter for Restriction in Upper Arteries
Novacor® Left Ventricular Assist Device	Implantable Heart Assist System in Heart and Great Vessels	Polyethylene socket	Synthetic Substitute, Polyethylene for Replacement in Lower Joints
Novation® Ceramic AHS® (Articulation Hip System)	Synthetic Substitute, Ceramic for Replacement in Lower Joints	Polymethylmethacrylate (PMMA)	Synthetic Substitute
Omnilink Elite® Vascular Balloon Expandable Stent System	Intraluminal Device	Polypropylene mesh	Synthetic Substitute
Open Pivot™ (mechanical) valve	Synthetic Substitute	Porcine (bioprosthetic) valve	Zooplastic Tissue in Heart and Great Vessels
Open Pivot™ Aortic Valve Graft (AVG)	Synthetic Substitute	PRECICE intramedullary limb lengthening system	Internal Fixation Device, Intramedullary Limb Lengthening for Insertion in Lower Bones
Optimizer™ III implantable pulse generator	Contractility Modulation Device for Insertion in Subcutaneous Tissue and Fascia		Internal Fixation Device, Intramedullary Limb Lengthening for Insertion in Upper Bones
Oropharyngeal airway (OPA)	Intraluminal Device, Airway in Mouth and Throat	PRESTIGE® Cervical Disc	Synthetic Substitute
Ovatio™ CRT-D	Cardiac Resynchronization Defibrillator Pulse Generator for Insertion in Subcutaneous Tissue and Fascia	PrimeAdvanced® neurostimulator (SureScan®) (MRI Safe)	Stimulator Generator, Multiple Array for Insertion in Subcutaneous Tissue and Fascia
		PROCEED™ Ventral Patch	Synthetic Substitute
OXINIUM™	Synthetic Substitute, Oxidized Zirconium on Polyethylene for Replacement in Lower Joints	Prodisc-C™	Synthetic Substitute
		Prodisc-L™	Synthetic Substitute
Paclitaxel-eluting coronary stent	Intraluminal Device, Drug-eluting in Heart and Great Vessels	PROLENE® Polypropylene Hernia System (PHS)	Synthetic Substitute
Paclitaxel-eluting peripheral stent	Intraluminal Device, Drug-eluting in Upper Arteries	Protecta™ XT CRT-D	Cardiac Resynchronization Defibrillator Pulse Generator for Insertion in Subcutaneous Tissue and Fascia
	Intraluminal Device, Drug-eluting in Lower Arteries	Protecta™ XT DR (XT VR)	Defibrillator Generator for Insertion in Subcutaneous Tissue and Fascia
Partially absorbable mesh	Synthetic Substitute	Protege® RX Carotid Stent System	Intraluminal Device
Pedicle-based dynamic stabilization device	Spinal Stabilization Device, Pedicle-Based for Insertion in Upper Joints	Pump reservoir	Infusion Device, Pump in Subcutaneous Tissue and Fascia
	Spinal Stabilization Device, Pedicle-Based for Insertion in Lower Joints	REALIZE® Adjustable Gastric Band	Extraluminal Device
		Rebound HRD® (Hernia Repair Device)	Synthetic Substitute
Perceval sutureless valve	Zooplastic Tissue, Rapid Deployment Technique in New Technology	RestoreAdvanced® neurostimulator (SureScan®) (MRI Safe)	Stimulator Generator, Multiple Array Rechargeable for Insertion in Subcutaneous Tissue and Fascia
Percutaneous endoscopic gastrojejunostomy (PEG/J) tube	Feeding Device in Gastrointestinal System	RestoreSensor® neurostimulator (SureScan®) (MRI Safe)	Stimulator Generator, Multiple Array Rechargeable for Insertion in Subcutaneous Tissue and Fascia

Device Term	ICD-10-PCS Value	Device Term	ICD-10-PCS Value
RestoreUltra® neurostimulator (SureScan®) (MRI Safe)	Stimulator Generator, Multiple Array Rechargeable for Insertion in Subcutaneous Tissue and Fascia	Single lead pacemaker (atrium) (ventricle)	Pacemaker, Single Chamber for Insertion in Subcutaneous Tissue and Fascia
Reveal® (LINQ) (DX) (XT)	Monitoring Device	Single lead rate responsive pacemaker (atrium) (ventricle)	Pacemaker, Single Chamber Rate Responsive for Insertion in Subcutaneous Tissue and Fascia
Reverse® Shoulder Prosthesis	Synthetic Substitute, Reverse Ball and Socket for Replacement in Upper Joints	Sirolimus-eluting coronary stent	Intraluminal Device, Drug-eluting in Heart and Great Vessels
Revo MRI™ SureScan® pacemaker	Pacemaker, Dual Chamber for Insertion in Subcutaneous Tissue and Fascia	SJM Biocor® Stented Valve System	Zooplastic Tissue in Heart and Great Vessels
Rheos® System device	Stimulator Generator in Subcutaneous Tissue and Fascia	Spacer, Articulating (Antibiotic)	Articulating Spacer in Lower Joints
Rheos® System lead	Stimulator Lead in Upper Arteries	Spacer, Static (Antibiotic)	Spacer in Lower Joints
RNS® System lead	Neurostimulator Lead in Central Nervous System and Cranial Nerves	Spinal cord neurostimulator lead	Neurostimulator Lead in Central Nervous System and Cranial Nerves
RNS® system neurostimulator generator	Neurostimulator Generator in Head and Facial Bones	Spinal growth rods, magnetically controlled	Magnetically Controlled Growth Rod(s) in New Technology
Sacral nerve modulation (SNM) lead	Stimulator Lead in Urinary System	Spiration IBV™ Valve System	Intraluminal Device, Endobronchial Valve in Respiratory System
S-ICD™ lead	Subcutaneous Defibrillator Lead in Subcutaneous Tissue and Fascia	Static Spacer (Antibiotic)	Spacer in Lower Joints
Sacral neuromodulation lead	Stimulator Lead in Urinary System	Stent, intraluminal (cardiovascular) (gastrointestinal) (hepatobiliary) (urinary)	Intraluminal Device
SAPIEN® transcatheter aortic valve	Zooplastic Tissue in Heart and Great Vessels	Stented tissue valve	Zooplastic Tissue in Heart and Great Vessels
SAVAL below-the-knee (BTK) drug-eluting stent system	Intraluminal Device, Sustained Release Drug-eluting in New Technology	Stratos LV®	Cardiac Resynchronization Pacemaker Pulse Generator for Insertion in Subcutaneous Tissue and Fascia
	Intraluminal Device, Sustained Release Drug-eluting, Two in New Technology	Subcutaneous injection reservoir, port	Vascular Access Device, Totally Implantable in Subcutaneous Tissue and Fascia
	Intraluminal Device, Sustained Release Drug-eluting, Three in New Technology	Subcutaneous injection reservoir, pump	Infusion Device, Pump in Subcutaneous Tissue and Fascia
	Intraluminal Device, Sustained Release Drug-eluting, Four or More in New Technology	Subdermal progesterone implant	Contraceptive Device in Subcutaneous Tissue and Fascia
Secura™ (DR) (VR)	Defibrillator Generator for Insertion in Subcutaneous Tissue and Fascia	Surpass Streamline™ Flow Diverter	Intraluminal Device, Flow Diverter for Restriction in Upper Arteries
Sheffield hybrid external fixator	External Fixation Device, Hybrid for Insertion in Upper Bones	Sutureless valve, Perceval™	Zooplastic Tissue, Rapid Deployment Technique in New Technology
	External Fixation Device, Hybrid for Reposition in Upper Bones	SynCardia™ Total Artificial Heart	Synthetic Substitute
	External Fixation Device, Hybrid for Insertion in Lower Bones	Synchra™ CRT-P	Cardiac Resynchronization Pacemaker Pulse Generator for Insertion in Subcutaneous Tissue and Fascia
	External Fixation Device, Hybrid for Reposition in Lower Bones	SynchroMed® pump	Infusion Device, Pump in Subcutaneous Tissue and Fascia
Sheffield ring external fixator	External Fixation Device, Ring for Insertion in Upper Bones	Talent® Converter	Intraluminal Device
	External Fixation Device, Ring for Reposition in Upper Bones	Talent® Occluder	Intraluminal Device
	External Fixation Device, Ring for Insertion in Lower Bones	Talent® Stent Graft (abdominal) (thoracic)	Intraluminal Device
	External Fixation Device, Ring for Reposition in Lower Bones	TandemHeart® System	Short-term External Heart Assist System in Heart and Great Vessels
		TAXUS® Liberte® Paclitaxel-eluting Coronary Stent System	Intraluminal Device, Drug-eluting in Heart and Great Vessels

Device Term	ICD-10-PCS Value
Therapeutic occlusion coil(s)	Intraluminal Device
Thoracostomy tube	Drainage Device
Thoratec® IVAD (Implantable Ventricular Assist Device)	Implantable Heart Assist System in Heart and Great Vessels
Thoratec Paracorporeal Ventricular Assist Device	Short-term External Heart Assist System in Heart and Great Vessels
Tibial insert	Liner in Lower Joints
Tissue bank graft	Nonautologous Tissue Substitute
Tissue expander (inflatable) (injectable)	Tissue Expander in Skin and Breast
	Tissue Expander in Subcutaneous Tissue and Fascia
Titanium Sternal Fixation System (TSFS)	Internal Fixation Device, Rigid Plate for Insertion in Upper Bones
	Internal Fixation Device, Rigid Plate for Reposition in Upper Bones
Total artificial (replacement) heart	Synthetic Substitute
Tracheostomy tube	Tracheostomy Device in Respiratory System
Trifecta™ Valve (aortic)	Zooplastic Tissue in Heart and Great Vessels
Tunneled central venous catheter	Vascular Access Device, Tunneled in Subcutaneous Tissue and Fascia
Tunneled spinal (intrathecal) catheter	Infusion Device
Two lead pacemaker	Pacemaker, Dual Chamber for Insertion in Subcutaneous Tissue and Fascia
Ultraflex™ Precision Colonic Stent System	Intraluminal Device
ULTRAPRO® Hernia System (UHS)	Synthetic Substitute
ULTRAPRO® Partially Absorbable Lightweight Mesh	Synthetic Substitute
ULTRAPRO® Plug	Synthetic Substitute
Ultrasonic osteogenic stimulator	Bone Growth Stimulator in Head and Facial Bones
	Bone Growth Stimulator in Upper Bones
	Bone Growth Stimulator in Lower Bones
Ultrasound bone healing system	Bone Growth Stimulator in Head and Facial Bones
	Bone Growth Stimulator in Upper Bones
	Bone Growth Stimulator in Lower Bones
Uniplanar external fixator	External Fixation Device, Monoplanar for Insertion in Upper Bones
	External Fixation Device, Monoplanar for Reposition in Upper Bones
	External Fixation Device, Monoplanar for Insertion in Lower Bones
	External Fixation Device, Monoplanar for Reposition in Lower Bones

Device Term	ICD-10-PCS Value
Urinary incontinence stimulator lead	Stimulator Lead in Urinary System
V-Wave Interatrial Shunt System	Synthetic Substitute
Vaginal pessary	Intraluminal Device, Pessary in Female Reproductive System
Valiant® Thoracic Stent Graft	Intraluminal Device
Vectra® Vascular Access Graft	Vascular Access Device, Tunneled in Subcutaneous Tissue and Fascia
Ventrio™ Hernia Patch	Synthetic Substitute
Versa®	Pacemaker, Dual Chamber for Insertion in Subcutaneous Tissue and Fascia
Virtuoso® (II) (DR) (VR)	Defibrillator Generator for Insertion in Subcutaneous Tissue and Fascia
Viva™ (XT) (S)	Cardiac Resynchronization Defibrillator Pulse Generator for Insertion in Subcutaneous Tissue and Fascia
WALLSTENT® Endoprosthesis	Intraluminal Device
X-STOP® Spacer	Spinal Stabilization Device, Interspinous Process for Insertion in Upper Joints
	Spinal Stabilization Device, Interspinous Process for Insertion in Lower Joints
Xact® Carotid Stent System	Intraluminal Device
Xenograft	Zooplastic Tissue in Heart and Great Vessels
XIENCE™ Everolimus Eluting Coronary Stent System	Intraluminal Device, Drug-eluting in Heart and Great Vessels
XLIF® System	Interbody Fusion Device in Lower Joints
Zenith AAA Endovascular Graft	Intraluminal Device
Zenith Flex® AAA Endovascular Graft	Intraluminal Device
Zenith TX2® TAA Endovascular Graft	Intraluminal Device
Zenith® Fenestrated AAA Endovascular Graft	Intraluminal Device, Branched or Fenestrated, One or Two Arteries for Restriction in Lower Arteries
	Intraluminal Device, Branched or Fenestrated, Three or More Arteries for Restriction in Lower Arteries
Zenith® Renu™ AAA Ancillary Graft	Intraluminal Device
Zilver® PTX® (paclitaxel) Drug-eluting Peripheral Stent	Intraluminal Device, Drug-eluting in Upper Arteries
	Intraluminal Device, Drug-eluting in Lower Arteries
Zimmer® NexGen® LPS Mobile Bearing Knee	Synthetic Substitute
Zimmer® NexGen® LPS-Flex Mobile Knee	Synthetic Substitute
Zotarolimus-eluting coronary stent	Intraluminal Device, Drug-eluting in Heart and Great Vessels

Appendix D: Device Aggregation Table

Specific Device	For Operation	In Body System	General Device
Autologous Arterial Tissue	All applicable	Heart and Great Vessels	**7** Autologous Tissue Substitute
		Lower Arteries	
		Lower Veins	
		Upper Arteries	
		Upper Veins	
Autologous Venous Tissue	All applicable	Heart and Great Vessels	**7** Autologous Tissue Substitute
		Lower Arteries	
		Lower Veins	
		Upper Arteries	
		Upper Veins	
Cardiac Lead, Defibrillator	Insertion	Heart and Great Vessels	**M** Cardiac Lead
Cardiac Lead, Pacemaker	Insertion	Heart and Great Vessels	**M** Cardiac Lead
Cardiac Resynchronization Defibrillator Pulse Generator	Insertion	Subcutaneous Tissue and Fascia	**P** Cardiac Rhythm Related Device
Cardiac Resynchronization Pacemaker Pulse Generator	Insertion	Subcutaneous Tissue and Fascia	**P** Cardiac Rhythm Related Device
Contractility Modulation Device	Insertion	Subcutaneous Tissue and Fascia	**P** Cardiac Rhythm Related Device
Defibrillator Generator	Insertion	Subcutaneous Tissue and Fascia	**P** Cardiac Rhythm Related Device
Epiretinal Visual Prosthesis	All applicable	Eye	**J** Synthetic Substitute
External Fixation Device, Hybrid	Insertion	Lower Bones	**5** External Fixation Device
		Upper Bones	
External Fixation Device, Hybrid	Reposition	Lower Bones	**5** External Fixation Device
		Upper Bones	
External Fixation Device, Limb Lengthening	Insertion	Lower Bones	**5** External Fixation Device
		Upper Bones	
External Fixation Device, Monoplanar	Insertion	Lower Bones	**5** External Fixation Device
		Upper Bones	
External Fixation Device, Monoplanar	Reposition	Lower Bones	**5** External Fixation Device
		Upper Bones	
External Fixation Device, Ring	Insertion	Lower Bones	**5** External Fixation Device
		Upper Bones	
External Fixation Device, Ring	Reposition	Lower Bones	**5** External Fixation Device
		Upper Bones	
Hearing Device, Bone Conduction	Insertion	Ear, Nose, Sinus	**S** Hearing Device
Hearing Device, Multiple Channel Cochlear Prosthesis	Insertion	Ear, Nose, Sinus	**S** Hearing Device
Hearing Device, Single Channel Cochlear Prosthesis	Insertion	Ear, Nose, Sinus	**S** Hearing Device
Internal Fixation Device, Intramedullary	All applicable	Lower Bones	**4** Internal Fixation Device
		Upper Bones	
Internal Fixation Device, Intramedullary Limb Lengthening	Insertion	Lower Bones	**6** Internal Fixation Device, Intramedullary
		Upper Bones	
Internal Fixation Device, Rigid Plate	Insertion	Upper Bones	**4** Internal Fixation Device
Internal Fixation Device, Rigid Plate	Reposition	Upper Bones	**4** Internal Fixation Device

Specific Device	For Operation	In Body System	General Device
Intraluminal Device, Airway	All applicable	Ear, Nose, Sinus Gastrointestinal System Mouth and Throat	**D** Intraluminal Device
Intraluminal Device, Bioactive	All applicable	Upper Arteries	**D** Intraluminal Device
Intraluminal Device, Branched or Fenestrated, One or Two Arteries	Restriction	Heart and Great Vessels	**D** Intraluminal Device
		Lower Arteries	
Intraluminal Device, Branched or Fenestrated, Three or More Arteries	Restriction	Heart and Great Vessels	**D** Intraluminal Device
		Lower Arteries	
Intraluminal Device, Drug-eluting	All applicable	Heart and Great Vessels	**D** Intraluminal Device
		Lower Arteries	
		Upper Arteries	
Intraluminal Device, Drug-eluting, Four or More	All applicable	Heart and Great Vessels	**D** Intraluminal Device
		Lower Arteries	
		Upper Arteries	
Intraluminal Device, Drug-eluting, Three	All applicable	Heart and Great Vessels	**D** Intraluminal Device
		Lower Arteries	
		Upper Arteries	
Intraluminal Device, Drug-eluting, Two	All applicable	Heart and Great Vessels	**D** Intraluminal Device
		Lower Arteries	
		Upper Arteries	
Intraluminal Device, Endobronchial Valve	All applicable	Respiratory System	**D** Intraluminal Device
Intraluminal Device, Endotracheal Airway	All applicable	Respiratory System	**D** Intraluminal Device
Intraluminal Device, Flow Diverter	Restriction	Upper Arteries	**D** Intraluminal Device
Intraluminal Device, Four or More	All applicable	Heart and Great Vessels	**D** Intraluminal Device
		Lower Arteries	
		Upper Arteries	
Intraluminal Device, Pessary	All applicable	Female Reproductive System	**D** Intraluminal Device
Intraluminal Device, Radioactive	All applicable	Heart and Great Vessels	**D** Intraluminal Device
Intraluminal Device, Three	All applicable	Heart and Great Vessels	**D** Intraluminal Device
		Lower Arteries	
		Upper Arteries	
Intraluminal Device, Two	All applicable	Heart and Great Vessels	**D** Intraluminal Device
		Lower Arteries	
		Upper Arteries	
Monitoring Device, Hemodynamic	Insertion	Subcutaneous Tissue and Fascia	**2** Monitoring Device
Monitoring Device, Pressure Sensor	Insertion	Heart and Great Vessels	**2** Monitoring Device
Pacemaker, Dual Chamber	Insertion	Subcutaneous Tissue and Fascia	**P** Cardiac Rhythm Related Device
Pacemaker, Single Chamber	Insertion	Subcutaneous Tissue and Fascia	**P** Cardiac Rhythm Related Device
Pacemaker, Single Chamber Rate Responsive	Insertion	Subcutaneous Tissue and Fascia	**P** Cardiac Rhythm Related Device
Spinal Stabilization Device, Facet Replacement	Insertion	Lower Joints	**4** Internal Fixation Device
		Upper Joints	
Spinal Stabilization Device, Interspinous Process	Insertion	Lower Joints	**4** Internal Fixation Device
		Upper Joints	
Spinal Stabilization Device, Pedicle-Based	Insertion	Lower Joints	**4** Internal Fixation Device
		Upper Joints	

Specific Device	For Operation	In Body System	General Device
Stimulator Generator, Multiple Array	Insertion	Subcutaneous Tissue and Fascia	**M** Stimulator Generator
Stimulator Generator, Multiple Array Rechargeable	Insertion	Subcutaneous Tissue and Fascia	**M** Stimulator Generator
Stimulator Generator, Single Array	Insertion	Subcutaneous Tissue and Fascia	**M** Stimulator Generator
Stimulator Generator, Single Array Rechargeable	Insertion	Subcutaneous Tissue and Fascia	**M** Stimulator Generator
Synthetic Substitute, Ceramic	Replacement	Lower Joints	**J** Synthetic Substitute
Synthetic Substitute, Ceramic on Polyethylene	Replacement	Lower Joints	**J** Synthetic Substitute
Synthetic Substitute, Intraocular Telescope	Replacement	Eye	**J** Synthetic Substitute
Synthetic Substitute, Metal	Replacement	Lower Joints	**J** Synthetic Substitute
Synthetic Substitute, Metal on Polyethylene	Replacement	Lower Joints	**J** Synthetic Substitute
Synthetic Substitute, Oxidized Zirconium on Polyethylene	Replacement	Lower Joints	**J** Synthetic Substitute
Synthetic Substitute, Polyethylene	Replacement	Lower Joints	**J** Synthetic Substitute
Synthetic Substitute, Reverse Ball and Socket	Replacement	Upper Joints	**J** Synthetic Substitute

This page intentionally left blank

Appendix E: Character Meaning

0: Medical and Surgical
0: Central Nervous System and Cranial Nerves

Operation-Character 3	Body Part-Character 4	Approach-Character 5	Device-Character 6	Qualifier-Character 7
1 Bypass	**0** Brain	**0** Open	**0** Drainage Device	**0** Nasopharynx
2 Change	**1** Cerebral Meninges	**3** Percutaneous	**1** Radioactive Element	**1** Mastoid Sinus
5 Destruction	**2** Dura Mater	**4** Percutaneous Endoscopic	**2** Monitoring Device	**2** Atrium
7 Dilation	**3** Epidural Space, Intracranial	**X** External	**3** Infusion Device	**3** Blood Vessel
8 Division	**4** Subdural Space, Intracranial		**4** Radioactive Element,Cesium-131 Collagen Implant	**4** Pleural Cavity
9 Drainage	**5** Subarachnoid Space, Intracranial		**7** Autologous Tissue Substitute	**5** Intestine
B Excision	**6** Cerebral Ventricle		**J** Synthetic Substitute	**6** Peritoneal Cavity
C Extirpation	**7** Cerebral Hemisphere		**K** Nonautologous Tissue Substitute	**7** Urinary Tract
D Extraction	**8** Basal Ganglia		**M** Neurostimulator Lead	**8** Bone Marrow
F Fragmentation	**9** Thalamus		**Y** Other Device	**9** Fallopian Tube
H Insertion	**A** Hypothalamus		**Z** No Device	**A** Subgaleal Space
J Inspection	**B** Pons			**B** Cerebral Cisterns
K Map	**C** Cerebellum			**F** Olfactory Nerve
N Release	**D** Medulla Oblongata			**G** Optic Nerve
P Removal	**E** Cranial Nerve			**H** Oculomotor Nerve
Q Repair	**F** Olfactory Nerve			**J** Trochlear Nerve
R Replacement	**G** Optic Nerve			**K** Trigeminal Nerve
S Reposition	**H** Oculomotor Nerve			**L** Abducens Nerve
T Resection	**J** Trochlear Nerve			**M** Facial Nerve
U Supplement	**K** Trigeminal Nerve			**N** Acoustic Nerve
W Revision	**L** Abducens Nerve			**P** Glossopharyngeal Nerve
X Transfer	**M** Facial Nerve			**Q** Vagus Nerve
	N Acoustic Nerve			**R** Accessory Nerve
	P Glossopharyngeal Nerve			**S** Hypoglossal Nerve
	Q Vagus Nerve			**X** Diagnostic
	R Accessory Nerve			**Z** No Qualifier
	S Hypoglossal Nerve			
	T Spinal Meninges			
	U Spinal Canal			
	V Spinal Cord			
	W Cervical Spinal Cord			
	X Thoracic Spinal Cord			
	Y Lumbar Spinal Cord			

0: Medical and Surgical
1: Peripheral Nervous System

Operation-Character 3	Body Part-Character 4	Approach-Character 5	Device-Character 6	Qualifier-Character 7
2 Change	**0** Cervical Plexus	**0** Open	**0** Drainage Device	**1** Cervical Nerve
5 Destruction	**1** Cervical Nerve	**3** Percutaneous	**1** Radioactive Element	**2** Phrenic Nerve
8 Division	**2** Phrenic Nerve	**4** Percutaneous Endoscopic	**2** Monitoring Device	**4** Ulnar Nerve
9 Drainage	**3** Brachial Plexus	**X** External	**7** Autologous Tissue Substitute	**5** Median Nerve
B Excision	**4** Ulnar Nerve		**J** Synthetic Substitute	**6** Radial Nerve
C Extirpation	**5** Median Nerve		**K** Nonautologous Tissue Substitute	**8** Thoracic Nerve
D Extraction	**6** Radial Nerve		**M** Neurostimulator Lead	**B** Lumbar Nerve
H Insertion	**8** Thoracic Nerve		**Y** Other Device	**C** Perineal Nerve
J Inspection	**9** Lumbar Plexus		**Z** No Device	**D** Femoral Nerve
N Release	**A** Lumbosacral Plexus			**F** Sciatic Nerve
P Removal	**B** Lumbar Nerve			**G** Tibial Nerve
Q Repair	**C** Pudendal Nerve			**H** Peroneal Nerve
R Replacement	**D** Femoral Nerve			**X** Diagnostic
S Reposition	**F** Sciatic Nerve			**Z** No Qualifier
U Supplement	**G** Tibial Nerve			
W Revision	**H** Peroneal Nerve			
X Transfer	**K** Head and Neck Sympathetic Nerve			
	L Thoracic Sympathetic Nerve			
	M Abdominal Sympathetic Nerve			
	N Lumbar Sympathetic Nerve			
	P Sacral Sympathetic Nerve			
	Q Sacral Plexus			
	R Sacral Nerve			
	Y Peripheral Nerve			

0: Medical and Surgical
2: Heart and Great Vessels

Operation-Character 3	Body Part-Character 4	Approach-Character 5	Device-Character 6	Qualifier-Character 7
1 Bypass	**0** Coronary Artery, One Artery	**0** Open	**0** Monitoring Device, Pressure Sensor	**0** Allogeneic
4 Creation	**1** Coronary Artery, Two Arteries	**3** Percutaneous	**2** Monitoring Device	**0** Ultrasonic
5 Destruction	**2** Coronary Artery, Three Arteries	**4** Percutaneous Endoscopic	**3** Infusion Device	**1** Syngeneic
7 Dilation	**3** Coronary Artery, Four or More Arteries	**X** External	**4** Intraluminal Device, Drug-eluting	**2** Zooplastic
8 Division	**4** Coronary Vein		**5** Intraluminal Device, Drug-eluting, Two	**2** Common Atrioventricular Valve
B Excision	**5** Atrial Septum		**6** Intraluminal Device, Drug-eluting, Three	**3** Coronary Artery
C Extirpation	**6** Atrium, Right		**7** Intraluminal Device, Drug-eluting, Four or More	**4** Coronary Vein
F Fragmentation	**7** Atrium, Left		**7** Autologous Tissue Substitute	**5** Coronary Circulation
H Insertion	**8** Conduction Mechanism		**8** Zooplastic Tissue	**6** Atrium, Right
J Inspection	**9** Chordae Tendineae		**9** Autologous Venous Tissue	**6** Bifurcation
K Map	**A** Heart		**A** Autologous Arterial Tissue	**7** Atrium, Left
L Occlusion	**B** Heart, Right		**C** Extraluminal Device	**8** Internal Mammary, Right
N Release	**C** Heart, Left		**D** Intraluminal Device	**9** Internal Mammary, Left
P Removal	**D** Papillary Muscle		**E** Intraluminal Device, Two	**A** Innominate Artery
Q Repair	**F** Aortic Valve		**E** Intraluminal Device, Branched or Fenestrated, One or Two Arteries	**B** Subclavian
R Replacement	**G** Mitral Valve		**F** Intraluminal Device, Three	**C** Thoracic Artery
S Reposition	**H** Pulmonary Valve		**F** Intraluminal Device, Branched or Fenestrated, Three or More Arteries	**D** Carotid
T Resection	**J** Tricuspid Valve		**G** Intraluminal Device, Four or More	**E** Atrioventricular Valve, Left
U Supplement	**K** Ventricle, Right		**J** Cardiac Lead, Pacemaker	**F** Abdominal Artery
V Restriction	**L** Ventricle, Left		**J** Synthetic Substitute	**G** Atrioventricular Valve, Right
W Revision	**M** Ventricular Septum		**K** Cardiac Lead, Defibrillator	**G** Axillary Artery
Y Transplantation	**N** Pericardium		**K** Nonautologous Tissue Substitute	**H** Transapical
	P Pulmonary Trunk		**M** Cardiac Lead	**H** Brachial Artery
	Q Pulmonary Artery, Right		**N** Intracardiac Pacemaker	**J** Intraoperative
	R Pulmonary Artery, Left		**Q** Implantable Heart Assist System	**J** Temporary
	S Pulmonary Vein, Right		**R** Short-term External Heart Assist System	**J** Truncal Valve
	T Pulmonary Vein, Left		**T** Intraluminal Device, Radioactive	**K** Left Atrial Appendage
	V Superior Vena Cava		**Y** Other Device	**P** Pulmonary Trunk
	W Thoracic Aorta, Descending		**Z** No Device	**Q** Pulmonary Artery, Right
	X Thoracic Aorta, Ascending/Arch			**R** Pulmonary Artery, Left
	Y Great Vessel			**S** Biventricular
				S Pulmonary Vein, Right
				T Pulmonary Vein, Left
				T Ductus Arteriosus
				U Pulmonary Vein, Confluence
				V Lower Extremity Artery
				W Aorta
				X Diagnostic
				Z No Qualifier

0: Medical and Surgical
3: Upper Arteries

Operation-Character 3	Body Part-Character 4	Approach-Character 5	Device-Character 6	Qualifier-Character 7
1 Bypass	**0** Internal Mammary Artery, Right	**0** Open	**0** Drainage Device	**0** Ultrasonic
5 Destruction	**1** Internal Mammary Artery, Left	**3** Percutaneous	**2** Monitoring Device	**0** Upper Arm Artery, Right
7 Dilation	**2** Innominate Artery	**4** Percutaneous Endoscopic	**3** Infusion Device	**1** Drug-Coated Balloon
9 Drainage	**3** Subclavian Artery, Right	**X** External	**4** Intraluminal Device, Drug-eluting	**1** Upper Arm Artery, Left
B Excision	**4** Subclavian Artery, Left		**5** Intraluminal Device, Drug-eluting, Two	**2** Upper Arm Artery, Bilateral
C Extirpation	**5** Axillary Artery, Right		**6** Intraluminal Device, Drug-eluting, Three	**3** Lower Arm Artery, Right
F Fragmentation	**6** Axillary Artery, Left		**7** Autologous Tissue Substitute	**4** Lower Arm Artery, Left
H Insertion	**7** Brachial Artery, Right		**7** Intraluminal Device, Drug-eluting, Four or More	**5** Lower Arm Artery, Bilateral
J Inspection	**8** Brachial Artery, Left		**9** Autologous Venous Tissue	**6** Bifurcation
L Occlusion	**9** Ulnar Artery, Right		**A** Autologous Arterial Tissue	**6** Upper Leg Artery, Right
N Release	**A** Ulnar Artery, Left		**B** Intraluminal Device, Bioactive	**7** Stent Retriever
P Removal	**B** Radial Artery, Right		**C** Extraluminal Device	**7** Upper Leg Artery, Left
Q Repair	**C** Radial Artery, Left		**D** Intraluminal Device	**8** Upper Leg Artery, Bilateral
R Replacement	**D** Hand Artery, Right		**E** Intraluminal Device, Two	**9** Lower Leg Artery, Right
S Reposition	**F** Hand Artery, Left		**F** Intraluminal Device, Three	**B** Lower Leg Artery, Left
U Supplement	**G** Intracranial Artery		**G** Intraluminal Device, Four or More	**C** Lower Leg Artery, Bilateral
V Restriction	**H** Common Carotid Artery, Right		**J** Synthetic Substitute	**D** Upper Arm Vein
W Revision	**J** Common Carotid Artery, Left		**K** Nonautologous Tissue Substitute	**F** Lower Arm Vein
	K Internal Carotid Artery, Right		**M** Stimulator Lead	**G** Intracranial Artery
	L Internal Carotid Artery, Left		**Y** Other Device	**J** Extracranial Artery, Right
	M External Carotid Artery, Right		**Z** No Device	**K** Extracranial Artery, Left
	N External Carotid Artery, Left			**M** Pulmonary Artery, Right
	P Vertebral Artery, Right			**N** Pulmonary Artery, Left
	Q Vertebral Artery, Left			**T** Abdominal Artery
	R Face Artery			**V** Superior Vena Cava
	S Temporal Artery, Right			**W** Lower Extremity Vein
	T Temporal Artery, Left			**X** Diagnostic
	U Thyroid Artery, Right			**Y** Upper Artery
	V Thyroid Artery, Left			**Z** No Qualifier
	Y Upper Artery			

0: Medical and Surgical
4: Lower Arteries

Operation-Character 3	Body Part-Character 4	Approach-Character 5	Device-Character 6	Qualifier-Character 7
1 Bypass	**0** Abdominal Aorta	**0** Open	**0** Drainage Device	**0** Abdominal Aorta
5 Destruction	**1** Celiac Artery	**3** Percutaneous	**1** Radioactive Element	**0** Ultrasonic
7 Dilation	**2** Gastric Artery	**4** Percutaneous Endoscopic	**2** Monitoring Device	**1** Celiac Artery
9 Drainage	**3** Hepatic Artery	**X** External	**3** Infusion Device	**1** Drug-Coated Balloon
B Excision	**4** Splenic Artery		**4** Intraluminal Device, Drug-eluting	**2** Mesenteric Artery
C Extirpation	**5** Superior Mesenteric Artery		**5** Intraluminal Device, Drug-eluting, Two	**3** Renal Artery, Right
F Fragmentation	**6** Colic Artery, Right		**6** Intraluminal Device, Drug-eluting, Three	**4** Renal Artery, Left
H Insertion	**7** Colic Artery, Left		**7** Autologous Tissue Substitute	**5** Renal Artery, Bilateral
J Inspection	**8** Colic Artery, Middle		**7** Intraluminal Device, Drug-eluting, Four or More	**6** Bifurcation
L Occlusion	**9** Renal Artery, Right		**9** Autologous Venous Tissue	**6** Common Iliac Artery, Right
N Release	**A** Renal Artery, Left		**A** Autologous Arterial Tissue	**7** Common Iliac Artery, Left
P Removal	**B** Inferior Mesenteric Artery		**C** Extraluminal Device	**8** Common Iliac Arteries, Bilateral
Q Repair	**C** Common Iliac Artery, Right		**D** Intraluminal Device	**9** Internal Iliac Artery, Right
R Replacement	**D** Common Iliac Artery, Left		**E** Intraluminal Device, Branched or Fenestrated, One or Two Arteries	**B** Internal Iliac Artery, Left
S Reposition	**E** Internal Iliac Artery, Right		**E** Intraluminal Device, Two	**C** Internal Iliac Arteries, Bilateral
U Supplement	**F** Internal Iliac Artery, Left		**F** Intraluminal Device, Branched or Fenestrated, Three or More Arteries	**D** External Iliac Artery, Right
V Restriction	**H** External Iliac Artery, Right		**F** Intraluminal Device, Three	**F** External Iliac Artery, Left
W Revision	**J** External Iliac Artery, Left		**G** Intraluminal Device, Four or More	**G** External Iliac Arteries, Bilateral
	K Femoral Artery, Right		**J** Synthetic Substitute	**H** Femoral Artery, Right
	L Femoral Artery, Left		**K** Nonautologous Tissue Substitute	**J** Femoral Artery, Left
	M Popliteal Artery, Right		**Y** Other Device	**J** Temporary
	N Popliteal Artery, Left		**Z** No Device	**K** Femoral Arteries, Bilateral
	P Anterior Tibial Artery, Right			**L** Popliteal Artery
	Q Anterior Tibial Artery, Left			**M** Peroneal Artery
	R Posterior Tibial Artery, Right			**N** Posterior Tibial Artery
	S Posterior Tibial Artery, Left			**P** Foot Artery
	T Peroneal Artery, Right			**Q** Lower Extremity Artery
	U Peroneal Artery, Left			**R** Lower Artery
	V Foot Artery, Right			**S** Lower Extremity Vein
	W Foot Artery, Left			**T** Uterine Artery, Right
	Y Lower Artery			**U** Uterine Artery, Left
				X Diagnostic
				Z No Qualifier

0: Medical and Surgical
5: Upper Veins

Operation-Character 3	Body Part-Character 4	Approach-Character 5	Device-Character 6	Qualifier-Character 7
1 Bypass	**0** Azygos Vein	**0** Open	**0** Drainage Device	**0** Ultrasonic
5 Destruction	**1** Hemiazygos Vein	**3** Percutaneous	**2** Monitoring Device	**1** Drug-Coated Balloon
7 Dilation	**3** Innominate Vein, Right	**4** Percutaneous Endoscopic	**3** Infusion Device	**X** Diagnostic
9 Drainage	**4** Innominate Vein, Left	**X** External	**7** Autologous Tissue Substitute	**Y** Upper Vein
B Excision	**5** Subclavian Vein, Right		**9** Autologous Venous Tissue	**Z** No Qualifier
C Extirpation	**6** Subclavian Vein, Left		**A** Autologous Arterial Tissue	
D Extraction	**7** Axillary Vein, Right		**C** Extraluminal Device	
F Fragmentation	**8** Axillary Vein, Left		**D** Intraluminal Device	
H Insertion	**9** Brachial Vein, Right		**J** Synthetic Substitute	
J Inspection	**A** Brachial Vein, Left		**K** Nonautologous Tissue Substitute	
L Occlusion	**B** Basilic Vein, Right		**M** Neurostimulator Lead	
N Release	**C** Basilic Vein, Left		**Y** Other Device	
P Removal	**D** Cephalic Vein, Right		**Z** No Device	
Q Repair	**F** Cephalic Vein, Left			
R Replacement	**G** Hand Vein, Right			
S Reposition	**H** Hand Vein, Left			
U Supplement	**L** Intracranial Vein			
V Restriction	**M** Internal Jugular Vein, Right			
W Revision	**N** Internal Jugular Vein, Left			
	P External Jugular Vein, Right			
	Q External Jugular Vein, Left			
	R Vertebral Vein, Right			
	S Vertebral Vein, Left			
	T Face Vein, Right			
	V Face Vein, Left			
	Y Upper Vein			

0: Medical and Surgical
6: Lower Veins

Operation-Character 3	Body Part-Character 4	Approach-Character 5	Device-Character 6	Qualifier-Character 7
1 Bypass	**0** Inferior Vena Cava	**0** Open	**0** Drainage Device	**0** Ultrasonic
5 Destruction	**1** Splenic Vein	**3** Percutaneous	**2** Monitoring Device	**4** Hepatic Vein
7 Dilation	**2** Gastric Vein	**4** Percutaneous Endoscopic	**3** Infusion Device	**5** Superior Mesenteric Vein
9 Drainage	**3** Esophageal Vein	**7** Via Natural or Artificial Opening	**7** Autologous Tissue Substitute	**6** Inferior Mesenteric Vein
B Excision	**4** Hepatic Vein	**8** Via Natural or Artificial Opening Endoscopic	**9** Autologous Venous Tissue	**9** Renal Vein, Right
C Extirpation	**5** Superior Mesenteric Vein	**X** External	**A** Autologous Arterial Tissue	**B** Renal Vein, Left
D Extraction	**6** Inferior Mesenteric Vein		**C** Extraluminal Device	**C** Hemorrhoidal Plexus
F Fragmentation	**7** Colic Vein		**D** Intraluminal Device	**P** Pulmonary Trunk
H Insertion	**8** Portal Vein		**J** Synthetic Substitute	**Q** Pulmonary Artery, Right
J Inspection	**9** Renal Vein, Right		**K** Nonautologous Tissue Substitute	**R** Pulmonary Artery, Left
L Occlusion	**B** Renal Vein, Left		**Y** Other Device	**T** Via Umbilical Vein
N Release	**C** Common Iliac Vein, Right		**Z** No Device	**X** Diagnostic
P Removal	**D** Common Iliac Vein, Left			**Y** Lower Vein
Q Repair	**F** External Iliac Vein, Right			**Z** No Qualifier
R Replacement	**G** External Iliac Vein, Left			
S Reposition	**H** Hypogastric Vein, Right			
U Supplement	**J** Hypogastric Vein, Left			
V Restriction	**M** Femoral Vein, Right			
W Revision	**N** Femoral Vein, Left			
	P Saphenous Vein, Right			
	Q Saphenous Vein, Left			
	T Foot Vein, Right			
	V Foot Vein, Left			
	Y Lower Vein			

0: Medical and Surgical
7: Lymphatic and Hemic Systems

Operation-Character 3	Body Part-Character 4	Approach-Character 5	Device-Character 6	Qualifier-Character 7
2 Change	**0** Lymphatic, Head	**0** Open	**0** Drainage Device	**0** Allogeneic
5 Destruction	**1** Lymphatic, Right Neck	**3** Percutaneous	**1** Radioactive Element	**1** Syngeneic
9 Drainage	**2** Lymphatic, Left Neck	**4** Percutaneous Endoscopic	**3** Infusion Device	**2** Zooplastic
B Excision	**3** Lymphatic, Right Upper Extremity	**8** Via Natural or Artificial Opening Endoscopic	**7** Autologous Tissue Substitute	**X** Diagnostic
C Extirpation	**4** Lymphatic, Left Upper Extremity	**X** External	**C** Extraluminal Device	**Z** No Qualifier
D Extraction	**5** Lymphatic, Right Axillary		**D** Intraluminal Device	
H Insertion	**6** Lymphatic, Left Axillary		**J** Synthetic Substitute	
J Inspection	**7** Lymphatic, Thorax		**K** Nonautologous Tissue Substitute	
L Occlusion	**8** Lymphatic, Internal Mammary, Right		**Y** Other Device	
N Release	**9** Lymphatic, Internal Mammary, Left		**Z** No Device	
P Removal	**B** Lymphatic, Mesenteric			
Q Repair	**C** Lymphatic, Pelvis			
S Reposition	**D** Lymphatic, Aortic			
T Resection	**F** Lymphatic, Right Lower Extremity			
U Supplement	**G** Lymphatic, Left Lower Extremity			
V Restriction	**H** Lymphatic, Right Inguinal			
W Revision	**J** Lymphatic, Left Inguinal			
Y Transplantation	**K** Thoracic Duct			
	L Cisterna Chyli			
	M Thymus			
	N Lymphatic			
	P Spleen			
	Q Bone Marrow, Sternum			
	R Bone Marrow, Iliac			
	S Bone Marrow, Vertebral			
	T Bone Marrow			

0: Medical and Surgical
8: Eye

Operation-Character 3	Body Part-Character 4	Approach-Character 5	Device-Character 6	Qualifier-Character 7
0 Alteration	**0** Eye, Right	**0** Open	**0** Drainage Device	**3** Nasal Cavity
1 Bypass	**1** Eye, Left	**3** Percutaneous	**0** Synthetic Substitute, Intraocular Telescope	**4** Sclera
2 Change	**2** Anterior Chamber, Right	**7** Via Natural or Artificial Opening	**1** Radioactive Element	**X** Diagnostic
5 Destruction	**3** Anterior Chamber, Left	**8** Via Natural or Artificial Opening Endoscopic	**3** Infusion Device	**Z** No Qualifier
7 Dilation	**4** Vitreous, Right	**X** External	**5** Epiretinal Visual Prosthesis	
9 Drainage	**5** Vitreous, Left		**7** Autologous Tissue Substitute	
B Excision	**6** Sclera, Right		**C** Extraluminal Device	
C Extirpation	**7** Sclera, Left		**D** Intraluminal Device	
D Extraction	**8** Cornea, Right		**J** Synthetic Substitute	
F Fragmentation	**9** Cornea, Left		**K** Nonautologous Tissue Substitute	
H Insertion	**A** Choroid, Right		**Y** Other Device	
J Inspection	**B** Choroid, Left		**Z** No Device	
L Occlusion	**C** Iris, Right			
M Reattachment	**D** Iris, Left			
N Release	**E** Retina, Right			
P Removal	**F** Retina, Left			
Q Repair	**G** Retinal Vessel, Right			
R Replacement	**H** Retinal Vessel, Left			
S Reposition	**J** Lens, Right			
T Resection	**K** Lens, Left			
U Supplement	**L** Extraocular Muscle, Right			
V Restriction	**M** Extraocular Muscle, Left			
W Revision	**N** Upper Eyelid, Right			
X Transfer	**P** Upper Eyelid, Left			
	Q Lower Eyelid, Right			
	R Lower Eyelid, Left			
	S Conjunctiva, Right			
	T Conjunctiva, Left			
	V Lacrimal Gland, Right			
	W Lacrimal Gland, Left			
	X Lacrimal Duct, Right			
	Y Lacrimal Duct, Left			

0: Medical and Surgical
9: Ear, Nose, Sinus

Operation-Character 3	Body Part-Character 4	Approach-Character 5	Device-Character 6	Qualifier-Character 7
0 Alteration	**0** External Ear, Right	**0** Open	**0** Drainage Device	**0** Endolymphatic
1 Bypass	**1** External Ear, Left	**3** Percutaneous	**1** Radioactive Element	**X** Diagnostic
2 Change	**2** External Ear, Bilateral	**4** Percutaneous Endoscopic	**4** Hearing Device, Bone Conduction	**Z** No Qualifier
3 Control	**3** External Auditory Canal, Right	**7** Via Natural or Artificial Opening	**5** Hearing Device, Single Channel Cochlear Prosthesis	
5 Destruction	**4** External Auditory Canal, Left	**8** Via Natural or Artificial Opening Endoscopic	**6** Hearing Device, Multiple Channel Cochlear Prosthesis	
7 Dilation	**5** Middle Ear, Right	**X** External	**7** Autologous Tissue Substitute	
8 Division	**6** Middle Ear, Left		**B** Intraluminal Device, Airway	
9 Drainage	**7** Tympanic Membrane, Right		**D** Intraluminal Device	
B Excision	**8** Tympanic Membrane, Left		**J** Synthetic Substitute	
C Extirpation	**9** Auditory Ossicle, Right		**K** Nonautologous Tissue Substitute	
D Extraction	**A** Auditory Ossicle, Left		**S** Hearing Device	
H Insertion	**B** Mastoid Sinus, Right		**Y** Other Device	
J Inspection	**C** Mastoid Sinus, Left		**Z** No Device	
M Reattachment	**D** Inner Ear, Right			
N Release	**E** Inner Ear, Left			
P Removal	**F** Eustachian Tube, Right			
Q Repair	**G** Eustachian Tube, Left			
R Replacement	**H** Ear, Right			
S Reposition	**J** Ear, Left			
T Resection	**K** Nasal Mucosa and Soft Tissue			
U Supplement	**L** Nasal Turbinate			
W Revision	**M** Nasal Septum			
	N Nasopharynx			
	P Accessory Sinus			
	Q Maxillary Sinus, Right			
	R Maxillary Sinus, Left			
	S Frontal Sinus, Right			
	T Frontal Sinus, Left			
	U Ethmoid Sinus, Right			
	V Ethmoid Sinus, Left			
	W Sphenoid Sinus, Right			
	X Sphenoid Sinus, Left			
	Y Sinus			

0: Medical and Surgical
B: Respiratory System

Operation-Character 3	Body Part-Character 4	Approach-Character 5	Device-Character 6	Qualifier-Character 7
1 Bypass	**0** Tracheobronchial Tree	**0** Open	**0** Drainage Device	**0** Allogeneic
2 Change	**1** Trachea	**3** Percutaneous	**1** Radioactive Element	**1** Syngeneic
5 Destruction	**2** Carina	**4** Percutaneous Endoscopic	**2** Monitoring Device	**2** Zooplastic
7 Dilation	**3** Main Bronchus, Right	**7** Via Natural or Artificial Opening	**3** Infusion Device	**4** Cutaneous
9 Drainage	**4** Upper Lobe Bronchus, Right	**8** Via Natural or Artificial Opening Endoscopic	**7** Autologous Tissue Substitute	**6** Esophagus
B Excision	**5** Middle Lobe Bronchus, Right	**X** External	**C** Extraluminal Device	**X** Diagnostic
C Extirpation	**6** Lower Lobe Bronchus, Right		**D** Intraluminal Device	**Z** No Qualifier
D Extraction	**7** Main Bronchus, Left		**E** Intraluminal Device, Endotracheal Airway	
F Fragmentation	**8** Upper Lobe Bronchus, Left		**F** Tracheostomy Device	
H Insertion	**9** Lingula Bronchus		**G** Intraluminal Device, Endobronchial Valve	
J Inspection	**B** Lower Lobe Bronchus, Left		**J** Synthetic Substitute	
L Occlusion	**C** Upper Lung Lobe, Right		**K** Nonautologous Tissue Substitute	
M Reattachment	**D** Middle Lung Lobe, Right		**M** Diaphragmatic Pacemaker Lead	
N Release	**F** Lower Lung Lobe, Right		**Y** Other Device	
P Removal	**G** Upper Lung Lobe, Left		**Z** No Device	
Q Repair	**H** Lung Lingula			
R Replacement	**J** Lower Lung Lobe, Left			
S Reposition	**K** Lung, Right			
T Resection	**L** Lung, Left			
U Supplement	**M** Lungs, Bilateral			
V Restriction	**N** Pleura, Right			
W Revision	**P** Pleura, Left			
Y Transplantation	**Q** Pleura			
	T Diaphragm			

0: Medical and Surgical
C: Mouth and Throat

Operation-Character 3	Body Part-Character 4	Approach-Character 5	Device-Character 6	Qualifier-Character 7
0 Alteration	**0** Upper Lip	**0** Open	**0** Drainage Device	**0** Single
2 Change	**1** Lower Lip	**3** Percutaneous	**1** Radioactive Element	**1** Multiple
5 Destruction	**2** Hard Palate	**4** Percutaneous Endoscopic	**5** External Fixation Device	**2** All
7 Dilation	**3** Soft Palate	**7** Via Natural or Artificial Opening	**7** Autologous Tissue Substitute	**X** Diagnostic
9 Drainage	**4** Buccal Mucosa	**8** Via Natural or Artificial Opening Endoscopic	**B** Intraluminal Device, Airway	**Z** No Qualifier
B Excision	**5** Upper Gingiva	**X** External	**C** Extraluminal Device	
C Extirpation	**6** Lower Gingiva		**D** Intraluminal Device	
D Extraction	**7** Tongue		**J** Synthetic Substitute	
F Fragmentation	**8** Parotid Gland, Right		**K** Nonautologous Tissue Substitute	
H Insertion	**9** Parotid Gland, Left		**Y** Other Device	
J Inspection	**A** Salivary Gland		**Z** No Device	
L Occlusion	**B** Parotid Duct, Right			
M Reattachment	**C** Parotid Duct, Left			
N Release	**D** Sublingual Gland, Right			
P Removal	**F** Sublingual Gland, Left			
Q Repair	**G** Submaxillary Gland, Right			
R Replacement	**H** Submaxillary Gland, Left			
S Reposition	**J** Minor Salivary Gland			
T Resection	**M** Pharynx			
U Supplement	**N** Uvula			
V Restriction	**P** Tonsils			
W Revision	**Q** Adenoids			
X Transfer	**R** Epiglottis			
	S Larynx			
	T Vocal Cord, Right			
	V Vocal Cord, Left			
	W Upper Tooth			
	X Lower Tooth			
	Y Mouth and Throat			

0: Medical and Surgical
D: Gastrointestinal System

Operation-Character 3	Body Part-Character 4	Approach-Character 5	Device-Character 6	Qualifier-Character 7
1 Bypass	**0** Upper Intestinal Tract	**0** Open	**0** Drainage Device	**0** Allogeneic
2 Change	**1** Esophagus, Upper	**3** Percutaneous	**1** Radioactive Element	**1** Syngeneic
5 Destruction	**2** Esophagus, Middle	**4** Percutaneous Endoscopic	**2** Monitoring Device	**2** Zooplastic
7 Dilation	**3** Esophagus, Lower	**7** Via Natural or Artificial Opening	**3** Infusion Device	**3** Vertical
8 Division	**4** Esophagogastric Junction	**8** Via Natural or Artificial Opening Endoscopic	**7** Autologous Tissue Substitute	**4** Cutaneous
9 Drainage	**5** Esophagus	**X** External	**B** Intraluminal Device, Airway	**5** Esophagus
B Excision	**6** Stomach		**C** Extraluminal Device	**6** Stomach
C Extirpation	**7** Stomach, Pylorus		**D** Intraluminal Device	**7** Vagina
D Extraction	**8** Small Intestine		**J** Synthetic Substitute	**8** Small Intestine
F Fragmentation	**9** Duodenum		**K** Nonautologous Tissue Substitute	**9** Duodenum
H Insertion	**A** Jejunum		**L** Artificial Sphincter	**A** Jejunum
J Inspection	**B** Ileum		**M** Stimulator Lead	**B** Ileum
L Occlusion	**C** Ileocecal Valve		**U** Feeding Device	**H** Cecum
M Reattachment	**D** Lower Intestinal Tract		**Y** Other Device	**K** Ascending Colon
N Release	**E** Large Intestine		**Z** No Device	**L** Transverse Colon
P Removal	**F** Large Intestine, Right			**M** Descending Colon
Q Repair	**G** Large Intestine, Left			**N** Sigmoid Colon
R Replacement	**H** Cecum			**P** Rectum
S Reposition	**J** Appendix			**Q** Anus
T Resection	**K** Ascending Colon			**X** Diagnostic
U Supplement	**L** Transverse Colon			**Z** No Qualifier
V Restriction	**M** Descending Colon			
W Revision	**N** Sigmoid Colon			
X Transfer	**P** Rectum			
Y Transplantation	**Q** Anus			
	R Anal Sphincter			
	U Omentum			
	V Mesentery			
	W Peritoneum			

0: Medical and Surgical
F: Hepatobiliary System and Pancreas

Operation-Character 3	Body Part-Character 4	Approach-Character 5	Device-Character 6	Qualifier-Character 7
1 Bypass	**0** Liver	**0** Open	**0** Drainage Device	**0** Allogeneic
2 Change	**1** Liver, Right Lobe	**3** Percutaneous	**1** Radioactive Element	**1** Syngeneic
5 Destruction	**2** Liver, Left Lobe	**4** Percutaneous Endoscopic	**2** Monitoring Device	**2** Zooplastic
7 Dilation	**4** Gallbladder	**7** Via Natural or Artificial Opening	**3** Infusion Device	**3** Duodenum
8 Division	**5** Hepatic Duct, Right	**8** Via Natural or Artificial Opening Endoscopic	**7** Autologous Tissue Substitute	**4** Stomach
9 Drainage	**6** Hepatic Duct, Left	**X** External	**C** Extraluminal Device	**5** Hepatic Duct, Right
B Excision	**7** Hepatic Duct, Common		**D** Intraluminal Device	**6** Hepatic Duct, Left
C Extirpation	**8** Cystic Duct		**J** Synthetic Substitute	**7** Hepatic Duct, Caudate
D Extraction	**9** Common Bile Duct		**K** Nonautologous Tissue Substitute	**8** Cystic Duct
F Fragmentation	**B** Hepatobiliary Duct		**Y** Other Device	**9** Common Bile Duct
H Insertion	**C** Ampulla of Vater		**Z** No Device	**B** Small Intestine
J Inspection	**D** Pancreatic Duct			**C** Large Intestine
L Occlusion	**F** Pancreatic Duct, Accessory			**F** Irreversible Electroporation
M Reattachment	**G** Pancreas			**X** Diagnostic
N Release				**Z** No Qualifier
P Removal				
Q Repair				
R Replacement				
S Reposition				
T Resection				
U Supplement				
V Restriction				
W Revision				
Y Transplantation				

0: Medical and Surgical
G: Endocrine System

Operation-Character 3	Body Part-Character 4	Approach-Character 5	Device-Character 6	Qualifier-Character 7
2 Change	**0** Pituitary Gland	**0** Open	**0** Drainage Device	**X** Diagnostic
5 Destruction	**1** Pineal Body	**3** Percutaneous	**1** Radioactive Element	**Z** No Qualifier
8 Division	**2** Adrenal Gland, Left	**4** Percutaneous Endoscopic	**2** Monitoring Device	
9 Drainage	**3** Adrenal Gland, Right	**X** External	**3** Infusion Device	
B Excision	**4** Adrenal Glands, Bilateral		**Y** Other Device	
C Extirpation	**5** Adrenal Gland		**Z** No Device	
H Insertion	**6** Carotid Body, Left			
J Inspection	**7** Carotid Body, Right			
M Reattachment	**8** Carotid Bodies, Bilateral			
N Release	**9** Para-aortic Body			
P Removal	**B** Coccygeal Glomus			
Q Repair	**C** Glomus Jugulare			
S Reposition	**D** Aortic Body			
T Resection	**F** Paraganglion Extremity			
W Revision	**G** Thyroid Gland Lobe, Left			
	H Thyroid Gland Lobe, Right			
	J Thyroid Gland Isthmus			
	K Thyroid Gland			
	L Superior Parathyroid Gland, Right			
	M Superior Parathyroid Gland, Left			
	N Inferior Parathyroid Gland, Right			
	P Inferior Parathyroid Gland, Left			
	Q Parathyroid Glands, Multiple			
	R Parathyroid Gland			
	S Endocrine Gland			

0: Medical and Surgical
H: Skin and Breast

Operation-Character 3	Body Part-Character 4	Approach-Character 5	Device-Character 6	Qualifier-Character 7
0 Alteration	**0** Skin, Scalp	**0** Open	**0** Drainage Device	**2** Cell Suspension Technique
2 Change	**1** Skin, Face	**3** Percutaneous	**1** Radioactive Element	**3** Full Thickness
5 Destruction	**2** Skin, Right Ear	**7** Via Natural or Artificial Opening	**7** Autologous Tissue Substitute	**4** Partial Thickness
8 Division	**3** Skin, Left Ear	**8** Via Natural or Artificial Opening Endoscopic	**J** Synthetic Substitute	**5** Latissimus Dorsi Myocutaneous Flap
9 Drainage	**4** Skin, Neck	**X** External	**K** Nonautologous Tissue Substitute	**6** Transverse Rectus Abdominis Myocutaneous Flap
B Excision	**5** Skin, Chest		**N** Tissue Expander	**7** Deep Inferior Epigastric Artery Perforator Flap
C Extirpation	**6** Skin, Back		**Y** Other Device	**8** Superficial Inferior Epigastric Artery Flap
D Extraction	**7** Skin, Abdomen		**Z** No Device	**9** Gluteal Artery Perforator Flap
H Insertion	**8** Skin, Buttock			**D** Multiple
J Inspection	**9** Skin, Perineum			**X** Diagnostic
M Reattachment	**A** Skin, Inguinal			**Z** No Qualifier
N Release	**B** Skin, Right Upper Arm			
P Removal	**C** Skin, Left Upper Arm			
Q Repair	**D** Skin, Right Lower Arm			
R Replacement	**E** Skin, Left Lower Arm			
S Reposition	**F** Skin, Right Hand			
T Resection	**G** Skin, Left Hand			
U Supplement	**H** Skin, Right Upper Leg			
W Revision	**J** Skin, Left Upper Leg			
X Transfer	**K** Skin, Right Lower Leg			
	L Skin, Left Lower Leg			
	M Skin, Right Foot			
	N Skin, Left Foot			
	P Skin			
	Q Finger Nail			
	R Toe Nail			
	S Hair			
	T Breast, Right			
	U Breast, Left			
	V Breast, Bilateral			
	W Nipple, Right			
	X Nipple, Left			
	Y Supernumerary Breast			

0: Medical and Surgical
J: Subcutaneous Tissue and Fascia

Operation-Character 3	Body Part-Character 4	Approach-Character 5	Device-Character 6	Qualifier-Character 7
0 Alteration	**0** Subcutaneous Tissue and Fascia, Scalp	**0** Open	**0** Drainage Device	**B** Skin and Subcutaneous Tissue
2 Change	**1** Subcutaneous Tissue and Fascia, Face	**3** Percutaneous	**0** Monitoring Device, Hemodynamic	**C** Skin, Subcutaneous Tissue and Fascia
5 Destruction	**4** Subcutaneous Tissue and Fascia, Right Neck	**X** External	**1** Radioactive Element	**X** Diagnostic
8 Division	**5** Subcutaneous Tissue and Fascia, Left Neck		**2** Monitoring Device	**Z** No Qualifier
9 Drainage	**6** Subcutaneous Tissue and Fascia, Chest		**3** Infusion Device	
B Excision	**7** Subcutaneous Tissue and Fascia, Back		**4** Pacemaker, Single Chamber	
C Extirpation	**8** Subcutaneous Tissue and Fascia, Abdomen		**5** Pacemaker, Single Chamber Rate Responsive	
D Extraction	**9** Subcutaneous Tissue and Fascia, Buttock		**6** Pacemaker, Dual Chamber	
H Insertion	**B** Subcutaneous Tissue and Fascia, Perineum		**7** Autologous Tissue Substitute	
J Inspection	**C** Subcutaneous Tissue and Fascia, Pelvic Region		**7** Cardiac Resynchronization Pacemaker Pulse Generator	
N Release	**D** Subcutaneous Tissue and Fascia, Right Upper Arm		**8** Defibrillator Generator	
P Removal	**F** Subcutaneous Tissue and Fascia, Left Upper Arm		**9** Cardiac Resynchronization Defibrillator Pulse Generator	
Q Repair	**G** Subcutaneous Tissue and Fascia, Right Lower Arm		**A** Contractility Modulation Device	
R Replacement	**H** Subcutaneous Tissue and Fascia, Left Lower Arm		**B** Stimulator Generator, Single Array	
U Supplement	**J** Subcutaneous Tissue and Fascia, Right Hand		**C** Stimulator Generator, Single Array Rechargeable	
W Revision	**K** Subcutaneous Tissue and Fascia, Left Hand		**D** Stimulator Generator, Multiple Array	
X Transfer	**L** Subcutaneous Tissue and Fascia, Right Upper Leg		**E** Stimulator Generator, Multiple Array Rechargeable	
	M Subcutaneous Tissue and Fascia, Left Upper Leg		**F** Subcutaneous Defibrillator Lead	
	N Subcutaneous Tissue and Fascia, Right Lower Leg		**H** Contraceptive Device	
	P Subcutaneous Tissue and Fascia, Left Lower Leg		**J** Synthetic Substitute	
	Q Subcutaneous Tissue and Fascia, Right Foot		**K** Nonautologous Tissue Substitute	
	R Subcutaneous Tissue and Fascia, Left Foot		**M** Stimulator Generator	
	S Subcutaneous Tissue and Fascia, Head and Neck		**N** Tissue Expander	
	T Subcutaneous Tissue and Fascia, Trunk		**P** Cardiac Rhythm Related Device	
	V Subcutaneous Tissue and Fascia, Upper Extremity		**V** Infusion Device, Pump	
	W Subcutaneous Tissue and Fascia, Lower Extremity		**W** Vascular Access Device, Totally Implantable	
			X Vascular Access Device, Tunneled	
			Y Other Device	
			Z No Device	

0: Medical and Surgical
K: Muscles

Operation-Character 3	Body Part-Character 4	Approach-Character 5	Device-Character 6	Qualifier-Character 7
2 Change	**0** Head Muscle	**0** Open	**0** Drainage Device	**0** Skin
5 Destruction	**1** Facial Muscle	**3** Percutaneous	**7** Autologous Tissue Substitute	**1** Subcutaneous Tissue
8 Division	**2** Neck Muscle, Right	**4** Percutaneous Endoscopic	**J** Synthetic Substitute	**2** Skin and Subcutaneous Tissue
9 Drainage	**3** Neck Muscle, Left	**X** External	**K** Nonautologous Tissue Substitute	**5** Latissimus Dorsi Myocutaneous Flap
B Excision	**4** Tongue, Palate, Pharynx Muscle		**M** Stimulator Lead	**6** Transverse Rectus Abdominis Myocutaneous Flap
C Extirpation	**5** Shoulder Muscle, Right		**Y** Other Device	**7** Deep Inferior Epigastric Artery Perforator Flap
D Extraction	**6** Shoulder Muscle, Left		**Z** No Device	**8** Superficial Inferior Epigastric Artery Flap
H Insertion	**7** Upper Arm Muscle, Right			**9** Gluteal Artery Perforator Flap
J Inspection	**8** Upper Arm Muscle, Left			**X** Diagnostic
M Reattachment	**9** Lower Arm and Wrist Muscle, Right			**Z** No Qualifier
N Release	**B** Lower Arm and Wrist Muscle, Left			
P Removal	**C** Hand Muscle, Right			
Q Repair	**D** Hand Muscle, Left			
R Replacement	**F** Trunk Muscle, Right			
S Reposition	**G** Trunk Muscle, Left			
T Resection	**H** Thorax Muscle, Right			
U Supplement	**J** Thorax Muscle, Left			
W Revision	**K** Abdomen Muscle, Right			
X Transfer	**L** Abdomen Muscle, Left			
	M Perineum Muscle			
	N Hip Muscle, Right			
	P Hip Muscle, Left			
	Q Upper Leg Muscle, Right			
	R Upper Leg Muscle, Left			
	S Lower Leg Muscle, Right			
	T Lower Leg Muscle, Left			
	V Foot Muscle, Right			
	W Foot Muscle, Left			
	X Upper Muscle			
	Y Lower Muscle			

0: Medical and Surgical
L: Tendons

Operation-Character 3	Body Part-Character 4	Approach-Character 5	Device-Character 6	Qualifier-Character 7
2 Change	**0** Head and Neck Tendon	**0** Open	**0** Drainage Device	**X** Diagnostic
5 Destruction	**1** Shoulder Tendon, Right	**3** Percutaneous	**7** Autologous Tissue Substitute	**Z** No Qualifier
8 Division	**2** Shoulder Tendon, Left	**4** Percutaneous Endoscopic	**J** Synthetic Substitute	
9 Drainage	**3** Upper Arm Tendon, Right	**X** External	**K** Nonautologous Tissue Substitute	
B Excision	**4** Upper Arm Tendon, Left		**Y** Other Device	
C Extirpation	**5** Lower Arm and Wrist Tendon, Right		**Z** No Device	
D Extraction	**6** Lower Arm and Wrist Tendon, Left			
H Insertion	**7** Hand Tendon, Right			
J Inspection	**8** Hand Tendon, Left			
M Reattachment	**9** Trunk Tendon, Right			
N Release	**B** Trunk Tendon, Left			
P Removal	**C** Thorax Tendon, Right			
Q Repair	**D** Thorax Tendon, Left			
R Replacement	**F** Abdomen Tendon, Right			
S Reposition	**G** Abdomen Tendon, Left			
T Resection	**H** Perineum Tendon			
U Supplement	**J** Hip Tendon, Right			
W Revision	**K** Hip Tendon, Left			
X Transfer	**L** Upper Leg Tendon, Right			
	M Upper Leg Tendon, Left			
	N Lower Leg Tendon, Right			
	P Lower Leg Tendon, Left			
	Q Knee Tendon, Right			
	R Knee Tendon, Left			
	S Ankle Tendon, Right			
	T Ankle Tendon, Left			
	V Foot Tendon, Right			
	W Foot Tendon, Left			
	X Upper Tendon			
	Y Lower Tendon			

0: Medical and Surgical
M: Bursae and Ligaments

Operation-Character 3	Body Part-Character 4	Approach-Character 5	Device-Character 6	Qualifier-Character 7
2 Change	**0** Head and Neck Bursa and Ligament	**0** Open	**0** Drainage Device	**X** Diagnostic
5 Destruction	**1** Shoulder Bursa and Ligament, Right	**3** Percutaneous	**7** Autologous Tissue Substitute	**Z** No Qualifier
8 Division	**2** Shoulder Bursa and Ligament, Left	**4** Percutaneous Endoscopic	**J** Synthetic Substitute	
9 Drainage	**3** Elbow Bursa and Ligament, Right	**X** External	**K** Nonautologous Tissue Substitute	
B Excision	**4** Elbow Bursa and Ligament, Left		**Y** Other Device	
C Extirpation	**5** Wrist Bursa and Ligament, Right		**Z** No Device	
D Extraction	**6** Wrist Bursa and Ligament, Left			
H Insertion	**7** Hand Bursa and Ligament, Right			
J Inspection	**8** Hand Bursa and Ligament, Left			
M Reattachment	**9** Upper Extremity Bursa and Ligament, Right			
N Release	**B** Upper Extremity Bursa and Ligament, Left			
P Removal	**C** Upper Spine Bursa and Ligament			
Q Repair	**D** Lower Spine Bursa and Ligament			
R Replacement	**F** Sternum Bursa and Ligament			
S Reposition	**G** Rib(s) Bursa and Ligament			
T Resection	**H** Abdomen Bursa and Ligament, Right			
U Supplement	**J** Abdomen Bursa and Ligament, Left			
W Revision	**K** Perineum Bursa and Ligament			
X Transfer	**L** Hip Bursa and Ligament, Right			
	M Hip Bursa and Ligament, Left			
	N Knee Bursa and Ligament, Right			
	P Knee Bursa and Ligament, Left			
	Q Ankle Bursa and Ligament, Right			
	R Ankle Bursa and Ligament, Left			
	S Foot Bursa and Ligament, Right			
	T Foot Bursa and Ligament, Left			
	V Lower Extremity Bursa and Ligament, Right			
	W Lower Extremity Bursa and Ligament, Left			
	X Upper Bursa and Ligament			
	Y Lower Bursa and Ligament			

0: Medical and Surgical
N: Head and Facial Bones

Operation-Character 3	Body Part-Character 4	Approach-Character 5	Device-Character 6	Qualifier-Character 7
2 Change	**0** Skull	**0** Open	**0** Drainage Device	**X** Diagnostic
5 Destruction	**1** Frontal Bone	**3** Percutaneous	**4** Internal Fixation Device	**Z** No Qualifier
8 Division	**3** Parietal Bone, Right	**4** Percutaneous Endoscopic	**5** External Fixation Device	
9 Drainage	**4** Parietal Bone, Left	**X** External	**7** Autologous Tissue Substitute	
B Excision	**5** Temporal Bone, Right		**J** Synthetic Substitute	
C Extirpation	**6** Temporal Bone, Left		**K** Nonautologous Tissue Substitute	
D Extraction	**7** Occipital Bone		**M** Bone Growth Stimulator	
H Insertion	**B** Nasal Bone		**N** Neurostimulator Generator	
J Inspection	**C** Sphenoid Bone		**S** Hearing Device	
N Release	**F** Ethmoid Bone, Right		**Y** Other Device	
P Removal	**G** Ethmoid Bone, Left		**Z** No Device	
Q Repair	**H** Lacrimal Bone, Right			
R Replacement	**J** Lacrimal Bone, Left			
S Reposition	**K** Palatine Bone, Right			
T Resection	**L** Palatine Bone, Left			
U Supplement	**M** Zygomatic Bone, Right			
W Revision	**N** Zygomatic Bone, Left			
	P Orbit, Right			
	Q Orbit, Left			
	R Maxilla			
	T Mandible, Right			
	V Mandible, Left			
	W Facial Bone			
	X Hyoid Bone			

0: Medical and Surgical
P: Upper Bones

Operation-Character 3	Body Part-Character 4	Approach-Character 5	Device-Character 6	Qualifier-Character 7
2 Change	0 Sternum	0 Open	0 Drainage Device	X Diagnostic
5 Destruction	1 Ribs, 1 to 2	3 Percutaneous	0 Internal Fixation Device, Rigid Plate	Z No Qualifier
8 Division	2 Ribs, 3 or More	4 Percutaneous Endoscopic	4 Internal Fixation Device	
9 Drainage	3 Cervical Vertebra	X External	5 External Fixation Device	
B Excision	4 Thoracic Vertebra		6 Internal Fixation Device, Intramedullary	
C Extirpation	5 Scapula, Right		7 Autologous Tissue Substitute	
D Extraction	6 Scapula, Left		8 External Fixation Device, Limb Lengthening	
H Insertion	7 Glenoid Cavity, Right		B External Fixation Device, Monoplanar	
J Inspection	8 Glenoid Cavity, Left		C External Fixation Device, Ring	
N Release	9 Clavicle, Right		D External Fixation Device, Hybrid	
P Removal	B Clavicle, Left		J Synthetic Substitute	
Q Repair	C Humeral Head, Right		K Nonautologous Tissue Substitute	
R Replacement	D Humeral Head, Left		M Bone Growth Stimulator	
S Reposition	F Humeral Shaft, Right		Y Other Device	
T Resection	G Humeral Shaft, Left		Z No Device	
U Supplement	H Radius, Right			
W Revision	J Radius, Left			
	K Ulna, Right			
	L Ulna, Left			
	M Carpal, Right			
	N Carpal, Left			
	P Metacarpal, Right			
	Q Metacarpal, Left			
	R Thumb Phalanx, Right			
	S Thumb Phalanx, Left			
	T Finger Phalanx, Right			
	V Finger Phalanx, Left			
	Y Upper Bone			

0: Medical and Surgical
Q: Lower Bones

Operation-Character 3	Body Part-Character 4	Approach-Character 5	Device-Character 6	Qualifier-Character 7
2 Change	**0** Lumbar Vertebra	**0** Open	**0** Drainage Device	**2** Sesamoid Bone(s) 1st Toe
5 Destruction	**1** Sacrum	**3** Percutaneous	**4** Internal Fixation Device	**X** Diagnostic
8 Division	**2** Pelvic Bone, Right	**4** Percutaneous Endoscopic	**5** External Fixation Device	**Z** No Qualifier
9 Drainage	**3** Pelvic Bone, Left	**X** External	**6** Internal Fixation Device, Intramedullary	
B Excision	**4** Acetabulum, Right		**7** Autologous Tissue Substitute	
C Extirpation	**5** Acetabulum, Left		**8** External Fixation Device, Limb Lengthening	
D Extraction	**6** Upper Femur, Right		**B** External Fixation Device, Monoplanar	
H Insertion	**7** Upper Femur, Left		**C** External Fixation Device, Ring	
J Inspection	**8** Femoral Shaft, Right		**D** External Fixation Device, Hybrid	
N Release	**9** Femoral Shaft, Left		**J** Synthetic Substitute	
P Removal	**B** Lower Femur, Right		**K** Nonautologous Tissue Substitute	
Q Repair	**C** Lower Femur, Left		**M** Bone Growth Stimulator	
R Replacement	**D** Patella, Right		**Y** Other Device	
S Reposition	**F** Patella, Left		**Z** No Device	
T Resection	**G** Tibia, Right			
U Supplement	**H** Tibia, Left			
W Revision	**J** Fibula, Right			
	K Fibula, Left			
	L Tarsal, Right			
	M Tarsal, Left			
	N Metatarsal, Right			
	P Metatarsal, Left			
	Q Toe Phalanx, Right			
	R Toe Phalanx, Left			
	S Coccyx			
	Y Lower Bone			

0: Medical and Surgical
R: Upper Joints

Operation-Character 3	Body Part-Character 4	Approach-Character 5	Device-Character 6	Qualifier-Character 7
2 Change	**0** Occipital-cervical Joint	**0** Open	**0** Drainage Device	**0** Anterior Approach, Anterior Column
5 Destruction	**1** Cervical Vertebral Joint	**3** Percutaneous	**0** Synthetic Substitute, Reverse Ball and Socket	**1** Posterior Approach, Posterior Column
9 Drainage	**2** Cervical Vertebral Joints, 2 or more	**4** Percutaneous Endoscopic	**3** Infusion Device	**6** Humeral Surface
B Excision	**3** Cervical Vertebral Disc	**X** External	**3** Internal Fixation Device, Sustained Compression	**7** Glenoid Surface
C Extirpation	**4** Cervicothoracic Vertebral Joint		**4** Internal Fixation Device	**J** Posterior Approach, Anterior Column
G Fusion	**5** Cervicothoracic Vertebral Disc		**5** External Fixation Device	**X** Diagnostic
H Insertion	**6** Thoracic Vertebral Joint		**7** Autologous Tissue Substitute	**Z** No Qualifier
J Inspection	**7** Thoracic Vertebral Joints, 2 to 7		**8** Spacer	
N Release	**8** Thoracic Vertebral Joints, 8 or more		**A** Interbody Fusion Device	
P Removal	**9** Thoracic Vertebral Disc		**B** Spinal Stabilization Device, Interspinous Process	
Q Repair	**A** Thoracolumbar Vertebral Joint		**C** Spinal Stabilization Device, Pedicle-Based	
R Replacement	**B** Thoracolumbar Vertebral Disc		**D** Spinal Stabilization Device, Facet Replacement	
S Reposition	**C** Temporomandibular Joint, Right		**J** Synthetic Substitute	
T Resection	**D** Temporomandibular Joint, Left		**K** Nonautologous Tissue Substitute	
U Supplement	**E** Sternoclavicular Joint, Right		**Y** Other Device	
W Revision	**F** Sternoclavicular Joint, Left		**Z** No Device	
	G Acromioclavicular Joint, Right			
	H Acromioclavicular Joint, Left			
	J Shoulder Joint, Right			
	K Shoulder Joint, Left			
	L Elbow Joint, Right			
	M Elbow Joint, Left			
	N Wrist Joint, Right			
	P Wrist Joint, Left			
	Q Carpal Joint, Right			
	R Carpal Joint, Left			
	S Carpometacarpal Joint, Right			
	T Carpometacarpal Joint, Left			
	U Metacarpophalangeal Joint, Right			
	V Metacarpophalangeal Joint, Left			
	W Finger Phalangeal Joint, Right			
	X Finger Phalangeal Joint, Left			
	Y Upper Joint			

0: Medical and Surgical
S: Lower Joints

Operation-Character 3	Body Part-Character 4	Approach-Character 5	Device-Character 6	Qualifier-Character 7
2 Change	**0** Lumbar Vertebral Joint	**0** Open	**0** Drainage Device	**0** Anterior Approach, Anterior Column
5 Destruction	**1** Lumbar Vertebral Joints, 2 or more	**3** Percutaneous	**0** Synthetic Substitute, Polyethylene	**1** Posterior Approach, Posterior Column
9 Drainage	**2** Lumbar Vertebral Disc	**4** Percutaneous Endoscopic	**1** Synthetic Substitute, Metal	**9** Cemented
B Excision	**3** Lumbosacral Joint	**X** External	**2** Synthetic Substitute, Metal on Polyethylene	**A** Uncemented
C Extirpation	**4** Lumbosacral Disc		**3** Infusion Device	**C** Patellar Surface
G Fusion	**5** Sacrococcygeal Joint		**3** Internal Fixation Device, Sustained Compression	**J** Posterior Approach, Anterior Column
H Insertion	**6** Coccygeal Joint		**3** Synthetic Substitute, Ceramic	**X** Diagnostic
J Inspection	**7** Sacroiliac Joint, Right		**4** Internal Fixation Device	**Z** No Qualifier
N Release	**8** Sacroiliac Joint, Left		**4** Synthetic Substitute, Ceramic on Polyethylene	
P Removal	**9** Hip Joint, Right		**5** External Fixation Device	
Q Repair	**A** Hip Joint, Acetabular Surface, Right		**6** Synthetic Substitute, Oxidized Zirconium on Polyethylene	
R Replacement	**B** Hip Joint, Left		**7** Autologous Tissue Substitute	
S Reposition	**C** Knee Joint, Right		**8** Spacer	
T Resection	**D** Knee Joint, Left		**9** Liner	
U Supplement	**E** Hip Joint, Acetabular Surface, Left		**A** Interbody Fusion Device	
W Revision	**F** Ankle Joint, Right		**B** Resurfacing Device	
	G Ankle Joint, Left		**B** Spinal Stabilization Device, Interspinous Process	
	H Tarsal Joint, Right		**C** Spinal Stabilization Device, Pedicle-Based	
	J Tarsal Joint, Left		**D** Spinal Stabilization Device, Facet Replacement	
	K Tarsometatarsal Joint, Right		**E** Articulating Spacer	
	L Tarsometatarsal Joint, Left		**J** Synthetic Substitute	
	M Metatarsal-Phalangeal Joint, Right		**K** Nonautologous Tissue Substitute	
	N Metatarsal-Phalangeal Joint, Left		**L** Synthetic Substitute, Unicondylar Medial	
	P Toe Phalangeal Joint, Right		**M** Synthetic Substitute, Unicondylar Lateral	
	Q Toe Phalangeal Joint, Left		**N** Synthetic Substitute, Patellofemoral	
	R Hip Joint, Femoral Surface, Right		**Y** Other Device	
	S Hip Joint, Femoral Surface, Left		**Z** No Device	
	T Knee Joint, Femoral Surface, Right			
	U Knee Joint, Femoral Surface, Left			
	V Knee Joint, Tibial Surface, Right			
	W Knee Joint, Tibial Surface, Left			
	Y Lower Joint			

0: Medical and Surgical
T: Urinary System

Operation-Character 3	Body Part-Character 4	Approach-Character 5	Device-Character 6	Qualifier-Character 7
1 Bypass	0 Kidney, Right	0 Open	0 Drainage Device	0 Allogeneic
2 Change	1 Kidney, Left	3 Percutaneous	1 Radioactive Element	1 Syngeneic
5 Destruction	2 Kidneys, Bilateral	4 Percutaneous Endoscopic	2 Monitoring Device	2 Zooplastic
7 Dilation	3 Kidney Pelvis, Right	7 Via Natural or Artificial Opening	3 Infusion Device	3 Kidney Pelvis, Right
8 Division	4 Kidney Pelvis, Left	8 Via Natural or Artificial Opening Endoscopic	7 Autologous Tissue Substitute	4 Kidney Pelvis, Left
9 Drainage	5 Kidney	X External	C Extraluminal Device	6 Ureter, Right
B Excision	6 Ureter, Right		D Intraluminal Device	7 Ureter, Left
C Extirpation	7 Ureter, Left		J Synthetic Substitute	8 Colon
D Extraction	8 Ureters, Bilateral		K Nonautologous Tissue Substitute	9 Colocutaneous
F Fragmentation	9 Ureter		L Artificial Sphincter	A Ileum
H Insertion	B Bladder		M Stimulator Lead	B Bladder
J Inspection	C Bladder Neck		Y Other Device	C Ileocutaneous
L Occlusion	D Urethra		Z No Device	D Cutaneous
M Reattachment				X Diagnostic
N Release				Z No Qualifier
P Removal				
Q Repair				
R Replacement				
S Reposition				
T Resection				
U Supplement				
V Restriction				
W Revision				
Y Transplantation				

0: Medical and Surgical
U: Female Reproductive System

Operation-Character 3	Body Part-Character 4	Approach-Character 5	Device-Character 6	Qualifier-Character 7
1 Bypass	**0** Ovary, Right	**0** Open	**0** Drainage Device	**0** Allogeneic
2 Change	**1** Ovary, Left	**3** Percutaneous	**1** Radioactive Element	**1** Syngeneic
5 Destruction	**2** Ovaries, Bilateral	**4** Percutaneous Endoscopic	**3** Infusion Device	**2** Zooplastic
7 Dilation	**3** Ovary	**7** Via Natural or Artificial Opening	**7** Autologous Tissue Substitute	**5** Fallopian Tube, Right
8 Division	**4** Uterine Supporting Structure	**8** Via Natural or Artificial Opening Endoscopic	**C** Extraluminal Device	**6** Fallopian Tube, Left
9 Drainage	**5** Fallopian Tube, Right	**F** Via Natural or Artificial Opening With Percutaneous Endoscopic Assistance	**D** Intraluminal Device	**9** Uterus
B Excision	**6** Fallopian Tube, Left	**X** External	**G** Intraluminal Device, Pessary	**L** Supracervical
C Extirpation	**7** Fallopian Tubes, Bilateral		**H** Contraceptive Device	**X** Diagnostic
D Extraction	**8** Fallopian Tube		**J** Synthetic Substitute	**Z** No Qualifier
F Fragmentation	**9** Uterus		**K** Nonautologous Tissue Substitute	
H Insertion	**B** Endometrium		**Y** Other Device	
J Inspection	**C** Cervix		**Z** No Device	
L Occlusion	**D** Uterus and Cervix			
M Reattachment	**F** Cul-de-sac			
N Release	**G** Vagina			
P Removal	**H** Vagina and Cul-de-sac			
Q Repair	**J** Clitoris			
S Reposition	**K** Hymen			
T Resection	**L** Vestibular Gland			
U Supplement	**M** Vulva			
V Restriction	**N** Ova			
W Revision				
Y Transplantation				

0: Medical and Surgical
V: Male Reproductive System

Operation-Character 3	Body Part-Character 4	Approach-Character 5	Device-Character 6	Qualifier-Character 7
1 Bypass	**0** Prostate	**0** Open	**0** Drainage Device	**0** Allogeneic
2 Change	**1** Seminal Vesicle, Right	**3** Percutaneous	**1** Radioactive Element	**1** Syngeneic
5 Destruction	**2** Seminal Vesicle, Left	**4** Percutaneous Endoscopic	**3** Infusion Device	**2** Zooplastic
7 Dilation	**3** Seminal Vesicles, Bilateral	**7** Via Natural or Artificial Opening	**7** Autologous Tissue Substitute	**D** Urethra
9 Drainage	**4** Prostate and Seminal Vesicles	**8** Via Natural or Artificial Opening Endoscopic	**C** Extraluminal Device	**J** Epididymis, Right
B Excision	**5** Scrotum	**X** External	**D** Intraluminal Device	**K** Epididymis, Left
C Extirpation	**6** Tunica Vaginalis, Right		**J** Synthetic Substitute	**N** Vas Deferens, Right
H Insertion	**7** Tunica Vaginalis, Left		**K** Nonautologous Tissue Substitute	**P** Vas Deferens, Left
J Inspection	**8** Scrotum and Tunica Vaginalis		**Y** Other Device	**S** Penis
L Occlusion	**9** Testis, Right		**Z** No Device	**X** Diagnostic
M Reattachment	**B** Testis, Left			**Z** No Qualifier
N Release	**C** Testes, Bilateral			
P Removal	**D** Testis			
Q Repair	**F** Spermatic Cord, Right			
R Replacement	**G** Spermatic Cord, Left			
S Reposition	**H** Spermatic Cords, Bilateral			
T Resection	**J** Epididymis, Right			
U Supplement	**K** Epididymis, Left			
W Revision	**L** Epididymis, Bilateral			
X Transfer	**M** Epididymis and Spermatic Cord			
Y Transplantation	**N** Vas Deferens, Right			
	P Vas Deferens, Left			
	Q Vas Deferens, Bilateral			
	R Vas Deferens			
	S Penis			
	T Prepuce			

0: Medical and Surgical
W: Anatomical Regions, General

Operation-Character 3	Body Part-Character 4	Approach-Character 5	Device-Character 6	Qualifier-Character 7
0 Alteration	**0** Head	**0** Open	**0** Drainage Device	**0** Allogeneic
1 Bypass	**1** Cranial Cavity	**3** Percutaneous	**1** Radioactive Element	**0** Vagina
2 Change	**2** Face	**4** Percutaneous Endoscopic	**3** Infusion Device	**1** Penis
3 Control	**3** Oral Cavity and Throat	**7** Via Natural or Artificial Opening	**7** Autologous Tissue Substitute	**1** Syngeneic
4 Creation	**4** Upper Jaw	**8** Via Natural or Artificial Opening Endoscopic	**J** Synthetic Substitute	**2** Stoma
8 Division	**5** Lower Jaw	**X** External	**K** Nonautologous Tissue Substitute	**4** Cutaneous
9 Drainage	**6** Neck		**Y** Other Device	**6** Bladder
B Excision	**8** Chest Wall		**Z** No Device	**9** Pleural Cavity, Right
C Extirpation	**9** Pleural Cavity, Right			**B** Pleural Cavity, Left
F Fragmentation	**B** Pleural Cavity, Left			**G** Peritoneal Cavity
H Insertion	**C** Mediastinum			**J** Pelvic Cavity
J Inspection	**D** Pericardial Cavity			**W** Upper Vein
M Reattachment	**F** Abdominal Wall			**X** Diagnostic
P Removal	**G** Peritoneal Cavity			**Y** Lower Vein
Q Repair	**H** Retroperitoneum			**Z** No Qualifier
U Supplement	**J** Pelvic Cavity			
W Revision	**K** Upper Back			
Y Transplantation	**L** Lower Back			
	M Perineum, Male			
	N Perineum, Female			
	P Gastrointestinal Tract			
	Q Respiratory Tract			
	R Genitourinary Tract			

0: Medical and Surgical
X: Anatomical Regions, Upper Extremities

Operation-Character 3	Body Part-Character 4	Approach-Character 5	Device-Character 6	Qualifier-Character 7
0 Alteration	**0** Forequarter, Right	**0** Open	**0** Drainage Device	**0** Allogeneic
2 Change	**1** Forequarter, Left	**3** Percutaneous	**1** Radioactive Element	**0** Complete
3 Control	**2** Shoulder Region, Right	**4** Percutaneous Endoscopic	**3** Infusion Device	**1** High
6 Detachment	**3** Shoulder Region, Left	**X** External	**7** Autologous Tissue Substitute	**1** Syngeneic
9 Drainage	**4** Axilla, Right		**J** Synthetic Substitute	**2** Mid
B Excision	**5** Axilla, Left		**K** Nonautologous Tissue Substitute	**3** Low
H Insertion	**6** Upper Extremity, Right		**Y** Other Device	**4** Complete 1st Ray
J Inspection	**7** Upper Extremity, Left		**Z** No Device	**5** Complete 2nd Ray
M Reattachment	**8** Upper Arm, Right			**6** Complete 3rd Ray
P Removal	**9** Upper Arm, Left			**7** Complete 4th Ray
Q Repair	**B** Elbow Region, Right			**8** Complete 5th Ray
R Replacement	**C** Elbow Region, Left			**9** Partial 1st Ray
U Supplement	**D** Lower Arm, Right			**B** Partial 2nd Ray
W Revision	**F** Lower Arm, Left			**C** Partial 3rd Ray
X Transfer	**G** Wrist Region, Right			**D** Partial 4th Ray
Y Transplantation	**H** Wrist Region, Left			**F** Partial 5th Ray
	J Hand, Right			**L** Thumb, Right
	K Hand, Left			**M** Thumb, Left
	L Thumb, Right			**N** Toe, Right
	M Thumb, Left			**P** Toe, Left
	N Index Finger, Right			**X** Diagnostic
	P Index Finger, Left			**Z** No Qualifier
	Q Middle Finger, Right			
	R Middle Finger, Left			
	S Ring Finger, Right			
	T Ring Finger, Left			
	V Little Finger, Right			
	W Little Finger, Left			

0: Medical and Surgical
Y: Anatomical Regions, Lower Extremities

Operation-Character 3	Body Part-Character 4	Approach-Character 5	Device-Character 6	Qualifier-Character 7
0 Alteration	**0** Buttock, Right	**0** Open	**0** Drainage Device	**0** Complete
2 Change	**1** Buttock, Left	**3** Percutaneous	**1** Radioactive Element	**1** High
3 Control	**2** Hindquarter, Right	**4** Percutaneous Endoscopic	**3** Infusion Device	**2** Mid
6 Detachment	**3** Hindquarter, Left	**X** External	**7** Autologous Tissue Substitute	**3** Low
9 Drainage	**4** Hindquarter, Bilateral		**J** Synthetic Substitute	**4** Complete 1st Ray
B Excision	**5** Inguinal Region, Right		**K** Nonautologous Tissue Substitute	**5** Complete 2nd Ray
H Insertion	**6** Inguinal Region, Left		**Y** Other Device	**6** Complete 3rd Ray
J Inspection	**7** Femoral Region, Right		**Z** No Device	**7** Complete 4th Ray
M Reattachment	**8** Femoral Region, Left			**8** Complete 5th Ray
P Removal	**9** Lower Extremity, Right			**9** Partial 1st Ray
Q Repair	**A** Inguinal Region, Bilateral			**B** Partial 2nd Ray
U Supplement	**B** Lower Extremity, Left			**C** Partial 3rd Ray
W Revision	**C** Upper Leg, Right			**D** Partial 4th Ray
	D Upper Leg, Left			**F** Partial 5th Ray
	E Femoral Region, Bilateral			**X** Diagnostic
	F Knee Region, Right			**Z** No Qualifier
	G Knee Region, Left			
	H Lower Leg, Right			
	J Lower Leg, Left			
	K Ankle Region, Right			
	L Ankle Region, Left			
	M Foot, Right			
	N Foot, Left			
	P 1st Toe, Right			
	Q 1st Toe, Left			
	R 2nd Toe, Right			
	S 2nd Toe, Left			
	T 3rd Toe, Right			
	U 3rd Toe, Left			
	V 4th Toe, Right			
	W 4th Toe, Left			
	X 5th Toe, Right			
	Y 5th Toe, Left			

1: Obstetrics
0: Pregnancy

Operation-Character 3	Body Part-Character 4	Approach-Character 5	Device-Character 6	Qualifier-Character 7
2 Change	**0** Products of Conception	**0** Open	**3** Monitoring Electrode	**0** High
9 Drainage	**1** Products of Conception, Retained	**3** Percutaneous	**Y** Other Device	**1** Low
A Abortion	**2** Products of Conception, Ectopic	**4** Percutaneous Endoscopic	**Z** No Device	**2** Extraperitoneal
D Extraction		**7** Via Natural or Artificial Opening		**3** Low Forceps
E Delivery		**8** Via Natural or Artificial Opening Endoscopic		**4** Mid Forceps
H Insertion		**X** External		**5** High Forceps
J Inspection				**6** Vacuum
P Removal				**7** Internal Version
Q Repair				**8** Other
S Reposition				**9** Fetal Blood
T Resection				**9** Manual
Y Transplantation				**A** Fetal Cerebrospinal Fluid
				B Fetal Fluid, Other
				C Amniotic Fluid, Therapeutic
				D Fluid, Other
				E Nervous System
				F Cardiovascular System
				G Lymphatics and Hemic
				H Eye
				J Ear, Nose and Sinus
				K Respiratory System
				L Mouth and Throat
				M Gastrointestinal System
				N Hepatobiliary and Pancreas
				P Endocrine System
				Q Skin
				R Musculoskeletal System
				S Urinary System
				T Female Reproductive System
				U Amniotic Fluid, Diagnostic
				V Male Reproductive System
				W Laminaria
				X Abortifacient
				Y Other Body System
				Z No Qualifier

3: Administration
E: Physiological Systems and Anatomical Regions

Operation-Character 3	Body System/Region-Character 4	Approach-Character 5	Substance-Character 6	Qualifier-Character 7
0 Introduction	**0** Skin and Mucous Membranes	**0** Open	**0** Antineoplastic	**0** Autologous
1 Irrigation	**1** Subcutaneous Tissue	**3** Percutaneous	**1** Thrombolytic	**0** Influenza Vaccine
	2 Muscle	**4** Percutaneous Endoscopic	**2** Anti-infective	**1** Nonautologous
	3 Peripheral Vein	**7** Via Natural or Artificial Opening	**3** Anti-inflammatory	**2** High-dose Interleukin-2
	4 Central Vein	**8** Via Natural or Artificial Opening Endoscopic	**4** Serum, Toxoid and Vaccine	**3** Low-dose Interleukin-2
	5 Peripheral Artery	**X** External	**5** Adhesion Barrier	**4** Liquid Brachytherapy Radioisotope
	6 Central Artery		**6** Nutritional Substance	**5** Other Antineoplastic
	7 Coronary Artery		**7** Electrolytic and Water Balance Substance	**6** Recombinant Human activated Protein C
	8 Heart		**8** Irrigating Substance	**7** Other Thrombolytic
	9 Nose		**9** Dialysate	**8** Oxazolidinones
	A Bone Marrow		**A** Stem Cells, Embryonic	**9** Other Anti-infective
	B Ear		**B** Anesthetic Agent	**A** Anti-Infective Envelope
	C Eye		**E** Stem Cells, Somatic	**B** Recombinant Bone Morphogenetic Protein
	D Mouth and Pharynx		**F** Intracirculatory Anesthetic	**C** Other Substance
	E Products of Conception		**G** Other Therapeutic Substance	**D** Nitric Oxide
	F Respiratory Tract		**H** Radioactive Substance	**F** Other Gas
	G Upper GI		**K** Other Diagnostic Substance	**G** Insulin
	H Lower GI		**L** Sperm	**H** Human B-type Natriuretic Peptide
	J Biliary and Pancreatic Tract		**M** Pigment	**J** Other Hormone
	K Genitourinary Tract		**N** Analgesics, Hypnotics, Sedatives	**K** Immunostimulator
	L Pleural Cavity		**P** Platelet Inhibitor	**L** Immunosuppressive
	M Peritoneal Cavity		**Q** Fertilized Ovum	**M** Monoclonal Antibody
	N Male Reproductive		**R** Antiarrhythmic	**N** Blood Brain Barrier Disruption
	P Female Reproductive		**S** Gas	**P** Clofarabine
	Q Cranial Cavity and Brain		**T** Destructive Agent	**Q** Glucarpidase
	R Spinal Canal		**U** Pancreatic Islet Cells	**X** Diagnostic
	S Epidural Space		**V** Hormone	**Y** Hyperthermic
	T Peripheral Nerves and Plexi		**W** Immunotherapeutic	**Z** No Qualifier
	U Joints		**X** Vasopressor	
	V Bones			
	W Lymphatics			
	X Cranial Nerves			
	Y Pericardial Cavity			

4: Measurement and Monitoring
A: Physiological Systems

Operation-Character 3	Body System-Character 4	Approach-Character 5	Function/Device-Character 6	Qualifier-Character 7
0 Measurement	0 Central Nervous	0 Open	0 Acuity	0 Central
1 Monitoring	1 Peripheral Nervous	3 Percutaneous	1 Capacity	1 Peripheral
	2 Cardiac	4 Percutaneous Endoscopic	2 Conductivity	2 Portal
	3 Arterial	7 Via Natural or Artificial Opening	3 Contractility	3 Pulmonary
	4 Venous	8 Via Natural or Artificial Opening Endoscopic	4 Electrical Activity	4 Stress
	5 Circulatory	X External	5 Flow	5 Ambulatory
	6 Lymphatic		6 Metabolism	6 Right Heart
	7 Visual		7 Mobility	7 Left Heart
	8 Olfactory		8 Motility	8 Bilateral
	9 Respiratory		9 Output	9 Sensory
	B Gastrointestinal		B Pressure	A Guidance
	C Biliary		C Rate	B Motor
	D Urinary		D Resistance	C Coronary
	F Musculoskeletal		F Rhythm	D Intracranial
	G Skin and Breast		G Secretion	E Compartment
	H Products of Conception, Cardiac		H Sound	F Other Thoracic
	J Products of Conception, Nervous		J Pulse	G Intraoperative
	Z None		K Temperature	H Indocyanine Green Dye
			L Volume	Z No Qualifier
			M Total Activity	
			N Sampling and Pressure	
			P Action Currents	
			Q Sleep	
			R Saturation	
			S Vascular Perfusion	

4: Measurement and Monitoring
B: Physiological Devices

Operation-Character 3	Body System-Character 4	Approach-Character 5	Function/Device-Character 6	Qualifier-Character 7
0 Measurement	0 Central Nervous	X External	S Pacemaker	Z No Qualifier
	1 Peripheral Nervous		T Defibrillator	
	2 Cardiac		V Stimulator	
	9 Respiratory			
	F Musculoskeletal			

5: Extracorporeal Assistance and Performance
A: Physiological Systems

Operation-Character 3	Body System-Character 4	Duration-Character 5	Function-Character 6	Qualifier-Character 7
0 Assistance	**2** Cardiac	**0** Single	**0** Filtration	**0** Balloon Pump
1 Performance	**5** Circulatory	**1** Intermittent	**1** Output	**1** Hyperbaric
2 Restoration	**9** Respiratory	**2** Continuous	**2** Oxygenation	**2** Manual
	C Biliary	**3** Less than 24 Consecutive Hours	**3** Pacing	**4** Nonmechanical
	D Urinary	**4** 24-96 Consecutive Hours	**4** Rhythm	**5** Pulsatile Compression
		5 Greater than 96 Consecutive Hours	**5** Ventilation	**6** Other Pump
		6 Multiple		**7** Continuous Positive Airway Pressure
		7 Intermittent, Less than 6 Hours Per Day		**8** Intermittent Positive Airway Pressure
		8 Prolonged Intermittent, 6-18 hours Per Day		**9** Continuous Negative Airway Pressure
		9 Continuous, Greater than18 hours Per Day		**A** High Nasal Flow/Velocity
		A Intraoperative		**B** Intermittent Negative Airway Pressure
				C Supersaturated
				D Impeller Pump
				F Membrane, Central
				G Membrane, Peripheral Veno-arterial
				H Membrane, Peripheral Veno-venous
				Z No Qualifier

6: Extracorporeal Therapies
A: Physiological Systems

Operation-Character 3	Body System-Character 4	Duration-Character 5	Qualifier-Character 6	Qualifier-Character 7
0 Atmospheric Control	**0** Skin	**0** Single	**B** Donor Organ	**0** Erythrocytes
1 Decompression	**1** Urinary	**1** Multiple	**Z** No Qualifier	**1** Leukocytes
2 Electromagnetic Therapy	**2** Central Nervous			**2** Platelets
3 Hyperthermia	**3** Musculoskeletal			**3** Plasma
4 Hypothermia	**5** Circulatory			**4** Head and Neck Vessels
5 Pheresis	**B** Respiratory System			**5** Heart
6 Phototherapy	**F** Hepatobiliary System and Pancreas			**6** Peripheral Vessels
7 Ultrasound Therapy	**T** Urinary System			**7** Other Vessels
8 Ultraviolet Light Therapy	**Z** None			**T** Stem Cells, Cord Blood
9 Shock Wave Therapy				**V** Stem Cells, Hematopoietic
B Perfusion				**Z** No Qualifier

7: Osteopathic
W: Anatomical Regions

Operation-Character 3	Body Region-Character 4	Approach-Character 5	Method-Character 6	Qualifier-Character 7
0 Treatment	**0** Head	**X** External	**0** Articulatory-Raising	**Z** None
	1 Cervical		**1** Fascial Release	
	2 Thoracic		**2** General Mobilization	
	3 Lumbar		**3** High Velocity-Low Amplitude	
	4 Sacrum		**4** Indirect	
	5 Pelvis		**5** Low Velocity-High Amplitude	
	6 Lower Extremities		**6** Lymphatic Pump	
	7 Upper Extremities		**7** Muscle Energy-Isometric	
	8 Rib Cage		**8** Muscle Energy-Isotonic	
	9 Abdomen		**9** Other Method	

8: Other Procedures
C: Indwelling Device

Operation-Character 3	Body Region-Character 4	Approach-Character 5	Method-Character 6	Qualifier-Character 7
0 Other Procedures	**1** Nervous System	**X** External	**6** Collection	**J** Cerebrospinal Fluid
	2 Circulatory System			**K** Blood
				L Other Fluid

8: Other Procedures
E: Physiological Systems and Anatomical Regions

Operation-Character 3	Body Region-Character 4	Approach-Character 5	Method-Character 6	Qualifier-Character 7
0 Other Procedures	**1** Nervous System	**0** Open	**0** Acupuncture	**0** Anesthesia
	2 Circulatory System	**3** Percutaneous	**1** Therapeutic Massage	**1** In Vitro Fertilization
	9 Head and Neck Region	**4** Percutaneous Endoscopic	**6** Collection	**2** Breast Milk
	H Integumentary System and Breast	**7** Via Natural or Artificial Opening	**B** Computer Assisted Procedure	**3** Sperm
	K Musculoskeletal System	**8** Via Natural or Artificial Opening Endoscopic	**C** Robotic Assisted Procedure	**4** Yoga Therapy
	U Female Reproductive System	**X** External	**D** Near Infrared Spectroscopy	**5** Meditation
	V Male Reproductive System		**E** Fluorescence Guided Procedure	**6** Isolation
	W Trunk Region		**Y** Other Method	**7** Examination
	X Upper Extremity			**8** Suture Removal
	Y Lower Extremity			**9** Piercing
	Z None			**C** Prostate
				D Rectum
				F With Fluoroscopy
				G With Computerized Tomography
				H With Magnetic Resonance Imaging
				M Aminolevulinic Acid
				Z No Qualifier

9: Chiropractic
W: Anatomical Regions

Operation-Character 3	Body Region-Character 4	Approach-Character 5	Method-Character 6	Qualifier-Character 7
B Manipulation	**0** Head	**X** External	**B** Non-Manual	**Z** None
	1 Cervical		**C** Indirect Visceral	
	2 Thoracic		**D** Extra-Articular	
	3 Lumbar		**F** Direct Visceral	
	4 Sacrum		**G** Long Lever Specific Contact	
	5 Pelvis		**H** Short Lever Specific Contact	
	6 Lower Extremities		**J** Long and Short Lever Specific Contact	
	7 Upper Extremities		**K** Mechanically Assisted	
	8 Rib Cage		**L** Other Method	
	9 Abdomen			

B: Imaging
0: Central Nervous System

Type-Character 3	Body Part-Character 4	Contrast-Character 5	Qualifier-Character 6	Qualifier-Character 7
0 Plain Radiography	**0** Brain	**0** High Osmolar	**0** Unenhanced and Enhanced	**Z** None
1 Fluoroscopy	**7** Cisterna	**1** Low Osmolar	**Z** None	
2 Computerized Tomography (CT Scan)	**8** Cerebral Ventricle(s)	**Y** Other Contrast		
3 Magnetic Resonance Imaging (MRI)	**9** Sella Turcica/Pituitary Gland	**Z** None		
4 Ultrasonography	**B** Spinal Cord			
	C Acoustic Nerves			

B: Imaging
2: Heart

Type-Character 3	Body Part-Character 4	Contrast-Character 5	Qualifier-Character 6	Qualifier-Character 7
0 Plain Radiography	**0** Coronary Artery, Single	**0** High Osmolar	**0** Unenhanced and Enhanced	**0** Intraoperative
1 Fluoroscopy	**1** Coronary Arteries, Multiple	**1** Low Osmolar	**1** Laser	**3** Intravascular
2 Computerized Tomography (CT Scan)	**2** Coronary Artery Bypass Graft, Single	**Y** Other Contrast	**2** Intravascular Optical Coherence	**4** Transesophageal
3 Magnetic Resonance Imaging (MRI)	**3** Coronary Artery Bypass Grafts, Multiple	**Z** None	**Z** None	**Z** None
4 Ultrasonography	**4** Heart, Right			
	5 Heart, Left			
	6 Heart, Right and Left			
	7 Internal Mammary Bypass Graft, Right			
	8 Internal Mammary Bypass Graft, Left			
	B Heart with Aorta			
	C Pericardium			
	D Pediatric Heart			
	F Bypass Graft, Other			

B: Imaging
3: Upper Arteries

Type-Character 3	Body Part-Character 4	Contrast-Character 5	Qualifier-Character 6	Qualifier-Character 7
0 Plain Radiography	**0** Thoracic Aorta	**0** High Osmolar	**0** Unenhanced and Enhanced	**0** Intraoperative
1 Fluoroscopy	**1** Brachiocephalic-Subclavian Artery, Right	**1** Low Osmolar	**1** Laser	**3** Intravascular
2 Computerized Tomography (CT Scan)	**2** Subclavian Artery, Left	**Y** Other Contrast	**2** Intravascular Optical Coherence	**Z** None
3 Magnetic Resonance Imaging (MRI)	**3** Common Carotid Artery, Right	**Z** None	**Z** None	
4 Ultrasonography	**4** Common Carotid Artery, Left			
	5 Common Carotid Arteries, Bilateral			
	6 Internal Carotid Artery, Right			
	7 Internal Carotid Artery, Left			
	8 Internal Carotid Arteries, Bilateral			
	9 External Carotid Artery, Right			
	B External Carotid Artery, Left			
	C External Carotid Arteries, Bilateral			
	D Vertebral Artery, Right			
	F Vertebral Artery, Left			
	G Vertebral Arteries, Bilateral			
	H Upper Extremity Arteries, Right			
	J Upper Extremity Arteries, Left			
	K Upper Extremity Arteries, Bilateral			
	L Intercostal and Bronchial Arteries			
	M Spinal Arteries			
	N Upper Arteries, Other			
	P Thoraco-Abdominal Aorta			
	Q Cervico-Cerebral Arch			
	R Intracranial Arteries			
	S Pulmonary Artery, Right			
	T Pulmonary Artery, Left			
	U Pulmonary Trunk			
	V Ophthalmic Arteries			

B: Imaging
4: Lower Arteries

Type-Character 3	Body Part-Character 4	Contrast-Character 5	Qualifier-Character 6	Qualifier-Character 7
0 Plain Radiography	**0** Abdominal Aorta	**0** High Osmolar	**0** Unenhanced and Enhanced	**0** Intraoperative
1 Fluoroscopy	**1** Celiac Artery	**1** Low Osmolar	**1** Laser	**3** Intravascular
2 Computerized Tomography (CT Scan)	**2** Hepatic Artery	**Y** Other Contrast	**2** Intravascular Optical Coherence	**Z** None
3 Magnetic Resonance Imaging (MRI)	**3** Splenic Arteries	**Z** None	**Z** None	
4 Ultrasonography	**4** Superior Mesenteric Artery			
	5 Inferior Mesenteric Artery			
	6 Renal Artery, Right			
	7 Renal Artery, Left			
	8 Renal Arteries, Bilateral			
	9 Lumbar Arteries			
	B Intra-Abdominal Arteries, Other			
	C Pelvic Arteries			
	D Aorta and Bilateral Lower Extremity Arteries			
	F Lower Extremity Arteries, Right			
	G Lower Extremity Arteries, Left			
	H Lower Extremity Arteries, Bilateral			
	J Lower Arteries, Other			
	K Celiac and Mesenteric Arteries			
	L Femoral Artery			
	M Renal Artery Transplant			
	N Penile Arteries			

B: Imaging
5: Veins

Type-Character 3	Body Part-Character 4	Contrast-Character 5	Qualifier-Character 6	Qualifier-Character 7
0 Plain Radiography	**0** Epidural Veins	**0** High Osmolar	**0** Unenhanced and Enhanced	**3** Intravascular
1 Fluoroscopy	**1** Cerebral and Cerebellar Veins	**1** Low Osmolar	**2** Intravascular Optical Coherence	**A** Guidance
2 Computerized Tomography (CT Scan)	**2** Intracranial Sinuses	**Y** Other Contrast	**Z** None	**Z** None
3 Magnetic Resonance Imaging (MRI)	**3** Jugular Veins, Right	**Z** None		
4 Ultrasonography	**4** Jugular Veins, Left			
	5 Jugular Veins, Bilateral			
	6 Subclavian Vein, Right			
	7 Subclavian Vein, Left			
	8 Superior Vena Cava			
	9 Inferior Vena Cava			
	B Lower Extremity Veins, Right			
	C Lower Extremity Veins, Left			
	D Lower Extremity Veins, Bilateral			
	F Pelvic (Iliac) Veins, Right			
	G Pelvic (Iliac) Veins, Left			
	H Pelvic (Iliac) Veins, Bilateral			
	J Renal Vein, Right			
	K Renal Vein, Left			
	L Renal Veins, Bilateral			
	M Upper Extremity Veins, Right			
	N Upper Extremity Veins, Left			
	P Upper Extremity Veins, Bilateral			
	Q Pulmonary Vein, Right			
	R Pulmonary Vein, Left			
	S Pulmonary Veins, Bilateral			
	T Portal and Splanchnic Veins			
	V Veins, Other			
	W Dialysis Shunt/Fistula			

B: Imaging
7: Lymphatic System

Type-Character 3	Body Part-Character 4	Contrast-Character 5	Qualifier-Character 6	Qualifier-Character 7
0 Plain Radiography	**0** Abdominal/Retroperitoneal Lymphatics, Unilateral	**0** High Osmolar	**Z** None	**Z** None
	1 Abdominal/Retroperitoneal Lymphatics, Bilateral	**1** Low Osmolar		
	4 Lymphatics, Head and Neck	**Y** Other Contrast		
	5 Upper Extremity Lymphatics, Right			
	6 Upper Extremity Lymphatics, Left			
	7 Upper Extremity Lymphatics, Bilateral			
	8 Lower Extremity Lymphatics, Right			
	9 Lower Extremity Lymphatics, Left			
	B Lower Extremity Lymphatics, Bilateral			
	C Lymphatics, Pelvic			

B: Imaging
8: Eye

Type-Character 3	Body Part-Character 4	Contrast-Character 5	Qualifier-Character 6	Qualifier-Character 7
0 Plain Radiography	**0** Lacrimal Duct, Right	**0** High Osmolar	**0** Unenhanced and Enhanced	**Z** None
2 Computerized Tomography (CT Scan)	**1** Lacrimal Duct, Left	**1** Low Osmolar	**Z** None	
3 Magnetic Resonance Imaging (MRI)	**2** Lacrimal Ducts, Bilateral	**Y** Other Contrast		
4 Ultrasonography	**3** Optic Foramina, Right	**Z** None		
	4 Optic Foramina, Left			
	5 Eye, Right			
	6 Eye, Left			
	7 Eyes, Bilateral			

B: Imaging
9: Ear, Nose, Mouth and Throat

Type-Character 3	Body Part-Character 4	Contrast-Character 5	Qualifier-Character 6	Qualifier-Character 7
0 Plain Radiography	**0** Ear	**0** High Osmolar	**0** Unenhanced and Enhanced	**Z** None
1 Fluoroscopy	**2** Paranasal Sinuses	**1** Low Osmolar	**Z** None	
2 Computerized Tomography (CT Scan)	**4** Parotid Gland, Right	**Y** Other Contrast		
3 Magnetic Resonance Imaging (MRI)	**5** Parotid Gland, Left	**Z** None		
	6 Parotid Glands, Bilateral			
	7 Submandibular Gland, Right			
	8 Submandibular Gland, Left			
	9 Submandibular Glands, Bilateral			
	B Salivary Gland, Right			
	C Salivary Gland, Left			
	D Salivary Glands, Bilateral			
	F Nasopharynx/Oropharynx			
	G Pharynx and Epiglottis			
	H Mastoids			
	J Larynx			

B: Imaging
B: Respiratory System

Type-Character 3	Body Part-Character 4	Contrast-Character 5	Qualifier-Character 6	Qualifier-Character 7
0 Plain Radiography	**2** Lung, Right	**0** High Osmolar	**0** Unenhanced and Enhanced	**Z** None
1 Fluoroscopy	**3** Lung, Left	**1** Low Osmolar	**Z** None	
2 Computerized Tomography (CT Scan)	**4** Lungs, Bilateral	**Y** Other Contrast		
3 Magnetic Resonance Imaging (MRI)	**6** Diaphragm	**Z** None		
4 Ultrasonography	**7** Tracheobronchial Tree, Right			
	8 Tracheobronchial Tree, Left			
	9 Tracheobronchial Trees, Bilateral			
	B Pleura			
	C Mediastinum			
	D Upper Airways			
	F Trachea/Airways			
	G Lung Apices			

B: Imaging
D: Gastrointestinal System

Type-Character 3	Body Part-Character 4	Contrast-Character 5	Qualifier-Character 6	Qualifier-Character 7
1 Fluoroscopy	**1** Esophagus	**0** High Osmolar	**0** Unenhanced and Enhanced	**Z** None
2 Computerized Tomography (CT Scan)	**2** Stomach	**1** Low Osmolar	**Z** None	
4 Ultrasonography	**3** Small Bowel	**Y** Other Contrast		
	4 Colon	**Z** None		
	5 Upper GI			
	6 Upper GI and Small Bowel			
	7 Gastrointestinal Tract			
	8 Appendix			
	9 Duodenum			
	B Mouth/Oropharynx			
	C Rectum			

B: Imaging
F: Hepatobiliary System and Pancreas

Type-Character 3	Body Part-Character 4	Contrast-Character 5	Qualifier-Character 6	Qualifier-Character 7
0 Plain Radiography	**0** Bile Ducts	**0** High Osmolar	**0** Unenhanced and Enhanced	**Z** None
1 Fluoroscopy	**1** Biliary and Pancreatic Ducts	**1** Low Osmolar	**Z** None	
2 Computerized Tomography (CT Scan)	**2** Gallbladder	**2** Fluorescing Agent		
3 Magnetic Resonance Imaging (MRI)	**3** Gallbladder and Bile Ducts	**Y** Other Contrast		
4 Ultrasonography	**4** Gallbladder, Bile Ducts and Pancreatic Ducts	**Z** None		
5 Other Imaging	**5** Liver			
	6 Liver and Spleen			
	7 Pancreas			
	8 Pancreatic Ducts			
	C Hepatobiliary System, All			

B: Imaging
G: Endocrine System

Type-Character 3	Body Part-Character 4	Contrast-Character 5	Qualifier-Character 6	Qualifier-Character 7
2 Computerized Tomography (CT Scan)	**0** Adrenal Gland, Right	**0** High Osmolar	**0** Unenhanced and Enhanced	**Z** None
3 Magnetic Resonance Imaging (MRI)	**1** Adrenal Gland, Left	**1** Low Osmolar	**Z** None	
4 Ultrasonography	**2** Adrenal Glands, Bilateral	**Y** Other Contrast		
	3 Parathyroid Glands	**Z** None		
	4 Thyroid Gland			

B: Imaging
H: Skin, Subcutaneous Tissue and Breast

Type-Character 3	Body Part-Character 4	Contrast-Character 5	Qualifier-Character 6	Qualifier-Character 7
0 Plain Radiography	**0** Breast, Right	**0** High Osmolar	**0** Unenhanced and Enhanced	**Z** None
3 Magnetic Resonance Imaging (MRI)	**1** Breast, Left	**1** Low Osmolar	**Z** None	
4 Ultrasonography	**2** Breasts, Bilateral	**Y** Other Contrast		
	3 Single Mammary Duct, Right	**Z** None		
	4 Single Mammary Duct, Left			
	5 Multiple Mammary Ducts, Right			
	6 Multiple Mammary Ducts, Left			
	7 Extremity, Upper			
	8 Extremity, Lower			
	9 Abdominal Wall			
	B Chest Wall			
	C Head and Neck			
	D Subcutaneous Tissue, Head/Neck			
	F Subcutaneous Tissue, Upper Extremity			
	G Subcutaneous Tissue, Thorax			
	H Subcutaneous Tissue, Abdomen and Pelvis			
	J Subcutaneous Tissue, Lower Extremity			

B: Imaging
L: Connective Tissue

Type-Character 3	Body Part-Character 4	Contrast-Character 5	Qualifier-Character 6	Qualifier-Character 7
3 Magnetic Resonance Imaging (MRI)	**0** Connective Tissue, Upper Extremity	**Y** Other Contrast	**0** Unenhanced and Enhanced	**Z** None
4 Ultrasonography	**1** Connective Tissue, Lower Extremity	**Z** None	**Z** None	
	2 Tendons, Upper Extremity			
	3 Tendons, Lower Extremity			

B: Imaging
N: Skull and Facial Bones

Type-Character 3	Body Part-Character 4	Contrast-Character 5	Qualifier-Character 6	Qualifier-Character 7
0 Plain Radiography	**0** Skull	**0** High Osmolar	**Z** None	**Z** None
1 Fluoroscopy	**1** Orbit, Right	**1** Low Osmolar		
2 Computerized Tomography (CT Scan)	**2** Orbit, Left	**Y** Other Contrast		
3 Magnetic Resonance Imaging (MRI)	**3** Orbits, Bilateral	**Z** None		
	4 Nasal Bones			
	5 Facial Bones			
	6 Mandible			
	7 Temporomandibular Joint, Right			
	8 Temporomandibular Joint, Left			
	9 Temporomandibular Joints, Bilateral			
	B Zygomatic Arch, Right			
	C Zygomatic Arch, Left			
	D Zygomatic Arches, Bilateral			
	F Temporal Bones			
	G Tooth, Single			
	H Teeth, Multiple			
	J Teeth, All			

B: Imaging
P: Non-Axial Upper Bones

Type-Character 3	Body Part-Character 4	Contrast-Character 5	Qualifier-Character 6	Qualifier-Character 7
0 Plain Radiography	**0** Sternoclavicular Joint, Right	**0** High Osmolar	**0** Unenhanced and Enhanced	**1** Densitometry
1 Fluoroscopy	**1** Sternoclavicular Joint, Left	**1** Low Osmolar	**Z** None	**Z** None
2 Computerized Tomography (CT Scan)	**2** Sternoclavicular Joints, Bilateral	**Y** Other Contrast		
3 Magnetic Resonance Imaging (MRI)	**3** Acromioclavicular Joints, Bilateral	**Z** None		
4 Ultrasonography	**4** Clavicle, Right			
	5 Clavicle, Left			
	6 Scapula, Right			
	7 Scapula, Left			
	8 Shoulder, Right			
	9 Shoulder, Left			
	A Humerus, Right			
	B Humerus, Left			
	C Hand/Finger Joint, Right			
	D Hand/Finger Joint, Left			
	E Upper Arm, Right			
	F Upper Arm, Left			
	G Elbow, Right			
	H Elbow, Left			
	J Forearm, Right			
	K Forearm, Left			
	L Wrist, Right			
	M Wrist, Left			
	N Hand, Right			
	P Hand, Left			
	Q Hands and Wrists, Bilateral			
	R Finger(s), Right			
	S Finger(s), Left			
	T Upper Extremity, Right			
	U Upper Extremity, Left			
	V Upper Extremities, Bilateral			
	W Thorax			
	X Ribs, Right			
	Y Ribs, Left			

B: Imaging
Q: Non-Axial Lower Bones

Type-Character 3	Body Part-Character 4	Contrast-Character 5	Qualifier-Character 6	Qualifier-Character 7
0 Plain Radiography	**0** Hip, Right	**0** High Osmolar	**0** Unenhanced and Enhanced	**1** Densitometry
1 Fluoroscopy	**1** Hip, Left	**1** Low Osmolar	**Z** None	**Z** None
2 Computerized Tomography (CT Scan)	**2** Hips, Bilateral	**Y** Other Contrast		
3 Magnetic Resonance Imaging (MRI)	**3** Femur, Right	**Z** None		
4 Ultrasonography	**4** Femur, Left			
	7 Knee, Right			
	8 Knee, Left			
	9 Knees, Bilateral			
	B Tibia/Fibula, Right			
	C Tibia/Fibula, Left			
	D Lower Leg, Right			
	F Lower Leg, Left			
	G Ankle, Right			
	H Ankle, Left			
	J Calcaneus, Right			
	K Calcaneus, Left			
	L Foot, Right			
	M Foot, Left			
	P Toe(s), Right			
	Q Toe(s), Left			
	R Lower Extremity, Right			
	S Lower Extremity, Left			
	V Patella, Right			
	W Patella, Left			
	X Foot/Toe Joint, Right			
	Y Foot/Toe Joint, Left			

B: Imaging
R: Axial Skeleton, Except Skull and Facial Bones

Type-Character 3	Body Part-Character 4	Contrast-Character 5	Qualifier-Character 6	Qualifier-Character 7
0 Plain Radiography	**0** Cervical Spine	**0** High Osmolar	**0** Unenhanced and Enhanced	**1** Densitometry
1 Fluoroscopy	**1** Cervical Disc(s)	**1** Low Osmolar	**Z** None	**Z** None
2 Computerized Tomography (CT Scan)	**2** Thoracic Disc(s)	**Y** Other Contrast		
3 Magnetic Resonance Imaging (MRI)	**3** Lumbar Disc(s)	**Z** None		
4 Ultrasonography	**4** Cervical Facet Joint(s)			
	5 Thoracic Facet Joint(s)			
	6 Lumbar Facet Joint(s)			
	7 Thoracic Spine			
	8 Thoracolumbar Joint			
	9 Lumbar Spine			
	B Lumbosacral Joint			
	C Pelvis			
	D Sacroiliac Joints			
	F Sacrum and Coccyx			
	G Whole Spine			
	H Sternum			

B: Imaging
T: Urinary System

Type-Character 3	Body Part-Character 4	Contrast-Character 5	Qualifier-Character 6	Qualifier-Character 7
0 Plain Radiography	**0** Bladder	**0** High Osmolar	**0** Unenhanced and Enhanced	**Z** None
1 Fluoroscopy	**1** Kidney, Right	**1** Low Osmolar	**Z** None	
2 Computerized Tomography (CT Scan)	**2** Kidney, Left	**Y** Other Contrast		
3 Magnetic Resonance Imaging (MRI)	**3** Kidneys, Bilateral	**Z** None		
4 Ultrasonography	**4** Kidneys, Ureters and Bladder			
	5 Urethra			
	6 Ureter, Right			
	7 Ureter, Left			
	8 Ureters, Bilateral			
	9 Kidney Transplant			
	B Bladder and Urethra			
	C Ileal Diversion Loop			
	D Kidney, Ureter and Bladder, Right			
	F Kidney, Ureter and Bladder, Left			
	G Ileal Loop, Ureters and Kidneys			
	J Kidneys and Bladder			

B: Imaging
U: Female Reproductive System

Type-Character 3	Body Part-Character 4	Contrast-Character 5	Qualifier-Character 6	Qualifier-Character 7
0 Plain Radiography	**0** Fallopian Tube, Right	**0** High Osmolar	**0** Unenhanced and Enhanced	**Z** None
1 Fluoroscopy	**1** Fallopian Tube, Left	**1** Low Osmolar	**Z** None	
3 Magnetic Resonance Imaging (MRI)	**2** Fallopian Tubes, Bilateral	**Y** Other Contrast		
4 Ultrasonography	**3** Ovary, Right	**Z** None		
	4 Ovary, Left			
	5 Ovaries, Bilateral			
	6 Uterus			
	8 Uterus and Fallopian Tubes			
	9 Vagina			
	B Pregnant Uterus			
	C Uterus and Ovaries			

B: Imaging
V: Male Reproductive System

Type-Character 3	Body Part-Character 4	Contrast-Character 5	Qualifier-Character 6	Qualifier-Character 7
0 Plain Radiography	**0** Corpora Cavernosa	**0** High Osmolar	**0** Unenhanced and Enhanced	**Z** None
1 Fluoroscopy	**1** Epididymis, Right	**1** Low Osmolar	**Z** None	
2 Computerized Tomography (CT Scan)	**2** Epididymis, Left	**Y** Other Contrast		
3 Magnetic Resonance Imaging (MRI)	**3** Prostate	**Z** None		
4 Ultrasonography	**4** Scrotum			
	5 Testicle, Right			
	6 Testicle, Left			
	7 Testicles, Bilateral			
	8 Vasa Vasorum			
	9 Prostate and Seminal Vesicles			
	B Penis			

B: Imaging
W: Anatomical Regions

Type-Character 3	Body Part-Character 4	Contrast-Character 5	Qualifier-Character 6	Qualifier-Character 7
0 Plain Radiography	**0** Abdomen	**0** High Osmolar	**0** Unenhanced and Enhanced	**Z** None
1 Fluoroscopy	**1** Abdomen and Pelvis	**1** Low Osmolar	**1** Bacterial Autofluorescence	
2 Computerized Tomography (CT Scan)	**2** Trunk	**Y** Other Contrast	**Z** None	
3 Magnetic Resonance Imaging (MRI)	**3** Chest	**Z** None		
4 Ultrasonography	**4** Chest and Abdomen			
5 Other Imaging	**5** Chest, Abdomen and Pelvis			
	8 Head			
	9 Head and Neck			
	B Long Bones, All			
	C Lower Extremity			
	F Neck			
	G Pelvic Region			
	H Retroperitoneum			
	J Upper Extremity			
	K Whole Body			
	L Whole Skeleton			
	M Whole Body, Infant			
	P Brachial Plexus			

B: Imaging
Y: Fetus and Obstetrical

Type-Character 3	Body Part-Character 4	Contrast-Character 5	Qualifier-Character 6	Qualifier-Character 7
3 Magnetic Resonance Imaging (MRI)	0 Fetal Head	Y Other Contrast	0 Unenhanced and Enhanced	Z None
4 Ultrasonography	1 Fetal Heart	Z None	Z None	
	2 Fetal Thorax			
	3 Fetal Abdomen			
	4 Fetal Spine			
	5 Fetal Extremities			
	6 Whole Fetus			
	7 Fetal Umbilical Cord			
	8 Placenta			
	9 First Trimester, Single Fetus			
	B First Trimester, Multiple Gestation			
	C Second Trimester, Single Fetus			
	D Second Trimester, Multiple Gestation			
	F Third Trimester, Single Fetus			
	G Third Trimester, Multiple Gestation			

C: Nuclear Medicine
0: Central Nervous System

Type-Character 3	Body Part-Character 4	Radionuclide-Character 5	Qualifier-Character 6	Qualifier-Character 7
1 Planar Nuclear Medicine Imaging	0 Brain	1 Technetium 99m (Tc-99m)	Z None	Z None
2 Tomographic (Tomo) Nuclear Medicine Imaging	5 Cerebrospinal Fluid	B Carbon 11 (C-11)		
3 Positron Emission Tomographic (PET) Imaging	Y Central Nervous System	D Indium 111 (In-111)		
5 Nonimaging Nuclear Medicine Probe		F Iodine 123 (I-123)		
		K Fluorine 18 (F-18)		
		M Oxygen 15 (O-15)		
		S Thallium 201 (Tl-201)		
		V Xenon 133 (Xe-133)		
		Y Other Radionuclide		

C: Nuclear Medicine
2: Heart

Type-Character 3	Body Part-Character 4	Radionuclide-Character 5	Qualifier-Character 6	Qualifier-Character 7
1 Planar Nuclear Medicine Imaging	6 Heart, Right and Left	1 Technetium 99m (Tc-99m)	Z None	Z None
2 Tomographic (Tomo) Nuclear Medicine Imaging	G Myocardium	D Indium 111 (In-111)		
3 Positron Emission Tomographic (PET) Imaging	Y Heart	K Fluorine 18 (F-18)		
5 Nonimaging Nuclear Medicine Probe		M Oxygen 15 (O-15)		
		Q Rubidium 82 (Rb-82)		
		R Nitrogen 13 (N-13)		
		S Thallium 201 (Tl-201)		
		Y Other Radionuclide		
		Z None		

C: Nuclear Medicine
5: Veins

Type-Character 3	Body Part-Character 4	Radionuclide-Character 5	Qualifier-Character 6	Qualifier-Character 7
1 Planar Nuclear Medicine Imaging	**B** Lower Extremity Veins, Right	**1** Technetium 99m (Tc-99m)	**Z** None	**Z** None
	C Lower Extremity Veins, Left	**Y** Other Radionuclide		
	D Lower Extremity Veins, Bilateral			
	N Upper Extremity Veins, Right			
	P Upper Extremity Veins, Left			
	Q Upper Extremity Veins, Bilateral			
	R Central Veins			
	Y Veins			

C: Nuclear Medicine
7: Lymphatic and Hematologic System

Type-Character 3	Body Part-Character 4	Radionuclide-Character 5	Qualifier-Character 6	Qualifier-Character 7
1 Planar Nuclear Medicine Imaging	**0** Bone Marrow	**1** Technetium 99m (Tc-99m)	**Z** None	**Z** None
2 Tomographic (Tomo) Nuclear Medicine Imaging	**2** Spleen	**7** Cobalt 58 (Co-58)		
5 Nonimaging Nuclear Medicine Probe	**3** Blood	**C** Cobalt 57 (Co-57)		
6 Nonimaging Nuclear Medicine Assay	**5** Lymphatics, Head and Neck	**D** Indium 111 (In-111)		
	D Lymphatics, Pelvic	**H** Iodine 125 (I-125)		
	J Lymphatics, Head	**W** Chromium (Cr-51)		
	K Lymphatics, Neck	**Y** Other Radionuclide		
	L Lymphatics, Upper Chest			
	M Lymphatics, Trunk			
	N Lymphatics, Upper Extremity			
	P Lymphatics, Lower Extremity			
	Y Lymphatic and Hematologic System			

C: Nuclear Medicine
8: Eye

Type-Character 3	Body Part-Character 4	Radionuclide-Character 5	Qualifier-Character 6	Qualifier-Character 7
1 Planar Nuclear Medicine Imaging	**9** Lacrimal Ducts, Bilateral	**1** Technetium 99m (Tc-99m)	**Z** None	**Z** None
	Y Eye	**Y** Other Radionuclide		

C: Nuclear Medicine
9: Ear, Nose, Mouth and Throat

Type-Character 3	Body Part-Character 4	Radionuclide-Character 5	Qualifier-Character 6	Qualifier-Character 7
1 Planar Nuclear Medicine Imaging	**B** Salivary Glands, Bilateral	**1** Technetium 99m (Tc-99m)	**Z** None	**Z** None
	Y Ear, Nose, Mouth and Throat	**Y** Other Radionuclide		

C: Nuclear Medicine
B: Respiratory System

Type-Character 3	Body Part-Character 4	Radionuclide-Character 5	Qualifier-Character 6	Qualifier-Character 7
1 Planar Nuclear Medicine Imaging	**2** Lungs and Bronchi	**1** Technetium 99m (Tc-99m)	**Z** None	**Z** None
2 Tomographic (Tomo) Nuclear Medicine Imaging	**Y** Respiratory System	**9** Krypton (Kr-81m)		
3 Positron Emission Tomographic (PET) Imaging		**K** Fluorine 18 (F-18)		
		T Xenon 127 (Xe-127)		
		V Xenon 133 (Xe-133)		
		Y Other Radionuclide		

C: Nuclear Medicine
D: Gastrointestinal System

Type-Character 3	Body Part-Character 4	Radionuclide-Character 5	Qualifier-Character 6	Qualifier-Character 7
1 Planar Nuclear Medicine Imaging	**5** Upper Gastrointestinal Tract	**1** Technetium 99m (Tc-99m)	**Z** None	**Z** None
2 Tomographic (Tomo) Nuclear Medicine Imaging	**7** Gastrointestinal Tract	**D** Indium 111 (In-111)		
	Y Digestive System	**Y** Other Radionuclide		

C: Nuclear Medicine
F: Hepatobiliary System and Pancreas

Type-Character 3	Body Part-Character 4	Radionuclide-Character 5	Qualifier-Character 6	Qualifier-Character 7
1 Planar Nuclear Medicine Imaging	**4** Gallbladder	**1** Technetium 99m (Tc-99m)	**Z** None	**Z** None
2 Tomographic (Tomo) Nuclear Medicine Imaging	**5** Liver	**Y** Other Radionuclide		
	6 Liver and Spleen			
	C Hepatobiliary System, All			
	Y Hepatobiliary System and Pancreas			

C: Nuclear Medicine
G: Endocrine System

Type-Character 3	Body Part-Character 4	Radionuclide-Character 5	Qualifier-Character 6	Qualifier-Character 7
1 Planar Nuclear Medicine Imaging	**1** Parathyroid Glands	**1** Technetium 99m (Tc-99m)	**Z** None	**Z** None
2 Tomographic (Tomo) Nuclear Medicine Imaging	**2** Thyroid Gland	**F** Iodine 123 (I-123)		
4 Nonimaging Nuclear Medicine Uptake	**4** Adrenal Glands, Bilateral	**G** Iodine 131 (I-131)		
	Y Endocrine System	**S** Thallium 201 (Tl-201)		
		Y Other Radionuclide		

C: Nuclear Medicine
H: Skin, Subcutaneous Tissue and Breast

Type-Character 3	Body Part-Character 4	Radionuclide-Character 5	Qualifier-Character 6	Qualifier-Character 7
1 Planar Nuclear Medicine Imaging	**0** Breast, Right	**1** Technetium 99m (Tc-99m)	**Z** None	**Z** None
2 Tomographic (Tomo) Nuclear Medicine Imaging	**1** Breast, Left	**S** Thallium 201 (Tl-201)		
	2 Breasts, Bilateral	**Y** Other Radionuclide		
	Y Skin, Subcutaneous Tissue and Breast			

C: Nuclear Medicine
P: Musculoskeletal System

Type-Character 3	Body Part-Character 4	Radionuclide-Character 5	Qualifier-Character 6	Qualifier-Character 7
1 Planar Nuclear Medicine Imaging	**1** Skull	**1** Technetium 99m (Tc-99m)	**Z** None	**Z** None
2 Tomographic (Tomo) Nuclear Medicine Imaging	**2** Cervical Spine	**Y** Other Radionuclide		
5 Nonimaging Nuclear Medicine Probe	**3** Skull and Cervical Spine	**Z** None		
	4 Thorax			
	5 Spine			
	6 Pelvis			
	7 Spine and Pelvis			
	8 Upper Extremity, Right			
	9 Upper Extremity, Left			
	B Upper Extremities, Bilateral			
	C Lower Extremity, Right			
	D Lower Extremity, Left			
	F Lower Extremities, Bilateral			
	G Thoracic Spine			
	H Lumbar Spine			
	J Thoracolumbar Spine			
	N Upper Extremities			
	P Lower Extremities			
	Y Musculoskeletal System, Other			
	Z Musculoskeletal System, All			

C: Nuclear Medicine
T: Urinary System

Type-Character 3	Body Part-Character 4	Radionuclide-Character 5	Qualifier-Character 6	Qualifier-Character 7
1 Planar Nuclear Medicine Imaging	**3** Kidneys, Ureters and Bladder	**1** Technetium 99m (Tc-99m)	**Z** None	**Z** None
2 Tomographic (Tomo) Nuclear Medicine Imaging	**H** Bladder and Ureters	**F** Iodine 123 (I-123)		
6 Nonimaging Nuclear Medicine Assay	**Y** Urinary System	**G** Iodine 131 (I-131)		
		H Iodine 125 (I-125)		
		Y Other Radionuclide		

C: Nuclear Medicine
V: Male Reproductive System

Type-Character 3	Body Part-Character 4	Radionuclide-Character 5	Qualifier-Character 6	Qualifier-Character 7
1 Planar Nuclear Medicine Imaging	**9** Testicles, Bilateral	**1** Technetium 99m (Tc-99m)	**Z** None	**Z** None
	Y Male Reproductive System	**Y** Other Radionuclide		

C: Nuclear Medicine
W: Anatomical Regions

Type-Character 3	Body Part-Character 4	Radionuclide-Character 5	Qualifier-Character 6	Qualifier-Character 7
1 Planar Nuclear Medicine Imaging	0 Abdomen	1 Technetium 99m (Tc-99m)	Z None	Z None
2 Tomographic (Tomo) Nuclear Medicine Imaging	1 Abdomen and Pelvis	8 Samarium 153 (Sm-153)		
3 Positron Emission Tomographic (PET) Imaging	3 Chest	D Indium 111 (In-111)		
5 Nonimaging Nuclear Medicine Probe	4 Chest and Abdomen	F Iodine 123 (I-123)		
7 Systemic Nuclear Medicine Therapy	6 Chest and Neck	G Iodine 131 (I-131)		
	B Head and Neck	K Fluorine 18 (F-18)		
	D Lower Extremity	L Gallium 67 (Ga-67)		
	G Thyroid	N Phosphorus 32 (P-32)		
	J Pelvic Region	P Strontium 89 (Sr-89)		
	M Upper Extremity	S Thallium 201 (Tl-201)		
	N Whole Body	Y Other Radionuclide		
	Y Anatomical Regions, Multiple	Z None		
	Z Anatomical Region, Other			

D: Radiation Therapy
0: Central and Peripheral Nervous System

Modality-Character 3	Treatment Site -Character 4	Modality Qualifier-Character 5	Isotope -Character 6	Qualifier-Character 7
0 Beam Radiation	0 Brain	0 Photons <1 MeV	6 Cesium 131 (Cs-131)	0 Intraoperative
1 Brachytherapy	1 Brain Stem	1 Photons 1 - 10 MeV	7 Cesium 137 (Cs-137)	1 Unidirectional Source
2 Stereotactic Radiosurgery	6 Spinal Cord	2 Photons >10 MeV	8 Iridium 192 (Ir-192)	Z None
Y Other Radiation	7 Peripheral Nerve	3 Electrons	9 Iodine 125 (I-125)	
		4 Heavy Particles (Protons, Ions)	B Palladium 103 (Pd-103)	
		5 Neutrons	C Californium 252 (Cf-252)	
		6 Neutron Capture	Y Other Isotope	
		7 Contact Radiation	Z None	
		8 Hyperthermia		
		9 High Dose Rate (HDR)		
		B Low Dose Rate (LDR)		
		C Intraoperative Radiation Therapy (IORT)		
		D Stereotactic Other Photon Radiosurgery		
		F Plaque Radiation		
		H Stereotactic Particulate Radiosurgery		
		J Stereotactic Gamma Beam Radiosurgery		
		K Laser Interstitial Thermal Therapy		

D: Radiation Therapy
7: Lymphatic and Hematologic System

Modality-Character 3	Treatment Site -Character 4	Modality Qualifier-Character 5	Isotope -Character 6	Qualifier-Character 7
0 Beam Radiation	**0** Bone Marrow	**0** Photons <1 MeV	**6** Cesium 131 (Cs-131)	**0** Intraoperative
1 Brachytherapy	**1** Thymus	**1** Photons 1 - 10 MeV	**7** Cesium 137 (Cs-137)	**1** Unidirectional Source
2 Stereotactic Radiosurgery	**2** Spleen	**2** Photons >10 MeV	**8** Iridium 192 (Ir-192)	**Z** None
Y Other Radiation	**3** Lymphatics, Neck	**3** Electrons	**9** Iodine 125 (I-125)	
	4 Lymphatics, Axillary	**4** Heavy Particles (Protons, Ions)	**B** Palladium 103 (Pd-103)	
	5 Lymphatics, Thorax	**5** Neutrons	**C** Californium 252 (Cf-252)	
	6 Lymphatics, Abdomen	**6** Neutron Capture	**Y** Other Isotope	
	7 Lymphatics, Pelvis	**8** Hyperthermia	**Z** None	
	8 Lymphatics, Inguinal	**9** High Dose Rate (HDR)		
		B Low Dose Rate (LDR)		
		D Stereotactic Other Photon Radiosurgery		
		F Plaque Radiation		
		H Stereotactic Particulate Radiosurgery		
		J Stereotactic Gamma Beam Radiosurgery		

D: Radiation Therapy
8: Eye

Modality-Character 3	Treatment Site -Character 4	Modality Qualifier-Character 5	Isotope -Character 6	Qualifier-Character 7
0 Beam Radiation	**0** Eye	**0** Photons <1 MeV	**6** Cesium 131 (Cs-131)	**0** Intraoperative
1 Brachytherapy		**1** Photons 1 - 10 MeV	**7** Cesium 137 (Cs-137)	**1** Unidirectional Source
2 Stereotactic Radiosurgery		**2** Photons >10 MeV	**8** Iridium 192 (Ir-192)	**Z** None
Y Other Radiation		**3** Electrons	**9** Iodine 125 (I-125)	
		4 Heavy Particles (Protons, Ions)	**B** Palladium 103 (Pd-103)	
		5 Neutrons	**C** Californium 252 (Cf-252)	
		6 Neutron Capture	**Y** Other Isotope	
		7 Contact Radiation	**Z** None	
		8 Hyperthermia		
		9 High Dose Rate (HDR)		
		B Low Dose Rate (LDR)		
		D Stereotactic Other Photon Radiosurgery		
		F Plaque Radiation		
		H Stereotactic Particulate Radiosurgery		
		J Stereotactic Gamma Beam Radiosurgery		

D: Radiation Therapy
9: Ear, Nose, Mouth and Throat

Modality-Character 3	Treatment Site -Character 4	Modality Qualifier-Character 5	Isotope -Character 6	Qualifier-Character 7
0 Beam Radiation	**0** Ear	**0** Photons <1 MeV	**6** Cesium 131 (Cs-131)	**0** Intraoperative
1 Brachytherapy	**1** Nose	**1** Photons 1 - 10 MeV	**7** Cesium 137 (Cs-137)	**1** Unidirectional Source
2 Stereotactic Radiosurgery	**3** Hypopharynx	**2** Photons >10 MeV	**8** Iridium 192 (Ir-192)	**Z** None
Y Other Radiation	**4** Mouth	**3** Electrons	**9** Iodine 125 (I-125)	
	5 Tongue	**4** Heavy Particles (Protons, Ions)	**B** Palladium 103 (Pd-103)	
	6 Salivary Glands	**5** Neutrons	**C** Californium 252 (Cf-252)	
	7 Sinuses	**6** Neutron Capture	**Y** Other Isotope	
	8 Hard Palate	**7** Contact Radiation	**Z** None	
	9 Soft Palate	**8** Hyperthermia		
	B Larynx	**9** High Dose Rate (HDR)		
	C Pharynx	**B** Low Dose Rate (LDR)		
	D Nasopharynx	**C** Intraoperative Radiation Therapy (IORT)		
	F Oropharynx	**D** Stereotactic Other Photon Radiosurgery		
		F Plaque Radiation		
		H Stereotactic Particulate Radiosurgery		
		J Stereotactic Gamma Beam Radiosurgery		

D: Radiation Therapy
B: Respiratory System

Modality-Character 3	Treatment Site -Character 4	Modality Qualifier-Character 5	Isotope -Character 6	Qualifier-Character 7
0 Beam Radiation	**0** Trachea	**0** Photons <1 MeV	**6** Cesium 131 (Cs-131)	**0** Intraoperative
1 Brachytherapy	**1** Bronchus	**1** Photons 1 - 10 MeV	**7** Cesium 137 (Cs-137)	**1** Unidirectional Source
2 Stereotactic Radiosurgery	**2** Lung	**2** Photons >10 MeV	**8** Iridium 192 (Ir-192)	**Z** None
Y Other Radiation	**5** Pleura	**3** Electrons	**9** Iodine 125 (I-125)	
	6 Mediastinum	**4** Heavy Particles (Protons, Ions)	**B** Palladium 103 (Pd-103)	
	7 Chest Wall	**5** Neutrons	**C** Californium 252 (Cf-252)	
	8 Diaphragm	**6** Neutron Capture	**Y** Other Isotope	
		7 Contact Radiation	**Z** None	
		8 Hyperthermia		
		9 High Dose Rate (HDR)		
		B Low Dose Rate (LDR)		
		D Stereotactic Other Photon Radiosurgery		
		F Plaque Radiation		
		H Stereotactic Particulate Radiosurgery		
		J Stereotactic Gamma Beam Radiosurgery		
		K Laser Interstitial Thermal Therapy		

D: Radiation Therapy
D: Gastrointestinal System

Modality-Character 3	Treatment Site -Character 4	Modality Qualifier-Character 5	Isotope -Character 6	Qualifier-Character 7
0 Beam Radiation	**0** Esophagus	**0** Photons <1 MeV	**6** Cesium 131 (Cs-131)	**0** Intraoperative
1 Brachytherapy	**1** Stomach	**1** Photons 1 - 10 MeV	**7** Cesium 137 (Cs-137)	**1** Unidirectional Source
2 Stereotactic Radiosurgery	**2** Duodenum	**2** Photons >10 MeV	**8** Iridium 192 (Ir-192)	**Z** None
Y Other Radiation	**3** Jejunum	**3** Electrons	**9** Iodine 125 (I-125)	
	4 Ileum	**4** Heavy Particles (Protons, Ions)	**B** Palladium 103 (Pd-103)	
	5 Colon	**5** Neutrons	**C** Californium 252 (Cf-252)	
	7 Rectum	**6** Neutron Capture	**Y** Other Isotope	
	8 Anus	**7** Contact Radiation	**Z** None	
		8 Hyperthermia		
		9 High Dose Rate (HDR)		
		B Low Dose Rate (LDR)		
		C Intraoperative Radiation Therapy (IORT)		
		D Stereotactic Other Photon Radiosurgery		
		F Plaque Radiation		
		H Stereotactic Particulate Radiosurgery		
		J Stereotactic Gamma Beam Radiosurgery		
		K Laser Interstitial Thermal Therapy		

D: Radiation Therapy
F: Hepatobiliary System and Pancreas

Modality-Character 3	Treatment Site -Character 4	Modality Qualifier-Character 5	Isotope -Character 6	Qualifier-Character 7
0 Beam Radiation	**0** Liver	**0** Photons <1 MeV	**6** Cesium 131 (Cs-131)	**0** Intraoperative
1 Brachytherapy	**1** Gallbladder	**1** Photons 1 - 10 MeV	**7** Cesium 137 (Cs-137)	**1** Unidirectional Source
2 Stereotactic Radiosurgery	**2** Bile Ducts	**2** Photons >10 MeV	**8** Iridium 192 (Ir-192)	**Z** None
Y Other Radiation	**3** Pancreas	**3** Electrons	**9** Iodine 125 (I-125)	
		4 Heavy Particles (Protons, Ions)	**B** Palladium 103 (Pd-103)	
		5 Neutrons	**C** Californium 252 (Cf-252)	
		6 Neutron Capture	**Y** Other Isotope	
		7 Contact Radiation	**Z** None	
		8 Hyperthermia		
		9 High Dose Rate (HDR)		
		B Low Dose Rate (LDR)		
		C Intraoperative Radiation Therapy (IORT)		
		D Stereotactic Other Photon Radiosurgery		
		F Plaque Radiation		
		H Stereotactic Particulate Radiosurgery		
		J Stereotactic Gamma Beam Radiosurgery		
		K Laser Interstitial Thermal Therapy		

D: Radiation Therapy
G: Endocrine System

Modality-Character 3	Treatment Site -Character 4	Modality Qualifier-Character 5	Isotope -Character 6	Qualifier-Character 7
0 Beam Radiation	**0** Pituitary Gland	**0** Photons <1 MeV	**6** Cesium 131 (Cs-131)	**0** Intraoperative
1 Brachytherapy	**1** Pineal Body	**1** Photons 1 - 10 MeV	**7** Cesium 137 (Cs-137)	**1** Unidirectional Source
2 Stereotactic Radiosurgery	**2** Adrenal Glands	**2** Photons >10 MeV	**8** Iridium 192 (Ir-192)	**Z** None
Y Other Radiation	**4** Parathyroid Glands	**3** Electrons	**9** Iodine 125 (I-125)	
	5 Thyroid	**5** Neutrons	**B** Palladium 103 (Pd-103)	
		6 Neutron Capture	**C** Californium 252 (Cf-252)	
		7 Contact Radiation	**Y** Other Isotope	
		8 Hyperthermia	**Z** None	
		9 High Dose Rate (HDR)		
		B Low Dose Rate (LDR)		
		D Stereotactic Other Photon Radiosurgery		
		F Plaque Radiation		
		H Stereotactic Particulate Radiosurgery		
		J Stereotactic Gamma Beam Radiosurgery		
		K Laser Interstitial Thermal Therapy		

D: Radiation Therapy
H: Skin

Modality- Character 3	Treatment Site -Character 4	Modality Qualifier- Character 5	Isotope -Character 6	Qualifier-Character 7
0 Beam Radiation	**2** Skin, Face	**0** Photons <1 MeV	**Z** None	**0** Intraoperative
Y Other Radiation	**3** Skin, Neck	**1** Photons 1 - 10 MeV		**Z** None
	4 Skin, Arm	**2** Photons >10 MeV		
	5 Skin, Hand	**3** Electrons		
	6 Skin, Chest	**4** Heavy Particles (Protons, Ions)		
	7 Skin, Back	**5** Neutrons		
	8 Skin, Abdomen	**6** Neutron Capture		
	9 Skin, Buttock	**7** Contact Radiation		
	B Skin, Leg	**8** Hyperthermia		
	C Skin, Foot	**F** Plaque Radiation		

D: Radiation Therapy
M: Breast

Modality- Character 3	Treatment Site -Character 4	Modality Qualifier- Character 5	Isotope -Character 6	Qualifier-Character 7
0 Beam Radiation	**0** Breast, Left	**0** Photons <1 MeV	**6** Cesium 131 (Cs-131)	**0** Intraoperative
1 Brachytherapy	**1** Breast, Right	**1** Photons 1 - 10 MeV	**7** Cesium 137 (Cs-137)	**1** Unidirectional Source
2 Stereotactic Radiosurgery		**2** Photons >10 MeV	**8** Iridium 192 (Ir-192)	**Z** None
Y Other Radiation		**3** Electrons	**9** Iodine 125 (I-125)	
		4 Heavy Particles (Protons, Ions)	**B** Palladium 103 (Pd-103)	
		5 Neutrons	**C** Californium 252 (Cf-252)	
		6 Neutron Capture	**Y** Other Isotope	
		7 Contact Radiation	**Z** None	
		8 Hyperthermia		
		9 High Dose Rate (HDR)		
		B Low Dose Rate (LDR)		
		D Stereotactic Other Photon Radiosurgery		
		F Plaque Radiation		
		H Stereotactic Particulate Radiosurgery		
		J Stereotactic Gamma Beam Radiosurgery		
		K Laser Interstitial Thermal Therapy		

D: Radiation Therapy
P: Musculoskeletal System

Modality- Character 3	Treatment Site -Character 4	Modality Qualifier- Character 5	Isotope -Character 6	Qualifier-Character 7
0 Beam Radiation	**0** Skull	**0** Photons <1 MeV	**Z** None	**0** Intraoperative
Y Other Radiation	**2** Maxilla	**1** Photons 1 - 10 MeV		**Z** None
	3 Mandible	**2** Photons >10 MeV		
	4 Sternum	**3** Electrons		
	5 Rib(s)	**4** Heavy Particles (Protons, Ions)		
	6 Humerus	**5** Neutrons		
	7 Radius/Ulna	**6** Neutron Capture		
	8 Pelvic Bones	**7** Contact Radiation		
	9 Femur	**8** Hyperthermia		
	B Tibia/Fibula	**F** Plaque Radiation		
	C Other Bone			

D: Radiation Therapy
T: Urinary System

Modality-Character 3	Treatment Site -Character 4	Modality Qualifier-Character 5	Isotope -Character 6	Qualifier-Character 7
0 Beam Radiation	0 Kidney	0 Photons <1 MeV	6 Cesium 131 (Cs-131)	0 Intraoperative
1 Brachytherapy	1 Ureter	1 Photons 1 - 10 MeV	7 Cesium 137 (Cs-137)	1 Unidirectional Source
2 Stereotactic Radiosurgery	2 Bladder	2 Photons >10 MeV	8 Iridium 192 (Ir-192)	Z None
Y Other Radiation	3 Urethra	3 Electrons	9 Iodine 125 (I-125)	
		4 Heavy Particles (Protons, Ions)	B Palladium 103 (Pd-103)	
		5 Neutrons	C Californium 252 (Cf-252)	
		6 Neutron Capture	Y Other Isotope	
		7 Contact Radiation	Z None	
		8 Hyperthermia		
		9 High Dose Rate (HDR)		
		B Low Dose Rate (LDR)		
		C Intraoperative Radiation Therapy (IORT)		
		D Stereotactic Other Photon Radiosurgery		
		F Plaque Radiation		
		H Stereotactic Particulate Radiosurgery		
		J Stereotactic Gamma Beam Radiosurgery		

D: Radiation Therapy
U: Female Reproductive System

Modality-Character 3	Treatment Site -Character 4	Modality Qualifier-Character 5	Isotope -Character 6	Qualifier-Character 7
0 Beam Radiation	0 Ovary	0 Photons <1 MeV	6 Cesium 131 (Cs-131)	0 Intraoperative
1 Brachytherapy	1 Cervix	1 Photons 1 - 10 MeV	7 Cesium 137 (Cs-137)	1 Unidirectional Source
2 Stereotactic Radiosurgery	2 Uterus	2 Photons >10 MeV	8 Iridium 192 (Ir-192)	Z None
Y Other Radiation		3 Electrons	9 Iodine 125 (I-125)	
		4 Heavy Particles (Protons, Ions)	B Palladium 103 (Pd-103)	
		5 Neutrons	C Californium 252 (Cf-252)	
		6 Neutron Capture	Y Other Isotope	
		7 Contact Radiation	Z None	
		8 Hyperthermia		
		9 High Dose Rate (HDR)		
		B Low Dose Rate (LDR)		
		C Intraoperative Radiation Therapy (IORT)		
		D Stereotactic Other Photon Radiosurgery		
		F Plaque Radiation		
		H Stereotactic Particulate Radiosurgery		
		J Stereotactic Gamma Beam Radiosurgery		

D: Radiation Therapy
V: Male Reproductive System

Modality- Character 3	Treatment Site -Character 4	Modality Qualifier- Character 5	Isotope -Character 6	Qualifier-Character 7
0 Beam Radiation	**0** Prostate	**0** Photons <1 MeV	**6** Cesium 131 (Cs-131)	**0** Intraoperative
1 Brachytherapy	**1** Testis	**1** Photons 1 - 10 MeV	**7** Cesium 137 (Cs-137)	**1** Unidirectional Source
2 Stereotactic Radiosurgery		**2** Photons >10 MeV	**8** Iridium 192 (Ir-192)	**Z** None
Y Other Radiation		**3** Electrons	**9** Iodine 125 (I-125)	
		4 Heavy Particles (Protons, Ions)	**B** Palladium 103 (Pd-103)	
		5 Neutrons	**C** Californium 252 (Cf-252)	
		6 Neutron Capture	**Y** Other Isotope	
		7 Contact Radiation	**Z** None	
		8 Hyperthermia		
		9 High Dose Rate (HDR)		
		B Low Dose Rate (LDR)		
		C Intraoperative Radiation Therapy (IORT)		
		D Stereotactic Other Photon Radiosurgery		
		F Plaque Radiation		
		H Stereotactic Particulate Radiosurgery		
		J Stereotactic Gamma Beam Radiosurgery		

D: Radiation Therapy
W: Anatomical Regions

Modality- Character 3	Treatment Site -Character 4	Modality Qualifier- Character 5	Isotope -Character 6	Qualifier-Character 7
0 Beam Radiation	**1** Head and Neck	**0** Photons <1 MeV	**6** Cesium 131 (Cs-131)	**0** Intraoperative
1 Brachytherapy	**2** Chest	**1** Photons 1 - 10 MeV	**7** Cesium 137 (Cs-137)	**1** Unidirectional Source
2 Stereotactic Radiosurgery	**3** Abdomen	**2** Photons >10 MeV	**8** Iridium 192 (Ir-192)	**Z** None
Y Other Radiation	**4** Hemibody	**3** Electrons	**9** Iodine 125 (I-125)	
	5 Whole Body	**4** Heavy Particles (Protons, Ions)	**B** Palladium 103 (Pd-103)	
	6 Pelvic Region	**5** Neutrons	**C** Californium 252 (Cf-252)	
		6 Neutron Capture	**D** Iodine 131 (I-131)	
		7 Contact Radiation	**F** Phosphorus 32 (P-32)	
		8 Hyperthermia	**G** Strontium 89 (Sr-89)	
		9 High Dose Rate (HDR)	**H** Strontium 90 (Sr-90)	
		B Low Dose Rate (LDR)	**Y** Other Isotope	
		D Stereotactic Other Photon Radiosurgery	**Z** None	
		F Plaque Radiation		
		G Isotope Administration		
		H Stereotactic Particulate Radiosurgery		
		J Stereotactic Gamma Beam Radiosurgery		

F: Physical Rehabilitation and Diagnostic Audiology
0: Rehabilitation

Type-Character 3	Body System/Region-Character 4	Type Qualifier-Character 5	Equipment-Character 6	Qualifier-Character 7
0 Speech Assessment	**0** Neurological System - Head and Neck	**0** Bathing/Showering	**1** Audiometer	**Z** None
1 Motor and/or Nerve Function Assessment	**1** Neurological System - Upper Back / Upper Extremity	**0** Bathing/Showering Technique	**2** Sound Field / Booth	
2 Activities of Daily Living Assessment	**2** Neurological System - Lower Back / Lower Extremity	**0** Bathing/Showering Techniques	**4** Electroacoustic Immittance / Acoustic Reflex	
6 Speech Treatment	**3** Neurological System - Whole Body	**0** Cochlear Implant Rehabilitation	**5** Hearing Aid Selection / Fitting / Test	
7 Motor Treatment	**4** Circulatory System - Head and Neck	**0** Filtered Speech	**7** Electrophysiologic	
8 Activities of Daily Living Treatment	**5** Circulatory System - Upper Back / Upper Extremity	**0** Hearing and Related Disorders Counseling	**8** Vestibular / Balance	
9 Hearing Treatment	**6** Circulatory System - Lower Back / Lower Extremity	**0** Muscle Performance	**9** Cochlear Implant	
B Cochlear Implant Treatment	**7** Circulatory System - Whole Body	**0** Nonspoken Language	**B** Physical Agents	
C Vestibular Treatment	**8** Respiratory System - Head and Neck	**0** Range of Motion and Joint Mobility	**C** Mechanical	
D Device Fitting	**9** Respiratory System - Upper Back / Upper Extremity	**0** Tinnitus Masker	**D** Electrotherapeutic	
F Caregiver Training	**B** Respiratory System - Lower Back / Lower Extremity	**0** Vestibular	**E** Orthosis	
	C Respiratory System - Whole Body	**1** Dressing	**F** Assistive, Adaptive, Supportive or Protective	
	D Integumentary System - Head and Neck	**1** Dressing Techniques	**G** Aerobic Endurance and Conditioning	
	F Integumentary System - Upper Back / Upper Extremity	**1** Hearing and Related Disorders Prevention	**H** Mechanical or Electromechanical	
	G Integumentary System -Lower Back / Lower Extremity	**1** Integumentary Integrity	**J** Somatosensory	
	H Integumentary System - Whole Body	**1** Monaural Hearing Aid	**K** Audiovisual	
	J Musculoskeletal System - Head and Neck	**1** Muscle Performance	**L** Assistive Listening	
	K Musculoskeletal System - Upper Back / Upper Extremity	**1** Perceptual Processing	**M** Augmentative / Alternative Communication	
	L Musculoskeletal System - Lower Back / Lower Extremity	**1** Speech Threshold	**N** Biosensory Feedback	
	M Musculoskeletal System - Whole Body	**1** Speech-Language Pathology and Related Disorders Counseling	**P** Computer	
	N Genitourinary System	**2** Auditory Processing	**Q** Speech Analysis	
	Z None	**2** Binaural Hearing Aid	**S** Voice Analysis	
		2 Coordination/Dexterity	**T** Aerodynamic Function	
		2 Feeding and Eating	**U** Prosthesis	
		2 Feeding/Eating	**V** Speech Prosthesis	
		2 Grooming/Personal Hygiene	**W** Swallowing	
		2 Speech/Word Recognition	**X** Cerumen Management	
		2 Speech-Language Pathology and Related Disorders Prevention	**Y** Other Equipment	
		2 Visual Motor Integration	**Z** None	
		3 Aphasia		
		3 Augmentative/Alternative Communication System		
		3 Cerumen Management		
		3 Coordination/Dexterity		

Table continued on next page

Table continued from previous page

Type-Character 3	Body System/Region-Character 4	Type Qualifier-Character 5	Equipment-Character 6	Qualifier-Character 7
		3 Feeding/Eating		
		3 Grooming/Personal Hygiene		
		3 Motor Function		
		3 Postural Control		
		3 Staggered Spondaic Word		
		4 Articulation/Phonology		
		4 Bed Mobility		
		4 Home Management		
		4 Motor Function		
		4 Sensorineural Acuity Level		
		4 Voice Prosthetic		
		4 Wheelchair Mobility		
		5 Assistive Listening Device		
		5 Aural Rehabilitation		
		5 Bed Mobility		
		5 Perceptual Processing		
		5 Range of Motion and Joint Integrity		
		5 Synthetic Sentence Identification		
		5 Transfer		
		5 Wound Management		
		6 Communicative/Cognitive Integration Skills		
		6 Dynamic Orthosis		
		6 Psychosocial Skills		
		6 Sensory Awareness/Processing/Integrity		
		6 Speech and/or Language Screening		
		6 Therapeutic Exercise		
		6 Wheelchair Mobility		
		7 Aerobic Capacity and Endurance		
		7 Facial Nerve Function		
		7 Fluency		
		7 Manual Therapy Techniques		
		7 Nonspoken Language		
		7 Static Orthosis		
		7 Therapeutic Exercise		
		7 Vocational Activities and Functional Community or Work Reintegration Skills		
		8 Airway Clearance Techniques		
		8 Anthropometric Characteristics		
		8 Motor Speech		
		8 Prosthesis		
		8 Receptive/Expressive Language		
		8 Transfer Training		
		9 Articulation/Phonology		
		9 Assistive, Adaptive, Supportive or Protective Devices		
		9 Cranial Nerve Integrity		
		9 Gait Training/Functional Ambulation		
		9 Orofacial Myofunctional		
		9 Somatosensory Evoked Potentials		

Table continued on next page

Table continued from previous page

Type-Character 3	Body System/Region-Character 4	Type Qualifier-Character 5	Equipment-Character 6	Qualifier-Character 7
		9 Wound Management		
		B Bed Mobility		
		B Environmental, Home and Work Barriers		
		B Motor Speech		
		B Receptive/Expressive Language		
		B Vocational Activities and Functional Community or Work Reintegration Skills		
		C Aphasia		
		C Ergonomics and Body Mechanics		
		C Gait Training/Functional Ambulation		
		C Transfer		
		C Voice		
		D Application, Proper Use and Care of Devices		
		D Fluency		
		D Gait and/or Balance		
		D Neuromotor Development		
		D Swallowing Dysfunction		
		F Application, Proper Use and Care of Orthoses		
		F Pain		
		F Voice		
		F Wheelchair Mobility		
		G Application, Proper Use and Care of Prosthesis		
		G Communicative/Cognitive Integration Skills		
		G Reflex Integrity		
		G Ventilation, Respiration and Circulation		
		H Bedside Swallowing and Oral Function		
		H Home Management		
		H Vocational Activities and Functional Community or Work Reintegration Skills		
		J Communication Skills		
		J Instrumental Swallowing and Oral Function		
		K Orofacial Myofunctional		
		L Augmentative/Alternative Communication System		
		M Voice Prosthetic		
		N Non-invasive Instrumental Status		
		P Oral Peripheral Mechanism		
		Q Performance Intensity Phonetically Balanced Speech Discrimination		
		R Brief Tone Stimuli		
		S Distorted Speech		
		T Dichotic Stimuli		
		V Temporal Ordering of Stimuli		
		W Masking Patterns		
		X Other Specified Central Auditory Processing		

F: Physical Rehabilitation and Diagnostic Audiology
1: Diagnostic Audiology

Type-Character 3	Body System/Region-Character 4	Type Qualifier-Character 5	Equipment-Character 6	Qualifier-Character 7
3 Hearing Assessment	**Z** None	**0** Bithermal, Binaural Caloric Irrigation	**0** Occupational Hearing	**Z** None
4 Hearing Aid Assessment		**0** Cochlear Implant	**1** Audiometer	
5 Vestibular Assessment		**0** Hearing Screening	**2** Sound Field / Booth	
		1 Bithermal, Monaural Caloric Irrigation	**3** Tympanometer	
		1 Ear Canal Probe Microphone	**4** Electroacoustic Immittance / Acoustic Reflex	
		1 Pure Tone Audiometry, Air	**5** Hearing Aid Selection / Fitting / Test	
		2 Monaural Hearing Aid	**6** Otoacoustic Emission (OAE)	
		2 Pure Tone Audiometry, Air and Bone	**7** Electrophysiologic	
		2 Unithermal Binaural Screen	**8** Vestibular / Balance	
		3 Bekesy Audiometry	**9** Cochlear Implant	
		3 Binaural Hearing Aid	**K** Audiovisual	
		3 Oscillating Tracking	**L** Assistive Listening	
		4 Assistive Listening System/Device Selection	**P** Computer	
		4 Conditioned Play Audiometry	**Y** Other Equipment	
		4 Sinusoidal Vertical Axis Rotational	**Z** None	
		5 Dix-Hallpike Dynamic		
		5 Select Picture Audiometry		
		5 Sensory Aids		
		6 Binaural Electroacoustic Hearing Aid Check		
		6 Computerized Dynamic Posturography		
		6 Visual Reinforcement Audiometry		
		7 Alternate Binaural or Monaural Loudness Balance		
		7 Ear Protector Attenuation		
		7 Tinnitus Masker		
		8 Monaural Electroacoustic Hearing Aid Check		
		8 Tone Decay		
		9 Short Increment Sensitivity Index		
		B Stenger		
		C Pure Tone Stenger		
		D Tympanometry		
		F Eustachian Tube Function		
		G Acoustic Reflex Patterns		
		H Acoustic Reflex Threshold		
		J Acoustic Reflex Decay		
		K Electrocochleography		
		L Auditory Evoked Potentials		
		M Evoked Otoacoustic Emissions, Screening		
		N Evoked Otoacoustic Emissions, Diagnostic		
		P Aural Rehabilitation Status		
		Q Auditory Processing		

G: Mental Health
Z: None

Type-Character 3	Qualifier-Character 4	Qualifier-Character 5	Qualifier-Character 6	Qualifier-Character 7
1 Psychological Tests	**0** Developmental	**Z** None	**Z** None	**Z** None
2 Crisis Intervention	**0** Educational			
3 Medication Management	**0** Interactive			
5 Individual Psychotherapy	**0** Unilateral-Single Seizure			
6 Counseling	**1** Behavioral			
7 Family Psychotherapy	**1** Personality and Behavioral			
B Electroconvulsive Therapy	**1** Unilateral-Multiple Seizure			
C Biofeedback	**1** Vocational			
F Hypnosis	**2** Bilateral-Single Seizure			
G Narcosynthesis	**2** Cognitive			
H Group Psychotherapy	**2** Intellectual and Psychoeducational			
J Light Therapy	**2** Other Family Psychotherapy			
	3 Bilateral-Multiple Seizure			
	3 Interpersonal			
	3 Neuropsychological			
	3 Other Counseling			
	4 Neurobehavioral and Cognitive Status			
	4 Other Electroconvulsive Therapy			
	4 Psychoanalysis			
	5 Psychodynamic			
	6 Supportive			
	8 Cognitive-Behavioral			
	9 Other Biofeedback			
	9 Psychophysiological			
	Z None			

H: Substance Abuse Treatment
Z: None

Type-Character 3	Qualifier-Character 4	Qualifier-Character 5	Qualifier-Character 6	Qualifier-Character 7
2 Detoxification Services	**0** Cognitive	**Z** None	**Z** None	**Z** None
3 Individual Counseling	**0** Nicotine Replacement			
4 Group Counseling	**1** Behavioral			
5 Individual Psychotherapy	**1** Methadone Maintenance			
6 Family Counseling	**2** Cognitive-Behavioral			
8 Medication Management	**2** Levo-alpha-acetylmethadol (LAAM)			
9 Pharmacotherapy	**3** 12-Step			
	3 Antabuse			
	3 Other Family Counseling			
	4 Interpersonal			
	4 Naltrexone			
	5 Interactive			
	5 Naloxone			
	5 Vocational			
	6 Clonidine			
	6 Psychoeducation			
	7 Bupropion			
	7 Motivational Enhancement			
	8 Confrontational			
	8 Psychiatric Medication			
	9 Continuing Care			
	9 Other Replacement Medication			
	9 Supportive			
	B Psychoanalysis			
	B Spiritual			
	C Pre/Post-Test Infectious Disease			
	C Psychodynamic			
	D Psychophysiological			
	Z None			

X: New Technology
2: Cardiovascular System

Operation-Character 3	Body Part-Character 4	Approach-Character 5	Device-Character 6	Qualifier-Character 7
7 Dilation	**0** Coronary Artery, One Artery	**0** Open	**1** Cerebral Embolic Filtration, Dual Filter	**1** New Technology Group 1
A Assistance	**1** Coronary Artery, Two Arteries	**3** Percutaneous	**3** Cerebral Embolic Filtration, Extracorporeal Flow Reversal Circuit	**2** New Technology Group 2
C Extirpation	**2** Coronary Artery, Three Arteries	**4** Percutaneous Endoscopic	**3** Zooplastic Tissue, Rapid Deployment Technique	**5** New Technology Group 5
R Replacement	**3** Coronary Artery, Four or More Arteries		**6** Orbital Atherectomy Technology	**6** New Technology Group 6
	5 Innominate Artery and Left Common Carotid Artery		**8** Intraluminal Device, Sustained Release Drug-eluting	
	6 Aortic Arch		**9** Intraluminal Device, Sustained Release Drug-eluting, Two	
	F Aortic Valve		**B** Intraluminal Device, Sustained Release Drug-eluting, Three	
	H Femoral Artery, Right		**C** Intraluminal Device, Sustained Release Drug-eluting, Four or More	
	H Common Carotid Artery, Right			
	J Common Carotid Artery, Left			
	J Femoral Artery, Left			
	K Popliteal Artery, Proximal Right			
	L Popliteal Artery, Proximal Left			
	M Popliteal Artery, Distal Right			
	N Popliteal Artery, Distal Left			
	P Anterior Tibial Artery, Right			
	Q Anterior Tibial Artery, Left			
	R Posterior Tibial Artery, Right			
	S Posterior Tibial Artery, Left			
	T Peroneal Artery, Right			
	U Peroneal Artery, Left			

X: New Technology
H: Skin, Subcutaneous Tissue, Fascia and Breast

Operation-Character 3	Body Part-Character 4	Approach-Character 5	Device-Character 6	Qualifier-Character 7
R Replacement	**P** Skin	**X** External	**L** Skin Substitute, Porcine Liver Derived	**2** New Technology Group 2

X: New Technology
K: Muscles, Tendons, Bursae and Ligaments

Operation-Character 3	Body Part-Character 4	Approach-Character 5	Device-Character 6	Qualifier-Character 7
0 Introduction	**2** Muscle	**3** Percutaneous	**0** Concentrated Bone Marrow Aspirate	**3** New Technology Group 3

X: New Technology
N: Bones

Operation-Character 3	Body Part-Character 4	Approach-Character 5	Device-Character 6	Qualifier-Character 7
S Reposition	**0** Lumbar Vertebra	**0** Open	**3** Magnetically Controlled Growth Rod(s)	**2** New Technology Group 2
U Supplement	**3** Cervical Vertebra	**3** Percutaneous	**5** Synthetic Substitute, Mechanically Expandable (Paired)	**6** New Technology Group 6
	4 Thoracic Vertebra			

X: New Technology
R: Joints

Operation-Character 3	Body Part-Character 4	Approach-Character 5	Device-Character 6	Qualifier-Character 7
2 Monitoring	**0** Occipital-cervical Joint	**0** Open	**2** Intraoperative Knee Replacement Sensor	**1** New Technology Group 1
G Fusion	**1** Cervical Vertebral Joint		**9** Interbody Fusion Device, Nanotextured Surface	**2** New Technology Group 2
	2 Cervical Vertebral Joints, 2 or more		**F** Interbody Fusion Device, Radiolucent Porous	**3** New Technology Group 3
	4 Cervicothoracic Vertebral Joint			
	6 Thoracic Vertebral Joint			
	7 Thoracic Vertebral Joints, 2 to 7			
	8 Thoracic Vertebral Joints, 8 or more			
	A Thoracolumbar Vertebral Joint			
	B Lumbar Vertebral Joint			
	C Lumbar Vertebral Joints, 2 or more			
	D Lumbosacral Joint			
	G Knee Joint, Right			
	H Knee Joint, Left			

X: New Technology
T: Urinary System

Operation-Character 3	Body Part-Character 4	Approach-Character 5	Device-Character 6	Qualifier-Character 7
2 Monitoring	**5** Kidney	**X** External	**E** Fluorescent Pyrazine	**5** New Technology Group 5

X: New Technology
V: Male Reproductive System

Operation-Character 3	Body Part-Character 4	Approach-Character 5	Device-Character 6	Qualifier-Character 7
5 Destruction	**0** Prostate	**8** Via Natural or Artificial Opening Endoscopic	**A** Robotic Waterjet Ablation	**4** New Technology Group 4

X: New Technology
W: Anatomical Regions

Operation-Character 3	Body Part-Character 4	Approach-Character 5	Device-Character 6	Qualifier-Character 7
0 Introduction	**1** Subcutaneous Tissue	**3** Percutaneous	**0** Brexanolone	**1** New Technology Group 1
1 Transfusion	**2** Muscle	**7** Via Natural or Artificial Opening	**2** Plasma, Convalescent (Nonautologous)	**2** New Technology Group 2
2 Transfusion	**3** Peripheral Vein	**8** Via Natural or Artificial Opening Endoscopic	**1** Eladocagene exuparvovec	**3** New Technology Group 3
	4 Central Vein	**X** External	**2** Ceftazidime-Avibactam Anti-infective	**4** New Technology Group 4
	9 Nose		**2** Nerinitide	**5** New Technology Group 5
	D Mouth and Pharynx		**3** Idarucizumab, Dabigatran Reversal Agent	**6** New Technology Group 6
	G Upper GI		**3** Durvalumab Antineoplastic	
	H Lower GI		**4** Brexucabtagene Autoleucel Immunotherapy	
	Q Cranial Cavity and Brain		**4** Isavuconazole Antiinfective	
			5 Blinatumomab Antineoplastic Immunotherapy	
			6 Lefamulin Anti-infective	
			7 Coagulation Factor Xa, Inactivated	
			7 Lisocabtagene Maraleucel Immunotherapy	
			8 Mineral-based Topical Hemostatic Agent	
			8 Uridine Triacetate	
			9 Defibrotide Sodium Anticoagulant	
			9 Ceftolozane/Tazobactam Anti-infective	
			A Bezlotoxumab Monoclonal Antibody	
			A Cefiderocol Anti-infective	
			B Cytarabine and Daunorubicin Liposome Antineoplastic	
			B Omadacycline Anti-infective	
			C Eculizumab	
			C Engineered Autologous Chimeric Antigen Receptor T-cell Immunotherapy	
			D Atezolizumab Antineoplastic	
			E Etesevimab Monoclonal Antibody	
			E Remdesivir Anti-infective	
			F Bamlanivimab Monoclonal Antibody	
			F Other New Technology Therapeutic Substance	
			G Plazomicin Anti-infective	
			G REGN-COV2 Monoclonal Antibody	
			G Sarilumab	
			H Other New Technology Monoclonal Antibody	

Table continued on next page

X: New Technology
W: Anatomical Regions

Table continued from previous page

Operation-Character 3	Body Part-Character 4	Approach-Character 5	Device-Character 6	Qualifier-Character 7
			H Synthetic Human Angiotensin II	
			H Tocilizumab	
			J Apalutamide Antineoplastic	
			K Fosfomycin Anti-infective	
			K Leronlimab Monoclonal Antibody	
			L CD24Fc Immunomodulator	
			L Erdafitinib Antineoplastic	
			M Baricitinib	
			M Esketamine Hydrochloride	
			N Meropenem-vaborbactam Anti-infective	
			Q Tagraxofusp-erzs Antineoplastic	
			R Venetoclax Antineoplastic	
			S COVID-19 Vaccine Dose 1	
			S Iobenguane I-131 Antineoplastic	
			T COVID-19 Vaccine Dose 2	
			T Ruxolitinib	
			U COVID-19 Vaccine	
			U Imipenem-cilastatin-relebactam Anti-infective	
			V Gilteritinib Antineoplastic	
			W Caplacizumab	

X: New Technology
X: Physiological Systems

Operation-Character 3	Body Part-Character 4	Approach-Character 5	Device-Character 6	Qualifier-Character 7
E Measurement	**5** Circulatory	**X** External	**M** Infection, Whole Blood Nucleic Acid-base Microbial Detection	**5** New Technology Group 5
	B Respiratory		**N** Infection, Positive Blood Culture Fluorescence Hybridization for Organism Identification, Concentration and Susceptibility	**6** New Technology Group 6
			Q Infection, Lower Respiratory Fluid Nucleic Acid-base Microbial Detection	

X: New Technology
Y: Extracorporeal

Operation-Character 3	Body Part-Character 4	Approach-Character 5	Device-Character 6	Qualifier-Character 7
0 Introduction	**V** Vein Graft	**X** External	**8** Endothelial Damage Inhibitor	**3** New Technology Group 3

This page intentionally left blank

Appendix F: Substance Key

Substance Term	ICD-10-PCS Value
ACTEMRA®	Tocilizumab
AIGISRx® Antibacterial Envelope	Anti-Infective Envelope
Andexanet Alfa, Factor Xa Inhibitor Reversal Agent	Coagulation Factor Xa, Inactivated
Andexxa®	Coagulation Factor Xa, Inactivated
Angiotensin II	Synthetic Human Angiotensin II
Antibacterial Envelope (TYRX™) (AIGISRx™)	Anti-Infective Envelope
Antimicrobial Envelope	Anti-Infective Envelope
Axicabtagene Ciloeucel	Engineered Autologous Chimeric Antigen Receptor T-cell Immunotherapy
AZEDRA®	Iobenguane I-131 Antineoplastic
Bone morphogenetic protein 2 (BMP 2)	Recombinant Bone Morphogenetic Protein
Brexucabtagene Autoleucel	Brexucabtagene Autoleucel Immunotherapy
CBMA (Concentrated Bone Marrow Aspirate)	Concentrated Bone Marrow Aspirate
Clolar®	Clofarabine
Coagulation Factor Xa, (Recombinant) Inactivated	Coagulation Factor Xa, Inactivated
CONTEPO™	Fosfomycin Anti-infective
Defitelio®	Defibrotide Sodium Anticoagulant
DuraGraft® Endothelial Damage Inhibitor	Endothelial Damage Inhibitor
ELZONRIS™	Tagraxofusp-erzs Antineoplastic
ERLEADA™	Apalutamide Antineoplastic
Factor Xa Inhibitor Reversal Agent, Andexanet Alfa	Coagulation Factor Xa, Inactivated
FETROJA®	Cefiderocol Anti-infective
Fosfomycin injection	Fosfomycin Anti-infective
GIAPREZA™	Synthetic Human Angiotensin II
GS-5734	Remdesivir Anti-infective
Hemospray® Endoscopic Hemostat	Mineral-based Topical Hemostatic Agent
Human angiotensin II, synthetic	Synthetic Human Angiotensin II
IMFINZI®	Durvalumab Antineoplastic
IMI/REL	Imipenem-cilastatin-relebactam Anti-infective
Iobenguane I-131, High Specific Activity (HSA)	Iobenguane I-131 Antineoplastic
Jakafi®	Ruxolitinib
Kcentra®	4-Factor Prothrombin Complex Concentrate
KEVZARA®	Sarilumab
KYMRIAH®	Engineered Autologous Chimeric Antigen Receptor T-cell Immunotherapy
Lisocabtagene Maraleucel	Lisocabtagene Maraleucel Immunotherapy
NA-1 (Nerinitide)	Nerinitide
Nesiritide®	Human B-type Natriuretic Peptide
NUZYRA™	Omadacycline Anti-infective
OTL-101	Hematopoietic Stem/Progenitor Cells, Genetically Modified
rhBMP-2	Recombinant Bone Morphogenetic Protein
Seprafilm®	Adhesion Barrier
Soliris®	Eculizumab
SPRAVATO™	Esketamine Hydrochloride
STELARA®	Other New Technology Therapeutic Substance

Substance Term	ICD-10-PCS Value
TECENTRIQ®	Atezolizumab Antineoplastic
Tisagenlecleucel	Engineered Autologous Chimeric Antigen Receptor T-cell Immunotherapy
Tissue Plasminogen Activator (tPA)(r- tPA)	Other Thrombolytic
TYRX™ Antibacterial Envelope	Anti-Infective Envelope
Ustekinumab	Other New Technology Therapeutic Substance
Vabomere™	Meropenem-vaborbactam Anti-infective
Veklury	Remdesivir Anti-infective
Venclexta®	Venetoclax Antineoplastic
Vistogard®	Uridine Triacetate
Voraxaze®	Glucarpidase
VYXEOS™	Cytarabine and Daunorubicin Liposome Antineoplastic
XENLETA™	Lefamulin Anti-infective
XOSPATA®	Gilteritinib Antineoplastic
ZERBAXA®	Ceftolozane/Tazobactam Anti-infective
ZINPLAVA™	Bezlotoxumab Monoclonal Antibody
ZULRESSO™	Brexanolone
Zyvox®	Oxazolidinones

Appendix G: Combination Clusters

Due to the nature of a specific procedure, the first code in the cluster needs to be reported with one or more of the additional codes listed for all codes to be considered valid. The example below is for insertion of a cardiac defibrillator lead into the right ventricle (highlighted code). The additional procedure describes the exact location of where the lead is inserted, which is required for correct reporting:

`02HK0KZ`

and   0JH609Z

You would need to review the first procedure in the combination/cluster to determine whether you need to report the additional code.

The CMS site also provides additional information on combinations/clusters.

02H60KZ and 0JH608Z	02H64KZ and 0JH638Z	02H74KZ and 0JH808Z	02HK0KZ and 0JH608Z	02HK3KZ and 0JH809Z	02HK4MZ and 0JH80AZ	02HL3KZ and 0JH839Z
02H60KZ and 0JH638Z	02H64KZ and 0JH808Z	02H74KZ and 0JH838Z	02HK0KZ and 0JH609Z	02HK3KZ and 0JH838Z	02HK4MZ and 0JH83AZ	02HL4KZ and 0JH608Z
02H60KZ and 0JH808Z	02H64KZ and 0JH838Z	02HA0RS and 02PA0RZ	02HK0KZ and 0JH638Z	02HK3KZ and 0JH839Z	02HL0KZ and 0JH608Z	02HL4KZ and 0JH609Z
02H60KZ and 0JH838Z	02H64MZ and 0JH60AZ	02HA0RS and 02PA3RZ	02HK0KZ and 0JH639Z	02HK3MZ and 0JH60AZ	02HL0KZ and 0JH609Z	02HL4KZ and 0JH638Z
02H60MZ and 0JH60AZ	02H64MZ and 0JH63AZ	02HA0RS and 02PA4RZ	02HK0KZ and 0JH808Z	02HK3MZ and 0JH63AZ	02HL0KZ and 0JH638Z	02HL4KZ and 0JH639Z
02H60MZ and 0JH63AZ	02H64MZ and 0JH80AZ	02HA0RZ and 02PA0RZ	02HK0KZ and 0JH809Z	02HK3MZ and 0JH80AZ	02HL0KZ and 0JH639Z	02HL4KZ and 0JH808Z
02H60MZ and 0JH80AZ	02H64MZ and 0JH83AZ	02HA0RZ and 02PA3RZ	02HK0KZ and 0JH838Z	02HK3MZ and 0JH83AZ	02HL0KZ and 0JH808Z	02HL4KZ and 0JH809Z
02H60MZ and 0JH83AZ	02H70KZ and 0JH608Z	02HA0RZ and 02PA4RZ	02HK0KZ and 0JH839Z	02HK4KZ and 0JH608Z	02HL0KZ and 0JH809Z	02HL4KZ and 0JH838Z
02H63KZ and 0JH608Z	02H70KZ and 0JH638Z	02HA3RS and 02PA0RZ	02HK0MZ and 0JH60AZ	02HK4KZ and 0JH609Z	02HL0KZ and 0JH838Z	02HL4KZ and 0JH839Z
02H63KZ and 0JH638Z	02H70KZ and 0JH808Z	02HA3RS and 02PA3RZ	02HK0MZ and 0JH63AZ	02HK4KZ and 0JH638Z	02HL0KZ and 0JH839Z	02RK0JZ and 02RL0JZ
02H63KZ and 0JH808Z	02H70KZ and 0JH838Z	02HA3RS and 02PA4RZ	02HK0MZ and 0JH80AZ	02HK4KZ and 0JH639Z	02HL3KZ and 0JH608Z	02WA0QZ and 02PA0RZ
02H63KZ and 0JH838Z	02H73KZ and 0JH608Z	02HA4RS and 02PA0RZ	02HK0MZ and 0JH83AZ	02HK4KZ and 0JH808Z	02HL3KZ and 0JH609Z	02WA0QZ and 02PA3RZ
02H63MZ and 0JH60AZ	02H73KZ and 0JH638Z	02HA4RS and 02PA3RZ	02HK3KZ and 0JH608Z	02HK4KZ and 0JH809Z	02HL3KZ and 0JH638Z	02WA0QZ and 02PA4RZ
02H63MZ and 0JH63AZ	02H73KZ and 0JH808Z	02HA4RS and 02PA4RZ	02HK3KZ and 0JH609Z	02HK4KZ and 0JH838Z	02HL3KZ and 0JH639Z	02WA0RZ and 02PA0RZ
02H63MZ and 0JH80AZ	02H73KZ and 0JH838Z	02HA4RZ and 02PA0RZ	02HK3KZ and 0JH638Z	02HK4KZ and 0JH839Z	02HL3KZ and 0JH808Z	02WA0RZ and 02PA3RZ
02H63MZ and 0JH83AZ	02H74KZ and 0JH608Z	02HA4RZ and 02PA3RZ	02HK3KZ and 0JH639Z	02HK4MZ and 0JH60AZ	02HL3KZ and 0JH809Z	02WA0RZ and 02PA4RZ
02H64KZ and 0JH608Z	02H74KZ and 0JH638Z	02HA4RZ and 02PA4RZ	02HK3KZ and 0JH808Z	02HK4MZ and 0JH63AZ	02HL3KZ and 0JH838Z	02WA3QZ and 02PA0RZ

02WA3QZ and 02PA3RZ	07T50ZZ and 07T60ZZ and 0HTV0ZZ	0DQM0ZZ and 0WQFXZ2	0JH604Z and 02H40MZ	0JH604Z and 02HK4MZ	0JH605Z and 02H63MZ	0JH605Z and 02HN0MZ
02WA3QZ and 02PA4RZ	07T50ZZ and 07T60ZZ and 0HTV0ZZ and 0KTH0ZZ and 0KTJ0ZZ	0DQN0ZZ and 0WQFXZ2	0JH604Z and 02H43JZ	0JH604Z and 02HL0JZ	0JH605Z and 02H64JZ	0JH605Z and 02HN3JZ
02WA3RZ and 02PA0RZ		0DT90ZZ and 0FTG0ZZ	0JH604Z and 02H43MZ	0JH604Z and 02HL0MZ	0JH605Z and 02H64MZ	0JH605Z and 02HN3MZ
02WA3RZ and 02PA3RZ	07T50ZZ and 07T70ZZ and 07T80ZZ and 0HTT0ZZ and 0KTH0ZZ	0HRT37Z and 0JD63ZZ	0JH604Z and 02H44JZ	0JH604Z and 02HL3JZ	0JH605Z and 02H70JZ	0JH605Z and 02HN4JZ
02WA3RZ and 02PA4RZ		0HRT37Z and 0JD73ZZ	0JH604Z and 02H44MZ	0JH604Z and 02HL3MZ	0JH605Z and 02H70MZ	0JH605Z and 02HN4MZ
02WA4QZ and 02PA0RZ	07T50ZZ and 0HTT0ZZ	0HRT37Z and 0JD83ZZ	0JH604Z and 02H60JZ	0JH604Z and 02HL4JZ	0JH605Z and 02H73JZ	0JH606Z and 02H40JZ
02WA4QZ and 02PA3RZ	07T50ZZ and 0HTT0ZZ and 0KTH0ZZ	0HRT37Z and 0JD93ZZ	0JH604Z and 02H60MZ	0JH604Z and 02HL4MZ	0JH605Z and 02H73MZ	0JH606Z and 02H40MZ
02WA4QZ and 02PA4RZ		0HRT37Z and 0JDL3ZZ	0JH604Z and 02H63JZ	0JH604Z and 02HN0JZ	0JH605Z and 02H74JZ	0JH606Z and 02H43JZ
02WA4RZ and 02PA0RZ	07T60ZZ and 07T70ZZ and 07T90ZZ and 0HTU0ZZ and 0KTJ0ZZ	0HRT37Z and 0JDM3ZZ	0JH604Z and 02H63MZ	0JH604Z and 02HN0MZ	0JH605Z and 02H74MZ	0JH606Z and 02H43MZ
02WA4RZ and 02PA3RZ		0HRU37Z and 0JD63ZZ	0JH604Z and 02H64JZ	0JH604Z and 02HN3JZ	0JH605Z and 02HK0JZ	0JH606Z and 02H44JZ
02WA4RZ and 02PA4RZ	07T60ZZ and 0HTU0ZZ and 0KTJ0ZZ	0HRU37Z and 0JD73ZZ	0JH604Z and 02H64MZ	0JH604Z and 02HN3MZ	0JH605Z and 02HK0MZ	0JH606Z and 02H44MZ
07BH0ZZ and 0UTM0ZZ	07T60ZZ and 0HTU0ZZ	0HRU37Z and 0JD83ZZ	0JH604Z and 02H70JZ	0JH604Z and 02HN4JZ	0JH605Z and 02HK3JZ	0JH606Z and 02H60JZ
07BH0ZZ and 0UTMXZZ	0DQ80ZZ and 0WQFXZ2	0HRU37Z and 0JD93ZZ	0JH604Z and 02H70MZ	0JH604Z and 02HN4MZ	0JH605Z and 02HK3MZ	0JH606Z and 02H60MZ
07BH4ZZ and 0UTM0ZZ	0DQ90ZZ and 0WQFXZ2	0HRU37Z and 0JDL3ZZ	0JH604Z and 02H73JZ	0JH605Z and 02H40JZ	0JH605Z and 02HK4JZ	0JH606Z and 02H63JZ
07BH4ZZ and 0UTMXZZ	0DQA0ZZ and 0WQFXZ2	0HRU37Z and 0JDM3ZZ	0JH604Z and 02H73MZ	0JH605Z and 02H40MZ	0JH605Z and 02HK4MZ	0JH606Z and 02H63MZ
07BJ0ZZ and 0UTM0ZZ	0DQB0ZZ and 0WQFXZ2	0HRV37Z and 0JD63ZZ	0JH604Z and 02H74JZ	0JH605Z and 02H43JZ	0JH605Z and 02HL0JZ	0JH606Z and 02H64JZ
07BJ0ZZ and 0UTMXZZ	0DQE0ZZ and 0WQFXZ2	0HRV37Z and 0JD73ZZ	0JH604Z and 02H74MZ	0JH605Z and 02H43MZ	0JH605Z and 02HL0MZ	0JH606Z and 02H64MZ
07BJ4ZZ and 0UTM0ZZ	0DQF0ZZ and 0WQFXZ2	0HRV37Z and 0JD83ZZ	0JH604Z and 02HK0JZ	0JH605Z and 02H44JZ	0JH605Z and 02HL3JZ	0JH606Z and 02H70JZ
07BJ4ZZ and 0UTMXZZ	0DQG0ZZ and 0WQFXZ2	0HRV37Z and 0JD93ZZ	0JH604Z and 02HK0MZ	0JH605Z and 02H44MZ	0JH605Z and 02HL3MZ	0JH606Z and 02H70MZ
07T50ZZ and 07T60ZZ and 07T70ZZ and 07T80ZZ and 07T90ZZ and 0HTV0ZZ and 0KTH0ZZ and 0KTJ0ZZ	0DQH0ZZ and 0WQFXZ2	0HRV37Z and 0JDL3ZZ	0JH604Z and 02HK3JZ	0JH605Z and 02H60JZ	0JH605Z and 02HL4JZ	0JH606Z and 02H73JZ
	0DQK0ZZ and 0WQFXZ2	0HRV37Z and 0JDM3ZZ	0JH604Z and 02HK3MZ	0JH605Z and 02H60MZ	0JH605Z and 02HL4MZ	0JH606Z and 02H73MZ
	0DQL0ZZ and 0WQFXZ2	0JH604Z and 02H40JZ	0JH604Z and 02HK4JZ	0JH605Z and 02H63JZ	0JH605Z and 02HN0JZ	0JH606Z and 02H74JZ

0JH606Z and 02H74MZ	0JH607Z and 02H43MZ	0JH607Z and 02HL0MZ	0JH609Z and 02H40KZ	0JH60BZ and 00HE4MZ	0JH60CZ and 00HE0MZ	0JH60CZ and 0DH63MZ
0JH606Z and 02HK0JZ	0JH607Z and 02H44JZ	0JH607Z and 02HL3JZ	0JH609Z and 02H43JZ	0JH60BZ and 00HU0MZ	0JH60CZ and 00HE3MZ	0JH60CZ and 0DH64MZ
0JH606Z and 02HK0MZ	0JH607Z and 02H44MZ	0JH607Z and 02HL3MZ	0JH609Z and 02H43KZ	0JH60BZ and 00HU3MZ	0JH60CZ and 00HE4MZ	0JH60DZ and 00H00MZ
0JH606Z and 02HK3JZ	0JH607Z and 02H60JZ	0JH607Z and 02HL4JZ	0JH609Z and 02H43MZ	0JH60BZ and 00HU4MZ	0JH60CZ and 00HU0MZ	0JH60DZ and 00H03MZ
0JH606Z and 02HK3MZ	0JH607Z and 02H60MZ	0JH607Z and 02HL4MZ	0JH609Z and 02H44KZ	0JH60BZ and 00HV0MZ	0JH60CZ and 00HU3MZ	0JH60DZ and 00H04MZ
0JH606Z and 02HK4JZ	0JH607Z and 02H63JZ	0JH607Z and 02HN0JZ	0JH609Z and 02H60KZ	0JH60BZ and 00HV3MZ	0JH60CZ and 00HU4MZ	0JH60DZ and 00H60MZ
0JH606Z and 02HK4MZ	0JH607Z and 02H63MZ	0JH607Z and 02HN0MZ	0JH609Z and 02H63KZ	0JH60BZ and 00HV4MZ	0JH60CZ and 00HV0MZ	0JH60DZ and 00H63MZ
0JH606Z and 02HL0JZ	0JH607Z and 02H64JZ	0JH607Z and 02HN3JZ	0JH609Z and 02H64KZ	0JH60BZ and 01HY0MZ	0JH60CZ and 00HV3MZ	0JH60DZ and 00H64MZ
0JH606Z and 02HL0MZ	0JH607Z and 02H64MZ	0JH607Z and 02HN3MZ	0JH609Z and 02H70KZ	0JH60BZ and 01HY3MZ	0JH60CZ and 00HV4MZ	0JH60DZ and 00HE0MZ
0JH606Z and 02HL3JZ	0JH607Z and 02H70JZ	0JH607Z and 02HN4JZ	0JH609Z and 02H73KZ	0JH60BZ and 01HY4MZ	0JH60CZ and 01HY0MZ	0JH60DZ and 00HE3MZ
0JH606Z and 02HL3MZ	0JH607Z and 02H70MZ	0JH607Z and 02HN4MZ	0JH609Z and 02H74KZ	0JH60BZ and 05H00MZ	0JH60CZ and 01HY3MZ	0JH60DZ and 00HE4MZ
0JH606Z and 02HL4JZ	0JH607Z and 02H73JZ	0JH608Z and 02H40KZ	0JH609Z and 02HN0JZ	0JH60BZ and 05H03MZ	0JH60CZ and 01HY4MZ	0JH60DZ and 00HU0MZ
0JH606Z and 02HL4MZ	0JH607Z and 02H73MZ	0JH608Z and 02H44KZ	0JH609Z and 02HN0KZ	0JH60BZ and 05H04MZ	0JH60CZ and 05H00MZ	0JH60DZ and 00HU3MZ
0JH606Z and 02HN0JZ	0JH607Z and 02H74JZ	0JH608Z and 02HN0JZ	0JH609Z and 02HN0MZ	0JH60BZ and 05H30MZ	0JH60CZ and 05H03MZ	0JH60DZ and 00HU4MZ
0JH606Z and 02HN0MZ	0JH607Z and 02H74MZ	0JH608Z and 02HN0KZ	0JH609Z and 02HN3JZ	0JH60BZ and 05H33MZ	0JH60CZ and 05H04MZ	0JH60DZ and 00HV0MZ
0JH606Z and 02HN3JZ	0JH607Z and 02HK0JZ	0JH608Z and 02HN0MZ	0JH609Z and 02HN3KZ	0JH60BZ and 05H34MZ	0JH60CZ and 05H30MZ	0JH60DZ and 00HV3MZ
0JH606Z and 02HN3MZ	0JH607Z and 02HK0MZ	0JH608Z and 02HN3JZ	0JH609Z and 02HN3MZ	0JH60BZ and 05H40MZ	0JH60CZ and 05H33MZ	0JH60DZ and 00HV4MZ
0JH606Z and 02HN4JZ	0JH607Z and 02HK3JZ	0JH608Z and 02HN3KZ	0JH609Z and 02HN4JZ	0JH60BZ and 05H43MZ	0JH60CZ and 05H34MZ	0JH60DZ and 01HY0MZ
0JH606Z and 02HN4MZ	0JH607Z and 02HK3MZ	0JH608Z and 02HN3MZ	0JH609Z and 02HN4KZ	0JH60BZ and 05H44MZ	0JH60CZ and 05H40MZ	0JH60DZ and 01HY3MZ
0JH607Z and 02H40JZ	0JH607Z and 02HK4JZ	0JH608Z and 02HN4JZ	0JH609Z and 02HN4MZ	0JH60BZ and 0DH60MZ	0JH60CZ and 05H43MZ	0JH60DZ and 01HY4MZ
0JH607Z and 02H40MZ	0JH607Z and 02HK4MZ	0JH608Z and 02HN4KZ	0JH60BZ and 00HE0MZ	0JH60BZ and 0DH63MZ	0JH60CZ and 05H44MZ	0JH60DZ and 05H00MZ
0JH607Z and 02H43JZ	0JH607Z and 02HL0JZ	0JH608Z and 02HN4MZ	0JH60BZ and 00HE3MZ	0JH60BZ and 0DH64MZ	0JH60CZ and 0DH60MZ	0JH60DZ and 05H03MZ

0JH60DZ and 05H04MZ	0JH60EZ and 00HV0MZ	0JH60FZ and 0JH808Z	0JH60PZ and 02HK0JZ	0JH634Z and 02H44JZ	0JH634Z and 02HL3JZ	0JH635Z and 02H70JZ
0JH60DZ and 05H30MZ	0JH60EZ and 00HV3MZ	0JH60FZ and 0JH809Z	0JH60PZ and 02HK0MZ	0JH634Z and 02H44MZ	0JH634Z and 02HL3MZ	0JH635Z and 02H70MZ
0JH60DZ and 05H33MZ	0JH60EZ and 00HV4MZ	0JH60FZ and 0JH838Z	0JH60PZ and 02HK3JZ	0JH634Z and 02H60JZ	0JH634Z and 02HL4JZ	0JH635Z and 02H73JZ
0JH60DZ and 05H34MZ	0JH60EZ and 01HY0MZ	0JH60FZ and 0JH839Z	0JH60PZ and 02HK3MZ	0JH634Z and 02H60MZ	0JH634Z and 02HL4MZ	0JH635Z and 02H73MZ
0JH60DZ and 05H40MZ	0JH60EZ and 01HY3MZ	0JH60PZ and 02H40JZ	0JH60PZ and 02HK4JZ	0JH634Z and 02H63JZ	0JH634Z and 02HN0JZ	0JH635Z and 02H74JZ
0JH60DZ and 05H43MZ	0JH60EZ and 01HY4MZ	0JH60PZ and 02H40MZ	0JH60PZ and 02HK4MZ	0JH634Z and 02H63MZ	0JH634Z and 02HN0MZ	0JH635Z and 02H74MZ
0JH60DZ and 05H44MZ	0JH60EZ and 05H00MZ	0JH60PZ and 02H43JZ	0JH60PZ and 02HL0JZ	0JH634Z and 02H64JZ	0JH634Z and 02HN3JZ	0JH635Z and 02HK0JZ
0JH60DZ and 0DH60MZ	0JH60EZ and 05H03MZ	0JH60PZ and 02H43MZ	0JH60PZ and 02HL0MZ	0JH634Z and 02H64MZ	0JH634Z and 02HN3MZ	0JH635Z and 02HK0MZ
0JH60DZ and 0DH63MZ	0JH60EZ and 05H04MZ	0JH60PZ and 02H44JZ	0JH60PZ and 02HL3JZ	0JH634Z and 02H70JZ	0JH634Z and 02HN4JZ	0JH635Z and 02HK3JZ
0JH60DZ and 0DH64MZ	0JH60EZ and 05H30MZ	0JH60PZ and 02H44MZ	0JH60PZ and 02HL3MZ	0JH634Z and 02H70MZ	0JH634Z and 02HN4MZ	0JH635Z and 02HK3MZ
0JH60EZ and 00H00MZ	0JH60EZ and 05H33MZ	0JH60PZ and 02H60JZ	0JH60PZ and 02HL4JZ	0JH634Z and 02H73JZ	0JH635Z and 02H40JZ	0JH635Z and 02HK4JZ
0JH60EZ and 00H03MZ	0JH60EZ and 05H34MZ	0JH60PZ and 02H60MZ	0JH60PZ and 02HL4MZ	0JH634Z and 02H73MZ	0JH635Z and 02H40MZ	0JH635Z and 02HK4MZ
0JH60EZ and 00H04MZ	0JH60EZ and 05H40MZ	0JH60PZ and 02H63JZ	0JH60PZ and 02HN0JZ	0JH634Z and 02H74JZ	0JH635Z and 02H43JZ	0JH635Z and 02HL0JZ
0JH60EZ and 00H60MZ	0JH60EZ and 05H43MZ	0JH60PZ and 02H63MZ	0JH60PZ and 02HN0MZ	0JH634Z and 02H74MZ	0JH635Z and 02H43MZ	0JH635Z and 02HL0MZ
0JH60EZ and 00H63MZ	0JH60EZ and 05H44MZ	0JH60PZ and 02H64JZ	0JH60PZ and 02HN3JZ	0JH634Z and 02HK0JZ	0JH635Z and 02H44JZ	0JH635Z and 02HL3JZ
0JH60EZ and 00H64MZ	0JH60EZ and 0DH60MZ	0JH60PZ and 02H64MZ	0JH60PZ and 02HN3MZ	0JH634Z and 02HK0MZ	0JH635Z and 02H44MZ	0JH635Z and 02HL3MZ
0JH60EZ and 00HE0MZ	0JH60EZ and 0DH63MZ	0JH60PZ and 02H70JZ	0JH60PZ and 02HN4JZ	0JH634Z and 02HK3JZ	0JH635Z and 02H60JZ	0JH635Z and 02HL4JZ
0JH60EZ and 00HE3MZ	0JH60EZ and 0DH64MZ	0JH60PZ and 02H70MZ	0JH60PZ and 02HN4MZ	0JH634Z and 02HK3MZ	0JH635Z and 02H60MZ	0JH635Z and 02HL4MZ
0JH60EZ and 00HE4MZ	0JH60FZ and 0JH608Z	0JH60PZ and 02H73JZ	0JH634Z and 02H40JZ	0JH634Z and 02HK4JZ	0JH635Z and 02H63JZ	0JH635Z and 02HN0JZ
0JH60EZ and 00HU0MZ	0JH60FZ and 0JH609Z	0JH60PZ and 02H73MZ	0JH634Z and 02H40MZ	0JH634Z and 02HK4MZ	0JH635Z and 02H63MZ	0JH635Z and 02HN0MZ
0JH60EZ and 00HU3MZ	0JH60FZ and 0JH638Z	0JH60PZ and 02H74JZ	0JH634Z and 02H43JZ	0JH634Z and 02HL0JZ	0JH635Z and 02H64JZ	0JH635Z and 02HN3JZ
0JH60EZ and 00HU4MZ	0JH60FZ and 0JH639Z	0JH60PZ and 02H74MZ	0JH634Z and 02H43MZ	0JH634Z and 02HL0MZ	0JH635Z and 02H64MZ	0JH635Z and 02HN3MZ

0JH635Z and 02HN4JZ	0JH636Z and 02HK3JZ	0JH637Z and 02H60JZ	0JH637Z and 02HL4JZ	0JH639Z and 02H43MZ	0JH63BZ and 00HU4MZ	0JH63CZ and 00HU0MZ
0JH635Z and 02HN4MZ	0JH636Z and 02HK3MZ	0JH637Z and 02H60MZ	0JH637Z and 02HL4MZ	0JH639Z and 02H44KZ	0JH63BZ and 00HV0MZ	0JH63CZ and 00HU3MZ
0JH636Z and 02H40JZ	0JH636Z and 02HK4JZ	0JH637Z and 02H63JZ	0JH637Z and 02HN0JZ	0JH639Z and 02H60KZ	0JH63BZ and 00HV3MZ	0JH63CZ and 00HU4MZ
0JH636Z and 02H40MZ	0JH636Z and 02HK4MZ	0JH637Z and 02H63MZ	0JH637Z and 02HN0MZ	0JH639Z and 02H63KZ	0JH63BZ and 00HV4MZ	0JH63CZ and 00HV0MZ
0JH636Z and 02H43JZ	0JH636Z and 02HL0JZ	0JH637Z and 02H64JZ	0JH637Z and 02HN3JZ	0JH639Z and 02H64KZ	0JH63BZ and 01HY0MZ	0JH63CZ and 00HV3MZ
0JH636Z and 02H43MZ	0JH636Z and 02HL0MZ	0JH637Z and 02H64MZ	0JH637Z and 02HN3MZ	0JH639Z and 02H70KZ	0JH63BZ and 01HY3MZ	0JH63CZ and 00HV4MZ
0JH636Z and 02H44JZ	0JH636Z and 02HL3JZ	0JH637Z and 02H70JZ	0JH637Z and 02HN4JZ	0JH639Z and 02H73KZ	0JH63BZ and 01HY4MZ	0JH63CZ and 01HY0MZ
0JH636Z and 02H44MZ	0JH636Z and 02HL3MZ	0JH637Z and 02H70MZ	0JH637Z and 02HN4MZ	0JH639Z and 02H74KZ	0JH63BZ and 05H00MZ	0JH63CZ and 01HY3MZ
0JH636Z and 02H60JZ	0JH636Z and 02HL4JZ	0JH637Z and 02H73JZ	0JH638Z and 02H40KZ	0JH639Z and 02HN0JZ	0JH63BZ and 05H03MZ	0JH63CZ and 01HY4MZ
0JH636Z and 02H60MZ	0JH636Z and 02HL4MZ	0JH637Z and 02H73MZ	0JH638Z and 02H44KZ	0JH639Z and 02HN0KZ	0JH63BZ and 05H04MZ	0JH63CZ and 05H00MZ
0JH636Z and 02H63JZ	0JH636Z and 02HN0JZ	0JH637Z and 02H74JZ	0JH638Z and 02HN0JZ	0JH639Z and 02HN0MZ	0JH63BZ and 05H30MZ	0JH63CZ and 05H03MZ
0JH636Z and 02H63MZ	0JH636Z and 02HN0MZ	0JH637Z and 02H74MZ	0JH638Z and 02HN0KZ	0JH639Z and 02HN3JZ	0JH63BZ and 05H33MZ	0JH63CZ and 05H04MZ
0JH636Z and 02H64JZ	0JH636Z and 02HN3JZ	0JH637Z and 02HK0JZ	0JH638Z and 02HN0MZ	0JH639Z and 02HN3KZ	0JH63BZ and 05H34MZ	0JH63CZ and 05H30MZ
0JH636Z and 02H64MZ	0JH636Z and 02HN3MZ	0JH637Z and 02HK0MZ	0JH638Z and 02HN3JZ	0JH639Z and 02HN3MZ	0JH63BZ and 05H40MZ	0JH63CZ and 05H33MZ
0JH636Z and 02H70JZ	0JH636Z and 02HN4JZ	0JH637Z and 02HK3JZ	0JH638Z and 02HN3KZ	0JH639Z and 02HN4JZ	0JH63BZ and 05H43MZ	0JH63CZ and 05H34MZ
0JH636Z and 02H70MZ	0JH636Z and 02HN4MZ	0JH637Z and 02HK3MZ	0JH638Z and 02HN3MZ	0JH639Z and 02HN4KZ	0JH63BZ and 05H44MZ	0JH63CZ and 05H40MZ
0JH636Z and 02H73JZ	0JH637Z and 02H40JZ	0JH637Z and 02HK4JZ	0JH638Z and 02HN4JZ	0JH639Z and 02HN4MZ	0JH63BZ and 0DH60MZ	0JH63CZ and 05H43MZ
0JH636Z and 02H73MZ	0JH637Z and 02H40MZ	0JH637Z and 02HK4MZ	0JH638Z and 02HN4KZ	0JH63BZ and 00HE0MZ	0JH63BZ and 0DH63MZ	0JH63CZ and 05H44MZ
0JH636Z and 02H74JZ	0JH637Z and 02H43JZ	0JH637Z and 02HL0JZ	0JH638Z and 02HN4MZ	0JH63BZ and 00HE3MZ	0JH63BZ and 0DH64MZ	0JH63CZ and 0DH60MZ
0JH636Z and 02H74MZ	0JH637Z and 02H43MZ	0JH637Z and 02HL0MZ	0JH639Z and 02H40KZ	0JH63BZ and 00HE4MZ	0JH63CZ and 00HE0MZ	0JH63CZ and 0DH63MZ
0JH636Z and 02HK0JZ	0JH637Z and 02H44JZ	0JH637Z and 02HL3JZ	0JH639Z and 02H43JZ	0JH63BZ and 00HU0MZ	0JH63CZ and 00HE3MZ	0JH63CZ and 0DH64MZ
0JH636Z and 02HK0MZ	0JH637Z and 02H44MZ	0JH637Z and 02HL3MZ	0JH639Z and 02H43KZ	0JH63BZ and 00HU3MZ	0JH63CZ and 00HE4MZ	0JH63DZ and 00H00MZ

0JH63DZ and 00H03MZ	0JH63DZ and 05H34MZ	0JH63EZ and 01HY0MZ	0JH63FZ and 0JH839Z	0JH63PZ and 02HK3MZ	0JH70BZ and 00HV3MZ	0JH70CZ and 00HU4MZ
0JH63DZ and 00H04MZ	0JH63DZ and 05H40MZ	0JH63EZ and 01HY3MZ	0JH63PZ and 02H40JZ	0JH63PZ and 02HK4JZ	0JH70BZ and 00HV4MZ	0JH70CZ and 00HV0MZ
0JH63DZ and 00H60MZ	0JH63DZ and 05H43MZ	0JH63EZ and 01HY4MZ	0JH63PZ and 02H40MZ	0JH63PZ and 02HK4MZ	0JH70BZ and 01HY0MZ	0JH70CZ and 00HV3MZ
0JH63DZ and 00H63MZ	0JH63DZ and 05H44MZ	0JH63EZ and 05H00MZ	0JH63PZ and 02H43JZ	0JH63PZ and 02HL0JZ	0JH70BZ and 01HY3MZ	0JH70CZ and 00HV4MZ
0JH63DZ and 00H64MZ	0JH63DZ and 0DH60MZ	0JH63EZ and 05H03MZ	0JH63PZ and 02H43MZ	0JH63PZ and 02HL0MZ	0JH70BZ and 01HY4MZ	0JH70CZ and 01HY0MZ
0JH63DZ and 00HE0MZ	0JH63DZ and 0DH63MZ	0JH63EZ and 05H04MZ	0JH63PZ and 02H44JZ	0JH63PZ and 02HL3JZ	0JH70BZ and 05H00MZ	0JH70CZ and 01HY3MZ
0JH63DZ and 00HE3MZ	0JH63DZ and 0DH64MZ	0JH63EZ and 05H30MZ	0JH63PZ and 02H44MZ	0JH63PZ and 02HL3MZ	0JH70BZ and 05H03MZ	0JH70CZ and 01HY4MZ
0JH63DZ and 00HE4MZ	0JH63EZ and 00H00MZ	0JH63EZ and 05H33MZ	0JH63PZ and 02H60JZ	0JH63PZ and 02HL4JZ	0JH70BZ and 05H04MZ	0JH70CZ and 05H00MZ
0JH63DZ and 00HU0MZ	0JH63EZ and 00H03MZ	0JH63EZ and 05H34MZ	0JH63PZ and 02H60MZ	0JH63PZ and 02HL4MZ	0JH70BZ and 05H30MZ	0JH70CZ and 05H03MZ
0JH63DZ and 00HU3MZ	0JH63EZ and 00H04MZ	0JH63EZ and 05H40MZ	0JH63PZ and 02H63JZ	0JH63PZ and 02HN0JZ	0JH70BZ and 05H33MZ	0JH70CZ and 05H04MZ
0JH63DZ and 00HU4MZ	0JH63EZ and 00H60MZ	0JH63EZ and 05H43MZ	0JH63PZ and 02H63MZ	0JH63PZ and 02HN0MZ	0JH70BZ and 05H34MZ	0JH70CZ and 05H30MZ
0JH63DZ and 00HV0MZ	0JH63EZ and 00H63MZ	0JH63EZ and 05H44MZ	0JH63PZ and 02H64JZ	0JH63PZ and 02HN3JZ	0JH70BZ and 05H40MZ	0JH70CZ and 05H33MZ
0JH63DZ and 00HV3MZ	0JH63EZ and 00H64MZ	0JH63EZ and 0DH60MZ	0JH63PZ and 02H64MZ	0JH63PZ and 02HN3MZ	0JH70BZ and 05H43MZ	0JH70CZ and 05H34MZ
0JH63DZ and 00HV4MZ	0JH63EZ and 00HE0MZ	0JH63EZ and 0DH63MZ	0JH63PZ and 02H70JZ	0JH63PZ and 02HN4JZ	0JH70BZ and 05H44MZ	0JH70CZ and 05H40MZ
0JH63DZ and 01HY0MZ	0JH63EZ and 00HE3MZ	0JH63EZ and 0DH64MZ	0JH63PZ and 02H70MZ	0JH63PZ and 02HN4MZ	0JH70BZ and 0DH60MZ	0JH70CZ and 05H43MZ
0JH63DZ and 01HY3MZ	0JH63EZ and 00HE4MZ	0JH63FZ and 0JH608Z	0JH63PZ and 02H73JZ	0JH70BZ and 00HE0MZ	0JH70BZ and 0DH63MZ	0JH70CZ and 05H44MZ
0JH63DZ and 01HY4MZ	0JH63EZ and 00HU0MZ	0JH63FZ and 0JH609Z	0JH63PZ and 02H73MZ	0JH70BZ and 00HE3MZ	0JH70BZ and 0DH64MZ	0JH70CZ and 0DH60MZ
0JH63DZ and 05H00MZ	0JH63EZ and 00HU3MZ	0JH63FZ and 0JH638Z	0JH63PZ and 02H74JZ	0JH70BZ and 00HE4MZ	0JH70CZ and 00HE0MZ	0JH70CZ and 0DH63MZ
0JH63DZ and 05H03MZ	0JH63EZ and 00HU4MZ	0JH63FZ and 0JH639Z	0JH63PZ and 02H74MZ	0JH70BZ and 00HU0MZ	0JH70CZ and 00HE3MZ	0JH70CZ and 0DH64MZ
0JH63DZ and 05H04MZ	0JH63EZ and 00HV0MZ	0JH63FZ and 0JH808Z	0JH63PZ and 02HK0JZ	0JH70BZ and 00HU3MZ	0JH70CZ and 00HE4MZ	0JH70DZ and 00H00MZ
0JH63DZ and 05H30MZ	0JH63EZ and 00HV3MZ	0JH63FZ and 0JH809Z	0JH63PZ and 02HK0MZ	0JH70BZ and 00HU4MZ	0JH70CZ and 00HU0MZ	0JH70DZ and 00H03MZ
0JH63DZ and 05H33MZ	0JH63EZ and 00HV4MZ	0JH63FZ and 0JH838Z	0JH63PZ and 02HK3JZ	0JH70BZ and 00HV0MZ	0JH70CZ and 00HU3MZ	0JH70DZ and 00H04MZ

0JH70DZ	0JH70DZ	0JH70EZ	0JH73BZ	0JH73CZ	0JH73DZ	0JH73DZ
and 00H60MZ	and 05H43MZ	and 01HY4MZ	and 01HY0MZ	and 00HV3MZ	and 00H64MZ	and 0DH60MZ
0JH70DZ	0JH70DZ	0JH70EZ	0JH73BZ	0JH73CZ	0JH73DZ	0JH73DZ
and 00H63MZ	and 05H44MZ	and 05H00MZ	and 01HY3MZ	and 00HV4MZ	and 00HE0MZ	and 0DH63MZ
0JH70DZ	0JH70DZ	0JH70EZ	0JH73BZ	0JH73CZ	0JH73DZ	0JH73DZ
and 00H64MZ	and 0DH60MZ	and 05H03MZ	and 01HY4MZ	and 01HY0MZ	and 00HE3MZ	and 0DH64MZ
0JH70DZ	0JH70DZ	0JH70EZ	0JH73BZ	0JH73CZ	0JH73DZ	0JH73EZ
and 00HE0MZ	and 0DH63MZ	and 05H04MZ	and 05H00MZ	and 01HY3MZ	and 00HE4MZ	and 00H00MZ
0JH70DZ	0JH70DZ	0JH70EZ	0JH73BZ	0JH73CZ	0JH73DZ	0JH73EZ
and 00HE3MZ	and 0DH64MZ	and 05H30MZ	and 05H03MZ	and 01HY4MZ	and 00HU0MZ	and 00H03MZ
0JH70DZ	0JH70EZ	0JH70EZ	0JH73BZ	0JH73CZ	0JH73DZ	0JH73EZ
and 00HE4MZ	and 00H00MZ	and 05H33MZ	and 05H04MZ	and 05H00MZ	and 00HU3MZ	and 00H04MZ
0JH70DZ	0JH70EZ	0JH70EZ	0JH73BZ	0JH73CZ	0JH73DZ	0JH73EZ
and 00HU0MZ	and 00H03MZ	and 05H34MZ	and 05H30MZ	and 05H03MZ	and 00HU4MZ	and 00H60MZ
0JH70DZ	0JH70EZ	0JH70EZ	0JH73BZ	0JH73CZ	0JH73DZ	0JH73EZ
and 00HU3MZ	and 00H04MZ	and 05H40MZ	and 05H33MZ	and 05H04MZ	and 00HV0MZ	and 00H63MZ
0JH70DZ	0JH70EZ	0JH70EZ	0JH73BZ	0JH73CZ	0JH73DZ	0JH73EZ
and 00HU4MZ	and 00H60MZ	and 05H43MZ	and 05H34MZ	and 05H30MZ	and 00HV3MZ	and 00H64MZ
0JH70DZ	0JH70EZ	0JH70EZ	0JH73BZ	0JH73CZ	0JH73DZ	0JH73EZ
and 00HV0MZ	and 00H63MZ	and 05H44MZ	and 05H40MZ	and 05H33MZ	and 00HV4MZ	and 00HE0MZ
0JH70DZ	0JH70EZ	0JH70EZ	0JH73BZ	0JH73CZ	0JH73DZ	0JH73EZ
and 00HV3MZ	and 00H64MZ	and 0DH60MZ	and 05H43MZ	and 05H34MZ	and 01HY0MZ	and 00HE3MZ
0JH70DZ	0JH70EZ	0JH70EZ	0JH73BZ	0JH73CZ	0JH73DZ	0JH73EZ
and 00HV4MZ	and 00HE0MZ	and 0DH63MZ	and 05H44MZ	and 05H40MZ	and 01HY3MZ	and 00HE4MZ
0JH70DZ	0JH70EZ	0JH70EZ	0JH73BZ	0JH73CZ	0JH73DZ	0JH73EZ
and 01HY0MZ	and 00HE3MZ	and 0DH64MZ	and 0DH60MZ	and 05H43MZ	and 01HY4MZ	and 00HU0MZ
0JH70DZ	0JH70EZ	0JH73BZ	0JH73BZ	0JH73CZ	0JH73DZ	0JH73EZ
and 01HY3MZ	and 00HE4MZ	and 00HE0MZ	and 0DH63MZ	and 05H44MZ	and 05H00MZ	and 00HU3MZ
0JH70DZ	0JH70EZ	0JH73BZ	0JH73BZ	0JH73CZ	0JH73DZ	0JH73EZ
and 01HY4MZ	and 00HU0MZ	and 00HE3MZ	and 0DH64MZ	and 0DH60MZ	and 05H03MZ	and 00HU4MZ
0JH70DZ	0JH70EZ	0JH73BZ	0JH73CZ	0JH73CZ	0JH73DZ	0JH73EZ
and 05H00MZ	and 00HU3MZ	and 00HE4MZ	and 00HE0MZ	and 0DH63MZ	and 05H04MZ	and 00HV0MZ
0JH70DZ	0JH70EZ	0JH73BZ	0JH73CZ	0JH73CZ	0JH73DZ	0JH73EZ
and 05H03MZ	and 00HU4MZ	and 00HU0MZ	and 00HE3MZ	and 0DH64MZ	and 05H30MZ	and 00HV3MZ
0JH70DZ	0JH70EZ	0JH73BZ	0JH73CZ	0JH73DZ	0JH73DZ	0JH73EZ
and 05H04MZ	and 00HV0MZ	and 00HU3MZ	and 00HE4MZ	and 00H00MZ	and 05H33MZ	and 00HV4MZ
0JH70DZ	0JH70EZ	0JH73BZ	0JH73CZ	0JH73DZ	0JH73DZ	0JH73EZ
and 05H30MZ	and 00HV3MZ	and 00HU4MZ	and 00HU0MZ	and 00H03MZ	and 05H34MZ	and 01HY0MZ
0JH70DZ	0JH70EZ	0JH73BZ	0JH73CZ	0JH73DZ	0JH73DZ	0JH73EZ
and 05H33MZ	and 00HV4MZ	and 00HV0MZ	and 00HU3MZ	and 00H04MZ	and 05H40MZ	and 01HY3MZ
0JH70DZ	0JH70EZ	0JH73BZ	0JH73CZ	0JH73DZ	0JH73DZ	0JH73EZ
and 05H34MZ	and 01HY0MZ	and 00HV3MZ	and 00HU4MZ	and 00H60MZ	and 05H43MZ	and 01HY4MZ
0JH70DZ	0JH70EZ	0JH73BZ	0JH73CZ	0JH73DZ	0JH73DZ	0JH73EZ
and 05H40MZ	and 01HY3MZ	and 00HV4MZ	and 00HV0MZ	and 00H63MZ	and 05H44MZ	and 05H00MZ

0JH73EZ and 05H03MZ	0JH804Z and 02H64MZ	0JH804Z and 02HN3MZ	0JH805Z and 02HK0MZ	0JH806Z and 02H44MZ	0JH806Z and 02HL3MZ	0JH807Z and 02H70MZ
0JH73EZ and 05H04MZ	0JH804Z and 02H70JZ	0JH804Z and 02HN4JZ	0JH805Z and 02HK3JZ	0JH806Z and 02H60JZ	0JH806Z and 02HL4JZ	0JH807Z and 02H73JZ
0JH73EZ and 05H30MZ	0JH804Z and 02H70MZ	0JH804Z and 02HN4MZ	0JH805Z and 02HK3MZ	0JH806Z and 02H60MZ	0JH806Z and 02HL4MZ	0JH807Z and 02H73MZ
0JH73EZ and 05H33MZ	0JH804Z and 02H73JZ	0JH805Z and 02H40JZ	0JH805Z and 02HK4JZ	0JH806Z and 02H63JZ	0JH806Z and 02HN0JZ	0JH807Z and 02H74JZ
0JH73EZ and 05H34MZ	0JH804Z and 02H73MZ	0JH805Z and 02H40MZ	0JH805Z and 02HK4MZ	0JH806Z and 02H63MZ	0JH806Z and 02HN0MZ	0JH807Z and 02H74MZ
0JH73EZ and 05H40MZ	0JH804Z and 02H74JZ	0JH805Z and 02H43JZ	0JH805Z and 02HL0JZ	0JH806Z and 02H64JZ	0JH806Z and 02HN3JZ	0JH807Z and 02HK0JZ
0JH73EZ and 05H43MZ	0JH804Z and 02H74MZ	0JH805Z and 02H43MZ	0JH805Z and 02HL0MZ	0JH806Z and 02H64MZ	0JH806Z and 02HN3MZ	0JH807Z and 02HK0MZ
0JH73EZ and 05H44MZ	0JH804Z and 02HK0JZ	0JH805Z and 02H44JZ	0JH805Z and 02HL3JZ	0JH806Z and 02H70JZ	0JH806Z and 02HN4JZ	0JH807Z and 02HK3JZ
0JH73EZ and 0DH60MZ	0JH804Z and 02HK0MZ	0JH805Z and 02H44MZ	0JH805Z and 02HL3MZ	0JH806Z and 02H70MZ	0JH806Z and 02HN4MZ	0JH807Z and 02HK3MZ
0JH73EZ and 0DH63MZ	0JH804Z and 02HK3JZ	0JH805Z and 02H60JZ	0JH805Z and 02HL4JZ	0JH806Z and 02H73JZ	0JH807Z and 02H40JZ	0JH807Z and 02HK4JZ
0JH73EZ and 0DH64MZ	0JH804Z and 02HK3MZ	0JH805Z and 02H60MZ	0JH805Z and 02HL4MZ	0JH806Z and 02H73MZ	0JH807Z and 02H40MZ	0JH807Z and 02HK4MZ
0JH804Z and 02H40JZ	0JH804Z and 02HK4JZ	0JH805Z and 02H63JZ	0JH805Z and 02HN0JZ	0JH806Z and 02H74JZ	0JH807Z and 02H43JZ	0JH807Z and 02HL0JZ
0JH804Z and 02H40MZ	0JH804Z and 02HK4MZ	0JH805Z and 02H63MZ	0JH805Z and 02HN0MZ	0JH806Z and 02H74MZ	0JH807Z and 02H43MZ	0JH807Z and 02HL0MZ
0JH804Z and 02H43JZ	0JH804Z and 02HL0JZ	0JH805Z and 02H64JZ	0JH805Z and 02HN3JZ	0JH806Z and 02HK0JZ	0JH807Z and 02H44JZ	0JH807Z and 02HL3JZ
0JH804Z and 02H43MZ	0JH804Z and 02HL0MZ	0JH805Z and 02H64MZ	0JH805Z and 02HN3MZ	0JH806Z and 02HK0MZ	0JH807Z and 02H44MZ	0JH807Z and 02HL3MZ
0JH804Z and 02H44JZ	0JH804Z and 02HL3JZ	0JH805Z and 02H70JZ	0JH805Z and 02HN4JZ	0JH806Z and 02HK3JZ	0JH807Z and 02H60JZ	0JH807Z and 02HL4JZ
0JH804Z and 02H44MZ	0JH804Z and 02HL3MZ	0JH805Z and 02H70MZ	0JH805Z and 02HN4MZ	0JH806Z and 02HK3MZ	0JH807Z and 02H60MZ	0JH807Z and 02HL4MZ
0JH804Z and 02H60JZ	0JH804Z and 02HL4JZ	0JH805Z and 02H73JZ	0JH806Z and 02H40JZ	0JH806Z and 02HK4JZ	0JH807Z and 02H63JZ	0JH807Z and 02HN0JZ
0JH804Z and 02H60MZ	0JH804Z and 02HL4MZ	0JH805Z and 02H73MZ	0JH806Z and 02H40MZ	0JH806Z and 02HK4MZ	0JH807Z and 02H63MZ	0JH807Z and 02HN0MZ
0JH804Z and 02H63JZ	0JH804Z and 02HN0JZ	0JH805Z and 02H74JZ	0JH806Z and 02H43JZ	0JH806Z and 02HL0JZ	0JH807Z and 02H64JZ	0JH807Z and 02HN3JZ
0JH804Z and 02H63MZ	0JH804Z and 02HN0MZ	0JH805Z and 02H74MZ	0JH806Z and 02H43MZ	0JH806Z and 02HL0MZ	0JH807Z and 02H64MZ	0JH807Z and 02HN3MZ
0JH804Z and 02H64JZ	0JH804Z and 02HN3JZ	0JH805Z and 02HK0JZ	0JH806Z and 02H44JZ	0JH806Z and 02HL3JZ	0JH807Z and 02H70JZ	0JH807Z and 02HN4JZ

0JH807Z and 02HN4MZ	0JH809Z and 02H74KZ	0JH80BZ and 05H00MZ	0JH80CZ and 01HY3MZ	0JH80DZ and 00HE4MZ	0JH80EZ and 00H00MZ	0JH80EZ and 05H33MZ
0JH808Z and 02H40KZ	0JH809Z and 02HN0JZ	0JH80BZ and 05H03MZ	0JH80CZ and 01HY4MZ	0JH80DZ and 00HU0MZ	0JH80EZ and 00H03MZ	0JH80EZ and 05H34MZ
0JH808Z and 02H44KZ	0JH809Z and 02HN0KZ	0JH80BZ and 05H04MZ	0JH80CZ and 05H00MZ	0JH80DZ and 00HU3MZ	0JH80EZ and 00H04MZ	0JH80EZ and 05H40MZ
0JH808Z and 02HN0JZ	0JH809Z and 02HN0MZ	0JH80BZ and 05H30MZ	0JH80CZ and 05H03MZ	0JH80DZ and 00HU4MZ	0JH80EZ and 00H60MZ	0JH80EZ and 05H43MZ
0JH808Z and 02HN0KZ	0JH809Z and 02HN3JZ	0JH80BZ and 05H33MZ	0JH80CZ and 05H04MZ	0JH80DZ and 00HV0MZ	0JH80EZ and 00H63MZ	0JH80EZ and 05H44MZ
0JH808Z and 02HN0MZ	0JH809Z and 02HN3KZ	0JH80BZ and 05H34MZ	0JH80CZ and 05H30MZ	0JH80DZ and 00HV3MZ	0JH80EZ and 00H64MZ	0JH80EZ and 0DH60MZ
0JH808Z and 02HN3JZ	0JH809Z and 02HN3MZ	0JH80BZ and 05H40MZ	0JH80CZ and 05H33MZ	0JH80DZ and 00HV4MZ	0JH80EZ and 00HE0MZ	0JH80EZ and 0DH63MZ
0JH808Z and 02HN3KZ	0JH809Z and 02HN4JZ	0JH80BZ and 05H43MZ	0JH80CZ and 05H34MZ	0JH80DZ and 01HY0MZ	0JH80EZ and 00HE3MZ	0JH80EZ and 0DH64MZ
0JH808Z and 02HN3MZ	0JH809Z and 02HN4KZ	0JH80BZ and 05H44MZ	0JH80CZ and 05H40MZ	0JH80DZ and 01HY3MZ	0JH80EZ and 00HE4MZ	0JH80PZ and 02H40JZ
0JH808Z and 02HN4JZ	0JH809Z and 02HN4MZ	0JH80BZ and 0DH60MZ	0JH80CZ and 05H43MZ	0JH80DZ and 01HY4MZ	0JH80EZ and 00HU0MZ	0JH80PZ and 02H40MZ
0JH808Z and 02HN4KZ	0JH80BZ and 00HE0MZ	0JH80BZ and 0DH63MZ	0JH80CZ and 05H44MZ	0JH80DZ and 05H00MZ	0JH80EZ and 00HU3MZ	0JH80PZ and 02H43JZ
0JH808Z and 02HN4MZ	0JH80BZ and 00HE3MZ	0JH80BZ and 0DH64MZ	0JH80CZ and 0DH60MZ	0JH80DZ and 05H03MZ	0JH80EZ and 00HU4MZ	0JH80PZ and 02H43MZ
0JH809Z and 02H40KZ	0JH80BZ and 00HE4MZ	0JH80CZ and 00HE0MZ	0JH80CZ and 0DH63MZ	0JH80DZ and 05H04MZ	0JH80EZ and 00HV0MZ	0JH80PZ and 02H44JZ
0JH809Z and 02H43JZ	0JH80BZ and 00HU0MZ	0JH80CZ and 00HE3MZ	0JH80CZ and 0DH64MZ	0JH80DZ and 05H30MZ	0JH80EZ and 00HV3MZ	0JH80PZ and 02H44MZ
0JH809Z and 02H43KZ	0JH80BZ and 00HU3MZ	0JH80CZ and 00HE4MZ	0JH80DZ and 00H00MZ	0JH80DZ and 05H33MZ	0JH80EZ and 00HV4MZ	0JH80PZ and 02H60JZ
0JH809Z and 02H43MZ	0JH80BZ and 00HU4MZ	0JH80CZ and 00HU0MZ	0JH80DZ and 00H03MZ	0JH80DZ and 05H34MZ	0JH80EZ and 01HY0MZ	0JH80PZ and 02H60MZ
0JH809Z and 02H44KZ	0JH80BZ and 00HV0MZ	0JH80CZ and 00HU3MZ	0JH80DZ and 00H04MZ	0JH80DZ and 05H40MZ	0JH80EZ and 01HY3MZ	0JH80PZ and 02H63JZ
0JH809Z and 02H60KZ	0JH80BZ and 00HV3MZ	0JH80CZ and 00HU4MZ	0JH80DZ and 00H60MZ	0JH80DZ and 05H43MZ	0JH80EZ and 01HY4MZ	0JH80PZ and 02H63MZ
0JH809Z and 02H63KZ	0JH80BZ and 00HV4MZ	0JH80CZ and 00HV0MZ	0JH80DZ and 00H63MZ	0JH80DZ and 05H44MZ	0JH80EZ and 05H00MZ	0JH80PZ and 02H64JZ
0JH809Z and 02H64KZ	0JH80BZ and 01HY0MZ	0JH80CZ and 00HV3MZ	0JH80DZ and 00H64MZ	0JH80DZ and 0DH60MZ	0JH80EZ and 05H03MZ	0JH80PZ and 02H64MZ
0JH809Z and 02H70KZ	0JH80BZ and 01HY3MZ	0JH80CZ and 00HV4MZ	0JH80DZ and 00HE0MZ	0JH80DZ and 0DH63MZ	0JH80EZ and 05H04MZ	0JH80PZ and 02H70JZ
0JH809Z and 02H73KZ	0JH80BZ and 01HY4MZ	0JH80CZ and 01HY0MZ	0JH80DZ and 00HE3MZ	0JH80DZ and 0DH64MZ	0JH80EZ and 05H30MZ	0JH80PZ and 02H70MZ

0JH80PZ and 02H73JZ	0JH834Z and 02H40JZ	0JH834Z and 02HK4JZ	0JH835Z and 02H63JZ	0JH835Z and 02HN0JZ	0JH836Z and 02H74JZ	0JH837Z and 02H43JZ
0JH80PZ and 02H73MZ	0JH834Z and 02H40MZ	0JH834Z and 02HK4MZ	0JH835Z and 02H63MZ	0JH835Z and 02HN0MZ	0JH836Z and 02H74MZ	0JH837Z and 02H43MZ
0JH80PZ and 02H74JZ	0JH834Z and 02H43JZ	0JH834Z and 02HL0JZ	0JH835Z and 02H64JZ	0JH835Z and 02HN3JZ	0JH836Z and 02HK0JZ	0JH837Z and 02H44JZ
0JH80PZ and 02H74MZ	0JH834Z and 02H43MZ	0JH834Z and 02HL0MZ	0JH835Z and 02H64MZ	0JH835Z and 02HN3MZ	0JH836Z and 02HK0MZ	0JH837Z and 02H44MZ
0JH80PZ and 02HK0JZ	0JH834Z and 02H44JZ	0JH834Z and 02HL3JZ	0JH835Z and 02H70JZ	0JH835Z and 02HN4JZ	0JH836Z and 02HK3JZ	0JH837Z and 02H60JZ
0JH80PZ and 02HK0MZ	0JH834Z and 02H44MZ	0JH834Z and 02HL3MZ	0JH835Z and 02H70MZ	0JH835Z and 02HN4MZ	0JH836Z and 02HK3MZ	0JH837Z and 02H60MZ
0JH80PZ and 02HK3JZ	0JH834Z and 02H60JZ	0JH834Z and 02HL4JZ	0JH835Z and 02H73JZ	0JH836Z and 02H40JZ	0JH836Z and 02HK4JZ	0JH837Z and 02H63JZ
0JH80PZ and 02HK3MZ	0JH834Z and 02H60MZ	0JH834Z and 02HL4MZ	0JH835Z and 02H73MZ	0JH836Z and 02H40MZ	0JH836Z and 02HK4MZ	0JH837Z and 02H63MZ
0JH80PZ and 02HK4JZ	0JH834Z and 02H63JZ	0JH834Z and 02HN0JZ	0JH835Z and 02H74JZ	0JH836Z and 02H43JZ	0JH836Z and 02HL0JZ	0JH837Z and 02H64JZ
0JH80PZ and 02HK4MZ	0JH834Z and 02H63MZ	0JH834Z and 02HN0MZ	0JH835Z and 02H74MZ	0JH836Z and 02H43MZ	0JH836Z and 02HL0MZ	0JH837Z and 02H64MZ
0JH80PZ and 02HL0JZ	0JH834Z and 02H64JZ	0JH834Z and 02HN3JZ	0JH835Z and 02HK0JZ	0JH836Z and 02H44JZ	0JH836Z and 02HL3JZ	0JH837Z and 02H70JZ
0JH80PZ and 02HL0MZ	0JH834Z and 02H64MZ	0JH834Z and 02HN3MZ	0JH835Z and 02HK0MZ	0JH836Z and 02H44MZ	0JH836Z and 02HL3MZ	0JH837Z and 02H70MZ
0JH80PZ and 02HL3JZ	0JH834Z and 02H70JZ	0JH834Z and 02HN4JZ	0JH835Z and 02HK3JZ	0JH836Z and 02H60JZ	0JH836Z and 02HL4JZ	0JH837Z and 02H73JZ
0JH80PZ and 02HL3MZ	0JH834Z and 02H70MZ	0JH834Z and 02HN4MZ	0JH835Z and 02HK3MZ	0JH836Z and 02H60MZ	0JH836Z and 02HL4MZ	0JH837Z and 02H73MZ
0JH80PZ and 02HL4JZ	0JH834Z and 02H73JZ	0JH835Z and 02H40JZ	0JH835Z and 02HK4JZ	0JH836Z and 02H63JZ	0JH836Z and 02HN0JZ	0JH837Z and 02H74JZ
0JH80PZ and 02HL4MZ	0JH834Z and 02H73MZ	0JH835Z and 02H40MZ	0JH835Z and 02HK4MZ	0JH836Z and 02H63MZ	0JH836Z and 02HN0MZ	0JH837Z and 02H74MZ
0JH80PZ and 02HN0JZ	0JH834Z and 02H74JZ	0JH835Z and 02H43JZ	0JH835Z and 02HL0JZ	0JH836Z and 02H64JZ	0JH836Z and 02HN3JZ	0JH837Z and 02HK0JZ
0JH80PZ and 02HN0MZ	0JH834Z and 02H74MZ	0JH835Z and 02H43MZ	0JH835Z and 02HL0MZ	0JH836Z and 02H64MZ	0JH836Z and 02HN3MZ	0JH837Z and 02HK0MZ
0JH80PZ and 02HN3JZ	0JH834Z and 02HK0JZ	0JH835Z and 02H44JZ	0JH835Z and 02HL3JZ	0JH836Z and 02H70JZ	0JH836Z and 02HN4JZ	0JH837Z and 02HK3JZ
0JH80PZ and 02HN3MZ	0JH834Z and 02HK0MZ	0JH835Z and 02H44MZ	0JH835Z and 02HL3MZ	0JH836Z and 02H70MZ	0JH836Z and 02HN4MZ	0JH837Z and 02HK3MZ
0JH80PZ and 02HN4JZ	0JH834Z and 02HK3JZ	0JH835Z and 02H60JZ	0JH835Z and 02HL4JZ	0JH836Z and 02H73JZ	0JH837Z and 02H40JZ	0JH837Z and 02HK4JZ
0JH80PZ and 02HN4MZ	0JH834Z and 02HK3MZ	0JH835Z and 02H60MZ	0JH835Z and 02HL4MZ	0JH836Z and 02H73MZ	0JH837Z and 02H40MZ	0JH837Z and 02HK4MZ

0JH837Z and 02HL0JZ	0JH838Z and 02HN4MZ	0JH83BZ and 00HE3MZ	0JH83BZ and 0DH64MZ	0JH83CZ and 0DH60MZ	0JH83DZ and 05H03MZ	0JH83EZ and 00HU4MZ
0JH837Z and 02HL0MZ	0JH839Z and 02H40KZ	0JH83BZ and 00HE4MZ	0JH83CZ and 00HE0MZ	0JH83CZ and 0DH63MZ	0JH83DZ and 05H04MZ	0JH83EZ and 00HV0MZ
0JH837Z and 02HL3JZ	0JH839Z and 02H43JZ	0JH83BZ and 00HU0MZ	0JH83CZ and 00HE3MZ	0JH83CZ and 0DH64MZ	0JH83DZ and 05H30MZ	0JH83EZ and 00HV3MZ
0JH837Z and 02HL3MZ	0JH839Z and 02H43KZ	0JH83BZ and 00HU3MZ	0JH83CZ and 00HE4MZ	0JH83DZ and 00H00MZ	0JH83DZ and 05H33MZ	0JH83EZ and 00HV4MZ
0JH837Z and 02HL4JZ	0JH839Z and 02H43MZ	0JH83BZ and 00HU4MZ	0JH83CZ and 00HU0MZ	0JH83DZ and 00H03MZ	0JH83DZ and 05H34MZ	0JH83EZ and 01HY0MZ
0JH837Z and 02HL4MZ	0JH839Z and 02H44KZ	0JH83BZ and 00HV0MZ	0JH83CZ and 00HU3MZ	0JH83DZ and 00H04MZ	0JH83DZ and 05H40MZ	0JH83EZ and 01HY3MZ
0JH837Z and 02HN0JZ	0JH839Z and 02H60KZ	0JH83BZ and 00HV3MZ	0JH83CZ and 00HU4MZ	0JH83DZ and 00H60MZ	0JH83DZ and 05H43MZ	0JH83EZ and 01HY4MZ
0JH837Z and 02HN0MZ	0JH839Z and 02H63KZ	0JH83BZ and 00HV4MZ	0JH83CZ and 00HV0MZ	0JH83DZ and 00H63MZ	0JH83DZ and 05H44MZ	0JH83EZ and 05H00MZ
0JH837Z and 02HN3JZ	0JH839Z and 02H64KZ	0JH83BZ and 01HY0MZ	0JH83CZ and 00HV3MZ	0JH83DZ and 00H64MZ	0JH83DZ and 0DH60MZ	0JH83EZ and 05H03MZ
0JH837Z and 02HN3MZ	0JH839Z and 02H70KZ	0JH83BZ and 01HY3MZ	0JH83CZ and 00HV4MZ	0JH83DZ and 00HE0MZ	0JH83DZ and 0DH63MZ	0JH83EZ and 05H04MZ
0JH837Z and 02HN4JZ	0JH839Z and 02H73KZ	0JH83BZ and 01HY4MZ	0JH83CZ and 01HY0MZ	0JH83DZ and 00HE3MZ	0JH83DZ and 0DH64MZ	0JH83EZ and 05H30MZ
0JH837Z and 02HN4MZ	0JH839Z and 02H74KZ	0JH83BZ and 05H00MZ	0JH83CZ and 01HY3MZ	0JH83DZ and 00HE4MZ	0JH83EZ and 00H00MZ	0JH83EZ and 05H33MZ
0JH838Z and 02H40KZ	0JH839Z and 02HN0JZ	0JH83BZ and 05H03MZ	0JH83CZ and 01HY4MZ	0JH83DZ and 00HU0MZ	0JH83EZ and 00H03MZ	0JH83EZ and 05H34MZ
0JH838Z and 02H44KZ	0JH839Z and 02HN0KZ	0JH83BZ and 05H04MZ	0JH83CZ and 05H00MZ	0JH83DZ and 00HU3MZ	0JH83EZ and 00H04MZ	0JH83EZ and 05H40MZ
0JH838Z and 02HN0JZ	0JH839Z and 02HN0MZ	0JH83BZ and 05H30MZ	0JH83CZ and 05H03MZ	0JH83DZ and 00HU4MZ	0JH83EZ and 00H60MZ	0JH83EZ and 05H43MZ
0JH838Z and 02HN0KZ	0JH839Z and 02HN3JZ	0JH83BZ and 05H33MZ	0JH83CZ and 05H04MZ	0JH83DZ and 00HV0MZ	0JH83EZ and 00H63MZ	0JH83EZ and 05H44MZ
0JH838Z and 02HN0MZ	0JH839Z and 02HN3KZ	0JH83BZ and 05H34MZ	0JH83CZ and 05H30MZ	0JH83DZ and 00HV3MZ	0JH83EZ and 00H64MZ	0JH83EZ and 0DH60MZ
0JH838Z and 02HN3JZ	0JH839Z and 02HN3MZ	0JH83BZ and 05H40MZ	0JH83CZ and 05H33MZ	0JH83DZ and 00HV4MZ	0JH83EZ and 00HE0MZ	0JH83EZ and 0DH63MZ
0JH838Z and 02HN3KZ	0JH839Z and 02HN4JZ	0JH83BZ and 05H43MZ	0JH83CZ and 05H34MZ	0JH83DZ and 01HY0MZ	0JH83EZ and 00HE3MZ	0JH83EZ and 0DH64MZ
0JH838Z and 02HN3MZ	0JH839Z and 02HN4KZ	0JH83BZ and 05H44MZ	0JH83CZ and 05H40MZ	0JH83DZ and 01HY3MZ	0JH83EZ and 00HE4MZ	0JH83PZ and 02H40JZ
0JH838Z and 02HN4JZ	0JH839Z and 02HN4MZ	0JH83BZ and 0DH60MZ	0JH83CZ and 05H43MZ	0JH83DZ and 01HY4MZ	0JH83EZ and 00HU0MZ	0JH83PZ and 02H40MZ
0JH838Z and 02HN4KZ	0JH83BZ and 00HE0MZ	0JH83BZ and 0DH63MZ	0JH83CZ and 05H44MZ	0JH83DZ and 05H00MZ	0JH83EZ and 00HU3MZ	0JH83PZ and 02H43JZ

0JH83PZ and 02H43MZ
0JH83PZ and 02H44JZ
0JH83PZ and 02H44MZ
0JH83PZ and 02H60JZ
0JH83PZ and 02H60MZ
0JH83PZ and 02H63JZ
0JH83PZ and 02H63MZ
0JH83PZ and 02H64JZ
0JH83PZ and 02H64MZ
0JH83PZ and 02H70JZ
0JH83PZ and 02H70MZ
0JH83PZ and 02H73JZ
0JH83PZ and 02H73MZ
0JH83PZ and 02H74JZ
0JH83PZ and 02H74MZ
0JH83PZ and 02HK0JZ
0JH83PZ and 02HK0MZ
0JH83PZ and 02HK3JZ
0JH83PZ and 02HK3MZ
0JH83PZ and 02HK4JZ
0JH83PZ and 02HK4MZ
0JH83PZ and 02HL0JZ

0JH83PZ and 02HL0MZ
0JH83PZ and 02HL3JZ
0JH83PZ and 02HL3MZ
0JH83PZ and 02HL4JZ
0JH83PZ and 02HL4MZ
0JH83PZ and 02HN0JZ
0JH83PZ and 02HN0MZ
0JH83PZ and 02HN3JZ
0JH83PZ and 02HN3MZ
0JH83PZ and 02HN4JZ
0JH83PZ and 02HN4MZ
0NH00NZ and 00H00MZ
0NH00NZ and 00H03MZ
0NH00NZ and 00H04MZ
0NH00NZ and 00H60MZ
0NH00NZ and 00H63MZ
0NH00NZ and 00H64MZ
0PS33ZZ and 0PU33JZ
0PS43ZZ and 0PU43JZ
0QS03ZZ and 0QU03JZ
0QS13ZZ and 0QU13JZ
0QSS3ZZ and 0QUS3JZ

One of
0RG7070
0RG70A0
0RG70J0
0RG70K0
0RG7370
0RG73A0
0RG73J0
0RG73K0
0RG7470
0RG74A0
0RG74J0
0RG74K0
XRG70F3

with one of
0SG1070
0SG10A0
0SG10J0
0SG10K0
0SG1370
0SG13A0
0SG13J0
0SG13K0
0SG1470
0SG14A0
0SG14J0
0SG14K0
XRGC0F3

One of
0RG7071
0RG707J
0RG70AJ
0RG70J1
0RG70JJ
0RG70K1
0RG70KJ
0RG7371
0RG737J
0RG73AJ
0RG73J1
0RG73JJ
0RG73K1
0RG73KJ
0RG7471
0RG747J
0RG74AJ
0RG74J1
0RG74JJ
0RG74K1
0RG74KJ
XRG7092
XRG70F3

with one of
0SG1071
0SG107J
0SG10AJ
0SG10J1
0SG10JJ
0SG10K1
0SG10KJ
0SG1371
0SG137J
0SG13AJ
0SG13J1
0SG13JJ
0SG13K1
0SG13KJ
0SG1471
0SG147J
0SG14AJ
0SG14J1
0SG14JJ
0SG14K1
0SG14KJ
XRGC092
XRGC0F3

0SP908Z and 0SR9019
0SP908Z and 0SR901A
0SP908Z and 0SR901Z
0SP908Z and 0SR9029
0SP908Z and 0SR902A
0SP908Z and 0SR902Z
0SP908Z and 0SR9039
0SP908Z and 0SR903A
0SP908Z and 0SR903Z
0SP908Z and 0SR9049
0SP908Z and 0SR904A
0SP908Z and 0SR904Z

0SP908Z and 0SR9069
0SP908Z and 0SR906A
0SP908Z and 0SR906Z
0SP908Z and 0SR90J9
0SP908Z and 0SR90JA
0SP908Z and 0SR90JZ
0SP908Z and 0SRA009
0SP908Z and 0SRA00A
0SP908Z and 0SRA00Z
0SP908Z and 0SRA019
0SP908Z and 0SRA01A
0SP908Z and 0SRA01Z
0SP908Z and 0SRA039
0SP908Z and 0SRA03A
0SP908Z and 0SRA03Z
0SP908Z and 0SRA0J9
0SP908Z and 0SRA0JA
0SP908Z and 0SRA0JZ
0SP908Z and 0SRR019
0SP908Z and 0SRR01A
0SP908Z and 0SRR01Z
0SP908Z and 0SRR039

0SP908Z and 0SRR03A
0SP908Z and 0SRR03Z
0SP908Z and 0SRR0J9
0SP908Z and 0SRR0JA
0SP908Z and 0SRR0JZ
0SP908Z and 0SU909Z
0SP908Z and 0SUA09Z
0SP908Z and 0SUR09Z
0SP909Z and 0SR9019
0SP909Z and 0SR901A
0SP909Z and 0SR901Z
0SP909Z and 0SR9029
0SP909Z and 0SR902A
0SP909Z and 0SR902Z
0SP909Z and 0SR9039
0SP909Z and 0SR903A
0SP909Z and 0SR903Z
0SP909Z and 0SR9049
0SP909Z and 0SR904A
0SP909Z and 0SR904Z
0SP909Z and 0SR9069
0SP909Z and 0SR906A

0SP909Z and 0SR906Z
0SP909Z and 0SR90J9
0SP909Z and 0SR90JA
0SP909Z and 0SR90JZ
0SP909Z and 0SRA009
0SP909Z and 0SRA00A
0SP909Z and 0SRA00Z
0SP909Z and 0SRA019
0SP909Z and 0SRA01A
0SP909Z and 0SRA01Z
0SP909Z and 0SRA039
0SP909Z and 0SRA03A
0SP909Z and 0SRA03Z
0SP909Z and 0SRA0J9
0SP909Z and 0SRA0JA
0SP909Z and 0SRA0JZ
0SP909Z and 0SRR019
0SP909Z and 0SRR01A
0SP909Z and 0SRR01Z
0SP909Z and 0SRR039
0SP909Z and 0SRR03A
0SP909Z and 0SRR03Z

0SP909Z and 0SRR0J9	0SP90BZ and 0SR90JA	0SP90BZ and 0SRR0JZ	0SP90EZ and 0SRR0J9	0SP90JZ and 0SRA009	0SP948Z and 0SR901A	0SP948Z and 0SRA01Z
0SP909Z and 0SRR0JA	0SP90BZ and 0SR90JZ	0SP90BZ and 0SU909Z	0SP90EZ and 0SRR0JZ	0SP90JZ and 0SRA00A	0SP948Z and 0SR901Z	0SP948Z and 0SRA039
0SP909Z and 0SRR0JZ	0SP90BZ and 0SRA009	0SP90BZ and 0SUA09Z	0SP90EZ and 0SU909Z	0SP90JZ and 0SRA00Z	0SP948Z and 0SR9029	0SP948Z and 0SRA03A
0SP909Z and 0SU909Z	0SP90BZ and 0SRA00A	0SP90BZ and 0SUR09Z	0SP90EZ and 0SUA09Z	0SP90JZ and 0SRA019	0SP948Z and 0SR902A	0SP948Z and 0SRA03Z
0SP909Z and 0SUA09Z	0SP90BZ and 0SRA00Z	0SP90EZ and 0SR901A	0SP90JZ and 0SR9019	0SP90JZ and 0SRA01A	0SP948Z and 0SR902Z	0SP948Z and 0SRA0J9
0SP909Z and 0SUR09Z	0SP90BZ and 0SRA019	0SP90EZ and 0SR9039	0SP90JZ and 0SR902A	0SP90JZ and 0SRA01Z	0SP948Z and 0SR9039	0SP948Z and 0SRA0JA
0SP90BZ and 0SR9019	0SP90BZ and 0SRA01A	0SP90EZ and 0SR903A	0SP90JZ and 0SR901Z	0SP90JZ and 0SRA039	0SP948Z and 0SR903A	0SP948Z and 0SRA0JZ
0SP90BZ and 0SR901A	0SP90BZ and 0SRA01Z	0SP90EZ and 0SR904A	0SP90JZ and 0SR9029	0SP90JZ and 0SRA03A	0SP948Z and 0SR903Z	0SP948Z and 0SRR019
0SP90BZ and 0SR901Z	0SP90BZ and 0SRA039	0SP90EZ and 0SR904Z	0SP90JZ and 0SR902A	0SP90JZ and 0SRA03Z	0SP948Z and 0SR9049	0SP948Z and 0SRR01A
0SP90BZ and 0SR9029	0SP90BZ and 0SRA03A	0SP90EZ and 0SR906A	0SP90JZ and 0SR902Z	0SP90JZ and 0SRA0J9	0SP948Z and 0SR904A	0SP948Z and 0SRR01Z
0SP90BZ and 0SR902A	0SP90BZ and 0SRA03Z	0SP90EZ and 0SR90J9	0SP90JZ and 0SR9039	0SP90JZ and 0SRA0JA	0SP948Z and 0SR904Z	0SP948Z and 0SRR039
0SP90BZ and 0SR902Z	0SP90BZ and 0SRA0J9	0SP90EZ and 0SR90JZ	0SP90JZ and 0SR903A	0SP90JZ and 0SRA0JZ	0SP948Z and 0SR9069	0SP948Z and 0SRR03A
0SP90BZ and 0SR9039	0SP90BZ and 0SRA0JA	0SP90EZ and 0SRA009	0SP90JZ and 0SR903Z	0SP90JZ and 0SRR019	0SP948Z and 0SR906A	0SP948Z and 0SRR03Z
0SP90BZ and 0SR903A	0SP90BZ and 0SRA0JZ	0SP90EZ and 0SRA00Z	0SP90JZ and 0SR9049	0SP90JZ and 0SRR01A	0SP948Z and 0SR906Z	0SP948Z and 0SRR0J9
0SP90BZ and 0SR903Z	0SP90BZ and 0SRR019	0SP90EZ and 0SRA019	0SP90JZ and 0SR904A	0SP90JZ and 0SRR01Z	0SP948Z and 0SR90J9	0SP948Z and 0SRR0JA
0SP90BZ and 0SR9049	0SP90BZ and 0SRR01A	0SP90EZ and 0SRA01Z	0SP90JZ and 0SR904Z	0SP90JZ and 0SRR039	0SP948Z and 0SR90JA	0SP948Z and 0SRR0JZ
0SP90BZ and 0SR904A	0SP90BZ and 0SRR01Z	0SP90EZ and 0SRA039	0SP90JZ and 0SR9069	0SP90JZ and 0SRR03A	0SP948Z and 0SR90JZ	0SP948Z and 0SU909Z
0SP90BZ and 0SR904Z	0SP90BZ and 0SRR039	0SP90EZ and 0SRA03Z	0SP90JZ and 0SR906A	0SP90JZ and 0SRR03Z	0SP948Z and 0SRA009	0SP948Z and 0SUA09Z
0SP90BZ and 0SR9069	0SP90BZ and 0SRR03A	0SP90EZ and 0SRA0JA	0SP90JZ and 0SR906Z	0SP90JZ and 0SRR0J9	0SP948Z and 0SRA00A	0SP948Z and 0SUR09Z
0SP90BZ and 0SR906A	0SP90BZ and 0SRR03Z	0SP90EZ and 0SRR01A	0SP90JZ and 0SR90J9	0SP90JZ and 0SRR0JA	0SP948Z and 0SRA00Z	0SP94JZ and 0SR9019
0SP90BZ and 0SR906Z	0SP90BZ and 0SRR0J9	0SP90EZ and 0SRR03A	0SP90JZ and 0SR90JA	0SP90JZ and 0SRR0JZ	0SP948Z and 0SRA019	0SP94JZ and 0SR901A
0SP90BZ and 0SR90J9	0SP90BZ and 0SRR0JA	0SP90EZ and 0SRR03A	0SP90JZ and 0SR90JZ	0SP948Z and 0SR9019	0SP948Z and 0SRA01A	0SP94JZ and 0SR901Z

0SP94JZ and 0SR9029	0SP94JZ and 0SRA03A	0SPA0JZ and 0SR902Z	0SPA0JZ and 0SRA0J9	0SPA4JZ and 0SR904A	0SPA4JZ and 0SRR01Z	0SPB08Z and 0SRB069
0SP94JZ and 0SR902A	0SP94JZ and 0SRA03Z	0SPA0JZ and 0SR9039	0SPA0JZ and 0SRA0JA	0SPA4JZ and 0SR904Z	0SPA4JZ and 0SRR039	0SPB08Z and 0SRB06A
0SP94JZ and 0SR902Z	0SP94JZ and 0SRA0J9	0SPA0JZ and 0SR903A	0SPA0JZ and 0SRA0JZ	0SPA4JZ and 0SR9069	0SPA4JZ and 0SRR03A	0SPB08Z and 0SRB06Z
0SP94JZ and 0SR9039	0SP94JZ and 0SRA0JA	0SPA0JZ and 0SR903Z	0SPA0JZ and 0SRR019	0SPA4JZ and 0SR906A	0SPA4JZ and 0SRR03Z	0SPB08Z and 0SRB0J9
0SP94JZ and 0SR903A	0SP94JZ and 0SRA0JZ	0SPA0JZ and 0SR9049	0SPA0JZ and 0SRR01A	0SPA4JZ and 0SR906Z	0SPA4JZ and 0SRR0J9	0SPB08Z and 0SRB0JA
0SP94JZ and 0SR903Z	0SP94JZ and 0SRR019	0SPA0JZ and 0SR904A	0SPA0JZ and 0SRR01Z	0SPA4JZ and 0SR90J9	0SPA4JZ and 0SRR0JA	0SPB08Z and 0SRB0JZ
0SP94JZ and 0SR9049	0SP94JZ and 0SRR01A	0SPA0JZ and 0SR904Z	0SPA0JZ and 0SRR039	0SPA4JZ and 0SR90JA	0SPA4JZ and 0SRR0JZ	0SPB08Z and 0SRE009
0SP94JZ and 0SR904A	0SP94JZ and 0SRR01Z	0SPA0JZ and 0SR9069	0SPA0JZ and 0SRR03A	0SPA4JZ and 0SR90JZ	0SPA4JZ and 0SU909Z	0SPB08Z and 0SRE00A
0SP94JZ and 0SR904Z	0SP94JZ and 0SRR039	0SPA0JZ and 0SR906A	0SPA0JZ and 0SRR03Z	0SPA4JZ and 0SRA009	0SPA4JZ and 0SUA09Z	0SPB08Z and 0SRE00Z
0SP94JZ and 0SR9069	0SP94JZ and 0SRR03A	0SPA0JZ and 0SR906Z	0SPA0JZ and 0SRR0J9	0SPA4JZ and 0SRA00A	0SPA4JZ and 0SUR09Z	0SPB08Z and 0SRE019
0SP94JZ and 0SR906A	0SP94JZ and 0SRR03Z	0SPA0JZ and 0SR90J9	0SPA0JZ and 0SRR0JA	0SPA4JZ and 0SRA00Z	0SPB08Z and 0SRB019	0SPB08Z and 0SRE01A
0SP94JZ and 0SR906Z	0SP94JZ and 0SRR0J9	0SPA0JZ and 0SR90JA	0SPA0JZ and 0SRR0JZ	0SPA4JZ and 0SRA019	0SPB08Z and 0SRB01A	0SPB08Z and 0SRE01Z
0SP94JZ and 0SR90J9	0SP94JZ and 0SRR0JA	0SPA0JZ and 0SR90JZ	0SPA4JZ and 0SR9019	0SPA4JZ and 0SRA01A	0SPB08Z and 0SRB01Z	0SPB08Z and 0SRE039
0SP94JZ and 0SR90JA	0SP94JZ and 0SRR0JZ	0SPA0JZ and 0SRA009	0SPA4JZ and 0SR901A	0SPA4JZ and 0SRA01Z	0SPB08Z and 0SRB029	0SPB08Z and 0SRE03A
0SP94JZ and 0SR90JZ	0SP94JZ and 0SU909Z	0SPA0JZ and 0SRA00A	0SPA4JZ and 0SR901Z	0SPA4JZ and 0SRA039	0SPB08Z and 0SRB02A	0SPB08Z and 0SRE03Z
0SP94JZ and 0SRA009	0SP94JZ and 0SUA09Z	0SPA0JZ and 0SRA00Z	0SPA4JZ and 0SR9029	0SPA4JZ and 0SRA03A	0SPB08Z and 0SRB02Z	0SPB08Z and 0SRE0J9
0SP94JZ and 0SRA00A	0SP94JZ and 0SUR09Z	0SPA0JZ and 0SRA019	0SPA4JZ and 0SR902A	0SPA4JZ and 0SRA03Z	0SPB08Z and 0SRB039	0SPB08Z and 0SRE0JA
0SP94JZ and 0SRA00Z	0SPA0JZ and 0SR9019	0SPA0JZ and 0SRA01A	0SPA4JZ and 0SR902Z	0SPA4JZ and 0SRA0J9	0SPB08Z and 0SRB03A	0SPB08Z and 0SRE0JZ
0SP94JZ and 0SRA019	0SPA0JZ and 0SR901A	0SPA0JZ and 0SRA01Z	0SPA4JZ and 0SR9039	0SPA4JZ and 0SRA0JA	0SPB08Z and 0SRB03Z	0SPB08Z and 0SRS019
0SP94JZ and 0SRA01A	0SPA0JZ and 0SR901Z	0SPA0JZ and 0SRA039	0SPA4JZ and 0SR903A	0SPA4JZ and 0SRA0JZ	0SPB08Z and 0SRB049	0SPB08Z and 0SRS01A
0SP94JZ and 0SRA01Z	0SPA0JZ and 0SR9029	0SPA0JZ and 0SRA03A	0SPA4JZ and 0SR903Z	0SPA4JZ and 0SRR019	0SPB08Z and 0SRB04A	0SPB08Z and 0SRS01Z
0SP94JZ and 0SRA039	0SPA0JZ and 0SR902A	0SPA0JZ and 0SRA03Z	0SPA4JZ and 0SR9049	0SPA4JZ and 0SRR01A	0SPB08Z and 0SRB04Z	0SPB08Z and 0SRS039

0SPB08Z and 0SRS03A	0SPB09Z and 0SRB06Z	0SPB09Z and 0SRS0J9	0SPB0BZ and 0SRB0J9	0SPB0BZ and 0SRS0JA	0SPB0EZ and 0SRE03A	0SPB0JZ and 0SRB04A
0SPB08Z and 0SRS03Z	0SPB09Z and 0SRB0J9	0SPB09Z and 0SRS0JA	0SPB0BZ and 0SRB0JA	0SPB0BZ and 0SRS0JZ	0SPB0EZ and 0SRE0J9	0SPB0JZ and 0SRB04Z
0SPB08Z and 0SRS0J9	0SPB09Z and 0SRB0JA	0SPB09Z and 0SRS0JZ	0SPB0BZ and 0SRB0JZ	0SPB0BZ and 0SRB0JZ	0SPB0EZ and 0SRE0JZ	0SPB0JZ and 0SRB069
0SPB08Z and 0SRS0JA	0SPB09Z and 0SRB0JZ	0SPB09Z and 0SUB09Z	0SPB0BZ and 0SRE009	0SPB0BZ and 0SUB09Z	0SPB0EZ and 0SRS01A	0SPB0JZ and 0SRB06A
0SPB08Z and 0SRS0JZ	0SPB09Z and 0SRE009	0SPB09Z and 0SUE09Z	0SPB0BZ and 0SRE00A	0SPB0BZ and 0SUE09Z	0SPB0EZ and 0SRS039	0SPB0JZ and 0SRB06Z
0SPB08Z and 0SUB09Z	0SPB09Z and 0SRE00A	0SPB09Z and 0SUS09Z	0SPB0BZ and 0SRE00Z	0SPB0BZ and 0SUS09Z	0SPB0EZ and 0SRS03A	0SPB0JZ and 0SRB0EZ
0SPB08Z and 0SUE09Z	0SPB09Z and 0SRE00Z	0SPB0BZ and 0SRB019	0SPB0BZ and 0SRE019	0SPB0EZ and 0SRB019	0SPB0EZ and 0SRS03Z	0SPB0JZ and 0SRB0J9
0SPB08Z and 0SUS09Z	0SPB09Z and 0SRE019	0SPB0BZ and 0SRB01A	0SPB0BZ and 0SRE01A	0SPB0EZ and 0SRB01Z	0SPB0EZ and 0SRS0J9	0SPB0JZ and 0SRB0JA
0SPB09Z and 0SRB019	0SPB09Z and 0SRE01A	0SPB0BZ and 0SRB01Z	0SPB0BZ and 0SRE01Z	0SPB0EZ and 0SRB029	0SPB0EZ and 0SRS0JA	0SPB0JZ and 0SRB0JZ
0SPB09Z and 0SRB01A	0SPB09Z and 0SRE01Z	0SPB0BZ and 0SRB029	0SPB0BZ and 0SRE039	0SPB0EZ and 0SRB039	0SPB0EZ and 0SRS0JZ	0SPB0JZ and 0SRE009
0SPB09Z and 0SRB01Z	0SPB09Z and 0SRE039	0SPB0BZ and 0SRB02A	0SPB0BZ and 0SRE03A	0SPB0EZ and 0SRB03A	0SPB0EZ and 0SUB09Z	0SPB0JZ and 0SRE00A
0SPB09Z and 0SRB029	0SPB09Z and 0SRE03A	0SPB0BZ and 0SRB02Z	0SPB0BZ and 0SRE03Z	0SPB0EZ and 0SRB03Z	0SPB0EZ and 0SUE09Z	0SPB0JZ and 0SRE00Z
0SPB09Z and 0SRB02A	0SPB09Z and 0SRE03Z	0SPB0BZ and 0SRB039	0SPB0BZ and 0SRE0J9	0SPB0EZ and 0SRB049	0SPB0JZ and 0SRB019	0SPB0JZ and 0SRE019
0SPB09Z and 0SRB02Z	0SPB09Z and 0SRE0J9	0SPB0BZ and 0SRB03A	0SPB0BZ and 0SRE0JA	0SPB0EZ and 0SRB04A	0SPB0JZ and 0SRB01A	0SPB0JZ and 0SRE01A
0SPB09Z and 0SRB039	0SPB09Z and 0SRE0JA	0SPB0BZ and 0SRB03Z	0SPB0BZ and 0SRE0JZ	0SPB0EZ and 0SRB04Z	0SPB0JZ and 0SRB01Z	0SPB0JZ and 0SRE01Z
0SPB09Z and 0SRB03A	0SPB09Z and 0SRE0JZ	0SPB0BZ and 0SRB049	0SPB0BZ and 0SRS019	0SPB0EZ and 0SRB069	0SPB0JZ and 0SRB029	0SPB0JZ and 0SRE039
0SPB09Z and 0SRB03Z	0SPB09Z and 0SRS019	0SPB0BZ and 0SRB04A	0SPB0BZ and 0SRS01A	0SPB0EZ and 0SRB06A	0SPB0JZ and 0SRB02A	0SPB0JZ and 0SRE03A
0SPB09Z and 0SRB049	0SPB09Z and 0SRS01A	0SPB0BZ and 0SRB04Z	0SPB0BZ and 0SRS01Z	0SPB0EZ and 0SRB06Z	0SPB0JZ and 0SRB02Z	0SPB0JZ and 0SRE03Z
0SPB09Z and 0SRB04A	0SPB09Z and 0SRS01Z	0SPB0BZ and 0SRB069	0SPB0BZ and 0SRS039	0SPB0EZ and 0SRB0JA	0SPB0JZ and 0SRB039	0SPB0JZ and 0SRE0J9
0SPB09Z and 0SRB04Z	0SPB09Z and 0SRS039	0SPB0BZ and 0SRB06A	0SPB0BZ and 0SRS03A	0SPB0EZ and 0SRE00A	0SPB0JZ and 0SRB03A	0SPB0JZ and 0SRE0JA
0SPB09Z and 0SRB069	0SPB09Z and 0SRS03A	0SPB0BZ and 0SRB06Z	0SPB0BZ and 0SRS03Z	0SPB0EZ and 0SRE00Z	0SPB0JZ and 0SRB03Z	0SPB0JZ and 0SRE0JZ
0SPB09Z and 0SRB06A	0SPB09Z and 0SRS03Z	0SPB0BZ and 0SRB0EZ	0SPB0BZ and 0SRS0J9	0SPB0EZ and 0SRE01A	0SPB0JZ and 0SRB049	0SPB0JZ and 0SRS019

0SPB0JZ and 0SRS01A	0SPB48Z and 0SRB06Z	0SPB48Z and 0SRS03Z	0SPB4JZ and 0SRB0EZ	0SPB4JZ and 0SRS0J9	0SPC09Z and 0SRC0J9	0SPC0JC and 0SRC0EZ
0SPB0JZ and 0SRS01Z	0SPB48Z and 0SRB0EZ	0SPB48Z and 0SRS0J9	0SPB4JZ and 0SRB0J9	0SPB4JZ and 0SRS0JA	0SPC09Z and 0SRC0JA	0SPC0JC and 0SRC0J9
0SPB0JZ and 0SRS039	0SPB48Z and 0SRB0J9	0SPB48Z and 0SRS0JA	0SPB4JZ and 0SRB0JA	0SPB4JZ and 0SRS0JZ	0SPC09Z and 0SRC0JZ	0SPC0JC and 0SRC0JA
0SPB0JZ and 0SRS03A	0SPB48Z and 0SRB0JA	0SPB48Z and 0SRS0JZ	0SPB4JZ and 0SRB0JZ	0SPB4JZ and 0SUB09Z	0SPC09Z and 0SRC0L9	0SPC0JC and 0SRC0JZ
0SPB0JZ and 0SRS03Z	0SPB48Z and 0SRB0JZ	0SPB48Z and 0SUB09Z	0SPB4JZ and 0SRE009	0SPB4JZ and 0SUE09Z	0SPC09Z and 0SRC0LA	0SPC0JC and 0SRC0N9
0SPB0JZ and 0SRS0J9	0SPB48Z and 0SRE009	0SPB48Z and 0SUE09Z	0SPB4JZ and 0SRE00A	0SPB4JZ and 0SUS09Z	0SPC09Z and 0SRC0LZ	0SPC0JC and 0SRC0NA
0SPB0JZ and 0SRS0JA	0SPB48Z and 0SRE00A	0SPB48Z and 0SUS09Z	0SPB4JZ and 0SRE00Z	0SPC08Z and 0SRC069	0SPC09Z and 0SRC0M9	0SPC0JC and 0SRC0NZ
0SPB0JZ and 0SRS0JZ	0SPB48Z and 0SRE00Z	0SPB4JZ and 0SRB019	0SPB4JZ and 0SRE019	0SPC08Z and 0SRC06A	0SPC09Z and 0SRC0MZ	0SPC0JC and 0SRT0J9
0SPB48Z and 0SRB019	0SPB48Z and 0SRE019	0SPB4JZ and 0SRB01A	0SPB4JZ and 0SRE01A	0SPC08Z and 0SRC06Z	0SPC09Z and 0SRC0NA	0SPC0JC and 0SRT0JA
0SPB48Z and 0SRB01A	0SPB48Z and 0SRE01A	0SPB4JZ and 0SRB01Z	0SPB4JZ and 0SRE01Z	0SPC08Z and 0SRC0J9	0SPC09Z and 0SRC0NZ	0SPC0JC and 0SRT0JZ
0SPB48Z and 0SRB01Z	0SPB48Z and 0SRE01Z	0SPB4JZ and 0SRB029	0SPB4JZ and 0SRE039	0SPC08Z and 0SRC0JA	0SPC09Z and 0SRT0J9	0SPC0JC and 0SRV0J9
0SPB48Z and 0SRB029	0SPB48Z and 0SRE039	0SPB4JZ and 0SRB02A	0SPB4JZ and 0SRE03A	0SPC08Z and 0SRC0JZ	0SPC09Z and 0SRT0JA	0SPC0JC and 0SRV0JA
0SPB48Z and 0SRB02A	0SPB48Z and 0SRE03A	0SPB4JZ and 0SRB02Z	0SPB4JZ and 0SRE03Z	0SPC08Z and 0SRC0NA	0SPC09Z and 0SRT0JZ	0SPC0JC and 0SRV0JZ
0SPB48Z and 0SRB02Z	0SPB48Z and 0SRE03Z	0SPB4JZ and 0SRB039	0SPB4JZ and 0SRE0J9	0SPC08Z and 0SRT0J9	0SPC09Z and 0SRV0J9	0SPC0JZ and 0SRC069
0SPB48Z and 0SRB039	0SPB48Z and 0SRE0J9	0SPB4JZ and 0SRB03A	0SPB4JZ and 0SRE0JA	0SPC08Z and 0SRT0JA	0SPC09Z and 0SRV0JA	0SPC0JZ and 0SRC06A
0SPB48Z and 0SRB03A	0SPB48Z and 0SRE0JA	0SPB4JZ and 0SRB03Z	0SPB4JZ and 0SRE0JZ	0SPC08Z and 0SRT0JZ	0SPC09Z and 0SRV0JZ	0SPC0JZ and 0SRC06Z
0SPB48Z and 0SRB03Z	0SPB48Z and 0SRE0JZ	0SPB4JZ and 0SRB049	0SPB4JZ and 0SRS019	0SPC08Z and 0SRV0J9	0SPC09Z and 0SUV09Z	0SPC0JZ and 0SRC0J9
0SPB48Z and 0SRB049	0SPB48Z and 0SRS019	0SPB4JZ and 0SRB04A	0SPB4JZ and 0SRS01A	0SPC08Z and 0SRV0JA	0SPC0EZ and 0SRC069	0SPC0JZ and 0SRC0JA
0SPB48Z and 0SRB04A	0SPB48Z and 0SRS01A	0SPB4JZ and 0SRB04Z	0SPB4JZ and 0SRS01Z	0SPC08Z and 0SRV0JZ	0SPC0EZ and 0SRT0J9	0SPC0JZ and 0SRC0JZ
0SPB48Z and 0SRB04Z	0SPB48Z and 0SRS01Z	0SPB4JZ and 0SRB069	0SPB4JZ and 0SRS039	0SPC09Z and 0SRC069	0SPC0JC and 0SRC069	0SPC0JZ and 0SRC0L9
0SPB48Z and 0SRB069	0SPB48Z and 0SRS039	0SPB4JZ and 0SRB06A	0SPB4JZ and 0SRS03A	0SPC09Z and 0SRC06A	0SPC0JC and 0SRC06A	0SPC0JZ and 0SRC0LA
0SPB48Z and 0SRB06A	0SPB48Z and 0SRS03A	0SPB4JZ and 0SRB06Z	0SPB4JZ and 0SRS03Z	0SPC09Z and 0SRC06Z	0SPC0JC and 0SRC06Z	0SPC0JZ and 0SRC0LZ

	and			and			and	
0SPC0JZ	and	0SRC0MZ	0SPC0NZ	and	0SRC069	0SPC48Z	and	0SRC069
0SPC0JZ	and	0SRC0NA	0SPC0NZ	and	0SRC06A	0SPC48Z	and	0SRC06A
0SPC0JZ	and	0SRT0J9	0SPC0NZ	and	0SRC0J9	0SPC48Z	and	0SRC06Z
0SPC0JZ	and	0SRT0JA	0SPC0NZ	and	0SRC0JZ	0SPC48Z	and	0SRC0J9
0SPC0JZ	and	0SRT0JZ	0SPC0NZ	and	0SRC0L9	0SPC48Z	and	0SRC0JA
0SPC0JZ	and	0SRV0J9	0SPC0NZ	and	0SRC0LZ	0SPC48Z	and	0SRC0JZ
0SPC0JZ	and	0SRV0JA	0SPC0NZ	and	0SRT0J9	0SPC48Z	and	0SRC0N9
0SPC0JZ	and	0SRV0JZ	0SPC0NZ	and	0SRT0JZ	0SPC48Z	and	0SRC0NA
0SPC0LZ	and	0SRC069	0SPC0NZ	and	0SRV0JA	0SPC48Z	and	0SRC0NZ
0SPC0LZ	and	0SRC0JZ	0SPC38Z	and	0SRC069	0SPC48Z	and	0SRT0J9
0SPC0LZ	and	0SRT0J9	0SPC38Z	and	0SRC06A	0SPC48Z	and	0SRT0JA
0SPC0LZ	and	0SRT0JZ	0SPC38Z	and	0SRC06Z	0SPC48Z	and	0SRT0JZ
0SPC0MZ	and	0SRC069	0SPC38Z	and	0SRC0J9	0SPC48Z	and	0SRV0J9
0SPC0MZ	and	0SRC06A	0SPC38Z	and	0SRC0JA	0SPC48Z	and	0SRV0JA
0SPC0MZ	and	0SRC0J9	0SPC38Z	and	0SRC0JZ	0SPC48Z	and	0SRV0JZ
0SPC0MZ	and	0SRC0JZ	0SPC38Z	and	0SRC0NA	0SPC4JC	and	0SRC069
0SPC0MZ	and	0SRC0L9	0SPC38Z	and	0SRT0J9	0SPC4JC	and	0SRC06A
0SPC0MZ	and	0SRC0LZ	0SPC38Z	and	0SRT0JA	0SPC4JC	and	0SRC06Z
0SPC0MZ	and	0SRT0J9	0SPC38Z	and	0SRT0JZ	0SPC4JC	and	0SRC0J9
0SPC0MZ	and	0SRT0JA	0SPC38Z	and	0SRV0J9	0SPC4JC	and	0SRC0JA
0SPC0MZ	and	0SRT0JZ	0SPC38Z	and	0SRV0JA	0SPC4JC	and	0SRC0JZ
0SPC0MZ	and	0SRV0JA	0SPC38Z	and	0SRV0JZ	0SPC4JC	and	0SRC0N9

	and			and			and	
0SPC4JC	and	0SRC0NA	0SPC4MZ	and	0SRC069	0SPD08Z	and	0SRW0J9
0SPC4JC	and	0SRC0NZ	0SPC4MZ	and	0SRC0J9	0SPD08Z	and	0SRW0JA
0SPC4JC	and	0SRT0J9	0SPC4MZ	and	0SRC0JZ	0SPD08Z	and	0SRW0JZ
0SPC4JC	and	0SRT0JA	0SPC4MZ	and	0SRC0L9	0SPD09Z	and	0SRD069
0SPC4JC	and	0SRV0J9	0SPC4MZ	and	0SRC0LZ	0SPD09Z	and	0SRD06A
0SPC4JC	and	0SRV0JA	0SPC4MZ	and	0SRT0J9	0SPD09Z	and	0SRD06Z
0SPC4JZ	and	0SRC069	0SPC4MZ	and	0SRT0JZ	0SPD09Z	and	0SRD0J9
0SPC4JZ	and	0SRC06A	0SPC4NZ	and	0SRC069	0SPD09Z	and	0SRD0JA
0SPC4JZ	and	0SRC06Z	0SPC4NZ	and	0SRC0J9	0SPD09Z	and	0SRD0JZ
0SPC4JZ	and	0SRC0J9	0SPC4NZ	and	0SRC0JZ	0SPD09Z	and	0SRD0L9
0SPC4JZ	and	0SRC0JA	0SPC4NZ	and	0SRC0LZ	0SPD09Z	and	0SRD0LA
0SPC4JZ	and	0SRC0JZ	0SPC4NZ	and	0SRT0J9	0SPD09Z	and	0SRD0LZ
0SPC4JZ	and	0SRC0L9	0SPC4NZ	and	0SRT0JZ	0SPD09Z	and	0SRD0MA
0SPC4JZ	and	0SRC0LA	0SPD08Z	and	0SRD069	0SPD09Z	and	0SRD0NA
0SPC4JZ	and	0SRC0LZ	0SPD08Z	and	0SRD06A	0SPD09Z	and	0SRU0J9
0SPC4JZ	and	0SRC0NA	0SPD08Z	and	0SRD06Z	0SPD09Z	and	0SRU0JA
0SPC4JZ	and	0SRT0J9	0SPD08Z	and	0SRD0J9	0SPD09Z	and	0SRU0JZ
0SPC4JZ	and	0SRT0JA	0SPD08Z	and	0SRD0JA	0SPD09Z	and	0SRW0J9
0SPC4JZ	and	0SRT0JZ	0SPD08Z	and	0SRD0JZ	0SPD09Z	and	0SRW0JA
0SPC4JZ	and	0SRV0J9	0SPD08Z	and	0SRU0J9	0SPD09Z	and	0SRW0JZ
0SPC4JZ	and	0SRV0JA	0SPD08Z	and	0SRU0JA	0SPD09Z	and	0SUW09Z
0SPC4JZ	and	0SRV0JZ	0SPD08Z	and	0SRU0JZ	0SPD0EZ	and	0SRD069

0SPD0EZ	and	0SRD06Z
0SPD0EZ	and	0SRD0JZ
0SPD0EZ	and	0SRW0J9
0SPD0JC	and	0SRD069
0SPD0JC	and	0SRD06A
0SPD0JC	and	0SRD06Z
0SPD0JC	and	0SRD0J9
0SPD0JC	and	0SRD0JA
0SPD0JC	and	0SRD0JZ
0SPD0JC	and	0SRD0N9
0SPD0JC	and	0SRD0NA
0SPD0JC	and	0SRD0NZ
0SPD0JC	and	0SRU0J9
0SPD0JC	and	0SRU0JA
0SPD0JC	and	0SRU0JZ
0SPD0JC	and	0SRW0J9
0SPD0JC	and	0SRW0JA
0SPD0JC	and	0SRW0JZ
0SPD0JZ	and	0SRD069
0SPD0JZ	and	0SRD06A
0SPD0JZ	and	0SRD06Z
0SPD0JZ	and	0SRD0J9

0SPD0JZ and 0SRD0JA	0SPD0LZ and 0SRW0JA	0SPD0NZ and 0SRW0JA	0SPD48Z and 0SRU0JA	0SPD4JZ and 0SRD0J9	0SPE0JZ and 0SRB02A	0SPE0JZ and 0SRE03A
0SPD0JZ and 0SRD0JZ	0SPD0MZ and 0SRD069	0SPD38Z and 0SRD069	0SPD48Z and 0SRU0JZ	0SPD4JZ and 0SRD0JA	0SPE0JZ and 0SRB02Z	0SPE0JZ and 0SRE03Z
0SPD0JZ and 0SRD0L9	0SPD0MZ and 0SRD06A	0SPD38Z and 0SRD06A	0SPD48Z and 0SRW0J9	0SPD4JZ and 0SRD0JZ	0SPE0JZ and 0SRB039	0SPE0JZ and 0SRE0J9
0SPD0JZ and 0SRD0LA	0SPD0MZ and 0SRD06Z	0SPD38Z and 0SRD06Z	0SPD48Z and 0SRW0JA	0SPD4JZ and 0SRD0L9	0SPE0JZ and 0SRB03A	0SPE0JZ and 0SRE0JA
0SPD0JZ and 0SRD0LZ	0SPD0MZ and 0SRD0J9	0SPD38Z and 0SRD0J9	0SPD48Z and 0SRW0JZ	0SPD4JZ and 0SRD0LA	0SPE0JZ and 0SRB03Z	0SPE0JZ and 0SRE0JZ
0SPD0JZ and 0SRD0MA	0SPD0MZ and 0SRD0JZ	0SPD38Z and 0SRD0JA	0SPD4JC and 0SRD069	0SPD4JZ and 0SRD0LZ	0SPE0JZ and 0SRB049	0SPE0JZ and 0SRS019
0SPD0JZ and 0SRD0NA	0SPD0MZ and 0SRD0L9	0SPD38Z and 0SRD0JZ	0SPD4JC and 0SRD06A	0SPD4JZ and 0SRD0MA	0SPE0JZ and 0SRB04A	0SPE0JZ and 0SRS01A
0SPD0JZ and 0SRU0J9	0SPD0MZ and 0SRD0LZ	0SPD38Z and 0SRD0NA	0SPD4JC and 0SRD06Z	0SPD4JZ and 0SRD0NA	0SPE0JZ and 0SRB04Z	0SPE0JZ and 0SRS01Z
0SPD0JZ and 0SRU0JA	0SPD0MZ and 0SRU0JA	0SPD38Z and 0SRU0J9	0SPD4JC and 0SRD0J9	0SPD4JZ and 0SRU0J9	0SPE0JZ and 0SRB069	0SPE0JZ and 0SRS039
0SPD0JZ and 0SRU0JZ	0SPD0MZ and 0SRW0J9	0SPD38Z and 0SRU0JA	0SPD4JC and 0SRD0JA	0SPD4JZ and 0SRU0JA	0SPE0JZ and 0SRB06A	0SPE0JZ and 0SRS03A
0SPD0JZ and 0SRW0J9	0SPD0MZ and 0SRW0JA	0SPD38Z and 0SRU0JZ	0SPD4JC and 0SRD0JZ	0SPD4JZ and 0SRU0JZ	0SPE0JZ and 0SRB06Z	0SPE0JZ and 0SRS03Z
0SPD0JZ and 0SRW0JA	0SPD0NZ and 0SRD069	0SPD38Z and 0SRW0J9	0SPD4JC and 0SRD0N9	0SPD4JZ and 0SRW0J9	0SPE0JZ and 0SRB0EZ	0SPE0JZ and 0SRS0J9
0SPD0JZ and 0SRW0JZ	0SPD0NZ and 0SRD06A	0SPD38Z and 0SRW0JA	0SPD4JC and 0SRD0NA	0SPD4JZ and 0SRW0JA	0SPE0JZ and 0SRB0J9	0SPE0JZ and 0SRS0JA
0SPD0LZ and 0SRD069	0SPD0NZ and 0SRD06Z	0SPD38Z and 0SRW0JZ	0SPD4JC and 0SRD0NZ	0SPD4JZ and 0SRW0JZ	0SPE0JZ and 0SRB0JA	0SPE0JZ and 0SRS0JZ
0SPD0LZ and 0SRD06A	0SPD0NZ and 0SRD0J9	0SPD48Z and 0SRD069	0SPD4JC and 0SRU0J9	0SPD4MZ and 0SRD06Z	0SPE0JZ and 0SRB0JZ	0SPE4JZ and 0SRB019
0SPD0LZ and 0SRD06Z	0SPD0NZ and 0SRD0JA	0SPD48Z and 0SRD06A	0SPD4JC and 0SRU0JA	0SPD4NZ and 0SRD069	0SPE0JZ and 0SRE009	0SPE4JZ and 0SRB01A
0SPD0LZ and 0SRD0J9	0SPD0NZ and 0SRD0JZ	0SPD48Z and 0SRD06Z	0SPD4JC and 0SRW0J9	0SPD4NZ and 0SRD06Z	0SPE0JZ and 0SRE00A	0SPE4JZ and 0SRB01Z
0SPD0LZ and 0SRD0JZ	0SPD0NZ and 0SRD0L9	0SPD48Z and 0SRD0J9	0SPD4JC and 0SRW0JA	0SPD4NZ and 0SRW0J9	0SPE0JZ and 0SRE00Z	0SPE4JZ and 0SRB029
0SPD0LZ and 0SRD0L9	0SPD0NZ and 0SRD0LZ	0SPD48Z and 0SRD0JA	0SPD4JC and 0SRW0JZ	0SPE0JZ and 0SRB019	0SPE0JZ and 0SRE019	0SPE4JZ and 0SRB02A
0SPD0LZ and 0SRD0LZ	0SPD0NZ and 0SRU0JA	0SPD48Z and 0SRD0JZ	0SPD4JZ and 0SRD069	0SPE0JZ and 0SRB01A	0SPE0JZ and 0SRE01A	0SPE4JZ and 0SRB02Z
0SPD0LZ and 0SRU0JA	0SPD0NZ and 0SRU0JZ	0SPD48Z and 0SRD0NA	0SPD4JZ and 0SRD06A	0SPE0JZ and 0SRB01Z	0SPE0JZ and 0SRE01Z	0SPE4JZ and 0SRB039
0SPD0LZ and 0SRW0J9	0SPD0NZ and 0SRW0J9	0SPD48Z and 0SRU0J9	0SPD4JZ and 0SRD06Z	0SPE0JZ and 0SRB029	0SPE0JZ and 0SRE039	0SPE4JZ and 0SRB03A

0SPE4JZ and 0SRB03Z	0SPE4JZ and 0SRE0JZ	0SPR0JZ and 0SR9049	0SPR0JZ and 0SRR01A	0SPR4JZ and 0SR906Z	0SPR4JZ and 0SRR0J9	0SPS0JZ and 0SRB0J9
0SPE4JZ and 0SRB049	0SPE4JZ and 0SRS019	0SPR0JZ and 0SR904A	0SPR0JZ and 0SRR01Z	0SPR4JZ and 0SR90J9	0SPR4JZ and 0SRR0JA	0SPS0JZ and 0SRB0JA
0SPE4JZ and 0SRB04A	0SPE4JZ and 0SRS01A	0SPR0JZ and 0SR904Z	0SPR0JZ and 0SRR039	0SPR4JZ and 0SR90JA	0SPR4JZ and 0SRR0JZ	0SPS0JZ and 0SRB0JZ
0SPE4JZ and 0SRB04Z	0SPE4JZ and 0SRS01Z	0SPR0JZ and 0SR9069	0SPR0JZ and 0SRR03A	0SPR4JZ and 0SR90JZ	0SPR4JZ and 0SU909Z	0SPS0JZ and 0SRE009
0SPE4JZ and 0SRB069	0SPE4JZ and 0SRS039	0SPR0JZ and 0SR906A	0SPR0JZ and 0SRR03Z	0SPR4JZ and 0SRA009	0SPR4JZ and 0SUA09Z	0SPS0JZ and 0SRE00A
0SPE4JZ and 0SRB06A	0SPE4JZ and 0SRS03A	0SPR0JZ and 0SR906Z	0SPR0JZ and 0SRR0J9	0SPR4JZ and 0SRA00A	0SPR4JZ and 0SUR09Z	0SPS0JZ and 0SRE00Z
0SPE4JZ and 0SRB06Z	0SPE4JZ and 0SRS03Z	0SPR0JZ and 0SR90J9	0SPR0JZ and 0SRR0JA	0SPR4JZ and 0SRA00Z	0SPS0JZ and 0SRB019	0SPS0JZ and 0SRE019
0SPE4JZ and 0SRB0EZ	0SPE4JZ and 0SRS0J9	0SPR0JZ and 0SR90JA	0SPR0JZ and 0SRR0JZ	0SPR4JZ and 0SRA019	0SPS0JZ and 0SRB01A	0SPS0JZ and 0SRE01A
0SPE4JZ and 0SRB0J9	0SPE4JZ and 0SRS0JA	0SPR0JZ and 0SR90JZ	0SPR4JZ and 0SR9019	0SPR4JZ and 0SRA01A	0SPS0JZ and 0SRB01Z	0SPS0JZ and 0SRE01Z
0SPE4JZ and 0SRB0JA	0SPE4JZ and 0SRS0JZ	0SPR0JZ and 0SRA009	0SPR4JZ and 0SR901A	0SPR4JZ and 0SRA01Z	0SPS0JZ and 0SRB029	0SPS0JZ and 0SRE039
0SPE4JZ and 0SRB0JZ	0SPE4JZ and 0SUB09Z	0SPR0JZ and 0SRA00A	0SPR4JZ and 0SR901Z	0SPR4JZ and 0SRA039	0SPS0JZ and 0SRB02A	0SPS0JZ and 0SRE03A
0SPE4JZ and 0SRE009	0SPE4JZ and 0SUE09Z	0SPR0JZ and 0SRA00Z	0SPR4JZ and 0SR9029	0SPR4JZ and 0SRA03A	0SPS0JZ and 0SRB02Z	0SPS0JZ and 0SRE03Z
0SPE4JZ and 0SRE00A	0SPE4JZ and 0SUS09Z	0SPR0JZ and 0SRA019	0SPR4JZ and 0SR902A	0SPR4JZ and 0SRA03Z	0SPS0JZ and 0SRB039	0SPS0JZ and 0SRE0J9
0SPE4JZ and 0SRE00Z	0SPR0JZ and 0SR9019	0SPR0JZ and 0SRA01A	0SPR4JZ and 0SR902Z	0SPR4JZ and 0SRA0J9	0SPS0JZ and 0SRB03A	0SPS0JZ and 0SRE0JA
0SPE4JZ and 0SRE019	0SPR0JZ and 0SR901A	0SPR0JZ and 0SRA01Z	0SPR4JZ and 0SR9039	0SPR4JZ and 0SRA0JA	0SPS0JZ and 0SRB03Z	0SPS0JZ and 0SRE0JZ
0SPE4JZ and 0SRE01A	0SPR0JZ and 0SR901Z	0SPR0JZ and 0SRA039	0SPR4JZ and 0SR903A	0SPR4JZ and 0SRA0JZ	0SPS0JZ and 0SRB049	0SPS0JZ and 0SRS019
0SPE4JZ and 0SRE01Z	0SPR0JZ and 0SR9029	0SPR0JZ and 0SRA03A	0SPR4JZ and 0SR903Z	0SPR4JZ and 0SRR019	0SPS0JZ and 0SRB04A	0SPS0JZ and 0SRS01A
0SPE4JZ and 0SRE039	0SPR0JZ and 0SR902A	0SPR0JZ and 0SRA03Z	0SPR4JZ and 0SR9049	0SPR4JZ and 0SRR01A	0SPS0JZ and 0SRB04Z	0SPS0JZ and 0SRS01Z
0SPE4JZ and 0SRE03A	0SPR0JZ and 0SR902Z	0SPR0JZ and 0SRA0J9	0SPR4JZ and 0SR904A	0SPR4JZ and 0SRR01Z	0SPS0JZ and 0SRB069	0SPS0JZ and 0SRS039
0SPE4JZ and 0SRE03Z	0SPR0JZ and 0SR9039	0SPR0JZ and 0SRA0JA	0SPR4JZ and 0SR904Z	0SPR4JZ and 0SRR039	0SPS0JZ and 0SRB06A	0SPS0JZ and 0SRS03A
0SPE4JZ and 0SRE0J9	0SPR0JZ and 0SR903A	0SPR0JZ and 0SRA0JZ	0SPR4JZ and 0SR9069	0SPR4JZ and 0SRR03A	0SPS0JZ and 0SRB06Z	0SPS0JZ and 0SRS03Z
0SPE4JZ and 0SRE0JA	0SPR0JZ and 0SR903Z	0SPR0JZ and 0SRR019	0SPR4JZ and 0SR906A	0SPR4JZ and 0SRR03Z	0SPS0JZ and 0SRB0EZ	0SPS0JZ and 0SRS0J9

0SPS0JZ and 0SRS0JA	0SPS4JZ and 0SRE00A	0SPS4JZ and 0SUS09Z	0SPT4JZ and 0SRC0N9	0SPU4JZ and 0SRD069	0SPV0JZ and 0SRT0J9	0SPW0JZ and 0SRD0J9
0SPS0JZ and 0SRS0JZ	0SPS4JZ and 0SRE00Z	0SPT0JZ and 0SRC069	0SPT4JZ and 0SRC0NA	0SPU4JZ and 0SRD06A	0SPV0JZ and 0SRT0JA	0SPW0JZ and 0SRD0JA
0SPS4JZ and 0SRB019	0SPS4JZ and 0SRE019	0SPT0JZ and 0SRC06A	0SPT4JZ and 0SRC0NZ	0SPU4JZ and 0SRD06Z	0SPV0JZ and 0SRT0JZ	0SPW0JZ and 0SRD0JZ
0SPS4JZ and 0SRB01A	0SPS4JZ and 0SRE01A	0SPT0JZ and 0SRC06Z	0SPT4JZ and 0SRT0J9	0SPU4JZ and 0SRD0EZ	0SPV0JZ and 0SRV0J9	0SPW0JZ and 0SRD0NA
0SPS4JZ and 0SRB01Z	0SPS4JZ and 0SRE01Z	0SPT0JZ and 0SRC0J9	0SPT4JZ and 0SRT0JA	0SPU4JZ and 0SRD0J9	0SPV0JZ and 0SRV0JA	0SPW0JZ and 0SRU0J9
0SPS4JZ and 0SRB029	0SPS4JZ and 0SRE039	0SPT0JZ and 0SRC0JA	0SPT4JZ and 0SRV0J9	0SPU4JZ and 0SRD0JA	0SPV0JZ and 0SRV0JZ	0SPW0JZ and 0SRU0JA
0SPS4JZ and 0SRB02A	0SPS4JZ and 0SRE03A	0SPT0JZ and 0SRC0JZ	0SPT4JZ and 0SRV0JA	0SPU4JZ and 0SRD0JZ	0SPV4JZ and 0SRC069	0SPW0JZ and 0SRU0JZ
0SPS4JZ and 0SRB02Z	0SPS4JZ and 0SRE03Z	0SPT0JZ and 0SRC0N9	0SPU0JZ and 0SRD069	0SPU4JZ and 0SRD0N9	0SPV4JZ and 0SRC06A	0SPW0JZ and 0SRW0J9
0SPS4JZ and 0SRB039	0SPS4JZ and 0SRE0J9	0SPT0JZ and 0SRC0NA	0SPU0JZ and 0SRD06A	0SPU4JZ and 0SRD0NA	0SPV4JZ and 0SRC06Z	0SPW0JZ and 0SRW0JA
0SPS4JZ and 0SRB03A	0SPS4JZ and 0SRE0JA	0SPT0JZ and 0SRC0NZ	0SPU0JZ and 0SRD06Z	0SPU4JZ and 0SRD0NZ	0SPV4JZ and 0SRC0J9	0SPW0JZ and 0SRW0JZ
0SPS4JZ and 0SRB03Z	0SPS4JZ and 0SRE0JZ	0SPT0JZ and 0SRT0J9	0SPU0JZ and 0SRD0J9	0SPU4JZ and 0SRU0J9	0SPV4JZ and 0SRC0JA	0SPW4JZ and 0SRD069
0SPS4JZ and 0SRB049	0SPS4JZ and 0SRS019	0SPT0JZ and 0SRT0JA	0SPU0JZ and 0SRD0JA	0SPU4JZ and 0SRU0JA	0SPV4JZ and 0SRC0JZ	0SPW4JZ and 0SRD06A
0SPS4JZ and 0SRB04A	0SPS4JZ and 0SRS01A	0SPT0JZ and 0SRT0JZ	0SPU0JZ and 0SRD0JZ	0SPU4JZ and 0SRW0J9	0SPV4JZ and 0SRC0N9	0SPW4JZ and 0SRD06Z
0SPS4JZ and 0SRB04Z	0SPS4JZ and 0SRS01Z	0SPT0JZ and 0SRV0J9	0SPU0JZ and 0SRD0N9	0SPU4JZ and 0SRW0JA	0SPV4JZ and 0SRC0NA	0SPW4JZ and 0SRD0J9
0SPS4JZ and 0SRB069	0SPS4JZ and 0SRS039	0SPT0JZ and 0SRV0JA	0SPU0JZ and 0SRD0NA	0SPU4JZ and 0SRW0JZ	0SPV4JZ and 0SRC0NZ	0SPW4JZ and 0SRD0JA
0SPS4JZ and 0SRB06A	0SPS4JZ and 0SRS03A	0SPT0JZ and 0SRV0JZ	0SPU0JZ and 0SRD0NZ	0SPV0JZ and 0SRC069	0SPV4JZ and 0SRT0J9	0SPW4JZ and 0SRD0JZ
0SPS4JZ and 0SRB06Z	0SPS4JZ and 0SRS03Z	0SPT4JZ and 0SRC069	0SPU0JZ and 0SRU0J9	0SPV0JZ and 0SRC06A	0SPV4JZ and 0SRT0JA	0SPW4JZ and 0SRD0NA
0SPS4JZ and 0SRB0EZ	0SPS4JZ and 0SRS0J9	0SPT4JZ and 0SRC06A	0SPU0JZ and 0SRU0JA	0SPV0JZ and 0SRC06Z	0SPV4JZ and 0SRV0J9	0SPW4JZ and 0SRD0NZ
0SPS4JZ and 0SRB0J9	0SPS4JZ and 0SRS0JA	0SPT4JZ and 0SRC06Z	0SPU0JZ and 0SRU0JZ	0SPV0JZ and 0SRC0J9	0SPV4JZ and 0SRV0JA	0SPW4JZ and 0SRU0J9
0SPS4JZ and 0SRB0JA	0SPS4JZ and 0SRS0JZ	0SPT4JZ and 0SRC0J9	0SPU0JZ and 0SRW0J9	0SPV0JZ and 0SRC0JA	0SPW0JZ and 0SRD069	0SPW4JZ and 0SRU0JA
0SPS4JZ and 0SRB0JZ	0SPS4JZ and 0SUB09Z	0SPT4JZ and 0SRC0JA	0SPU0JZ and 0SRW0JA	0SPV0JZ and 0SRC0JZ	0SPW0JZ and 0SRD06A	0SPW4JZ and 0SRW0J9
0SPS4JZ and 0SRE009	0SPS4JZ and 0SUE09Z	0SPT4JZ and 0SRC0JZ	0SPU0JZ and 0SRW0JZ	0SPV0JZ and 0SRC0NA	0SPW0JZ and 0SRD06Z	0SPW4JZ and 0SRW0JA

0SPW4JZ and 0SRW0JZ	0SRA03A and 0SP90EZ	0SRC0EZ and 0SPC08Z	0SRC0JZ and 0SPC4LZ	0SRC0N9 and 0SPC4JZ	0SRD0EZ and 0SPU0JZ	0SRD0LA and 0SPD4LZ
0SR9019 and 0SP90EZ	0SRA0J9 and 0SP90EZ	0SRC0EZ and 0SPC09Z	0SRC0L9 and 0SPC0LZ	0SRC0N9 and 0SPV0JZ	0SRD0EZ and 0SPW0JZ	0SRD0LA and 0SPD4MZ
0SR901Z and 0SP90EZ	0SRA0JZ and 0SP90EZ	0SRC0EZ and 0SPC0JZ	0SRC0L9 and 0SPC4LZ	0SRC0NZ and 0SPC08Z	0SRD0EZ and 0SPW4JZ	0SRD0LA and 0SPD4NZ
0SR9029 and 0SP90EZ	0SRB01A and 0SPB0EZ	0SRC0EZ and 0SPC38Z	0SRC0L9 and 0SPC4NZ	0SRC0NZ and 0SPC0JZ	0SRD0J9 and 0SPD0EZ	0SRD0LZ and 0SPD4LZ
0SR902Z and 0SP90EZ	0SRB02A and 0SPB0EZ	0SRC0EZ and 0SPC48Z	0SRC0LA and 0SPC0LZ	0SRC0NZ and 0SPC38Z	0SRD0J9 and 0SPD4LZ	0SRD0LZ and 0SPD4MZ
0SR903Z and 0SP90EZ	0SRB0EZ and 0SPB08Z	0SRC0EZ and 0SPC4JC	0SRC0LA and 0SPC0MZ	0SRC0NZ and 0SPC4JZ	0SRD0J9 and 0SPD4MZ	0SRD0LZ and 0SPD4NZ
0SR9049 and 0SP90EZ	0SRB0EZ and 0SPB09Z	0SRC0EZ and 0SPC4JZ	0SRC0LA and 0SPC0NZ	0SRC0NZ and 0SPV0JZ	0SRD0J9 and 0SPD4NZ	0SRD0M9 and 0SPD09Z
0SR9069 and 0SP90EZ	0SRB0J9 and 0SPB0EZ	0SRC0EZ and 0SPT0JZ	0SRC0LA and 0SPC4LZ	0SRD069 and 0SPD4LZ	0SRD0JA and 0SPD0EZ	0SRD0M9 and 0SPD0JZ
0SR906Z and 0SP90EZ	0SRB0JZ and 0SPB0EZ	0SRC0EZ and 0SPT4JZ	0SRC0LA and 0SPC4MZ	0SRD069 and 0SPD4MZ	0SRD0JA and 0SPD0LZ	0SRD0M9 and 0SPD4JZ
0SR90EZ and 0SP908Z	0SRC069 and 0SPC4LZ	0SRC0EZ and 0SPV0JZ	0SRC0LA and 0SPC4NZ	0SRD06A and 0SPD0EZ	0SRD0JA and 0SPD0MZ	0SRD0MZ and 0SPD09Z
0SR90EZ and 0SP909Z	0SRC06A and 0SPC0EZ	0SRC0EZ and 0SPV4JZ	0SRC0LZ and 0SPC0LZ	0SRD06A and 0SPD4LZ	0SRD0JA and 0SPD4LZ	0SRD0MZ and 0SPD0JZ
0SR90EZ and 0SP90BZ	0SRC06A and 0SPC0LZ	0SRC0J9 and 0SPC0EZ	0SRC0LZ and 0SPC4LZ	0SRD06A and 0SPD4MZ	0SRD0JA and 0SPD4MZ	0SRD0MZ and 0SPD4JZ
0SR90EZ and 0SP90JZ	0SRC06A and 0SPC4LZ	0SRC0J9 and 0SPC0LZ	0SRC0M9 and 0SPC0JZ	0SRD06A and 0SPD4NZ	0SRD0JA and 0SPD4NZ	0SRD0N9 and 0SPD08Z
0SR90EZ and 0SP948Z	0SRC06A and 0SPC4MZ	0SRC0J9 and 0SPC4LZ	0SRC0M9 and 0SPC4JZ	0SRD06Z and 0SPD4LZ	0SRD0JZ and 0SPD4LZ	0SRD0N9 and 0SPD09Z
0SR90EZ and 0SP94JZ	0SRC06A and 0SPC4NZ	0SRC0JA and 0SPC0EZ	0SRC0MA and 0SPC09Z	0SRD0EZ and 0SPD08Z	0SRD0JZ and 0SPD4MZ	0SRD0N9 and 0SPD0JZ
0SR90EZ and 0SPA0JZ	0SRC06Z and 0SPC0EZ	0SRC0JA and 0SPC0LZ	0SRC0MA and 0SPC0JZ	0SRD0EZ and 0SPD09Z	0SRD0JZ and 0SPD4NZ	0SRD0N9 and 0SPD38Z
0SR90EZ and 0SPA4JZ	0SRC06Z and 0SPC0LZ	0SRC0JA and 0SPC0MZ	0SRC0MA and 0SPC4JZ	0SRD0EZ and 0SPD0JC	0SRD0L9 and 0SPD4LZ	0SRD0N9 and 0SPD48Z
0SR90EZ and 0SPR0JZ	0SRC06Z and 0SPC0MZ	0SRC0JA and 0SPC0NZ	0SRC0MZ and 0SPC4JZ	0SRD0EZ and 0SPD0JZ	0SRD0L9 and 0SPD4MZ	0SRD0N9 and 0SPD4JZ
0SR90EZ and 0SPR4JZ	0SRC06Z and 0SPC0NZ	0SRC0JA and 0SPC4LZ	0SRC0N9 and 0SPC08Z	0SRD0EZ and 0SPD38Z	0SRD0L9 and 0SPD4NZ	0SRD0N9 and 0SPW0JZ
0SR90JA and 0SP90EZ	0SRC06Z and 0SPC4LZ	0SRC0JA and 0SPC4MZ	0SRC0N9 and 0SPC09Z	0SRD0EZ and 0SPD48Z	0SRD0LA and 0SPD0LZ	0SRD0N9 and 0SPW4JZ
0SRA00A and 0SP90EZ	0SRC06Z and 0SPC4MZ	0SRC0JA and 0SPC4NZ	0SRC0N9 and 0SPC0JZ	0SRD0EZ and 0SPD4JC	0SRD0LA and 0SPD0MZ	0SRD0NA and 0SPD08Z
0SRA01A and 0SP90EZ	0SRC06Z and 0SPC4NZ	0SRC0JZ and 0SPC0EZ	0SRC0N9 and 0SPC38Z	0SRD0EZ and 0SPD4JZ	0SRD0LA and 0SPD0NZ	0SRD0NZ and 0SPD08Z

0SRD0NZ and 0SPD09Z	0SRT0J9 and 0SPC4LZ	0SRU0JA and 0SPD4NZ	0SRV0JZ and 0SPC0EZ	0SRW0JZ and 0SPD4NZ	0TY00Z2 and 0FYG0Z1	0UT47ZZ and 0UT98ZZ and 0UTC8ZZ
0SRD0NZ and 0SPD0JZ	0SRT0JA and 0SPC0EZ	0SRU0JZ and 0SPD0EZ	0SRV0JZ and 0SPC0LZ	0SUR09Z and 0SP90EZ	0TY00Z2 and 0FYG0Z2	0UT48ZZ and 0UT97ZZ and 0UTC7ZZ
0SRD0NZ and 0SPD38Z	0SRT0JA and 0SPC0LZ	0SRU0JZ and 0SPD0LZ	0SRV0JZ and 0SPC0MZ	0SUS09Z and 0SPB0EZ	0TY10Z0 and 0FYG0Z0	0UT48ZZ and 0UT97ZZ and 0UTC8ZZ
0SRD0NZ and 0SPD48Z	0SRT0JA and 0SPC0NZ	0SRU0JZ and 0SPD0MZ	0SRV0JZ and 0SPC0NZ	0TQB0ZZ and 0WQFXZ2	0TY10Z0 and 0FYG0Z1	0UT48ZZ and 0UT98ZZ and 0UTC7ZZ
0SRD0NZ and 0SPD4JZ	0SRT0JA and 0SPC4LZ	0SRU0JZ and 0SPD4LZ	0SRV0JZ and 0SPC4LZ	0TQB0ZZ and 0WQFXZZ	0TY10Z0 and 0FYG0Z2	0UT48ZZ and 0UT98ZZ and 0UTC8ZZ
0SRD0NZ and 0SPW0JZ	0SRT0JA and 0SPC4MZ	0SRU0JZ and 0SPD4MZ	0SRV0JZ and 0SPC4MZ	0TQB3ZZ and 0WQFXZ2	0TY10Z1 and 0FYG0Z0	0VT00ZZ and 0VT30ZZ
0SRE009 and 0SPB0EZ	0SRT0JA and 0SPC4NZ	0SRU0JZ and 0SPD4NZ	0SRV0JZ and 0SPC4NZ	0TQB3ZZ and 0WQFXZZ	0TY10Z1 and 0FYG0Z1	0VT00ZZ and 0VT34ZZ
0SRE019 and 0SPB0EZ	0SRT0JZ and 0SPC0EZ	0SRV0J9 and 0SPC0EZ	0SRW0J9 and 0SPD4LZ	0TQB4ZZ and 0WQFXZ2	0TY10Z1 and 0FYG0Z2	0VT04ZZ and 0VT30ZZ
0SRE01Z and 0SPB0EZ	0SRT0JZ and 0SPC4LZ	0SRV0J9 and 0SPC0LZ	0SRW0J9 and 0SPD4MZ	0TQB4ZZ and 0WQFXZZ	0TY10Z2 and 0FYG0Z0	0VT04ZZ and 0VT34ZZ
0SRE039 and 0SPB0EZ	0SRU0J9 and 0SPD0EZ	0SRV0J9 and 0SPC0MZ	0SRW0JA and 0SPD0EZ	0TTB0ZZ and 0TTD0ZZ and 0UT20ZZ and 0UT70ZZ and 0UT90ZZ and 0UTC0ZZ and 0UTG0ZZ	0TY10Z2 and 0FYG0Z1	0VT07ZZ and 0VT30ZZ
0SRE03Z and 0SPB0EZ	0SRU0J9 and 0SPD0LZ	0SRV0J9 and 0SPC0NZ	0SRW0JA and 0SPD4LZ		0TY10Z2 and 0FYG0Z2	0VT07ZZ and 0VT34ZZ
0SRE0JA and 0SPB0EZ	0SRU0J9 and 0SPD0MZ	0SRV0J9 and 0SPC4LZ	0SRW0JA and 0SPD4MZ		0UT40ZZ and 0UT90ZZ and 0UTC0ZZ	0VT08ZZ and 0VT30ZZ
0SRR019 and 0SP90EZ	0SRU0J9 and 0SPD0NZ	0SRV0J9 and 0SPC4MZ	0SRW0JA and 0SPD4NZ	0TY00Z0 and 0FYG0Z0	0UT44ZZ and 0UT94ZZ and 0UTC4ZZ	0VT08ZZ and 0VT34ZZ
0SRR01Z and 0SP90EZ	0SRU0J9 and 0SPD4LZ	0SRV0J9 and 0SPC4NZ	0SRW0JZ and 0SPD0EZ	0TY00Z0 and 0FYG0Z1	0UT44ZZ and 0UT9FZZ and 0UTC4ZZ	
0SRR039 and 0SP90EZ	0SRU0J9 and 0SPD4MZ	0SRV0JA and 0SPC0EZ	0SRW0JZ and 0SPD0LZ	0TY00Z0 and 0FYG0Z2	0UT47ZZ and 0UT97ZZ and 0UTC7ZZ	
0SRR03Z and 0SP90EZ	0SRU0J9 and 0SPD4NZ	0SRV0JA and 0SPC0LZ	0SRW0JZ and 0SPD0MZ	0TY00Z1 and 0FYG0Z0	0UT47ZZ and 0UT97ZZ and 0UTC8ZZ	
0SRR0JA and 0SP90EZ	0SRU0JA and 0SPD0EZ	0SRV0JA and 0SPC4LZ	0SRW0JZ and 0SPD0NZ	0TY00Z1 and 0FYG0Z1	0UT47ZZ and 0UT98ZZ and 0UTC7ZZ	
0SRS019 and 0SPB0EZ	0SRU0JA and 0SPD4LZ	0SRV0JA and 0SPC4MZ	0SRW0JZ and 0SPD4LZ	0TY00Z1 and 0FYG0Z2		
0SRS01Z and 0SPB0EZ	0SRU0JA and 0SPD4MZ	0SRV0JA and 0SPC4NZ	0SRW0JZ and 0SPD4MZ	0TY00Z2 and 0FYG0Z0		

Appendix H: Non-OR Procedure Not Affecting MS-DRG Assignment

0020X0Z	00974ZX	00BG3ZX	00JV3ZZ	00W6X0Z	015C0ZZ	019A3ZZ	01B64ZX	02B84ZX
0020XYZ	00983ZX	00BG4ZX	00P030Z	00W6X2Z	015C3ZZ	019A4ZX	01B83ZX	02B90ZX
002EX0Z	00984ZX	00BH3ZX	00P032Z	00W6X3Z	015C4ZZ	019B30Z	01B84ZX	02B93ZX
002EXYZ	00993ZX	00BH4ZX	00P033Z	00W6XJZ	015D0ZZ	019B3ZX	01B93ZX	02B94ZX
002UX0Z	00994ZX	00BJ3ZX	00P03YZ	00W6XMZ	015D3ZZ	019B3ZZ	01B94ZX	02BD0ZX
002UXYZ	009A3ZX	00BJ4ZX	00P04YZ	00WE3YZ	015D4ZZ	019B4ZX	01BA3ZX	02BD3ZX
005F0ZZ	009A4ZX	00BK3ZX	00P0X0Z	00WE4YZ	015F0ZZ	019C30Z	01BA4ZX	02BD4ZX
005F3ZZ	009B3ZX	00BK4ZX	00P0X2Z	00WEX0Z	015F3ZZ	019C3ZX	01BB3ZX	02BF0ZX
005F4ZZ	009B4ZX	00BL3ZX	00P0X3Z	00WEX2Z	015F4ZZ	019C3ZZ	01BB4ZX	02BF3ZX
005G0ZZ	009C3ZX	00BL4ZX	00P0XMZ	00WEX3Z	015G0ZZ	019C4ZX	01BC3ZX	02BF4ZX
005G3ZZ	009C4ZX	00BM3ZX	00P630Z	00WEX7Z	015G3ZZ	019D30Z	01BC4ZX	02BG0ZX
005G4ZZ	009D3ZX	00BM4ZX	00P632Z	00WEXMZ	015G4ZZ	019D3ZX	01BD3ZX	02BG3ZX
005H0ZZ	009D4ZX	00BN3ZX	00P633Z	00WU3YZ	015H0ZZ	019D3ZZ	01BD4ZX	02BG4ZX
005H3ZZ	009F3ZX	00BN4ZX	00P63YZ	00WU4YZ	015H3ZZ	019D4ZX	01BF3ZX	02BH0ZX
005H4ZZ	009F4ZX	00BP3ZX	00P64YZ	00WUX0Z	015H4ZZ	019F30Z	01BF4ZX	02BH3ZX
005J0ZZ	009G3ZX	00BP4ZX	00P6X0Z	00WUX2Z	015Q0ZZ	019F3ZX	01BG3ZX	02BH4ZX
005J3ZZ	009G4ZX	00BQ3ZX	00P6X2Z	00WUX3Z	015Q3ZZ	019F3ZZ	01BG4ZX	02BJ0ZX
005J4ZZ	009H3ZX	00BQ4ZX	00P6X3Z	00WUXJZ	015Q4ZZ	019F4ZX	01BH3ZX	02BJ3ZX
005K0ZZ	009H4ZX	00BR3ZX	00P6XMZ	00WUXMZ	015R3ZZ	019G30Z	01BH4ZX	02BJ4ZX
005K3ZZ	009J3ZX	00BR4ZX	00PE30Z	00WV3YZ	019030Z	019G3ZX	01BQ3ZX	02BK0ZX
005K4ZZ	009J4ZX	00BS3ZX	00PE32Z	00WV4YZ	01903ZX	019G3ZZ	01BQ4ZX	02BK3ZX
005L0ZZ	009K3ZX	00BS4ZX	00PE33Z	00WVX0Z	01903ZZ	019G4ZX	01BR3ZX	02BK4ZX
005L3ZZ	009K4ZX	00F3XZZ	00PE3YZ	00WVX2Z	01904ZX	019H30Z	01BR4ZX	02BL0ZX
005L4ZZ	009L3ZX	00F4XZZ	00PE4YZ	00WVX3Z	019130Z	019H3ZX	01HY01Z	02BL3ZX
005M0ZZ	009L4ZX	00F5XZZ	00PEX0Z	00WVX7Z	01913ZX	019H3ZZ	01HY31Z	02BL4ZX
005M3ZZ	009M3ZX	00F6XZZ	00PEX2Z	00WVXJZ	01913ZZ	019H4ZX	01HY3YZ	02BM0ZX
005M4ZZ	009M4ZX	00H001Z	00PEX3Z	00WVXKZ	01914ZX	019K30Z	01HY41Z	02BM3ZX
005N0ZZ	009N3ZX	00H031Z	00PEXMZ	00WVXMZ	019230Z	019K3ZZ	01HY4YZ	02BM4ZX
005N3ZZ	009N4ZX	00H041Z	00PU30Z	012YX0Z	01923ZX	019L30Z	01JY3ZZ	02FNXZZ
005N4ZZ	009P3ZX	00H601Z	00PU32Z	012YXYZ	01923ZZ	019L3ZZ	01PY30Z	02H432Z
005P0ZZ	009P4ZX	00H631Z	00PU33Z	01500ZZ	01924ZX	019M30Z	01PY32Z	02H433Z
005P3ZZ	009Q3ZX	00H641Z	00PU3YZ	01503ZZ	019330Z	019M3ZZ	01PY3YZ	02H632Z
005P4ZZ	009Q4ZX	00HE01Z	00PU4YZ	01504ZZ	01933ZX	019N30Z	01PY4YZ	02H633Z
005Q0ZZ	009R3ZX	00HE31Z	00PUX0Z	01513ZZ	01933ZZ	019N3ZZ	01PYX0Z	02H732Z
005Q3ZZ	009R4ZX	00HE32Z	00PUX2Z	01520ZZ	01934ZX	019P30Z	01PYX2Z	02H733Z
005Q4ZZ	009S3ZX	00HE3YZ	00PUX3Z	01523ZZ	019430Z	019P3ZZ	01PYXMZ	02HK30Z
005R0ZZ	009S4ZX	00HE41Z	00PUXMZ	01524ZZ	01943ZX	019Q30Z	01WY3YZ	02HK33Z
005R3ZZ	009T30Z	00HE4YZ	00PV30Z	01530ZZ	01943ZZ	019Q3ZX	01WY4YZ	02HL32Z
005R4ZZ	009T3ZX	00HU01Z	00PV32Z	01533ZZ	01944ZX	019Q3ZZ	01WYX0Z	02HL33Z
005S0ZZ	009T3ZZ	00HU03Z	00PV33Z	01534ZZ	019530Z	019Q4ZX	01WYX2Z	02HN32Z
005S3ZZ	009U30Z	00HU31Z	00PV3YZ	01540ZZ	01953ZX	019R30Z	01WYX7Z	02HP00Z
005S4ZZ	009U3ZX	00HU32Z	00PV4YZ	01543ZZ	01953ZZ	019R3ZX	01WYXMZ	02HP02Z
00903ZX	009U3ZZ	00HU33Z	00PVX0Z	01544ZZ	01954ZX	019R3ZZ	02173J6	02HP03Z
00904ZX	009U40Z	00HU3YZ	00PVX2Z	01550ZZ	019630Z	019R4ZX	02B40ZX	02HP30Z
00913ZX	009U4ZX	00HU41Z	00PVX3Z	01553ZZ	01963ZX	01B03ZX	02B43ZX	02HP32Z
00914ZX	009U4ZZ	00HU43Z	00PVXMZ	01554ZZ	01963ZZ	01B04ZX	02B44ZX	02HP33Z
00923ZX	009W30Z	00HU4YZ	00W03YZ	01560ZZ	01964ZX	01B13ZX	02B50ZX	02HP40Z
00924ZX	009W3ZX	00HV01Z	00W04YZ	01563ZZ	019830Z	01B14ZX	02B53ZX	02HP42Z
00933ZX	009W3ZZ	00HV03Z	00W0X0Z	01564ZZ	01983ZX	01B23ZX	02B54ZX	02HP43Z
00934ZX	009X30Z	00HV31Z	00W0X2Z	01583ZZ	01983ZZ	01B24ZX	02B60ZX	02HQ02Z
00943ZX	009X3ZX	00HV32Z	00W0X3Z	01590ZZ	01984ZX	01B33ZX	02B63ZX	02HQ03Z
00944ZX	009X3ZZ	00HV33Z	00W0X7Z	01593ZZ	019930Z	01B34ZX	02B64ZX	02HQ32Z
00953ZX	009Y30Z	00HV41Z	00W0XJZ	01594ZZ	01993ZX	01B43ZX	02B70ZX	02HQ33Z
00954ZX	009Y3ZX	00HV43Z	00W0XKZ	015A0ZZ	01993ZZ	01B44ZX	02B73ZX	02HQ42Z
00963ZX	009Y3ZZ	00J03ZZ	00W0XMZ	015A3ZZ	01994ZX	01B53ZX	02B74ZX	02HQ43Z
00964ZX	00BF3ZX	00JE3ZZ	00W63YZ	015A4ZZ	019A30Z	01B54ZX	02B80ZX	02HR02Z
00973ZX	00BF4ZX	00JU3ZZ	00W64YZ	015B3ZZ	019A3ZX	01B63ZX	02B83ZX	02HR03Z

02HR32Z	02WAXJZ	039540Z	039F30Z	039P4ZZ	03H333Z	03HQ33Z	04910ZZ	049940Z
02HR33Z	02WAXKZ	03954ZZ	039F3ZX	039Q00Z	03H343Z	03HQ43Z	049130Z	04994ZZ
02HR42Z	02WAXMZ	039600Z	039F3ZZ	039Q0ZZ	03H403Z	03HR03Z	04913ZX	049A00Z
02HR43Z	02WAXNZ	03960ZZ	039F40Z	039Q30Z	03H433Z	03HR33Z	04913ZZ	049A0ZZ
02HS03Z	02WAXQZ	039630Z	039F4ZZ	039Q3ZX	03H443Z	03HR43Z	049140Z	049A30Z
02HS32Z	02WAXRS	03963ZX	039G00Z	039Q3ZZ	03H503Z	03HS03Z	04914ZZ	049A3ZX
02HS33Z	02WAXRZ	03963ZZ	039G0ZZ	039Q40Z	03H533Z	03HS33Z	049200Z	049A3ZZ
02HS43Z	02WY32Z	039640Z	039G30Z	039Q4ZZ	03H543Z	03HS43Z	04920ZZ	049A40Z
02HT03Z	02WY33Z	03964ZZ	039G3ZX	039R00Z	03H603Z	03HT03Z	049230Z	049A4ZZ
02HT32Z	02WY3DZ	039700Z	039G3ZZ	039R0ZZ	03H633Z	03HT33Z	04923ZX	049B00Z
02HT33Z	02WY3YZ	03970ZZ	039G40Z	039R30Z	03H643Z	03HT43Z	04923ZZ	049B0ZZ
02HT43Z	02WY4YZ	039730Z	039G4ZZ	039R3ZX	03H703Z	03HU03Z	049240Z	049B30Z
02HV03Z	02WYX2Z	03973ZX	039H00Z	039R3ZZ	03H733Z	03HU33Z	04924ZZ	049B3ZX
02HV32Z	02WYX3Z	03973ZZ	039H0ZZ	039R40Z	03H743Z	03HU43Z	049300Z	049B3ZZ
02HV33Z	02WYX7Z	039740Z	039H30Z	039R4ZZ	03H803Z	03HV03Z	04930ZZ	049B40Z
02HV43Z	02WYX8Z	03974ZZ	039H3ZX	039S00Z	03H833Z	03HV33Z	049330Z	049B4ZZ
02HW00Z	02WYXCZ	039800Z	039H3ZZ	039S0ZZ	03H843Z	03HV43Z	04933ZX	049C00Z
02HW03Z	02WYXDZ	03980ZZ	039H40Z	039S30Z	03H903Z	03HY03Z	04933ZZ	049C0ZZ
02HW30Z	02WYXJZ	039830Z	039H4ZZ	039S3ZX	03H933Z	03HY32Z	049340Z	049C30Z
02HW32Z	02WYXKZ	03983ZX	039J00Z	039S3ZZ	03H943Z	03HY33Z	04934ZZ	049C3ZX
02HW33Z	039000Z	03983ZZ	039J0ZZ	039S40Z	03HA03Z	03HY3YZ	049400Z	049C3ZZ
02HW40Z	03900ZZ	039840Z	039J30Z	039S4ZZ	03HA33Z	03HY43Z	04940ZZ	049C40Z
02HW43Z	039030Z	03984ZZ	039J3ZX	039T00Z	03HA43Z	03HY4YZ	049430Z	049C4ZZ
02HX00Z	03903ZX	039900Z	039J3ZZ	039T0ZZ	03HB03Z	03JY3ZZ	04943ZX	049D00Z
02HX03Z	03903ZZ	03990ZZ	039J40Z	039T30Z	03HB33Z	03JY4ZZ	04943ZZ	049D0ZZ
02HX30Z	039040Z	039930Z	039J4ZZ	039T3ZX	03HB43Z	03JYXZZ	049440Z	049D30Z
02HX33Z	03904ZZ	03993ZX	039K00Z	039T3ZZ	03HC03Z	03PY30Z	04944ZZ	049D3ZX
02HX40Z	039100Z	03993ZZ	039K0ZZ	039T40Z	03HC33Z	03PY32Z	049500Z	049D3ZZ
02HX43Z	03910ZZ	039940Z	039K30Z	039T4ZZ	03HC43Z	03PY33Z	04950ZZ	049D40Z
02JA3ZZ	039130Z	03994ZZ	039K3ZX	039U00Z	03HD03Z	03PY3DZ	049530Z	049D4ZZ
02JY3ZZ	03913ZX	039A00Z	039K3ZZ	039U0ZZ	03HD33Z	03PY3YZ	04953ZX	049E00Z
02PA32Z	03913ZZ	039A0ZZ	039K40Z	039U30Z	03HD43Z	03PY4YZ	04953ZZ	049E0ZZ
02PA33Z	039140Z	039A30Z	039K4ZZ	039U3ZX	03HF03Z	03PYX0Z	049540Z	049E30Z
02PA3DZ	03914ZZ	039A3ZX	039L00Z	039U3ZZ	03HF33Z	03PYX2Z	04954ZZ	049E3ZX
02PA3YZ	039200Z	039A3ZZ	039L0ZZ	039U40Z	03HF43Z	03PYX3Z	049600Z	049E3ZZ
02PA4YZ	03920ZZ	039A40Z	039L30Z	039U4ZZ	03HG03Z	03PYXDZ	04960ZZ	049E40Z
02PAX2Z	039230Z	039A4ZZ	039L3ZX	039V00Z	03HG33Z	03PYXMZ	049630Z	049E4ZZ
02PAX3Z	03923ZX	039B00Z	039L3ZZ	039V0ZZ	03HG43Z	03WY30Z	04963ZX	049F00Z
02PAXDZ	03923ZZ	039B0ZZ	039L40Z	039V30Z	03HH03Z	03WY32Z	04963ZZ	049F0ZZ
02PAXMZ	039240Z	039B30Z	039L4ZZ	039V3ZX	03HH33Z	03WY33Z	049640Z	049F30Z
02PY32Z	03924ZZ	039B3ZX	039M00Z	039V3ZZ	03HH43Z	03WY3DZ	04964ZZ	049F3ZX
02PY33Z	039300Z	039B3ZZ	039M0ZZ	039V40Z	03HJ03Z	03WY3YZ	049700Z	049F3ZZ
02PY3DZ	03930ZZ	039B40Z	039M30Z	039V4ZZ	03HJ33Z	03WY4YZ	04970ZZ	049F40Z
02PY3YZ	039330Z	039B4ZZ	039M3ZX	039Y00Z	03HJ43Z	03WYX0Z	049730Z	049F4ZZ
02PY4YZ	03933ZX	039C00Z	039M3ZZ	039Y0ZZ	03HK03Z	03WYX2Z	04973ZX	049H00Z
02PYX2Z	03933ZZ	039C0ZZ	039M40Z	039Y30Z	03HK33Z	03WYX3Z	04973ZZ	049H0ZZ
02PYX3Z	039340Z	039C30Z	039M4ZZ	039Y3ZX	03HK43Z	03WYX7Z	049740Z	049H30Z
02PYXDZ	03934ZZ	039C3ZX	039N00Z	039Y3ZZ	03HL03Z	03WYXCZ	04974ZZ	049H3ZX
02UG3JH	039400Z	039C3ZZ	039N0ZZ	039Y40Z	03HL33Z	03WYXDZ	049800Z	049H3ZZ
02WA32Z	03940ZZ	039C40Z	039N30Z	039Y4ZZ	03HL43Z	03WYXJZ	04980ZZ	049H40Z
02WA33Z	039430Z	039C4ZZ	039N3ZX	03H003Z	03HM03Z	03WYXKZ	049830Z	049H4ZZ
02WA3DZ	03943ZX	039D00Z	039N3ZZ	03H033Z	03HM33Z	03WYXMZ	04983ZX	049J00Z
02WA3YZ	03943ZZ	039D0ZZ	039N40Z	03H043Z	03HM43Z	049000Z	04983ZZ	049J0ZZ
02WA4YZ	039440Z	039D30Z	039N4ZZ	03H103Z	03HN03Z	04900ZZ	049840Z	049J30Z
02WAX2Z	03944ZZ	039D3ZX	039P00Z	03H133Z	03HN33Z	049030Z	04984ZZ	049J3ZX
02WAX3Z	039500Z	039D3ZZ	039P0ZZ	03H143Z	03HN43Z	04903ZX	049900Z	049J3ZZ
02WAX7Z	03950ZZ	039D40Z	039P30Z	03H203Z	03HP03Z	04903ZZ	04990ZZ	049J40Z
02WAX8Z	039530Z	039D4ZZ	039P3ZX	03H233Z	03HP33Z	049040Z	049930Z	049J4ZZ
02WAXCZ	03953ZX	039F00Z	039P3ZZ	03H243Z	03HP43Z	04904ZZ	04993ZX	049K00Z
02WAXDZ	03953ZZ	039F0ZZ	039P40Z	03H303Z	03HQ03Z	049100Z	04993ZZ	049K0ZZ

049K30Z	049T4ZZ	04H933Z	04HW33Z	05943ZX	059D00Z	059Q3ZZ	05H833Z	05JYXZZ
049K3ZX	049U00Z	04H943Z	04HW43Z	05943ZZ	059D0ZZ	059Q40Z	05H843Z	05P002Z
049K3ZZ	049U0ZZ	04HA03Z	04HY03Z	059440Z	059D30Z	059Q4ZZ	05H903Z	05P032Z
049K40Z	049U30Z	04HA33Z	04HY32Z	05944ZZ	059D3ZX	059R00Z	05H933Z	05P042Z
049K4ZZ	049U3ZX	04HA43Z	04HY33Z	059500Z	059D3ZZ	059R0ZZ	05H943Z	05P0X2Z
049L00Z	049U3ZZ	04HB03Z	04HY3YZ	05950ZZ	059D40Z	059R30Z	05HA03Z	05PY30Z
049L0ZZ	049U40Z	04HB33Z	04HY43Z	059530Z	059D4ZZ	059R3ZX	05HA33Z	05PY32Z
049L30Z	049U4ZZ	04HB43Z	04HY4YZ	05953ZX	059F00Z	059R3ZZ	05HA43Z	05PY33Z
049L3ZX	049V00Z	04HC03Z	04JY3ZZ	05953ZZ	059F0ZZ	059R40Z	05HB03Z	05PY3DZ
049L3ZZ	049V0ZZ	04HC33Z	04JY4ZZ	059540Z	059F30Z	059R4ZZ	05HB33Z	05PY3YZ
049L40Z	049V30Z	04HC43Z	04JYXZZ	05954ZZ	059F3ZX	059S00Z	05HB43Z	05PY4YZ
049L4ZZ	049V3ZX	04HD03Z	04PY30Z	059600Z	059F3ZZ	059S0ZZ	05HC03Z	05PYX0Z
049M00Z	049V3ZZ	04HD33Z	04PY32Z	05960ZZ	059F40Z	059S30Z	05HC33Z	05PYX2Z
049M0ZZ	049V40Z	04HD43Z	04PY33Z	059630Z	059F4ZZ	059S3ZX	05HC43Z	05PYX3Z
049M30Z	049V4ZZ	04HE03Z	04PY3DZ	05963ZX	059G00Z	059S3ZZ	05HD03Z	05PYXDZ
049M3ZX	049W00Z	04HE33Z	04PY3YZ	05963ZZ	059G0ZZ	059S40Z	05HD33Z	05W0XMZ
049M3ZZ	049W0ZZ	04HE43Z	04PY4YZ	059640Z	059G30Z	059S4ZZ	05HD43Z	05W3XMZ
049M40Z	049W30Z	04HF03Z	04PYX0Z	05964ZZ	059G3ZX	059T00Z	05HF03Z	05W4XMZ
049M4ZZ	049W3ZX	04HF33Z	04PYX1Z	059700Z	059G3ZZ	059T0ZZ	05HF33Z	05WY30Z
049N00Z	049W3ZZ	04HF43Z	04PYX2Z	05970ZZ	059G40Z	059T30Z	05HF43Z	05WY32Z
049N0ZZ	049W40Z	04HH03Z	04PYX3Z	059730Z	059G4ZZ	059T3ZX	05HG03Z	05WY33Z
049N30Z	049W4ZZ	04HH33Z	04PYXDZ	05973ZX	059H00Z	059T3ZZ	05HG33Z	05WY3DZ
049N3ZX	049Y00Z	04HH43Z	04WY30Z	05973ZZ	059H0ZZ	059T40Z	05HG43Z	05WY3YZ
049N3ZZ	049Y0ZZ	04HJ03Z	04WY32Z	059740Z	059H30Z	059T4ZZ	05HH03Z	05WY4YZ
049N40Z	049Y30Z	04HJ33Z	04WY33Z	05974ZZ	059H3ZX	059V00Z	05HH33Z	05WYX0Z
049N4ZZ	049Y3ZX	04HJ43Z	04WY3DZ	059800Z	059H3ZZ	059V0ZZ	05HH43Z	05WYX2Z
049P00Z	049Y3ZZ	04HK03Z	04WY3YZ	05980ZZ	059H40Z	059V30Z	05HL03Z	05WYX3Z
049P0ZZ	049Y40Z	04HK33Z	04WY4YZ	059830Z	059H4ZZ	059V3ZX	05HL33Z	05WYX7Z
049P30Z	049Y4ZZ	04HK43Z	04WYX0Z	05983ZX	059L00Z	059V3ZZ	05HL43Z	05WYXCZ
049P3ZX	04H002Z	04HL03Z	04WYX2Z	05983ZZ	059L0ZZ	059V40Z	05HM03Z	05WYXDZ
049P3ZZ	04H003Z	04HL33Z	04WYX3Z	059840Z	059L30Z	059V4ZZ	05HM33Z	05WYXJZ
049P40Z	04H032Z	04HL43Z	04WYX7Z	05984ZZ	059L3ZX	059Y00Z	05HM43Z	05WYXKZ
049P4ZZ	04H033Z	04HM03Z	04WYXCZ	059900Z	059L3ZZ	059Y0ZZ	05HN03Z	069000Z
049Q00Z	04H042Z	04HM33Z	04WYXDZ	05990ZZ	059L40Z	059Y30Z	05HN33Z	06900ZZ
049Q0ZZ	04H043Z	04HM43Z	04WYXJZ	059930Z	059L4ZZ	059Y3ZX	05HN43Z	069030Z
049Q30Z	04H103Z	04HN03Z	04WYXKZ	05993ZX	059M00Z	059Y3ZZ	05HP03Z	06903ZX
049Q3ZX	04H133Z	04HN33Z	059000Z	05993ZZ	059M0ZZ	059Y40Z	05HP33Z	06903ZZ
049Q3ZZ	04H143Z	04HN43Z	05900ZZ	059940Z	059M30Z	059Y4ZZ	05HP43Z	069040Z
049Q40Z	04H203Z	04HP03Z	059030Z	05994ZZ	059M3ZX	05H003Z	05HQ03Z	06904ZZ
049Q4ZZ	04H233Z	04HP33Z	05903ZX	059A00Z	059M3ZZ	05H033Z	05HQ33Z	069100Z
049R00Z	04H243Z	04HP43Z	05903ZZ	059A0ZZ	059M40Z	05H043Z	05HQ43Z	06910ZZ
049R0ZZ	04H303Z	04HQ03Z	059040Z	059A30Z	059M4ZZ	05H103Z	05HR03Z	069130Z
049R30Z	04H333Z	04HQ33Z	05904ZZ	059A3ZX	059N00Z	05H133Z	05HR33Z	06913ZX
049R3ZX	04H343Z	04HQ43Z	059100Z	059A3ZZ	059N0ZZ	05H143Z	05HR43Z	06913ZZ
049R3ZZ	04H403Z	04HR03Z	05910ZZ	059A40Z	059N30Z	05H303Z	05HS03Z	069140Z
049R40Z	04H433Z	04HR33Z	059130Z	059A4ZZ	059N3ZX	05H333Z	05HS33Z	06914ZZ
049R4ZZ	04H443Z	04HR43Z	05913ZX	059B00Z	059N3ZZ	05H343Z	05HS43Z	069200Z
049S00Z	04H503Z	04HS03Z	05913ZZ	059B0ZZ	059N40Z	05H403Z	05HT03Z	06920ZZ
049S0ZZ	04H533Z	04HS33Z	059140Z	059B30Z	059N4ZZ	05H433Z	05HT33Z	069230Z
049S30Z	04H543Z	04HS43Z	05914ZZ	059B3ZX	059P00Z	05H443Z	05HT43Z	06923ZX
049S3ZX	04H603Z	04HT03Z	059300Z	059B3ZZ	059P0ZZ	05H503Z	05HV03Z	06923ZZ
049S3ZZ	04H633Z	04HT33Z	05930ZZ	059B40Z	059P30Z	05H533Z	05HV33Z	069240Z
049S40Z	04H643Z	04HT43Z	059330Z	059B4ZZ	059P3ZX	05H543Z	05HV43Z	06924ZZ
049S4ZZ	04H703Z	04HU03Z	05933ZX	059C00Z	059P3ZZ	05H603Z	05HY03Z	069330Z
049T00Z	04H733Z	04HU33Z	05933ZZ	059C0ZZ	059P40Z	05H633Z	05HY32Z	06933ZX
049T0ZZ	04H743Z	04HU43Z	059340Z	059C30Z	059P4ZZ	05H643Z	05HY33Z	06933ZZ
049T30Z	04H803Z	04HV03Z	05934ZZ	059C3ZX	059Q00Z	05H703Z	05HY3YZ	069400Z
049T3ZX	04H833Z	04HV33Z	059400Z	059C3ZZ	059Q0ZZ	05H733Z	05HY43Z	06940ZZ
049T3ZZ	04H843Z	04HV43Z	05940ZZ	059C40Z	059Q30Z	05H743Z	05HY4YZ	069430Z
049T40Z	04H903Z	04HW03Z	059430Z	059C4ZZ	059Q3ZX	05H803Z	05JY3ZZ	06943ZX

06943ZZ	069F0ZZ	069T40Z	06HF03Z	06PY3YZ	07958ZX	079K8ZX	07DB8ZX	07HM41Z
069440Z	069F30Z	069T4ZZ	06HF33Z	06PY4YZ	07958ZZ	079K8ZZ	07DC3ZX	07HM43Z
06944ZZ	069F3ZX	069V00Z	06HF43Z	06PYX0Z	079630Z	079L30Z	07DC4ZX	07HN01Z
069500Z	069F3ZZ	069V0ZZ	06HG03Z	06PYX2Z	07963ZZ	079L3ZZ	07DC8ZX	07HN03Z
06950ZZ	069F40Z	069V30Z	06HG33Z	06PYX3Z	079680Z	079L80Z	07DD3ZX	07HN31Z
069530Z	069F4ZZ	069V3ZX	06HG43Z	06PYXDZ	07968ZX	079L8ZX	07DD4ZX	07HN33Z
06953ZX	069G00Z	069V3ZZ	06HH03Z	06WY30Z	07968ZZ	079L8ZZ	07DD8ZX	07HN3YZ
06953ZZ	069G0ZZ	069V40Z	06HH33Z	06WY32Z	079730Z	079M30Z	07DF3ZX	07HN41Z
069540Z	069G30Z	069V4ZZ	06HH43Z	06WY33Z	07973ZZ	079M3ZZ	07DF4ZX	07HN43Z
06954ZZ	069G3ZX	069Y00Z	06HJ03Z	06WY3DZ	079780Z	079P30Z	07DF8ZX	07HN4YZ
069600Z	069G3ZZ	069Y0ZZ	06HJ33Z	06WY3YZ	07978ZX	079P3ZX	07DG3ZX	07HP01Z
06960ZZ	069G40Z	069Y30Z	06HJ43Z	06WY4YZ	07978ZZ	079P3ZZ	07DG4ZX	07HP03Z
069630Z	069G4ZZ	069Y3ZX	06HM03Z	06WYX0Z	079830Z	079P40Z	07DG8ZX	07HP31Z
06963ZX	069H00Z	069Y3ZZ	06HM33Z	06WYX2Z	07983ZZ	079P4ZX	07DH3ZX	07HP33Z
06963ZZ	069H0ZZ	069Y40Z	06HM43Z	06WYX3Z	079880Z	079P4ZZ	07DH4ZX	07HP3YZ
069640Z	069H30Z	069Y4ZZ	06HN03Z	06WYX7Z	07988ZX	079T00Z	07DH8ZX	07HP41Z
06964ZZ	069H3ZX	06H003T	06HN33Z	06WYXCZ	07988ZZ	079T0ZX	07DJ3ZX	07HP43Z
069700Z	069H3ZZ	06H003Z	06HN43Z	06WYXDZ	079930Z	079T0ZZ	07DJ4ZX	07HP4YZ
06970ZZ	069H40Z	06H00DZ	06HP03Z	06WYXJZ	07993ZZ	079T30Z	07DJ8ZX	07HT01Z
069730Z	069H4ZZ	06H033T	06HP33Z	06WYXKZ	079980Z	079T3ZX	07DK3ZX	07HT03Z
06973ZX	069J00Z	06H033Z	06HP43Z	072KX0Z	07998ZX	079T3ZZ	07DK4ZX	07HT0YZ
06973ZZ	069J0ZZ	06H03DZ	06HQ03Z	072KXYZ	07998ZZ	079T40Z	07DK8ZX	07HT31Z
069740Z	069J30Z	06H043Z	06HQ33Z	072LX0Z	079B30Z	079T4ZX	07DL3ZX	07HT33Z
06974ZZ	069J3ZX	06H04DZ	06HQ43Z	072LXYZ	079B3ZZ	079T4ZZ	07DL4ZX	07HT3YZ
069800Z	069J3ZZ	06H103Z	06HT03Z	072MX0Z	079B80Z	07BP3ZX	07DL8ZX	07HT41Z
06980ZZ	069J40Z	06H133Z	06HT33Z	072MXYZ	079B8ZX	07BP4ZX	07DM3ZX	07HT43Z
069830Z	069J4ZZ	06H143Z	06HT43Z	072NX0Z	079B8ZZ	07CP3ZX	07DM4ZX	07HT4YZ
06983ZX	069M00Z	06H203Z	06HV03Z	072NXYZ	079C30Z	07CP4ZX	07DP3ZX	07JK3ZZ
06983ZZ	069M0ZZ	06H233Z	06HV33Z	072PX0Z	079C3ZZ	07D03ZX	07DP4ZX	07JL3ZZ
069840Z	069M30Z	06H243Z	06HV43Z	072PXYZ	079C80Z	07D04ZX	07DQ0ZX	07JM3ZZ
06984ZZ	069M3ZX	06H303Z	06HY03Z	072TX0Z	079C8ZX	07D08ZX	07DQ0ZZ	07JN3ZZ
069900Z	069M3ZZ	06H333Z	06HY32Z	072TXYZ	079C8ZZ	07D13ZX	07DQ3ZX	07JN8ZZ
06990ZZ	069M40Z	06H343Z	06HY33Z	079030Z	079D30Z	07D14ZX	07DQ3ZZ	07JNXZZ
069930Z	069M4ZZ	06H403Z	06HY3YZ	07903ZZ	079D3ZZ	07D18ZX	07DR0ZX	07JP3ZZ
06993ZX	069N00Z	06H433Z	06HY43Z	079080Z	079D80Z	07D23ZX	07DR0ZZ	07JP4ZZ
06993ZZ	069N0ZZ	06H443Z	06HY4YZ	07908ZX	079D8ZX	07D24ZX	07DR3ZX	07JPXZZ
069940Z	069N30Z	06H503Z	06JY3ZZ	07908ZZ	079D8ZZ	07D28ZX	07DR3ZZ	07JT0ZZ
06994ZZ	069N3ZX	06H533Z	06JYXZZ	079130Z	079F30Z	07D33ZX	07DS0ZX	07JT3ZZ
069B00Z	069N3ZZ	06H543Z	06L27CZ	07913ZZ	079F3ZZ	07D34ZX	07DS0ZZ	07JT4ZZ
069B0ZZ	069N40Z	06H603Z	06L27DZ	079180Z	079F80Z	07D38ZX	07DS3ZX	07PK3YZ
069B30Z	069N4ZZ	06H633Z	06L27ZZ	07918ZX	079F8ZX	07D43ZX	07DS3ZZ	07PK4YZ
069B3ZX	069P00Z	06H643Z	06L28CZ	07918ZZ	079F8ZZ	07D44ZX	07HK01Z	07PKX0Z
069B3ZZ	069P0ZZ	06H703Z	06L28DZ	079230Z	079G30Z	07D48ZX	07HK03Z	07PKX3Z
069B40Z	069P30Z	06H733Z	06L28ZZ	07923ZZ	079G3ZZ	07D53ZX	07HK31Z	07PKXDZ
069B4ZZ	069P3ZX	06H743Z	06L33CZ	079280Z	079G80Z	07D54ZX	07HK33Z	07PL3YZ
069C00Z	069P3ZZ	06H803Z	06L33DZ	07928ZX	079G8ZX	07D58ZX	07HK3YZ	07PL4YZ
069C0ZZ	069P40Z	06H833Z	06L33ZZ	07928ZZ	079G8ZZ	07D63ZX	07HK41Z	07PLX0Z
069C30Z	069P4ZZ	06H843Z	06L34CZ	079330Z	079H30Z	07D64ZX	07HK43Z	07PLX3Z
069C3ZX	069Q00Z	06H903Z	06L34DZ	07933ZZ	079H3ZZ	07D68ZX	07HL01Z	07PLXDZ
069C3ZZ	069Q0ZZ	06H933Z	06L34ZZ	079380Z	079H80Z	07D73ZX	07HL03Z	07PM3YZ
069C40Z	069Q30Z	06H943Z	06L37CZ	07938ZX	079H8ZX	07D74ZX	07HL31Z	07PM4YZ
069C4ZZ	069Q3ZX	06HB03Z	06L37DZ	07938ZZ	079H8ZZ	07D78ZX	07HL33Z	07PMX0Z
069D00Z	069Q3ZZ	06HB33Z	06L37ZZ	079430Z	079J30Z	07D83ZX	07HL3YZ	07PMX3Z
069D0ZZ	069Q40Z	06HB43Z	06L38CZ	07943ZZ	079J3ZZ	07D84ZX	07HL41Z	07PN3YZ
069D30Z	069Q4ZZ	06HC03Z	06L38DZ	079480Z	079J80Z	07D88ZX	07HL43Z	07PN4YZ
069D3ZX	069T00Z	06HC33Z	06L38ZZ	07948ZX	079J8ZX	07D93ZX	07HM01Z	07PNX0Z
069D3ZZ	069T0ZZ	06HC43Z	06PY30Z	07948ZZ	079J8ZZ	07D94ZX	07HM03Z	07PNX3Z
069D40Z	069T30Z	06HD03Z	06PY32Z	079530Z	079K30Z	07D98ZX	07HM31Z	07PNXDZ
069D4ZZ	069T3ZX	06HD33Z	06PY33Z	07953ZZ	079K3ZZ	07DB3ZX	07HM33Z	07PP3YZ
069F00Z	069T3ZZ	06HD43Z	06PY3DZ	079580Z	079K80Z	07DB4ZX	07HM3YZ	07PP4YZ

07PPX0Z	080P0ZZ	089P0ZZ	08JMXZZ	08W1X0Z	095M4ZZ	099400Z	099B7ZZ	099K80Z
07PPX3Z	080P37Z	089P30Z	08P03YZ	08W1X3Z	095M8ZZ	09940ZX	099B80Z	099K8ZX
07PT00Z	080P3JZ	089P3ZX	08P070Z	08W1X7Z	097F0DZ	09940ZZ	099B8ZX	099K8ZZ
07PT30Z	080P3KZ	089P3ZZ	08P073Z	08W1XCZ	097F0ZZ	099430Z	099B8ZZ	099KX0Z
07PT40Z	080P3ZZ	089PX0Z	08P07DZ	08W1XDZ	097F3ZZ	09943ZX	099C30Z	099KXZX
07PTX0Z	080PX7Z	089PXZX	08P07YZ	08W1XJZ	097F4ZZ	09943ZZ	099C3ZZ	099KXZX
07WK3YZ	080PXJZ	089PXZZ	08P080Z	08W1XKZ	097F7DZ	099440Z	099C70Z	099L00Z
07WK4YZ	080PXKZ	089Q00Z	08P083Z	08WJ3YZ	097F7ZZ	09944ZX	099C7ZX	099L0ZX
07WKX0Z	080PXZZ	089Q0ZZ	08P08DZ	08WJXJZ	097F8DZ	09944ZZ	099C7ZZ	099L0ZZ
07WKX3Z	080Q07Z	089Q30Z	08P08YZ	08WK3YZ	097F8ZZ	099470Z	099C80Z	099L30Z
07WKX7Z	080Q0JZ	089Q3ZX	08P0X0Z	08WKXJZ	097G0DZ	09947ZX	099C8ZX	099L3ZX
07WKXCZ	080Q0KZ	089Q3ZZ	08P0X1Z	08WL3YZ	097G0ZZ	09947ZZ	099C8ZZ	099L3ZZ
07WKXDZ	080Q0ZZ	089QX0Z	08P0X3Z	08WM3YZ	097G3ZZ	099480Z	099D70Z	099L40Z
07WKXJZ	080Q37Z	089QXZX	08P0XCZ	092HX0Z	097G4ZZ	09948ZX	099D7ZX	099L4ZX
07WKXKZ	080Q3JZ	089QXZZ	08P0XDZ	092HXYZ	097G7DZ	09948ZZ	099D7ZZ	099L4ZZ
07WL3YZ	080Q3KZ	089R00Z	08P0XJZ	092JX0Z	097G7ZZ	0994X0Z	099D80Z	099L70Z
07WL4YZ	080Q3ZZ	089R0ZZ	08P13YZ	092JXYZ	097G8DZ	0994XZX	099D8ZX	099L7ZX
07WLX0Z	080QX7Z	089R30Z	08P170Z	092KX0Z	097G8ZZ	0994XZZ	099D8ZZ	099L7ZZ
07WLX3Z	080QXJZ	089R3ZX	08P173Z	092KXYZ	099000Z	09950ZZ	099E70Z	099L80Z
07WLX7Z	080QXKZ	089R3ZZ	08P17DZ	092YX0Z	09900ZX	09957ZX	099E7ZX	099L8ZX
07WLXCZ	080QXZZ	089RX0Z	08P17YZ	092YXYZ	09900ZZ	09957ZZ	099E7ZZ	099L8ZZ
07WLXDZ	080R07Z	089RXZX	08P180Z	093K7ZZ	099030Z	099580Z	099E80Z	099M00Z
07WLXJZ	080R0JZ	089RXZZ	08P183Z	093K8ZZ	09903ZX	09958ZX	099E8ZX	099M0ZX
07WLXKZ	080R0KZ	089SXZX	08P18DZ	09500ZZ	09903ZZ	09958ZZ	099E8ZZ	099M0ZZ
07WM3YZ	080R0ZZ	089SXZZ	08P18YZ	09503ZZ	099040Z	099600Z	099F00Z	099M30Z
07WM4YZ	080R37Z	089TXZX	08P1X0Z	09504ZZ	09904ZX	09967ZX	099F0ZZ	099M3ZX
07WMX0Z	080R3JZ	089TXZZ	08P1X1Z	0950XZZ	09904ZZ	09967ZZ	099F30Z	099M3ZZ
07WMX3Z	080R3KZ	08C0XZZ	08P1X3Z	09510ZZ	0990X0Z	099680Z	099F3ZZ	099M40Z
07WN3YZ	080R3ZZ	08C1XZZ	08P1XCZ	09513ZZ	0990XZX	09968ZX	099F40Z	099M4ZX
07WN4YZ	080RX7Z	08C2XZZ	08P1XDZ	09514ZZ	0990XZZ	09968ZZ	099F4ZZ	099M4ZZ
07WNX0Z	080RXJZ	08C3XZZ	08P1XJZ	0951XZZ	099100Z	09970ZZ	099F70Z	099M70Z
07WNX3Z	080RXKZ	08C6XZZ	08PJ3YZ	09530ZZ	09910ZX	09973ZZ	099F7ZX	099M7ZX
07WNX7Z	080RXZZ	08C7XZZ	08PK3YZ	09533ZZ	09910ZZ	09974ZZ	099F7ZZ	099M7ZZ
07WNXCZ	0820X0Z	08CN0ZZ	08PL3YZ	09534ZZ	099130Z	09977ZX	099F80Z	099M80Z
07WNXDZ	0820XYZ	08CN3ZZ	08PM3YZ	09537ZZ	09913ZX	09977ZZ	099F8ZX	099M8ZX
07WNXJZ	0821X0Z	08CNXZZ	08QN0ZZ	09538ZZ	09913ZZ	09978ZX	099F8ZZ	099M8ZZ
07WNXKZ	0821XYZ	08CP0ZZ	08QN3ZZ	0953XZZ	099140Z	09978ZZ	099G00Z	099N0ZX
07WP3YZ	085E3ZZ	08CP3ZZ	08QNXZZ	09540ZZ	09914ZX	09980ZZ	099G0ZZ	099N30Z
07WP4YZ	085F3ZZ	08CPXZZ	08QP0ZZ	09543ZZ	09914ZZ	09983ZZ	099G30Z	099N3ZX
07WPX0Z	0890XZX	08CQ0ZZ	08QP3ZZ	09544ZZ	0991X0Z	09984ZZ	099G3ZZ	099N3ZZ
07WPX3Z	0890XZZ	08CQ3ZZ	08QPXZZ	09547ZZ	0991XZX	09987ZX	099G40Z	099N4ZX
07WT00Z	0891XZZ	08CQXZZ	08QQ0ZZ	09548ZZ	0991XZZ	09987ZZ	099G4ZZ	099N7ZX
07WT30Z	0891XZZ	08CR0ZZ	08QQ3ZZ	0954XZZ	099300Z	09988ZX	099G70Z	099N8ZX
07WT40Z	0896XZX	08CR3ZZ	08QQXZZ	095F0ZZ	09930ZX	09988ZZ	099G7ZX	099P30Z
07WTX0Z	0896XZZ	08CRXZZ	08QR0ZZ	095F3ZZ	09930ZZ	099970Z	099G7ZZ	099P3ZX
080N07Z	0897XZX	08CSXZZ	08QR3ZZ	095F4ZZ	099330Z	09997ZX	099G80Z	099P3ZZ
080N0JZ	0897XZZ	08CTXZZ	08QRXZZ	095F7ZZ	09933ZX	09997ZZ	099G8ZX	099P40Z
080N0KZ	0898XZX	08F4XZZ	08W03YZ	095F8ZZ	09933ZZ	099980Z	099G8ZZ	099P4ZX
080N0ZZ	0898XZZ	08F5XZZ	08W07YZ	095G0ZZ	099340Z	09998ZX	099K00Z	099P4ZZ
080N37Z	0899XZX	08H03YZ	08W08YZ	095G3ZZ	09934ZX	09998ZZ	099K0ZX	099P70Z
080N3JZ	0899XZZ	08H07YZ	08W0X0Z	095G4ZZ	09934ZZ	099A70Z	099K0ZZ	099P7ZX
080N3KZ	089N00Z	08H08YZ	08W0X3Z	095G7ZZ	099370Z	099A7ZX	099K30Z	099P7ZZ
080N3ZZ	089N0ZZ	08H13YZ	08W0X7Z	095G8ZZ	09937ZX	099A7ZZ	099K3ZX	099P80Z
080NX7Z	089N30Z	08H17YZ	08W0XCZ	095K0ZZ	09937ZZ	099A80Z	099K3ZZ	099P8ZX
080NXJZ	089N3ZX	08H18YZ	08W0XDZ	095K3ZZ	099380Z	099A8ZX	099K40Z	099P8ZZ
080NXKZ	089N3ZZ	08J0XZZ	08W0XJZ	095K4ZZ	09938ZX	099A8ZZ	099K4ZX	099Q30Z
080NXZZ	089NX0Z	08J1XZZ	08W0XKZ	095K8ZZ	09938ZZ	099B30Z	099K4ZZ	099Q3ZX
080P07Z	089NXZX	08JJXZZ	08W13YZ	095KXZZ	0993X0Z	099B3ZZ	099K70Z	099Q3ZZ
080P0JZ	089NXZZ	08JKXZZ	08W17YZ	095M0ZZ	0993XZX	099B70Z	099K7ZX	099Q40Z
080P0KZ	089P00Z	08JLXZZ	08W18YZ	095M3ZZ	0993XZZ	099B7ZX	099K7ZZ	099Q4ZX

099Q4ZZ	099V4ZZ	09B40ZZ	09BQ8ZX	09CG7ZZ	09HY7YZ	09NL4ZZ	09PK37Z	09TF4ZZ
099Q70Z	099V70Z	09B43ZX	09BR3ZX	09CG8ZZ	09HY81Z	09NL7ZZ	09PK3DZ	09TF7ZZ
099Q7ZX	099V7ZX	09B43ZZ	09BR4ZX	09CK0ZZ	09HY8YZ	09NL8ZZ	09PK3JZ	09TF8ZZ
099Q7ZZ	099V7ZZ	09B44ZX	09BR8ZX	09CK3ZZ	09J73ZZ	09NM0ZZ	09PK3KZ	09TG0ZZ
099Q80Z	099V80Z	09B44ZZ	09BS3ZX	09CK4ZZ	09J77ZZ	09NM3ZZ	09PK3YZ	09TG4ZZ
099Q8ZX	099V8ZX	09B47ZX	09BS4ZX	09CK8ZZ	09J78ZZ	09NM4ZZ	09PK40Z	09TG7ZZ
099Q8ZZ	099V8ZZ	09B47ZZ	09BS8ZX	09CKXZZ	09J7XZZ	09NM8ZZ	09PK47Z	09TG8ZZ
099R30Z	099W30Z	09B48ZX	09BT3ZX	09CL0ZZ	09J83ZZ	09P700Z	09PK4DZ	09WH3JZ
099R3ZX	099W3ZX	09B48ZZ	09BT4ZX	09CL3ZZ	09J87ZZ	09P770Z	09PK4JZ	09WH3KZ
099R3ZZ	099W3ZZ	09B4XZX	09BT8ZX	09CL4ZZ	09J88ZZ	09P780Z	09PK4KZ	09WH3YZ
099R40Z	099W40Z	09B4XZZ	09BU3ZX	09CL7ZZ	09J8XZZ	09P7X0Z	09PK4YZ	09WH4JZ
099R4ZX	099W4ZX	09BF0ZX	09BU4ZX	09CL8ZZ	09JD3ZZ	09P800Z	09PK70Z	09WH4KZ
099R4ZZ	099W4ZZ	09BF0ZZ	09BU8ZX	09CM0ZZ	09JD8ZZ	09P870Z	09PK77Z	09WH4YZ
099R70Z	099W70Z	09BF3ZX	09BV3ZX	09CM3ZZ	09JDXZZ	09P880Z	09PK7DZ	09WH7DZ
099R7ZX	099W7ZX	09BF3ZZ	09BV4ZX	09CM4ZZ	09JE3ZZ	09P8X0Z	09PK7JZ	09WH7YZ
099R7ZZ	099W7ZZ	09BF4ZX	09BV8ZX	09CM8ZZ	09JE8ZZ	09PH30Z	09PK7KZ	09WH8DZ
099R80Z	099W80Z	09BF4ZZ	09BW3ZX	09HD01Z	09JEXZZ	09PH3JZ	09PK7YZ	09WH8YZ
099R8ZX	099W8ZX	09BF7ZX	09BW4ZX	09HD31Z	09JH0ZZ	09PH3KZ	09PK80Z	09WHX0Z
099R8ZZ	099W8ZZ	09BF7ZZ	09BW8ZX	09HD41Z	09JH3ZZ	09PH3YZ	09PK87Z	09WHX7Z
099S30Z	099X30Z	09BF8ZX	09BX3ZX	09HE01Z	09JH4ZZ	09PH40Z	09PK8DZ	09WHXDZ
099S3ZX	099X3ZX	09BF8ZZ	09BX4ZX	09HE31Z	09JH7ZZ	09PH4JZ	09PK8JZ	09WHXJZ
099S3ZZ	099X3ZZ	09BG0ZX	09BX8ZX	09HE41Z	09JH8ZZ	09PH4KZ	09PK8KZ	09WHXKZ
099S40Z	099X40Z	09BG0ZZ	09C00ZZ	09HH01Z	09JHXZZ	09PH4YZ	09PK8YZ	09WJ3JZ
099S4ZX	099X4ZX	09BG3ZX	09C03ZZ	09HH31Z	09JJ0ZZ	09PH70Z	09PKX0Z	09WJ3KZ
099S4ZZ	099X4ZZ	09BG3ZZ	09C04ZZ	09HH3YZ	09JJ3ZZ	09PH7DZ	09PKX7Z	09WJ3YZ
099S70Z	099X70Z	09BG4ZX	09C0XZZ	09HH41Z	09JJ4ZZ	09PH7YZ	09PKXDZ	09WJ4JZ
099S7ZX	099X7ZX	09BG4ZZ	09C10ZZ	09HH4YZ	09JJ7ZZ	09PH80Z	09PKXJZ	09WJ4KZ
099S7ZZ	099X7ZZ	09BG7ZX	09C13ZZ	09HH71Z	09JJ8ZZ	09PH8DZ	09PKXKZ	09WJ4YZ
099S80Z	099X80Z	09BG7ZZ	09C14ZZ	09HH7YZ	09JJXZZ	09PH8YZ	09PY3YZ	09WJ7DZ
099S8ZX	099X8ZX	09BG8ZX	09C1XZZ	09HH81Z	09JK0ZZ	09PHX0Z	09PY4YZ	09WJ7YZ
099S8ZZ	099X8ZZ	09BG8ZZ	09C30ZZ	09HH8YZ	09JK3ZZ	09PHX7Z	09PY7YZ	09WJ8DZ
099T30Z	09B00ZX	09BK0ZX	09C33ZZ	09HJ01Z	09JK4ZZ	09PHXDZ	09PY8YZ	09WJ8YZ
099T3ZX	09B00ZZ	09BK0ZZ	09C34ZZ	09HJ31Z	09JK8ZZ	09PHXJZ	09PYX0Z	09WJX0Z
099T3ZZ	09B03ZX	09BK3ZX	09C37ZZ	09HJ3YZ	09JKXZZ	09PHXKZ	09Q0XZZ	09WJX7Z
099T40Z	09B03ZZ	09BK3ZZ	09C38ZZ	09HJ41Z	09JY0ZZ	09PJ30Z	09Q1XZZ	09WJXDZ
099T4ZX	09B04ZX	09BK4ZX	09C3XZZ	09HJ4YZ	09JY3ZZ	09PJ3JZ	09Q2XZZ	09WJXJZ
099T4ZZ	09B04ZZ	09BK4ZZ	09C40ZZ	09HJ71Z	09JY4ZZ	09PJ3KZ	09Q3XZZ	09WJXKZ
099T70Z	09B0XZX	09BK8ZX	09C43ZZ	09HJ7YZ	09JY8ZZ	09PJ3YZ	09Q4XZZ	09WK00Z
099T7ZX	09B0XZX	09BK8ZZ	09C44ZZ	09HJ81Z	09JYXZZ	09PJ40Z	09QF0ZZ	09WK07Z
099T7ZZ	09B10ZX	09BKXZX	09C47ZZ	09HJ8YZ	09N0XZZ	09PJ4JZ	09QF3ZZ	09WK0DZ
099T80Z	09B10ZZ	09BKXZZ	09C48ZZ	09HK01Z	09N1XZZ	09PJ4KZ	09QF4ZZ	09WK0JZ
099T8ZX	09B13ZX	09BL0ZX	09C4XZZ	09HK0YZ	09N3XZZ	09PJ4YZ	09QF7ZZ	09WK0KZ
099T8ZZ	09B13ZZ	09BL3ZX	09C70ZZ	09HK31Z	09N4XZZ	09PJ70Z	09QF8ZZ	09WK0YZ
099U30Z	09B14ZX	09BL4ZX	09C73ZZ	09HK3YZ	09NF0ZZ	09PJ7DZ	09QFXZZ	09WK30Z
099U3ZX	09B14ZZ	09BL7ZX	09C74ZZ	09HK41Z	09NF3ZZ	09PJ7YZ	09QG0ZZ	09WK37Z
099U3ZZ	09B1XZX	09BL8ZX	09C77ZZ	09HK4YZ	09NF4ZZ	09PJ80Z	09QG3ZZ	09WK3DZ
099U40Z	09B1XZZ	09BM0ZX	09C78ZZ	09HK71Z	09NF7ZZ	09PJ8DZ	09QG4ZZ	09WK3JZ
099U4ZX	09B30ZX	09BM3ZX	09C80ZZ	09HK7YZ	09NF8ZZ	09PJ8YZ	09QG7ZZ	09WK3KZ
099U4ZZ	09B30ZZ	09BM4ZX	09C83ZZ	09HK81Z	09NG0ZZ	09PJX0Z	09QG8ZZ	09WK3YZ
099U70Z	09B33ZX	09BM8ZX	09C84ZZ	09HK8YZ	09NG3ZZ	09PJX7Z	09QGXZZ	09WK40Z
099U7ZX	09B33ZZ	09BN0ZX	09C87ZZ	09HN71Z	09NG4ZZ	09PJXDZ	09QKXZZ	09WK47Z
099U7ZZ	09B34ZX	09BN3ZX	09C88ZZ	09HN7BZ	09NG7ZZ	09PJXJZ	09SF0ZZ	09WK4DZ
099U80Z	09B34ZZ	09BN4ZX	09CF0ZZ	09HN81Z	09NG8ZZ	09PJXKZ	09SF4ZZ	09WK4JZ
099U8ZX	09B37ZX	09BN7ZX	09CF3ZZ	09HN8BZ	09NK0ZZ	09PK00Z	09SF7ZZ	09WK4KZ
099U8ZZ	09B37ZZ	09BN8ZX	09CF4ZZ	09HY01Z	09NK3ZZ	09PK07Z	09SF8ZZ	09WK4YZ
099V30Z	09B38ZX	09BP3ZX	09CF7ZZ	09HY31Z	09NK4ZZ	09PK0DZ	09SG0ZZ	09WK70Z
099V3ZX	09B38ZZ	09BP4ZX	09CF8ZZ	09HY3YZ	09NK8ZZ	09PK0JZ	09SG4ZZ	09WK77Z
099V3ZZ	09B3XZX	09BP8ZX	09CG0ZZ	09HY41Z	09NKXZZ	09PK0KZ	09SG7ZZ	09WK7DZ
099V40Z	09B3XZZ	09BQ3ZX	09CG3ZZ	09HY4YZ	09NL0ZZ	09PK0YZ	09SG8ZZ	09WK7JZ
099V4ZX	09B40ZX	09BQ4ZX	09CG4ZZ	09HY71Z	09NL3ZZ	09PK30Z	09TF0ZZ	09WK7KZ

09WK7YZ	0B740ZZ	0B7B0ZZ	0B977ZX	0B9K4ZX	0BB53ZX	0BC18ZZ	0BF2XZZ	0BHT8YZ
09WK80Z	0B743DZ	0B7B3DZ	0B977ZZ	0B9K7ZX	0BB54ZX	0BC27ZZ	0BF37ZZ	0BJ03ZZ
09WK87Z	0B743ZZ	0B7B3ZZ	0B9780Z	0B9K8ZX	0BB54ZZ	0BC28ZZ	0BF38ZZ	0BJ07ZZ
09WK8DZ	0B744DZ	0B7B4DZ	0B978ZX	0B9K8ZZ	0BB57ZX	0BC37ZZ	0BF3XZZ	0BJ08ZZ
09WK8JZ	0B744ZZ	0B7B4ZZ	0B978ZZ	0B9L3ZX	0BB58ZX	0BC38ZZ	0BF47ZZ	0BJ0XZZ
09WK8KZ	0B747DZ	0B7B7DZ	0B983ZX	0B9L4ZX	0BB58ZZ	0BC47ZZ	0BF48ZZ	0BJ13ZZ
09WK8YZ	0B747ZZ	0B7B7ZZ	0B984ZX	0B9L7ZX	0BB63ZX	0BC48ZZ	0BF4XZZ	0BJ14ZZ
09WKX0Z	0B748DZ	0B7B8DZ	0B9870Z	0B9L8ZX	0BB64ZX	0BC57ZZ	0BF57ZZ	0BJ17ZZ
09WKX7Z	0B748ZZ	0B7B8ZZ	0B987ZX	0B9L8ZZ	0BB64ZZ	0BC58ZZ	0BF58ZZ	0BJ18ZZ
09WKXDZ	0B750DZ	0B913ZX	0B987ZZ	0B9M3ZX	0BB67ZX	0BC67ZZ	0BF5XZZ	0BJ1XZZ
09WKXJZ	0B750ZZ	0B914ZX	0B9880Z	0B9M4ZX	0BB68ZX	0BC68ZZ	0BF67ZZ	0BJK3ZZ
09WKXKZ	0B753DZ	0B9170Z	0B988ZX	0B9M7ZX	0BB68ZZ	0BC77ZZ	0BF68ZZ	0BJK7ZZ
09WY3YZ	0B753ZZ	0B917ZX	0B988ZZ	0B9M8ZX	0BB73ZX	0BC78ZZ	0BF6XZZ	0BJK8ZZ
09WY4YZ	0B754DZ	0B917ZZ	0B993ZX	0B9M8ZZ	0BB74ZX	0BC87ZZ	0BF77ZZ	0BJKXZZ
09WY7YZ	0B754ZZ	0B9180Z	0B994ZX	0B9N00Z	0BB74ZZ	0BC88ZZ	0BF78ZZ	0BJL3ZZ
09WY8YZ	0B757DZ	0B918ZX	0B9970Z	0B9N0ZX	0BB77ZX	0BC97ZZ	0BF7XZZ	0BJL7ZZ
09WYX0Z	0B757ZZ	0B918ZZ	0B997ZX	0B9N0ZZ	0BB78ZX	0BC98ZZ	0BF87ZZ	0BJL8ZZ
0B110D6	0B758DZ	0B923ZX	0B997ZZ	0B9N30Z	0BB78ZZ	0BCB7ZZ	0BF88ZZ	0BJLXZZ
0B20X0Z	0B758ZZ	0B924ZX	0B9980Z	0B9N3ZX	0BB83ZX	0BCB8ZZ	0BF8XZZ	0BJQ3ZZ
0B20XYZ	0B760DZ	0B9270Z	0B998ZX	0B9N3ZZ	0BB84ZX	0BCN3ZZ	0BF97ZZ	0BJQ7ZZ
0B21X0Z	0B760ZZ	0B927ZX	0B998ZZ	0B9N4ZX	0BB84ZZ	0BCP3ZZ	0BF98ZZ	0BJQ8ZZ
0B21XEZ	0B763DZ	0B927ZZ	0B9B3ZX	0B9N80Z	0BB87ZX	0BD14ZX	0BF9XZZ	0BJQXZZ
0B21XFZ	0B763ZZ	0B9280Z	0B9B4ZX	0B9N8ZX	0BB88ZX	0BD18ZX	0BFB7ZZ	0BJT3ZZ
0B21XYZ	0B764DZ	0B928ZX	0B9B70Z	0B9N8ZZ	0BB88ZZ	0BD24ZX	0BFB8ZZ	0BJT7ZZ
0B2KX0Z	0B764ZZ	0B928ZZ	0B9B7ZX	0B9P00Z	0BB93ZX	0BD28ZX	0BFBXZZ	0BJT8ZZ
0B2KXYZ	0B767DZ	0B933ZX	0B9B7ZZ	0B9P0ZX	0BB94ZX	0BD34ZX	0BH03YZ	0BJTXZZ
0B2LX0Z	0B767ZZ	0B934ZX	0B9B80Z	0B9P0ZZ	0BB94ZZ	0BD38ZX	0BH072Z	0BP03YZ
0B2LXYZ	0B768DZ	0B9370Z	0B9B8ZX	0B9P30Z	0BB97ZX	0BD44ZX	0BH073Z	0BP04YZ
0B2QX0Z	0B768ZZ	0B937ZX	0B9B8ZZ	0B9P3ZX	0BB98ZX	0BD48ZX	0BH07DZ	0BP070Z
0B2QXYZ	0B770DZ	0B937ZZ	0B9C3ZX	0B9P3ZZ	0BB98ZZ	0BD54ZX	0BH07YZ	0BP072Z
0B2TX0Z	0B770ZZ	0B9380Z	0B9C4ZX	0B9P4ZX	0BBB3ZX	0BD58ZX	0BH082Z	0BP073Z
0B2TXYZ	0B773DZ	0B938ZX	0B9C7ZX	0B9P80Z	0BBB4ZX	0BD64ZX	0BH083Z	0BP07DZ
0B534ZZ	0B773ZZ	0B938ZZ	0B9C8ZX	0B9P8ZX	0BBB4ZZ	0BD68ZX	0BH08DZ	0BP07YZ
0B544ZZ	0B774DZ	0B943ZX	0B9C8ZZ	0B9P8ZZ	0BBB7ZX	0BD74ZX	0BH08YZ	0BP080Z
0B554ZZ	0B774ZZ	0B944ZX	0B9D3ZX	0B9T30Z	0BBB8ZX	0BD78ZX	0BH13EZ	0BP082Z
0B564ZZ	0B777DZ	0B9470Z	0B9D4ZX	0B9T3ZX	0BBB8ZZ	0BD84ZX	0BH13YZ	0BP083Z
0B574ZZ	0B777ZZ	0B947ZX	0B9D7ZX	0B9T3ZZ	0BBC3ZX	0BD88ZX	0BH172Z	0BP08DZ
0B584ZZ	0B778DZ	0B947ZZ	0B9D8ZX	0B9T40Z	0BBC8ZZ	0BD94ZX	0BH17DZ	0BP08YZ
0B594ZZ	0B778ZZ	0B9480Z	0B9D8ZZ	0B9T4ZX	0BBD3ZX	0BD98ZX	0BH17EZ	0BP0X0Z
0B5B4ZZ	0B780DZ	0B948ZX	0B9F3ZX	0B9T4ZZ	0BBD8ZZ	0BDB4ZX	0BH17YZ	0BP0X1Z
0B5C8ZZ	0B780ZZ	0B948ZZ	0B9F4ZX	0BB13ZX	0BBF3ZX	0BDB8ZX	0BH182Z	0BP0X2Z
0B5D8ZZ	0B783DZ	0B953ZX	0B9F7ZX	0BB14ZX	0BBF8ZZ	0BDC4ZX	0BH18DZ	0BP0X3Z
0B5F8ZZ	0B783ZZ	0B954ZX	0B9F8ZX	0BB17ZX	0BBG3ZX	0BDC8ZX	0BH18EZ	0BP0XDZ
0B5G8ZZ	0B784DZ	0B9570Z	0B9F8ZZ	0BB18ZX	0BBG8ZZ	0BDD4ZX	0BH18YZ	0BP10FZ
0B5H8ZZ	0B784ZZ	0B957ZX	0B9G3ZX	0BB23ZX	0BBH3ZX	0BDD8ZX	0BHK3YZ	0BP13FZ
0B5J8ZZ	0B787DZ	0B957ZZ	0B9G4ZX	0BB24ZX	0BBH8ZZ	0BDF4ZX	0BHK72Z	0BP14FZ
0B5K8ZZ	0B787ZZ	0B9580Z	0B9G7ZX	0BB27ZX	0BBJ3ZX	0BDF8ZX	0BHK73Z	0BP170Z
0B5L8ZZ	0B788DZ	0B958ZX	0B9G8ZX	0BB28ZX	0BBJ8ZZ	0BDG4ZX	0BHK7YZ	0BP172Z
0B5M8ZZ	0B788ZZ	0B958ZZ	0B9G8ZZ	0BB33ZX	0BBK3ZX	0BDG8ZX	0BHK82Z	0BP17DZ
0B730DZ	0B790DZ	0B963ZX	0B9H3ZX	0BB34ZX	0BBK8ZZ	0BDH4ZX	0BHK83Z	0BP17FZ
0B730ZZ	0B790ZZ	0B964ZX	0B9H4ZX	0BB34ZZ	0BBL3ZX	0BDH8ZX	0BHL3YZ	0BP180Z
0B733DZ	0B793DZ	0B9670Z	0B9H7ZX	0BB37ZX	0BBL8ZZ	0BDJ4ZX	0BHL72Z	0BP182Z
0B733ZZ	0B793ZZ	0B967ZX	0B9H8ZX	0BB38ZX	0BBM3ZX	0BDJ8ZX	0BHL73Z	0BP18DZ
0B734DZ	0B794DZ	0B967ZZ	0B9H8ZZ	0BB38ZZ	0BBM4ZZ	0BDK4ZX	0BHL7YZ	0BP18FZ
0B734ZZ	0B794ZZ	0B9680Z	0B9J3ZX	0BB43ZX	0BBM8ZZ	0BDK8ZX	0BHL82Z	0BP1X0Z
0B737DZ	0B797DZ	0B968ZX	0B9J4ZX	0BB44ZX	0BBN0ZX	0BDL4ZX	0BHL83Z	0BP1X2Z
0B737ZZ	0B797ZZ	0B968ZZ	0B9J7ZX	0BB44ZZ	0BBN3ZX	0BDL8ZX	0BHQ3YZ	0BP1XDZ
0B738DZ	0B798DZ	0B973ZX	0B9J8ZX	0BB47ZX	0BBP0ZX	0BDM4ZX	0BHQ7YZ	0BP1XFZ
0B738ZZ	0B798ZZ	0B974ZX	0B9J8ZZ	0BB48ZX	0BBP3ZX	0BDM8ZX	0BHT3YZ	0BPK3YZ
0B740DZ	0B7B0DZ	0B9770Z	0B9K3ZX	0BB48ZZ	0BC17ZZ	0BF1XZZ	0BHT7YZ	0BPK70Z

0BPK71Z	0BW082Z	0BWTX0Z	0C940ZX	0C9H30Z	0C9X0Z0	0CBV7ZX	0CDWXZ1	0CMX0Z1
0BPK72Z	0BW083Z	0BWTX2Z	0C9430Z	0C9H3ZX	0C9X0Z1	0CBV8ZX	0CDWXZ2	0CMX0Z2
0BPK73Z	0BW08DZ	0BWTX7Z	0C943ZX	0C9H3ZZ	0C9X0Z2	0CBW0Z0	0CDXXZ0	0CMXXZ0
0BPK7YZ	0BW08YZ	0BWTXJZ	0C943ZZ	0C9J00Z	0C9XX00	0CBW0Z1	0CDXXZ1	0CMXXZ1
0BPK80Z	0BW0X0Z	0BWTXKZ	0C94XZX	0C9J0ZZ	0C9XX01	0CBW0Z2	0CDXXZ2	0CMXXZ2
0BPK81Z	0BW0X2Z	0BWTXMZ	0C9500Z	0C9J30Z	0C9XX02	0CBWXZ0	0CFB0ZZ	0CN00ZZ
0BPK82Z	0BW0X3Z	0C2AX0Z	0C950ZX	0C9J3ZX	0C9XXZ0	0CBWXZ1	0CFB3ZZ	0CN03ZZ
0BPK83Z	0BW0X7Z	0C2AXYZ	0C950ZZ	0C9J3ZZ	0C9XXZ1	0CBWXZ2	0CFB7ZZ	0CN0XZZ
0BPKX0Z	0BW0XCZ	0C2SX0Z	0C9530Z	0C9M0ZX	0C9XXZ2	0CBX0Z0	0CFBXZZ	0CN10ZZ
0BPKX1Z	0BW0XDZ	0C2SXYZ	0C953ZX	0C9M30Z	0CB00ZX	0CBX0Z1	0CFC0ZZ	0CN13ZZ
0BPKX2Z	0BW0XJZ	0C2YX0Z	0C953ZZ	0C9M3ZX	0CB03ZX	0CBX0Z2	0CFC3ZZ	0CN1XZZ
0BPKX3Z	0BW0XKZ	0C2YXYZ	0C95X0Z	0C9M3ZZ	0CB0XZX	0CBXXZ0	0CFC7ZZ	0CN4XZZ
0BPL3YZ	0BW1X0Z	0C550ZZ	0C95XZX	0C9M4ZX	0CB10ZX	0CBXXZ1	0CFCXZZ	0CN50ZZ
0BPL70Z	0BW1X2Z	0C553ZZ	0C95XZZ	0C9M7ZX	0CB13ZX	0CBXXZ2	0CHA01Z	0CN53ZZ
0BPL72Z	0BW1X7Z	0C55XZZ	0C9600Z	0C9M8ZX	0CB1XZX	0CC0XZZ	0CHA31Z	0CN5XZZ
0BPL73Z	0BW1XCZ	0C560ZZ	0C960ZX	0C9N30Z	0CB40ZX	0CC1XZZ	0CHA3YZ	0CN60ZZ
0BPL7YZ	0BW1XDZ	0C563ZZ	0C960ZZ	0C9N3ZZ	0CB43ZX	0CC2XZZ	0CHA71Z	0CN63ZZ
0BPL80Z	0BW1XFZ	0C56XZZ	0C9630Z	0C9P30Z	0CB4XZX	0CC3XZZ	0CHA7YZ	0CN6XZZ
0BPL82Z	0BW1XJZ	0C5W0Z0	0C963ZX	0C9P3ZZ	0CB50ZX	0CC4XZZ	0CHA81Z	0CN70ZZ
0BPL83Z	0BW1XKZ	0C5W0Z1	0C963ZZ	0C9Q30Z	0CB50ZZ	0CC50ZZ	0CHA8YZ	0CN73ZZ
0BPLX0Z	0BWK3YZ	0C5W0Z2	0C96X0Z	0C9Q3ZZ	0CB53ZX	0CC53ZZ	0CHS01Z	0CN7XZZ
0BPLX1Z	0BWK70Z	0C5WXZ0	0C96XZX	0C9R30Z	0CB53ZZ	0CC5XZZ	0CHS0YZ	0CNW0Z0
0BPLX2Z	0BWK72Z	0C5WXZ1	0C96XZZ	0C9R3ZX	0CB5XZX	0CC60ZZ	0CHS31Z	0CNW0Z1
0BPLX3Z	0BWK73Z	0C5WXZ2	0C9730Z	0C9R3ZZ	0CB5XZZ	0CC63ZZ	0CHS3YZ	0CNW0Z2
0BPQ00Z	0BWK7YZ	0C5X0Z0	0C973ZX	0C9R4ZX	0CB60ZX	0CC6XZZ	0CHS71Z	0CNWXZ0
0BPQ01Z	0BWK80Z	0C5X0Z1	0C973ZZ	0C9R7ZX	0CB60ZZ	0CC7XZZ	0CHS7YZ	0CNWXZ1
0BPQ02Z	0BWK82Z	0C5X0Z2	0C97XZZ	0C9R8ZX	0CB63ZX	0CC83ZZ	0CHS81Z	0CNWXZ2
0BPQ30Z	0BWK83Z	0C5XXZ0	0C9800Z	0C9S30Z	0CB63ZZ	0CC93ZZ	0CHS8YZ	0CNX0Z0
0BPQ31Z	0BWKX0Z	0C5XXZ1	0C9830Z	0C9S3ZX	0CB6XZX	0CCB0ZZ	0CHY01Z	0CNX0Z1
0BPQ32Z	0BWKX2Z	0C5XXZ2	0C983ZX	0C9S3ZZ	0CB6XZZ	0CCB3ZZ	0CHY0YZ	0CNX0Z2
0BPQ3YZ	0BWKX3Z	0C7B0DZ	0C983ZZ	0C9S4ZX	0CB73ZX	0CCC0ZZ	0CHY31Z	0CNXXZ0
0BPQ40Z	0BWL3YZ	0C7B0ZZ	0C9900Z	0C9S7ZX	0CB7XZX	0CCC3ZZ	0CHY3YZ	0CNXXZ1
0BPQ41Z	0BWL70Z	0C7B3DZ	0C9930Z	0C9S8ZX	0CB83ZX	0CCD0ZZ	0CHY71Z	0CNXXZ2
0BPQ42Z	0BWL72Z	0C7B3ZZ	0C993ZX	0C9T30Z	0CB93ZX	0CCD3ZZ	0CHY7BZ	0CPA00Z
0BPQ70Z	0BWL73Z	0C7B7DZ	0C993ZZ	0C9T3ZX	0CBB3ZX	0CCF0ZZ	0CHY7YZ	0CPA0CZ
0BPQ71Z	0BWL7YZ	0C7B7ZZ	0C9B00Z	0C9T3ZZ	0CBC3ZX	0CCF3ZZ	0CHY81Z	0CPA0YZ
0BPQ72Z	0BWL80Z	0C7C0DZ	0C9B0ZZ	0C9T4ZX	0CBD3ZX	0CCG3ZZ	0CHY8BZ	0CPA30Z
0BPQ7YZ	0BWL82Z	0C7C0ZZ	0C9B30Z	0C9T7ZX	0CBF3ZX	0CCH3ZZ	0CHY8YZ	0CPA3CZ
0BPQ80Z	0BWL83Z	0C7C3DZ	0C9B3ZX	0C9T8ZX	0CBG3ZX	0CCJ0ZZ	0CJA0ZZ	0CPA3YZ
0BPQ81Z	0BWLX0Z	0C7C3ZZ	0C9B3ZZ	0C9V30Z	0CBH3ZX	0CCJ3ZZ	0CJA3ZZ	0CPA7YZ
0BPQ82Z	0BWLX2Z	0C7C7DZ	0C9C00Z	0C9V3ZX	0CBJ3ZX	0CCM7ZZ	0CJAXZZ	0CPA8YZ
0BPQX0Z	0BWLX3Z	0C7C7ZZ	0C9C0ZZ	0C9V3ZZ	0CBM0ZX	0CCM8ZZ	0CJS0ZZ	0CPS3YZ
0BPQX1Z	0BWQ00Z	0C7M7DZ	0C9C30Z	0C9V4ZX	0CBM3ZX	0CCNXZZ	0CJS3ZZ	0CPS70Z
0BPQX2Z	0BWQ02Z	0C7M7ZZ	0C9C3ZX	0C9V7ZX	0CBM4ZX	0CCPXZZ	0CJS4ZZ	0CPS7DZ
0BPT3YZ	0BWQ0YZ	0C7M8DZ	0C9C3ZZ	0C9V8ZX	0CBM7ZX	0CCQXZZ	0CJS7ZZ	0CPS7YZ
0BPT70Z	0BWQ30Z	0C7M8ZZ	0C9D00Z	0C9W000	0CBM8ZX	0CCS7ZZ	0CJS8ZZ	0CPS80Z
0BPT72Z	0BWQ32Z	0C900ZX	0C9D0ZZ	0C9W001	0CBR3ZX	0CCS8ZZ	0CJSXZZ	0CPS8DZ
0BPT7YZ	0BWQ3YZ	0C9030Z	0C9D30Z	0C9W002	0CBR4ZX	0CCW0Z0	0CJY0ZZ	0CPS8YZ
0BPT80Z	0BWQ40Z	0C903ZX	0C9D3ZX	0C9W0Z0	0CBR7ZX	0CCW0Z1	0CJY3ZZ	0CPSX0Z
0BPT82Z	0BWQ42Z	0C903ZZ	0C9D3ZZ	0C9W0Z1	0CBR8ZX	0CCW0Z2	0CJY4ZZ	0CPSX7Z
0BPT8YZ	0BWQ70Z	0C90XZX	0C9F00Z	0C9W0Z2	0CBS3ZX	0CCWXZ0	0CJY7ZZ	0CPSXDZ
0BPTX0Z	0BWQ72Z	0C910ZX	0C9F0ZZ	0C9WX00	0CBS4ZX	0CCWXZ1	0CJY8ZZ	0CPSXJZ
0BPTX2Z	0BWQ7YZ	0C9130Z	0C9F30Z	0C9WX01	0CBS7ZX	0CCWXZ2	0CJYXZZ	0CPSXKZ
0BPTXMZ	0BWQ80Z	0C913ZX	0C9F3ZX	0C9WX02	0CBS8ZX	0CCX0Z0	0CMW0Z0	0CPY3YZ
0BW03YZ	0BWQ82Z	0C913ZZ	0C9F3ZZ	0C9WXZ0	0CBT3ZX	0CCX0Z1	0CMW0Z1	0CPY70Z
0BW04YZ	0BWQX0Z	0C91XZZ	0C9G00Z	0C9WXZ1	0CBT4ZX	0CCX0Z2	0CMW0Z2	0CPY7DZ
0BW072Z	0BWQX2Z	0C9230Z	0C9G30Z	0C9WXZ2	0CBT7ZX	0CCXXZ0	0CMWXZ0	0CPY7YZ
0BW073Z	0BWT3YZ	0C923ZZ	0C9G3ZX	0C9X000	0CBT8ZX	0CCXXZ1	0CMWXZ1	0CPY80Z
0BW07DZ	0BWT7YZ	0C9330Z	0C9G3ZZ	0C9X001	0CBV3ZX	0CCXXZ2	0CMWXZ2	0CPY8DZ
0BW07YZ	0BWT8YZ	0C933ZZ	0C9H00Z	0C9X002	0CBV4ZX	0CDWXZ0	0CMX0Z0	0CPY8YZ

0CPYX0Z	0CRXXJ2	0CWYX7Z	0D5L8ZZ	0D7A7ZZ	0D7M3DZ	0D973ZX	0D9F8ZX	0D9Q30Z
0CPYX1Z	0CRXXK0	0CWYXDZ	0D5M4ZZ	0D7A8DZ	0D7M4DZ	0D973ZZ	0D9G30Z	0D9Q3ZX
0CPYX7Z	0CRXXK1	0CWYXJZ	0D5M8ZZ	0D7A8ZZ	0D7M7DZ	0D974ZX	0D9G3ZX	0D9Q3ZZ
0CPYXDZ	0CRXXK2	0CWYXKZ	0D5N4ZZ	0D7B0DZ	0D7M7ZZ	0D9770Z	0D9G3ZZ	0D9Q4ZX
0CPYXJZ	0CSW050	0D16074	0D5N8ZZ	0D7B3DZ	0D7M8DZ	0D977ZX	0D9G4ZX	0D9Q7ZX
0CPYXKZ	0CSW051	0D160J4	0D5P0ZZ	0D7B4DZ	0D7M8ZZ	0D9780Z	0D9G70Z	0D9Q8ZX
0CQ0XZZ	0CSW052	0D160K4	0D5P3ZZ	0D7B7DZ	0D7N0DZ	0D978ZX	0D9G7ZX	0D9QXZX
0CQ1XZZ	0CSW0Z0	0D160Z4	0D5P4ZZ	0D7B7ZZ	0D7N3DZ	0D9830Z	0D9G80Z	0D9R0ZX
0CQ4XZZ	0CSW0Z1	0D163J4	0D5P7ZZ	0D7B8DZ	0D7N4DZ	0D983ZX	0D9G8ZX	0D9R30Z
0CQ50ZZ	0CSW0Z2	0D16474	0D5P8ZZ	0D7B8ZZ	0D7N7DZ	0D983ZZ	0D9H30Z	0D9R3ZX
0CQ53ZZ	0CSWX50	0D164J4	0D5Q4ZZ	0D7C0DZ	0D7N7ZZ	0D984ZX	0D9H3ZX	0D9R3ZZ
0CQ5XZZ	0CSWX51	0D164K4	0D5Q8ZZ	0D7C3DZ	0D7N8DZ	0D9870Z	0D9H3ZZ	0D9R4ZX
0CQ60ZZ	0CSWX52	0D164Z4	0D5R4ZZ	0D7C4DZ	0D7N8ZZ	0D987ZX	0D9H4ZX	0D9U30Z
0CQ63ZZ	0CSWXZ0	0D16874	0D717DZ	0D7C7DZ	0D7P7DZ	0D9880Z	0D9H70Z	0D9U3ZX
0CQ6XZZ	0CSWXZ1	0D168J4	0D717ZZ	0D7C7ZZ	0D7P7ZZ	0D988ZX	0D9H7ZX	0D9U3ZZ
0CQ7XZZ	0CSWXZ2	0D168K4	0D718DZ	0D7C8DZ	0D7P8DZ	0D9930Z	0D9H80Z	0D9U40Z
0CQW0Z0	0CSX050	0D168Z4	0D718ZZ	0D7C8ZZ	0D7P8ZZ	0D993ZX	0D9H8ZX	0D9U4ZZ
0CQW0Z1	0CSX051	0D20X0Z	0D727DZ	0D7E0DZ	0D7Q7DZ	0D993ZZ	0D9J30Z	0D9V30Z
0CQW0Z2	0CSX052	0D20XUZ	0D727ZZ	0D7E3DZ	0D7Q7ZZ	0D994ZX	0D9J3ZZ	0D9V3ZX
0CQWXZ0	0CSX0Z0	0D20XYZ	0D728DZ	0D7E4DZ	0D7Q8DZ	0D9970Z	0D9K30Z	0D9V3ZZ
0CQWXZ1	0CSX0Z1	0D2DX0Z	0D728ZZ	0D7E7DZ	0D7Q8ZZ	0D997ZX	0D9K3ZX	0D9V40Z
0CQWXZ2	0CSX0Z2	0D2DXUZ	0D737DZ	0D7E7ZZ	0D9130Z	0D9980Z	0D9K3ZZ	0D9V4ZZ
0CQX0Z0	0CSXX50	0D2DXYZ	0D737ZZ	0D7E8DZ	0D913ZX	0D998ZX	0D9K4ZX	0D9W30Z
0CQX0Z1	0CSXX51	0D2UX0Z	0D738DZ	0D7E8ZZ	0D913ZZ	0D9A30Z	0D9K70Z	0D9W3ZX
0CQX0Z2	0CSXX52	0D2UXYZ	0D738ZZ	0D7F0DZ	0D914ZX	0D9A3ZX	0D9K7ZX	0D9W3ZZ
0CQXXZ0	0CSXXZ0	0D2VX0Z	0D747DZ	0D7F3DZ	0D917ZX	0D9A3ZZ	0D9K80Z	0DB13ZX
0CQXXZ1	0CSXXZ1	0D2VXYZ	0D747ZZ	0D7F4DZ	0D918ZX	0D9A70Z	0D9K8ZX	0DB14ZX
0CQXXZ2	0CSXXZ2	0D2WX0Z	0D748DZ	0D7F7DZ	0D9230Z	0D9A7ZX	0D9L30Z	0DB14ZZ
0CRW070	0CTW0Z0	0D2WXYZ	0D748ZZ	0D7F7ZZ	0D923ZX	0D9A80Z	0D9L3ZX	0DB17ZX
0CRW071	0CTW0Z1	0D514ZZ	0D757DZ	0D7F8DZ	0D923ZZ	0D9A8ZX	0D9L3ZZ	0DB18ZX
0CRW072	0CTW0Z2	0D518ZZ	0D757ZZ	0D7F8ZZ	0D924ZX	0D9B30Z	0D9L4ZX	0DB18ZZ
0CRW0J0	0CTX0Z0	0D524ZZ	0D758DZ	0D7G0DZ	0D927ZX	0D9B3ZX	0D9L70Z	0DB23ZX
0CRW0J1	0CTX0Z1	0D528ZZ	0D758ZZ	0D7G3DZ	0D928ZX	0D9B3ZZ	0D9L7ZX	0DB24ZX
0CRW0J2	0CTX0Z2	0D534ZZ	0D767DZ	0D7G4DZ	0D9330Z	0D9B4ZX	0D9L80Z	0DB24ZZ
0CRW0K0	0CU20JZ	0D538ZZ	0D767ZZ	0D7G7DZ	0D933ZX	0D9B70Z	0D9L8ZX	0DB27ZX
0CRW0K1	0CU23JZ	0D544ZZ	0D768DZ	0D7G7ZZ	0D933ZZ	0D9B7ZX	0D9M30Z	0DB28ZX
0CRW0K2	0CWA00Z	0D548ZZ	0D768ZZ	0D7G8DZ	0D934ZX	0D9B80Z	0D9M3ZX	0DB28ZZ
0CRWX70	0CWA0CZ	0D554ZZ	0D774DZ	0D7G8ZZ	0D937ZX	0D9B8ZX	0D9M3ZZ	0DB33ZX
0CRWX71	0CWA0YZ	0D558ZZ	0D777DZ	0D7H0DZ	0D938ZX	0D9C30Z	0D9M4ZX	0DB34ZX
0CRWX72	0CWA30Z	0D564ZZ	0D777ZZ	0D7H3DZ	0D9430Z	0D9C3ZX	0D9M70Z	0DB34ZZ
0CRWXJ0	0CWA3CZ	0D568ZZ	0D778DZ	0D7H4DZ	0D943ZX	0D9C3ZZ	0D9M7ZX	0DB37ZX
0CRWXJ1	0CWA3YZ	0D574ZZ	0D778ZZ	0D7H7DZ	0D943ZZ	0D9C4ZX	0D9M80Z	0DB38ZX
0CRWXJ2	0CWA7YZ	0D578ZZ	0D780DZ	0D7H7ZZ	0D944ZX	0D9C7ZX	0D9M8ZX	0DB38ZZ
0CRWXK0	0CWA8YZ	0D588ZZ	0D783DZ	0D7H8DZ	0D947ZX	0D9C8ZX	0D9N30Z	0DB43ZX
0CRWXK1	0CWAX0Z	0D594ZZ	0D784DZ	0D7H8ZZ	0D948ZX	0D9E30Z	0D9N3ZX	0DB44ZX
0CRWXK2	0CWAXCZ	0D598ZZ	0D787DZ	0D7K0DZ	0D9530Z	0D9E3ZX	0D9N3ZZ	0DB47ZX
0CRX070	0CWS3YZ	0D5A8ZZ	0D787ZZ	0D7K3DZ	0D953ZX	0D9E3ZZ	0D9N4ZX	0DB48ZX
0CRX071	0CWS7YZ	0D5B8ZZ	0D788DZ	0D7K4DZ	0D953ZZ	0D9E4ZX	0D9N70Z	0DB48ZZ
0CRX072	0CWS8YZ	0D5C8ZZ	0D788ZZ	0D7K7DZ	0D954ZX	0D9E70Z	0D9N7ZX	0DB53ZX
0CRX0J0	0CWSX0Z	0D5E4ZZ	0D790DZ	0D7K7ZZ	0D957ZX	0D9E7ZX	0D9N80Z	0DB54ZX
0CRX0J1	0CWSX7Z	0D5E8ZZ	0D793DZ	0D7K8DZ	0D958ZX	0D9E80Z	0D9N8ZX	0DB54ZZ
0CRX0J2	0CWSXDZ	0D5F4ZZ	0D794DZ	0D7K8ZZ	0D9630Z	0D9E8ZX	0D9P30Z	0DB57ZX
0CRX0K0	0CWSXJZ	0D5F8ZZ	0D797DZ	0D7L0DZ	0D963ZX	0D9F30Z	0D9P3ZX	0DB58ZX
0CRX0K1	0CWSXKZ	0D5G4ZZ	0D797ZZ	0D7L3DZ	0D963ZZ	0D9F3ZX	0D9P3ZZ	0DB58ZZ
0CRX0K2	0CWY07Z	0D5G8ZZ	0D798DZ	0D7L4DZ	0D964ZX	0D9F3ZZ	0D9P4ZX	0DB63Z3
0CRXX70	0CWY3YZ	0D5H4ZZ	0D798ZZ	0D7L7DZ	0D9670Z	0D9F4ZX	0D9P70Z	0DB63ZX
0CRXX71	0CWY7YZ	0D5H8ZZ	0D7A0DZ	0D7L7ZZ	0D967ZX	0D9F70Z	0D9P7ZX	0DB63ZZ
0CRXX72	0CWY8YZ	0D5K4ZZ	0D7A3DZ	0D7L8DZ	0D9680Z	0D9F7ZX	0D9P80Z	0DB67Z3
0CRXXJ0	0CWYX0Z	0D5K8ZZ	0D7A4DZ	0D7L8ZZ	0D968ZX	0D9F80Z	0D9P8ZX	0DB67ZX
0CRXXJ1	0CWYX1Z	0D5L4ZZ	0D7A7DZ	0D7M0DZ	0D9730Z	0D9F80Z	0D9Q0ZX	0DB67ZZ

0DB68Z3	0DBL8ZZ	0DCG7ZZ	0DDG4ZX	0DH582Z	0DH983Z	0DHP8DZ	0DL40ZZ	0DP08UZ
0DB68ZX	0DBM3ZX	0DCG8ZZ	0DDG8ZX	0DH583Z	0DH98DZ	0DJ03ZZ	0DL43CZ	0DP08YZ
0DB68ZZ	0DBM4ZX	0DCH7ZZ	0DDH3ZX	0DH58BZ	0DH98UZ	0DJ07ZZ	0DL43DZ	0DP0X0Z
0DB73ZX	0DBM7ZX	0DCH8ZZ	0DDH4ZX	0DH58DZ	0DHA01Z	0DJ08ZZ	0DL43ZZ	0DP0X2Z
0DB74ZX	0DBM8ZX	0DCK7ZZ	0DDH8ZX	0DH58UZ	0DHA0DZ	0DJ0XZZ	0DL44CZ	0DP0X3Z
0DB74ZZ	0DBM8ZZ	0DCK8ZZ	0DDK3ZX	0DH58YZ	0DHA0UZ	0DJ63ZZ	0DL44DZ	0DP0XDZ
0DB77ZX	0DBN3ZX	0DCL7ZZ	0DDK4ZX	0DH601Z	0DHA31Z	0DJ67ZZ	0DL44ZZ	0DP0XUZ
0DB78ZX	0DBN4ZX	0DCL8ZZ	0DDK8ZX	0DH631Z	0DHA3DZ	0DJ68ZZ	0DL47DZ	0DP53YZ
0DB78ZZ	0DBN7ZX	0DCM7ZZ	0DDL3ZX	0DH63UZ	0DHA3UZ	0DJ6XZZ	0DL47ZZ	0DP54YZ
0DB83ZX	0DBN8ZX	0DCM8ZZ	0DDL4ZX	0DH63YZ	0DHA41Z	0DJD3ZZ	0DL48DZ	0DP571Z
0DB84ZX	0DBN8ZZ	0DCN7ZZ	0DDL8ZX	0DH641Z	0DHA4DZ	0DJD7ZZ	0DL48ZZ	0DP57DZ
0DB87ZX	0DBP3ZX	0DCN8ZZ	0DDM3ZX	0DH64UZ	0DHA4UZ	0DJD8ZZ	0DL50CZ	0DP57YZ
0DB88ZX	0DBP4ZX	0DCP7ZZ	0DDM4ZX	0DH64YZ	0DHA71Z	0DJDXZZ	0DL50DZ	0DP581Z
0DB93ZX	0DBP7ZX	0DCP8ZZ	0DDM8ZX	0DH671Z	0DHA72Z	0DJU3ZZ	0DL50ZZ	0DP58DZ
0DB94ZX	0DBP8ZX	0DCQ7ZZ	0DDN3ZX	0DH672Z	0DHA73Z	0DJUXZZ	0DL53CZ	0DP58YZ
0DB94ZZ	0DBP8ZZ	0DCQ8ZZ	0DDN4ZX	0DH673Z	0DHA7DZ	0DJV3ZZ	0DL53DZ	0DP5X1Z
0DB97ZX	0DBQ0ZX	0DCQXZZ	0DDN8ZX	0DH67DZ	0DHA7UZ	0DJVXZZ	0DL53ZZ	0DP5X2Z
0DB98ZX	0DBQ3ZX	0DD13ZX	0DDP3ZX	0DH67UZ	0DHA81Z	0DJW3ZZ	0DL54CZ	0DP5X3Z
0DB98ZZ	0DBQ4ZX	0DD14ZX	0DDP4ZX	0DH67YZ	0DHA82Z	0DJWXZZ	0DL54DZ	0DP5XDZ
0DBA3ZX	0DBQ7ZX	0DD18ZX	0DDP8ZX	0DH681Z	0DHA83Z	0DL10CZ	0DL54ZZ	0DP5XUZ
0DBA4ZX	0DBQ8ZX	0DD23ZX	0DDQ3ZX	0DH682Z	0DHA8DZ	0DL10DZ	0DL57DZ	0DP63YZ
0DBA7ZX	0DBQ8ZZ	0DD24ZX	0DDQ4ZX	0DH683Z	0DHA8UZ	0DL10ZZ	0DL57ZZ	0DP64YZ
0DBA8ZX	0DBQXZX	0DD28ZX	0DDQ8ZX	0DH68DZ	0DHB01Z	0DL13CZ	0DL58DZ	0DP670Z
0DBB3ZX	0DBR0ZX	0DD33ZX	0DDQXZX	0DH68UZ	0DHB0DZ	0DL13DZ	0DL58ZZ	0DP672Z
0DBB4ZX	0DBR3ZX	0DD34ZX	0DF5XZZ	0DH68YZ	0DHB0UZ	0DL13ZZ	0DN87ZZ	0DP673Z
0DBB7ZX	0DBR4ZX	0DD38ZX	0DF6XZZ	0DH801Z	0DHB31Z	0DL14CZ	0DN88ZZ	0DP67DZ
0DBB8ZX	0DBU3ZX	0DD43ZX	0DF8XZZ	0DH80DZ	0DHB3DZ	0DL14DZ	0DN97ZZ	0DP67UZ
0DBC3ZX	0DBU4ZX	0DD44ZX	0DF9XZZ	0DH80UZ	0DHB3UZ	0DL14ZZ	0DN98ZZ	0DP67YZ
0DBC4ZX	0DBV3ZX	0DD48ZX	0DFAXZZ	0DH831Z	0DHB41Z	0DL17DZ	0DNA7ZZ	0DP680Z
0DBC7ZX	0DBV4ZX	0DD53ZX	0DFBXZZ	0DH83DZ	0DHB4DZ	0DL17ZZ	0DNA8ZZ	0DP682Z
0DBC8ZX	0DBW3ZX	0DD54ZX	0DFEXZZ	0DH83UZ	0DHB4UZ	0DL18DZ	0DNB7ZZ	0DP683Z
0DBE3ZX	0DBW4ZX	0DD58ZX	0DFFXZZ	0DH841Z	0DHB71Z	0DL18ZZ	0DNB8ZZ	0DP68DZ
0DBE4ZX	0DC17ZZ	0DD63ZX	0DFGXZZ	0DH84DZ	0DHB72Z	0DL20CZ	0DNE7ZZ	0DP68UZ
0DBE7ZX	0DC18ZZ	0DD64ZX	0DFHXZZ	0DH84UZ	0DHB73Z	0DL20DZ	0DNE8ZZ	0DP68YZ
0DBE8ZX	0DC27ZZ	0DD68ZX	0DFJXZZ	0DH871Z	0DHB7DZ	0DL20ZZ	0DNF7ZZ	0DP6X0Z
0DBE8ZZ	0DC28ZZ	0DD73ZX	0DFKXZZ	0DH872Z	0DHB7UZ	0DL23CZ	0DNF8ZZ	0DP6X2Z
0DBF3ZX	0DC37ZZ	0DD74ZX	0DFLXZZ	0DH873Z	0DHB81Z	0DL23DZ	0DNG7ZZ	0DP6X3Z
0DBF4ZX	0DC38ZZ	0DD78ZX	0DFMXZZ	0DH87DZ	0DHB82Z	0DL23ZZ	0DNG8ZZ	0DP6XDZ
0DBF7ZX	0DC47ZZ	0DD83ZX	0DFNXZZ	0DH87UZ	0DHB83Z	0DL24CZ	0DNH7ZZ	0DP6XUZ
0DBF8ZX	0DC48ZZ	0DD84ZX	0DFPXZZ	0DH881Z	0DHB8DZ	0DL24DZ	0DNH8ZZ	0DPD3YZ
0DBF8ZZ	0DC57ZZ	0DD88ZX	0DFQXZZ	0DH882Z	0DHB8UZ	0DL24ZZ	0DNK7ZZ	0DPD4YZ
0DBG3ZX	0DC58ZZ	0DD93ZX	0DH00YZ	0DH883Z	0DHD0YZ	0DL27DZ	0DNK8ZZ	0DPD70Z
0DBG4ZX	0DC67ZZ	0DD94ZX	0DH03YZ	0DH88DZ	0DHD3YZ	0DL27ZZ	0DNL7ZZ	0DPD72Z
0DBG7ZX	0DC68ZZ	0DD98ZX	0DH04YZ	0DH88UZ	0DHD4YZ	0DL28DZ	0DNL8ZZ	0DPD73Z
0DBG8ZX	0DC77ZZ	0DDA3ZX	0DH07YZ	0DH901Z	0DHD7YZ	0DL28ZZ	0DNM7ZZ	0DPD7DZ
0DBG8ZZ	0DC78ZZ	0DDA4ZX	0DH08YZ	0DH90DZ	0DHD8YZ	0DL30CZ	0DNM8ZZ	0DPD7UZ
0DBH3ZX	0DC87ZZ	0DDA8ZX	0DH50DZ	0DH90UZ	0DHE01Z	0DL30DZ	0DNN7ZZ	0DPD7YZ
0DBH4ZX	0DC88ZZ	0DDB3ZX	0DH50UZ	0DH931Z	0DHE0DZ	0DL30ZZ	0DNN8ZZ	0DPD80Z
0DBH7ZX	0DC97ZZ	0DDB4ZX	0DH53DZ	0DH93DZ	0DHE31Z	0DL33CZ	0DP03YZ	0DPD82Z
0DBH8ZX	0DC98ZZ	0DDB8ZX	0DH53UZ	0DH93UZ	0DHE3DZ	0DL33DZ	0DP04YZ	0DPD83Z
0DBH8ZZ	0DCA7ZZ	0DDC3ZX	0DH53YZ	0DH941Z	0DHE41Z	0DL33ZZ	0DP070Z	0DPD8DZ
0DBK3ZX	0DCA8ZZ	0DDC4ZX	0DH54DZ	0DH94DZ	0DHE4DZ	0DL34CZ	0DP072Z	0DPD8UZ
0DBK4ZX	0DCB7ZZ	0DDC8ZX	0DH54UZ	0DH94UZ	0DHE71Z	0DL34DZ	0DP073Z	0DPD8YZ
0DBK7ZX	0DCB8ZZ	0DDE3ZX	0DH54YZ	0DH971Z	0DHE7DZ	0DL34ZZ	0DP07DZ	0DPDX0Z
0DBK8ZX	0DCC7ZZ	0DDE4ZX	0DH572Z	0DH972Z	0DHE81Z	0DL37DZ	0DP07UZ	0DPDX2Z
0DBK8ZZ	0DCC8ZZ	0DDE8ZX	0DH573Z	0DH973Z	0DHE8DZ	0DL37ZZ	0DP07YZ	0DPDX3Z
0DBL3ZX	0DCE7ZZ	0DDF3ZX	0DH57BZ	0DH97DZ	0DHP0DZ	0DL38DZ	0DP080Z	0DPDXDZ
0DBL4ZX	0DCE8ZZ	0DDF4ZX	0DH57DZ	0DH97UZ	0DHP3DZ	0DL38ZZ	0DP082Z	0DPDXUZ
0DBL7ZX	0DCF7ZZ	0DDF8ZX	0DH57UZ	0DH981Z	0DHP4DZ	0DL40CZ	0DP083Z	0DPP71Z
0DBL8ZX	0DCF8ZZ	0DDG3ZX	0DH57YZ	0DH982Z	0DHP7DZ	0DL40DZ	0DP08DZ	0DPP81Z

0DPPX1Z	0DWDX7Z	0F764DZ	0F948ZZ	0F9D4ZX	0FBC8ZX	0FD83ZX	0FHB3YZ	0FL64DZ
0DQU0ZZ	0DWDXCZ	0F764ZZ	0F9530Z	0F9D7ZX	0FBC8ZZ	0FD84ZX	0FHB43Z	0FL64ZZ
0DQU3ZZ	0DWDXDZ	0F767DZ	0F953ZX	0F9D80Z	0FBD3ZX	0FD88ZX	0FHB4DZ	0FL67DZ
0DQU4ZZ	0DWDXJZ	0F768DZ	0F953ZZ	0F9D8ZX	0FBD4ZX	0FD93ZX	0FHB4YZ	0FL67ZZ
0DS5XZZ	0DWDXKZ	0F768ZZ	0F954ZX	0F9D8ZZ	0FBD4ZZ	0FD94ZX	0FHB72Z	0FL68DZ
0DS6XZZ	0DWDXUZ	0F773DZ	0F957ZX	0F9F30Z	0FBD7ZX	0FD98ZX	0FHB73Z	0FL68ZZ
0DS9XZZ	0DWU00Z	0F773ZZ	0F9580Z	0F9F3ZX	0FBD8ZX	0FDC3ZX	0FHB7YZ	0FL73CZ
0DSAXZZ	0DWU30Z	0F774DZ	0F958ZX	0F9F3ZZ	0FBD8ZZ	0FDC4ZX	0FHB82Z	0FL73DZ
0DSBXZZ	0DWU40Z	0F774ZZ	0F958ZZ	0F9F4ZX	0FBF3ZX	0FDC8ZX	0FHB83Z	0FL73ZZ
0DSHXZZ	0DWV00Z	0F777DZ	0F9630Z	0F9F7ZX	0FBF4ZX	0FDD3ZX	0FHB8DZ	0FL74CZ
0DSKXZZ	0DWV30Z	0F778DZ	0F963ZX	0F9F80Z	0FBF4ZZ	0FDD4ZX	0FHB8YZ	0FL74DZ
0DSLXZZ	0DWV40Z	0F778ZZ	0F963ZZ	0F9F8ZX	0FBF7ZX	0FDD8ZX	0FHD03Z	0FL74ZZ
0DSMXZZ	0DWW00Z	0F783DZ	0F964ZX	0F9F8ZZ	0FBF8ZX	0FDF3ZX	0FHD33Z	0FL77DZ
0DSNXZZ	0DWW30Z	0F783ZZ	0F967ZX	0F9G30Z	0FBF8ZZ	0FDF4ZX	0FHD3YZ	0FL77ZZ
0DSPXZZ	0DWW40Z	0F784DZ	0F9680Z	0F9G3ZX	0FBG3ZX	0FDF8ZX	0FHD43Z	0FL78DZ
0DSQXZZ	0DY50Z0	0F784ZZ	0F968ZX	0F9G3ZZ	0FBG4ZX	0FDG3ZX	0FHD4DZ	0FL78ZZ
0DV67DZ	0DY50Z1	0F787DZ	0F968ZZ	0F9G4ZX	0FBG8ZX	0FDG4ZX	0FHD4YZ	0FL83CZ
0DV68DZ	0DY50Z2	0F788DZ	0F9730Z	0F9G80Z	0FC53ZZ	0FDG8ZX	0FHD72Z	0FL83DZ
0DW03YZ	0F1D0D4	0F788ZZ	0F973ZX	0F9G8ZX	0FC54ZZ	0FF48ZZ	0FHD73Z	0FL83ZZ
0DW04YZ	0F1D0Z4	0F793DZ	0F973ZZ	0F9G8ZZ	0FC57ZZ	0FF4XZZ	0FHD7YZ	0FL84CZ
0DW07YZ	0F1D4D4	0F793ZZ	0F9740Z	0FB03ZX	0FC58ZZ	0FF58ZZ	0FHD82Z	0FL84DZ
0DW08UZ	0F1D4Z4	0F794DZ	0F974ZX	0FB13ZX	0FC63ZZ	0FF5XZZ	0FHD83Z	0FL84ZZ
0DW08YZ	0F20X0Z	0F794ZZ	0F974ZZ	0FB23ZX	0FC64ZZ	0FF68ZZ	0FHD8DZ	0FL87DZ
0DW0X0Z	0F20XYZ	0F797DZ	0F9770Z	0FB43ZX	0FC67ZZ	0FF6XZZ	0FHD8YZ	0FL87ZZ
0DW0X2Z	0F24X0Z	0F798DZ	0F977ZX	0FB44ZX	0FC68ZZ	0FF78ZZ	0FHG01Z	0FL88DZ
0DW0X3Z	0F24XYZ	0F798ZZ	0F977ZZ	0FB48ZX	0FC73ZZ	0FF7XZZ	0FHG03Z	0FL88ZZ
0DW0X7Z	0F2BX0Z	0F7C8DZ	0F9780Z	0FB53ZX	0FC74ZZ	0FF88ZZ	0FHG31Z	0FL93CZ
0DW0XCZ	0F2BXYZ	0F7C8ZZ	0F978ZX	0FB54ZX	0FC77ZZ	0FF8XZZ	0FHG33Z	0FL93DZ
0DW0XDZ	0F2DX0Z	0F7D4DZ	0F978ZZ	0FB54ZZ	0FC78ZZ	0FF98ZZ	0FHG3YZ	0FL93ZZ
0DW0XJZ	0F2DXYZ	0F7D4ZZ	0F9830Z	0FB57ZX	0FC83ZZ	0FF9XZZ	0FHG41Z	0FL94CZ
0DW0XKZ	0F2GX0Z	0F7D7DZ	0F983ZX	0FB58ZX	0FC84ZZ	0FFC8ZZ	0FHG43Z	0FL94DZ
0DW0XUZ	0F2GXYZ	0F7D8DZ	0F983ZZ	0FB58ZZ	0FC87ZZ	0FFCXZZ	0FHG4YZ	0FL94ZZ
0DW50YZ	0F554ZZ	0F7D8ZZ	0F984ZX	0FB63ZX	0FC88ZZ	0FFD8ZZ	0FJ03ZZ	0FL97DZ
0DW53YZ	0F558ZZ	0F7F4DZ	0F987ZX	0FB64ZX	0FC93ZZ	0FFDXZZ	0FJ0XZZ	0FL97ZZ
0DW54YZ	0F564ZZ	0F7F4ZZ	0F9880Z	0FB64ZZ	0FC94ZZ	0FFF8ZZ	0FJ43ZZ	0FL98DZ
0DW57YZ	0F568ZZ	0F7F8DZ	0F988ZX	0FB67ZX	0FC97ZZ	0FFFXZZ	0FJ48ZZ	0FL98ZZ
0DW58YZ	0F574ZZ	0F7F8ZZ	0F988ZZ	0FB68ZX	0FC98ZZ	0FH001Z	0FJ4XZZ	0FM44ZZ
0DW5XDZ	0F578ZZ	0F9030Z	0F9930Z	0FB68ZZ	0FCC4ZZ	0FH003Z	0FJB3ZZ	0FM54ZZ
0DW63YZ	0F584ZZ	0F903ZX	0F993ZX	0FB73ZX	0FCC8ZZ	0FH031Z	0FJB7ZZ	0FM64ZZ
0DW64YZ	0F588ZZ	0F903ZZ	0F993ZZ	0FB74ZX	0FCD3ZZ	0FH033Z	0FJB8ZZ	0FM74ZZ
0DW67YZ	0F594ZZ	0F9040Z	0F994ZX	0FB74ZZ	0FCD4ZZ	0FH03YZ	0FJD3ZZ	0FM84ZZ
0DW68UZ	0F598ZZ	0F904ZX	0F994ZZ	0FB77ZX	0FCD8ZZ	0FH041Z	0FJD7ZZ	0FM94ZZ
0DW68YZ	0F5C4ZZ	0F904ZZ	0F997ZX	0FB78ZX	0FCF3ZZ	0FH043Z	0FJD8ZZ	0FP03YZ
0DW6X0Z	0F5C8ZZ	0F9130Z	0F997ZZ	0FB78ZZ	0FCF4ZZ	0FH04YZ	0FJG3ZZ	0FP04YZ
0DW6X2Z	0F5D4ZZ	0F913ZX	0F9980Z	0FB83ZX	0FCF8ZZ	0FH103Z	0FJG8ZZ	0FP0X0Z
0DW6X3Z	0F5D8ZZ	0F913ZZ	0F998ZX	0FB84ZX	0FD03ZX	0FH133Z	0FJGXZZ	0FP0X2Z
0DW6X7Z	0F5F4ZZ	0F9140Z	0F998ZZ	0FB84ZZ	0FD13ZX	0FH143Z	0FL53CZ	0FP0X3Z
0DW6XCZ	0F5F8ZZ	0F914ZX	0F9C30Z	0FB87ZX	0FD23ZX	0FH203Z	0FL53DZ	0FP43YZ
0DW6XDZ	0F5G4ZF	0F914ZZ	0F9C3ZX	0FB88ZX	0FD43ZX	0FH233Z	0FL53ZZ	0FP44YZ
0DW6XJZ	0F5G4ZZ	0F9230Z	0F9C3ZZ	0FB88ZZ	0FD44ZX	0FH243Z	0FL54CZ	0FP4X0Z
0DW6XKZ	0F5G8ZZ	0F923ZX	0F9C40Z	0FB93ZX	0FD48ZX	0FH401Z	0FL54DZ	0FP4X2Z
0DW6XUZ	0F753DZ	0F923ZZ	0F9C4ZX	0FB94ZX	0FD53ZX	0FH403Z	0FL54ZZ	0FP4X3Z
0DWD3YZ	0F753ZZ	0F9240Z	0F9C4ZZ	0FB94ZZ	0FD54ZX	0FH431Z	0FL57DZ	0FP4XDZ
0DWD4YZ	0F754DZ	0F924ZX	0F9C7ZX	0FB97ZX	0FD58ZX	0FH433Z	0FL57ZZ	0FPB3YZ
0DWD7YZ	0F754ZZ	0F924ZZ	0F9C80Z	0FB98ZX	0FD63ZX	0FH43YZ	0FL58DZ	0FPB4YZ
0DWD8UZ	0F757DZ	0F9430Z	0F9C8ZX	0FB98ZZ	0FD64ZX	0FH441Z	0FL58ZZ	0FPB70Z
0DWD8YZ	0F758DZ	0F943ZX	0F9C8ZZ	0FBC3ZX	0FD68ZX	0FH443Z	0FL63CZ	0FPB72Z
0DWDX0Z	0F758ZZ	0F943ZZ	0F9D30Z	0FBC4ZX	0FD73ZX	0FH44YZ	0FL63DZ	0FPB73Z
0DWDX2Z	0F763DZ	0F9480Z	0F9D3ZX	0FBC4ZZ	0FD74ZX	0FHB03Z	0FL63ZZ	0FPB7DZ
0DWDX3Z	0F763ZZ	0F948ZX	0F9D3ZZ	0FBC7ZX	0FD78ZX	0FHB33Z	0FL64CZ	0FPB7YZ

0FPB80Z	0FV74CZ	0FWDX0Z	0G9G3ZZ	0GJK3ZZ	0H90XZX	0H9MX0Z	0H9X7ZX	0HBU3ZX
0FPB82Z	0FV74DZ	0FWDX2Z	0G9G40Z	0GJR3ZZ	0H90XZZ	0H9MXZX	0H9X7ZZ	0HBU7ZX
0FPB83Z	0FV74ZZ	0FWDX3Z	0G9G4ZX	0GJS3ZZ	0H91X0Z	0H9MXZZ	0H9X80Z	0HBU8ZX
0FPB8DZ	0FV77DZ	0FWDX7Z	0G9G4ZZ	0GP0X0Z	0H91XZX	0H9NX0Z	0H9X8ZX	0HBV3ZX
0FPB8YZ	0FV77ZZ	0FWDXCZ	0G9H30Z	0GP1X0Z	0H91XZZ	0H9NXZX	0H9X8ZZ	0HBV7ZX
0FPBX0Z	0FV78DZ	0FWDXDZ	0G9H3ZX	0GP5X0Z	0H92X0Z	0H9NXZZ	0H9XX0Z	0HBV8ZX
0FPBX1Z	0FV78ZZ	0FWDXJZ	0G9H3ZZ	0GPKX0Z	0H92XZX	0H9QX0Z	0H9XXZX	0HBW3ZX
0FPBX2Z	0FV83CZ	0FWDXKZ	0G9H40Z	0GPRX0Z	0H92XZZ	0H9QXZX	0H9XXZZ	0HBW7ZX
0FPBX3Z	0FV83DZ	0FWG3YZ	0G9H4ZX	0GPS3YZ	0H93X0Z	0H9QXZZ	0HB0XZX	0HBW8ZX
0FPBXDZ	0FV83ZZ	0FWG4YZ	0G9H4ZZ	0GPS4YZ	0H93XZX	0H9RX0Z	0HB0XZZ	0HBWXZX
0FPD3YZ	0FV84CZ	0FWGX0Z	0G9K30Z	0GPSX0Z	0H93XZZ	0H9RXZX	0HB1XZX	0HBX3ZX
0FPD4YZ	0FV84DZ	0FWGX2Z	0G9K3ZX	0GPSX2Z	0H94X0Z	0H9RXZZ	0HB1XZZ	0HBX7ZX
0FPD70Z	0FV84ZZ	0FWGX3Z	0G9K3ZZ	0GPSX3Z	0H94XZX	0H9T00Z	0HB2XZX	0HBX8ZX
0FPD72Z	0FV87DZ	0FWGXDZ	0G9K40Z	0GW0X0Z	0H94XZZ	0H9T30Z	0HB2XZZ	0HBXXZX
0FPD73Z	0FV87ZZ	0G20X0Z	0G9K4ZX	0GW1X0Z	0H95X0Z	0H9T3ZX	0HB3XZX	0HBY3ZX
0FPD7DZ	0FV88DZ	0G20XYZ	0G9K4ZZ	0GW5X0Z	0H95XZX	0H9T3ZZ	0HB3XZZ	0HBY7ZX
0FPD7YZ	0FV88ZZ	0G21X0Z	0G9L30Z	0GWKX0Z	0H95XZZ	0H9T70Z	0HB4XZX	0HBY8ZX
0FPD80Z	0FV93CZ	0G21XYZ	0G9L3ZZ	0GWRX0Z	0H96X0Z	0H9T7ZX	0HB4XZZ	0HC0XZZ
0FPD82Z	0FV93DZ	0G25X0Z	0G9L40Z	0GWS3YZ	0H96XZX	0H9T7ZZ	0HB5XZX	0HC1XZZ
0FPD83Z	0FV93ZZ	0G25XYZ	0G9L4ZZ	0GWS4YZ	0H96XZZ	0H9T80Z	0HB5XZZ	0HC2XZZ
0FPD8DZ	0FV94CZ	0G2KX0Z	0G9M30Z	0GWSX0Z	0H97X0Z	0H9T8ZX	0HB6XZX	0HC3XZZ
0FPD8YZ	0FV94DZ	0G2KXYZ	0G9M3ZZ	0GWSX2Z	0H97XZX	0H9T8ZZ	0HB6XZZ	0HC4XZZ
0FPDX0Z	0FV94ZZ	0G2RX0Z	0G9M40Z	0GWSX3Z	0H97XZZ	0H9U00Z	0HB7XZX	0HC5XZZ
0FPDX1Z	0FV97DZ	0G2RXYZ	0G9M4ZZ	0H0T3JZ	0H98X0Z	0H9U30Z	0HB7XZZ	0HC6XZZ
0FPDX2Z	0FV97ZZ	0G2SX0Z	0G9N30Z	0H0U3JZ	0H98XZX	0H9U3ZX	0HB8XZX	0HC7XZZ
0FPDX3Z	0FV98DZ	0G2SXYZ	0G9N3ZZ	0H0V3JZ	0H98XZZ	0H9U3ZZ	0HB8XZZ	0HC8XZZ
0FPDXDZ	0FV98ZZ	0G9030Z	0G9N40Z	0H2PX0Z	0H99XZX	0H9U70Z	0HB9XZX	0HC9XZZ
0FPG30Z	0FW03YZ	0G903ZZ	0G9N4ZZ	0H2PXYZ	0H9AX0Z	0H9U7ZX	0HBAXZX	0HCAXZZ
0FPG3YZ	0FW04YZ	0G9130Z	0G9P30Z	0H2TX0Z	0H9AXZX	0H9U7ZZ	0HBAXZZ	0HCBXZZ
0FPG4YZ	0FW0X0Z	0G913ZZ	0G9P3ZZ	0H2TXYZ	0H9AXZZ	0H9U80Z	0HBBXZX	0HCCXZZ
0FPGX0Z	0FW0X2Z	0G9230Z	0G9P40Z	0H2UX0Z	0H9BX0Z	0H9U8ZX	0HBBXZZ	0HCDXZZ
0FPGX2Z	0FW0X3Z	0G923ZX	0G9P4ZZ	0H2UXYZ	0H9BXZX	0H9U8ZZ	0HBCXZX	0HCEXZZ
0FPGX3Z	0FW43YZ	0G923ZZ	0G9Q30Z	0H52XZD	0H9BXZZ	0H9V00Z	0HBCXZZ	0HCFXZZ
0FTD4ZZ	0FW44YZ	0G924ZX	0G9Q3ZZ	0H52XZZ	0H9CX0Z	0H9V30Z	0HBDXZX	0HCGXZZ
0FTD8ZZ	0FW4X0Z	0G9330Z	0G9Q40Z	0H53XZD	0H9CXZX	0H9V3ZX	0HBDXZZ	0HCHXZZ
0FTF4ZZ	0FW4X2Z	0G933ZX	0G9Q4ZZ	0H53XZZ	0H9CXZZ	0H9V3ZZ	0HBEXZX	0HCJXZZ
0FTF8ZZ	0FW4X3Z	0G933ZZ	0G9R30Z	0H80XZZ	0H9DX0Z	0H9V70Z	0HBEXZZ	0HCKXZZ
0FV53CZ	0FW4XDZ	0G934ZX	0G9R3ZZ	0H81XZZ	0H9DXZX	0H9V7ZX	0HBFXZX	0HCLXZZ
0FV53DZ	0FWB3YZ	0G9430Z	0G9R40Z	0H82XZZ	0H9DXZZ	0H9V7ZZ	0HBFXZZ	0HCMXZZ
0FV53ZZ	0FWB4YZ	0G943ZX	0G9R4ZZ	0H83XZZ	0H9EX0Z	0H9V80Z	0HBGXZX	0HCNXZZ
0FV54CZ	0FWB7YZ	0G943ZZ	0GB23ZX	0H84XZZ	0H9EXZX	0H9V8ZX	0HBGXZZ	0HCQXZZ
0FV54DZ	0FWB80Z	0G944ZX	0GB24ZX	0H85XZZ	0H9EXZZ	0H9V8ZZ	0HBHXZX	0HCRXZZ
0FV54ZZ	0FWB82Z	0G9630Z	0GB33ZX	0H86XZZ	0H9FX0Z	0H9W00Z	0HBHXZZ	0HCT3ZZ
0FV57DZ	0FWB8DZ	0G963ZZ	0GB34ZX	0H87XZZ	0H9FXZX	0H9W30Z	0HBJXZX	0HCT7ZZ
0FV57ZZ	0FWB8YZ	0G9730Z	0GB43ZX	0H88XZZ	0H9FXZZ	0H9W3ZX	0HBJXZZ	0HCT8ZZ
0FV58DZ	0FWBX0Z	0G973ZZ	0GB44ZX	0H89XZZ	0H9GX0Z	0H9W3ZZ	0HBKXZX	0HCU3ZZ
0FV58ZZ	0FWBX2Z	0G9830Z	0GBG3ZX	0H8AXZZ	0H9GXZX	0H9W70Z	0HBKXZZ	0HCU7ZZ
0FV63CZ	0FWBX3Z	0G983ZZ	0GBG4ZX	0H8BXZZ	0H9GXZZ	0H9W7ZX	0HBLXZX	0HCU8ZZ
0FV63DZ	0FWBX7Z	0G9930Z	0GBH3ZX	0H8CXZZ	0H9HX0Z	0H9W7ZZ	0HBLXZZ	0HCV3ZZ
0FV63ZZ	0FWBXCZ	0G993ZZ	0GBH4ZX	0H8DXZZ	0H9HXZX	0H9W80Z	0HBMXZX	0HCV7ZZ
0FV64CZ	0FWBXDZ	0G9B30Z	0GBJ3ZX	0H8EXZZ	0H9HXZZ	0H9W8ZX	0HBMXZZ	0HCV8ZZ
0FV64DZ	0FWBXJZ	0G9B3ZZ	0GBJ4ZX	0H8FXZZ	0H9JX0Z	0H9W8ZZ	0HBNXZX	0HCW3ZZ
0FV64ZZ	0FWBXKZ	0G9C30Z	0GHS01Z	0H8GXZZ	0H9JXZX	0H9WX0Z	0HBNXZZ	0HCW7ZZ
0FV67DZ	0FWD3YZ	0G9C3ZZ	0GHS31Z	0H8HXZZ	0H9JXZZ	0H9WXZX	0HBQXZX	0HCW8ZZ
0FV67ZZ	0FWD4YZ	0G9D30Z	0GHS3YZ	0H8JXZZ	0H9KX0Z	0H9WXZZ	0HBQXZZ	0HCWXZZ
0FV68DZ	0FWD7YZ	0G9D3ZZ	0GHS41Z	0H8KXZZ	0H9KXZX	0H9X00Z	0HBRXZX	0HCX3ZZ
0FV68ZZ	0FWD80Z	0G9F30Z	0GHS4YZ	0H8LXZZ	0H9KXZZ	0H9X30Z	0HBRXZZ	0HCX7ZZ
0FV73CZ	0FWD82Z	0G9F3ZZ	0GJ03ZZ	0H8MXZZ	0H9LX0Z	0H9X3ZX	0HBT3ZX	0HCX8ZZ
0FV73DZ	0FWD8DZ	0G9G30Z	0GJ13ZZ	0H8NXZZ	0H9LXZX	0H9X3ZZ	0HBT7ZX	0HCXXZZ
0FV73ZZ	0FWD8YZ	0G9G3ZX	0GJ53ZZ	0H90X0Z	0H9LXZZ	0H9X70Z	0HBT8ZX	0HD0XZZ

0HD1XZZ	0HPT00Z	0HQFXZZ	0HWU3YZ	0J993ZZ	0J9P3ZZ	0JC43ZZ	0JH83YZ	0JPS00Z
0HD2XZZ	0HPT01Z	0HQGXZZ	0HWU70Z	0J9B00Z	0J9Q00Z	0JC50ZZ	0JHD0HZ	0JPS01Z
0HD3XZZ	0HPT07Z	0HQHXZZ	0HWU77Z	0J9B0ZZ	0J9Q0ZX	0JC53ZZ	0JHD3HZ	0JPS03Z
0HD4XZZ	0HPT0KZ	0HQJXZZ	0HWU7JZ	0J9B30Z	0J9Q30Z	0JC60ZZ	0JHF0HZ	0JPS07Z
0HD5XZZ	0HPT30Z	0HQKXZZ	0HWU7KZ	0J9B3ZX	0J9Q3ZX	0JC63ZZ	0JHF3HZ	0JPS0JZ
0HD6XZZ	0HPT31Z	0HQLXZZ	0HWU7NZ	0J9B3ZZ	0J9Q3ZZ	0JC70ZZ	0JHG0HZ	0JPS0KZ
0HD7XZZ	0HPT37Z	0HQMXZZ	0HWU7YZ	0J9C00Z	0J9R00Z	0JC73ZZ	0JHG3HZ	0JPS0NZ
0HD8XZZ	0HPT3KZ	0HQNXZZ	0HWU80Z	0J9C0ZX	0J9R0ZX	0JC80ZZ	0JHH0HZ	0JPS0YZ
0HD9XZZ	0HPT3YZ	0HRSX7Z	0HWU87Z	0J9C30Z	0J9R30Z	0JC83ZZ	0JHH3HZ	0JPS30Z
0HDAXZZ	0HPT70Z	0HSSXZZ	0HWU8JZ	0J9C3ZX	0J9R3ZX	0JC90ZZ	0JHL0HZ	0JPS31Z
0HDBXZZ	0HPT71Z	0HTQXZZ	0HWU8KZ	0J9C3ZZ	0J9R3ZZ	0JC93ZZ	0JHL3HZ	0JPS33Z
0HDCXZZ	0HPT77Z	0HTRXZZ	0HWU8NZ	0J9D00Z	0JB00ZX	0JCB0ZZ	0JHM0HZ	0JPS37Z
0HDDXZZ	0HPT7JZ	0HUT3JZ	0HWU8YZ	0J9D0ZX	0JB03ZX	0JCB3ZZ	0JHM3HZ	0JPS3JZ
0HDEXZZ	0HPT7KZ	0HUU3JZ	0J2SX0Z	0J9D30Z	0JB10ZX	0JCC0ZZ	0JHN0HZ	0JPS3KZ
0HDFXZZ	0HPT7NZ	0HUV3JZ	0J2SXYZ	0J9D3ZX	0JB13ZX	0JCC3ZZ	0JHS03Z	0JPS3NZ
0HDGXZZ	0HPT7YZ	0HWPX0Z	0J2TX0Z	0J9D3ZZ	0JB40ZX	0JCD0ZZ	0JHS33Z	0JPS3YZ
0HDHXZZ	0HPT80Z	0HWPX7Z	0J2TXYZ	0J9F00Z	0JB43ZX	0JCD3ZZ	0JHS3YZ	0JPSX0Z
0HDJXZZ	0HPT81Z	0HWPXJZ	0J2VX0Z	0J9F0ZX	0JB50ZX	0JCF0ZZ	0JHT03Z	0JPSX1Z
0HDKXZZ	0HPT87Z	0HWPXKZ	0J2VXYZ	0J9F30Z	0JB53ZX	0JCF3ZZ	0JHT33Z	0JPSX3Z
0HDLXZZ	0HPT8JZ	0HWPXYZ	0J2WX0Z	0J9F3ZX	0JB60ZX	0JCG0ZZ	0JHT3YZ	0JPT00Z
0HDMXZZ	0HPT8KZ	0HWQX0Z	0J2WXYZ	0J9F3ZZ	0JB63ZX	0JCG3ZZ	0JHV03Z	0JPT01Z
0HDNXZZ	0HPT8NZ	0HWQX7Z	0J9000Z	0J9G00Z	0JB70ZX	0JCH0ZZ	0JHV33Z	0JPT02Z
0HDQXZZ	0HPT8YZ	0HWQXJZ	0J900ZX	0J9G0ZX	0JB73ZX	0JCH3ZZ	0JHV3YZ	0JPT03Z
0HDRXZZ	0HPU00Z	0HWQXKZ	0J9030Z	0J9G30Z	0JB80ZX	0JCJ0ZZ	0JHW03Z	0JPT07Z
0HDSXZZ	0HPU01Z	0HWRX0Z	0J903ZX	0J9G3ZX	0JB83ZX	0JCJ3ZZ	0JHW33Z	0JPT0HZ
0HHPXYZ	0HPU07Z	0HWRX7Z	0J903ZZ	0J9G3ZZ	0JB90ZX	0JCK0ZZ	0JHW3YZ	0JPT0JZ
0HHT3YZ	0HPU0KZ	0HWRXJZ	0J9100Z	0J9H00Z	0JB93ZX	0JCK3ZZ	0JJS0ZZ	0JPT0KZ
0HHT7YZ	0HPU30Z	0HWRXKZ	0J910ZX	0J9H0ZX	0JBB0ZX	0JCL0ZZ	0JJS3ZZ	0JPT0MZ
0HHT8YZ	0HPU31Z	0HWSX7Z	0J9130Z	0J9H30Z	0JBB3ZX	0JCL3ZZ	0JJSXZZ	0JPT0NZ
0HHU3YZ	0HPU37Z	0HWSXJZ	0J913ZX	0J9H3ZX	0JBC0ZX	0JCM0ZZ	0JJT0ZZ	0JPT0VZ
0HHU7YZ	0HPU3KZ	0HWSXKZ	0J913ZZ	0J9H3ZZ	0JBC3ZX	0JCM3ZZ	0JJT3ZZ	0JPT0WZ
0HHU8YZ	0HPU3YZ	0HWT00Z	0J9400Z	0J9J00Z	0JBD0ZX	0JCN0ZZ	0JJTXZZ	0JPT0XZ
0HJPXZZ	0HPU70Z	0HWT07Z	0J940ZX	0J9J0ZX	0JBD3ZX	0JCN3ZZ	0JJV0ZZ	0JPT0YZ
0HJQXZZ	0HPU71Z	0HWT0KZ	0J9430Z	0J9J30Z	0JBF0ZX	0JCP0ZZ	0JJV3ZZ	0JPT30Z
0HJRXZZ	0HPU77Z	0HWT0NZ	0J943ZX	0J9J3ZX	0JBF3ZX	0JCP3ZZ	0JJVXZZ	0JPT31Z
0HJT0ZZ	0HPU7JZ	0HWT30Z	0J943ZZ	0J9J3ZZ	0JBG0ZX	0JCQ0ZZ	0JJW0ZZ	0JPT32Z
0HJT3ZZ	0HPU7KZ	0HWT37Z	0J9500Z	0J9K00Z	0JBG3ZX	0JCQ3ZZ	0JJW3ZZ	0JPT33Z
0HJT7ZZ	0HPU7NZ	0HWT3KZ	0J950ZX	0J9K0ZX	0JBH0ZX	0JCR0ZZ	0JJWXZZ	0JPT37Z
0HJT8ZZ	0HPU7YZ	0HWT3NZ	0J9530Z	0J9K30Z	0JBH3ZX	0JCR3ZZ	0JN0XZZ	0JPT3HZ
0HJU0ZZ	0HPU80Z	0HWT3YZ	0J953ZX	0J9K3ZX	0JBJ0ZX	0JD03ZZ	0JN1XZZ	0JPT3JZ
0HJU3ZZ	0HPU81Z	0HWT70Z	0J953ZZ	0J9K3ZZ	0JBJ3ZX	0JD13ZZ	0JN4XZZ	0JPT3KZ
0HJU7ZZ	0HPU87Z	0HWT77Z	0J9600Z	0J9L00Z	0JBK0ZX	0JD43ZZ	0JN5XZZ	0JPT3MZ
0HJU8ZZ	0HPU8JZ	0HWT7JZ	0J960ZX	0J9L0ZX	0JBK3ZX	0JD53ZZ	0JN6XZZ	0JPT3NZ
0HM0XZZ	0HPU8KZ	0HWT7KZ	0J9630Z	0J9L30Z	0JBL0ZX	0JDB3ZZ	0JN7XZZ	0JPT3VZ
0HPPX0Z	0HPU8NZ	0HWT7NZ	0J963ZX	0J9L3ZX	0JBL3ZX	0JDC3ZZ	0JN8XZZ	0JPT3WZ
0HPPX7Z	0HPU8YZ	0HWT7YZ	0J963ZZ	0J9L3ZZ	0JBM0ZX	0JDD3ZZ	0JN9XZZ	0JPT3XZ
0HPPXJZ	0HQ0XZZ	0HWT80Z	0J9700Z	0J9M00Z	0JBM3ZX	0JDF3ZZ	0JNBXZZ	0JPT3YZ
0HPPXKZ	0HQ1XZZ	0HWT87Z	0J970ZX	0J9M0ZX	0JBN0ZX	0JDG3ZZ	0JNCXZZ	0JPTX0Z
0HPPXYZ	0HQ2XZZ	0HWT8JZ	0J9730Z	0J9M30Z	0JBN3ZX	0JDH3ZZ	0JNDXZZ	0JPTX1Z
0HPQX0Z	0HQ3XZZ	0HWT8KZ	0J973ZX	0J9M3ZX	0JBP0ZX	0JDJ3ZZ	0JNFXZZ	0JPTX2Z
0HPQX7Z	0HQ4XZZ	0HWT8NZ	0J973ZZ	0J9M3ZZ	0JBP3ZX	0JDK3ZZ	0JNGXZZ	0JPTX3Z
0HPQXJZ	0HQ5XZZ	0HWT8YZ	0J9800Z	0J9N00Z	0JBQ0ZX	0JDN3ZZ	0JNHXZZ	0JPTXHZ
0HPQXKZ	0HQ6XZZ	0HWU00Z	0J980ZX	0J9N0ZX	0JBQ3ZX	0JDP3ZZ	0JNJXZZ	0JPTXVZ
0HPRX0Z	0HQ7XZZ	0HWU07Z	0J9830Z	0J9N30Z	0JBR0ZX	0JDQ3ZZ	0JNKXZZ	0JPTXXZ
0HPRX7Z	0HQ8XZZ	0HWU0KZ	0J983ZX	0J9N3ZX	0JBR3ZX	0JDR3ZZ	0JNLXZZ	0JPV00Z
0HPRXJZ	0HQAXZZ	0HWU0NZ	0J983ZZ	0J9N3ZZ	0JC00ZZ	0JH60YZ	0JNMXZZ	0JPV01Z
0HPRXKZ	0HQBXZZ	0HWU30Z	0J9900Z	0J9P00Z	0JC03ZZ	0JH63YZ	0JNNXZZ	0JPV03Z
0HPSX7Z	0HQCXZZ	0HWU37Z	0J990ZX	0J9P0ZX	0JC10ZZ	0JH70YZ	0JNPXZZ	0JPV07Z
0HPSXJZ	0HQDXZZ	0HWU3KZ	0J9930Z	0J9P30Z	0JC13ZZ	0JH73YZ	0JNQXZZ	0JPV0HZ
0HPSXKZ	0HQEXZZ	0HWU3NZ	0J993ZX	0J9P3ZX	0JC40ZZ	0JH80YZ	0JNRXZZ	0JPV0JZ

0JPV0KZ	0JQ83ZZ	0K9030Z	0KHY3YZ	0L9030Z	0LHY3YZ	0M903ZX	0M9B40Z	0M9P0ZX
0JPV0NZ	0JQ93ZZ	0K903ZZ	0KHY4YZ	0L903ZZ	0LHY4YZ	0M903ZZ	0M9B4ZZ	0M9P30Z
0JPV0VZ	0JQB3ZZ	0K9130Z	0KJX3ZZ	0L9130Z	0LJX3ZZ	0M904ZX	0M9C0ZX	0M9P3ZX
0JPV0WZ	0JQC3ZZ	0K913ZZ	0KJXXZZ	0L913ZZ	0LJXXZZ	0M904ZZ	0M9C30Z	0M9P3ZX
0JPV0XZ	0JQD3ZZ	0K9230Z	0KJY3ZZ	0L9230Z	0LJY3ZZ	0M910ZX	0M9C3ZX	0M9P4ZX
0JPV0YZ	0JQF3ZZ	0K923ZZ	0KJYXZZ	0L923ZZ	0LJYXZZ	0M9130Z	0M9C3ZZ	0M9P4ZZ
0JPV30Z	0JQG3ZZ	0K9330Z	0KN0XZZ	0L9330Z	0LN0XZZ	0M913ZX	0M9C40Z	0M9Q0ZX
0JPV31Z	0JQH3ZZ	0K933ZZ	0KN1XZZ	0L933ZZ	0LN1XZZ	0M913ZZ	0M9C4ZX	0M9Q30Z
0JPV33Z	0JQJ3ZZ	0K9430Z	0KN2XZZ	0L9430Z	0LN2XZZ	0M9140Z	0M9C4ZZ	0M9Q3ZX
0JPV37Z	0JQK3ZZ	0K943ZZ	0KN3XZZ	0L943ZZ	0LN3XZZ	0M914ZX	0M9D0ZX	0M9Q3ZZ
0JPV3HZ	0JQL3ZZ	0K9530Z	0KN4XZZ	0L9530Z	0LN4XZZ	0M920ZX	0M9D30Z	0M9Q4ZX
0JPV3JZ	0JQM3ZZ	0K953ZZ	0KN5XZZ	0L953ZZ	0LN5XZZ	0M9230Z	0M9D3ZX	0M9Q4ZZ
0JPV3KZ	0JQN3ZZ	0K9630Z	0KN6XZZ	0L9630Z	0LN6XZZ	0M923ZX	0M9D3ZZ	0M9R0ZX
0JPV3NZ	0JQP3ZZ	0K963ZZ	0KN7XZZ	0L963ZZ	0LN7XZZ	0M923ZZ	0M9D40Z	0M9R30Z
0JPV3VZ	0JQQ3ZZ	0K9730Z	0KN8XZZ	0L9730Z	0LN8XZZ	0M9240Z	0M9D4ZX	0M9R3ZZ
0JPV3WZ	0JQR3ZZ	0K973ZZ	0KN9XZZ	0L973ZZ	0LN9XZZ	0M924ZX	0M9D4ZZ	0M9R4ZX
0JPV3XZ	0JWSX0Z	0K9830Z	0KNBXZZ	0L974ZZ	0LNBXZZ	0M930ZX	0M9F0ZX	0M9R4ZZ
0JPV3YZ	0JWSX3Z	0K983ZZ	0KNCXZZ	0L9830Z	0LNCXZZ	0M9330Z	0M9F30Z	0M9S0ZX
0JPVX0Z	0JWSX7Z	0K9930Z	0KNDXZZ	0L983ZZ	0LNDXZZ	0M933ZX	0M9F3ZX	0M9S30Z
0JPVX1Z	0JWSXJZ	0K993ZZ	0KNFXZZ	0L984ZZ	0LNFXZZ	0M933ZZ	0M9F3ZZ	0M9S3ZX
0JPVX3Z	0JWSXKZ	0K9B30Z	0KNGXZZ	0L9930Z	0LNGXZZ	0M9340Z	0M9F40Z	0M9S3ZZ
0JPVXHZ	0JWSXNZ	0K9B3ZZ	0KNHXZZ	0L993ZZ	0LNHXZZ	0M934ZX	0M9F4ZX	0M9S4ZX
0JPVXVZ	0JWT3YZ	0K9C30Z	0KNJXZZ	0L9B30Z	0LNJXZZ	0M940ZX	0M9F4ZZ	0M9S4ZZ
0JPVXXZ	0JWTX0Z	0K9C3Z	0KNKXZZ	0L9B3ZZ	0LNKXZZ	0M9430Z	0M9G0ZX	0M9T0ZX
0JPW00Z	0JWTX2Z	0K9C4ZZ	0KNLXZZ	0L9C30Z	0LNLXZZ	0M943ZX	0M9G30Z	0M9T30Z
0JPW01Z	0JWTX3Z	0K9D30Z	0KNMXZZ	0L9C3ZZ	0LNMXZZ	0M943ZZ	0M9G3ZX	0M9T3ZX
0JPW03Z	0JWTX7Z	0K9D3ZZ	0KNNXZZ	0L9D30Z	0LNNXZZ	0M9440Z	0M9G3ZZ	0M9T3ZZ
0JPW07Z	0JWTXFZ	0K9D4ZZ	0KNPXZZ	0L9D3ZZ	0LNPXZZ	0M944ZX	0M9G40Z	0M9T4ZX
0JPW0HZ	0JWTXHZ	0K9F30Z	0KNQXZZ	0L9F30Z	0LNQXZZ	0M950ZX	0M9G4ZX	0M9T4ZZ
0JPW0JZ	0JWTXJZ	0K9F3ZZ	0KNRXZZ	0L9F3ZZ	0LNRXZZ	0M9530Z	0M9G4ZZ	0M9V30Z
0JPW0KZ	0JWTXKZ	0K9G30Z	0KNSXZZ	0L9G30Z	0LNSXZZ	0M953ZX	0M9H30Z	0M9V3ZZ
0JPW0NZ	0JWTXNZ	0K9G3ZZ	0KNTXZZ	0L9G3ZZ	0LNTXZZ	0M953ZZ	0M9H3ZZ	0M9V40Z
0JPW0VZ	0JWTXPZ	0K9H30Z	0KNVXZZ	0L9H30Z	0LNVXZZ	0M954ZX	0M9H40Z	0M9V4ZZ
0JPW0WZ	0JWTXVZ	0K9H3ZZ	0KNWXZZ	0L9H3ZZ	0LNWXZZ	0M954ZZ	0M9H4ZZ	0M9W30Z
0JPW0XZ	0JWTXWZ	0K9J30Z	0KPX3YZ	0L9J30Z	0LPX30Z	0M960ZX	0M9J30Z	0M9W30Z
0JPW0YZ	0JWTXXZ	0K9J3ZZ	0KPX4YZ	0L9J3ZZ	0LPX3YZ	0M9630Z	0M9J3ZZ	0M9W3ZZ
0JPW30Z	0JWVX0Z	0K9K30Z	0KPXX0Z	0L9K30Z	0LPX4YZ	0M963ZX	0M9J40Z	0M9W40Z
0JPW31Z	0JWVX3Z	0K9K3ZZ	0KPXXMZ	0L9K3ZZ	0LPXX0Z	0M963ZZ	0M9J4ZZ	0M9W4ZZ
0JPW33Z	0JWVX7Z	0K9L30Z	0KPY3YZ	0L9L30Z	0LPY30Z	0M964ZX	0M9K30Z	0MB00ZX
0JPW37Z	0JWVXHZ	0K9L3ZZ	0KPY4YZ	0L9L3ZZ	0LPY3YZ	0M964ZZ	0M9K3ZZ	0MB03ZX
0JPW3HZ	0JWVXJZ	0K9M30Z	0KPYX0Z	0L9M30Z	0LPY4YZ	0M970ZX	0M9K40Z	0MB04ZX
0JPW3JZ	0JWVXKZ	0K9M3ZZ	0KPYXMZ	0L9M3ZZ	0LPYX0Z	0M9730Z	0M9K4ZZ	0MB10ZX
0JPW3KZ	0JWVXNZ	0K9N30Z	0KWX3YZ	0L9N30Z	0LWX3YZ	0M973ZX	0M9L0ZX	0MB13ZX
0JPW3NZ	0JWVXVZ	0K9N3ZZ	0KWX4YZ	0L9N3ZZ	0LWX4YZ	0M973ZZ	0M9L30Z	0MB14ZX
0JPW3VZ	0JWVXWZ	0K9P30Z	0KWXX0Z	0L9P30Z	0LWXX0Z	0M9740Z	0M9L3ZX	0MB20ZX
0JPW3WZ	0JWVXXZ	0K9P3ZZ	0KWXX7Z	0L9P3ZZ	0LWXX7Z	0M974ZX	0M9L3ZZ	0MB23ZX
0JPW3XZ	0JWWX0Z	0K9Q30Z	0KWXXJZ	0L9Q30Z	0LWXXJZ	0M974ZZ	0M9L40Z	0MB24ZX
0JPW3YZ	0JWWX3Z	0K9Q3ZZ	0KWXXKZ	0L9Q3ZZ	0LWXXKZ	0M980ZX	0M9L4ZX	0MB30ZX
0JPWX0Z	0JWWX7Z	0K9R30Z	0KWXXMZ	0L9R30Z	0LWY3YZ	0M9830Z	0M9M0ZX	0MB33ZX
0JPWX1Z	0JWWXHZ	0K9R3ZZ	0KWY3YZ	0L9R3ZZ	0LWY4YZ	0M983ZX	0M9M30Z	0MB34ZX
0JPWX3Z	0JWWXJZ	0K9S30Z	0KWY4YZ	0L9S30Z	0LWYX0Z	0M983ZZ	0M9M3ZX	0MB40ZX
0JPWXHZ	0JWWXKZ	0K9S3ZZ	0KWYX0Z	0L9S3ZZ	0LWYX7Z	0M9840Z	0M9M3ZZ	0MB43ZX
0JPWXVZ	0JWWXNZ	0K9T30Z	0KWYX7Z	0L9T30Z	0LWYXJZ	0M984ZX	0M9M40Z	0MB44ZX
0JPWXXZ	0JWWXVZ	0K9T3ZZ	0KWYXJZ	0L9T3ZZ	0LWYXKZ	0M984ZZ	0M9M4ZX	0MB50ZX
0JQ03ZZ	0JWWXWZ	0K9V30Z	0KWYXKZ	0L9V30Z	0M2XX0Z	0M9930Z	0M9N0ZX	0MB53ZX
0JQ13ZZ	0JWWXXZ	0K9V3ZZ	0KWYXMZ	0L9V3ZZ	0M2XXYZ	0M993ZZ	0M9N30Z	0MB54ZX
0JQ43ZZ	0K2XX0Z	0K9W30Z	0L2XX0Z	0L9W30Z	0M2YX0Z	0M9940Z	0M9N3ZX	0MB60ZX
0JQ53ZZ	0K2XXYZ	0K9W3ZZ	0L2XXYZ	0L9W3ZZ	0M2YXYZ	0M994ZZ	0M9N3ZZ	0MB63ZX
0JQ63ZZ	0K2YX0Z	0KHX3YZ	0L2YX0Z	0LHX3YZ	0M900ZX	0M9B30Z	0M9N4ZX	0MB64ZX
0JQ73ZZ	0K2YXYZ	0KHX4YZ	0L2YXYZ	0LHX4YZ	0M9030Z	0M9B3ZZ	0M9N4ZZ	0MB70ZX

0MB73ZX	0MN7XZZ	0N9630Z	0NBR4ZX	0NPBX4Z	0NSJ3ZZ	0NW0X0Z	0P9B30Z	0PP0X4Z
0MB74ZX	0MN8XZZ	0N963ZZ	0NBT0ZX	0NPBXMZ	0NSJ44Z	0NW0X4Z	0P9B3ZZ	0PP1X4Z
0MB80ZX	0MN9XZZ	0N9730Z	0NBT3ZX	0NPWX0Z	0NSJ4ZZ	0NW0X5Z	0P9C30Z	0PP2X4Z
0MB83ZX	0MNBXZZ	0N973ZZ	0NBT4ZX	0NPWXMZ	0NSJXZZ	0NW0X7Z	0P9C3ZZ	0PP3X4Z
0MB84ZX	0MNCXZZ	0N9B00Z	0NBV0ZX	0NQ0XZZ	0NSK34Z	0NW0XJZ	0P9D30Z	0PP4X4Z
0MB94ZX	0MNDXZZ	0N9B0ZX	0NBV3ZX	0NQ1XZZ	0NSK3ZZ	0NW0XKZ	0P9D3ZZ	0PP5X4Z
0MBB0ZX	0MNFXZZ	0N9B0ZZ	0NBV4ZX	0NQ3XZZ	0NSK44Z	0NW0XMZ	0P9F30Z	0PP6X4Z
0MBB3ZX	0MNGXZZ	0N9B30Z	0NCB0ZZ	0NQ4XZZ	0NSK4ZZ	0NW0XSZ	0P9F3ZZ	0PP7X4Z
0MBB4ZX	0MNHXZZ	0N9B3ZX	0NCB3ZZ	0NQ5XZZ	0NSKXZZ	0NWB00Z	0P9G30Z	0PP8X4Z
0MBC0ZX	0MNJXZZ	0N9B3ZZ	0NCB4ZZ	0NQ6XZZ	0NSL34Z	0NWB04Z	0P9G3ZZ	0PP9X4Z
0MBC3ZX	0MNKXZZ	0N9B40Z	0NCR0ZZ	0NQ7XZZ	0NSL3ZZ	0NWB07Z	0P9H30Z	0PPBX4Z
0MBC4ZX	0MNLXZZ	0N9B4ZX	0NCR3ZZ	0NQBXZZ	0NSL44Z	0NWB0JZ	0P9H3ZZ	0PPCX4Z
0MBD0ZX	0MNMXZZ	0N9B4ZZ	0NCR4ZZ	0NQCXZZ	0NSL4ZZ	0NWB0KZ	0P9J30Z	0PPCX5Z
0MBD3ZX	0MNNXZZ	0N9C30Z	0NCT0ZZ	0NQFXZZ	0NSLXZZ	0NWB0MZ	0P9J3ZZ	0PPDX4Z
0MBD4ZX	0MNPXZZ	0N9C3ZZ	0NCT3ZZ	0NQGXZZ	0NSM34Z	0NWB30Z	0P9K30Z	0PPDX5Z
0MBF0ZX	0MNQXZZ	0N9F30Z	0NCT4ZZ	0NQHXZZ	0NSM3ZZ	0NWB34Z	0P9K3ZZ	0PPFX4Z
0MBF3ZX	0MNRXZZ	0N9F3ZZ	0NCV0ZZ	0NQJXZZ	0NSM44Z	0NWB37Z	0P9L30Z	0PPFX5Z
0MBF4ZX	0MNSXZZ	0N9G30Z	0NCV3ZZ	0NQKXZZ	0NSM4ZZ	0NWB3JZ	0P9L3ZZ	0PPGX4Z
0MBG0ZX	0MNTXZZ	0N9G3ZZ	0NCV4ZZ	0NQLXZZ	0NSMXZZ	0NWB3KZ	0P9M30Z	0PPGX5Z
0MBG3ZX	0MNVXZZ	0N9H30Z	0NH005Z	0NQMXZZ	0NSN34Z	0NWB3MZ	0P9M3ZZ	0PPHX4Z
0MBG4ZX	0MNWXZZ	0N9H3ZZ	0NH035Z	0NQNXZZ	0NSN3ZZ	0NWB40Z	0P9N30Z	0PPHX5Z
0MBL0ZX	0MPX30Z	0N9J30Z	0NH045Z	0NQPXZZ	0NSN44Z	0NWB44Z	0P9N3ZZ	0PPJX4Z
0MBL3ZX	0MPX3YZ	0N9J3ZZ	0NHB04Z	0NQQXZZ	0NSN4ZZ	0NWB47Z	0P9P30Z	0PPJX5Z
0MBL4ZX	0MPX4YZ	0N9K30Z	0NHB0MZ	0NQRXZZ	0NSNXZZ	0NWB4JZ	0P9P3ZZ	0PPKX4Z
0MBM0ZX	0MPXX0Z	0N9K3ZZ	0NHB34Z	0NQTXZZ	0NSP34Z	0NWB4KZ	0P9Q30Z	0PPKX5Z
0MBM3ZX	0MPY30Z	0N9L30Z	0NHB3MZ	0NQVXZZ	0NSP3ZZ	0NWB4MZ	0P9Q3ZZ	0PPLX4Z
0MBM4ZX	0MPY3YZ	0N9L3ZZ	0NHB44Z	0NQXXZZ	0NSP44Z	0NWBX0Z	0P9R30Z	0PPLX5Z
0MBN0ZX	0MPY4YZ	0N9M30Z	0NHB4MZ	0NS0XZZ	0NSP4Z	0NWBX4Z	0P9R3ZZ	0PPMX4Z
0MBN3ZX	0MPYX0Z	0N9M3ZZ	0NJ03ZZ	0NS1XZZ	0NSPXZZ	0NWBX7Z	0P9S30Z	0PPMX5Z
0MBN4ZX	0MWX3YZ	0N9N30Z	0NJ0XZZ	0NS3XZZ	0NSQ34Z	0NWBXJZ	0P9S3ZZ	0PPNX4Z
0MBP0ZX	0MWX4YZ	0N9N3ZZ	0NJB3ZZ	0NS4XZZ	0NSQ3ZZ	0NWBXKZ	0P9T30Z	0PPNX5Z
0MBP3ZX	0MWXX0Z	0N9P30Z	0NJBXZZ	0NS5XZZ	0NSQ44Z	0NWBXMZ	0P9T3ZZ	0PPPX4Z
0MBP4ZX	0MWXX7Z	0N9P3ZZ	0NJW3ZZ	0NS6XZZ	0NSQ4ZZ	0NWWX0Z	0P9V30Z	0PPPX5Z
0MBQ0ZX	0MWXXJZ	0N9Q30Z	0NJWXZZ	0NS7XZZ	0NSQXZZ	0NWWX4Z	0P9V3ZZ	0PPQX4Z
0MBQ3ZX	0MWXXKZ	0N9Q3ZZ	0NNB0ZZ	0NSB34Z	0NSR34Z	0NWWX7Z	0PHC08Z	0PPQX5Z
0MBQ4ZX	0MWY3YZ	0N9R00Z	0NNB3ZZ	0NSB3ZZ	0NSR35Z	0NWWXJZ	0PHC38Z	0PPRX4Z
0MBR0ZX	0MWY4YZ	0N9R0ZZ	0NNB4ZZ	0NSB44Z	0NSR3ZZ	0NWWXKZ	0PHC48Z	0PPRX5Z
0MBR3ZX	0MWYX0Z	0N9R30Z	0NP035Z	0NSB4ZZ	0NSR44Z	0NWWXMZ	0PHD08Z	0PPSX4Z
0MBR4ZX	0MWYX7Z	0N9R3ZZ	0NP045Z	0NSBXZZ	0NSR45Z	0P2YX0Z	0PHD38Z	0PPSX5Z
0MBS0ZX	0MWYXJZ	0N9R40Z	0NP0X0Z	0NSC34Z	0NSR4ZZ	0P2YXYZ	0PHD48Z	0PPTX4Z
0MBS3ZX	0MWYXKZ	0N9R4ZZ	0NP0X5Z	0NSC3ZZ	0NSRXZZ	0P9030Z	0PHF08Z	0PPTX5Z
0MBS4ZX	0N20X0Z	0N9T00Z	0NPB00Z	0NSC44Z	0NST34Z	0P903ZZ	0PHF38Z	0PPVX4Z
0MBT0ZX	0N20XYZ	0N9T0ZZ	0NPB04Z	0NSC4ZZ	0NST35Z	0P9130Z	0PHF48Z	0PPVX5Z
0MBT3ZX	0N2BX0Z	0N9T30Z	0NPB07Z	0NSCXZZ	0NST3ZZ	0P913ZZ	0PHG08Z	0PPY30Z
0MBT4ZX	0N2BXYZ	0N9T3ZZ	0NPB0JZ	0NST44Z	0NST44Z	0P9230Z	0PHG38Z	0PPYX0Z
0MHX3YZ	0N2WX0Z	0N9T40Z	0NPB0KZ	0NSF34Z	0NST45Z	0P923ZZ	0PHG48Z	0PPYXMZ
0MHX4YZ	0N2WXYZ	0N9T4ZZ	0NPB0MZ	0NSF3ZZ	0NST4ZZ	0P9330Z	0PHH08Z	0PQ0XZZ
0MHY3YZ	0N8B0ZZ	0N9V00Z	0NPB30Z	0NSF44Z	0NSTXZZ	0P933ZZ	0PHH38Z	0PQ1XZZ
0MHY4YZ	0N8B3ZZ	0N9V0ZZ	0NPB34Z	0NSF4ZZ	0NSV34Z	0P9430Z	0PHH48Z	0PQ2XZZ
0MJX3ZZ	0N8B4ZZ	0N9V30Z	0NPB37Z	0NSFXZZ	0NSV35Z	0P943ZZ	0PHJ08Z	0PQ3XZZ
0MJXXZZ	0N9030Z	0N9V3ZZ	0NPB3JZ	0NSG34Z	0NSV3ZZ	0P9530Z	0PHJ38Z	0PQ4XZZ
0MJY3ZZ	0N903ZZ	0N9V40Z	0NPB3KZ	0NSG3ZZ	0NSV44Z	0P953ZZ	0PHJ48Z	0PQ5XZZ
0MJYXZZ	0N9130Z	0N9V4ZZ	0NPB3MZ	0NSG44Z	0NSV45Z	0P9630Z	0PHK08Z	0PQ6XZZ
0MN0XZZ	0N913ZZ	0N9X30Z	0NPB40Z	0NSG4ZZ	0NSV4ZZ	0P963ZZ	0PHK38Z	0PQ7XZZ
0MN1XZZ	0N9330Z	0N9X3ZZ	0NPB44Z	0NSGXZZ	0NSVXZZ	0P9730Z	0PHK48Z	0PQ8XZZ
0MN2XZZ	0N933ZZ	0NBB0ZX	0NPB47Z	0NSH34Z	0NSX34Z	0P973ZZ	0PHL08Z	0PQ9XZZ
0MN3XZZ	0N9430Z	0NBB3ZX	0NPB4JZ	0NSH3ZZ	0NSX3ZZ	0P9830Z	0PHL38Z	0PQBXZZ
0MN4XZZ	0N943ZZ	0NBB4ZX	0NPB4KZ	0NSH44Z	0NSX44Z	0P983ZZ	0PHL48Z	0PQCXZZ
0MN5XZZ	0N9530Z	0NBR0ZX	0NPB4MZ	0NSH4ZZ	0NSX4ZZ	0P9930Z	0PJY3ZZ	0PQDXZZ
0MN6XZZ	0N953ZZ	0NBR3ZX	0NPBX0Z	0NSJ34Z	0NSXXZZ	0P993ZZ	0PJYXZZ	0PQFXZZ

0PQGXZZ	0PSK3ZZ	0PW7XJZ	0PWNX5Z	0Q9C30Z	0QP005Z	0QPS05Z	0QSB4ZZ	0QW2XKZ
0PQHXZZ	0PSK4ZZ	0PW7XKZ	0PWNX7Z	0Q9C3Z	0QP035Z	0QPS35Z	0QSBXZZ	0QW3X4Z
0PQJXZZ	0PSKXZZ	0PW8X4Z	0PWNXJZ	0Q9D30Z	0QP045Z	0QPS45Z	0QSC3ZZ	0QW3X5Z
0PQKXZZ	0PSL3ZZ	0PW8X7Z	0PWNXKZ	0Q9D3Z	0QP0X4Z	0QPSX4Z	0QSC4ZZ	0QW3X7Z
0PQLXZZ	0PSL4ZZ	0PW8XJZ	0PWPX4Z	0Q9F30Z	0QP0X5Z	0QPSX5Z	0QSCXZZ	0QW3XJZ
0PQMXZZ	0PSLXZZ	0PW8XKZ	0PWPX5Z	0Q9F3Z	0QP105Z	0QPY30Z	0QSD3ZZ	0QW3XKZ
0PQNXZZ	0PSM3ZZ	0PW9X4Z	0PWPX7Z	0Q9G30Z	0QP135Z	0QPYX0Z	0QSD4ZZ	0QW4X4Z
0PQPXZZ	0PSM4ZZ	0PW9X7Z	0PWPXJZ	0Q9G3Z	0QP145Z	0QPYXMZ	0QSDXZZ	0QW4X7Z
0PQQXZZ	0PSMXZZ	0PW9XJZ	0PWPXKZ	0Q9H30Z	0QP1X4Z	0QQ0XZZ	0QSF3ZZ	0QW4XJZ
0PQRXZZ	0PSN3ZZ	0PW9XKZ	0PWQX4Z	0Q9H3Z	0QP1X5Z	0QQ1XZZ	0QSF4ZZ	0QW4XKZ
0PQSXZZ	0PSN4ZZ	0PWBX4Z	0PWQX5Z	0Q9J30Z	0QP2X4Z	0QQ2XZZ	0QSFXZZ	0QW5X4Z
0PQTXZZ	0PSNXZZ	0PWBX7Z	0PWQX7Z	0Q9J3Z	0QP2X5Z	0QQ3XZZ	0QSG3ZZ	0QW5X7Z
0PQVXZZ	0PSP3ZZ	0PWBXJZ	0PWQXJZ	0Q9K30Z	0QP3X4Z	0QQ4XZZ	0QSG4ZZ	0QW5XJZ
0PS03ZZ	0PSP4ZZ	0PWBXKZ	0PWQXKZ	0Q9K3Z	0QP3X5Z	0QQ5XZZ	0QSGXZZ	0QW5XKZ
0PS04ZZ	0PSPXZZ	0PWCX4Z	0PWRX4Z	0Q9L30Z	0QP405Z	0QQ6XZZ	0QSH3ZZ	0QW6X4Z
0PS0XZZ	0PSQ3ZZ	0PWCX5Z	0PWRX5Z	0Q9L3Z	0QP435Z	0QQ7XZZ	0QSH4ZZ	0QW6X5Z
0PS13ZZ	0PSQ4ZZ	0PWCX7Z	0PWRX7Z	0Q9M30Z	0QP445Z	0QQ8XZZ	0QSHXZZ	0QW6X7Z
0PS14ZZ	0PSQXZZ	0PWCXJZ	0PWRXJZ	0Q9M3Z	0QP4X4Z	0QQ9XZZ	0QSJ3ZZ	0QW6XJZ
0PS1XZZ	0PSR3ZZ	0PWCXKZ	0PWRXKZ	0Q9N30Z	0QP4X5Z	0QQBXZZ	0QSJ4ZZ	0QW6XKZ
0PS23ZZ	0PSR4ZZ	0PWDX4Z	0PWSX4Z	0Q9N3Z	0QP505Z	0QQCXZZ	0QSJXZZ	0QW7X4Z
0PS24ZZ	0PSRXZZ	0PWDX5Z	0PWSX5Z	0Q9P30Z	0QP535Z	0QQDXZZ	0QSK3ZZ	0QW7X5Z
0PS2XZZ	0PSS3ZZ	0PWDX7Z	0PWSX7Z	0Q9P3Z	0QP545Z	0QQFXZZ	0QSK4ZZ	0QW7X7Z
0PS3XZZ	0PSS4ZZ	0PWDXJZ	0PWSXJZ	0Q9Q30Z	0QP5X4Z	0QQGXZZ	0QSKXZZ	0QW7XJZ
0PS4XZZ	0PSSXZZ	0PWDXKZ	0PWSXKZ	0Q9Q3Z	0QP5X5Z	0QQHXZZ	0QSL3ZZ	0QW7XKZ
0PS53ZZ	0PST3ZZ	0PWFX4Z	0PWTX4Z	0Q9R30Z	0QP6X4Z	0QQJXZZ	0QSL4ZZ	0QW8X4Z
0PS54ZZ	0PST4ZZ	0PWFX5Z	0PWTX5Z	0Q9R3Z	0QP6X5Z	0QQKXZZ	0QSLXZZ	0QW8X5Z
0PS5XZZ	0PSTXZZ	0PWFX7Z	0PWTX7Z	0Q9S30Z	0QP7X4Z	0QQLXZZ	0QSM3ZZ	0QW8X7Z
0PS63ZZ	0PSV3ZZ	0PWFXJZ	0PWTXJZ	0Q9S3Z	0QP7X5Z	0QQMXZZ	0QSM4ZZ	0QW8XJZ
0PS64ZZ	0PSV4ZZ	0PWFXKZ	0PWTXKZ	0QH608Z	0QP8X4Z	0QQNXZZ	0QSMXZZ	0QW8XKZ
0PS6XZZ	0PSVXZZ	0PWGX4Z	0PWVX4Z	0QH638Z	0QP8X5Z	0QQPXZZ	0QSN3Z2	0QW9X4Z
0PS73ZZ	0PW0X4Z	0PWGX5Z	0PWVX5Z	0QH648Z	0QP9X4Z	0QQQXZZ	0QSN3ZZ	0QW9X5Z
0PS74ZZ	0PW0X7Z	0PWGX7Z	0PWVX7Z	0QH708Z	0QP9X5Z	0QQRXZZ	0QSN4Z2	0QW9X7Z
0PS7XZZ	0PW0XJZ	0PWGXJZ	0PWVXJZ	0QH738Z	0QPBX4Z	0QQSXZZ	0QSN4ZZ	0QW9XJZ
0PS83ZZ	0PW0XKZ	0PWGXKZ	0PWVXKZ	0QH748Z	0QPBX5Z	0QS0XZZ	0QSNXZ2	0QW9XKZ
0PS84ZZ	0PW1X4Z	0PWHX4Z	0PWYX0Z	0QH808Z	0QPCX4Z	0QS1XZZ	0QSNXZZ	0QWBX4Z
0PS8XZZ	0PW1X7Z	0PWHX5Z	0PWYXMZ	0QH838Z	0QPCX5Z	0QS23ZZ	0QSP3Z2	0QWBX5Z
0PS93ZZ	0PW1XJZ	0PWHX7Z	0Q2YX0Z	0QH848Z	0QPDX4Z	0QS24ZZ	0QSP3ZZ	0QWBX7Z
0PS94ZZ	0PW1XKZ	0PWHXJZ	0Q2YXYZ	0QH908Z	0QPDX5Z	0QS2XZZ	0QSP4Z2	0QWBXJZ
0PS9XZZ	0PW2X4Z	0PWHXKZ	0Q9030Z	0QH938Z	0QPFX4Z	0QS33ZZ	0QSP4ZZ	0QWBXKZ
0PSB3ZZ	0PW2X7Z	0PWJX4Z	0Q903ZZ	0QH948Z	0QPFX5Z	0QS34ZZ	0QSPXZ2	0QWCX4Z
0PSB4ZZ	0PW2XJZ	0PWJX5Z	0Q9130Z	0QHB08Z	0QPGX4Z	0QS3XZZ	0QSPXZZ	0QWCX5Z
0PSBXZZ	0PW2XKZ	0PWJX7Z	0Q913ZZ	0QHB38Z	0QPGX5Z	0QS43ZZ	0QSQ3ZZ	0QWCX7Z
0PSC3ZZ	0PW3X4Z	0PWJXJZ	0Q9230Z	0QHB48Z	0QPHX4Z	0QS44ZZ	0QSQ4ZZ	0QWCXJZ
0PSC4ZZ	0PW3X7Z	0PWJXKZ	0Q923ZZ	0QHC08Z	0QPHX5Z	0QS4XZZ	0QSQXZZ	0QWCXKZ
0PSCXZZ	0PW3XJZ	0PWKX4Z	0Q9330Z	0QHC38Z	0QPJX4Z	0QS53ZZ	0QSR3ZZ	0QWDX4Z
0PSD3ZZ	0PW3XKZ	0PWKX5Z	0Q933ZZ	0QHC48Z	0QPJX5Z	0QS54ZZ	0QSR4ZZ	0QWDX5Z
0PSD4ZZ	0PW4X4Z	0PWKX7Z	0Q9430Z	0QHG08Z	0QPKX4Z	0QS5XZZ	0QSRXZZ	0QWDX7Z
0PSDXZZ	0PW4X7Z	0PWKXJZ	0Q943ZZ	0QHG38Z	0QPKX5Z	0QS63ZZ	0QSSXZZ	0QWDXJZ
0PSF3ZZ	0PW4XJZ	0PWKXKZ	0Q9530Z	0QHG48Z	0QPLX4Z	0QS64ZZ	0QW0X4Z	0QWDXKZ
0PSF4ZZ	0PW4XKZ	0PWLX4Z	0Q953ZZ	0QHH08Z	0QPLX5Z	0QS6XZZ	0QW0X7Z	0QWFX4Z
0PSFXZZ	0PW5X4Z	0PWLX5Z	0Q9630Z	0QHH38Z	0QPMX4Z	0QS73ZZ	0QW0XJZ	0QWFX5Z
0PSG3ZZ	0PW5X7Z	0PWLX7Z	0Q963ZZ	0QHH48Z	0QPMX5Z	0QS74ZZ	0QW0XKZ	0QWFX7Z
0PSG4ZZ	0PW5XJZ	0PWLXJZ	0Q9730Z	0QHJ08Z	0QPNX4Z	0QS7XZZ	0QW1X4Z	0QWFXJZ
0PSGXZZ	0PW5XKZ	0PWLXKZ	0Q973ZZ	0QHJ38Z	0QPNX5Z	0QS83ZZ	0QW1X7Z	0QWFXKZ
0PSH3ZZ	0PW6X4Z	0PWMX4Z	0Q9830Z	0QHJ48Z	0QPPX4Z	0QS84ZZ	0QW1XJZ	0QWGX4Z
0PSH4ZZ	0PW6X7Z	0PWMX5Z	0Q983ZZ	0QHK08Z	0QPPX5Z	0QS8XZZ	0QW1XKZ	0QWGX5Z
0PSHXZZ	0PW6XJZ	0PWMX7Z	0Q9930Z	0QHK38Z	0QPQX4Z	0QS93ZZ	0QW2X4Z	0QWGX7Z
0PSJ3ZZ	0PW6XKZ	0PWMXJZ	0Q993ZZ	0QHK48Z	0QPQX5Z	0QS94ZZ	0QW2X5Z	0QWGXJZ
0PSJ4ZZ	0PW7X4Z	0PWMXKZ	0Q9B30Z	0QJY3ZZ	0QPRX4Z	0QS9XZZ	0QW2X7Z	0QWGXKZ
0PSJXZZ	0PW7X7Z	0PWNX4Z	0Q9B3ZZ	0QJYXZZ	0QPRX5Z	0QSB3ZZ	0QW2XJZ	0QWHX4Z

0QWHX5Z	0R900ZX	0R9B40Z	0R9M40Z	0R9W30Z	0RBL4ZX	0RGU43Z	0RHE03Z	0RHQ03Z
0QWHX7Z	0R9030Z	0R9B4ZX	0R9M4ZX	0R9W3ZX	0RBM0ZX	0RGV03Z	0RHE08Z	0RHQ08Z
0QWHXJZ	0R903ZX	0R9B4ZZ	0R9M4ZZ	0R9W3ZZ	0RBM3ZX	0RGV33Z	0RHE33Z	0RHQ33Z
0QWHXKZ	0R903ZZ	0R9C30Z	0R9N0ZX	0R9W40Z	0RBM4ZX	0RGV43Z	0RHE38Z	0RHQ38Z
0QWJX4Z	0R9040Z	0R9C3ZZ	0R9N30Z	0R9W4ZX	0RBN0ZX	0RGW03Z	0RHE43Z	0RHQ43Z
0QWJX5Z	0R904ZX	0R9D30Z	0R9N3ZX	0R9W4ZZ	0RBN3ZX	0RGW33Z	0RHE48Z	0RHQ48Z
0QWJX7Z	0R904ZZ	0R9D3ZZ	0R9N3ZZ	0R9X0ZX	0RBN4ZX	0RGW43Z	0RHF03Z	0RHR03Z
0QWJXJZ	0R910ZX	0R9E0ZX	0R9N40Z	0R9X30Z	0RBP0ZX	0RGX03Z	0RHF08Z	0RHR08Z
0QWJXKZ	0R9130Z	0R9E30Z	0R9N4ZX	0R9X3ZX	0RBP3ZX	0RGX33Z	0RHF33Z	0RHR33Z
0QWKX4Z	0R913ZX	0R9E3ZX	0R9N4ZZ	0R9X3ZZ	0RBP4ZX	0RGX43Z	0RHF38Z	0RHR38Z
0QWKX5Z	0R913ZZ	0R9E3ZZ	0R9P0ZX	0R9X40Z	0RBQ0ZX	0RH003Z	0RHF43Z	0RHR43Z
0QWKX7Z	0R9140Z	0R9E40Z	0R9P30Z	0R9X4ZX	0RBQ3ZX	0RH008Z	0RHF48Z	0RHR48Z
0QWKXJZ	0R914ZX	0R9E4ZX	0R9P3ZX	0R9X4ZZ	0RBQ4ZX	0RH033Z	0RHG03Z	0RHS03Z
0QWKXKZ	0R914ZZ	0R9E4ZZ	0R9P3ZZ	0RB00ZX	0RBR0ZX	0RH038Z	0RHG08Z	0RHS08Z
0QWLX4Z	0R930ZX	0R9F0ZX	0R9P40Z	0RB03ZX	0RBR3ZX	0RH043Z	0RHG33Z	0RHS33Z
0QWLX5Z	0R9330Z	0R9F30Z	0R9P4ZX	0RB04ZX	0RBR4ZX	0RH048Z	0RHG38Z	0RHS38Z
0QWLX7Z	0R933ZX	0R9F3ZX	0R9P4ZZ	0RB10ZX	0RBS0ZX	0RH103Z	0RHG43Z	0RHS43Z
0QWLXJZ	0R933ZZ	0R9F3ZZ	0R9Q0ZX	0RB13ZX	0RBS3ZX	0RH108Z	0RHG48Z	0RHS48Z
0QWLXKZ	0R9340Z	0R9F40Z	0R9Q30Z	0RB14ZX	0RBS4ZX	0RH133Z	0RHH03Z	0RHT03Z
0QWMX4Z	0R934ZX	0R9F4ZX	0R9Q3ZX	0RB30ZX	0RBT0ZX	0RH138Z	0RHH08Z	0RHT08Z
0QWMX5Z	0R934ZZ	0R9F4ZZ	0R9Q3ZZ	0RB33ZX	0RBT3ZX	0RH143Z	0RHH33Z	0RHT33Z
0QWMX7Z	0R940ZX	0R9G0ZX	0R9Q40Z	0RB34ZX	0RBT4ZX	0RH148Z	0RHH38Z	0RHT38Z
0QWMXJZ	0R9430Z	0R9G30Z	0R9Q4ZX	0RB40ZX	0RBU0ZX	0RH303Z	0RHH43Z	0RHT43Z
0QWMXKZ	0R943ZX	0R9G3ZX	0R9Q4ZZ	0RB43ZX	0RBU3ZX	0RH333Z	0RHH48Z	0RHT48Z
0QWNX4Z	0R943ZZ	0R9G3ZZ	0R9R0ZX	0RB44ZX	0RBU4ZX	0RH343Z	0RHJ03Z	0RHU03Z
0QWNX5Z	0R9440Z	0R9G40Z	0R9R30Z	0RB50ZX	0RBV0ZX	0RH403Z	0RHJ08Z	0RHU08Z
0QWNX7Z	0R944ZX	0R9G4ZX	0R9R3ZX	0RB53ZX	0RBV3ZX	0RH408Z	0RHJ33Z	0RHU33Z
0QWNXJZ	0R944ZZ	0R9G4ZZ	0R9R3ZZ	0RB54ZX	0RBV4ZX	0RH433Z	0RHJ38Z	0RHU38Z
0QWNXKZ	0R950ZX	0R9H0ZX	0R9R40Z	0RB60ZX	0RBW0ZX	0RH438Z	0RHJ43Z	0RHU43Z
0QWPX4Z	0R9530Z	0R9H30Z	0R9R4ZX	0RB63ZX	0RBW3ZX	0RH443Z	0RHJ48Z	0RHU48Z
0QWPX5Z	0R953ZX	0R9H3ZX	0R9R4ZZ	0RB64ZX	0RBW4ZX	0RH448Z	0RHK03Z	0RHV03Z
0QWPX7Z	0R953ZZ	0R9H3ZZ	0R9S0ZX	0RB90ZX	0RBX0ZX	0RH503Z	0RHK08Z	0RHV08Z
0QWPXJZ	0R9540Z	0R9H40Z	0R9S30Z	0RB93ZX	0RBX3ZX	0RH533Z	0RHK33Z	0RHV33Z
0QWPXKZ	0R954ZX	0R9H4ZX	0R9S3ZX	0RB94ZX	0RBX4ZX	0RH543Z	0RHK38Z	0RHV38Z
0QWQX4Z	0R954ZZ	0R9H4ZZ	0R9S3ZZ	0RBA0ZX	0RGL03Z	0RH603Z	0RHK43Z	0RHV43Z
0QWQX5Z	0R960ZX	0R9J0ZX	0R9S40Z	0RBA3ZX	0RGL33Z	0RH608Z	0RHK48Z	0RHV48Z
0QWQX7Z	0R9630Z	0R9J30Z	0R9S4ZX	0RBA4ZX	0RGL43Z	0RH633Z	0RHL03Z	0RHW03Z
0QWQXJZ	0R963ZX	0R9J3ZX	0R9S4ZZ	0RBB0ZX	0RGM03Z	0RH638Z	0RHL08Z	0RHW08Z
0QWQXKZ	0R963ZZ	0R9J3ZZ	0R9T0ZX	0RBB3ZX	0RGM33Z	0RH643Z	0RHL33Z	0RHW33Z
0QWRX4Z	0R9640Z	0R9J40Z	0R9T30Z	0RBB4ZX	0RGM43Z	0RH648Z	0RHL38Z	0RHW38Z
0QWRX5Z	0R964ZX	0R9J4ZX	0R9T3ZX	0RBE0ZX	0RGN03Z	0RH903Z	0RHL43Z	0RHW43Z
0QWRX7Z	0R964ZZ	0R9J4ZZ	0R9T3ZZ	0RBE3ZX	0RGN33Z	0RH933Z	0RHL48Z	0RHW48Z
0QWRXJZ	0R990ZX	0R9K0ZX	0R9T40Z	0RBE4ZX	0RGN43Z	0RH943Z	0RHM03Z	0RHX03Z
0QWRXKZ	0R9930Z	0R9K30Z	0R9T4ZX	0RBF0ZX	0RGP03Z	0RHA03Z	0RHM08Z	0RHX08Z
0QWSX4Z	0R993ZX	0R9K3ZX	0R9T4ZZ	0RBF3ZX	0RGP33Z	0RHA08Z	0RHM33Z	0RHX33Z
0QWSX7Z	0R993ZZ	0R9K3ZZ	0R9U0ZX	0RBF4ZX	0RGP43Z	0RHA33Z	0RHM38Z	0RHX38Z
0QWSXJZ	0R9940Z	0R9K40Z	0R9U30Z	0RBG0ZX	0RGQ03Z	0RHA38Z	0RHM43Z	0RHX43Z
0QWSXKZ	0R994ZX	0R9K4ZX	0R9U3ZX	0RBG3ZX	0RGQ33Z	0RHA43Z	0RHM48Z	0RHX48Z
0QWYX0Z	0R994ZZ	0R9K4ZZ	0R9U3ZZ	0RBG4ZX	0RGQ43Z	0RHA48Z	0RHN03Z	0RJ03ZZ
0QWYXMZ	0R9A0ZX	0R9L0ZX	0R9U40Z	0RBH0ZX	0RGR03Z	0RHB03Z	0RHN08Z	0RJ0XZZ
0R2YX0Z	0R9A30Z	0R9L30Z	0R9U4ZX	0RBH3ZX	0RGR33Z	0RHB33Z	0RHN33Z	0RJ13ZZ
0R2YXYZ	0R9A3ZX	0R9L3ZX	0R9U4ZZ	0RBH4ZX	0RGR43Z	0RHB43Z	0RHN38Z	0RJ1XZZ
0R533ZZ	0R9A3ZZ	0R9L3ZZ	0R9V0ZX	0RBJ0ZX	0RGS03Z	0RHC08Z	0RHN43Z	0RJ33ZZ
0R534ZZ	0R9A40Z	0R9L40Z	0R9V30Z	0RBJ3ZX	0RGS33Z	0RHC33Z	0RHN48Z	0RJ3XZZ
0R553ZZ	0R9A4ZX	0R9L4ZX	0R9V3ZX	0RBJ4ZX	0RGS43Z	0RHC38Z	0RHP03Z	0RJ43ZZ
0R554ZZ	0R9A4ZZ	0R9L4ZZ	0R9V3ZZ	0RBK0ZX	0RGT03Z	0RHC48Z	0RHP08Z	0RJ4XZZ
0R593ZZ	0R9B0ZX	0R9M0ZX	0R9V40Z	0RBK3ZX	0RGT33Z	0RHD08Z	0RHP33Z	0RJ53ZZ
0R594ZZ	0R9B30Z	0R9M30Z	0R9V4ZX	0RBK4ZX	0RGT43Z	0RHD33Z	0RHP38Z	0RJ5XZZ
0R5B3ZZ	0R9B3ZX	0R9M3ZX	0R9V4ZZ	0RBL0ZX	0RGU03Z	0RHD38Z	0RHP43Z	0RJ63ZZ
0R5B4ZZ	0R9B3ZZ	0R9M3ZZ	0R9W0ZX	0RBL3ZX	0RGU33Z	0RHD48Z	0RHP48Z	0RJ6XZZ

0RJ93ZZ	0RNHXZZ	0RPA30Z	0RPJ38Z	0RPR33Z	0RPXX5Z	0RSC34Z	0RSM44Z	0RSU34Z	
0RJ9XZZ	0RNJXZZ	0RPA33Z	0RPJ48Z	0RPR38Z	0RQ0XZZ	0RSC3ZZ	0RSM45Z	0RSU35Z	
0RJA3ZZ	0RNKXZZ	0RPA38Z	0RPJX0Z	0RPR48Z	0RQ1XZZ	0RSC44Z	0RSM4ZZ	0RSU3ZZ	
0RJAXZZ	0RNLXZZ	0RPA48Z	0RPJX3Z	0RPRX0Z	0RQ3XZZ	0RSC4ZZ	0RSMX4Z	0RSU44Z	
0RJB3ZZ	0RNMXZZ	0RPAX0Z	0RPJX4Z	0RPRX3Z	0RQ4XZZ	0RSCX4Z	0RSMX5Z	0RSU45Z	
0RJBXZZ	0RNNXZZ	0RPAX3Z	0RPK08Z	0RPRX4Z	0RQ5XZZ	0RSCXZZ	0RSMXZZ	0RSU4ZZ	
0RJC3ZZ	0RNPXZZ	0RPAX4Z	0RPK30Z	0RPRX5Z	0RQ6XZZ	0RSD34Z	0RSN34Z	0RSUX4Z	
0RJCXZZ	0RNQXZZ	0RPB30Z	0RPK33Z	0RPS08Z	0RQ9XZZ	0RSD3ZZ	0RSN35Z	0RSUX5Z	
0RJD3ZZ	0RNRXZZ	0RPB33Z	0RPK38Z	0RPS30Z	0RQAXZZ	0RSD44Z	0RSN3ZZ	0RSUXZZ	
0RJDXZZ	0RNSXZZ	0RPBX0Z	0RPK48Z	0RPS33Z	0RQBXZZ	0RSD4ZZ	0RSN44Z	0RSV34Z	
0RJE3ZZ	0RNTXZZ	0RPBX3Z	0RPKX0Z	0RPS38Z	0RQCXZZ	0RSDX4Z	0RSN45Z	0RSV35Z	
0RJEXZZ	0RNUXZZ	0RPC08Z	0RPKX3Z	0RPS48Z	0RQDXZZ	0RSDXZZ	0RSN4ZZ	0RSV3ZZ	
0RJF3ZZ	0RNVXZZ	0RPC30Z	0RPKX4Z	0RPSX0Z	0RQEXZZ	0RSE34Z	0RSNX4Z	0RSV44Z	
0RJFXZZ	0RNWXZZ	0RPC33Z	0RPL08Z	0RPSX3Z	0RQFXZZ	0RSE3ZZ	0RSNX5Z	0RSV45Z	
0RJG3ZZ	0RNXXZZ	0RPC38Z	0RPL30Z	0RPSX4Z	0RQGXZZ	0RSE44Z	0RSNXZZ	0RSV4ZZ	
0RJGXZZ	0RP008Z	0RPC48Z	0RPL33Z	0RPSX5Z	0RQHXZZ	0RSE4ZZ	0RSP34Z	0RSVX4Z	
0RJH3ZZ	0RP030Z	0RPCX0Z	0RPL38Z	0RPT08Z	0RQJXZZ	0RSEX4Z	0RSP35Z	0RSVX5Z	
0RJHXZZ	0RP033Z	0RPCX3Z	0RPL48Z	0RPT30Z	0RQKXZZ	0RSEXZZ	0RSP3ZZ	0RSVXZZ	
0RJJ3ZZ	0RP038Z	0RPD08Z	0RPLX0Z	0RPT33Z	0RQLXZZ	0RSF34Z	0RSP44Z	0RSW34Z	
0RJJXZZ	0RP048Z	0RPD30Z	0RPLX3Z	0RPT38Z	0RQMXZZ	0RSF3ZZ	0RSP45Z	0RSW35Z	
0RJK3ZZ	0RP0X0Z	0RPD33Z	0RPLX4Z	0RPT48Z	0RQNXZZ	0RSF44Z	0RSP4ZZ	0RSW3ZZ	
0RJKXZZ	0RP0X3Z	0RPD38Z	0RPLX5Z	0RPTX0Z	0RQPXZZ	0RSF4ZZ	0RSPX4Z	0RSW44Z	
0RJL3ZZ	0RP0X4Z	0RPD48Z	0RPM08Z	0RPTX3Z	0RQQXZZ	0RSFX4Z	0RSPX5Z	0RSW45Z	
0RJLXZZ	0RP108Z	0RPDX0Z	0RPM30Z	0RPTX4Z	0RQRXZZ	0RSFXZZ	0RSPXZZ	0RSW4ZZ	
0RJM3ZZ	0RP130Z	0RPDX3Z	0RPM33Z	0RPTX5Z	0RQSXZZ	0RSG34Z	0RSQ34Z	0RSWX4Z	
0RJMXZZ	0RP133Z	0RPE08Z	0RPM38Z	0RPU08Z	0RQTXZZ	0RSG3ZZ	0RSQ35Z	0RSWX5Z	
0RJN3ZZ	0RP138Z	0RPE30Z	0RPM48Z	0RPU30Z	0RQUXZZ	0RSG44Z	0RSQ3ZZ	0RSWXZZ	
0RJNXZZ	0RP148Z	0RPE33Z	0RPMX0Z	0RPU33Z	0RQVXZZ	0RSG4ZZ	0RSQ44Z	0RSX34Z	
0RJP3ZZ	0RP1X0Z	0RPE38Z	0RPMX3Z	0RPU38Z	0RQWXZZ	0RSGX4Z	0RSQ45Z	0RSX35Z	
0RJPXZZ	0RP1X3Z	0RPE48Z	0RPMX4Z	0RPU48Z	0RQXXZZ	0RSGXZZ	0RSQ4ZZ	0RSX3ZZ	
0RJQ3ZZ	0RP1X4Z	0RPEX0Z	0RPMX5Z	0RPUX0Z	0RS034Z	0RSH34Z	0RSQX4Z	0RSX44Z	
0RJQXZZ	0RP330Z	0RPEX3Z	0RPN08Z	0RPUX3Z	0RS03ZZ	0RSH3ZZ	0RSQX5Z	0RSX45Z	
0RJR3ZZ	0RP333Z	0RPEX4Z	0RPN30Z	0RPUX4Z	0RS044Z	0RSH44Z	0RSQXZZ	0RSX4ZZ	
0RJRXZZ	0RP3X0Z	0RPF08Z	0RPN33Z	0RPUX5Z	0RS04ZZ	0RSH4ZZ	0RSR34Z	0RSXX4Z	
0RJS3ZZ	0RP3X3Z	0RPF30Z	0RPN38Z	0RPV08Z	0RS0X4Z	0RSHX4Z	0RSR35Z	0RSXX5Z	
0RJSXZZ	0RP408Z	0RPF33Z	0RPN48Z	0RPV30Z	0RS0XZZ	0RSHXZZ	0RSR3ZZ	0RSXXZZ	
0RJT3ZZ	0RP430Z	0RPF38Z	0RPNX0Z	0RPV33Z	0RS134Z	0RSJ34Z	0RSR44Z	0RW0X0Z	
0RJTXZZ	0RP433Z	0RPF48Z	0RPNX3Z	0RPV38Z	0RS13ZZ	0RSJ3ZZ	0RSR45Z	0RW0X3Z	
0RJU3ZZ	0RP438Z	0RPFX0Z	0RPNX4Z	0RPV48Z	0RS144Z	0RSJ44Z	0RSR4ZZ	0RW0X4Z	
0RJUXZZ	0RP448Z	0RPFX3Z	0RPNX5Z	0RPVX0Z	0RS14ZZ	0RSJ4ZZ	0RSRX4Z	0RW0X7Z	
0RJV3ZZ	0RP4X0Z	0RPFX4Z	0RPP08Z	0RPVX3Z	0RS1X4Z	0RSJX4Z	0RSRX5Z	0RW0X8Z	
0RJVXZZ	0RP4X3Z	0RPG08Z	0RPP30Z	0RPVX4Z	0RS1XZZ	0RSJXZZ	0RSRXZZ	0RW0XAZ	
0RJW3ZZ	0RP4X4Z	0RPG30Z	0RPP33Z	0RPVX5Z	0RS434Z	0RSK34Z	0RSS34Z	0RW0XJZ	
0RJWXZZ	0RP530Z	0RPG33Z	0RPP38Z	0RPW08Z	0RS43ZZ	0RSK3ZZ	0RSS35Z	0RW0XKZ	
0RJX3ZZ	0RP533Z	0RPG38Z	0RPP48Z	0RPW30Z	0RS444Z	0RSK44Z	0RSS3ZZ	0RW1X0Z	
0RJXXZZ	0RP5X0Z	0RPG48Z	0RPPX0Z	0RPW33Z	0RS44ZZ	0RSK4ZZ	0RSS44Z	0RW1X3Z	
0RN0XZZ	0RP5X3Z	0RPGX0Z	0RPPX3Z	0RPW38Z	0RS4X4Z	0RSKX4Z	0RSS45Z	0RW1X4Z	
0RN1XZZ	0RP608Z	0RPGX3Z	0RPPX4Z	0RPW48Z	0RS4XZZ	0RSKXZZ	0RSS4ZZ	0RW1X7Z	
0RN3XZZ	0RP630Z	0RPGX4Z	0RPPX5Z	0RPWX0Z	0RS634Z	0RSL34Z	0RSSX4Z	0RW1X8Z	
0RN4XZZ	0RP633Z	0RPH08Z	0RPQ08Z	0RPWX3Z	0RS63ZZ	0RSL35Z	0RSSX5Z	0RW1XAZ	
0RN5XZZ	0RP638Z	0RPH30Z	0RPQ30Z	0RPWX4Z	0RS644Z	0RSL3ZZ	0RSSXZZ	0RW1XJZ	
0RN6XZZ	0RP648Z	0RPH33Z	0RPQ33Z	0RPWX5Z	0RS64ZZ	0RSL44Z	0RST34Z	0RW1XKZ	
0RN9XZZ	0RP6X0Z	0RPH38Z	0RPQ38Z	0RPX08Z	0RS6X4Z	0RSL45Z	0RST35Z	0RW3X0Z	
0RNAXZZ	0RP6X3Z	0RPH48Z	0RPQ48Z	0RPX30Z	0RS6XZZ	0RSL4ZZ	0RST3ZZ	0RW3X3Z	
0RNBXZZ	0RP6X4Z	0RPHX0Z	0RPQX0Z	0RPX33Z	0RSA34Z	0RSLX4Z	0RST44Z	0RW3X7Z	
0RNCXZZ	0RP930Z	0RPHX3Z	0RPQX3Z	0RPX38Z	0RSA3ZZ	0RSLX5Z	0RST45Z	0RW3XJZ	
0RNDXZZ	0RP933Z	0RPHX4Z	0RPQX4Z	0RPX48Z	0RSA44Z	0RSLXZZ	0RST4ZZ	0RW3XKZ	
0RNEXZZ	0RP9X0Z	0RPJ08Z	0RPQX5Z	0RPXX0Z	0RSA4ZZ	0RSM34Z	0RSTX4Z	0RW4X0Z	
0RNFXZZ	0RP9X3Z	0RPJ30Z	0RPR08Z	0RPXX3Z	0RSAX4Z	0RSM35Z	0RSTX5Z	0RW4X3Z	
0RNGXZZ	0RPA08Z	0RPJ33Z	0RPR30Z	0RPXX4Z	0RSAXZZ	0RSM3ZZ	0RSTXZZ	0RW4X4Z	

0RW4X7Z	0RWFX7Z	0RWPX7Z	0RWXX0Z	0S9830Z	0S9J4ZX	0SB63ZX	0SGD33Z	0SH543Z
0RW4X8Z	0RWFX8Z	0RWPX8Z	0RWXX3Z	0S983ZX	0S9J4ZZ	0SB64ZX	0SGD43Z	0SH548Z
0RW4XAZ	0RWFXJZ	0RWPXJZ	0RWXX4Z	0S983ZZ	0S9K0ZX	0SB70ZX	0SGF03Z	0SH603Z
0RW4XJZ	0RWFXKZ	0RWPXKZ	0RWXX5Z	0S9840Z	0S9K30Z	0SB73ZX	0SGF33Z	0SH608Z
0RW4XKZ	0RWGX0Z	0RWQX0Z	0RWXX7Z	0S984ZX	0S9K3ZX	0SB74ZX	0SGF43Z	0SH633Z
0RW5X0Z	0RWGX3Z	0RWQX3Z	0RWXX8Z	0S984ZZ	0S9K3ZZ	0SB80ZX	0SGG03Z	0SH638Z
0RW5X3Z	0RWGX4Z	0RWQX4Z	0RWXXJZ	0S990ZX	0S9K40Z	0SB83ZX	0SGG33Z	0SH643Z
0RW5X7Z	0RWGX7Z	0RWQX5Z	0RWXXKZ	0S9930Z	0S9K4ZX	0SB84ZX	0SGG43Z	0SH648Z
0RW5XJZ	0RWGX8Z	0RWQX7Z	0S2YX0Z	0S993ZX	0S9K4ZZ	0SB90ZX	0SGH03Z	0SH703Z
0RW5XKZ	0RWGXJZ	0RWQX8Z	0S2YXYZ	0S993ZZ	0S9L0ZX	0SB93ZX	0SGH33Z	0SH708Z
0RW6X0Z	0RWGXKZ	0RWQXJZ	0S900ZX	0S9940Z	0S9L30Z	0SB94ZX	0SGH43Z	0SH733Z
0RW6X3Z	0RWHX0Z	0RWQXKZ	0S9030Z	0S994ZX	0S9L3ZX	0SBB0ZX	0SGJ03Z	0SH738Z
0RW6X4Z	0RWHX3Z	0RWRX0Z	0S903ZX	0S994ZZ	0S9L3ZZ	0SBB3ZX	0SGJ33Z	0SH743Z
0RW6X7Z	0RWHX4Z	0RWRX3Z	0S903ZZ	0S9B0ZX	0S9L40Z	0SBB4ZX	0SGJ43Z	0SH748Z
0RW6X8Z	0RWHX7Z	0RWRX4Z	0S9040Z	0S9B30Z	0S9L4ZX	0SBC0ZX	0SGK03Z	0SH803Z
0RW6XAZ	0RWHX8Z	0RWRX5Z	0S904ZX	0S9B3ZX	0S9L4ZZ	0SBC3ZX	0SGK33Z	0SH808Z
0RW6XJZ	0RWHXJZ	0RWRX7Z	0S904ZZ	0S9B3ZZ	0S9M0ZX	0SBC4ZX	0SGK43Z	0SH833Z
0RW6XKZ	0RWHXKZ	0RWRX8Z	0S920ZX	0S9B40Z	0S9M30Z	0SBD0ZX	0SGL03Z	0SH838Z
0RW9X0Z	0RWJX0Z	0RWRXJZ	0S9230Z	0S9B4ZX	0S9M3ZX	0SBD3ZX	0SGL33Z	0SH843Z
0RW9X3Z	0RWJX3Z	0RWRXKZ	0S923ZX	0S9B4ZZ	0S9M3ZZ	0SBD4ZX	0SGL43Z	0SH848Z
0RW9X7Z	0RWJX4Z	0RWSX0Z	0S923ZZ	0S9C0ZX	0S9M40Z	0SBF0ZX	0SGM03Z	0SH903Z
0RW9XJZ	0RWJX7Z	0RWSX3Z	0S9240Z	0S9C30Z	0S9M4ZX	0SBF3ZX	0SGM33Z	0SH933Z
0RW9XKZ	0RWJX8Z	0RWSX4Z	0S924ZX	0S9C3ZX	0S9M4ZZ	0SBF4ZX	0SGM43Z	0SH938Z
0RWAX0Z	0RWJXJZ	0RWSX5Z	0S924ZZ	0S9C3ZZ	0S9N0ZX	0SBG0ZX	0SGN03Z	0SH943Z
0RWAX3Z	0RWJXKZ	0RWSX7Z	0S930ZX	0S9C40Z	0S9N30Z	0SBG3ZX	0SGN33Z	0SH948Z
0RWAX4Z	0RWKX0Z	0RWSX8Z	0S9330Z	0S9C4ZX	0S9N3ZX	0SBG4ZX	0SGN43Z	0SHB03Z
0RWAX7Z	0RWKX3Z	0RWSXJZ	0S933ZX	0S9C4ZZ	0S9N3ZZ	0SBH0ZX	0SGP03Z	0SHB33Z
0RWAX8Z	0RWKX4Z	0RWSXKZ	0S933ZZ	0S9D0ZX	0S9N40Z	0SBH3ZX	0SGP33Z	0SHB38Z
0RWAXAZ	0RWKX7Z	0RWTX0Z	0S9340Z	0S9D30Z	0S9N4ZX	0SBH4ZX	0SGP43Z	0SHB43Z
0RWAXJZ	0RWKX8Z	0RWTX3Z	0S934ZX	0S9D3ZX	0S9N4ZZ	0SBJ0ZX	0SGQ03Z	0SHB48Z
0RWAXKZ	0RWKXJZ	0RWTX4Z	0S934ZZ	0S9D3ZZ	0S9P0ZX	0SBJ3ZX	0SGQ33Z	0SHC03Z
0RWBX0Z	0RWKXKZ	0RWTX5Z	0S940ZX	0S9D40Z	0S9P30Z	0SBJ4ZX	0SGQ43Z	0SHC33Z
0RWBX3Z	0RWLX0Z	0RWTX7Z	0S9430Z	0S9D4ZX	0S9P3ZX	0SBK0ZX	0SH003Z	0SHC38Z
0RWBX7Z	0RWLX3Z	0RWTX8Z	0S943ZX	0S9D4ZZ	0S9P3ZZ	0SBK3ZX	0SH008Z	0SHC43Z
0RWBXJZ	0RWLX4Z	0RWTXJZ	0S943ZZ	0S9F0ZX	0S9P40Z	0SBK4ZX	0SH033Z	0SHC48Z
0RWBXKZ	0RWLX5Z	0RWTXKZ	0S9440Z	0S9F30Z	0S9P4ZX	0SBL0ZX	0SH038Z	0SHD03Z
0RWCX0Z	0RWLX7Z	0RWUX0Z	0S944ZX	0S9F3ZX	0S9P4ZZ	0SBL3ZX	0SH043Z	0SHD33Z
0RWCX3Z	0RWLX8Z	0RWUX3Z	0S944ZZ	0S9F3ZZ	0S9Q0ZX	0SBL4ZX	0SH048Z	0SHD38Z
0RWCX4Z	0RWLXJZ	0RWUX4Z	0S950ZX	0S9F40Z	0S9Q30Z	0SBM0ZX	0SH203Z	0SHD43Z
0RWCX7Z	0RWLXKZ	0RWUX5Z	0S9530Z	0S9F4ZX	0S9Q3ZX	0SBM3ZX	0SH208Z	0SHD48Z
0RWCX8Z	0RWMX0Z	0RWUX7Z	0S953ZX	0S9F4ZZ	0S9Q3ZZ	0SBM4ZX	0SH233Z	0SHF03Z
0RWCXJZ	0RWMX3Z	0RWUX8Z	0S953ZZ	0S9G0ZX	0S9Q40Z	0SBN0ZX	0SH238Z	0SHF08Z
0RWCXKZ	0RWMX4Z	0RWUXJZ	0S9540Z	0S9G30Z	0S9Q4ZX	0SBN3ZX	0SH243Z	0SHF33Z
0RWDX0Z	0RWMX5Z	0RWUXKZ	0S954ZX	0S9G3ZX	0S9Q4ZZ	0SBN4ZX	0SH248Z	0SHF38Z
0RWDX3Z	0RWMX7Z	0RWVX0Z	0S954ZZ	0S9G3ZZ	0SB00ZX	0SBP0ZX	0SH303Z	0SHF43Z
0RWDX4Z	0RWMX8Z	0RWVX3Z	0S960ZX	0S9G40Z	0SB03ZX	0SBP3ZX	0SH308Z	0SHF48Z
0RWDX7Z	0RWMXJZ	0RWVX4Z	0S9630Z	0S9G4ZX	0SB04ZX	0SBP4ZX	0SH333Z	0SHG03Z
0RWDX8Z	0RWMXKZ	0RWVX5Z	0S963ZX	0S9G4ZZ	0SB20ZX	0SBQ0ZX	0SH338Z	0SHG08Z
0RWDXJZ	0RWNX0Z	0RWVX7Z	0S963ZZ	0S9H0ZX	0SB23ZX	0SBQ3ZX	0SH343Z	0SHG33Z
0RWDXKZ	0RWNX3Z	0RWVX8Z	0S9640Z	0S9H30Z	0SB24ZX	0SBQ4ZX	0SH348Z	0SHG38Z
0RWEX0Z	0RWNX4Z	0RWVXJZ	0S964ZX	0S9H3ZX	0SB30ZX	0SG903Z	0SH403Z	0SHG43Z
0RWEX3Z	0RWNX5Z	0RWVXKZ	0S964ZZ	0S9H3ZZ	0SB33ZX	0SG933Z	0SH408Z	0SHG48Z
0RWEX4Z	0RWNX7Z	0RWWX0Z	0S970ZX	0S9H40Z	0SB34ZX	0SG943Z	0SH433Z	0SHH03Z
0RWEX7Z	0RWNX8Z	0RWWX3Z	0S9730Z	0S9H4ZX	0SB40ZX	0SGB03Z	0SH438Z	0SHH08Z
0RWEX8Z	0RWNXJZ	0RWWX4Z	0S973ZX	0S9H4ZZ	0SB43ZX	0SGB33Z	0SH443Z	0SHH33Z
0RWEXJZ	0RWNXKZ	0RWWX5Z	0S973ZZ	0S9J0ZX	0SB44ZX	0SGB43Z	0SH448Z	0SHH38Z
0RWEXKZ	0RWPX0Z	0RWWX7Z	0S9740Z	0S9J30Z	0SB50ZX	0SGC03Z	0SH503Z	0SHH43Z
0RWFX0Z	0RWPX3Z	0RWWX8Z	0S974ZX	0S9J3ZX	0SB53ZX	0SGC33Z	0SH508Z	0SHH48Z
0RWFX3Z	0RWPX4Z	0RWWXJZ	0S974ZZ	0S9J3ZZ	0SB54ZX	0SGC43Z	0SH533Z	0SHJ03Z
0RWFX4Z	0RWPX5Z	0RWWXKZ	0S980ZX	0S9J40Z	0SB60ZX	0SGD03Z	0SH538Z	0SHJ08Z

0SHJ33Z	0SJC3ZZ	0SP333Z	0SPCX4Z	0SPLX4Z	0SS034Z	0SSCX4Z	0SSL44Z	0SW3XAZ
0SHJ38Z	0SJCXZZ	0SP338Z	0SPCX5Z	0SPLX5Z	0SS03ZZ	0SSCX5Z	0SSL45Z	0SW3XJS
0SHJ43Z	0SJD3ZZ	0SP348Z	0SPD30Z	0SPM08Z	0SS044Z	0SSCXZZ	0SSL4ZZ	0SW3XKZ
0SHJ48Z	0SJDXZZ	0SP3X0Z	0SPD33Z	0SPM30Z	0SS04ZZ	0SSD34Z	0SSLX4Z	0SW4X0Z
0SHK03Z	0SJF3ZZ	0SP3X3Z	0SPDX0Z	0SPM33Z	0SS0X4Z	0SSD35Z	0SSLX5Z	0SW4X3Z
0SHK08Z	0SJFXZZ	0SP3X4Z	0SPDX3Z	0SPM38Z	0SS0XZZ	0SSD3ZZ	0SSLXZZ	0SW4X7Z
0SHK33Z	0SJG3ZZ	0SP430Z	0SPDX4Z	0SPM48Z	0SS334Z	0SSD44Z	0SSM34Z	0SW4XJZ
0SHK38Z	0SJGXZZ	0SP433Z	0SPDX5Z	0SPMX0Z	0SS33Z	0SSD45Z	0SSM35Z	0SW4XKZ
0SHK43Z	0SJH3ZZ	0SP4X0Z	0SPF08Z	0SPMX3Z	0SS344Z	0SSD4ZZ	0SSM3ZZ	0SW5X0Z
0SHK48Z	0SJHXZZ	0SP4X3Z	0SPF30Z	0SPMX4Z	0SS34ZZ	0SSDX4Z	0SSM44Z	0SW5X3Z
0SHL03Z	0SJJ3ZZ	0SP508Z	0SPF33Z	0SPMX5Z	0SS3X4Z	0SSDX5Z	0SSM45Z	0SW5X4Z
0SHL08Z	0SJJXZZ	0SP530Z	0SPF38Z	0SPN08Z	0SS3XZZ	0SSDXZZ	0SSM4ZZ	0SW5X7Z
0SHL33Z	0SJK3ZZ	0SP533Z	0SPF48Z	0SPN30Z	0SS534Z	0SSF34Z	0SSMX4Z	0SW5X8Z
0SHL38Z	0SJKXZZ	0SP538Z	0SPFX0Z	0SPN33Z	0SS53ZZ	0SSF35Z	0SSMX5Z	0SW5XJZ
0SHL43Z	0SJL3ZZ	0SP548Z	0SPFX3Z	0SPN38Z	0SS544Z	0SSF3ZZ	0SSMXZZ	0SW5XKZ
0SHL48Z	0SJLXZZ	0SP5X0Z	0SPFX4Z	0SPN48Z	0SS54ZZ	0SSF44Z	0SSN34Z	0SW6X0Z
0SHM03Z	0SJM3ZZ	0SP5X3Z	0SPFX5Z	0SPNX0Z	0SS5X4Z	0SSF45Z	0SSN35Z	0SW6X3Z
0SHM08Z	0SJMXZZ	0SP5X4Z	0SPG08Z	0SPNX3Z	0SS5XZZ	0SSF4ZZ	0SSN3ZZ	0SW6X4Z
0SHM33Z	0SJN3ZZ	0SP608Z	0SPG30Z	0SPNX4Z	0SS634Z	0SSFX4Z	0SSN44Z	0SW6X7Z
0SHM38Z	0SJNXZZ	0SP630Z	0SPG33Z	0SPNX5Z	0SS63ZZ	0SSFX5Z	0SSN45Z	0SW6X8Z
0SHM43Z	0SJP3ZZ	0SP633Z	0SPG38Z	0SPP08Z	0SS644Z	0SSFXZZ	0SSN4ZZ	0SW6XJZ
0SHM48Z	0SJPXZZ	0SP638Z	0SPG48Z	0SPP30Z	0SS64ZZ	0SSG34Z	0SSNX4Z	0SW6XKZ
0SHN03Z	0SJQ3ZZ	0SP648Z	0SPGX0Z	0SPP33Z	0SS6X4Z	0SSG35Z	0SSNX5Z	0SW7X0Z
0SHN08Z	0SJQXZZ	0SP6X0Z	0SPGX3Z	0SPP38Z	0SS6XZZ	0SSG3ZZ	0SSNXZZ	0SW7X3Z
0SHN33Z	0SN0XZZ	0SP6X3Z	0SPGX4Z	0SPP48Z	0SS734Z	0SSG44Z	0SSP34Z	0SW7X4Z
0SHN38Z	0SN2XZZ	0SP6X4Z	0SPGX5Z	0SPPX0Z	0SS73ZZ	0SSG45Z	0SSP35Z	0SW7X7Z
0SHN43Z	0SN3XZZ	0SP708Z	0SPH08Z	0SPPX3Z	0SS744Z	0SSG4ZZ	0SSP3ZZ	0SW7X8Z
0SHN48Z	0SN4XZZ	0SP730Z	0SPH30Z	0SPPX4Z	0SS74ZZ	0SSGX4Z	0SSP44Z	0SW7XJZ
0SHP03Z	0SN5XZZ	0SP733Z	0SPH33Z	0SPPX5Z	0SS7X4Z	0SSGX5Z	0SSP45Z	0SW7XKZ
0SHP08Z	0SN6XZZ	0SP738Z	0SPH38Z	0SPQ08Z	0SS7XZZ	0SSGXZZ	0SSP4ZZ	0SW8X0Z
0SHP33Z	0SN7XZZ	0SP748Z	0SPH48Z	0SPQ30Z	0SS834Z	0SSH34Z	0SSPX4Z	0SW8X3Z
0SHP38Z	0SN8XZZ	0SP7X0Z	0SPHX0Z	0SPQ33Z	0SS83ZZ	0SSH35Z	0SSPX5Z	0SW8X4Z
0SHP43Z	0SN9XZZ	0SP7X3Z	0SPHX3Z	0SPQ38Z	0SS844Z	0SSH3ZZ	0SSPXZZ	0SW8X7Z
0SHP48Z	0SNBXZZ	0SP7X4Z	0SPHX4Z	0SPQ48Z	0SS84ZZ	0SSH44Z	0SSQ34Z	0SW8X8Z
0SHQ03Z	0SNCXZZ	0SP808Z	0SPHX5Z	0SPQX0Z	0SS8X4Z	0SSH45Z	0SSQ35Z	0SW8XJZ
0SHQ08Z	0SNDXZZ	0SP830Z	0SPJ08Z	0SPQX3Z	0SS8XZZ	0SSH4ZZ	0SSQ3ZZ	0SW8XKZ
0SHQ33Z	0SNFXZZ	0SP833Z	0SPJ30Z	0SPQX4Z	0SS934Z	0SSHX4Z	0SSQ44Z	0SW9X0Z
0SHQ38Z	0SNGXZZ	0SP838Z	0SPJ33Z	0SPQX5Z	0SS935Z	0SSHX5Z	0SSQ45Z	0SW9X3Z
0SHQ43Z	0SNHXZZ	0SP848Z	0SPJ38Z	0SQ0XZZ	0SS93ZZ	0SSHXZZ	0SSQ4ZZ	0SW9X4Z
0SHQ48Z	0SNJXZZ	0SP8X0Z	0SPJ48Z	0SQ2XZZ	0SS944Z	0SSJ34Z	0SSQX4Z	0SW9X5Z
0SJ03ZZ	0SNKXZZ	0SP8X3Z	0SPJX0Z	0SQ3XZZ	0SS945Z	0SSJ35Z	0SSQX5Z	0SW9X7Z
0SJ0XZZ	0SNLXZZ	0SP8X4Z	0SPJX3Z	0SQ4XZZ	0SS94ZZ	0SSJ3ZZ	0SSQXZZ	0SW9X8Z
0SJ23ZZ	0SNMXZZ	0SP930Z	0SPJX4Z	0SQ5XZZ	0SS9X4Z	0SSJ44Z	0SW0X0Z	0SW9XJZ
0SJ2XZZ	0SNNXZZ	0SP933Z	0SPJX5Z	0SQ6XZZ	0SS9X5Z	0SSJ45Z	0SW0X3Z	0SW9XKZ
0SJ33ZZ	0SNPXZZ	0SP938Z	0SPK08Z	0SQ7XZZ	0SS9XZZ	0SSJ4ZZ	0SW0X4Z	0SWAXJZ
0SJ3XZZ	0SNQXZZ	0SP9X0Z	0SPK30Z	0SQ8XZZ	0SSB34Z	0SSJX4Z	0SW0X7Z	0SWBX0Z
0SJ43ZZ	0SP008Z	0SP9X3Z	0SPK33Z	0SQ9XZZ	0SSB35Z	0SSJX5Z	0SW0X8Z	0SWBX3Z
0SJ4XZZ	0SP030Z	0SP9X4Z	0SPK38Z	0SQBXZZ	0SSB3ZZ	0SSJXZZ	0SW0XAZ	0SWBX4Z
0SJ53ZZ	0SP033Z	0SP9X5Z	0SPK48Z	0SQCXZZ	0SSB44Z	0SSK34Z	0SW0XJZ	0SWBX5Z
0SJ5XZZ	0SP038Z	0SPB30Z	0SPKX0Z	0SQDXZZ	0SSB45Z	0SSK35Z	0SW0XKZ	0SWBX7Z
0SJ63ZZ	0SP048Z	0SPB33Z	0SPKX3Z	0SQFXZZ	0SSB4ZZ	0SSK3ZZ	0SW2X0Z	0SWBX8Z
0SJ6XZZ	0SP0X0Z	0SPB38Z	0SPKX4Z	0SQGXZZ	0SSBX4Z	0SSK44Z	0SW2X3Z	0SWBXJZ
0SJ73ZZ	0SP0X3Z	0SPBX0Z	0SPKX5Z	0SQHXZZ	0SSBX5Z	0SSK45Z	0SW2X7Z	0SWBXKZ
0SJ7XZZ	0SP0X4Z	0SPBX3Z	0SPL08Z	0SQJXZZ	0SSBXZZ	0SSK4ZZ	0SW2XJZ	0SWCX0Z
0SJ83ZZ	0SP230Z	0SPBX4Z	0SPL30Z	0SQKXZZ	0SSC34Z	0SSKX4Z	0SW2XKZ	0SWCX3Z
0SJ8XZZ	0SP233Z	0SPBX5Z	0SPL33Z	0SQLXZZ	0SSC35Z	0SSKX5Z	0SW3X0Z	0SWCX4Z
0SJ93ZZ	0SP2X0Z	0SPC30Z	0SPL38Z	0SQMXZZ	0SSC3ZZ	0SSKXZZ	0SW3X3Z	0SWCX5Z
0SJ9XZZ	0SP2X3Z	0SPC33Z	0SPL48Z	0SQNXZZ	0SSC44Z	0SSL34Z	0SW3X4Z	0SWCX7Z
0SJB3ZZ	0SP308Z	0SPCX0Z	0SPLX0Z	0SQPXZZ	0SSC45Z	0SSL35Z	0SW3X7Z	0SWCX8Z
0SJBXZZ	0SP330Z	0SPCX3Z	0SPLX3Z	0SQQXZZ	0SSC4ZZ	0SSL3ZZ	0SW3X8Z	0SWCXJC

0SWCXJZ	0SWMX0Z	0T777DZ	0T964ZX	0TB38ZX	0TFD4ZZ	0THD7YZ	0TPB7DZ	0TWBXCZ
0SWCXKZ	0SWMX3Z	0T777ZZ	0T9670Z	0TB43ZX	0TFD7ZZ	0THD81Z	0TPB7YZ	0TWBXDZ
0SWDX0Z	0SWMX4Z	0T780DZ	0T967ZX	0TB44ZX	0TFD8ZZ	0THD82Z	0TPB80Z	0TWBXJZ
0SWDX3Z	0SWMX5Z	0T783DZ	0T9680Z	0TB47ZX	0TFDXZZ	0THD83Z	0TPB82Z	0TWBXKZ
0SWDX4Z	0SWMX7Z	0T784DZ	0T968ZX	0TB48ZX	0TH501Z	0THD8YZ	0TPB83Z	0TWBXLZ
0SWDX5Z	0SWMX8Z	0T787DZ	0T9700Z	0TB63ZX	0TH503Z	0THDX3Z	0TPB8DZ	0TWBXMZ
0SWDX7Z	0SWMXJZ	0T787ZZ	0T9730Z	0TB64ZX	0TH531Z	0THD8YZ	0TPBX0Z	0TWD3YZ
0SWDX8Z	0SWMXKZ	0T788ZZ	0T973ZX	0TB67ZX	0TH533Z	0TJ53ZZ	0TPBX2Z	0TWD4YZ
0SWDXJC	0SWNX0Z	0T7B7DZ	0T973ZZ	0TB68ZX	0TH53YZ	0TJ54ZZ	0TPBX3Z	0TWD7YZ
0SWDXJZ	0SWNX3Z	0T7B7ZZ	0T9740Z	0TB73ZX	0TH541Z	0TJ57ZZ	0TPBXDZ	0TWD8YZ
0SWDXKZ	0SWNX4Z	0T7C0DZ	0T974ZX	0TB74ZX	0TH543Z	0TJ58ZZ	0TPBXLZ	0TWDX0Z
0SWEXJZ	0SWNX5Z	0T7C0ZZ	0T9770Z	0TB77ZX	0TH54YZ	0TJ5XZZ	0TPD3YZ	0TWDX2Z
0SWFX0Z	0SWNX7Z	0T7C3DZ	0T977ZX	0TB78ZX	0TH571Z	0TJ93ZZ	0TPD4YZ	0TWDX3Z
0SWFX3Z	0SWNX8Z	0T7C3ZZ	0T9780Z	0TBD0ZX	0TH572Z	0TJ94ZZ	0TPD70Z	0TWDX7Z
0SWFX4Z	0SWNXJZ	0T7C4DZ	0T978ZX	0TBD3ZX	0TH573Z	0TJ97ZZ	0TPD72Z	0TWDXCZ
0SWFX5Z	0SWNXKZ	0T7C4ZZ	0T9800Z	0TBD4ZX	0TH57YZ	0TJ98ZZ	0TPD73Z	0TWDXDZ
0SWFX7Z	0SWPX0Z	0T7C7DZ	0T9830Z	0TBD7ZX	0TH581Z	0TJ9XZZ	0TPD7DZ	0TWDXJZ
0SWFX8Z	0SWPX3Z	0T7C7ZZ	0T983ZX	0TBD8ZX	0TH582Z	0TJB3ZZ	0TPD7YZ	0TWDXKZ
0SWFXJZ	0SWPX4Z	0T7C8DZ	0T983ZZ	0TBDXZX	0TH583Z	0TJB7ZZ	0TPD80Z	0TWDXLZ
0SWFXKZ	0SWPX5Z	0T7C8ZZ	0T9840Z	0TCB7ZZ	0TH901Z	0TJB8ZZ	0TPD82Z	0U23X0Z
0SWGX0Z	0SWPX7Z	0T7D0DZ	0T984ZX	0TCB8ZZ	0TH903Z	0TJBXZZ	0TPD83Z	0U23XYZ
0SWGX3Z	0SWPX8Z	0T7D3DZ	0T9870Z	0TCC7ZZ	0TH931Z	0TJD3ZZ	0TPD8DZ	0U28X0Z
0SWGX4Z	0SWPXJZ	0T7D4DZ	0T987ZX	0TCC8ZZ	0TH933Z	0TJD4ZZ	0TPD8YZ	0U28XYZ
0SWGX5Z	0SWPXKZ	0T7D7DZ	0T9880Z	0TCD7ZZ	0TH93YZ	0TJD7ZZ	0TPDX0Z	0U2DX0Z
0SWGX7Z	0SWQX0Z	0T7D7ZZ	0T988ZX	0TCD8ZZ	0TH941Z	0TJD8ZZ	0TPDX2Z	0U2DXHZ
0SWGX8Z	0SWQX3Z	0T7D8DZ	0T9B30Z	0TCDXZZ	0TH943Z	0TJDXZZ	0TPDX3Z	0U2DXYZ
0SWGXJZ	0SWQX4Z	0T7D8ZZ	0T9B3ZZ	0TF30ZZ	0TH94YZ	0TP53YZ	0TPDXDZ	0U2HX0Z
0SWGXKZ	0SWQX5Z	0T9030Z	0T9B40Z	0TF37ZZ	0TH971Z	0TP54YZ	0TTD4ZZ	0U2HXGZ
0SWHX0Z	0SWQX7Z	0T903ZX	0T9B4ZZ	0TF38ZZ	0TH972Z	0TP570Z	0TTD7ZZ	0U2HXYZ
0SWHX3Z	0SWQX8Z	0T903ZZ	0T9B70Z	0TF3XZZ	0TH973Z	0TP572Z	0TTD8ZZ	0U2MX0Z
0SWHX4Z	0SWQXJZ	0T904ZX	0T9B7ZZ	0TF40ZZ	0TH97YZ	0TP573Z	0TW53YZ	0U2MXYZ
0SWHX5Z	0SWQXKZ	0T904ZZ	0T9B80Z	0TF47ZZ	0TH981Z	0TP57DZ	0TW54YZ	0U7C0DZ
0SWHX7Z	0SWRXJZ	0T907ZX	0T9B8ZZ	0TF48ZZ	0TH982Z	0TP57YZ	0TW57YZ	0U7C0ZZ
0SWHX8Z	0SWSXJZ	0T908ZX	0T9C30Z	0TF4XZZ	0TH983Z	0TP580Z	0TW5X0Z	0U7C3DZ
0SWHXJZ	0SWTXJZ	0T9130Z	0T9C3ZZ	0TF60ZZ	0THB01Z	0TP582Z	0TW5X2Z	0U7C3ZZ
0SWHXKZ	0SWUXJZ	0T913ZX	0T9C40Z	0TF63ZZ	0THB03Z	0TP583Z	0TW5X3Z	0U7C4DZ
0SWJX0Z	0SWVXJZ	0T913ZZ	0T9C4ZZ	0TF64ZZ	0THB31Z	0TP58DZ	0TW5X7Z	0U7C4ZZ
0SWJX3Z	0SWWXJZ	0T914ZX	0T9C70Z	0TF67ZZ	0THB33Z	0TP5X0Z	0TW5XCZ	0U7C7DZ
0SWJX4Z	0T25X0Z	0T914ZZ	0T9C7ZZ	0TF68ZZ	0THB3YZ	0TP5X2Z	0TW5XDZ	0U7C7ZZ
0SWJX5Z	0T25XYZ	0T917ZX	0T9C80Z	0TF6XZZ	0THB41Z	0TP5X3Z	0TW5XJZ	0U7C8DZ
0SWJX7Z	0T29X0Z	0T918ZX	0T9C8ZZ	0TF70ZZ	0THB43Z	0TP5XDZ	0TW5XKZ	0U7C8ZZ
0SWJX8Z	0T29XYZ	0T9330Z	0T9D0ZX	0TF73ZZ	0THB4YZ	0TP93YZ	0TW93YZ	0U7G7DZ
0SWJXJZ	0T2BX0Z	0T933ZX	0T9D30Z	0TF74ZZ	0THB71Z	0TP94YZ	0TW94YZ	0U7G7ZZ
0SWJXKZ	0T2BXYZ	0T933ZZ	0T9D3ZX	0TF77ZZ	0THB72Z	0TP970Z	0TW97YZ	0U7G8DZ
0SWKX0Z	0T2DX0Z	0T934ZX	0T9D3ZZ	0TF78ZZ	0THB73Z	0TP972Z	0TW9X0Z	0U7G8ZZ
0SWKX3Z	0T2DXYZ	0T934ZZ	0T9D4ZX	0TF7XZZ	0THB7YZ	0TP973Z	0TW9X2Z	0U8K7ZZ
0SWKX4Z	0T5D0ZZ	0T937ZX	0T9D7ZX	0TFB0ZZ	0THB81Z	0TP97DZ	0TW9X3Z	0U8K8ZZ
0SWKX5Z	0T5D3ZZ	0T938ZX	0T9D8ZX	0TFB3ZZ	0THB82Z	0TP97YZ	0TW9X7Z	0U8KXZZ
0SWKX7Z	0T5D4ZZ	0T9430Z	0T9DXZX	0TFB4ZZ	0THB83Z	0TP980Z	0TW9XCZ	0U9030Z
0SWKX8Z	0T5D7ZZ	0T943ZX	0TB03ZX	0TFB7ZZ	0THD01Z	0TP982Z	0TW9XDZ	0U903ZZ
0SWKXJZ	0T5D8ZZ	0T943ZZ	0TB04ZX	0TFB8ZZ	0THD03Z	0TP983Z	0TW9XJZ	0U9080Z
0SWKXKZ	0T5DXZZ	0T944ZX	0TB07ZX	0TFBXZZ	0THD31Z	0TP98DZ	0TW9XKZ	0U908ZX
0SWLX0Z	0T760DZ	0T944ZZ	0TB08ZX	0TFC0ZZ	0THD33Z	0TP9X0Z	0TW9XMZ	0U908ZZ
0SWLX3Z	0T763DZ	0T947ZX	0TB13ZX	0TFC3ZZ	0THD3YZ	0TP9X2Z	0TWB3YZ	0U9130Z
0SWLX4Z	0T764DZ	0T948ZX	0TB14ZX	0TFC4ZZ	0THD41Z	0TP9X3Z	0TWB4YZ	0U913ZZ
0SWLX5Z	0T767DZ	0T9600Z	0TB17ZX	0TFC7ZZ	0THD43Z	0TP9XDZ	0TWB7YZ	0U9180Z
0SWLX7Z	0T767ZZ	0T9630Z	0TB18ZX	0TFC8ZZ	0THD4YZ	0TPB3YZ	0TWBX0Z	0U918ZX
0SWLX8Z	0T770DZ	0T963ZX	0TB33ZX	0TFCXZZ	0THD71Z	0TPB4YZ	0TWBX2Z	0U918ZZ
0SWLXJZ	0T773DZ	0T963ZZ	0TB34ZX	0TFD0ZZ	0THD72Z	0TPB70Z	0TWBX3Z	0U9230Z
0SWLXKZ	0T774DZ	0T9640Z	0TB37ZX	0TFD3ZZ	0THD73Z	0TPB73Z	0TWBX7Z	0U923ZZ

0U9280Z	0UCMXZZ	0UJ87ZZ	0UPH8YZ	0V2MX0Z	0V960ZX	0V9H4ZX	0VB53ZZ	0VBQ3ZZ
0U928ZX	0UF5XZZ	0UJ88ZZ	0UPHX0Z	0V2MXYZ	0V960ZZ	0V9H4ZZ	0VB54ZX	0VBQ4ZX
0U928ZZ	0UF6XZZ	0UJ8XZZ	0UPHX1Z	0V2RX0Z	0V9630Z	0V9J0ZX	0VB54ZZ	0VBQ4ZZ
0U9430Z	0UF7XZZ	0UJD3ZZ	0UPHX3Z	0V2RXYZ	0V963ZX	0V9J30Z	0VB5XZX	0VBQ8ZX
0U943ZZ	0UF9XZZ	0UJD7ZZ	0UPHXDZ	0V2SX0Z	0V963ZZ	0V9J3ZX	0VB5XZZ	0VBQ8ZZ
0U9480Z	0UH301Z	0UJD8ZZ	0UPMX0Z	0V2SXYZ	0V9640Z	0V9J3ZZ	0VB60ZX	0VC53ZZ
0U948ZX	0UH303Z	0UJDXZZ	0UQG7ZZ	0V550ZZ	0V964ZX	0V9J4ZX	0VB63ZX	0VC54ZZ
0U948ZZ	0UH30YZ	0UJH3ZZ	0UQGXZZ	0V553ZZ	0V964ZZ	0V9K0ZX	0VB64ZX	0VC5XZZ
0U9530Z	0UH331Z	0UJH7ZZ	0UQKXZZ	0V554ZZ	0V9700Z	0V9K30Z	0VB70ZX	0VC60ZZ
0U953ZZ	0UH333Z	0UJH8ZZ	0UQMXZZ	0V55XZZ	0V970ZX	0V9K3ZX	0VB73ZX	0VC63ZZ
0U954ZZ	0UH33YZ	0UJHXZZ	0US9XZZ	0V5N0ZZ	0V970ZZ	0V9K3ZZ	0VB74ZX	0VC64ZZ
0U957ZZ	0UH341Z	0UJMXZZ	0UW33YZ	0V5N3ZZ	0V9730Z	0V9K4ZX	0VB93ZX	0VC70ZZ
0U958ZZ	0UH343Z	0UP33YZ	0UW34YZ	0V5N4ZZ	0V973ZX	0V9L0ZX	0VB94ZX	0VC73ZZ
0U9630Z	0UH34YZ	0UP34YZ	0UW37YZ	0V5N8ZZ	0V973ZZ	0V9L30Z	0VBB3ZX	0VC74ZZ
0U963ZZ	0UH371Z	0UP37YZ	0UW38YZ	0V5P0ZZ	0V9740Z	0V9L3ZX	0VBB4ZX	0VCN0ZZ
0U964ZZ	0UH37YZ	0UP38YZ	0UW3X0Z	0V5P3ZZ	0V974ZX	0V9L3ZZ	0VBC3ZX	0VCN3ZZ
0U967ZZ	0UH381Z	0UP3X0Z	0UW3X3Z	0V5P4ZZ	0V974ZZ	0V9L4ZX	0VBC4ZX	0VCN4ZZ
0U968ZZ	0UH38YZ	0UP3X3Z	0UW83YZ	0V5P8ZZ	0V9930Z	0V9N00Z	0VBF0ZX	0VCP0ZZ
0U9730Z	0UH803Z	0UP83YZ	0UW84YZ	0V5Q0ZZ	0V993ZX	0V9N0ZX	0VBF3ZX	0VCP3ZZ
0U973ZZ	0UH80YZ	0UP84YZ	0UW87YZ	0V5Q3ZZ	0V993ZZ	0V9N0ZZ	0VBF4ZX	0VCP4ZZ
0U974ZZ	0UH833Z	0UP870Z	0UW88YZ	0V5Q4ZZ	0V9940Z	0V9N30Z	0VBF8ZX	0VCQ0ZZ
0U977ZZ	0UH83YZ	0UP873Z	0UW8X0Z	0V5Q8ZZ	0V994ZX	0V9N3ZX	0VBG0ZX	0VCQ3ZZ
0U978ZZ	0UH843Z	0UP87DZ	0UW8X3Z	0V9030Z	0V994ZZ	0V9N3ZZ	0VBG3ZX	0VCQ4ZZ
0U9930Z	0UH84YZ	0UP87YZ	0UW8X7Z	0V903ZX	0V9B30Z	0V9N40Z	0VBG4ZX	0VCSXZZ
0U993ZZ	0UH873Z	0UP880Z	0UW8XCZ	0V903ZZ	0V9B3ZX	0V9N4ZX	0VBG8ZX	0VH403Z
0U9C30Z	0UH87YZ	0UP883Z	0UW8XDZ	0V9040Z	0V9B3ZZ	0V9N4ZZ	0VBH0ZX	0VH40YZ
0U9C3ZZ	0UH883Z	0UP88DZ	0UW8XJZ	0V904ZX	0V9B40Z	0V9P00Z	0VBH3ZX	0VH433Z
0U9F30Z	0UH88YZ	0UP88YZ	0UW8XKZ	0V904ZZ	0V9B4ZX	0V9P0ZX	0VBH4ZX	0VH43YZ
0U9F3ZZ	0UH901Z	0UP8X0Z	0UWD3YZ	0V907ZX	0V9B4ZZ	0V9P0ZZ	0VBH8ZX	0VH443Z
0U9F40Z	0UH90HZ	0UP8X3Z	0UWD4YZ	0V908ZX	0V9C30Z	0V9P30Z	0VBJ0ZX	0VH44YZ
0U9F4ZZ	0UH971Z	0UP8XDZ	0UWD7YZ	0V9130Z	0V9C3ZX	0V9P3ZX	0VBJ3ZX	0VH473Z
0U9G30Z	0UH97HZ	0UPD3CZ	0UWD8YZ	0V913ZX	0V9C3ZZ	0V9P3ZZ	0VBJ4ZX	0VH47YZ
0U9G3ZZ	0UH981Z	0UPD3YZ	0UWDX0Z	0V913ZZ	0V9C40Z	0V9P40Z	0VBJ8ZX	0VH483Z
0U9K00Z	0UH98HZ	0UPD4CZ	0UWDX3Z	0V9140Z	0V9C4ZX	0V9P4ZX	0VBK0ZX	0VH48YZ
0U9K0ZZ	0UHC7HZ	0UPD4YZ	0UWDX7Z	0V914ZX	0V9C4ZZ	0V9P4ZZ	0VBK3ZX	0VH803Z
0U9K30Z	0UHC8HZ	0UPD70Z	0UWDXCZ	0V914ZZ	0V9F00Z	0V9Q00Z	0VBK4ZX	0VH80YZ
0U9K3ZZ	0UHD03Z	0UPD73Z	0UWDXDZ	0V9230Z	0V9F0ZX	0V9Q0ZX	0VBK8ZX	0VH833Z
0U9K40Z	0UHD0YZ	0UPD7CZ	0UWDXHZ	0V923ZX	0V9F0ZZ	0V9Q0ZZ	0VBL0ZX	0VH83YZ
0U9K4ZZ	0UHD33Z	0UPD7DZ	0UWDXJZ	0V923ZZ	0V9F30Z	0V9Q30Z	0VBL3ZX	0VH843Z
0U9K70Z	0UHD3YZ	0UPD7HZ	0UWDXKZ	0V9240Z	0V9F3ZX	0V9Q3ZX	0VBL4ZX	0VH84YZ
0U9K7ZZ	0UHD43Z	0UPD7YZ	0UWH3YZ	0V924ZX	0V9F3ZZ	0V9Q3ZZ	0VBL8ZX	0VH873Z
0U9K80Z	0UHD4YZ	0UPD80Z	0UWH4YZ	0V924ZZ	0V9F40Z	0V9Q40Z	0VBN0ZX	0VH87YZ
0U9K8ZZ	0UHD73Z	0UPD83Z	0UWH7YZ	0V9330Z	0V9F4ZX	0V9Q4ZX	0VBN0ZZ	0VH883Z
0U9KX0Z	0UHD7YZ	0UPD8CZ	0UWH8YZ	0V933ZX	0V9F4ZZ	0V9Q4ZZ	0VBN3ZX	0VH88YZ
0U9KXZZ	0UHD83Z	0UPD8DZ	0UWHX0Z	0V933ZZ	0V9G00Z	0V9S30Z	0VBN3ZZ	0VHD01Z
0U9L00Z	0UHD8YZ	0UPD8HZ	0UWHX3Z	0V9340Z	0V9G0ZX	0V9S3ZZ	0VBN4ZX	0VHD03Z
0U9L0ZZ	0UHF7GZ	0UPD8YZ	0UWHX7Z	0V934ZX	0V9G0ZZ	0V9T30Z	0VBN4ZZ	0VHD0YZ
0U9LX0Z	0UHF8GZ	0UPDX0Z	0UWHXDZ	0V934ZZ	0V9G30Z	0V9T3ZZ	0VBN8ZX	0VHD31Z
0U9LXZZ	0UHG7GZ	0UPDX3Z	0UWHXJZ	0V9500Z	0V9G3ZX	0VB03ZX	0VBN8ZZ	0VHD33Z
0UC97ZZ	0UHG8GZ	0UPDXDZ	0UWHXKZ	0V950ZX	0V9G3ZZ	0VB04ZX	0VBP0ZX	0VHD3YZ
0UC98ZZ	0UHH3YZ	0UPDXHZ	0UWMX0Z	0V9530Z	0V9G40Z	0VB07ZX	0VBP0ZZ	0VHD41Z
0UCG7ZZ	0UHH4YZ	0UPH3YZ	0UWMX7Z	0V953ZX	0V9G4ZX	0VB08ZX	0VBP3ZX	0VHD43Z
0UCG8ZZ	0UHH73Z	0UPH4YZ	0UWMXJZ	0V953ZZ	0V9G4ZZ	0VB13ZX	0VBP3ZZ	0VHD4YZ
0UCGXZZ	0UHH7YZ	0UPH70Z	0UWMXKZ	0V9540Z	0V9H00Z	0VB14ZX	0VBP4ZX	0VHD71Z
0UCK0ZZ	0UHH83Z	0UPH73Z	0V24X0Z	0V954ZX	0V9H0ZX	0VB23ZX	0VBP4ZZ	0VHD73Z
0UCK3ZZ	0UHH8YZ	0UPH7DZ	0V24XYZ	0V954ZZ	0V9H0ZZ	0VB24ZX	0VBP8ZX	0VHD7YZ
0UCK4ZZ	0UJ33ZZ	0UPH7YZ	0V28X0Z	0V95X0Z	0V9H30Z	0VB33ZX	0VBP8ZZ	0VHD81Z
0UCK7ZZ	0UJ38ZZ	0UPH80Z	0V28XYZ	0V95XZX	0V9H3ZX	0VB34ZX	0VBQ0ZX	0VHD83Z
0UCK8ZZ	0UJ3XZZ	0UPH83Z	0V2DX0Z	0V95XZZ	0V9H3ZZ	0VB50ZX	0VBQ0ZZ	0VHD8YZ
0UCKXZZ	0UJ83ZZ	0UPH8DZ	0V2DXYZ	0V9600Z	0V9H40Z	0VB53ZX	0VBQ3ZX	0VHM03Z

0VHM0YZ	0VLG3ZZ	0VP47YZ	0VPR03Z	0VT54ZZ	0VWD7YZ	0VWRXCZ	0W1J0JY	0W914ZX
0VHM33Z	0VLG4CZ	0VP480Z	0VPR07Z	0VT5XZZ	0VWD8YZ	0VWRXDZ	0W1J3J4	0W914ZZ
0VHM3YZ	0VLG4DZ	0VP483Z	0VPR0CZ	0VTN0ZZ	0VWDX0Z	0VWRXJZ	0W1J3JW	0W920ZX
0VHM43Z	0VLG4ZZ	0VP48YZ	0VPR0JZ	0VTN4ZZ	0VWDX3Z	0VWRXKZ	0W1J3JY	0W9230Z
0VHM4YZ	0VLG8CZ	0VP4X0Z	0VPR0KZ	0VTP0ZZ	0VWDX7Z	0VWS3YZ	0W1J4J4	0W923ZX
0VHM73Z	0VLG8DZ	0VP4X1Z	0VPR0YZ	0VTP4ZZ	0VWDXJZ	0VWS4YZ	0W1J4JW	0W923ZZ
0VHM7YZ	0VLG8ZZ	0VP4X3Z	0VPR30Z	0VTQ0ZZ	0VWDXKZ	0VWS7YZ	0W1J4JY	0W924ZX
0VHM83Z	0VLH0CZ	0VP800Z	0VPR33Z	0VTQ4ZZ	0VWM3YZ	0VWS8YZ	0W20X0Z	0W930ZX
0VHM8YZ	0VLH0DZ	0VP803Z	0VPR37Z	0VTT0ZZ	0VWM4YZ	0VWSX0Z	0W20XYZ	0W9330Z
0VHR03Z	0VLH0ZZ	0VP807Z	0VPR3CZ	0VTT4ZZ	0VWM7YZ	0VWSX3Z	0W21X0Z	0W933ZX
0VHR0YZ	0VLH3CZ	0VP80JZ	0VPR3JZ	0VTTXZZ	0VWM8YZ	0VWSX7Z	0W21XYZ	0W933ZZ
0VHR33Z	0VLH3DZ	0VP80KZ	0VPR3KZ	0VUSX7Z	0VWMX0Z	0VWSXJZ	0W22X0Z	0W934ZX
0VHR3YZ	0VLH3ZZ	0VP80YZ	0VPR3YZ	0VUSXJZ	0VWMX3Z	0VWSXKZ	0W22XYZ	0W940ZX
0VHR43Z	0VLH4CZ	0VP830Z	0VPR40Z	0VUSXKZ	0VWMX7Z	0VY50Z0	0W24X0Z	0W9430Z
0VHR4YZ	0VLH4DZ	0VP833Z	0VPR43Z	0VW43YZ	0VWMXCZ	0VY50Z1	0W24XYZ	0W943ZX
0VHR73Z	0VLH4ZZ	0VP837Z	0VPR47Z	0VW44YZ	0VWMXJZ	0VY50Z2	0W25X0Z	0W943ZZ
0VHR7YZ	0VLH8CZ	0VP83JZ	0VPR4CZ	0VW47YZ	0VWMXKZ	0VYS0Z0	0W25XYZ	0W944ZX
0VHR83Z	0VLH8DZ	0VP83KZ	0VPR4JZ	0VW48YZ	0VWR00Z	0VYS0Z1	0W26X0Z	0W950ZX
0VHR8YZ	0VLH8ZZ	0VP83YZ	0VPR4KZ	0VW4X0Z	0VWR03Z	0VYS0Z2	0W26XYZ	0W9530Z
0VHS03Z	0VLN0CZ	0VP840Z	0VPR4YZ	0VW4X3Z	0VWR07Z	0W190J4	0W28X0Z	0W953ZX
0VHS0YZ	0VLN0ZZ	0VP843Z	0VPR70Z	0VW4X7Z	0VWR0CZ	0W190JG	0W28XYZ	0W953ZZ
0VHS33Z	0VLN3CZ	0VP847Z	0VPR73Z	0VW4XJZ	0VWR0DZ	0W190JW	0W29X0Z	0W954ZX
0VHS3YZ	0VLN3ZZ	0VP84JZ	0VPR77Z	0VW4XKZ	0VWR0JZ	0W190JY	0W29XYZ	0W960ZX
0VHS43Z	0VLN4CZ	0VP84KZ	0VPR7CZ	0VW800Z	0VWR0KZ	0W193J4	0W2BX0Z	0W9630Z
0VHS4YZ	0VLN4ZZ	0VP84YZ	0VPR7DZ	0VW803Z	0VWR0YZ	0W193JG	0W2BXYZ	0W963ZX
0VHS7YZ	0VLN8CZ	0VP870Z	0VPR7JZ	0VW807Z	0VWR30Z	0W193JW	0W2CX0Z	0W963ZZ
0VHS8YZ	0VLN8ZZ	0VP873Z	0VPR7KZ	0VW80JZ	0VWR33Z	0W193JY	0W2CXYZ	0W964ZX
0VHSX3Z	0VLP0CZ	0VP877Z	0VPR7YZ	0VW80KZ	0VWR37Z	0W194J4	0W2DX0Z	0W9800Z
0VJ43ZZ	0VLP0ZZ	0VP87JZ	0VPR80Z	0VW80YZ	0VWR3CZ	0W194JG	0W2DXYZ	0W980ZX
0VJ4XZZ	0VLP3CZ	0VP87KZ	0VPR83Z	0VW830Z	0VWR3DZ	0W194JW	0W2FX0Z	0W980ZZ
0VJ80ZZ	0VLP3ZZ	0VP87YZ	0VPR87Z	0VW833Z	0VWR3JZ	0W194JY	0W2FXYZ	0W9830Z
0VJ83ZZ	0VLP4CZ	0VP880Z	0VPR8CZ	0VW837Z	0VWR3KZ	0W1B0J4	0W2GX0Z	0W983ZX
0VJ84ZZ	0VLP4ZZ	0VP883Z	0VPR8DZ	0VW83JZ	0VWR3YZ	0W1B0JG	0W2GXYZ	0W983ZZ
0VJ8XZZ	0VLP8CZ	0VP887Z	0VPR8JZ	0VW83KZ	0VWR40Z	0W1B0JW	0W2HX0Z	0W9840Z
0VJD3ZZ	0VLP8ZZ	0VP88JZ	0VPR8KZ	0VW83YZ	0VWR43Z	0W1B0JY	0W2HXYZ	0W984ZX
0VJDXZZ	0VLQ0CZ	0VP88KZ	0VPR8YZ	0VW840Z	0VWR47Z	0W1B3J4	0W2JX0Z	0W984ZZ
0VJM3ZZ	0VLQ0ZZ	0VP88YZ	0VPRX0Z	0VW843Z	0VWR4CZ	0W1B3JG	0W2JXYZ	0W9900Z
0VJMXZZ	0VLQ3CZ	0VP8X0Z	0VPRX3Z	0VW847Z	0VWR4DZ	0W1B3JW	0W2KX0Z	0W990ZX
0VJR3ZZ	0VLQ3ZZ	0VP8X3Z	0VPRXDZ	0VW84JZ	0VWR4JZ	0W1B3JY	0W2KXYZ	0W990ZZ
0VJRXZZ	0VLQ4CZ	0VPD3YZ	0VPS3YZ	0VW84KZ	0VWR4KZ	0W1B4J4	0W2LX0Z	0W9930Z
0VJS3ZZ	0VLQ4ZZ	0VPD4YZ	0VPS4YZ	0VW84YZ	0VWR4YZ	0W1B4JG	0W2LXYZ	0W993ZX
0VJS4ZZ	0VLQ8CZ	0VPD70Z	0VPS70Z	0VW870Z	0VWR70Z	0W1B4JW	0W2MX0Z	0W993ZZ
0VJSXZZ	0VLQ8ZZ	0VPD73Z	0VPS73Z	0VW873Z	0VWR73Z	0W1B4JY	0W2MXYZ	0W9B00Z
0VLF0CZ	0VN90ZZ	0VPD7YZ	0VPS7YZ	0VW877Z	0VWR77Z	0W1G0J6	0W2NX0Z	0W9B0ZX
0VLF0DZ	0VN93ZZ	0VPD80Z	0VPS80Z	0VW87JZ	0VWR7CZ	0W1G0J9	0W2NXYZ	0W9B0ZZ
0VLF0ZZ	0VN94ZZ	0VPD83Z	0VPS83Z	0VW87KZ	0VWR7DZ	0W1G0JB	0W3P8ZZ	0W9B30Z
0VLF3CZ	0VNB0ZZ	0VPD8YZ	0VPS8YZ	0VW87YZ	0VWR7JZ	0W1G0JG	0W8NXZZ	0W9B3ZX
0VLF3DZ	0VNB3ZZ	0VPDX0Z	0VPSX0Z	0VW880Z	0VWR7KZ	0W1G0JJ	0W9000Z	0W9B3ZZ
0VLF3ZZ	0VNB4ZZ	0VPDX3Z	0VPSX3Z	0VW883Z	0VWR7YZ	0W1G3J6	0W900ZX	0W9C30Z
0VLF4CZ	0VNC0ZZ	0VPM3YZ	0VQ50ZZ	0VW887Z	0VWR80Z	0W1G3J9	0W900ZZ	0W9C3ZX
0VLF4DZ	0VNC3ZZ	0VPM4YZ	0VQ53ZZ	0VW88JZ	0VWR83Z	0W1G3JB	0W9030Z	0W9C3ZZ
0VLF4ZZ	0VNC4ZZ	0VPM70Z	0VQ54ZZ	0VW88KZ	0VWR87Z	0W1G3JG	0W903ZX	0W9C4ZX
0VLF8CZ	0VNT0ZZ	0VPM73Z	0VQ5XZZ	0VW88YZ	0VWR8CZ	0W1G3JJ	0W903ZZ	0W9D30Z
0VLF8DZ	0VNT3ZZ	0VPM7YZ	0VQ60ZZ	0VW8X0Z	0VWR8DZ	0W1G4J6	0W9040Z	0W9D3ZX
0VLF8ZZ	0VNT4ZZ	0VPM80Z	0VQ63ZZ	0VW8X3Z	0VWR8JZ	0W1G4J9	0W904ZX	0W9D3ZZ
0VLG0CZ	0VNTXZZ	0VPM83Z	0VQ64ZZ	0VW8X7Z	0VWR8KZ	0W1G4JB	0W904ZZ	0W9F30Z
0VLG0DZ	0VP43YZ	0VPM8YZ	0VQ70ZZ	0VW8XJZ	0VWR8YZ	0W1G4JG	0W9130Z	0W9F3ZZ
0VLG0ZZ	0VP44YZ	0VPMX0Z	0VQ73ZZ	0VW8XKZ	0VWRX0Z	0W1G4JJ	0W913ZX	0W9F40Z
0VLG3CZ	0VP470Z	0VPMX3Z	0VQ74ZZ	0VWD3YZ	0VWRX3Z	0W1J0J4	0W913ZZ	0W9F4ZZ
0VLG3DZ	0VP473Z	0VPR00Z	0VT50ZZ	0VWD4YZ	0VWRX7Z	0W1J0JW	0W9140Z	0W9G30Z

0W9G3ZX	0WB5XZX	0WFJ0ZZ	0WHR73Z	0WP00YZ	0WP40JZ	0WP631Z	0WP943Z	0WPJ4JZ
0W9G3ZZ	0WB60ZX	0WFJ3ZZ	0WHR7YZ	0WP030Z	0WP40KZ	0WP633Z	0WP94JZ	0WPJ4YZ
0W9H30Z	0WB63ZX	0WFJ4ZZ	0WHR83Z	0WP031Z	0WP40YZ	0WP637Z	0WP94YZ	0WPJX0Z
0W9H3ZZ	0WB64ZX	0WFJXZZ	0WHR8YZ	0WP033Z	0WP430Z	0WP63JZ	0WP9X0Z	0WPJX1Z
0W9J30Z	0WB6XZX	0WFP0ZZ	0WJ03ZZ	0WP037Z	0WP431Z	0WP63KZ	0WP9X1Z	0WPJX3Z
0W9J3ZX	0WB80ZX	0WFP3ZZ	0WJ04ZZ	0WP03JZ	0WP433Z	0WP63YZ	0WP9X3Z	0WPK00Z
0W9J3ZZ	0WB83ZX	0WFP4ZZ	0WJ0XZZ	0WP03KZ	0WP437Z	0WP640Z	0WPB00Z	0WPK01Z
0W9J70Z	0WB84ZX	0WFP7ZZ	0WJ13ZZ	0WP03YZ	0WP43JZ	0WP641Z	0WPB01Z	0WPK03Z
0W9J7ZX	0WB8XZX	0WFP8ZZ	0WJ23ZZ	0WP040Z	0WP43KZ	0WP643Z	0WPB03Z	0WPK07Z
0W9J7ZZ	0WBH3ZX	0WFPXZZ	0WJ24ZZ	0WP041Z	0WP43YZ	0WP647Z	0WPB0JZ	0WPK0JZ
0W9J80Z	0WBH4ZX	0WFQXZZ	0WJ2XZZ	0WP043Z	0WP440Z	0WP64JZ	0WPB0YZ	0WPK0KZ
0W9J8ZZ	0WBK0ZX	0WFR0ZZ	0WJ30ZZ	0WP047Z	0WP441Z	0WP64KZ	0WPB30Z	0WPK0YZ
0W9K00Z	0WBK3ZX	0WFR3ZZ	0WJ33ZZ	0WP04JZ	0WP443Z	0WP64YZ	0WPB31Z	0WPK30Z
0W9K0ZX	0WBK4ZX	0WFR4ZZ	0WJ34ZZ	0WP04KZ	0WP447Z	0WP6X0Z	0WPB33Z	0WPK31Z
0W9K0ZZ	0WBKXZX	0WFR7ZZ	0WJ3XZZ	0WP04YZ	0WP44JZ	0WP6X1Z	0WPB3JZ	0WPK33Z
0W9K30Z	0WBL0ZX	0WFR8ZZ	0WJ43ZZ	0WP0X0Z	0WP44KZ	0WP6X3Z	0WPB3YZ	0WPK37Z
0W9K3ZX	0WBL3ZX	0WFRXZZ	0WJ44ZZ	0WP0X1Z	0WP44YZ	0WP6X7Z	0WPB40Z	0WPK3JZ
0W9K3ZZ	0WBL4ZX	0WH103Z	0WJ4XZZ	0WP0X3Z	0WP4X0Z	0WP6XJZ	0WPB41Z	0WPK3KZ
0W9K40Z	0WBLXZX	0WH133Z	0WJ53ZZ	0WP0X7Z	0WP4X1Z	0WP6XKZ	0WPB43Z	0WPK3YZ
0W9K4ZX	0WBM0ZX	0WH143Z	0WJ54ZZ	0WP0XJZ	0WP4X3Z	0WP6XYZ	0WPB4JZ	0WPK40Z
0W9K4ZZ	0WBM3ZX	0WH803Z	0WJ5XZZ	0WP0XKZ	0WP4X7Z	0WP800Z	0WPB4YZ	0WPK41Z
0W9L00Z	0WBM4ZX	0WH80YZ	0WJ63ZZ	0WP0XYZ	0WP4XJZ	0WP801Z	0WPBX0Z	0WPK43Z
0W9L0ZX	0WBMXZX	0WH833Z	0WJ6XZZ	0WP103Z	0WP4XKZ	0WP803Z	0WPBX1Z	0WPK47Z
0W9L0ZZ	0WC1XZZ	0WH83YZ	0WJ83ZZ	0WP133Z	0WP4XYZ	0WP807Z	0WPBX3Z	0WPK4JZ
0W9L30Z	0WC3XZZ	0WH843Z	0WJ8XZZ	0WP143Z	0WP500Z	0WP80JZ	0WPCX0Z	0WPK4KZ
0W9L3ZX	0WC40ZZ	0WH84YZ	0WJ93ZZ	0WP1X0Z	0WP501Z	0WP80KZ	0WPCX1Z	0WPK4YZ
0W9L3ZZ	0WC43ZZ	0WH903Z	0WJB3ZZ	0WP1X1Z	0WP503Z	0WP80YZ	0WPCX3Z	0WPKX0Z
0W9L40Z	0WC44ZZ	0WH90YZ	0WJC3ZZ	0WP1X3Z	0WP507Z	0WP830Z	0WPCX7Z	0WPKX1Z
0W9L4ZX	0WC50ZZ	0WH933Z	0WJD0ZZ	0WP200Z	0WP50JZ	0WP831Z	0WPCXJZ	0WPKX3Z
0W9L4ZZ	0WC53ZZ	0WH93YZ	0WJD3ZZ	0WP201Z	0WP50KZ	0WP833Z	0WPCXKZ	0WPKX7Z
0W9M00Z	0WC54ZZ	0WH943Z	0WJF3ZZ	0WP203Z	0WP50YZ	0WP837Z	0WPCXYZ	0WPKXJZ
0W9M0ZX	0WC90ZZ	0WH94YZ	0WJFXZZ	0WP207Z	0WP530Z	0WP83JZ	0WPDX0Z	0WPKXKZ
0W9M0ZZ	0WC93ZZ	0WHB03Z	0WJG3ZZ	0WP20JZ	0WP531Z	0WP83KZ	0WPDX1Z	0WPKXYZ
0W9M30Z	0WC94ZZ	0WHB0YZ	0WJH3ZZ	0WP20KZ	0WP533Z	0WP83YZ	0WPDX3Z	0WPL00Z
0W9M3ZX	0WC9XZZ	0WHB33Z	0WJJ3ZZ	0WP20YZ	0WP537Z	0WP840Z	0WPFX0Z	0WPL01Z
0W9M3ZZ	0WCB0ZZ	0WHB3YZ	0WJK3ZZ	0WP230Z	0WP53JZ	0WP841Z	0WPFX1Z	0WPL03Z
0W9M40Z	0WCB3ZZ	0WHB43Z	0WJK4ZZ	0WP231Z	0WP53KZ	0WP843Z	0WPFX3Z	0WPL07Z
0W9M4ZX	0WCB4ZZ	0WHB4YZ	0WJKXZZ	0WP233Z	0WP53YZ	0WP847Z	0WPFX7Z	0WPL0JZ
0W9M4ZZ	0WCBXZZ	0WHG33Z	0WJL3ZZ	0WP237Z	0WP540Z	0WP84JZ	0WPFXJZ	0WPL0KZ
0W9N0ZX	0WCCXZZ	0WHP0YZ	0WJL4ZZ	0WP23JZ	0WP541Z	0WP84KZ	0WPFXKZ	0WPL0YZ
0W9N30Z	0WCDXZZ	0WHP33Z	0WJLXZZ	0WP23KZ	0WP543Z	0WP84YZ	0WPFXYZ	0WPL30Z
0W9N3ZX	0WCGXZZ	0WHP3YZ	0WJM3ZZ	0WP23YZ	0WP547Z	0WP8X0Z	0WPGX0Z	0WPL31Z
0W9N3ZZ	0WCHXZZ	0WHP43Z	0WJMXZZ	0WP240Z	0WP54JZ	0WP8X1Z	0WPGX1Z	0WPL33Z
0W9N4ZX	0WCJXZZ	0WHP4YZ	0WJN3ZZ	0WP241Z	0WP54KZ	0WP8X3Z	0WPGX3Z	0WPL37Z
0WB00ZX	0WCP7ZZ	0WHP73Z	0WJNXZZ	0WP243Z	0WP54YZ	0WP8X7Z	0WPHX0Z	0WPL3JZ
0WB03ZX	0WCP8ZZ	0WHP7YZ	0WJP3ZZ	0WP247Z	0WP5X0Z	0WP8XJZ	0WPHX1Z	0WPL3KZ
0WB04ZX	0WCPXZZ	0WHP83Z	0WJP7ZZ	0WP24JZ	0WP5X1Z	0WP8XKZ	0WPHX3Z	0WPL3YZ
0WB0XZX	0WCQ0ZZ	0WHP8YZ	0WJP8ZZ	0WP24KZ	0WP5X3Z	0WP8XYZ	0WPJ00Z	0WPL40Z
0WB20ZX	0WCQ3ZZ	0WHQ03Z	0WJQ3ZZ	0WP24YZ	0WP5X7Z	0WP900Z	0WPJ01Z	0WPL41Z
0WB23ZX	0WCQ4ZZ	0WHQ0YZ	0WJQ7ZZ	0WP2X0Z	0WP5XJZ	0WP901Z	0WPJ03Z	0WPL43Z
0WB24ZX	0WCQXZZ	0WHQ73Z	0WJQ8ZZ	0WP2X1Z	0WP5XKZ	0WP903Z	0WPJ0JZ	0WPL47Z
0WB2XZX	0WCR7ZZ	0WHQ7YZ	0WJR3ZZ	0WP2X3Z	0WP5XYZ	0WP90JZ	0WPJ0YZ	0WPL4JZ
0WB40ZX	0WCR8ZZ	0WHQ83Z	0WJR7ZZ	0WP2X7Z	0WP600Z	0WP90YZ	0WPJ30Z	0WPL4KZ
0WB43ZX	0WCRXZZ	0WHQ8YZ	0WJR8ZZ	0WP2XJZ	0WP601Z	0WP930Z	0WPJ31Z	0WPL4YZ
0WB44ZX	0WF1XZZ	0WHR03Z	0WP000Z	0WP2XKZ	0WP603Z	0WP931Z	0WPJ33Z	0WPLX0Z
0WB4XZX	0WF3XZZ	0WHR0YZ	0WP001Z	0WP2XYZ	0WP607Z	0WP933Z	0WPJ3JZ	0WPLX1Z
0WB50ZX	0WF9XZZ	0WHR33Z	0WP003Z	0WP400Z	0WP60JZ	0WP93JZ	0WPJ3YZ	0WPLX3Z
0WB53ZX	0WFBXZZ	0WHR3YZ	0WP007Z	0WP401Z	0WP60KZ	0WP93YZ	0WPJ40Z	0WPLX7Z
0WB54ZX	0WFCXZZ	0WHR43Z	0WP00JZ	0WP403Z	0WP60YZ	0WP940Z	0WPJ41Z	0WPLXJZ
	0WFGXZZ	0WHR4YZ	0WP00KZ	0WP407Z	0WP630Z	0WP941Z	0WPJ43Z	0WPLXKZ

0WPLXYZ	0WPR71Z	0WW837Z	0WWCX3Z	0WWP3YZ	0X940ZX	0X9B4ZX	0X9K3ZX	0XJ44ZZ
0WPM00Z	0WPR73Z	0WW83JZ	0WWCX7Z	0WWP41Z	0X940ZZ	0X9B4ZZ	0X9K3ZZ	0XJ4XZZ
0WPM01Z	0WPR7YZ	0WW83KZ	0WWCXJZ	0WWP43Z	0X9430Z	0X9C00Z	0X9K40Z	0XJ53ZZ
0WPM03Z	0WPR81Z	0WW83YZ	0WWCXKZ	0WWP4YZ	0X943ZX	0X9C0ZX	0X9K4ZX	0XJ54ZZ
0WPM0JZ	0WPR83Z	0WW840Z	0WWCXYZ	0WWP71Z	0X943ZZ	0X9C0ZZ	0X9K4ZZ	0XJ5XZZ
0WPM0YZ	0WPR8YZ	0WW841Z	0WWDX0Z	0WWP73Z	0X9440Z	0X9C30Z	0XB20ZX	0XJ63ZZ
0WPM30Z	0WPRX1Z	0WW843Z	0WWDX1Z	0WWP7YZ	0X944ZX	0X9C3ZX	0XB23ZX	0XJ64ZZ
0WPM31Z	0WPRX3Z	0WW847Z	0WWDX3Z	0WWP81Z	0X944ZZ	0X9C3ZZ	0XB24ZX	0XJ6XZZ
0WPM33Z	0WPRXYZ	0WW84JZ	0WWDXYZ	0WWP83Z	0X9500Z	0X9C40Z	0XB30ZX	0XJ73ZZ
0WPM3JZ	0WQNXZZ	0WW84KZ	0WWFX0Z	0WWP8YZ	0X950ZX	0X9C4ZX	0XB33ZX	0XJ74ZZ
0WPM3YZ	0WW0X0Z	0WW84YZ	0WWFX1Z	0WWPX1Z	0X950ZZ	0X9C4ZZ	0XB34ZX	0XJ7XZZ
0WPM40Z	0WW0X1Z	0WW8X0Z	0WWFX3Z	0WWPX3Z	0X9530Z	0X9D00Z	0XB40ZX	0XJ83ZZ
0WPM41Z	0WW0X3Z	0WW8X1Z	0WWFX7Z	0WWPXYZ	0X953ZX	0X9D0ZX	0XB43ZX	0XJ84ZZ
0WPM43Z	0WW0X7Z	0WW8X3Z	0WWFXJZ	0WWQ01Z	0X953ZZ	0X9D0ZZ	0XB44ZX	0XJ8XZZ
0WPM4JZ	0WW0XJZ	0WW8X7Z	0WWFXKZ	0WWQ03Z	0X9540Z	0X9D30Z	0XB50ZX	0XJ93ZZ
0WPM4YZ	0WW0XKZ	0WW8XJZ	0WWFXYZ	0WWQ0YZ	0X954ZX	0X9D3ZX	0XB53ZX	0XJ94ZZ
0WPMX0Z	0WW0XYZ	0WW8XKZ	0WWGX0Z	0WWQX1Z	0X954ZZ	0X9D3ZZ	0XB54ZX	0XJ9XZZ
0WPMX1Z	0WW1X0Z	0WW8XYZ	0WWGX1Z	0WWQX3Z	0X9600Z	0X9D40Z	0XB60ZX	0XJB3ZZ
0WPMX3Z	0WW1X1Z	0WW900Z	0WWGX3Z	0WWQXYZ	0X960ZX	0X9D4ZX	0XB63ZX	0XJB4ZZ
0WPMXYZ	0WW1X3Z	0WW901Z	0WWGXJZ	0WWR01Z	0X960ZZ	0X9D4ZZ	0XB64ZX	0XJBXZZ
0WPNX0Z	0WW1XJZ	0WW903Z	0WWGXYZ	0WWR03Z	0X9630Z	0X9F00Z	0XB70ZX	0XJC3ZZ
0WPNX1Z	0WW1XYZ	0WW90JZ	0WWHX0Z	0WWR0YZ	0X963ZX	0X9F0ZX	0XB73ZX	0XJC4ZZ
0WPNX3Z	0WW2X0Z	0WW90YZ	0WWHX1Z	0WWR31Z	0X963ZZ	0X9F0ZZ	0XB74ZX	0XJCXZZ
0WPNX7Z	0WW2X1Z	0WW930Z	0WWHX3Z	0WWR33Z	0X9640Z	0X9F30Z	0XB80ZX	0XJD3ZZ
0WPNXJZ	0WW2X3Z	0WW931Z	0WWHXYZ	0WWR3YZ	0X964ZX	0X9F3ZX	0XB83ZX	0XJD4ZZ
0WPNXKZ	0WW2X7Z	0WW933Z	0WWJX0Z	0WWR41Z	0X964ZZ	0X9F3ZZ	0XB84ZX	0XJDXZZ
0WPNXYZ	0WW2XJZ	0WW93JZ	0WWJX1Z	0WWR43Z	0X9700Z	0X9F40Z	0XB90ZX	0XJF3ZZ
0WPP31Z	0WW2XKZ	0WW93YZ	0WWJX3Z	0WWR4YZ	0X970ZX	0X9F4ZX	0XB93ZX	0XJF4ZZ
0WPP33Z	0WW2XYZ	0WW940Z	0WWJXJZ	0WWR71Z	0X970ZZ	0X9F4ZZ	0XB94ZX	0XJFXZZ
0WPP3YZ	0WW4X0Z	0WW941Z	0WWJXYZ	0WWR73Z	0X9730Z	0X9G00Z	0XBB0ZX	0XJG3ZZ
0WPP41Z	0WW4X1Z	0WW943Z	0WWKX0Z	0WWR7YZ	0X973ZX	0X9G0ZX	0XBB3ZX	0XJG4ZZ
0WPP43Z	0WW4X3Z	0WW94JZ	0WWKX1Z	0WWR81Z	0X973ZZ	0X9G0ZZ	0XBB4ZX	0XJGXZZ
0WPP4YZ	0WW4X7Z	0WW94YZ	0WWKX3Z	0WWR83Z	0X9740Z	0X9G30Z	0XBC0ZX	0XJH3ZZ
0WPP71Z	0WW4XJZ	0WW9X0Z	0WWKX7Z	0WWR8YZ	0X974ZX	0X9G3ZX	0XBC3ZX	0XJH4ZZ
0WPP73Z	0WW4XKZ	0WW9X1Z	0WWKXJZ	0WWRX1Z	0X974ZZ	0X9G3ZZ	0XBC4ZX	0XJHXZZ
0WPP7YZ	0WW4XYZ	0WW9X3Z	0WWKXKZ	0WWRX3Z	0X9800Z	0X9G40Z	0XBD0ZX	0XJJ3ZZ
0WPP81Z	0WW5X0Z	0WW9XJZ	0WWKXYZ	0WWRXYZ	0X980ZX	0X9G4ZX	0XBD3ZX	0XJJXZZ
0WPP83Z	0WW5X1Z	0WW9XYZ	0WWLX0Z	0X26X0Z	0X980ZZ	0X9G4ZZ	0XBD4ZX	0XJK3ZZ
0WPP8YZ	0WW5X3Z	0WWB00Z	0WWLX1Z	0X26XYZ	0X9830Z	0X9H00Z	0XBF0ZX	0XJKXZZ
0WPPX1Z	0WW5X7Z	0WWB01Z	0WWLX3Z	0X27X0Z	0X983ZX	0X9H0ZX	0XBF3ZX	0XP600Z
0WPPX3Z	0WW5XJZ	0WWB03Z	0WWLX7Z	0X27XYZ	0X983ZZ	0X9H0ZZ	0XBF4ZX	0XP601Z
0WPPXYZ	0WW5XKZ	0WWB0JZ	0WWLXJZ	0X9200Z	0X9840Z	0X9H30Z	0XBG0ZX	0XP603Z
0WPQ01Z	0WW5XYZ	0WWB0YZ	0WWLXKZ	0X920ZX	0X984ZX	0X9H3ZX	0XBG3ZX	0XP607Z
0WPQ03Z	0WW6X0Z	0WWB30Z	0WWLXYZ	0X920ZZ	0X984ZZ	0X9H3ZZ	0XBG4ZX	0XP60JZ
0WPQ0YZ	0WW6X1Z	0WWB31Z	0WWMX0Z	0X9230Z	0X9900Z	0X9H40Z	0XBH0ZX	0XP60KZ
0WPQ73Z	0WW6X3Z	0WWB33Z	0WWMX1Z	0X923ZX	0X990ZX	0X9H4ZX	0XBH3ZX	0XP60YZ
0WPQ83Z	0WW6X7Z	0WWB3JZ	0WWMX3Z	0X923ZZ	0X990ZZ	0X9H4ZZ	0XBH4ZX	0XP630Z
0WPQ8YZ	0WW6XJZ	0WWB3YZ	0WWMX7Z	0X9240Z	0X9930Z	0X9J00Z	0XBJ0ZX	0XP631Z
0WPQX1Z	0WW6XKZ	0WWB40Z	0WWMXJZ	0X924ZX	0X993ZX	0X9J0ZX	0XBJ3ZX	0XP633Z
0WPQX3Z	0WW6XYZ	0WWB41Z	0WWMXKZ	0X924ZZ	0X993ZZ	0X9J0ZZ	0XBJ4ZX	0XP637Z
0WPQXYZ	0WW800Z	0WWB43Z	0WWMXYZ	0X9300Z	0X9940Z	0X9J30Z	0XBK0ZX	0XP63JZ
0WPR01Z	0WW801Z	0WWB4JZ	0WWNX0Z	0X930ZX	0X994ZX	0X9J3ZX	0XBK3ZX	0XP63KZ
0WPR03Z	0WW803Z	0WWB4YZ	0WWNX1Z	0X930ZZ	0X994ZZ	0X9J3ZZ	0XBK4ZX	0XP63YZ
0WPR0YZ	0WW807Z	0WWBX0Z	0WWNX3Z	0X9330Z	0X9B00Z	0X9J40Z	0XJ23ZZ	0XP640Z
0WPR31Z	0WW80JZ	0WWBX1Z	0WWNX7Z	0X933ZX	0X9B0ZX	0X9J4ZX	0XJ24ZZ	0XP641Z
0WPR33Z	0WW80KZ	0WWBX3Z	0WWNXJZ	0X933ZZ	0X9B0ZZ	0X9J4ZZ	0XJ2XZZ	0XP643Z
0WPR3YZ	0WW80YZ	0WWBXJZ	0WWNXKZ	0X9340Z	0X9B30Z	0X9K00Z	0XJ33ZZ	0XP647Z
0WPR41Z	0WW830Z	0WWBXYZ	0WWNXYZ	0X934ZX	0X9B3ZX	0X9K0ZX	0XJ34ZZ	0XP64JZ
0WPR43Z	0WW831Z	0WWCX0Z	0WWP31Z	0X934ZZ	0X9B3ZZ	0X9K0ZZ	0XJ3XZZ	0XP64KZ
0WPR4YZ	0WW833Z	0WWCX1Z	0WWP33Z	0X9400Z	0X9B40Z	0X9K30Z	0XJ43ZZ	0XP64YZ

0XP6X0Z	0Y9100Z	0Y9D0ZZ	0Y9L4ZZ	0YBN4ZX	0YP90KZ	0YW9XJZ	10J18ZZ	10Q03ZE
0XP6X1Z	0Y910ZX	0Y9D30Z	0Y9M00Z	0YJ03ZZ	0YP90YZ	0YW9XKZ	10J1XZZ	10Q03ZF
0XP6X3Z	0Y910ZZ	0Y9D3ZX	0Y9M0ZX	0YJ04ZZ	0YP930Z	0YW9XYZ	10J20ZZ	10Q03ZG
0XP6X7Z	0Y9130Z	0Y9D3ZX	0Y9M0ZZ	0YJ0XZZ	0YP931Z	0YWBX0Z	10J23ZZ	10Q03ZH
0XP6XJZ	0Y913ZX	0Y9D40Z	0Y9M30Z	0YJ13ZZ	0YP933Z	0YWBX3Z	10J24ZZ	10Q03ZJ
0XP6XKZ	0Y913ZZ	0Y9D4ZX	0Y9M3ZX	0YJ14ZZ	0YP937Z	0YWBX7Z	10J27ZZ	10Q03ZK
0XP6XYZ	0Y9140Z	0Y9D4ZZ	0Y9M3ZZ	0YJ1XZZ	0YP93JZ	0YWBXJZ	10J28ZZ	10Q03ZL
0XP700Z	0Y914ZX	0Y9F00Z	0Y9M40Z	0YJ53ZZ	0YP93KZ	0YWBXKZ	10J2XZZ	10Q03ZM
0XP701Z	0Y914ZZ	0Y9F0ZX	0Y9M4ZX	0YJ5XZZ	0YP93YZ	0YWBXYZ	10P003Z	10Q03ZN
0XP703Z	0Y9530Z	0Y9F0ZZ	0Y9M4ZZ	0YJ63ZZ	0YP940Z	102073Z	10P00YZ	10Q03ZP
0XP707Z	0Y953ZZ	0Y9F30Z	0Y9N00Z	0YJ6XZZ	0YP941Z	10207YZ	10P073Z	10Q03ZQ
0XP70JZ	0Y9630Z	0Y9F3ZX	0Y9N0ZX	0YJ73ZZ	0YP943Z	10900Z9	10P07YZ	10Q03ZR
0XP70KZ	0Y963ZZ	0Y9F3ZZ	0Y9N0ZZ	0YJ7XZZ	0YP947Z	10900ZA	10Q00YE	10Q03ZS
0XP70YZ	0Y9700Z	0Y9F40Z	0Y9N30Z	0YJ83ZZ	0YP94JZ	10900ZB	10Q00YF	10Q03ZT
0XP730Z	0Y970ZX	0Y9F4ZX	0Y9N3ZX	0YJ8XZZ	0YP94KZ	10900ZC	10Q00YG	10Q03ZV
0XP731Z	0Y970ZZ	0Y9F4ZZ	0Y9N3ZZ	0YJ93ZZ	0YP94YZ	10900ZD	10Q00YH	10Q03ZY
0XP733Z	0Y9730Z	0Y9G00Z	0Y9N40Z	0YJ94ZZ	0YP9X0Z	10900ZU	10Q00YJ	10Q04YE
0XP737Z	0Y973ZX	0Y9G0ZX	0Y9N4ZX	0YJ9XZZ	0YP9X1Z	10903Z9	10Q00YK	10Q04YF
0XP73JZ	0Y973ZZ	0Y9G0ZZ	0Y9N4ZZ	0YJA3ZZ	0YP9X3Z	10903ZA	10Q00YL	10Q04YG
0XP73KZ	0Y9740Z	0Y9G30Z	0YB00ZX	0YJAXZZ	0YP9X7Z	10903ZB	10Q00YM	10Q04YH
0XP73YZ	0Y974ZX	0Y9G3ZX	0YB03ZX	0YJB3ZZ	0YP9XJZ	10903ZC	10Q00YN	10Q04YJ
0XP740Z	0Y974ZZ	0Y9G3ZZ	0YB04ZX	0YJB4ZZ	0YP9XKZ	10903ZD	10Q00YP	10Q04YK
0XP741Z	0Y9800Z	0Y9G40Z	0YB10ZX	0YJBXZZ	0YP9XYZ	10903ZU	10Q00YQ	10Q04YL
0XP743Z	0Y980ZX	0Y9G4ZX	0YB13ZX	0YJC3ZZ	0YPB00Z	10904Z9	10Q00YR	10Q04YM
0XP747Z	0Y980ZZ	0Y9G4ZZ	0YB14ZX	0YJC4ZZ	0YPB01Z	10904ZA	10Q00YS	10Q04YN
0XP74JZ	0Y9830Z	0Y9H00Z	0YB90ZX	0YJCXZZ	0YPB03Z	10904ZB	10Q00YT	10Q04YP
0XP74KZ	0Y983ZX	0Y9H0ZX	0YB93ZX	0YJD3ZZ	0YPB07Z	10904ZC	10Q00YV	10Q04YQ
0XP74YZ	0Y983ZZ	0Y9H0ZZ	0YB94ZX	0YJD4ZZ	0YPB0JZ	10904ZD	10Q00YY	10Q04YR
0XP7X0Z	0Y9840Z	0Y9H30Z	0YBB0ZX	0YJDXZZ	0YPB0KZ	10904ZU	10Q00ZE	10Q04YS
0XP7X1Z	0Y984ZX	0Y9H3ZX	0YBB3ZX	0YJE3ZZ	0YPB0YZ	10907Z9	10Q00ZF	10Q04YT
0XP7X3Z	0Y984ZZ	0Y9H3ZZ	0YBB4ZX	0YJEXZZ	0YPB30Z	10907ZA	10Q00ZG	10Q04YV
0XP7X7Z	0Y9900Z	0Y9H40Z	0YBC0ZX	0YJF3ZZ	0YPB31Z	10907ZB	10Q00ZH	10Q04YY
0XP7XJZ	0Y990ZX	0Y9H4ZX	0YBC3ZX	0YJF4ZZ	0YPB33Z	10907ZC	10Q00ZJ	10Q04ZE
0XP7XKZ	0Y990ZZ	0Y9H4ZZ	0YBC4ZX	0YJFXZZ	0YPB37Z	10907ZD	10Q00ZK	10Q04ZF
0XP7XYZ	0Y9930Z	0Y9J00Z	0YBD0ZX	0YJG3ZZ	0YPB3JZ	10907ZU	10Q00ZL	10Q04ZG
0XW6X0Z	0Y993ZX	0Y9J0ZX	0YBD3ZX	0YJG4ZZ	0YPB3KZ	10908Z9	10Q00ZM	10Q04ZH
0XW6X3Z	0Y993ZZ	0Y9J0ZZ	0YBD4ZX	0YJGXZZ	0YPB3YZ	10908ZA	10Q00ZN	10Q04ZJ
0XW6X7Z	0Y9940Z	0Y9J30Z	0YBF0ZX	0YJH3ZZ	0YPB40Z	10908ZB	10Q00ZP	10Q04ZK
0XW6XJZ	0Y994ZX	0Y9J3ZX	0YBF3ZX	0YJH4ZZ	0YPB41Z	10908ZC	10Q00ZQ	10Q04ZL
0XW6XKZ	0Y994ZZ	0Y9J3ZZ	0YBF4ZX	0YJHXZZ	0YPB43Z	10908ZD	10Q00ZR	10Q04ZM
0XW6XYZ	0Y9B00Z	0Y9J40Z	0YBG0ZX	0YJJ3ZZ	0YPB47Z	10908ZU	10Q00ZS	10Q04ZN
0XW7X0Z	0Y9B0ZX	0Y9J4ZX	0YBG3ZX	0YJJ4ZZ	0YPB4JZ	10A07Z6	10Q00ZT	10Q04ZP
0XW7X3Z	0Y9B0ZZ	0Y9J4ZZ	0YBG4ZX	0YJJXZZ	0YPB4KZ	10A07ZW	10Q00ZV	10Q04ZQ
0XW7X7Z	0Y9B30Z	0Y9K00Z	0YBH0ZX	0YJK3ZZ	0YPB4YZ	10A07ZX	10Q00ZY	10Q04ZR
0XW7XJZ	0Y9B3ZX	0Y9K0ZX	0YBH3ZX	0YJK4ZZ	0YPBX0Z	10D20ZZ	10Q03YE	10Q04ZS
0XW7XKZ	0Y9B3ZZ	0Y9K0ZZ	0YBH4ZX	0YJKXZZ	0YPBX1Z	10D24ZZ	10Q03YF	10Q04ZT
0XW7XYZ	0Y9B40Z	0Y9K30Z	0YBJ0ZX	0YJL3ZZ	0YPBX3Z	10H003Z	10Q03YG	10Q04ZV
0Y29X0Z	0Y9B4ZX	0Y9K3ZX	0YBJ3ZX	0YJL4ZZ	0YPBX7Z	10H00YZ	10Q03YH	10Q04ZY
0Y29XYZ	0Y9B4ZZ	0Y9K3ZZ	0YBJ4ZX	0YJLXZZ	0YPBXJZ	10H073Z	10Q03YJ	10Q07YE
0Y2BX0Z	0Y9C00Z	0Y9K40Z	0YBK0ZX	0YJM3ZZ	0YPBXKZ	10H07YZ	10Q03YK	10Q07YF
0Y2BXYZ	0Y9C0ZX	0Y9K4ZX	0YBK3ZX	0YJM4ZZ	0YPBXYZ	10J00ZZ	10Q03YL	10Q07YG
0Y9000Z	0Y9C0ZZ	0Y9K4ZZ	0YBK4ZX	0YJMXZZ	0YQ5XZZ	10J03ZZ	10Q03YM	10Q07YH
0Y900ZX	0Y9C30Z	0Y9L00Z	0YBL0ZX	0YJN3ZZ	0YQ6XZZ	10J04ZZ	10Q03YN	10Q07YJ
0Y900ZZ	0Y9C3ZX	0Y9L0ZX	0YBL3ZX	0YJN4ZZ	0YQ7XZZ	10J07ZZ	10Q03YP	10Q07YK
0Y9030Z	0Y9C3ZZ	0Y9L0ZZ	0YBL4ZX	0YJNXZZ	0YQ8XZZ	10J08ZZ	10Q03YQ	10Q07YL
0Y903ZX	0Y9C40Z	0Y9L30Z	0YBM0ZX	0YP900Z	0YQAXZZ	10J0XZZ	10Q03YR	10Q07YM
0Y903ZZ	0Y9C4ZX	0Y9L3ZX	0YBM3ZX	0YP901Z	0YQEXZZ	10J10ZZ	10Q03YS	10Q07YN
0Y9040Z	0Y9C4ZZ	0Y9L3ZZ	0YBM4ZX	0YP903Z	0YW9X0Z	10J13ZZ	10Q03YT	10Q07YP
0Y904ZX	0Y9D00Z	0Y9L40Z	0YBN0ZX	0YP907Z	0YW9X3Z	10J14ZZ	10Q03YV	10Q07YQ
0Y904ZZ	0Y9D0ZX	0Y9L4ZX	0YBN3ZX	0YP90JZ	0YW9X7Z	10J17ZZ	10Q03YY	10Q07YR

10Q07YS	10Y03ZL	2W01XYZ	2W08X5Z	2W0FX2Z	2W0MXYZ	2W0UX5Z	2W1PX7Z	2W34X1Z
10Q07YT	10Y03ZM	2W02X0Z	2W08X6Z	2W0FX3Z	2W0NX0Z	2W0UX6Z	2W1QX6Z	2W34X2Z
10Q07YV	10Y03ZN	2W02X1Z	2W08X7Z	2W0FX4Z	2W0NX1Z	2W0UX7Z	2W1QX7Z	2W34X3Z
10Q07YY	10Y03ZP	2W02X2Z	2W08XYZ	2W0FX5Z	2W0NX2Z	2W0UXYZ	2W1RX6Z	2W34XYZ
10Q07ZE	10Y03ZQ	2W02X3Z	2W09X0Z	2W0FX6Z	2W0NX3Z	2W0VX0Z	2W1RX7Z	2W35X1Z
10Q07ZF	10Y03ZR	2W02X4Z	2W09X1Z	2W0FX7Z	2W0NX4Z	2W0VX1Z	2W1SX6Z	2W35X2Z
10Q07ZG	10Y03ZS	2W02X5Z	2W09X2Z	2W0FXYZ	2W0NX5Z	2W0VX2Z	2W1SX7Z	2W35X3Z
10Q07ZH	10Y03ZT	2W02X6Z	2W09X3Z	2W0GX0Z	2W0NX6Z	2W0VX3Z	2W1TX6Z	2W35XYZ
10Q07ZJ	10Y03ZV	2W02X7Z	2W09X4Z	2W0GX1Z	2W0NX7Z	2W0VX4Z	2W1TX7Z	2W36X1Z
10Q07ZK	10Y03ZY	2W02XYZ	2W09X5Z	2W0GX2Z	2W0NXYZ	2W0VX5Z	2W1UX6Z	2W36X2Z
10Q07ZL	10Y04ZE	2W03X0Z	2W09X6Z	2W0GX3Z	2W0PX0Z	2W0VX6Z	2W1UX7Z	2W36X3Z
10Q07ZM	10Y04ZF	2W03X1Z	2W09X7Z	2W0GX4Z	2W0PX1Z	2W0VX7Z	2W1VX6Z	2W36XYZ
10Q07ZN	10Y04ZG	2W03X2Z	2W09XYZ	2W0GX5Z	2W0PX2Z	2W0VXYZ	2W1VX7Z	2W37X1Z
10Q07ZP	10Y04ZH	2W03X3Z	2W0AX0Z	2W0GX6Z	2W0PX3Z	2W10X6Z	2W20X4Z	2W37X2Z
10Q07ZQ	10Y04ZJ	2W03X4Z	2W0AX1Z	2W0GX7Z	2W0PX4Z	2W10X7Z	2W21X4Z	2W37X3Z
10Q07ZR	10Y04ZK	2W03X5Z	2W0AX2Z	2W0GXYZ	2W0PX5Z	2W11X6Z	2W22X4Z	2W37XYZ
10Q07ZS	10Y04ZL	2W03X6Z	2W0AX3Z	2W0HX0Z	2W0PX6Z	2W11X7Z	2W23X4Z	2W38X1Z
10Q07ZT	10Y04ZM	2W03X7Z	2W0AX4Z	2W0HX1Z	2W0PX7Z	2W12X6Z	2W24X4Z	2W38X2Z
10Q07ZV	10Y04ZN	2W03XYZ	2W0AX5Z	2W0HX2Z	2W0PXYZ	2W12X7Z	2W25X4Z	2W38X3Z
10Q07ZY	10Y04ZP	2W04X0Z	2W0AX6Z	2W0HX3Z	2W0QX0Z	2W13X6Z	2W26X4Z	2W38XYZ
10Q08YE	10Y04ZQ	2W04X1Z	2W0AX7Z	2W0HX4Z	2W0QX1Z	2W13X7Z	2W27X4Z	2W39X1Z
10Q08YF	10Y04ZR	2W04X2Z	2W0AXYZ	2W0HX5Z	2W0QX2Z	2W14X6Z	2W28X4Z	2W39X2Z
10Q08YG	10Y04ZS	2W04X3Z	2W0BX0Z	2W0HX6Z	2W0QX3Z	2W14X7Z	2W29X4Z	2W39X3Z
10Q08YH	10Y04ZT	2W04X4Z	2W0BX1Z	2W0HX7Z	2W0QX4Z	2W15X6Z	2W2AX4Z	2W39XYZ
10Q08YJ	10Y04ZV	2W04X5Z	2W0BX2Z	2W0HXYZ	2W0QX5Z	2W15X7Z	2W2BX4Z	2W3AX1Z
10Q08YK	10Y04ZY	2W04X6Z	2W0BX3Z	2W0JX0Z	2W0QX6Z	2W16X6Z	2W2CX4Z	2W3AX2Z
10Q08YL	10Y07ZE	2W04X7Z	2W0BX4Z	2W0JX1Z	2W0QX7Z	2W16X7Z	2W2DX4Z	2W3AX3Z
10Q08YM	10Y07ZF	2W04XYZ	2W0BX5Z	2W0JX2Z	2W0QXYZ	2W17X6Z	2W2EX4Z	2W3AXYZ
10Q08YN	10Y07ZG	2W05X0Z	2W0BX6Z	2W0JX3Z	2W0RX0Z	2W17X7Z	2W2FX4Z	2W3BX1Z
10Q08YP	10Y07ZH	2W05X1Z	2W0BX7Z	2W0JX4Z	2W0RX1Z	2W18X6Z	2W2GX4Z	2W3BX2Z
10Q08YQ	10Y07ZJ	2W05X2Z	2W0BXYZ	2W0JX5Z	2W0RX2Z	2W18X7Z	2W2HX4Z	2W3BX3Z
10Q08YR	10Y07ZK	2W05X3Z	2W0CX0Z	2W0JX6Z	2W0RX3Z	2W19X6Z	2W2JX4Z	2W3BXYZ
10Q08YS	10Y07ZL	2W05X4Z	2W0CX1Z	2W0JX7Z	2W0RX4Z	2W19X7Z	2W2KX4Z	2W3CX1Z
10Q08YT	10Y07ZM	2W05X5Z	2W0CX2Z	2W0JXYZ	2W0RX5Z	2W1AX6Z	2W2LX4Z	2W3CX2Z
10Q08YV	10Y07ZN	2W05X6Z	2W0CX3Z	2W0KX0Z	2W0RX6Z	2W1AX7Z	2W2MX4Z	2W3CX3Z
10Q08YY	10Y07ZP	2W05X7Z	2W0CX4Z	2W0KX1Z	2W0RX7Z	2W1BX6Z	2W2NX4Z	2W3CXYZ
10Q08ZE	10Y07ZQ	2W05XYZ	2W0CX5Z	2W0KX2Z	2W0RXYZ	2W1BX7Z	2W2PX4Z	2W3DX1Z
10Q08ZF	10Y07ZR	2W06X0Z	2W0CX6Z	2W0KX3Z	2W0SX0Z	2W1CX6Z	2W2QX4Z	2W3DX2Z
10Q08ZG	10Y07ZS	2W06X1Z	2W0CX7Z	2W0KX4Z	2W0SX1Z	2W1CX7Z	2W2RX4Z	2W3DX3Z
10Q08ZH	10Y07ZT	2W06X2Z	2W0CXYZ	2W0KX5Z	2W0SX2Z	2W1DX6Z	2W2SX4Z	2W3DXYZ
10Q08ZJ	10Y07ZV	2W06X3Z	2W0DX0Z	2W0KX6Z	2W0SX3Z	2W1DX7Z	2W2TX4Z	2W3EX1Z
10Q08ZK	10Y07ZY	2W06X4Z	2W0DX1Z	2W0KX7Z	2W0SX4Z	2W1EX6Z	2W2UX4Z	2W3EX2Z
10Q08ZL	2W00X0Z	2W06X5Z	2W0DX2Z	2W0KXYZ	2W0SX5Z	2W1EX7Z	2W2VX4Z	2W3EX3Z
10Q08ZM	2W00X1Z	2W06X6Z	2W0DX3Z	2W0LX0Z	2W0SX6Z	2W1FX6Z	2W30X1Z	2W3EXYZ
10Q08ZN	2W00X2Z	2W06X7Z	2W0DX4Z	2W0LX1Z	2W0SX7Z	2W1FX7Z	2W30X2Z	2W3FX1Z
10Q08ZP	2W00X3Z	2W06XYZ	2W0DX5Z	2W0LX2Z	2W0SXYZ	2W1GX6Z	2W30X3Z	2W3FX2Z
10Q08ZQ	2W00X4Z	2W07X0Z	2W0DX6Z	2W0LX3Z	2W0TX0Z	2W1GX7Z	2W30XYZ	2W3FX3Z
10Q08ZR	2W00X5Z	2W07X1Z	2W0DX7Z	2W0LX4Z	2W0TX1Z	2W1HX6Z	2W31X1Z	2W3FXYZ
10Q08ZS	2W00X6Z	2W07X2Z	2W0DXYZ	2W0LX5Z	2W0TX2Z	2W1HX7Z	2W31X2Z	2W3GX1Z
10Q08ZT	2W00X7Z	2W07X3Z	2W0EX0Z	2W0LX6Z	2W0TX3Z	2W1JX6Z	2W31X3Z	2W3GX2Z
10Q08ZV	2W00XYZ	2W07X4Z	2W0EX1Z	2W0LX7Z	2W0TX4Z	2W1JX7Z	2W31X9Z	2W3GX3Z
10Q08ZY	2W01X0Z	2W07X5Z	2W0EX2Z	2W0LXYZ	2W0TX5Z	2W1KX6Z	2W31XYZ	2W3GXYZ
10S07ZZ	2W01X1Z	2W07X6Z	2W0EX3Z	2W0MX0Z	2W0TX6Z	2W1KX7Z	2W32X1Z	2W3HX1Z
10S0XZZ	2W01X2Z	2W07X7Z	2W0EX4Z	2W0MX1Z	2W0TX7Z	2W1LX6Z	2W32X2Z	2W3HX2Z
10Y03ZE	2W01X3Z	2W07XYZ	2W0EX5Z	2W0MX2Z	2W0TXYZ	2W1LX7Z	2W32X3Z	2W3HX3Z
10Y03ZF	2W01X4Z	2W08X0Z	2W0EX6Z	2W0MX3Z	2W0UX0Z	2W1MX6Z	2W32XYZ	2W3HXYZ
10Y03ZG	2W01X5Z	2W08X1Z	2W0EX7Z	2W0MX4Z	2W0UX1Z	2W1MX7Z	2W33X1Z	2W3JX1Z
10Y03ZH	2W01X6Z	2W08X2Z	2W0EXYZ	2W0MX5Z	2W0UX2Z	2W1NX6Z	2W33X2Z	2W3JX2Z
10Y03ZJ	2W01X7Z	2W08X3Z	2W0FX0Z	2W0MX6Z	2W0UX3Z	2W1NX7Z	2W33X3Z	2W3JX3Z
10Y03ZK	2W01X9Z	2W08X4Z	2W0FX1Z	2W0MX7Z	2W0UX4Z	2W1PX6Z	2W33XYZ	2W3JXYZ

2W3KX1Z	2W4GX5Z	2W55X0Z	2W5BX6Z	2W5JX3Z	2W5RX0Z	2W67XZZ	2Y53X5Z	30240J0
2W3KX2Z	2W4HX5Z	2W55X1Z	2W5BX7Z	2W5JX4Z	2W5RX1Z	2W68X0Z	2Y54X5Z	30240J1
2W3KX3Z	2W4JX5Z	2W55X2Z	2W5BXYZ	2W5JX5Z	2W5RX2Z	2W68XZZ	2Y55X5Z	30240K0
2W3KXYZ	2W4KX5Z	2W55X3Z	2W5CX0Z	2W5JX6Z	2W5RX3Z	2W69X0Z	30230C0	30240K1
2W3LX1Z	2W4LX5Z	2W55X4Z	2W5CX1Z	2W5JX7Z	2W5RX4Z	2W69XZZ	30230H0	30240L0
2W3LX2Z	2W4MX5Z	2W55X5Z	2W5CX2Z	2W5JXYZ	2W5RX5Z	2W6AX0Z	30230H1	30240L1
2W3LX3Z	2W4NX5Z	2W55X6Z	2W5CX3Z	2W5KX0Z	2W5RX6Z	2W6AXZZ	30230J0	30240M0
2W3LXYZ	2W4PX5Z	2W55X7Z	2W5CX4Z	2W5KX1Z	2W5RX7Z	2W6BX0Z	30230J1	30240M1
2W3MX1Z	2W4QX5Z	2W55XYZ	2W5CX5Z	2W5KX2Z	2W5RXYZ	2W6BXZZ	30230K0	30240N0
2W3MX2Z	2W4RX5Z	2W56X0Z	2W5CX6Z	2W5KX3Z	2W5SX0Z	2W6CX0Z	30230K1	30240N1
2W3MX3Z	2W4SX5Z	2W56X1Z	2W5CX7Z	2W5KX4Z	2W5SX1Z	2W6CXZZ	30230L0	30240P0
2W3MXYZ	2W4TX5Z	2W56X2Z	2W5CXYZ	2W5KX5Z	2W5SX2Z	2W6DX0Z	30230L1	30240P1
2W3NX1Z	2W4UX5Z	2W56X3Z	2W5DX0Z	2W5KX6Z	2W5SX3Z	2W6DXZZ	30230M0	30240Q0
2W3NX2Z	2W4VX5Z	2W56X4Z	2W5DX1Z	2W5KX7Z	2W5SX4Z	2W6EX0Z	30230M1	30240Q1
2W3NX3Z	2W50X0Z	2W56X5Z	2W5DX2Z	2W5KXYZ	2W5SX5Z	2W6EXZZ	30230N0	30240R0
2W3NXYZ	2W50X1Z	2W56X6Z	2W5DX3Z	2W5LX0Z	2W5SX6Z	2W6FX0Z	30230N1	30240R1
2W3PX1Z	2W50X2Z	2W56X7Z	2W5DX4Z	2W5LX1Z	2W5SX7Z	2W6FXZZ	30230P0	30240S0
2W3PX2Z	2W50X3Z	2W56XYZ	2W5DX5Z	2W5LX2Z	2W5SXYZ	2W6GX0Z	30230P1	30240S1
2W3PX3Z	2W50X4Z	2W57X0Z	2W5DX6Z	2W5LX3Z	2W5TX0Z	2W6GXZZ	30230Q0	30240T0
2W3PXYZ	2W50X5Z	2W57X1Z	2W5DX7Z	2W5LX4Z	2W5TX1Z	2W6HX0Z	30230Q1	30240T1
2W3QX1Z	2W50X6Z	2W57X2Z	2W5DXYZ	2W5LX5Z	2W5TX2Z	2W6HXZZ	30230R0	30240V0
2W3QX2Z	2W50X7Z	2W57X3Z	2W5EX0Z	2W5LX6Z	2W5TX3Z	2W6JX0Z	30230R1	30240V1
2W3QX3Z	2W50XYZ	2W57X4Z	2W5EX1Z	2W5LX7Z	2W5TX4Z	2W6JXZZ	30230S0	30240W0
2W3QXYZ	2W51X0Z	2W57X5Z	2W5EX2Z	2W5LXYZ	2W5TX5Z	2W6KX0Z	30230S1	30240W1
2W3RX1Z	2W51X1Z	2W57X6Z	2W5EX3Z	2W5MX0Z	2W5TX6Z	2W6KXZZ	30230T0	30243C0
2W3RX2Z	2W51X2Z	2W57X7Z	2W5EX4Z	2W5MX1Z	2W5TX7Z	2W6LX0Z	30230T1	30243H0
2W3RX3Z	2W51X3Z	2W57XYZ	2W5EX5Z	2W5MX2Z	2W5TXYZ	2W6LXZZ	30230V0	30243H1
2W3RXYZ	2W51X4Z	2W58X0Z	2W5EX6Z	2W5MX3Z	2W5UX0Z	2W6MX0Z	30230V1	30243J0
2W3SX1Z	2W51X5Z	2W58X1Z	2W5EX7Z	2W5MX4Z	2W5UX1Z	2W6MXZZ	30230W0	30243J1
2W3SX2Z	2W51X6Z	2W58X2Z	2W5EXYZ	2W5MX5Z	2W5UX2Z	2W6NX0Z	30230W1	30243K0
2W3SX3Z	2W51X7Z	2W58X3Z	2W5FX0Z	2W5MX6Z	2W5UX3Z	2W6NXZZ	30233C0	30243K1
2W3SXYZ	2W51X9Z	2W58X4Z	2W5FX1Z	2W5MX7Z	2W5UX4Z	2W6PX0Z	30233H0	30243L0
2W3TX1Z	2W51XYZ	2W58X5Z	2W5FX2Z	2W5MXYZ	2W5UX5Z	2W6PXZZ	30233H1	30243L1
2W3TX2Z	2W52X0Z	2W58X6Z	2W5FX3Z	2W5NX0Z	2W5UX6Z	2W6QX0Z	30233J0	30243M0
2W3TX3Z	2W52X1Z	2W58X7Z	2W5FX4Z	2W5NX1Z	2W5UX7Z	2W6QXZZ	30233J1	30243M1
2W3TXYZ	2W52X2Z	2W58XYZ	2W5FX5Z	2W5NX2Z	2W5UXYZ	2W6RX0Z	30233K0	30243N0
2W3UX1Z	2W52X3Z	2W59X0Z	2W5FX6Z	2W5NX3Z	2W5VX0Z	2W6RXZZ	30233K1	30243N1
2W3UX2Z	2W52X4Z	2W59X1Z	2W5FX7Z	2W5NX4Z	2W5VX1Z	2W6SX0Z	30233L0	30243P0
2W3UX3Z	2W52X5Z	2W59X2Z	2W5FXYZ	2W5NX5Z	2W5VX2Z	2W6SXZZ	30233L1	30243P1
2W3UXYZ	2W52X6Z	2W59X3Z	2W5GX0Z	2W5NX6Z	2W5VX3Z	2W6TX0Z	30233M0	30243Q0
2W3VX1Z	2W52X7Z	2W59X4Z	2W5GX1Z	2W5NX7Z	2W5VX4Z	2W6TXZZ	30233M1	30243Q1
2W3VX2Z	2W52XYZ	2W59X5Z	2W5GX2Z	2W5NXYZ	2W5VX5Z	2W6UX0Z	30233N0	30243R0
2W3VX3Z	2W53X0Z	2W59X6Z	2W5GX3Z	2W5PX0Z	2W5VX6Z	2W6UXZZ	30233N1	30243R1
2W3VXYZ	2W53X1Z	2W59X7Z	2W5GX4Z	2W5PX1Z	2W5VX7Z	2W6VX0Z	30233P0	30243S0
2W40X5Z	2W53X2Z	2W59XYZ	2W5GX5Z	2W5PX2Z	2W5VXYZ	2W6VXZZ	30233P1	30243S1
2W41X5Z	2W53X3Z	2W5AX0Z	2W5GX6Z	2W5PX3Z	2W60X0Z	2Y00X5Z	30233Q0	30243T0
2W42X5Z	2W53X4Z	2W5AX1Z	2W5GX7Z	2W5PX4Z	2W60XZZ	2Y01X5Z	30233Q1	30243T1
2W43X5Z	2W53X5Z	2W5AX2Z	2W5GXYZ	2W5PX5Z	2W61X0Z	2Y02X5Z	30233R0	30243V0
2W44X5Z	2W53X6Z	2W5AX3Z	2W5HX0Z	2W5PX6Z	2W61XZZ	2Y03X5Z	30233R1	30243V1
2W45X5Z	2W53X7Z	2W5AX4Z	2W5HX1Z	2W5PX7Z	2W62X0Z	2Y04X5Z	30233S0	30243W0
2W46X5Z	2W53XYZ	2W5AX5Z	2W5HX2Z	2W5PXYZ	2W62XZZ	2Y05X5Z	30233S1	30243W1
2W47X5Z	2W54X0Z	2W5AX6Z	2W5HX3Z	2W5QX0Z	2W63X0Z	2Y40X5Z	30233T0	30273H1
2W48X5Z	2W54X1Z	2W5AX7Z	2W5HX4Z	2W5QX1Z	2W63XZZ	2Y41X5Z	30233T1	30273J1
2W49X5Z	2W54X2Z	2W5AXYZ	2W5HX5Z	2W5QX2Z	2W64X0Z	2Y42X5Z	30233V0	30273K1
2W4AX5Z	2W54X3Z	2W5BX0Z	2W5HX6Z	2W5QX3Z	2W64XZZ	2Y43X5Z	30233V1	30273L1
2W4BX5Z	2W54X4Z	2W5BX1Z	2W5HX7Z	2W5QX4Z	2W65X0Z	2Y44X5Z	30233W0	30273M1
2W4CX5Z	2W54X5Z	2W5BX2Z	2W5HXYZ	2W5QX5Z	2W65XZZ	2Y45X5Z	30233W1	30273N1
2W4DX5Z	2W54X6Z	2W5BX3Z	2W5JX0Z	2W5QX6Z	2W66X0Z	2Y50X5Z	30240C0	30273P1
2W4EX5Z	2W54X7Z	2W5BX4Z	2W5JX1Z	2W5QX7Z	2W66XZZ	2Y51X5Z	30240H0	30273Q1
2W4FX5Z	2W54XYZ	2W5BX5Z	2W5JX2Z	2W5QXYZ	2W67X0Z	2Y52X5Z	30240H1	30273R1

30273S1	3E023BZ	3E0400M	3E0507Z	3E060RZ	3E093BZ	3E0BX28	3E0D3BZ	3E0E73Z
30273T1	3E023GC	3E0400P	3E050FZ	3E060TZ	3E093GC	3E0BX29	3E0D3GC	3E0E76Z
30273V1	3E023HZ	3E04016	3E050GC	3E060VG	3E093HZ	3E0BX3Z	3E0D3HZ	3E0E77Z
30273W1	3E023KZ	3E04028	3E050GN	3E060VH	3E093KZ	3E0BXBZ	3E0D3KZ	3E0E7BZ
30277H1	3E023NZ	3E04029	3E050HZ	3E060VJ	3E093NZ	3E0BXGC	3E0D3NZ	3E0E7GC
30277J1	3E023TZ	3E0403Z	3E050KZ	3E060WK	3E093TZ	3E0BXHZ	3E0D3RZ	3E0E7HZ
30277K1	3E03003	3E0404Z	3E050NZ	3E060WL	3E09705	3E0BXKZ	3E0D3TZ	3E0E7KZ
30277L1	3E03005	3E0406Z	3E050PZ	3E060XZ	3E0970M	3E0BXNZ	3E0D704	3E0E7NZ
30277M1	3E0300M	3E0407Z	3E050RZ	3E06303	3E09728	3E0BXTZ	3E0D705	3E0E7SF
30277N1	3E0300P	3E040FZ	3E050TZ	3E06305	3E09729	3E0C304	3E0D70M	3E0E7TZ
30277P1	3E03016	3E040GC	3E050VG	3E0630M	3E0973Z	3E0C305	3E0D728	3E0E804
30277Q1	3E03028	3E040GN	3E050VH	3E0630P	3E0974Z	3E0C30M	3E0D729	3E0E805
30277R1	3E03029	3E040HZ	3E050VJ	3E06316	3E097BZ	3E0C328	3E0D73Z	3E0E80M
30277S1	3E0303Z	3E040KZ	3E050WK	3E06328	3E097GC	3E0C329	3E0D74Z	3E0E828
30277T1	3E0304Z	3E040NZ	3E050WL	3E06329	3E097HZ	3E0C33Z	3E0D76Z	3E0E829
30277V1	3E0306Z	3E040PZ	3E050XZ	3E0633Z	3E097KZ	3E0C3BZ	3E0D77Z	3E0E83Z
30277W1	3E0307Z	3E040RZ	3E05303	3E0634Z	3E097NZ	3E0C3GC	3E0D7BZ	3E0E86Z
30280B1	3E030FZ	3E040VG	3E05305	3E0636Z	3E097TZ	3E0C3HZ	3E0D7GC	3E0E87Z
30283B1	3E030GC	3E040VH	3E0530M	3E0637Z	3E09X05	3E0C3KZ	3E0D7HZ	3E0E8BZ
3C1ZX8Z	3E030GN	3E040VJ	3E0530P	3E063FZ	3E09X0M	3E0C3MZ	3E0D7KZ	3E0E8GC
3E00X05	3E030HZ	3E040WK	3E05316	3E063GC	3E09X28	3E0C3NZ	3E0D7NZ	3E0E8HZ
3E00X0M	3E030KZ	3E040WL	3E05328	3E063GN	3E09X29	3E0C3SF	3E0D7RZ	3E0E8KZ
3E00X28	3E030NZ	3E040XZ	3E05329	3E063HZ	3E09X3Z	3E0C3TZ	3E0D7TZ	3E0E8NZ
3E00X29	3E030PZ	3E04303	3E0533Z	3E063KZ	3E09X4Z	3E0C704	3E0DX04	3E0E8SF
3E00X3Z	3E030RZ	3E04305	3E0534Z	3E063NZ	3E09XBZ	3E0C705	3E0DX05	3E0E8TZ
3E00X4Z	3E030VG	3E0430M	3E0536Z	3E063PZ	3E09XGC	3E0C70M	3E0DX0M	3E0F304
3E00XBZ	3E030VH	3E0430P	3E0537Z	3E063RZ	3E09XHZ	3E0C728	3E0DX28	3E0F305
3E00XGC	3E030VJ	3E04316	3E053FZ	3E063TZ	3E09XKZ	3E0C729	3E0DX29	3E0F30M
3E00XKZ	3E030WK	3E04328	3E053GC	3E063VG	3E09XNZ	3E0C73Z	3E0DX3Z	3E0F328
3E00XMZ	3E030WL	3E04329	3E053GN	3E063VH	3E09XTZ	3E0C7BZ	3E0DX4Z	3E0F329
3E00XNZ	3E030XZ	3E0433Z	3E053HZ	3E063VJ	3E0A305	3E0C7GC	3E0DX6Z	3E0F33Z
3E00XTZ	3E03303	3E0434Z	3E053KZ	3E063WK	3E0A30M	3E0C7HZ	3E0DX7Z	3E0F36Z
3E0102A	3E03305	3E0436Z	3E053NZ	3E063WL	3E0A3GC	3E0C7KZ	3E0DXBZ	3E0F37Z
3E01305	3E0330M	3E0437Z	3E053PZ	3E063XZ	3E0B304	3E0C7MZ	3E0DXGC	3E0F3BZ
3E0130M	3E0330P	3E043FZ	3E053RZ	3E07016	3E0B305	3E0C7NZ	3E0DXHZ	3E0F3GC
3E01328	3E03316	3E043GC	3E053TZ	3E07017	3E0B30M	3E0C7SF	3E0DXKZ	3E0F3HZ
3E01329	3E03328	3E043GN	3E053VG	3E070GC	3E0B328	3E0C7TZ	3E0DXNZ	3E0F3KZ
3E0132A	3E03329	3E043GQ	3E053VH	3E070KZ	3E0B329	3E0CX04	3E0DXRZ	3E0F3NZ
3E0133Z	3E0333Z	3E043HZ	3E053VJ	3E070PZ	3E0B33Z	3E0CX05	3E0DXTZ	3E0F3SD
3E01340	3E0334Z	3E043KZ	3E053WK	3E07316	3E0B3BZ	3E0CX0M	3E0E304	3E0F3SF
3E0134Z	3E0336Z	3E043NZ	3E053WL	3E07317	3E0B3GC	3E0CX28	3E0E305	3E0F3TZ
3E0136Z	3E0337Z	3E043PZ	3E053XZ	3E073GC	3E0B3HZ	3E0CX29	3E0E30M	3E0F4GC
3E0137Z	3E033FZ	3E043RZ	3E06003	3E073KZ	3E0B3KZ	3E0CX3Z	3E0E328	3E0F704
3E013BZ	3E033GC	3E043TZ	3E06005	3E073PZ	3E0B3NZ	3E0CXBZ	3E0E329	3E0F705
3E013GC	3E033GN	3E043VG	3E0600M	3E074GC	3E0B3TZ	3E0CXGC	3E0E33Z	3E0F70M
3E013HZ	3E033GQ	3E043VH	3E0600P	3E08016	3E0B704	3E0CXHZ	3E0E36Z	3E0F728
3E013KZ	3E033HZ	3E043VJ	3E06016	3E080GC	3E0B705	3E0CXKZ	3E0E37Z	3E0F729
3E013NZ	3E033KZ	3E043WK	3E06028	3E080KZ	3E0B70M	3E0CXMZ	3E0E3BZ	3E0F73Z
3E013TZ	3E033NZ	3E043WL	3E06029	3E080PZ	3E0B728	3E0CXNZ	3E0E3GC	3E0F76Z
3E013VG	3E033PZ	3E043XZ	3E0603Z	3E08316	3E0B729	3E0CXSF	3E0E3HZ	3E0F77Z
3E013VJ	3E033RZ	3E05003	3E0604Z	3E083GC	3E0B73Z	3E0CXTZ	3E0E3KZ	3E0F7BZ
3E02305	3E033TZ	3E05005	3E0606Z	3E083KZ	3E0B7BZ	3E0D304	3E0E3NZ	3E0F7GC
3E0230M	3E033VG	3E0500M	3E0607Z	3E083PZ	3E0B7GC	3E0D305	3E0E3SF	3E0F7HZ
3E02328	3E033VH	3E0500P	3E060FZ	3E084GC	3E0B7HZ	3E0D30M	3E0E3TZ	3E0F7KZ
3E02329	3E033VJ	3E05016	3E060GC	3E09305	3E0B7KZ	3E0D328	3E0E4GC	3E0F7NZ
3E0233Z	3E033WK	3E05028	3E060GN	3E0930M	3E0B7NZ	3E0D329	3E0E704	3E0F7SD
3E02340	3E033WL	3E05029	3E060HZ	3E09328	3E0B7TZ	3E0D33Z	3E0E705	3E0F7SF
3E0234Z	3E033XZ	3E0503Z	3E060KZ	3E09329	3E0BX04	3E0D34Z	3E0E70M	3E0F7TZ
3E0236Z	3E04003	3E0504Z	3E060NZ	3E0933Z	3E0BX05	3E0D36Z	3E0E728	3E0F804
3E0237Z	3E04005	3E0506Z	3E060PZ	3E0934Z	3E0BX0M	3E0D37Z	3E0E729	3E0F805

3E0F80M	3E0H304	3E0J3TZ	3E0K7NZ	3E0M704	3E0P3BZ	3E0Q304	3E0T33Z	3E0Y329
3E0F828	3E0H305	3E0J4GC	3E0K7SF	3E0M705	3E0P3GC	3E0Q30M	3E0T3BZ	3E0Y33Z
3E0F829	3E0H30M	3E0J704	3E0K7TZ	3E0M70M	3E0P3HZ	3E0Q328	3E0T3GC	3E0Y36Z
3E0F83Z	3E0H328	3E0J705	3E0K804	3E0M7SF	3E0P3KZ	3E0Q329	3E0T3TZ	3E0Y37Z
3E0F86Z	3E0H329	3E0J70M	3E0K805	3E0N304	3E0P3LZ	3E0Q33Z	3E0U028	3E0Y3BZ
3E0F87Z	3E0H33Z	3E0J728	3E0K80M	3E0N305	3E0P3NZ	3E0Q36Z	3E0U029	3E0Y3GC
3E0F8BZ	3E0H36Z	3E0J729	3E0K828	3E0N30M	3E0P3SF	3E0Q37Z	3E0U0GB	3E0Y3HZ
3E0F8GC	3E0H37Z	3E0J73Z	3E0K829	3E0N328	3E0P3TZ	3E0Q3AZ	3E0U304	3E0Y3KZ
3E0F8HZ	3E0H3BZ	3E0J76Z	3E0K83Z	3E0N329	3E0P3VZ	3E0Q3BZ	3E0U305	3E0Y3NZ
3E0F8KZ	3E0H3GC	3E0J77Z	3E0K86Z	3E0N33Z	3E0P45Z	3E0Q3E0	3E0U30M	3E0Y3SF
3E0F8NZ	3E0H3HZ	3E0J7BZ	3E0K87Z	3E0N36Z	3E0P4GC	3E0Q3E1	3E0U328	3E0Y3TZ
3E0F8SD	3E0H3KZ	3E0J7GC	3E0K8BZ	3E0N37Z	3E0P704	3E0Q3GC	3E0U329	3E0Y4GC
3E0F8SF	3E0H3NZ	3E0J7HZ	3E0K8GC	3E0N3BZ	3E0P705	3E0Q3HZ	3E0U33Z	3E0Y704
3E0F8TZ	3E0H3SF	3E0J7KZ	3E0K8HZ	3E0N3GC	3E0P70M	3E0Q3KZ	3E0U36Z	3E0Y705
3E0G304	3E0H3TZ	3E0J7NZ	3E0K8KZ	3E0N3HZ	3E0P728	3E0Q3NZ	3E0U37Z	3E0Y70M
3E0G305	3E0H4GC	3E0J7SF	3E0K8NZ	3E0N3KZ	3E0P729	3E0Q3SF	3E0U3BZ	3E0Y7SF
3E0G30M	3E0H704	3E0J7TZ	3E0K8SF	3E0N3NZ	3E0P73Z	3E0Q3TZ	3E0U3GB	3E1038X
3E0G328	3E0H705	3E0J804	3E0K8TZ	3E0N3SF	3E0P76Z	3E0Q704	3E0U3GC	3E1038X
3E0G329	3E0H70M	3E0J805	3E0L05Z	3E0N3TZ	3E0P77Z	3E0Q70M	3E0U3HZ	3E10X8X
3E0G33Z	3E0H728	3E0J80M	3E0L304	3E0N4GC	3E0P7BZ	3E0Q7SF	3E0U3KZ	3E10X8X
3E0G36Z	3E0H729	3E0J828	3E0L305	3E0N704	3E0P7GC	3E0R0AZ	3E0U3NZ	3E1938X
3E0G37Z	3E0H73Z	3E0J829	3E0L30M	3E0N705	3E0P7HZ	3E0R0E0	3E0U3SF	3E1938Z
3E0G3BZ	3E0H76Z	3E0J83Z	3E0L328	3E0N70M	3E0P7KZ	3E0R0E1	3E0U3TZ	3E1978X
3E0G3GC	3E0H77Z	3E0J86Z	3E0L329	3E0N728	3E0P7LZ	3E0R303	3E0U4GC	3E1978Z
3E0G3HZ	3E0H7BZ	3E0J87Z	3E0L33Z	3E0N729	3E0P7NZ	3E0R304	3E0V0GB	3E1988X
3E0G3KZ	3E0H7GC	3E0J8BZ	3E0L35Z	3E0N73Z	3E0P7SF	3E0R305	3E0V305	3E1988Z
3E0G3NZ	3E0H7HZ	3E0J8GC	3E0L36Z	3E0N76Z	3E0P7TZ	3E0R30M	3E0V30M	3E1B38X
3E0G3SF	3E0H7KZ	3E0J8HZ	3E0L37Z	3E0N77Z	3E0P7VZ	3E0R328	3E0V328	3E1B38Z
3E0G3TZ	3E0H7NZ	3E0J8KZ	3E0L3BZ	3E0N7BZ	3E0P804	3E0R329	3E0V329	3E1B78X
3E0G4GC	3E0H7SF	3E0J8NZ	3E0L3GC	3E0N7GC	3E0P805	3E0R33Z	3E0V33Z	3E1B78Z
3E0G704	3E0H7TZ	3E0J8SF	3E0L3HZ	3E0N7HZ	3E0P80M	3E0R36Z	3E0V36Z	3E1B88X
3E0G705	3E0H804	3E0J8TZ	3E0L3KZ	3E0N7KZ	3E0P828	3E0R37Z	3E0V37Z	3E1B88Z
3E0G70M	3E0H805	3E0K304	3E0L3NZ	3E0N7NZ	3E0P829	3E0R3AZ	3E0V3BZ	3E1C38X
3E0G728	3E0H80M	3E0K305	3E0L3SF	3E0N7SF	3E0P83Z	3E0R3BZ	3E0V3GB	3E1C38Z
3E0G729	3E0H828	3E0K30M	3E0L3TZ	3E0N7TZ	3E0P86Z	3E0R3E0	3E0V3GC	3E1CX8X
3E0G73Z	3E0H829	3E0K328	3E0L45Z	3E0N804	3E0P87Z	3E0R3E1	3E0V3HZ	3E1CX8Z
3E0G76Z	3E0H83Z	3E0K329	3E0L704	3E0N805	3E0P8BZ	3E0R3GC	3E0V3KZ	3E1F38X
3E0G77Z	3E0H86Z	3E0K33Z	3E0L705	3E0N80M	3E0P8GC	3E0R3HZ	3E0V3NZ	3E1F38Z
3E0G7BZ	3E0H87Z	3E0K36Z	3E0L70M	3E0N828	3E0P8HZ	3E0R3KZ	3E0V3TZ	3E1F78X
3E0G7GC	3E0H8BZ	3E0K37Z	3E0L7SF	3E0N829	3E0P8KZ	3E0R3NZ	3E0W305	3E1F78Z
3E0G7HZ	3E0H8GC	3E0K3BZ	3E0M05Z	3E0N83Z	3E0P8NZ	3E0R3SF	3E0W30M	3E1F88X
3E0G7KZ	3E0H8HZ	3E0K3GC	3E0M304	3E0N86Z	3E0P8SF	3E0R3TZ	3E0W328	3E1F88Z
3E0G7NZ	3E0H8KZ	3E0K3HZ	3E0M305	3E0N87Z	3E0P8TZ	3E0R7SF	3E0W329	3E1G38X
3E0G7SF	3E0H8NZ	3E0K3KZ	3E0M30M	3E0N8BZ	3E0Q004	3E0S303	3E0W33Z	3E1G38Z
3E0G7TZ	3E0H8SF	3E0K3NZ	3E0M30Y	3E0N8GC	3E0Q00M	3E0S304	3E0W36Z	3E1G78X
3E0G804	3E0H8TZ	3E0K3SF	3E0M328	3E0N8HZ	3E0Q028	3E0S305	3E0W37Z	3E1G78Z
3E0G805	3E0J304	3E0K3TZ	3E0M329	3E0N8KZ	3E0Q029	3E0S30M	3E0W3BZ	3E1G88X
3E0G80M	3E0J305	3E0K4GC	3E0M33Z	3E0N8NZ	3E0Q03Z	3E0S328	3E0W3GC	3E1G88Z
3E0G828	3E0J30M	3E0K704	3E0M35Z	3E0N8SF	3E0Q06Z	3E0S329	3E0W3HZ	3E1H38X
3E0G829	3E0J328	3E0K705	3E0M36Z	3E0N8TZ	3E0Q07Z	3E0S33Z	3E0W3KZ	3E1H38Z
3E0G83Z	3E0J329	3E0K70M	3E0M37Z	3E0P05Z	3E0Q0AZ	3E0S36Z	3E0W3NZ	3E1H78X
3E0G86Z	3E0J33Z	3E0K728	3E0M3BZ	3E0P304	3E0Q0BZ	3E0S37Z	3E0W3TZ	3E1H78Z
3E0G87Z	3E0J36Z	3E0K729	3E0M3GC	3E0P305	3E0Q0E0	3E0S3BZ	3E0X33Z	3E1H88X
3E0G8BZ	3E0J37Z	3E0K73Z	3E0M3HZ	3E0P30M	3E0Q0E1	3E0S3GC	3E0X3BZ	3E1H88Z
3E0G8GC	3E0J3BZ	3E0K76Z	3E0M3KZ	3E0P328	3E0Q0GC	3E0S3HZ	3E0X3GC	3E1J38X
3E0G8HZ	3E0J3GC	3E0K77Z	3E0M3NZ	3E0P329	3E0Q0HZ	3E0S3KZ	3E0X3TZ	3E1J38Z
3E0G8KZ	3E0J3HZ	3E0K7BZ	3E0M3SF	3E0P33Z	3E0Q0KZ	3E0S3NZ	3E0Y304	3E1J78X
3E0G8NZ	3E0J3KZ	3E0K7GC	3E0M3TZ	3E0P35Z	3E0Q0NZ	3E0S3SF	3E0Y305	3E1J78Z
3E0G8SF	3E0J3NZ	3E0K7HZ	3E0M45Z	3E0P36Z	3E0Q0SF	3E0S3TZ	3E0Y30M	3E1J88X
3E0G8TZ	3E0J3SF	3E0K7KZ	3E0M4GC	3E0P37Z	3E0Q0TZ	3E0S7SF	3E0Y328	3E1J88Z

3E1K38X	4A0174Z	4A03X51	4A09X1Z	4A100BZ	4A12X4Z	4A143J3	4A1J82Z	6A3Z1ZZ
3E1K38Z	4A01829	4A03X5D	4A09X5Z	4A1034G	4A12X9Z	4A143R0	4A1J84Z	6A4Z0ZZ
3E1K78X	4A0182B	4A03XB1	4A09XCZ	4A1034Z	4A12XCZ	4A143R2	4A1J8BZ	6A4Z1ZZ
3E1K78Z	4A0184Z	4A03XH1	4A09XDZ	4A103BD	4A12XFZ	4A143R3	4A1JX2Z	6A550Z0
3E1K88X	4A01X29	4A03XJ1	4A09XLZ	4A103KD	4A12XHZ	4A14X51	4A1JX4Z	6A550Z1
3E1K88Z	4A01X2B	4A03XR1	4A09XMZ	4A103RD	4A12XM4	4A14XB1	4A1JXBZ	6A550Z2
3E1L38X	4A01X4Z	4A04050	4A0B78Z	4A1074G	4A12XSH	4A14XJ1	4A1Z7KZ	6A550Z3
3E1L38Z	4A0204Z	4A04051	4A0B7BZ	4A1074Z	4A13051	4A1605H	4A1ZXKZ	6A550ZT
3E1M38X	4A0209Z	4A04052	4A0B7GZ	4A107BD	4A13053	4A1635H	4A1ZXQZ	6A550ZV
3E1M38Z	4A020CZ	4A04053	4A0B88Z	4A107KD	4A1305C	4A1635Z	4B00XVZ	6A551Z0
3E1M39Z	4A020FZ	4A040B0	4A0B8BZ	4A107RD	4A130B1	4A163BZ	4B01XVZ	6A551Z1
3E1N38X	4A020HZ	4A040B1	4A0B8GZ	4A1084G	4A130B3	4A1675H	4B02XSZ	6A551Z2
3E1N38Z	4A020PZ	4A040B2	4A0C35Z	4A1084Z	4A130BC	4A1675Z	4B02XTZ	6A551Z3
3E1N78X	4A0234Z	4A040B3	4A0C3BZ	4A108BD	4A130H1	4A167BZ	4B09XSZ	6A551ZT
3E1N78Z	4A0239Z	4A040J0	4A0C75Z	4A108KD	4A130J1	4A1685H	4B0FXVZ	6A551ZV
3E1N88X	4A023CZ	4A040J1	4A0C7BZ	4A108RD	4A130J3	4A1685Z	5A02115	6A600ZZ
3E1N88Z	4A023HZ	4A040J2	4A0C85Z	4A10X2Z	4A130JC	4A168BZ	5A02215	6A601ZZ
3E1P38X	4A023PZ	4A040J3	4A0C8BZ	4A10X4G	4A130R1	4A1971Z	5A05121	6A650ZZ
3E1P38Z	4A0274Z	4A040R1	4A0D73Z	4A10X4Z	4A13351	4A1975Z	5A0512C	6A651ZZ
3E1P78X	4A0279Z	4A04350	4A0D75Z	4A11029	4A13353	4A197CZ	5A05221	6A750Z4
3E1P78Z	4A027CZ	4A04351	4A0D7BZ	4A1102B	4A1335C	4A197DZ	5A0522C	6A750Z5
3E1P88X	4A027HZ	4A04352	4A0D7DZ	4A1104G	4A133B1	4A197LZ	5A0920Z	6A750Z6
3E1P88Z	4A027PZ	4A04353	4A0D7LZ	4A1104Z	4A133B3	4A19X1Z	5A09357	6A750Z7
3E1Q38X	4A0284Z	4A043B0	4A0D83Z	4A11329	4A133BC	4A19X5Z	5A09358	6A750ZZ
3E1Q38Z	4A0289Z	4A043B1	4A0D85Z	4A1132B	4A133H1	4A19XCZ	5A09359	6A751Z4
3E1R38X	4A028CZ	4A043B2	4A0D8BZ	4A1134G	4A133J1	4A19XDZ	5A0935A	6A751Z5
3E1R38Z	4A028HZ	4A043B3	4A0D8DZ	4A1134Z	4A133J3	4A19XLZ	5A0935B	6A751Z6
3E1S38X	4A028PZ	4A043J0	4A0D8LZ	4A11729	4A133JC	4A1B78Z	5A0935Z	6A751Z7
3E1S38Z	4A02X4A	4A043J1	4A0F33Z	4A1172B	4A133R1	4A1B7BZ	5A09457	6A751ZZ
3E1U38X	4A02X4Z	4A043J2	4A0F3BE	4A1174G	4A13X51	4A1B7GZ	5A09458	6A800ZZ
3E1U38Z	4A02X9Z	4A043J3	4A0FX3Z	4A1174Z	4A13XB1	4A1B88Z	5A09459	6A801ZZ
3E1U48X	4A02XCZ	4A043R1	4A0H74Z	4A11829	4A13XH1	4A1B8BZ	5A0945A	6A930ZZ
3E1U48Z	4A02XFZ	4A044B2	4A0H7CZ	4A1182B	4A13XJ1	4A1B8GZ	5A0945B	6A931ZZ
3E1Y38X	4A02XHZ	4A04X51	4A0H7FZ	4A1184G	4A13XR1	4A1BXSH	5A0945Z	6AB50BZ
3E1Y38Z	4A02XM4	4A04XB1	4A0H7HZ	4A1184Z	4A14050	4A1D73Z	5A09557	6ABB0BZ
4A0002Z	4A02XPZ	4A04XJ1	4A0H84Z	4A11X29	4A14051	4A1D75Z	5A09558	6ABF0BZ
4A0004Z	4A03051	4A04XR1	4A0H8CZ	4A11X2B	4A14052	4A1D7BZ	5A09559	6ABT0BZ
4A000BZ	4A03053	4A05XLZ	4A0H8FZ	4A11X4G	4A14053	4A1D7DZ	5A0955A	7W00X0Z
4A0034Z	4A0305C	4A0635Z	4A0H8HZ	4A11X4Z	4A140B0	4A1D7LZ	5A0955B	7W00X1Z
4A003BD	4A030B1	4A063BZ	4A0HX4Z	4A1204Z	4A140B1	4A1D83Z	5A0955Z	7W00X2Z
4A003KD	4A030B3	4A0675Z	4A0HXCZ	4A1209Z	4A140B2	4A1D85Z	5A12012	7W00X3Z
4A003RD	4A030BC	4A067BZ	4A0HXFZ	4A120CZ	4A140B3	4A1D8BZ	5A1213Z	7W00X4Z
4A0074Z	4A030BF	4A0685Z	4A0HXHZ	4A120FZ	4A140J0	4A1D8DZ	5A1221Z	7W00X5Z
4A007BD	4A030H1	4A068BZ	4A0J72Z	4A120HZ	4A140J1	4A1D8LZ	5A1223Z	7W00X6Z
4A007KD	4A030J1	4A07X0Z	4A0J74Z	4A1234Z	4A140J2	4A1GXSH	5A15A2F	7W00X7Z
4A007RD	4A030J3	4A07X7Z	4A0J7BZ	4A1239Z	4A140J3	4A1H74Z	5A15A2G	7W00X8Z
4A0084Z	4A030JC	4A07XBZ	4A0J82Z	4A123CZ	4A140R0	4A1H7CZ	5A15A2H	7W00X9Z
4A008BD	4A030R1	4A08X0Z	4A0J84Z	4A123FZ	4A140R2	4A1H7FZ	5A19054	7W01X0Z
4A008KD	4A03351	4A0971Z	4A0J8BZ	4A123HZ	4A140R3	4A1H7HZ	5A1C00Z	7W01X1Z
4A008RD	4A03353	4A0975Z	4A0JX2Z	4A1274Z	4A14350	4A1H84Z	5A1C60Z	7W01X2Z
4A00X2Z	4A0335C	4A097CZ	4A0JX4Z	4A1279Z	4A14351	4A1H8CZ	5A2204Z	7W01X3Z
4A00X4Z	4A033B1	4A097DZ	4A0JXBZ	4A127CZ	4A14352	4A1H8FZ	6A0Z0ZZ	7W01X4Z
4A01029	4A033B3	4A097LZ	4A0Z76Z	4A127FZ	4A14353	4A1H8HZ	6A0Z1ZZ	7W01X5Z
4A0102B	4A033BC	4A097MZ	4A0Z7KZ	4A127HZ	4A143B0	4A1HX4Z	6A150ZZ	7W01X6Z
4A0104Z	4A033BF	4A0981Z	4A0ZX6Z	4A1284Z	4A143B1	4A1HXCZ	6A151ZZ	7W01X7Z
4A01329	4A033H1	4A0985Z	4A0ZXKZ	4A1289Z	4A143B2	4A1HXFZ	6A210ZZ	7W01X8Z
4A0132B	4A033J1	4A098CZ	4A0ZXQZ	4A128CZ	4A143B3	4A1HXHZ	6A211ZZ	7W01X9Z
4A0134Z	4A033J3	4A098DZ	4A1002Z	4A128FZ	4A143J0	4A1J72Z	6A220ZZ	7W02X0Z
4A01729	4A033JC	4A098LZ	4A1004G	4A128HZ	4A143J1	4A1J74Z	6A221ZZ	7W02X1Z
4A0172B	4A033R1	4A098MZ	4A1004Z	4A12X45	4A143J2	4A1J7BZ	6A3Z0ZZ	7W02X2Z

DRG ASSIGN

7W02X3Z	7W08X3Z	8E0W8EZ	9WB2XKZ	9WB9XGZ	B040ZZZ	B245ZZ3	B30B1ZZ	B30T1ZZ
7W02X4Z	7W08X4Z	8E0WXBF	9WB2XLZ	9WB9XHZ	B04BZZZ	B245ZZ4	B30BYZZ	B30TYZZ
7W02X5Z	7W08X5Z	8E0WXBG	9WB3XBZ	9WB9XJZ	B210010	B245ZZZ	B30BZZZ	B30TZZZ
7W02X6Z	7W08X6Z	8E0WXBH	9WB3XCZ	9WB9XKZ	B210110	B246YZZ	B30C0ZZ	B310010
7W02X7Z	7W08X7Z	8E0WXBZ	9WB3XDZ	9WB9XLZ	B210Y10	B246ZZ3	B30C1ZZ	B3100ZZ
7W02X8Z	7W08X8Z	8E0WXCZ	9WB3XFZ	B00B0ZZ	B211010	B246ZZ4	B30CYZZ	B310110
7W02X9Z	7W08X9Z	8E0WXY8	9WB3XGZ	B00B1ZZ	B211110	B246ZZZ	B30CZZZ	B3101ZZ
7W03X0Z	7W09X0Z	8E0X0CZ	9WB3XHZ	B00BYZZ	B211Y10	B24BYZZ	B30D0ZZ	B310Y10
7W03X1Z	7W09X1Z	8E0X0EZ	9WB3XJZ	B00BZZZ	B212010	B24BZZ3	B30D1ZZ	B310YZZ
7W03X2Z	7W09X2Z	8E0X3CZ	9WB3XKZ	B01B0ZZ	B212110	B24BZZ4	B30DYZZ	B310ZZZ
7W03X3Z	7W09X3Z	8E0X3EZ	9WB3XLZ	B01B1ZZ	B212Y10	B24BZZZ	B30DZZZ	B311010
7W03X4Z	7W09X4Z	8E0X4CZ	9WB4XBZ	B01BYZZ	B213010	B24CYZZ	B30F0ZZ	B3110ZZ
7W03X5Z	7W09X5Z	8E0X4EZ	9WB4XCZ	B01BZZZ	B213110	B24CZZ3	B30F1ZZ	B311110
7W03X6Z	7W09X6Z	8E0XXBF	9WB4XDZ	B02000Z	B213Y10	B24CZZ4	B30FYZZ	B3111ZZ
7W03X7Z	7W09X7Z	8E0XXBG	9WB4XFZ	B0200ZZ	B22100Z	B24CZZZ	B30FZZZ	B311Y10
7W03X8Z	7W09X8Z	8E0XXBH	9WB4XGZ	B02010Z	B2210ZZ	B24DYZZ	B30G0ZZ	B311YZZ
7W03X9Z	7W09X9Z	8E0XXBZ	9WB4XHZ	B0201ZZ	B22110Z	B24DZZ3	B30G1ZZ	B311ZZZ
7W04X0Z	8C01X6J	8E0XXCZ	9WB4XJZ	B020Y0Z	B2211ZZ	B24DZZ4	B30GYZZ	B312010
7W04X1Z	8C01X6L	8E0XXY8	9WB4XKZ	B020YZZ	B221Y0Z	B24DZZZ	B30GZZZ	B3120ZZ
7W04X2Z	8C02X6K	8E0Y0CZ	9WB4XLZ	B020ZZZ	B221YZZ	B3000ZZ	B30H0ZZ	B312110
7W04X3Z	8C02X6L	8E0Y0EZ	9WB5XBZ	B02700Z	B221Z2Z	B3001ZZ	B30H1ZZ	B3121ZZ
7W04X4Z	8E01XY7	8E0Y3CZ	9WB5XCZ	B0270ZZ	B221ZZZ	B300YZZ	B30HYZZ	B312Y10
7W04X5Z	8E023DZ	8E0Y3EZ	9WB5XDZ	B02710Z	B22300Z	B300ZZZ	B30HZZZ	B312YZZ
7W04X6Z	8E02XDZ	8E0Y4CZ	9WB5XFZ	B0271ZZ	B2230ZZ	B3010ZZ	B30J0ZZ	B312ZZZ
7W04X7Z	8E090CZ	8E0Y4EZ	9WB5XGZ	B027Y0Z	B22310Z	B3011ZZ	B30J1ZZ	B313010
7W04X8Z	8E090EM	8E0YXBF	9WB5XHZ	B027YZZ	B2231ZZ	B301YZZ	B30JYZZ	B3130ZZ
7W04X9Z	8E090EZ	8E0YXBG	9WB5XJZ	B027ZZZ	B223Y0Z	B301ZZZ	B30JZZZ	B313110
7W05X0Z	8E093CZ	8E0YXBH	9WB5XKZ	B02800Z	B223YZZ	B3020ZZ	B30K0ZZ	B3131ZZ
7W05X1Z	8E093EZ	8E0YXBZ	9WB5XLZ	B0280ZZ	B223Z2Z	B3021ZZ	B30K1ZZ	B313Y10
7W05X2Z	8E094CZ	8E0YXCZ	9WB6XBZ	B02810Z	B223ZZZ	B302YZZ	B30KYZZ	B313YZZ
7W05X3Z	8E094EZ	8E0YXY8	9WB6XCZ	B0281ZZ	B22600Z	B302ZZZ	B30KZZZ	B313ZZZ
7W05X4Z	8E097CZ	8E0ZXY1	9WB6XDZ	B028Y0Z	B2260ZZ	B3030ZZ	B30L0ZZ	B314010
7W05X5Z	8E097EZ	8E0ZXY4	9WB6XFZ	B028YZZ	B22610Z	B3031ZZ	B30L1ZZ	B3140ZZ
7W05X6Z	8E098CZ	8E0ZXY5	9WB6XGZ	B028ZZZ	B2261ZZ	B303YZZ	B30LYZZ	B314110
7W05X7Z	8E098EZ	8E0ZXY6	9WB6XHZ	B02900Z	B226Y0Z	B303ZZZ	B30LZZZ	B3141ZZ
7W05X8Z	8E09XBF	9WB0XBZ	9WB6XJZ	B0290ZZ	B226YZZ	B3040ZZ	B30M0ZZ	B314Y10
7W05X9Z	8E09XBG	9WB0XCZ	9WB6XKZ	B02910Z	B226Z2Z	B3041ZZ	B30M1ZZ	B314YZZ
7W06X0Z	8E09XBH	9WB0XDZ	9WB6XLZ	B0291ZZ	B226ZZZ	B304YZZ	B30MYZZ	B314ZZZ
7W06X1Z	8E09XBZ	9WB0XFZ	9WB7XBZ	B029Y0Z	B231Y0Z	B304ZZZ	B30MZZZ	B315010
7W06X2Z	8E09XCZ	9WB0XGZ	9WB7XCZ	B029YZZ	B231YZZ	B3050ZZ	B30N0ZZ	B3150ZZ
7W06X3Z	8E09XY8	9WB0XHZ	9WB7XDZ	B029ZZZ	B231ZZZ	B3051ZZ	B30N1ZZ	B315110
7W06X4Z	8E0H300	9WB0XJZ	9WB7XFZ	B02B00Z	B233Y0Z	B305YZZ	B30NYZZ	B3151ZZ
7W06X5Z	8E0H30Z	9WB0XKZ	9WB7XGZ	B02B0ZZ	B233YZZ	B305ZZZ	B30NZZZ	B315Y10
7W06X6Z	8E0HX62	9WB0XLZ	9WB7XHZ	B02B10Z	B233ZZZ	B3060ZZ	B30P0ZZ	B315YZZ
7W06X7Z	8E0HXY9	9WB1XBZ	9WB7XJZ	B02B1ZZ	B236Y0Z	B3061ZZ	B30P1ZZ	B315ZZZ
7W06X8Z	8E0KX1Z	9WB1XCZ	9WB7XKZ	B02BY0Z	B236YZZ	B306YZZ	B30PYZZ	B316010
7W06X9Z	8E0KXY7	9WB1XDZ	9WB7XLZ	B02BYZZ	B236ZZZ	B306ZZZ	B30PZZZ	B3160ZZ
7W07X0Z	8E0UXY7	9WB1XFZ	9WB8XBZ	B02BZZZ	B240YZZ	B3070ZZ	B30Q0ZZ	B316110
7W07X1Z	8E0VX1C	9WB1XGZ	9WB8XCZ	B030Y0Z	B240ZZ3	B3071ZZ	B30Q1ZZ	B3161ZZ
7W07X2Z	8E0VX1D	9WB1XHZ	9WB8XDZ	B030YZZ	B240ZZ4	B307YZZ	B30QYZZ	B316Y10
7W07X3Z	8E0VX63	9WB1XJZ	9WB8XFZ	B030ZZZ	B240ZZZ	B307ZZZ	B30QZZZ	B316YZZ
7W07X4Z	8E0W0CZ	9WB1XKZ	9WB8XGZ	B039Y0Z	B241YZZ	B3080ZZ	B30R0ZZ	B316ZZZ
7W07X5Z	8E0W0EZ	9WB1XLZ	9WB8XHZ	B039YZZ	B241ZZ3	B3081ZZ	B30R1ZZ	B317010
7W07X6Z	8E0W3CZ	9WB2XBZ	9WB8XJZ	B039ZZZ	B241ZZ4	B308YZZ	B30RYZZ	B3170ZZ
7W07X7Z	8E0W3EZ	9WB2XCZ	9WB8XKZ	B03BY0Z	B241ZZZ	B308ZZZ	B30RZZZ	B317110
7W07X8Z	8E0W4CZ	9WB2XDZ	9WB8XLZ	B03BYZZ	B244YZZ	B3090ZZ	B30S0ZZ	B3171ZZ
7W07X9Z	8E0W4EZ	9WB2XFZ	9WB9XBZ	B03BZZZ	B244ZZ3	B3091ZZ	B30S1ZZ	B317Y10
7W08X0Z	8E0W7CZ	9WB2XGZ	9WB9XCZ	B03CY0Z	B244ZZ4	B309YZZ	B30SYZZ	B317YZZ
7W08X1Z	8E0W7EZ	9WB2XHZ	9WB9XDZ	B03CYZZ	B244ZZZ	B309ZZZ	B30SZZZ	B317ZZZ
7W08X2Z	8E0W8CZ	9WB2XJZ	9WB9XFZ	B03CZZZ	B245YZZ	B30B0ZZ	B30T0ZZ	B318010

B3180ZZ	B31JYZZ	B31T110	B33HYZZ	B404YZZ	B414110	B41DZZZ	B42HZ2Z	B5010ZZ
B318110	B31JZZZ	B31T1ZZ	B33HZZZ	B4050ZZ	B4141ZZ	B41F010	B42HZZZ	B5011ZZ
B3181ZZ	B31K010	B31TY10	B33JY0Z	B4051ZZ	B414Y10	B41F0ZZ	B42M0ZZ	B501YZZ
B318Y10	B31K0ZZ	B31TYZZ	B33JYZZ	B405YZZ	B414YZZ	B41F110	B42M1ZZ	B5020ZZ
B318YZZ	B31K110	B31TZZZ	B33JZZZ	B4060ZZ	B414ZZZ	B41F1ZZ	B42MYZZ	B5021ZZ
B318ZZZ	B31K1ZZ	B31U010	B33KY0Z	B4061ZZ	B415010	B41FY10	B42MZ2Z	B502YZZ
B319010	B31KY10	B31U0ZZ	B33KYZZ	B406YZZ	B4150ZZ	B41FYZZ	B42MZZZ	B5030ZZ
B3190ZZ	B31KYZZ	B31U110	B33KZZZ	B4070ZZ	B415110	B41FZZZ	B430Y0Z	B5031ZZ
B319110	B31KZZZ	B31U1ZZ	B33MY0Z	B4071ZZ	B4151ZZ	B41G010	B430YZZ	B503YZZ
B3191ZZ	B31L010	B31UY10	B33MYZZ	B407YZZ	B415Y10	B41G0ZZ	B430ZZZ	B5040ZZ
B319Y10	B31L0ZZ	B31UYZZ	B33MZZZ	B4080ZZ	B415YZZ	B41G110	B431Y0Z	B5041ZZ
B319YZZ	B31L110	B31UZZZ	B33QY0Z	B4081ZZ	B415ZZZ	B41G1ZZ	B431YZZ	B504YZZ
B319ZZZ	B31L1ZZ	B3200ZZ	B33QYZZ	B408YZZ	B416010	B41GY10	B431ZZZ	B5050ZZ
B31B010	B31LY10	B3201ZZ	B33QZZZ	B4090ZZ	B4160ZZ	B41GYZZ	B434Y0Z	B5051ZZ
B31B0ZZ	B31LYZZ	B320YZZ	B33RY0Z	B4091ZZ	B416110	B41GZZZ	B434YZZ	B505YZZ
B31B110	B31LZZZ	B320Z2Z	B33RYZZ	B409YZZ	B4161ZZ	B41J010	B434ZZZ	B5060ZZ
B31B1ZZ	B31M010	B320ZZZ	B33RZZZ	B40B0ZZ	B416Y10	B41J0ZZ	B438Y0Z	B5061ZZ
B31BY10	B31M0ZZ	B3250ZZ	B340ZZ3	B40B1ZZ	B416YZZ	B41J110	B438YZZ	B506YZZ
B31BYZZ	B31M110	B3251ZZ	B340ZZZ	B40BYZZ	B416ZZZ	B41J1ZZ	B438ZZZ	B5070ZZ
B31BZZZ	B31M1ZZ	B325YZZ	B341ZZ3	B40C0ZZ	B417010	B41JY10	B43CY0Z	B5071ZZ
B31C010	B31MY10	B325Z2Z	B341ZZZ	B40C1ZZ	B4170ZZ	B41JYZZ	B43CYZZ	B507YZZ
B31C0ZZ	B31MYZZ	B325ZZZ	B342ZZ3	B40CYZZ	B417110	B41JZZZ	B43CZZZ	B5080ZZ
B31C110	B31MZZZ	B3280ZZ	B342ZZZ	B40D0ZZ	B4171ZZ	B4200ZZ	B43FY0Z	B5081ZZ
B31C1ZZ	B31N010	B3281ZZ	B343ZZ3	B40D1ZZ	B417Y10	B4201ZZ	B43FYZZ	B508YZZ
B31CY10	B31N0ZZ	B328YZZ	B343ZZZ	B40DYZZ	B417YZZ	B420YZZ	B43FZZZ	B5090ZZ
B31CYZZ	B31N110	B328Z2Z	B344ZZ3	B40F0ZZ	B417ZZZ	B420Z2Z	B43GY0Z	B5091ZZ
B31CZZZ	B31N1ZZ	B328ZZZ	B344ZZZ	B40F1ZZ	B418010	B420ZZZ	B43GYZZ	B509YZZ
B31D010	B31NY10	B32G0ZZ	B345ZZ3	B40FYZZ	B4180ZZ	B4210ZZ	B43GZZZ	B50B0ZZ
B31D0ZZ	B31NYZZ	B32G1ZZ	B345ZZZ	B40G0ZZ	B418110	B4211ZZ	B43HY0Z	B50B1ZZ
B31D110	B31NZZZ	B32GYZZ	B346ZZ3	B40G1ZZ	B4181ZZ	B421YZZ	B43HYZZ	B50BYZZ
B31D1ZZ	B31P010	B32GZ2Z	B346ZZZ	B40GYZZ	B418Y10	B421Z2Z	B43HZZZ	B50C0ZZ
B31DY10	B31P0ZZ	B32GZZZ	B347ZZ3	B40J0ZZ	B418YZZ	B421ZZZ	B440ZZ3	B50C1ZZ
B31DYZZ	B31P110	B32R0ZZ	B347ZZZ	B40J1ZZ	B418ZZZ	B4240ZZ	B440ZZZ	B50CYZZ
B31DZZZ	B31P1ZZ	B32R1ZZ	B348ZZ3	B40JYZZ	B419010	B4241ZZ	B444ZZ3	B50D0ZZ
B31F010	B31PY10	B32RYZZ	B348ZZZ	B40M0ZZ	B4190ZZ	B424YZZ	B444ZZZ	B50D1ZZ
B31F0ZZ	B31PYZZ	B32RZ2Z	B34HZZ3	B40M1ZZ	B419110	B424Z2Z	B445ZZ3	B50DYZZ
B31F110	B31PZZZ	B32RZZZ	B34HZZZ	B40MYZZ	B4191ZZ	B424ZZZ	B445ZZZ	B50F0ZZ
B31F1ZZ	B31Q010	B32S0ZZ	B34JZZ3	B410010	B419Y10	B4280ZZ	B446ZZ3	B50F1ZZ
B31FY10	B31Q0ZZ	B32S1ZZ	B34JZZZ	B4100ZZ	B419YZZ	B4281ZZ	B446ZZZ	B50FYZZ
B31FYZZ	B31Q110	B32SYZZ	B34KZZ3	B410110	B419ZZZ	B428YZZ	B447ZZ3	B50G0ZZ
B31FZZZ	B31Q1ZZ	B32SZ2Z	B34KZZZ	B4101ZZ	B41B010	B428Z2Z	B447ZZZ	B50G1ZZ
B31G010	B31QY10	B32SZZZ	B34RZZ3	B410Y10	B41B0ZZ	B428ZZZ	B448ZZ3	B50GYZZ
B31G0ZZ	B31QYZZ	B32T0ZZ	B34RZZZ	B410YZZ	B41B110	B42C0ZZ	B448ZZZ	B50H0ZZ
B31G110	B31QZZZ	B32T1ZZ	B34SZZ3	B410ZZZ	B41B1ZZ	B42C1ZZ	B44BZZ3	B50H1ZZ
B31G1ZZ	B31R010	B32TYZZ	B34SZZZ	B412010	B41BY10	B42CYZZ	B44BZZZ	B50HYZZ
B31GY10	B31R0ZZ	B32TZ2Z	B34TZZ3	B4120ZZ	B41BYZZ	B42CZ2Z	B44FZZ3	B50J0ZZ
B31GYZZ	B31R110	B32TZZZ	B34TZZZ	B412110	B41BZZZ	B42CZZZ	B44FZZZ	B50J1ZZ
B31GZZZ	B31R1ZZ	B330Y0Z	B34VZZ3	B4121ZZ	B41C010	B42F0ZZ	B44GZZ3	B50JYZZ
B31H010	B31RY10	B330YZZ	B34VZZZ	B412Y10	B41C0ZZ	B42F1ZZ	B44GZZZ	B50K0ZZ
B31H0ZZ	B31RYZZ	B330ZZZ	B4000ZZ	B412YZZ	B41C110	B42FYZZ	B44HZZ3	B50K1ZZ
B31H110	B31RZZZ	B335Y0Z	B4001ZZ	B412ZZZ	B41C1ZZ	B42FZ2Z	B44HZZZ	B50KYZZ
B31H1ZZ	B31S010	B335YZZ	B400YZZ	B413010	B41CY10	B42FZZZ	B44KZZ3	B50L0ZZ
B31HY10	B31S0ZZ	B335ZZZ	B4020ZZ	B4130ZZ	B41CYZZ	B42G0ZZ	B44KZZZ	B50L1ZZ
B31HYZZ	B31S110	B338Y0Z	B4021ZZ	B413110	B41CZZZ	B42G1ZZ	B44LZZ3	B50LYZZ
B31HZZZ	B31S1ZZ	B338YZZ	B402YZZ	B4131ZZ	B41D010	B42GYZZ	B44LZZZ	B50M0ZZ
B31J010	B31SY10	B338ZZZ	B4030ZZ	B413Y10	B41D0ZZ	B42GZ2Z	B44NZZ3	B50M1ZZ
B31J0ZZ	B31SYZZ	B33GY0Z	B4031ZZ	B413YZZ	B41D110	B42GZZZ	B44NZZZ	B50MYZZ
B31J110	B31SZZZ	B33GYZZ	B403YZZ	B413ZZZ	B41D1ZZ	B42H0ZZ	B5000ZZ	B50N0ZZ
B31J1ZZ	B31T010	B33GZZZ	B4040ZZ	B414010	B41DY10	B42H1ZZ	B5001ZZ	B50N1ZZ
B31JY10	B31T0ZZ	B33HY0Z	B4041ZZ	B4140ZZ	B41DYZZ	B42HYZZ	B500YZZ	B50NYZZ

B50P0ZZ	B514ZZZ	B51D1ZZ	B51MZZZ	B51W1ZZ	B52JZZZ	B538ZZZ	B54CZZZ	B801YZZ
B50P1ZZ	B5150ZA	B51DYZA	B51N0ZA	B51WYZA	B52K00Z	B539Y0Z	B54DZZ3	B8020ZZ
B50PYZZ	B5150ZZ	B51DYZZ	B51N0ZZ	B51WYZZ	B52K0ZZ	B539YZZ	B54DZZA	B8021ZZ
B50Q0ZZ	B5151ZA	B51DZZA	B51N1ZA	B51WZZA	B52K10Z	B539ZZZ	B54DZZZ	B802YZZ
B50Q1ZZ	B5151ZZ	B51DZZZ	B51N1ZZ	B51WZZZ	B52K1ZZ	B53BY0Z	B54JZZ3	B803ZZZ
B50QYZZ	B515YZA	B51F0ZA	B51NYZA	B52200Z	B52KY0Z	B53BYZZ	B54JZZA	B804ZZZ
B50R0ZZ	B515YZZ	B51F0ZZ	B51NYZZ	B52200ZZ	B52KYZZ	B53BZZZ	B54JZZZ	B805ZZZ
B50R1ZZ	B515ZZA	B51F1ZA	B51NZZA	B52210Z	B52KZ2Z	B53CY0Z	B54KZZ3	B806ZZZ
B50RYZZ	B515ZZZ	B51F1ZZ	B51NZZZ	B5221ZZ	B52KZZZ	B53CYZZ	B54KZZA	B807ZZZ
B50S0ZZ	B5160ZA	B51FYZA	B51P0ZA	B522Y0Z	B52L00Z	B53CZZZ	B54KZZZ	B82500Z
B50S1ZZ	B5160ZZ	B51FYZZ	B51P0ZZ	B522YZZ	B52L0ZZ	B53DY0Z	B54LZZ3	B8250ZZ
B50SYZZ	B5161ZA	B51FZZA	B51P1ZA	B522Z2Z	B52L10Z	B53DYZZ	B54LZZA	B82510Z
B50T0ZZ	B5161ZZ	B51FZZZ	B51P1ZZ	B522ZZZ	B52L1ZZ	B53DZZZ	B54LZZZ	B8251ZZ
B50T1ZZ	B516YZA	B51G0ZA	B51PYZA	B52800Z	B52LY0Z	B53HY0Z	B54MZZ3	B825Y0Z
B50TYZZ	B516YZZ	B51G0ZZ	B51PYZZ	B5280ZZ	B52LYZZ	B53HYZZ	B54MZZA	B825YZZ
B50V0ZZ	B516ZZA	B51G1ZA	B51PZZA	B52810Z	B52LZ2Z	B53HZZZ	B54MZZZ	B825ZZZ
B50V1ZZ	B516ZZZ	B51G1ZZ	B51PZZZ	B5281ZZ	B52LZZZ	B53LY0Z	B54NZZ3	B82600Z
B50VYZZ	B5170ZA	B51GYZA	B51Q0ZA	B528Y0Z	B52Q00Z	B53LYZZ	B54NZZA	B8260ZZ
B50W0ZZ	B5170ZZ	B51GYZZ	B51Q0ZZ	B528YZZ	B52Q0ZZ	B53LZZZ	B54NZZZ	B82610Z
B50W1ZZ	B5171ZA	B51GZZA	B51Q1ZA	B528Z2Z	B52Q10Z	B53MY0Z	B54PZZ3	B8261ZZ
B50WYZZ	B5171ZZ	B51GZZZ	B51Q1ZZ	B528ZZZ	B52Q1ZZ	B53MYZZ	B54PZZA	B826Y0Z
B5100ZA	B517YZA	B51H0ZA	B51QYZA	B52900Z	B52QY0Z	B53MZZZ	B54PZZZ	B826YZZ
B5100ZZ	B517YZZ	B51H0ZZ	B51QYZZ	B5290ZZ	B52QYZZ	B53NY0Z	B54TZZ3	B826ZZZ
B5101ZA	B517ZZA	B51H1ZA	B51QZZA	B52910Z	B52QZ2Z	B53NYZZ	B54TZZA	B82700Z
B5101ZZ	B517ZZZ	B51H1ZZ	B51QZZZ	B5291ZZ	B52QZZZ	B53NZZZ	B54TZZZ	B8270ZZ
B510YZA	B5180ZA	B51HYZA	B51R0ZA	B529Y0Z	B52R00Z	B53PY0Z	B7000ZZ	B82710Z
B510YZZ	B5180ZZ	B51HYZZ	B51R0ZZ	B529YZZ	B52R0ZZ	B53PYZZ	B7001ZZ	B8271ZZ
B510ZZA	B5181ZA	B51HZZA	B51R1ZA	B529Z2Z	B52R10Z	B53PZZZ	B700YZZ	B827Y0Z
B510ZZZ	B5181ZZ	B51HZZZ	B51R1ZZ	B529ZZZ	B52R1ZZ	B53SY0Z	B7010ZZ	B827YZZ
B5110ZA	B518YZA	B51J0ZA	B51RYZA	B52F00Z	B52RY0Z	B53SYZZ	B7011ZZ	B827ZZZ
B5110ZZ	B518YZZ	B51J0ZZ	B51RYZZ	B52F0ZZ	B52RYZZ	B53SZZZ	B701YZZ	B835Y0Z
B5111ZA	B518ZZA	B51J1ZA	B51RZZA	B52F10Z	B52RZ2Z	B53TY0Z	B7040ZZ	B835YZZ
B5111ZZ	B518ZZZ	B51J1ZZ	B51RZZZ	B52F1ZZ	B52RZZZ	B53TYZZ	B7041ZZ	B835ZZZ
B511YZA	B5190ZA	B51JYZA	B51S0ZA	B52FY0Z	B52S00Z	B53TZZZ	B704YZZ	B836Y0Z
B511YZZ	B5190ZZ	B51JYZZ	B51S0ZZ	B52FYZZ	B52S0ZZ	B53VY0Z	B7050ZZ	B836YZZ
B511ZZA	B5191ZA	B51JZZA	B51S1ZA	B52FZ2Z	B52S10Z	B53VYZZ	B7051ZZ	B836ZZZ
B511ZZZ	B5191ZZ	B51JZZZ	B51S1ZZ	B52FZZZ	B52S1ZZ	B53VZZZ	B705YZZ	B837Y0Z
B5120ZA	B519YZA	B51K0ZA	B51SYZA	B52G00Z	B52SY0Z	B543ZZ3	B7060ZZ	B837YZZ
B5120ZZ	B519YZZ	B51K0ZZ	B51SYZZ	B52G0ZZ	B52SYZZ	B543ZZA	B7061ZZ	B837ZZZ
B5121ZA	B519ZZA	B51K1ZA	B51SZZA	B52G10Z	B52SZ2Z	B543ZZZ	B706YZZ	B845ZZZ
B5121ZZ	B519ZZZ	B51K1ZZ	B51SZZZ	B52G1ZZ	B52SZZZ	B544ZZ3	B7070ZZ	B846ZZZ
B512YZA	B51B0ZA	B51KYZA	B51T0ZA	B52GY0Z	B52T00Z	B544ZZA	B7071ZZ	B847ZZZ
B512YZZ	B51B0ZZ	B51KYZZ	B51T0ZZ	B52GYZZ	B52T0ZZ	B544ZZZ	B707YZZ	B902ZZZ
B512ZZA	B51B1ZA	B51KZZA	B51T1ZA	B52GZ2Z	B52T10Z	B546ZZ3	B7080ZZ	B9040ZZ
B512ZZZ	B51B1ZZ	B51KZZZ	B51T1ZZ	B52GZZZ	B52T1ZZ	B546ZZA	B7081ZZ	B9041ZZ
B5130ZA	B51BYZA	B51L0ZA	B51TYZA	B52H00Z	B52TY0Z	B546ZZZ	B708YZZ	B904YZZ
B5130ZZ	B51BYZZ	B51L0ZZ	B51TYZZ	B52H0ZZ	B52TYZZ	B547ZZ3	B7090ZZ	B9050ZZ
B5131ZA	B51BZZA	B51L1ZA	B51TZZA	B52H10Z	B52TZ2Z	B547ZZA	B7091ZZ	B9051ZZ
B5131ZZ	B51BZZZ	B51L1ZZ	B51TZZZ	B52H1ZZ	B52TZZZ	B547ZZZ	B709YZZ	B905YZZ
B513YZA	B51C0ZA	B51LYZA	B51V0ZA	B52HY0Z	B531Y0Z	B548ZZ3	B70B0ZZ	B9060ZZ
B513YZZ	B51C0ZZ	B51LYZZ	B51V0ZZ	B52HYZZ	B531YZZ	B548ZZA	B70B1ZZ	B9061ZZ
B513ZZA	B51C1ZA	B51LZZA	B51V1ZA	B52HZ2Z	B531ZZZ	B548ZZZ	B70BYZZ	B906YZZ
B513ZZZ	B51C1ZZ	B51LZZZ	B51V1ZZ	B52HZZZ	B532Y0Z	B549ZZ3	B70C0ZZ	B9070ZZ
B5140ZA	B51CYZA	B51M0ZA	B51VYZA	B52J00Z	B532YZZ	B549ZZA	B70C1ZZ	B9071ZZ
B5140ZZ	B51CYZZ	B51M0ZZ	B51VYZZ	B52J0ZZ	B532ZZZ	B549ZZZ	B70CYZZ	B907YZZ
B5141ZA	B51CZZA	B51M1ZA	B51VZZA	B52J10Z	B535Y0Z	B54BZZ3	B8000ZZ	B9080ZZ
B5141ZZ	B51CZZZ	B51M1ZZ	B51VZZZ	B52J1ZZ	B535YZZ	B54BZZA	B8001ZZ	B9081ZZ
B514YZA	B51D0ZA	B51MYZA	B51W0ZA	B52JY0Z	B535ZZZ	B54BZZZ	B800YZZ	B908YZZ
B514YZZ	B51D0ZZ	B51MYZZ	B51W0ZZ	B52JYZZ	B538Y0Z	B54CZZ3	B8010ZZ	B9090ZZ
B514ZZA	B51D1ZA	B51MZZA	B51W1ZA	B52JZ2Z	B538YZZ	B54CZZA	B8011ZZ	B9091ZZ

B909YZZ	B92J10Z	BB2900Z	BF110ZZ	BF5020Z	BG43ZZZ	BL32YZZ	BN26YZZ	BP0RZZZ
B90B0ZZ	B92J1ZZ	BB290ZZ	BF111ZZ	BF502Z0	BG44ZZZ	BL32ZZZ	BN26ZZZ	BP0SZZZ
B90B1ZZ	B92JY0Z	BB2910Z	BF11YZZ	BF502ZZ	BH00ZZZ	BL33Y0Z	BN290ZZ	BP0XZZZ
B90BYZZ	B92JYZZ	BB291ZZ	BF120ZZ	BF52200	BH01ZZZ	BL33YZZ	BN291ZZ	BP0YZZZ
B90C0ZZ	B92JZZZ	BB29Y0Z	BF121ZZ	BF5220Z	BH02ZZZ	BL33ZZZ	BN29YZZ	BP10ZZZ
B90C1ZZ	B930Y0Z	BB29YZZ	BF12YZZ	BF522Z0	BH030ZZ	BL40ZZZ	BN29ZZZ	BP11ZZZ
B90CYZZ	B930YZZ	BB29ZZZ	BF130ZZ	BF522ZZ	BH031ZZ	BL41ZZZ	BN2F0ZZ	BP12ZZZ
B90D0ZZ	B930ZZZ	BB2F00Z	BF131ZZ	BF53200	BH03YZZ	BL42ZZZ	BN2F1ZZ	BP13ZZZ
B90D1ZZ	B932Y0Z	BB2F0ZZ	BF13YZZ	BF5320Z	BH03ZZZ	BL43ZZZ	BN2FYZZ	BP14ZZZ
B90DYZZ	B932YZZ	BB2F10Z	BF140ZZ	BF532Z0	BH040ZZ	BN00ZZZ	BN2FZZZ	BP15ZZZ
B90FZZZ	B932ZZZ	BB2F1ZZ	BF141ZZ	BF532ZZ	BH041ZZ	BN01ZZZ	BN39YZZ	BP16ZZZ
B90HZZZ	B936Y0Z	BB2FY0Z	BF14YZZ	BF55200	BH04YZZ	BN02ZZZ	BN39ZZZ	BP17ZZZ
B91GYZZ	B936YZZ	BB2FYZZ	BF180ZZ	BF5520Z	BH04ZZZ	BN03ZZZ	BP00ZZZ	BP180ZZ
B91GZZZ	B936ZZZ	BB2FZZZ	BF181ZZ	BF552Z0	BH050ZZ	BN04ZZZ	BP01ZZZ	BP181ZZ
B91JYZZ	B939Y0Z	BB3GY0Z	BF18YZZ	BF552ZZ	BH051ZZ	BN05ZZZ	BP02ZZZ	BP18YZZ
B91JZZZ	B939YZZ	BB3GYZZ	BF2500Z	BF56200	BH05YZZ	BN06ZZZ	BP03ZZZ	BP18ZZZ
B92000Z	B939ZZZ	BB3GZZZ	BF250ZZ	BF5620Z	BH05ZZZ	BN070ZZ	BP04ZZZ	BP190ZZ
B9200ZZ	B93DY0Z	BB4BZZZ	BF2510Z	BF562Z0	BH060ZZ	BN071ZZ	BP05ZZZ	BP191ZZ
B92010Z	B93DYZZ	BB4CZZZ	BF251ZZ	BF562ZZ	BH061ZZ	BN07YZZ	BP06ZZZ	BP19YZZ
B9201ZZ	B93DZZZ	BD11YZZ	BF25Y0Z	BF57200	BH06YZZ	BN07ZZZ	BP07ZZZ	BP19ZZZ
B920Y0Z	B93FY0Z	BD11ZZZ	BF25YZZ	BF5720Z	BH06ZZZ	BN080ZZ	BP080ZZ	BP1AZZZ
B920YZZ	B93FYZZ	BD12YZZ	BF25ZZZ	BF572Z0	BH30Y0Z	BN081ZZ	BP081ZZ	BP1BZZZ
B920ZZZ	B93FZZZ	BD12ZZZ	BF2600Z	BF572ZZ	BH30YZZ	BN08YZZ	BP08YZZ	BP1C0ZZ
B92200Z	B93JY0Z	BD13YZZ	BF260ZZ	BF5C200	BH30ZZZ	BN08ZZZ	BP08ZZZ	BP1C1ZZ
B9220ZZ	B93JYZZ	BD13ZZZ	BF2610Z	BF5C20Z	BH31Y0Z	BN090ZZ	BP090ZZ	BP1CYZZ
B92210Z	B93JZZZ	BD14YZZ	BF261ZZ	BF5C2Z0	BH31YZZ	BN091ZZ	BP091ZZ	BP1D0ZZ
B9221ZZ	BB07YZZ	BD14ZZZ	BF26Y0Z	BF5C2ZZ	BH31ZZZ	BN09YZZ	BP09YZZ	BP1D1ZZ
B922Y0Z	BB08YZZ	BD15YZZ	BF26YZZ	BG2200Z	BH32Y0Z	BN09ZZZ	BP09ZZZ	BP1DYZZ
B922YZZ	BB09YZZ	BD15ZZZ	BF26ZZZ	BG220ZZ	BH32YZZ	BN0BZZZ	BP0AZZZ	BP1EZZZ
B922ZZZ	BB0DZZZ	BD16YZZ	BF2700Z	BG2210Z	BH32ZZZ	BN0CZZZ	BP0BZZZ	BP1FZZZ
B92600Z	BB12ZZZ	BD16ZZZ	BF270ZZ	BG221ZZ	BH3DY0Z	BN0DZZZ	BP0C0ZZ	BP1G0ZZ
B9260ZZ	BB13ZZZ	BD19YZZ	BF2710Z	BG22Y0Z	BH3DYZZ	BN0GZZZ	BP0C1ZZ	BP1G1ZZ
B92610Z	BB14ZZZ	BD19ZZZ	BF271ZZ	BG22YZZ	BH3DZZZ	BN0HZZZ	BP0CYZZ	BP1GYZZ
B9261ZZ	BB16ZZZ	BD1BYZZ	BF27Y0Z	BG22ZZZ	BH3FY0Z	BN0JZZZ	BP0CZZZ	BP1H0ZZ
B926Y0Z	BB17YZZ	BD1BZZZ	BF27YZZ	BG2300Z	BH3FYZZ	BN170ZZ	BP0D0ZZ	BP1H1ZZ
B926YZZ	BB18YZZ	BD2400Z	BF27ZZZ	BG230ZZ	BH3FZZZ	BN171ZZ	BP0D1ZZ	BP1HYZZ
B926ZZZ	BB19YZZ	BD240ZZ	BF2C00Z	BG2310Z	BH3GY0Z	BN17YZZ	BP0DYZZ	BP1JZZZ
B92900Z	BB1CZZZ	BD2410Z	BF2C0ZZ	BG231ZZ	BH3GYZZ	BN17ZZZ	BP0DZZZ	BP1KZZZ
B9290ZZ	BB1DZZZ	BD241ZZ	BF2C10Z	BG23Y0Z	BH3GZZZ	BN180ZZ	BP0EZZZ	BP1L0ZZ
B92910Z	BB2400Z	BD24Y0Z	BF2C1ZZ	BG23YZZ	BH3HY0Z	BN181ZZ	BP0FZZZ	BP1L1ZZ
B9291ZZ	BB240ZZ	BD24YZZ	BF2CY0Z	BG23ZZZ	BH3HYZZ	BN18YZZ	BP0G0ZZ	BP1LYZZ
B929Y0Z	BB2410Z	BD24ZZZ	BF2CYZZ	BG2400Z	BH3HZZZ	BN18ZZZ	BP0G1ZZ	BP1LZZZ
B929YZZ	BB241ZZ	BD41ZZZ	BF2CZZZ	BG240ZZ	BH3JY0Z	BN190ZZ	BP0GYZZ	BP1M0ZZ
B929ZZZ	BB24Y0Z	BD42ZZZ	BF35Y0Z	BG2410Z	BH3JYZZ	BN191ZZ	BP0GZZZ	BP1M1ZZ
B92D00Z	BB24YZZ	BD47ZZZ	BF35YZZ	BG241ZZ	BH3JZZZ	BN19YZZ	BP0H0ZZ	BP1MYZZ
B92D0ZZ	BB24ZZZ	BD48ZZZ	BF35ZZZ	BG24Y0Z	BH40ZZZ	BN19ZZZ	BP0H1ZZ	BP1MZZZ
B92D10Z	BB2700Z	BD49ZZZ	BF36Y0Z	BG24YZZ	BH41ZZZ	BN200ZZ	BP0HYZZ	BP1NZZZ
B92D1ZZ	BB270ZZ	BD4CZZZ	BF36YZZ	BG24ZZZ	BH42ZZZ	BN201ZZ	BP0HZZZ	BP1PZZZ
B92DY0Z	BB2710Z	BF000ZZ	BF36ZZZ	BG32Y0Z	BH47ZZZ	BN20YZZ	BP0JZZZ	BP1RZZZ
B92DYZZ	BB271ZZ	BF001ZZ	BF37Y0Z	BG32YZZ	BH48ZZZ	BN20ZZZ	BP0KZZZ	BP1SZZZ
B92DZZZ	BB27Y0Z	BF00YZZ	BF37YZZ	BG32ZZZ	BH49ZZZ	BN230ZZ	BP0L0ZZ	BP1XZZZ
B92F00Z	BB27YZZ	BF030ZZ	BF37ZZZ	BG33Y0Z	BH4BZZZ	BN231ZZ	BP0L1ZZ	BP1YZZZ
B92F0ZZ	BB27ZZZ	BF031ZZ	BF40ZZZ	BG33YZZ	BH4CZZZ	BN23YZZ	BP0LYZZ	BP200ZZ
B92F10Z	BB2800Z	BF03YZZ	BF42ZZZ	BG33ZZZ	BL30Y0Z	BN23ZZZ	BP0LZZZ	BP201ZZ
B92F1ZZ	BB280ZZ	BF0C0ZZ	BF43ZZZ	BG34Y0Z	BL30YZZ	BN250ZZ	BP0M0ZZ	BP20YZZ
B92FY0Z	BB2810Z	BF0C1ZZ	BF45ZZZ	BG34YZZ	BL30ZZZ	BN251ZZ	BP0M1ZZ	BP210ZZ
B92FYZZ	BB281ZZ	BF0CYZZ	BF46ZZZ	BG34ZZZ	BL31Y0Z	BN25YZZ	BP0MYZZ	BP211ZZ
B92FZZZ	BB28Y0Z	BF100ZZ	BF47ZZZ	BG40ZZZ	BL31YZZ	BN25ZZZ	BP0MZZZ	BP21YZZ
B92J00Z	BB28YZZ	BF101ZZ	BF4CZZZ	BG41ZZZ	BL31ZZZ	BN260ZZ	BP0NZZZ	BP220ZZ
B92J0ZZ	BB28ZZZ	BF10YZZ	BF50200	BG42ZZZ	BL32Y0Z	BN261ZZ	BP0PZZZ	BP221ZZ

BP22YZZ	BP2K0ZZ	BP39ZZZ	BQ04ZZZ	BQ1HZZZ	BQ2H1ZZ	BQ34Y0Z	BR02ZZZ	BR170ZZ
BP22ZZZ	BP2K1ZZ	BP3CY0Z	BQ070ZZ	BQ1JZZZ	BQ2HYZZ	BQ34YZZ	BR030ZZ	BR171ZZ
BP230ZZ	BP2KYZZ	BP3CYZZ	BQ071ZZ	BQ1KZZZ	BQ2HZZZ	BQ34ZZZ	BR031ZZ	BR17YZZ
BP231ZZ	BP2KZZZ	BP3CZZZ	BQ07YZZ	BQ1LZZZ	BQ2J0ZZ	BQ37Y0Z	BR03YZZ	BR17ZZZ
BP23YZZ	BP2L0ZZ	BP3DY0Z	BQ07ZZZ	BQ1MZZZ	BQ2J1ZZ	BQ37YZZ	BR03ZZZ	BR180ZZ
BP23ZZZ	BP2L1ZZ	BP3DYZZ	BQ080ZZ	BQ1PZZZ	BQ2JYZZ	BQ37ZZZ	BR040ZZ	BR181ZZ
BP240ZZ	BP2LYZZ	BP3DZZZ	BQ081ZZ	BQ1QZZZ	BQ2JZZZ	BQ38Y0Z	BR041ZZ	BR18YZZ
BP241ZZ	BP2LZZZ	BP3EY0Z	BQ08YZZ	BQ1VZZZ	BQ2K0ZZ	BQ38YZZ	BR04YZZ	BR18ZZZ
BP24YZZ	BP2M0ZZ	BP3EYZZ	BQ08ZZZ	BQ1WZZZ	BQ2K1ZZ	BQ38ZZZ	BR04ZZZ	BR190ZZ
BP24ZZZ	BP2M1ZZ	BP3EZZZ	BQ0DZZZ	BQ1X0ZZ	BQ2KYZZ	BQ3DY0Z	BR050ZZ	BR191ZZ
BP250ZZ	BP2MYZZ	BP3FY0Z	BQ0FZZZ	BQ1X1ZZ	BQ2KZZZ	BQ3DYZZ	BR051ZZ	BR19YZZ
BP251ZZ	BP2MZZZ	BP3FYZZ	BQ0G0ZZ	BQ1XYZZ	BQ2L0ZZ	BQ3DZZZ	BR05YZZ	BR19ZZZ
BP25YZZ	BP2N0ZZ	BP3FZZZ	BQ0G1ZZ	BQ1XZZZ	BQ2L1ZZ	BQ3FY0Z	BR05ZZZ	BR1B0ZZ
BP25ZZZ	BP2N1ZZ	BP3GY0Z	BQ0GYZZ	BQ1Y0ZZ	BQ2LYZZ	BQ3FYZZ	BR060ZZ	BR1B1ZZ
BP260ZZ	BP2NYZZ	BP3GYZZ	BQ0GZZZ	BQ1Y1ZZ	BQ2LZZZ	BQ3FZZZ	BR061ZZ	BR1BYZZ
BP261ZZ	BP2NZZZ	BP3GZZZ	BQ0H0ZZ	BQ1YYZZ	BQ2M0ZZ	BQ3GY0Z	BR06YZZ	BR1BZZZ
BP26YZZ	BP2P0ZZ	BP3HY0Z	BQ0H1ZZ	BQ1YZZZ	BQ2M1ZZ	BQ3GYZZ	BR06ZZZ	BR1C0ZZ
BP26ZZZ	BP2P1ZZ	BP3HYZZ	BQ0HYZZ	BQ200ZZ	BQ2MYZZ	BQ3GZZZ	BR07ZZ1	BR1C1ZZ
BP270ZZ	BP2PYZZ	BP3HZZZ	BQ0HZZZ	BQ201ZZ	BQ2MZZZ	BQ3HY0Z	BR07ZZZ	BR1CYZZ
BP271ZZ	BP2PZZZ	BP3JY0Z	BQ0JZZZ	BQ20YZZ	BQ2P0ZZ	BQ3HYZZ	BR08ZZZ	BR1CZZZ
BP27YZZ	BP2Q0ZZ	BP3JYZZ	BQ0KZZZ	BQ20ZZZ	BQ2P1ZZ	BQ3HZZZ	BR09ZZ1	BR1D0ZZ
BP27ZZZ	BP2Q1ZZ	BP3JZZZ	BQ0LZZZ	BQ210ZZ	BQ2PYZZ	BQ3JY0Z	BR09ZZZ	BR1D1ZZ
BP280ZZ	BP2QYZZ	BP3KY0Z	BQ0MZZZ	BQ211ZZ	BQ2PZZZ	BQ3JYZZ	BR0BZZZ	BR1DYZZ
BP281ZZ	BP2QZZZ	BP3KYZZ	BQ0PZZZ	BQ21YZZ	BQ2Q0ZZ	BQ3JZZZ	BR0CZZZ	BR1DZZZ
BP28YZZ	BP2R0ZZ	BP3KZZZ	BQ0QZZZ	BQ21ZZZ	BQ2Q1ZZ	BQ3KY0Z	BR0D0ZZ	BR1F0ZZ
BP28ZZZ	BP2R1ZZ	BP3LY0Z	BQ0VZZZ	BQ230ZZ	BQ2QYZZ	BQ3KYZZ	BR0D1ZZ	BR1F1ZZ
BP290ZZ	BP2RYZZ	BP3LYZZ	BQ0WZZZ	BQ231ZZ	BQ2QZZZ	BQ3KZZZ	BR0DYZZ	BR1FYZZ
BP291ZZ	BP2RZZZ	BP3LZZZ	BQ0X0ZZ	BQ23YZZ	BQ2R0ZZ	BQ3LY0Z	BR0DZZZ	BR1FZZZ
BP29YZZ	BP2S0ZZ	BP3MY0Z	BQ0X1ZZ	BQ23ZZZ	BQ2R1ZZ	BQ3LYZZ	BR0FZZZ	BR1G0ZZ
BP29ZZZ	BP2S1ZZ	BP3MYZZ	BQ0XYZZ	BQ240ZZ	BQ2RYZZ	BQ3LZZZ	BR0GZZ1	BR1G1ZZ
BP2A0ZZ	BP2SYZZ	BP3MZZZ	BQ0Y0ZZ	BQ241ZZ	BQ2RZZZ	BQ3MY0Z	BR0GZZZ	BR1GYZZ
BP2A1ZZ	BP2SZZZ	BP48ZZ1	BQ0Y1ZZ	BQ24YZZ	BQ2S0ZZ	BQ3MYZZ	BR0HZZZ	BR1GZZZ
BP2AYZZ	BP2T0ZZ	BP48ZZZ	BQ0YYZZ	BQ24ZZZ	BQ2S1ZZ	BQ3MZZZ	BR100ZZ	BR1H0ZZ
BP2AZZZ	BP2T1ZZ	BP49ZZ1	BQ100ZZ	BQ270ZZ	BQ2SYZZ	BQ3PY0Z	BR101ZZ	BR1H1ZZ
BP2B0ZZ	BP2TYZZ	BP49ZZZ	BQ101ZZ	BQ271ZZ	BQ2SZZZ	BQ3PYZZ	BR10YZZ	BR1HYZZ
BP2B1ZZ	BP2TZZZ	BP4GZZ1	BQ10YZZ	BQ27YZZ	BQ2V0ZZ	BQ3PZZZ	BR10ZZZ	BR1HZZZ
BP2BYZZ	BP2U0ZZ	BP4GZZZ	BQ10ZZZ	BQ27ZZZ	BQ2V1ZZ	BQ3QY0Z	BR110ZZ	BR200ZZ
BP2BZZZ	BP2U1ZZ	BP4HZZ1	BQ110ZZ	BQ280ZZ	BQ2VYZZ	BQ3QYZZ	BR111ZZ	BR201ZZ
BP2CZZZ	BP2UYZZ	BP4HZZZ	BQ111ZZ	BQ281ZZ	BQ2VZZZ	BQ3QZZZ	BR11YZZ	BR20YZZ
BP2DZZZ	BP2UZZZ	BP4LZZ1	BQ11YZZ	BQ28YZZ	BQ2W0ZZ	BQ3VY0Z	BR11ZZZ	BR20ZZZ
BP2E0ZZ	BP2V0ZZ	BP4LZZZ	BQ11ZZZ	BQ28ZZZ	BQ2W1ZZ	BQ3VYZZ	BR120ZZ	BR270ZZ
BP2E1ZZ	BP2V1ZZ	BP4MZZ1	BQ13ZZZ	BQ2B0ZZ	BQ2WYZZ	BQ3VZZZ	BR121ZZ	BR271ZZ
BP2EYZZ	BP2VYZZ	BP4MZZZ	BQ14ZZZ	BQ2B1ZZ	BQ2WZZZ	BQ3WY0Z	BR12YZZ	BR27YZZ
BP2EZZZ	BP2VZZZ	BP4NZZ1	BQ170ZZ	BQ2BYZZ	BQ2X0ZZ	BQ3WYZZ	BR12ZZZ	BR27ZZZ
BP2F0ZZ	BP2W0ZZ	BP4NZZZ	BQ171ZZ	BQ2C0ZZ	BQ2X1ZZ	BQ3WZZZ	BR130ZZ	BR290ZZ
BP2F1ZZ	BP2W1ZZ	BP4PZZ1	BQ17YZZ	BQ2C1ZZ	BQ2XYZZ	BQ40ZZZ	BR131ZZ	BR291ZZ
BP2FYZZ	BP2WYZZ	BP4PZZZ	BQ17ZZZ	BQ2CYZZ	BQ2XZZZ	BQ41ZZZ	BR13YZZ	BR29YZZ
BP2FZZZ	BP2X0ZZ	BQ000ZZ	BQ180ZZ	BQ2D0ZZ	BQ2Y0ZZ	BQ42ZZZ	BR13ZZZ	BR29ZZZ
BP2G0ZZ	BP2X1ZZ	BQ001ZZ	BQ181ZZ	BQ2D1ZZ	BQ2Y1ZZ	BQ47ZZZ	BR140ZZ	BR2C0ZZ
BP2G1ZZ	BP2XYZZ	BQ00YZZ	BQ18YZZ	BQ2DYZZ	BQ2YYZZ	BQ48ZZZ	BR141ZZ	BR2C1ZZ
BP2GYZZ	BP2XZZZ	BQ00ZZ1	BQ18ZZZ	BQ2DZZZ	BQ2YZZZ	BQ49ZZZ	BR14YZZ	BR2CYZZ
BP2GZZZ	BP2Y0ZZ	BQ00ZZZ	BQ1DZZZ	BQ2F0ZZ	BQ30Y0Z	BR00ZZ1	BR14ZZZ	BR2CZZZ
BP2H0ZZ	BP2Y1ZZ	BQ010ZZ	BQ1FZZZ	BQ2F1ZZ	BQ30YZZ	BR00ZZZ	BR150ZZ	BR2D0ZZ
BP2H1ZZ	BP2YYZZ	BQ011ZZ	BQ1G0ZZ	BQ2FYZZ	BQ30ZZZ	BR010ZZ	BR151ZZ	BR2D1ZZ
BP2HYZZ	BP2YZZZ	BQ01YZZ	BQ1G1ZZ	BQ2FZZZ	BQ31Y0Z	BR011ZZ	BR15YZZ	BR2DYZZ
BP2HZZZ	BP38Y0Z	BQ01ZZ1	BQ1GYZZ	BQ2G0ZZ	BQ31YZZ	BR01YZZ	BR15ZZZ	BR2DZZZ
BP2J0ZZ	BP38YZZ	BQ01ZZZ	BQ1GZZZ	BQ2G1ZZ	BQ31ZZZ	BR01ZZZ	BR160ZZ	BR2F0ZZ
BP2J1ZZ	BP38ZZZ	BQ03ZZ1	BQ1H0ZZ	BQ2GYZZ	BQ33Y0Z	BR020ZZ	BR161ZZ	BR2F1ZZ
BP2JYZZ	BP39Y0Z	BQ03ZZZ	BQ1H1ZZ	BQ2GZZZ	BQ33YZZ	BR021ZZ	BR16YZZ	BR2FYZZ
BP2JZZZ	BP39YZZ	BQ04ZZ1	BQ1HYZZ	BQ2H0ZZ	BQ33ZZZ	BR02YZZ	BR16ZZZ	BR2FZZZ

BR30Y0Z	BT080ZZ	BT1G0ZZ	BT47ZZZ	BU39ZZZ	BV30YZZ	BW240ZZ	BW3PZZZ	C21G1ZZ
BR30YZZ	BT081ZZ	BT1G1ZZ	BT48ZZZ	BU3BY0Z	BV30ZZZ	BW2410Z	BW40ZZZ	C21GDZZ
BR30ZZZ	BT08YZZ	BT1GYZZ	BT49ZZZ	BU3BYZZ	BV33Y0Z	BW241ZZ	BW41ZZZ	C21GSZZ
BR31Y0Z	BT08ZZZ	BT1GZZZ	BT4JZZZ	BU3BZZZ	BV33YZZ	BW24Y0Z	BW4FZZZ	C21GYZZ
BR31YZZ	BT0B0ZZ	BT2000Z	BU000ZZ	BU3CY0Z	BV33ZZZ	BW24YZZ	BW4GZZZ	C21GZZZ
BR31ZZZ	BT0B1ZZ	BT200ZZ	BU001ZZ	BU3CYZZ	BV34Y0Z	BW24ZZZ	BW52Z1Z	C21YYZZ
BR32Y0Z	BT0BYZZ	BT2010Z	BU00YZZ	BU3CZZZ	BV34YZZ	BW2500Z	BW59Z1Z	C2261ZZ
BR32YZZ	BT0BZZZ	BT201ZZ	BU010ZZ	BU40YZZ	BV34ZZZ	BW250ZZ	BW5CZ1Z	C226YZZ
BR32ZZZ	BT0C0ZZ	BT20Y0Z	BU011ZZ	BU40ZZZ	BV35Y0Z	BW2510Z	BW5JZ1Z	C22G1ZZ
BR33Y0Z	BT0C1ZZ	BT20YZZ	BU01YZZ	BU41YZZ	BV35YZZ	BW251ZZ	BY30Y0Z	C22GDZZ
BR33YZZ	BT0CYZZ	BT20ZZZ	BU020ZZ	BU41ZZZ	BV35ZZZ	BW25Y0Z	BY30YZZ	C22GKZZ
BR33ZZZ	BT0CZZZ	BT2100Z	BU021ZZ	BU42YZZ	BV36Y0Z	BW25YZZ	BY30ZZZ	C22GSZZ
BR37Y0Z	BT100ZZ	BT210ZZ	BU02YZZ	BU42ZZZ	BV36YZZ	BW25ZZZ	BY31Y0Z	C22GYZZ
BR37YZZ	BT101ZZ	BT2110Z	BU060ZZ	BU43YZZ	BV36ZZZ	BW2800Z	BY31YZZ	C22GZZZ
BR37ZZZ	BT10YZZ	BT211ZZ	BU061ZZ	BU43ZZZ	BV37Y0Z	BW280ZZ	BY31ZZZ	C22YYZZ
BR39Y0Z	BT10ZZZ	BT21Y0Z	BU06YZZ	BU44YZZ	BV37YZZ	BW2810Z	BY32Y0Z	C23GKZZ
BR39YZZ	BT110ZZ	BT21YZZ	BU080ZZ	BU44ZZZ	BV37ZZZ	BW281ZZ	BY32YZZ	C23GMZZ
BR39ZZZ	BT111ZZ	BT21ZZZ	BU081ZZ	BU45YZZ	BV44ZZZ	BW28Y0Z	BY32ZZZ	C23GQZZ
BR3CY0Z	BT11YZZ	BT2200Z	BU08YZZ	BU45ZZZ	BV49ZZZ	BW28YZZ	BY33Y0Z	C23GRZZ
BR3CYZZ	BT11ZZZ	BT220ZZ	BU090ZZ	BU46YZZ	BV4BZZZ	BW28ZZZ	BY33YZZ	C23GYZZ
BR3CZZZ	BT120ZZ	BT2210Z	BU091ZZ	BU46ZZZ	BW00ZZZ	BW2900Z	BY33ZZZ	C23YYZZ
BR3FY0Z	BT121ZZ	BT221ZZ	BU09YZZ	BU4CYZZ	BW01ZZZ	BW290ZZ	BY34Y0Z	C2561ZZ
BR3FYZZ	BT12YZZ	BT22Y0Z	BU100ZZ	BU4CZZZ	BW03ZZZ	BW2910Z	BY34YZZ	C256YZZ
BR3FZZZ	BT12ZZZ	BT22YZZ	BU101ZZ	BV000ZZ	BW0BZZZ	BW291ZZ	BY34ZZZ	C25YYZZ
BR40ZZZ	BT130ZZ	BT22ZZZ	BU10YZZ	BV001ZZ	BW0CZZZ	BW29Y0Z	BY35Y0Z	C51B1ZZ
BR47ZZZ	BT131ZZ	BT2300Z	BU10ZZZ	BV00YZZ	BW0JZZZ	BW29YZZ	BY35YZZ	C51BYZZ
BR49ZZZ	BT13YZZ	BT230ZZ	BU110ZZ	BV010ZZ	BW0KZZZ	BW29ZZZ	BY35ZZZ	C51C1ZZ
BR4FZZZ	BT13ZZZ	BT2310Z	BU111ZZ	BV011ZZ	BW0LZZZ	BW2F00Z	BY36Y0Z	C51CYZZ
BT000ZZ	BT140ZZ	BT231ZZ	BU11YZZ	BV01YZZ	BW0MZZZ	BW2F0ZZ	BY36YZZ	C51D1ZZ
BT001ZZ	BT141ZZ	BT23Y0Z	BU11ZZZ	BV020ZZ	BW110ZZ	BW2F10Z	BY36ZZZ	C51DYZZ
BT00YZZ	BT14YZZ	BT23YZZ	BU120ZZ	BV021ZZ	BW111ZZ	BW2F1ZZ	BY47ZZZ	C51N1ZZ
BT00ZZZ	BT14ZZZ	BT23ZZZ	BU121ZZ	BV02YZZ	BW11YZZ	BW2FY0Z	BY48ZZZ	C51NYZZ
BT010ZZ	BT150ZZ	BT2900Z	BU12YZZ	BV030ZZ	BW11ZZZ	BW2FYZZ	BY49ZZZ	C51P1ZZ
BT011ZZ	BT151ZZ	BT290ZZ	BU12ZZZ	BV031ZZ	BW190ZZ	BW2FZZZ	BY4BZZZ	C51PYZZ
BT01YZZ	BT15YZZ	BT2910Z	BU160ZZ	BV03YZZ	BW191ZZ	BW2G00Z	BY4CZZZ	C51Q1ZZ
BT01ZZZ	BT15ZZZ	BT291ZZ	BU161ZZ	BV050ZZ	BW19YZZ	BW2G0ZZ	BY4DZZZ	C51QYZZ
BT020ZZ	BT160ZZ	BT29Y0Z	BU16YZZ	BV051ZZ	BW19ZZZ	BW2G10Z	BY4FZZZ	C51R1ZZ
BT021ZZ	BT161ZZ	BT29YZZ	BU16ZZZ	BV05YZZ	BW1C0ZZ	BW2G1ZZ	BY4GZZZ	C51RYZZ
BT02YZZ	BT16YZZ	BT29ZZZ	BU180ZZ	BV060ZZ	BW1C1ZZ	BW2GY0Z	C0101ZZ	C51YYZZ
BT02ZZZ	BT16ZZZ	BT30Y0Z	BU181ZZ	BV061ZZ	BW1CYZZ	BW2GYZZ	C010YZZ	C7101ZZ
BT030ZZ	BT170ZZ	BT30YZZ	BU18YZZ	BV06YZZ	BW1CZZZ	BW2GZZZ	C015DZZ	C710DZZ
BT031ZZ	BT171ZZ	BT30ZZZ	BU18ZZZ	BV080ZZ	BW1J0ZZ	BW30Y0Z	C015YZZ	C710YZZ
BT03YZZ	BT17YZZ	BT31Y0Z	BU190ZZ	BV081ZZ	BW1J1ZZ	BW30YZZ	C01YYZZ	C7121ZZ
BT03ZZZ	BT17ZZZ	BT31YZZ	BU191ZZ	BV08YZZ	BW1JYZZ	BW30ZZZ	C0201ZZ	C712YZZ
BT040ZZ	BT1B0ZZ	BT31ZZZ	BU19YZZ	BV100ZZ	BW1JZZZ	BW33Y0Z	C020FZZ	C713DZZ
BT041ZZ	BT1B1ZZ	BT32Y0Z	BU19ZZZ	BV101ZZ	BW2000Z	BW33YZZ	C020SZZ	C713YZZ
BT04YZZ	BT1BYZZ	BT32YZZ	BU33Y0Z	BV10YZZ	BW200ZZ	BW38Y0Z	C020YZZ	C7151ZZ
BT04ZZZ	BT1BZZZ	BT32ZZZ	BU33YZZ	BV10ZZZ	BW2010Z	BW38YZZ	C025DZZ	C715YZZ
BT050ZZ	BT1C0ZZ	BT33Y0Z	BU33ZZZ	BV180ZZ	BW201ZZ	BW38ZZZ	C025YZZ	C71D1ZZ
BT051ZZ	BT1C1ZZ	BT33YZZ	BU34Y0Z	BV181ZZ	BW20Y0Z	BW3FY0Z	C02YYZZ	C71DYZZ
BT05YZZ	BT1CYZZ	BT33ZZZ	BU34YZZ	BV18YZZ	BW20YZZ	BW3FYZZ	C030BZZ	C71J1ZZ
BT05ZZZ	BT1CZZZ	BT39Y0Z	BU34ZZZ	BV18ZZZ	BW20ZZZ	BW3FZZZ	C030KZZ	C71JYZZ
BT060ZZ	BT1D0ZZ	BT39YZZ	BU35Y0Z	BV2300Z	BW2100Z	BW3GY0Z	C030MZZ	C71K1ZZ
BT061ZZ	BT1D1ZZ	BT39ZZZ	BU35YZZ	BV230ZZ	BW210ZZ	BW3GYZZ	C030YZZ	C71KYZZ
BT06YZZ	BT1DYZZ	BT40ZZZ	BU35ZZZ	BV2310Z	BW2110Z	BW3GZZZ	C03YYZZ	C71L1ZZ
BT06ZZZ	BT1DZZZ	BT41ZZZ	BU36Y0Z	BV231ZZ	BW211ZZ	BW3HY0Z	C050VZZ	C71LYZZ
BT070ZZ	BT1F0ZZ	BT42ZZZ	BU36YZZ	BV23Y0Z	BW21Y0Z	BW3HYZZ	C050YZZ	C71M1ZZ
BT071ZZ	BT1F1ZZ	BT43ZZZ	BU36ZZZ	BV23YZZ	BW21YZZ	BW3HZZZ	C05YYZZ	C71MYZZ
BT07YZZ	BT1FYZZ	BT45ZZZ	BU39Y0Z	BV23ZZZ	BW21ZZZ	BW3PY0Z	C2161ZZ	C71N1ZZ
BT07ZZZ	BT1FZZZ	BT46ZZZ	BU39YZZ	BV30Y0Z	BW2400Z	BW3PYZZ	C216YZZ	C71NYZZ

C71P1ZZ	CD2YYZZ	CP151ZZ	CT1H1ZZ	CW1DFZZ	CW261ZZ	CW5D1ZZ	D010B7Z	D0Y6FZZ
C71PYZZ	CF141ZZ	CP15YZZ	CT1HYZZ	CW1DGZZ	CW26DZZ	CW5DDZZ	D010B8Z	D0Y77ZZ
C71YYZZ	CF14YZZ	CP161ZZ	CT1YYZZ	CW1DLZZ	CW26FZZ	CW5DYZZ	D010B9Z	D0Y78ZZ
C7221ZZ	CF151ZZ	CP16YZZ	CT231ZZ	CW1DSZZ	CW26GZZ	CW5J1ZZ	D010BB1	D0Y7CZZ
C722YZZ	CF15YZZ	CP171ZZ	CT23YZZ	CW1DYZZ	CW26KZZ	CW5JDZZ	D010BBZ	D0Y7FZZ
C72YYZZ	CF161ZZ	CP17YZZ	CT2YYZZ	CW1J1ZZ	CW26LZZ	CW5JYZZ	D010BCZ	D7000ZZ
C7551ZZ	CF16YZZ	CP181ZZ	CT631ZZ	CW1JDZZ	CW26SZZ	CW5M1ZZ	D010BYZ	D7001ZZ
C755YZZ	CF1C1ZZ	CP18YZZ	CT63FZZ	CW1JFZZ	CW26YZZ	CW5MDZZ	D01197Z	D7002ZZ
C75D1ZZ	CF1CYZZ	CP191ZZ	CT63GZZ	CW1JGZZ	CW2B1ZZ	CW5MYZZ	D01198Z	D7003Z0
C75DYZZ	CF1YYZZ	CP19YZZ	CT63HZZ	CW1JLZZ	CW2BDZZ	CW70NZZ	D01199Z	D7003ZZ
C75J1ZZ	CF241ZZ	CP1B1ZZ	CT63YZZ	CW1JSZZ	CW2BFZZ	CW70YZZ	D0119BZ	D7004ZZ
C75JYZZ	CF24YZZ	CP1BYZZ	CT6YYZZ	CW1JYZZ	CW2BGZZ	CW73NZZ	D0119CZ	D7005ZZ
C75K1ZZ	CF251ZZ	CP1C1ZZ	CV191ZZ	CW1M1ZZ	CW2BKZZ	CW73YZZ	D0119YZ	D7006ZZ
C75KYZZ	CF25YZZ	CP1CYZZ	CV19YZZ	CW1MDZZ	CW2BLZZ	CW7GGZZ	D011B6Z	D7010ZZ
C75L1ZZ	CF261ZZ	CP1D1ZZ	CV1YYZZ	CW1MFZZ	CW2BSZZ	CW7GYZZ	D011B7Z	D7011ZZ
C75LYZZ	CF26YZZ	CP1DYZZ	CW101ZZ	CW1MGZZ	CW2BYZZ	CW7N8ZZ	D011B8Z	D7012ZZ
C75M1ZZ	CF2YYZZ	CP1F1ZZ	CW10DZZ	CW1MLZZ	CW2D1ZZ	CW7NGZZ	D011B9Z	D7013Z0
C75MYZZ	CG111ZZ	CP1FYZZ	CW10FZZ	CW1MSZZ	CW2DDZZ	CW7NNZZ	D011BB1	D7013ZZ
C75N1ZZ	CG11SZZ	CP1YYZZ	CW10GZZ	CW1MYZZ	CW2DFZZ	CW7NPZZ	D011BBZ	D7014ZZ
C75NYZZ	CG11YZZ	CP1Z1ZZ	CW10LZZ	CW1N1ZZ	CW2DGZZ	CW7NYZZ	D011BCZ	D7015ZZ
C75P1ZZ	CG121ZZ	CP1ZYZZ	CW10SZZ	CW1NDZZ	CW2DKZZ	CW7YYZZ	D011BYZ	D7016ZZ
C75PYZZ	CG12FZZ	CP211ZZ	CW10YZZ	CW1NFZZ	CW2DLZZ	D0000ZZ	D01697Z	D7020ZZ
C75YYZZ	CG12GZZ	CP21YZZ	CW111ZZ	CW1NGZZ	CW2DSZZ	D0001ZZ	D01698Z	D7021ZZ
C7631ZZ	CG12YZZ	CP221ZZ	CW11DZZ	CW1NLZZ	CW2DYZZ	D0002ZZ	D01699Z	D7022ZZ
C7637ZZ	CG14GZZ	CP22YZZ	CW11FZZ	CW1NSZZ	CW2J1ZZ	D0003Z0	D0169BZ	D7023Z0
C763CZZ	CG14YZZ	CP231ZZ	CW11GZZ	CW1NYZZ	CW2JDZZ	D0003ZZ	D0169CZ	D7023ZZ
C763DZZ	CG1YYZZ	CP23YZZ	CW11LZZ	CW1YYZZ	CW2JFZZ	D0004ZZ	D0169YZ	D7024ZZ
C763HZZ	CG211ZZ	CP241ZZ	CW11SZZ	CW1ZZZZ	CW2JGZZ	D0005ZZ	D016B6Z	D7025ZZ
C763WZZ	CG21SZZ	CP24YZZ	CW11YZZ	CW201ZZ	CW2JKZZ	D0006ZZ	D016B7Z	D7026ZZ
C763YZZ	CG21YZZ	CP261ZZ	CW131ZZ	CW20DZZ	CW2JLZZ	D0010ZZ	D016B8Z	D7030ZZ
C76YYZZ	CG2YYZZ	CP26YZZ	CW13DZZ	CW20FZZ	CW2JSZZ	D0011ZZ	D016B9Z	D7031ZZ
C8191ZZ	CG421ZZ	CP271ZZ	CW13FZZ	CW20GZZ	CW2JYZZ	D0012ZZ	D016BB1	D7032ZZ
C819YZZ	CG42FZZ	CP27YZZ	CW13GZZ	CW20KZZ	CW2M1ZZ	D0013Z0	D016BBZ	D7033Z0
C81YYZZ	CG42GZZ	CP281ZZ	CW13KZZ	CW20LZZ	CW2MDZZ	D0013ZZ	D016BCZ	D7033ZZ
C91B1ZZ	CG42YZZ	CP28YZZ	CW13LZZ	CW20SZZ	CW2MFZZ	D0014ZZ	D016BYZ	D7034ZZ
C91BYZZ	CG4YYZZ	CP291ZZ	CW13SZZ	CW20YZZ	CW2MGZZ	D0015ZZ	D01797Z	D7035ZZ
C91YYZZ	CH101ZZ	CP29YZZ	CW13YZZ	CW211ZZ	CW2MKZZ	D0016ZZ	D01798Z	D7036ZZ
CB121ZZ	CH10SZZ	CP2B1ZZ	CW141ZZ	CW21DZZ	CW2MLZZ	D0060ZZ	D01799Z	D7040ZZ
CB129ZZ	CH10YZZ	CP2BYZZ	CW14DZZ	CW21FZZ	CW2MSZZ	D0061ZZ	D0179BZ	D7041ZZ
CB12TZZ	CH111ZZ	CP2C1ZZ	CW14FZZ	CW21GZZ	CW2MYZZ	D0062ZZ	D0179CZ	D7042ZZ
CB12VZZ	CH11SZZ	CP2CYZZ	CW14GZZ	CW21KZZ	CW2YYZZ	D0063Z0	D0179YZ	D7043Z0
CB12YZZ	CH11YZZ	CP2D1ZZ	CW14LZZ	CW21LZZ	CW3NYZZ	D0063ZZ	D017B6Z	D7043ZZ
CB1YYZZ	CH121ZZ	CP2DYZZ	CW14SZZ	CW21SZZ	CW501ZZ	D0064ZZ	D017B7Z	D7044ZZ
CB221ZZ	CH12SZZ	CP2F1ZZ	CW14YZZ	CW21YZZ	CW50DZZ	D0065ZZ	D017B8Z	D7045ZZ
CB229ZZ	CH12YZZ	CP2FYZZ	CW161ZZ	CW231ZZ	CW50YZZ	D0066ZZ	D017B9Z	D7046ZZ
CB22YZZ	CH1YYZZ	CP2G1ZZ	CW16DZZ	CW23DZZ	CW511ZZ	D0070ZZ	D017BB1	D7050ZZ
CB2YYZZ	CH201ZZ	CP2GYZZ	CW16FZZ	CW23FZZ	CW51DZZ	D0071ZZ	D017BBZ	D7051ZZ
CB32KZZ	CH20SZZ	CP2H1ZZ	CW16GZZ	CW23GZZ	CW51YZZ	D0072ZZ	D017BCZ	D7052ZZ
CB32YZZ	CH20YZZ	CP2HYZZ	CW16LZZ	CW23KZZ	CW531ZZ	D0073Z0	D017BYZ	D7053Z0
CB3YYZZ	CH211ZZ	CP2J1ZZ	CW16SZZ	CW23LZZ	CW53DZZ	D0073ZZ	D0Y07ZZ	D7053ZZ
CD151ZZ	CH21SZZ	CP2JYZZ	CW16YZZ	CW23SZZ	CW53YZZ	D0074ZZ	D0Y08ZZ	D7054ZZ
CD15DZZ	CH21YZZ	CP2YYZZ	CW1B1ZZ	CW23YZZ	CW541ZZ	D0075ZZ	D0Y0CZZ	D7055ZZ
CD15YZZ	CH221ZZ	CP55ZZZ	CW1BDZZ	CW241ZZ	CW54DZZ	D0076ZZ	D0Y0FZZ	D7056ZZ
CD171ZZ	CH22SZZ	CP5NZZZ	CW1BFZZ	CW24DZZ	CW54YZZ	D01097Z	D0Y17ZZ	D7060ZZ
CD17DZZ	CH22YZZ	CP5PZZZ	CW1BGZZ	CW24FZZ	CW561ZZ	D01098Z	D0Y18ZZ	D7061ZZ
CD17YZZ	CH2YYZZ	CP5YYZZ	CW1BLZZ	CW24GZZ	CW56DZZ	D01099Z	D0Y1CZZ	D7062ZZ
CD1YYZZ	CP111ZZ	CT131ZZ	CW1BSZZ	CW24KZZ	CW56YZZ	D0109BZ	D0Y1FZZ	D7063Z0
CD271ZZ	CP11YZZ	CT13FZZ	CW1BYZZ	CW24LZZ	CW5B1ZZ	D0109CZ	D0Y67ZZ	D7063ZZ
CD27DZZ	CP141ZZ	CT13GZZ	CW1D1ZZ	CW24SZZ	CW5BDZZ	D0109YZ	D0Y68ZZ	D7064ZZ
CD27YZZ	CP14YZZ	CT13YZZ	CW1DDZZ	CW24YZZ	CW5BYZZ	D010B6Z	D0Y6CZZ	D7065ZZ

D7066ZZ	D71398Z	D7179YZ	D810BBZ	D9075ZZ	D9119CZ	D916B8Z	D91BBCZ	D9YBFZZ
D7070ZZ	D71399Z	D717B6Z	D810BCZ	D9076ZZ	D9119YZ	D916B9Z	D91BBYZ	D9YCCZZ
D7071ZZ	D7139BZ	D717B7Z	D810BYZ	D9080ZZ	D911B6Z	D916BB1	D91D97Z	D9YCFZZ
D7072ZZ	D7139CZ	D717B8Z	D8Y07ZZ	D9081ZZ	D911B7Z	D916BBZ	D91D98Z	D9YD7ZZ
D7073Z0	D7139YZ	D717B9Z	D8Y08ZZ	D9082ZZ	D911B8Z	D916BCZ	D91D99Z	D9YD8ZZ
D7073ZZ	D713B6Z	D717BB1	D8Y0FZZ	D9083Z0	D911B9Z	D916BYZ	D91D9BZ	D9YDCZZ
D7074ZZ	D713B7Z	D717BBZ	D9000ZZ	D9083ZZ	D911BB1	D91797Z	D91D9CZ	D9YDFZZ
D7075ZZ	D713B8Z	D717BCZ	D9001ZZ	D9084ZZ	D911BBZ	D91798Z	D91D9YZ	D9YF7ZZ
D7076ZZ	D713B9Z	D717BYZ	D9002ZZ	D9085ZZ	D911BCZ	D91799Z	D91DB6Z	D9YF8ZZ
D7080ZZ	D713BB1	D71897Z	D9003Z0	D9086ZZ	D911BYZ	D9179BZ	D91DB7Z	DB000ZZ
D7081ZZ	D713BBZ	D71898Z	D9003ZZ	D9090ZZ	D91397Z	D9179CZ	D91DB8Z	DB001ZZ
D7082ZZ	D713BCZ	D71899Z	D9004ZZ	D9091ZZ	D91398Z	D9179YZ	D91DB9Z	DB002ZZ
D7083Z0	D713BYZ	D7189BZ	D9005ZZ	D9092ZZ	D91399Z	D917B6Z	D91DBB1	DB003Z0
D7083ZZ	D71497Z	D7189CZ	D9006ZZ	D9093Z0	D9139BZ	D917B7Z	D91DBBZ	DB003ZZ
D7084ZZ	D71498Z	D7189YZ	D9010ZZ	D9093ZZ	D9139CZ	D917B8Z	D91DBCZ	DB004ZZ
D7085ZZ	D71499Z	D718B6Z	D9011ZZ	D9094ZZ	D9139YZ	D917B9Z	D91DBYZ	DB005ZZ
D7086ZZ	D7149BZ	D718B7Z	D9012ZZ	D9095ZZ	D913B6Z	D917BB1	D91F97Z	DB006ZZ
D71097Z	D7149CZ	D718B8Z	D9013Z0	D9096ZZ	D913B7Z	D917BBZ	D91F98Z	DB010ZZ
D71098Z	D7149YZ	D718B9Z	D9013ZZ	D90B0ZZ	D913B8Z	D917BCZ	D91F99Z	DB011ZZ
D71099Z	D714B6Z	D718BB1	D9014ZZ	D90B1ZZ	D913B9Z	D917BYZ	D91F9BZ	DB012ZZ
D7109BZ	D714B7Z	D718BBZ	D9015ZZ	D90B2ZZ	D913BB1	D91897Z	D91F9CZ	DB013Z0
D7109CZ	D714B8Z	D718BCZ	D9016ZZ	D90B3Z0	D913BBZ	D91898Z	D91F9YZ	DB013ZZ
D7109YZ	D714B9Z	D718BYZ	D9030ZZ	D90B3ZZ	D913BCZ	D91899Z	D91FB6Z	DB014ZZ
D710B6Z	D714BB1	D7Y08ZZ	D9031ZZ	D90B4ZZ	D913BYZ	D9189BZ	D91FB7Z	DB015ZZ
D710B7Z	D714BBZ	D7Y0FZZ	D9032ZZ	D90B5ZZ	D91497Z	D9189CZ	D91FB8Z	DB016ZZ
D710B8Z	D714BCZ	D7Y18ZZ	D9033Z0	D90B6ZZ	D91498Z	D9189YZ	D91FB9Z	DB020ZZ
D710B9Z	D714BYZ	D7Y1FZZ	D9033ZZ	D90D0ZZ	D91499Z	D918B6Z	D91FBB1	DB021ZZ
D710BB1	D71597Z	D7Y28ZZ	D9034ZZ	D90D1ZZ	D9149BZ	D918B7Z	D91FBBZ	DB022ZZ
D710BBZ	D71598Z	D7Y2FZZ	D9035ZZ	D90D2ZZ	D9149CZ	D918B8Z	D91FBCZ	DB023Z0
D710BCZ	D71599Z	D7Y38ZZ	D9036ZZ	D90D3Z0	D9149YZ	D918B9Z	D91FBYZ	DB023ZZ
D710BYZ	D7159BZ	D7Y3FZZ	D9040ZZ	D90D3ZZ	D914B6Z	D918BB1	D9Y07ZZ	DB024ZZ
D71197Z	D7159CZ	D7Y48ZZ	D9041ZZ	D90D4ZZ	D914B7Z	D918BBZ	D9Y08ZZ	DB025ZZ
D71198Z	D7159YZ	D7Y4FZZ	D9042ZZ	D90D5ZZ	D914B8Z	D918BCZ	D9Y0FZZ	DB026ZZ
D71199Z	D715B6Z	D7Y58ZZ	D9043Z0	D90D6ZZ	D914B9Z	D918BYZ	D9Y17ZZ	DB050ZZ
D7119BZ	D715B7Z	D7Y5FZZ	D9043ZZ	D90F0ZZ	D914BB1	D91997Z	D9Y18ZZ	DB051ZZ
D7119CZ	D715B8Z	D7Y68ZZ	D9044ZZ	D90F1ZZ	D914BBZ	D91998Z	D9Y1FZZ	DB052ZZ
D7119YZ	D715B9Z	D7Y6FZZ	D9045ZZ	D90F2ZZ	D914BCZ	D91999Z	D9Y37ZZ	DB053Z0
D711B6Z	D715BB1	D7Y78ZZ	D9046ZZ	D90F3Z0	D914BYZ	D9199BZ	D9Y38ZZ	DB053ZZ
D711B7Z	D715BBZ	D7Y7FZZ	D9050ZZ	D90F3ZZ	D91597Z	D9199CZ	D9Y47ZZ	DB054ZZ
D711B8Z	D715BCZ	D7Y88ZZ	D9051ZZ	D90F4ZZ	D91598Z	D9199YZ	D9Y48ZZ	DB055ZZ
D711B9Z	D715BYZ	D7Y8FZZ	D9052ZZ	D90F5ZZ	D91599Z	D919B6Z	D9Y4CZZ	DB056ZZ
D711BB1	D71697Z	D8000ZZ	D9053Z0	D90F6ZZ	D9159BZ	D919B7Z	D9Y4FZZ	DB060ZZ
D711BBZ	D71698Z	D8001ZZ	D9053ZZ	D91097Z	D9159CZ	D919B8Z	D9Y57ZZ	DB061ZZ
D711BCZ	D71699Z	D8002ZZ	D9054ZZ	D91098Z	D9159YZ	D919B9Z	D9Y58ZZ	DB062ZZ
D711BYZ	D7169BZ	D8003Z0	D9055ZZ	D91099Z	D915B6Z	D919BB1	D9Y5FZZ	DB063Z0
D71297Z	D7169CZ	D8003ZZ	D9056ZZ	D9109BZ	D915B7Z	D919BBZ	D9Y67ZZ	DB063ZZ
D71298Z	D7169YZ	D8004ZZ	D9060ZZ	D9109CZ	D915B8Z	D919BCZ	D9Y68ZZ	DB064ZZ
D71299Z	D716B6Z	D8005ZZ	D9061ZZ	D9109YZ	D915B9Z	D919BYZ	D9Y6FZZ	DB065ZZ
D7129BZ	D716B7Z	D8006ZZ	D9062ZZ	D910B6Z	D915BB1	D91B97Z	D9Y77ZZ	DB066ZZ
D7129CZ	D716B8Z	D81097Z	D9063Z0	D910B7Z	D915BBZ	D91B98Z	D9Y78ZZ	DB070ZZ
D7129YZ	D716B9Z	D81098Z	D9063ZZ	D910B8Z	D915BCZ	D91B99Z	D9Y7FZZ	DB071ZZ
D712B6Z	D716BB1	D81099Z	D9064ZZ	D910B9Z	D915BYZ	D91B9BZ	D9Y87ZZ	DB072ZZ
D712B7Z	D716BBZ	D8109BZ	D9065ZZ	D910BB1	D91697Z	D91B9CZ	D9Y88ZZ	DB073Z0
D712B8Z	D716BCZ	D8109CZ	D9066ZZ	D910BBZ	D91698Z	D91B9YZ	D9Y8FZZ	DB073ZZ
D712B9Z	D716BYZ	D8109YZ	D9070ZZ	D910BCZ	D91699Z	D91BB6Z	D9Y97ZZ	DB074ZZ
D712BB1	D71797Z	D810B6Z	D9071ZZ	D910BYZ	D9169BZ	D91BB7Z	D9Y98ZZ	DB075ZZ
D712BBZ	D71798Z	D810B7Z	D9072ZZ	D91197Z	D9169CZ	D91BB8Z	D9Y9FZZ	DB076ZZ
D712BCZ	D71799Z	D810B8Z	D9073Z0	D91198Z	D9169YZ	D91BB9Z	D9YB7ZZ	DB080ZZ
D712BYZ	D7179BZ	D810B9Z	D9073ZZ	D91199Z	D916B6Z	D91BBB1	D9YB8ZZ	DB081ZZ
D71397Z	D7179CZ	D810BB1	D9074ZZ	D9119BZ	D916B7Z	D91BBBZ	D9YBCZZ	DB082ZZ

DB083Z0	DB15BYZ	DBY7FZZ	DD1097Z	DD149CZ	DDY5FZZ	DF11B7Z	DG012ZZ	DG12B6Z
DB083ZZ	DB1697Z	DBY87ZZ	DD1098Z	DD149YZ	DDY77ZZ	DF11B8Z	DG013Z0	DG12B7Z
DB084ZZ	DB1698Z	DBY88ZZ	DD1099Z	DD14B6Z	DDY78ZZ	DF11B9Z	DG013ZZ	DG12B8Z
DB085ZZ	DB1699Z	DBY8FZZ	DD109BZ	DD14B7Z	DDY7CZZ	DF11BB1	DG015ZZ	DG12B9Z
DB086ZZ	DB169BZ	DD000ZZ	DD109CZ	DD14B8Z	DDY7FZZ	DF11BBZ	DG016ZZ	DG12BB1
DB1097Z	DB169CZ	DD001ZZ	DD109YZ	DD14B9Z	DDY8CZZ	DF11BCZ	DG020ZZ	DG12BBZ
DB1098Z	DB169YZ	DD002ZZ	DD10B6Z	DD14BB1	DDY8FZZ	DF11BYZ	DG021ZZ	DG12BCZ
DB1099Z	DB16B6Z	DD003Z0	DD10B7Z	DD14BBZ	DF000ZZ	DF1297Z	DG022ZZ	DG12BYZ
DB109BZ	DB16B7Z	DD003ZZ	DD10B8Z	DD14BCZ	DF001ZZ	DF1298Z	DG023Z0	DG1497Z
DB109CZ	DB16B8Z	DD004ZZ	DD10B9Z	DD14BYZ	DF002ZZ	DF1299Z	DG023ZZ	DG1498Z
DB109YZ	DB16B9Z	DD005ZZ	DD10BB1	DD1597Z	DF003Z0	DF129BZ	DG025ZZ	DG1499Z
DB10B6Z	DB16BB1	DD006ZZ	DD10BBZ	DD1598Z	DF003ZZ	DF129CZ	DG026ZZ	DG149BZ
DB10B7Z	DB16BBZ	DD010ZZ	DD10BCZ	DD1599Z	DF004ZZ	DF129YZ	DG040ZZ	DG149CZ
DB10B8Z	DB16BCZ	DD011ZZ	DD10BYZ	DD159BZ	DF005ZZ	DF12B6Z	DG041ZZ	DG149YZ
DB10B9Z	DB16BYZ	DD012ZZ	DD1197Z	DD159CZ	DF006ZZ	DF12B7Z	DG042ZZ	DG14B6Z
DB10BB1	DB1797Z	DD013Z0	DD1198Z	DD159YZ	DF010ZZ	DF12B8Z	DG043Z0	DG14B7Z
DB10BBZ	DB1798Z	DD013ZZ	DD1199Z	DD15B6Z	DF011ZZ	DF12B9Z	DG043ZZ	DG14B8Z
DB10BCZ	DB1799Z	DD014ZZ	DD119BZ	DD15B7Z	DF012ZZ	DF12BB1	DG045ZZ	DG14B9Z
DB10BYZ	DB179BZ	DD015ZZ	DD119CZ	DD15B8Z	DF013Z0	DF12BBZ	DG046ZZ	DG14BB1
DB1197Z	DB179CZ	DD016ZZ	DD119YZ	DD15B9Z	DF013ZZ	DF12BCZ	DG050ZZ	DG14BBZ
DB1198Z	DB179YZ	DD020ZZ	DD11B6Z	DD15BB1	DF014ZZ	DF12BYZ	DG051ZZ	DG14BCZ
DB1199Z	DB17B6Z	DD021ZZ	DD11B7Z	DD15BBZ	DF015ZZ	DF1397Z	DG052ZZ	DG14BYZ
DB119BZ	DB17B7Z	DD022ZZ	DD11B8Z	DD15BCZ	DF016ZZ	DF1398Z	DG053Z0	DG1597Z
DB119CZ	DB17B8Z	DD023Z0	DD11B9Z	DD15BYZ	DF020ZZ	DF1399Z	DG053ZZ	DG1598Z
DB119YZ	DB17B9Z	DD023ZZ	DD11BB1	DD1797Z	DF021ZZ	DF139BZ	DG055ZZ	DG1599Z
DB11B6Z	DB17BB1	DD024ZZ	DD11BBZ	DD1798Z	DF022ZZ	DF139CZ	DG056ZZ	DG159BZ
DB11B7Z	DB17BBZ	DD025ZZ	DD11BCZ	DD1799Z	DF023Z0	DF139YZ	DG1097Z	DG159CZ
DB11B8Z	DB17BCZ	DD026ZZ	DD11BYZ	DD179BZ	DF023ZZ	DF13B6Z	DG1098Z	DG159YZ
DB11B9Z	DB17BYZ	DD030ZZ	DD1297Z	DD179CZ	DF024ZZ	DF13B7Z	DG1099Z	DG15B6Z
DB11BB1	DB1897Z	DD031ZZ	DD1298Z	DD179YZ	DF025ZZ	DF13B8Z	DG109BZ	DG15B7Z
DB11BBZ	DB1898Z	DD032ZZ	DD1299Z	DD17B6Z	DF026ZZ	DF13B9Z	DG109CZ	DG15B8Z
DB11BCZ	DB1899Z	DD033Z0	DD129BZ	DD17B7Z	DF030ZZ	DF13BB1	DG109YZ	DG15B9Z
DB11BYZ	DB189BZ	DD033ZZ	DD129CZ	DD17B8Z	DF031ZZ	DF13BBZ	DG10B6Z	DG15BB1
DB1297Z	DB189CZ	DD034ZZ	DD129YZ	DD17B9Z	DF032ZZ	DF13BCZ	DG10B7Z	DG15BBZ
DB1298Z	DB189YZ	DD035ZZ	DD12B6Z	DD17BB1	DF033Z0	DF13BYZ	DG10B8Z	DG15BCZ
DB1299Z	DB18B6Z	DD036ZZ	DD12B7Z	DD17BBZ	DF033ZZ	DFY07ZZ	DG10B9Z	DG15BYZ
DB129BZ	DB18B7Z	DD040ZZ	DD12B8Z	DD17BCZ	DF034ZZ	DFY08ZZ	DG10BB1	DGY07ZZ
DB129CZ	DB18B8Z	DD041ZZ	DD12B9Z	DD17BYZ	DF035ZZ	DFY0CZZ	DG10BBZ	DGY08ZZ
DB129YZ	DB18B9Z	DD042ZZ	DD12BB1	DDY07ZZ	DF036ZZ	DFY0FZZ	DG10BCZ	DGY0FZZ
DB12B6Z	DB18BB1	DD043Z0	DD12BBZ	DDY08ZZ	DF1097Z	DFY17ZZ	DG10BYZ	DGY17ZZ
DB12B7Z	DB18BBZ	DD043ZZ	DD12BCZ	DDY0FZZ	DF1098Z	DFY18ZZ	DG1197Z	DGY18ZZ
DB12B8Z	DB18BCZ	DD044ZZ	DD12BYZ	DDY17ZZ	DF1099Z	DFY1CZZ	DG1198Z	DGY1FZZ
DB12B9Z	DB18BYZ	DD045ZZ	DD1397Z	DDY18ZZ	DF109BZ	DFY1FZZ	DG1199Z	DGY27ZZ
DB12BB1	DBY07ZZ	DD046ZZ	DD1398Z	DDY1CZZ	DF109CZ	DFY27ZZ	DG119BZ	DGY28ZZ
DB12BBZ	DBY08ZZ	DD050ZZ	DD1399Z	DDY1FZZ	DF109YZ	DFY28ZZ	DG119CZ	DGY2FZZ
DB12BCZ	DBY0FZZ	DD051ZZ	DD139BZ	DDY27ZZ	DF10B6Z	DFY2CZZ	DG119YZ	DGY47ZZ
DB12BYZ	DBY17ZZ	DD052ZZ	DD139CZ	DDY28ZZ	DF10B7Z	DFY2FZZ	DG11B6Z	DGY48ZZ
DB1597Z	DBY18ZZ	DD053Z0	DD139YZ	DDY2CZZ	DF10B8Z	DFY37ZZ	DG11B7Z	DGY4FZZ
DB1598Z	DBY1FZZ	DD053ZZ	DD13B6Z	DDY2FZZ	DF10B9Z	DFY38ZZ	DG11B8Z	DGY57ZZ
DB1599Z	DBY27ZZ	DD054ZZ	DD13B7Z	DDY37ZZ	DF10BB1	DFY3CZZ	DG11B9Z	DGY58ZZ
DB159BZ	DBY28ZZ	DD055ZZ	DD13B8Z	DDY38ZZ	DF10BBZ	DFY3FZZ	DG11BB1	DGY5FZZ
DB159CZ	DBY2FZZ	DD056ZZ	DD13B9Z	DDY3CZZ	DF10BCZ	DG000ZZ	DG11BBZ	DH020ZZ
DB159YZ	DBY57ZZ	DD070ZZ	DD13BB1	DDY3FZZ	DF10BYZ	DG001ZZ	DG11BCZ	DH021ZZ
DB15B6Z	DBY58ZZ	DD071ZZ	DD13BBZ	DDY47ZZ	DF1197Z	DG002ZZ	DG11BYZ	DH022ZZ
DB15B7Z	DBY5FZZ	DD072ZZ	DD13BCZ	DDY48ZZ	DF1198Z	DG003Z0	DG1297Z	DH023Z0
DB15B8Z	DBY67ZZ	DD073Z0	DD13BYZ	DDY4CZZ	DF1199Z	DG003ZZ	DG1298Z	DH023ZZ
DB15B9Z	DBY68ZZ	DD073ZZ	DD1497Z	DDY4FZZ	DF119BZ	DG005ZZ	DG1299Z	DH024ZZ
DB15BB1	DBY6FZZ	DD074ZZ	DD1498Z	DDY57ZZ	DF119CZ	DG006ZZ	DG129BZ	DH025ZZ
DB15BBZ	DBY77ZZ	DD075ZZ	DD1499Z	DDY58ZZ	DF119YZ	DG010ZZ	DG129CZ	DH026ZZ
DB15BCZ	DBY78ZZ	DD076ZZ	DD149BZ	DDY5CZZ	DF11B6Z	DG011ZZ	DG129YZ	DH030ZZ

DH031ZZ	DHY3FZZ	DM11B9Z	DP071ZZ	DPY87ZZ	DT1199Z	DU003ZZ	DU12BCZ	DVY0CZZ
DH032ZZ	DHY47ZZ	DM11BB1	DP072ZZ	DPY88ZZ	DT119BZ	DU004ZZ	DU12BYZ	DVY0FZZ
DH033Z0	DHY48ZZ	DM11BBZ	DP073Z0	DPY8FZZ	DT119CZ	DU005ZZ	DUY07ZZ	DVY17ZZ
DH033ZZ	DHY4FZZ	DM11BCZ	DP073ZZ	DPY97ZZ	DT119YZ	DU006ZZ	DUY08ZZ	DVY18ZZ
DH034ZZ	DHY5FZZ	DM11BYZ	DP074ZZ	DPY98ZZ	DT11B6Z	DU010ZZ	DUY0CZZ	DVY1FZZ
DH035ZZ	DHY67ZZ	DMY07ZZ	DP075ZZ	DPY9FZZ	DT11B7Z	DU011ZZ	DUY0FZZ	DW010ZZ
DH036ZZ	DHY68ZZ	DMY08ZZ	DP076ZZ	DPYB7ZZ	DT11B8Z	DU012ZZ	DUY17ZZ	DW011ZZ
DH040ZZ	DHY6FZZ	DMY0FZZ	DP080ZZ	DPYB8ZZ	DT11B9Z	DU013Z0	DUY18ZZ	DW012ZZ
DH041ZZ	DHY77ZZ	DMY17ZZ	DP081ZZ	DPYBFZZ	DT11BB1	DU013ZZ	DUY1CZZ	DW013Z0
DH042ZZ	DHY78ZZ	DMY18ZZ	DP082ZZ	DPYC7ZZ	DT11BBZ	DU014ZZ	DUY1FZZ	DW013ZZ
DH043Z0	DHY7FZZ	DMY1FZZ	DP083Z0	DPYC8ZZ	DT11BCZ	DU015ZZ	DUY27ZZ	DW014ZZ
DH043ZZ	DHY87ZZ	DP000ZZ	DP083ZZ	DPYCFZZ	DT11BYZ	DU016ZZ	DUY28ZZ	DW015ZZ
DH044ZZ	DHY88ZZ	DP001ZZ	DP084ZZ	DT000ZZ	DT1297Z	DU020ZZ	DUY2CZZ	DW016ZZ
DH045ZZ	DHY8FZZ	DP002ZZ	DP085ZZ	DT001ZZ	DT1298Z	DU021ZZ	DUY2FZZ	DW020ZZ
DH046ZZ	DHY97ZZ	DP003Z0	DP086ZZ	DT002ZZ	DT1299Z	DU022ZZ	DV000ZZ	DW021ZZ
DH060ZZ	DHY98ZZ	DP003ZZ	DP090ZZ	DT003Z0	DT129BZ	DU023Z0	DV001ZZ	DW022ZZ
DH061ZZ	DHY9FZZ	DP004ZZ	DP091ZZ	DT003ZZ	DT129CZ	DU023ZZ	DV002ZZ	DW023Z0
DH062ZZ	DHYB7ZZ	DP005ZZ	DP092ZZ	DT004ZZ	DT129YZ	DU024ZZ	DV003Z0	DW023ZZ
DH063Z0	DHYB8ZZ	DP006ZZ	DP093Z0	DT005ZZ	DT12B6Z	DU025ZZ	DV003ZZ	DW024ZZ
DH063ZZ	DHYBFZZ	DP020ZZ	DP093ZZ	DT006ZZ	DT12B7Z	DU026ZZ	DV004ZZ	DW025ZZ
DH064ZZ	DHYCFZZ	DP021ZZ	DP094ZZ	DT010ZZ	DT12B8Z	DU1097Z	DV005ZZ	DW026ZZ
DH065ZZ	DM000ZZ	DP022ZZ	DP095ZZ	DT011ZZ	DT12B9Z	DU1098Z	DV006ZZ	DW030ZZ
DH066ZZ	DM001ZZ	DP023Z0	DP096ZZ	DT012ZZ	DT12BB1	DU1099Z	DV010ZZ	DW031ZZ
DH070ZZ	DM002ZZ	DP023ZZ	DP0B0ZZ	DT013Z0	DT12BBZ	DU109BZ	DV011ZZ	DW032ZZ
DH071ZZ	DM003Z0	DP024ZZ	DP0B1ZZ	DT013ZZ	DT12BCZ	DU109CZ	DV012ZZ	DW033Z0
DH072ZZ	DM003ZZ	DP025ZZ	DP0B2ZZ	DT014ZZ	DT12BYZ	DU109YZ	DV013Z0	DW033ZZ
DH073Z0	DM004ZZ	DP026ZZ	DP0B3Z0	DT015ZZ	DT1397Z	DU10B6Z	DV013ZZ	DW034ZZ
DH073ZZ	DM005ZZ	DP030ZZ	DP0B3ZZ	DT016ZZ	DT1398Z	DU10B7Z	DV014ZZ	DW035ZZ
DH074ZZ	DM006ZZ	DP031ZZ	DP0B4ZZ	DT020ZZ	DT1399Z	DU10B8Z	DV015ZZ	DW036ZZ
DH075ZZ	DM010ZZ	DP032ZZ	DP0B5ZZ	DT021ZZ	DT139BZ	DU10B9Z	DV016ZZ	DW040ZZ
DH076ZZ	DM011ZZ	DP033Z0	DP0B6ZZ	DT022ZZ	DT139CZ	DU10BB1	DV1097Z	DW041ZZ
DH080ZZ	DM012ZZ	DP033ZZ	DP0C0ZZ	DT023Z0	DT139YZ	DU10BBZ	DV1098Z	DW042ZZ
DH081ZZ	DM013Z0	DP034ZZ	DP0C1ZZ	DT023ZZ	DT13B6Z	DU10BCZ	DV1099Z	DW043Z0
DH082ZZ	DM013ZZ	DP035ZZ	DP0C2ZZ	DT024ZZ	DT13B7Z	DU10BYZ	DV109BZ	DW043ZZ
DH083Z0	DM014ZZ	DP036ZZ	DP0C3Z0	DT025ZZ	DT13B8Z	DU1197Z	DV109CZ	DW044ZZ
DH083ZZ	DM015ZZ	DP040ZZ	DP0C3ZZ	DT026ZZ	DT13B9Z	DU1198Z	DV109YZ	DW045ZZ
DH084ZZ	DM016ZZ	DP041ZZ	DP0C4ZZ	DT030ZZ	DT13BB1	DU1199Z	DV10B6Z	DW046ZZ
DH085ZZ	DM1097Z	DP042ZZ	DP0C5ZZ	DT031ZZ	DT13BBZ	DU119BZ	DV10B7Z	DW050ZZ
DH086ZZ	DM1098Z	DP043Z0	DP0C6ZZ	DT032ZZ	DT13BCZ	DU119CZ	DV10B8Z	DW051ZZ
DH090ZZ	DM1099Z	DP043ZZ	DPY07ZZ	DT033Z0	DT13BYZ	DU119YZ	DV10B9Z	DW052ZZ
DH091ZZ	DM109BZ	DP044ZZ	DPY08ZZ	DT033ZZ	DTY07ZZ	DU11B6Z	DV10BB1	DW053Z0
DH092ZZ	DM109CZ	DP045ZZ	DPY0FZZ	DT034ZZ	DTY08ZZ	DU11B7Z	DV10BBZ	DW053ZZ
DH093Z0	DM109YZ	DP046ZZ	DPY27ZZ	DT035ZZ	DTY0CZZ	DU11B8Z	DV10BCZ	DW054ZZ
DH093ZZ	DM10B6Z	DP050ZZ	DPY28ZZ	DT036ZZ	DTY0FZZ	DU11B9Z	DV10BYZ	DW055ZZ
DH094ZZ	DM10B7Z	DP051ZZ	DPY2FZZ	DT1097Z	DTY17ZZ	DU11BB1	DV1197Z	DW056ZZ
DH095ZZ	DM10B8Z	DP052ZZ	DPY37ZZ	DT1098Z	DTY18ZZ	DU11BBZ	DV1198Z	DW060ZZ
DH096ZZ	DM10B9Z	DP053Z0	DPY38ZZ	DT1099Z	DTY1CZZ	DU11BCZ	DV1199Z	DW061ZZ
DH0B0ZZ	DM10BB1	DP053ZZ	DPY3FZZ	DT109BZ	DTY1FZZ	DU11BYZ	DV119BZ	DW062ZZ
DH0B1ZZ	DM10BBZ	DP054ZZ	DPY47ZZ	DT109CZ	DTY27ZZ	DU1297Z	DV119CZ	DW063Z0
DH0B2ZZ	DM10BCZ	DP055ZZ	DPY48ZZ	DT109YZ	DTY28ZZ	DU1298Z	DV119YZ	DW063ZZ
DH0B3Z0	DM10BYZ	DP056ZZ	DPY4FZZ	DT10B6Z	DTY2CZZ	DU1299Z	DV11B6Z	DW064ZZ
DH0B3ZZ	DM1197Z	DP060ZZ	DPY57ZZ	DT10B7Z	DTY2FZZ	DU129BZ	DV11B7Z	DW065ZZ
DH0B4ZZ	DM1198Z	DP061ZZ	DPY58ZZ	DT10B8Z	DTY37ZZ	DU129CZ	DV11B8Z	DW066ZZ
DH0B5ZZ	DM1199Z	DP062ZZ	DPY5FZZ	DT10B9Z	DTY38ZZ	DU129YZ	DV11B9Z	DW10BB1
DH0B6ZZ	DM119BZ	DP063Z0	DPY67ZZ	DT10BB1	DTY3CZZ	DU12B6Z	DV11BB1	DW10BBZ
DHY27ZZ	DM119CZ	DP063ZZ	DPY68ZZ	DT10BBZ	DTY3FZZ	DU12B7Z	DV11BBZ	DW1197Z
DHY28ZZ	DM119YZ	DP064ZZ	DPY6FZZ	DT10BCZ	DU000ZZ	DU12B8Z	DV11BCZ	DW1198Z
DHY2FZZ	DM11B6Z	DP065ZZ	DPY77ZZ	DT10BYZ	DU001ZZ	DU12B9Z	DV11BYZ	DW1199Z
DHY37ZZ	DM11B7Z	DP066ZZ	DPY78ZZ	DT1197Z	DU002ZZ	DU12BB1	DVY07ZZ	DW119BZ
DHY38ZZ	DM11B8Z	DP070ZZ	DPY7FZZ	DT1198Z	DU003Z0	DU12BBZ	DVY08ZZ	DW119CZ

DW119YZ	DW1RBBZ	F13Z62Z	F14Z0LZ	F15Z7ZZ	XNU0356	XW0DXL5
DW11B6Z	DW1XBB1	F13Z6ZZ	F14Z0PZ	GZ10ZZZ	XNU4356	XW0DXR5
DW11B7Z	DW1XBBZ	F13Z71Z	F14Z0YZ	GZ11ZZZ	XT25XE5	XW0DXT5
DW11B8Z	DW1YBB1	F13Z7KZ	F14Z0ZZ	GZ12ZZZ	XW013W5	XW0DXV5
DW11B9Z	DW1YBBZ	F13Z7ZZ	F14Z15Z	GZ13ZZZ	XW03306	XW0G886
DW11BB1	DWY17ZZ	F13Z83Z	F14Z1ZZ	GZ14ZZZ	XW03321	XW0H886
DW11BBZ	DWY18ZZ	F13Z84Z	F14Z21Z	GZ2ZZZZ	XW03326	XW0Q316
DW11BCZ	DWY1FZZ	F13Z8ZZ	F14Z22Z	GZ3ZZZZ	XW03331	XW23346
DW11BYZ	DWY27ZZ	F13Z91Z	F14Z23Z	GZ50ZZZ	XW03336	XW23376
DW1297Z	DWY28ZZ	F13Z92Z	F14Z24Z	GZ51ZZZ	XW03341	XW24346
DW1298Z	DWY2FZZ	F13Z9ZZ	F14Z25Z	GZ52ZZZ	XW03351	XW24376
DW1299Z	DWY37ZZ	F13ZB1Z	F14Z2KZ	GZ53ZZZ	XW03366	XXE5XM5
DW129BZ	DWY38ZZ	F13ZB2Z	F14Z2LZ	GZ54ZZZ	XW03372	XXE5XN6
DW129CZ	DWY3FZZ	F13ZBZZ	F14Z2PZ	GZ55ZZZ	XW03392	XXEBXQ6
DW129YZ	DWY47ZZ	F13ZC1Z	F14Z2ZZ	GZ56ZZZ	XW03396	XY0VX83
DW12B6Z	DWY48ZZ	F13ZC2Z	F14Z31Z	GZ58ZZZ	XW033A3	
DW12B7Z	DWY4FZZ	F13ZCZZ	F14Z32Z	GZ59ZZZ	XW033A6	
DW12B8Z	DWY57ZZ	F13ZD3Z	F14Z33Z	GZ60ZZZ	XW033B3	
DW12B9Z	DWY58ZZ	F13ZD4Z	F14Z34Z	GZ61ZZZ	XW033B6	
DW12BB1	DWY5FZZ	F13ZDZZ	F14Z35Z	GZ63ZZZ	XW033C6	
DW12BBZ	DWY5GDZ	F13ZF3Z	F14Z3KZ	GZ72ZZZ	XW033D6	
DW12BCZ	DWY5GFZ	F13ZF4Z	F14Z3LZ	GZB0ZZZ	XW033F3	
DW12BYZ	DWY5GGZ	F13ZFZZ	F14Z3PZ	GZB1ZZZ	XW033G4	
DW1397Z	DWY5GHZ	F13ZG3Z	F14Z3ZZ	GZB2ZZZ	XW033H4	
DW1398Z	DWY5GYZ	F13ZG4Z	F14Z41Z	GZB3ZZZ	XW033K5	
DW1399Z	DWY67ZZ	F13ZGZZ	F14Z42Z	GZB4ZZZ	XW033N5	
DW139BZ	DWY68ZZ	F13ZH3Z	F14Z43Z	GZC9ZZZ	XW033Q5	
DW139CZ	DWY6FZZ	F13ZH4Z	F14Z44Z	GZFZZZZ	XW033S5	
DW139YZ	F0DZ8ZZ	F13ZHZZ	F14Z4KZ	GZGZZZZ	XW033U5	
DW13B6Z	F0DZ9EZ	F13ZJ3Z	F14Z4LZ	GZHZZZZ	XW033W5	
DW13B7Z	F0DZ9FZ	F13ZJ4Z	F14Z4ZZ	GZJZZZZ	XW04306	
DW13B8Z	F0DZ9UZ	F13ZJZZ	F14Z51Z	HZ2ZZZZ	XW04321	
DW13B9Z	F0DZ9ZZ	F13ZK7Z	F14Z52Z	HZ3CZZZ	XW04326	
DW13BB1	F13Z00Z	F13ZKZZ	F14Z53Z	HZ4CZZZ	XW04331	
DW13BBZ	F13Z01Z	F13ZL7Z	F14Z54Z	HZ63ZZZ	XW04336	
DW13BCZ	F13Z02Z	F13ZLZZ	F14Z55Z	HZ80ZZZ	XW04341	
DW13BYZ	F13Z03Z	F13ZM6Z	F14Z5KZ	HZ81ZZZ	XW04351	
DW1697Z	F13Z08Z	F13ZMZZ	F14Z5LZ	HZ82ZZZ	XW04366	
DW1698Z	F13Z09Z	F13ZN6Z	F14Z5ZZ	HZ83ZZZ	XW04372	
DW1699Z	F13Z0ZZ	F13ZNZZ	F14Z65Z	HZ84ZZZ	XW04392	
DW169BZ	F13Z10Z	F13ZP1Z	F14Z6ZZ	HZ85ZZZ	XW04396	
DW169CZ	F13Z11Z	F13ZP2Z	F14Z70Z	HZ86ZZZ	XW043A3	
DW169YZ	F13Z12Z	F13ZP4Z	F14Z7ZZ	HZ87ZZZ	XW043A6	
DW16B6Z	F13Z1ZZ	F13ZP9Z	F14Z85Z	HZ88ZZZ	XW043B3	
DW16B7Z	F13Z20Z	F13ZPKZ	F14Z8ZZ	HZ89ZZZ	XW043B6	
DW16B8Z	F13Z21Z	F13ZPLZ	F15Z08Z	HZ90ZZZ	XW043C6	
DW16B9Z	F13Z22Z	F13ZPPZ	F15Z0ZZ	HZ91ZZZ	XW043D6	
DW16BB1	F13Z2ZZ	F13ZPZZ	F15Z18Z	HZ92ZZZ	XW043F3	
DW16BBZ	F13Z31Z	F13ZQKZ	F15Z1ZZ	HZ93ZZZ	XW043G4	
DW16BCZ	F13Z32Z	F13ZQPZ	F15Z28Z	HZ94ZZZ	XW043H4	
DW16BYZ	F13Z3ZZ	F13ZQYZ	F15Z2ZZ	HZ95ZZZ	XW043K5	
DW1KBB1	F13Z41Z	F13ZQZZ	F15Z38Z	HZ96ZZZ	XW043N5	
DW1KBBZ	F13Z42Z	F14Z01Z	F15Z3ZZ	HZ97ZZZ	XW043Q5	
DW1LBB1	F13Z4KZ	F14Z02Z	F15Z48Z	HZ98ZZZ	XW043S5	
DW1LBBZ	F13Z4ZZ	F14Z03Z	F15Z4ZZ	HZ99ZZZ	XW043U5	
DW1PBB1	F13Z51Z	F14Z04Z	F15Z58Z	X2A5312	XW043W5	
DW1PBBZ	F13Z52Z	F14Z05Z	F15Z5ZZ	X2A6325	XW097M5	
DW1QBB1	F13Z5KZ	F14Z07Z	F15Z68Z	X2AH336	XW0DX66	
DW1QBBZ	F13Z5ZZ	F14Z09Z	F15Z6ZZ	X2AJ336	XW0DX82	
DW1RBB1	F13Z61Z	F14Z0KZ	F15Z75Z	XK02303	XW0DXJ5	

Land Your Dream Job

Accelerate your career and remove your apprentice designation with Practicode.

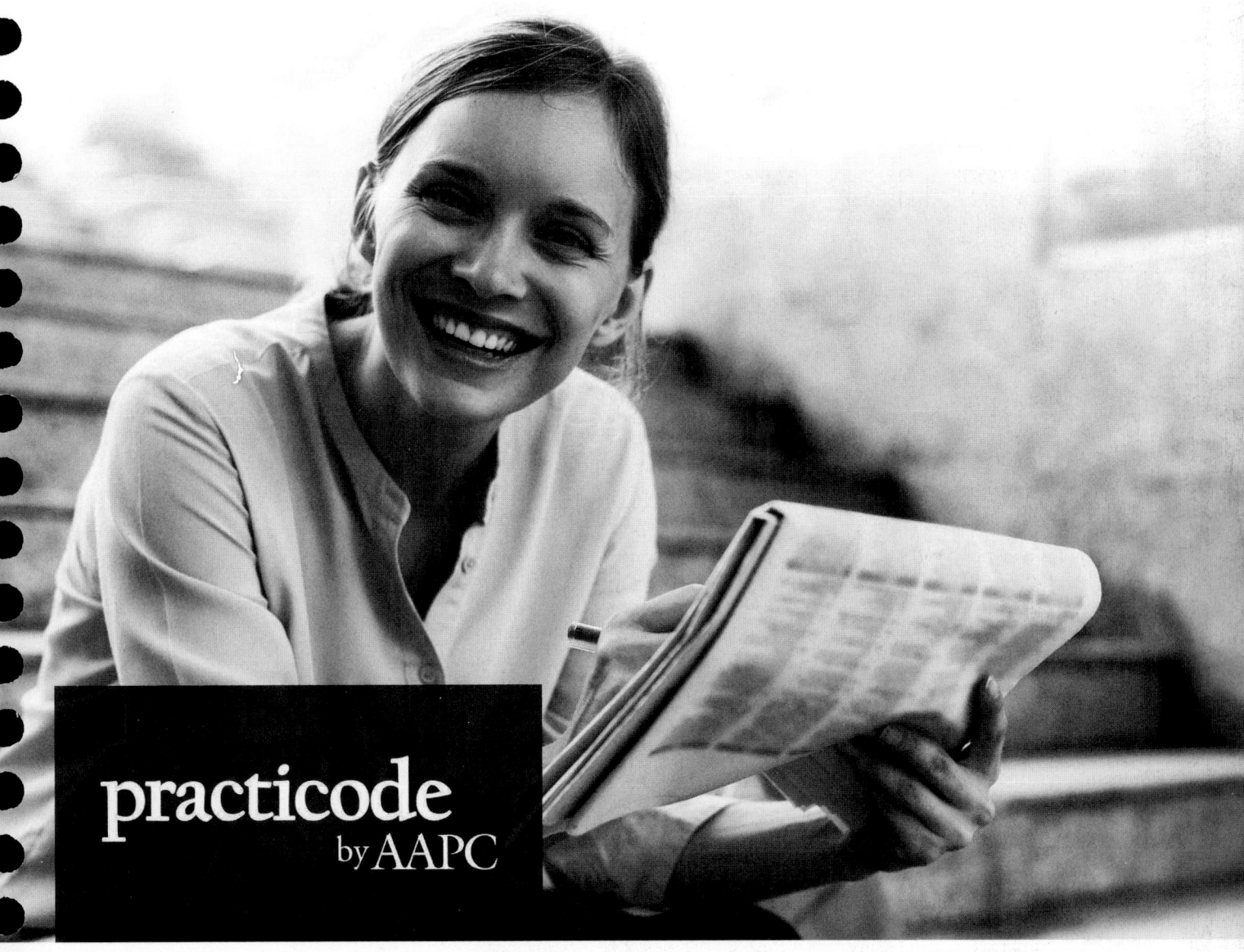

practicode by AAPC

Practicode gives you the experience you need to get the job you want. With over 600 real-world coding exercises, you'll earn one year of coding experience and get closer to removing your apprentice status. It's your career. Take control of it.

ADVANCE YOUR CREDENTIALS
ADVANCE YOUR CAREER

The more you learn, the more you can earn.

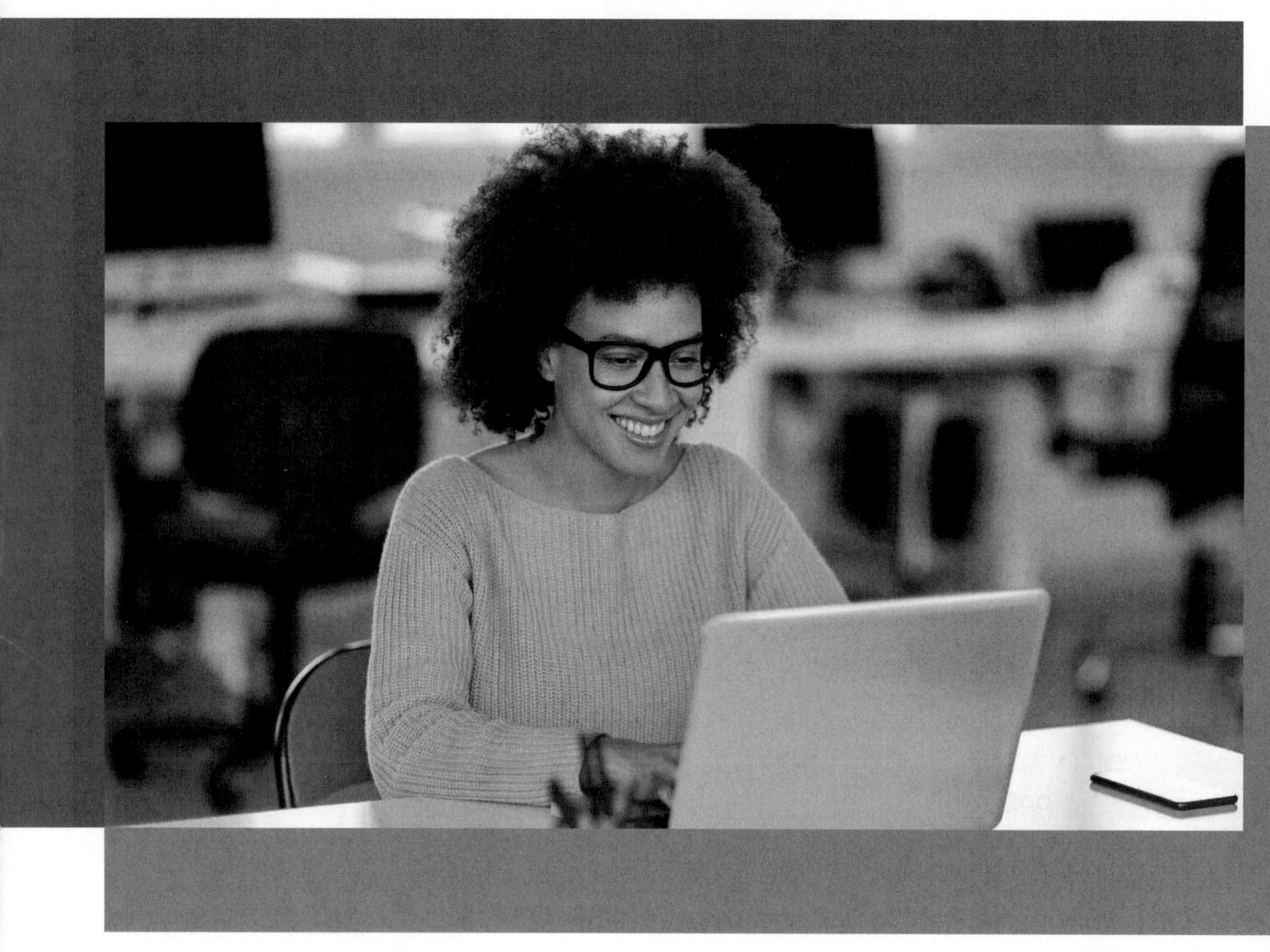

Learn more
Visit: https://www.aapc.com/training

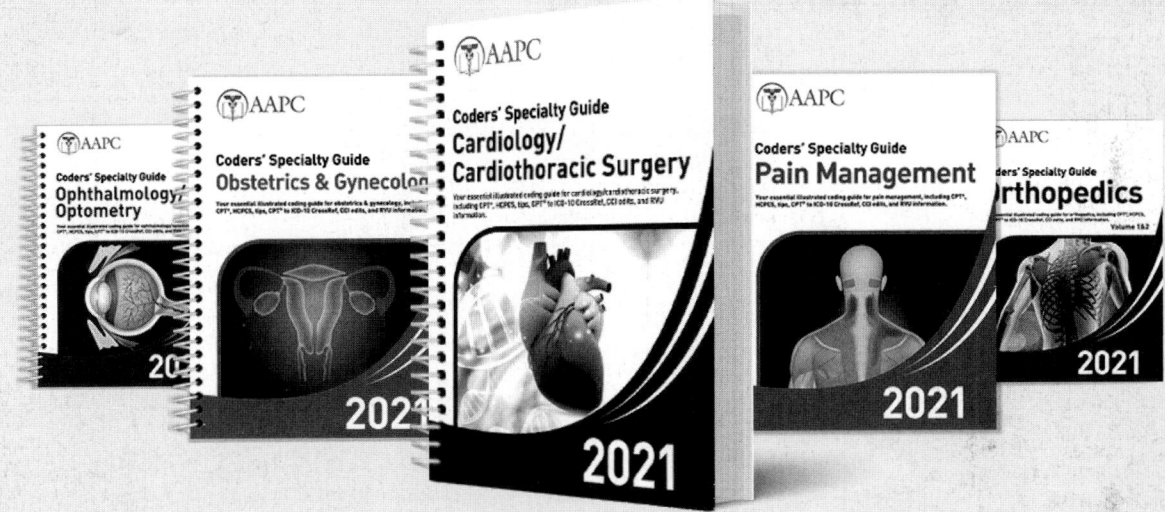

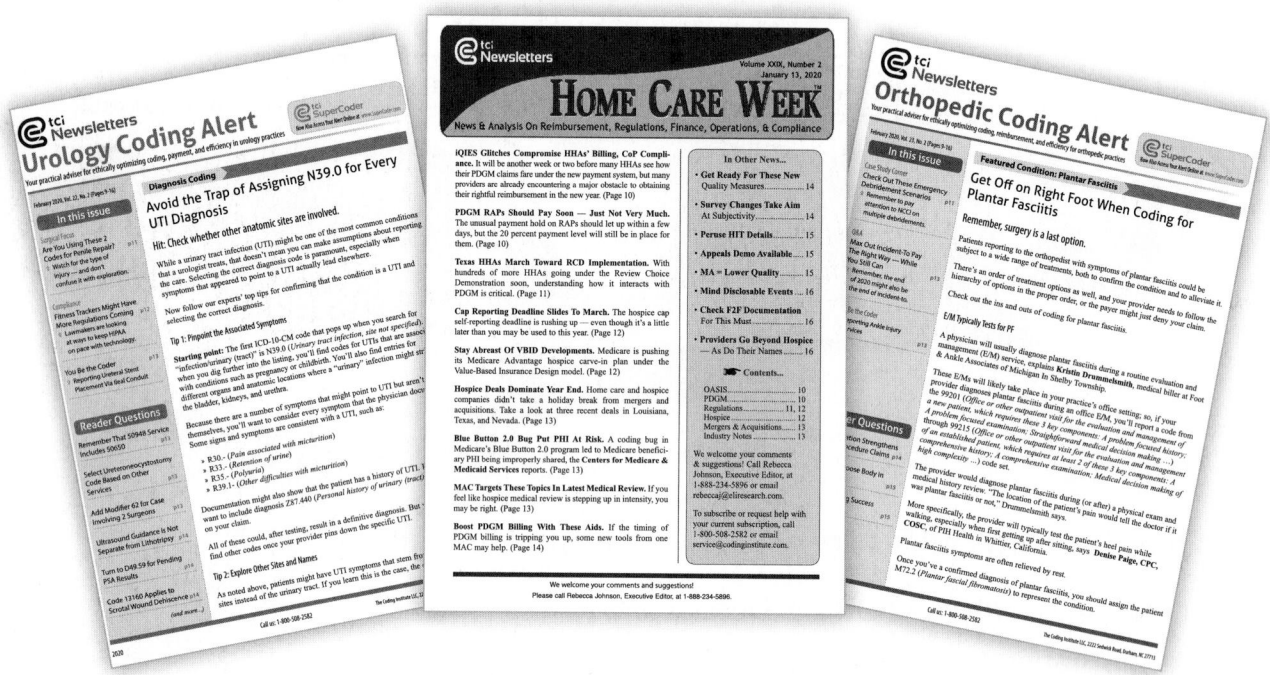
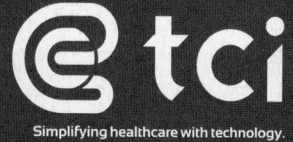